Scott-Conner & Dawson

ESSENTIAL OPERATIVE
TECHNIQUES and ANATOMY

FOURTH EDITION

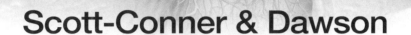

Scott-Conner & Dawson

ESSENTIAL OPERATIVE TECHNIQUES and ANATOMY

FOURTH EDITION

Carol E. H. Scott-Conner, M.D., Ph.D., M.B.A.

Professor
Department of Surgery
University of Iowa Roy J. and Lucille A. Carver College of Medicine
Iowa City, Iowa

. Wolters Kluwer | Lippincott Williams & Wilkins
Health

Philadelphia · Baltimore · New York · London
Buenos Aires · Hong Kong · Sydney · Tokyo

Acquisitions Editor: Keith Donnellan
Product Manager: Brendan Huffman
Production Project Manager: David Orzechowski
Senior Manufacturing Coordinator: Beth Welsh
Senior Design Coordinator: Teresa Mallon
Production Service: Aptara, Inc.

Library of Congress Cataloging-in-Publication Data

Scott-Conner, Carol E. H., author.
  [Operative anatomy]
  Scott-Conner & Dawson essential operative techniques and anatomy /
Carol E. H. Scott-Conner, David L. Dawson.—Fourth Edition.
      p. ; cm.
  Preceded by: Operative anatomy / Carol E. H. Scott-Conner, David L.
Dawson. 3rd ed. 2009.
  Includes bibliographical references and index.
    ISBN 978-1-4511-5172-5 (hardback : alk. paper)
  I. Dawson, David L., author. II. Title. III. Title: Essential
operative techniques and anatomy.
  [DNLM: 1. Surgical Procedures, Operative–methods. 2. Anatomy,
Regional. WO 500]
  QM531
  611–dc23
                          2013025967

Care has been taken to confirm the accuracy of the information presented and to describe generally accepted
practices. However, the authors, editors, and publisher are not responsible for errors or omissions or for any
consequences from application of the information in this book and make no warranty, expressed or implied,
with respect to the currency, completeness, or accuracy of the contents of the publication. Application of the
information in a particular situation remains the professional responsibility of the practitioner.

The authors, editors, and publisher have exerted every effort to ensure that drug selection and dosage set
forth in this text are in accordance with current recommendations and practice at the time of publication.
However, in view of ongoing research, changes in government regulations, and the constant flow of information
relating to drug therapy and drug reactions, the reader is urged to check the package insert for each drug for any
change in indications and dosage and for added warnings and precautions. This is particularly important when
the recommended agent is a new or infrequently employed drug.

Some drugs and medical devices presented in the publication have Food and Drug Administration (FDA)
clearance for limited use in restricted research settings. It is the responsibility of the health care provider to
ascertain the FDA status of each drug or device planned for use in their clinical practice.

To purchase additional copies of this book, call our customer service department at (800) 638-3030 or fax
orders to (301) 223-2320. International customers should call (301) 223-2300.

Visit Lippincott Williams & Wilkins on the Internet: at LWW.com. Lippincott Williams & Wilkins customer
service representatives are available from 8:30 am to 6 pm, EST.

10 9 8 7 6 5 4 3 2 1

CCS0913

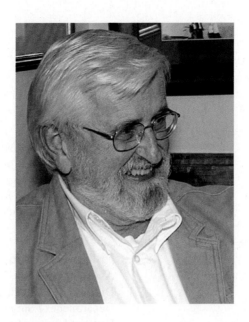

Dedicated to the memory of
David L. Dawson, PhD
1942–2011

David Lynn Dawson received his graduate training at the Southern Illinois University and devoted his life to the teaching of human gross anatomy. In 1975, he joined the faculty of Marshall University School of Medicine in Huntington, West Virginia. There he helped to establish a new medical school and wrote the anatomic portions of the first edition of this text. Throughout a long and productive teaching career that spanned three continents and almost four decades, he was a staunch and true advocate for anatomical education of students and residents—especially surgical residents. He was a founding member of the American Association of Clinical Anatomists and a mentor and friend to innumerable trainees. His contributions to this textbook were enormous and he is greatly missed.

Contributors

Laura A. Adam, MD
Critical Care Surgeon
Private Practice
St. Louis, Missouri

Parth B. Amin, MD
Clinical Assistant Professor of Vascular Surgery
Department of Surgery
University of Iowa Roy J. and Lucille A. Carver
   College of Medicine
Iowa City, Iowa

Evgeny V. Arshava, MD
Clinical Assistant Professor of Acute Care Surgery
Department of Surgery
University of Iowa Roy J. and Lucille A. Carver
   College of Medicine
Iowa City, Iowa

Frederick P. Beavers, MD
Associate Professor
Department of Surgery
Georgetown University
Interim Chief
Division of Vascular Surgery
Washington Hospital Center
Washington, DC

Anuradha R. Bhama, MD
Resident in General Surgery
Department of Surgery
University of Iowa Roy J. and Lucille A. Carver
   College of Medicine
Iowa City, Iowa

Lilja Thyri Bjornsdottir, MD
Chair, Division of Vascular Surgery
Department of Surgery
Landspitali University Hospital
Reykjavik, Iceland

Kevin A. Bridge, MD
Resident in General Surgery
Department of Surgery
University of Iowa Roy J. and Lucille A. Carver
   College of Medicine
Iowa City, Iowa

John C. Byrn, MD
Clinical Assistant Professor
Department of Surgery
University of Iowa Roy J. and Lucille A. Carver
   College of Medicine
Iowa City, Iowa

Phillip C. Camp, Jr., MD
Assistant Professor
Division of Thoracic Surgery
Department of Surgery
Harvard Medical School
Associate Surgeon
Brigham and Women's Hospital
Director, Transplant Administration
Director, Lung Transplantation
Director, ECMO Program
Boston, Massachusetts

J.C. Carr, MD
Resident in General Surgery
Department of Surgery
University of Iowa Roy J. and Lucille A. Carver
   College of Medicine
Iowa City, Iowa

Kent Choi, MD
Clinical Professor of Acute Care Surgery
Department of Surgery
University of Iowa Roy J. and Lucille A. Carver
   College of Medicine
Iowa City, Iowa

Hui Sen Chong, MD
Assistant Professor of Gastrointestinal Minimally
   Invasive Surgery
Department of Surgery
University of Iowa Roy J. and Lucille A. Carver
   College of Medicine
Iowa City, Iowa

Thomas E. Collins, MD
Clinical Associate Professor of Transplant Surgery
Department of Surgery
University of Iowa Roy J. and Lucille A. Carver
   College of Medicine
Iowa City, Iowa

James P. De Andrade, MD
Resident in General Surgery
Department of Surgery
University of Iowa Roy J. and Lucille A. Carver
 College of Medicine
Iowa City, Iowa

Jesse L. Dirksen, MD
Surgical Director
Edith Sanford Breast Cancer Center
Sioux Falls, South Dakota

Tamsin Durand, MD, MPH
General Surgeon
Surgical Associates of Rochester
Frisbie Memorial Hospital
Rochester, New Hampshire

Joss D. Fernandez, MD
Cardiothoracic and Vascular Surgeon
Missouri Heart Center
Columbia, Missouri

M. Victoria Gerken, MD
General Surgeon
Mineral King Surgical Associates
Visalia, California

Kevin D. Helling, MD
General Surgery Resident
Department of Surgery
Stanford University Medical Center
Palo Alto, California

Jamal J. Hoballah, MD, MBA
Professor & Chairman
Department of Surgery
American University of Beirut Medical Center
Beirut, Lebanon

Hisakazu Hoshi, MD
Clinical Associate Professor of Endocrine and Surgical
 Oncology
Department of Surgery
University of Iowa Roy J. and Lucille A. Carver
 College of Medicine
Iowa City, Iowa

James R. Howe, MD
Professor of Endocrine and Surgical Oncology
Department of Surgery
University of Iowa Roy J. and Lucille A. Carver
 College of Medicine
Iowa City, Iowa

Jennifer Hrabe, MD
Resident in General Surgery
Department of Surgery
University of Iowa Roy J. and Lucille A. Carver
 College of Medicine
Iowa City, Iowa

Andreas M. Kaiser, MD
Professor of Clinical Surgery
USC Division of Colorectal Surgery
Keck School of Medicine of USC
University of Southern California
Los Angeles, California

Daniel A. Katz, MD
Associate Professor of Transplant Surgery
Department of Surgery
University of Iowa Roy J. and Lucille A. Carver
 College of Medicine
Iowa City, Iowa

Kemp H. Kernstine, Sr., MD, PhD
Professor and Chairman
Division of Thoracic Surgery
University of Texas Southwestern Medical Center
Dallas, Texas

Prashant Khullar, MD
Clinical Assistant Professor of Acute Care Surgery
Department of Surgery
University of Iowa Roy J. and Lucille A. Carver
 College of Medicine
Iowa City, Iowa

Timothy F. Kresowik, MD
Professor of Vascular Surgery
Department of Surgery
University of Iowa Roy J. and Lucille A. Carver
 College of Medicine
Iowa City, Iowa

Geeta Lal, MD, MSc
Associate Professor of Endocrine and Surgical Oncology
Department of Surgery
University of Iowa Roy J. and Lucille A. Carver
 College of Medicine
Iowa City, Iowa

Grant O. Lee, MD
Resident in General Surgery
Department of Surgery
University of Iowa Roy J. and Lucille A. Carver
 College of Medicine
Iowa City, Iowa

Samy Mokhtar Maklad, MD
Clinical Assistant Professor of Acute Care Surgery
Department of Surgery
University of Iowa Roy J. and Lucille A. Carver
    College of Medicine
Iowa City, Iowa

James J. Mezhir, MD
Assistant Professor of Endocrine and Surgical Oncology
Department of Surgery
University of Iowa Roy J. and Lucille A. Carver
    College of Medicine
Iowa City, Iowa

Rachael Nicholson, MD
Clinical Assistant Professor of Vascular Surgery
Department of Surgery
University of Iowa Roy J. and Lucille A. Carver
    College of Medicine
Iowa City, Iowa

Courtney L. Olmsted, BSE, MD
Resident in General Surgery
Department of Surgery
University of Iowa Roy J. and Lucille A. Carver
    College of Medicine
Iowa City, Iowa

Kristine Clodfelter Orion, MD
Resident in General Surgery
Department of Surgery
University of Iowa Roy J. and Lucille A. Carver
    College of Medicine
Iowa City, Iowa

Carlos A. Pelaez, MD
Clinical Assistant Professor of Acute Care Surgery
Department of Surgery
University of Iowa Roy J. and Lucille A. Carver
    College of Medicine
Iowa City, Iowa

Graeme J. Pitcher, MD
Clinical Associate Professor Pediatric Surgery
University of Iowa Roy J. and Lucille A. Carver
    College of Medicine
Iowa City, Iowa

Isaac Samuel, MD
Associate Professor of Bariatric and Gastrointestinal Surgery
Department of Surgery
University of Iowa Roy J. and Lucille A. Carver
    College of Medicine
Iowa City, Iowa

Virginia Oliva Shaffer, MD
Assistant Professor
Department of General and GI Surgery
Colorectal Surgery
Emory University School of Medicine
Atlanta, Georgia

Melhem J. Sharafuddin, MD
Associate Clinical Professor of Surgery and Radiology
Director of Endovascular Surgery
University of Iowa Roy J. And Lucille A. Carver
    College of Medicine
Iowa City, Iowa

W. John Sharp
Professor
Department of Surgery
University of Iowa
Iowa City, Iowa

Scott K. Sherman, MD
Resident in General Surgery
Department of Surgery
University of Iowa Carver College of Medicine
Iowa City, Iowa

Rajesh Shetty, DNB (Gen.Surg)
Formerly, Fellow, Abdominal Transplant Surgery
University of Iowa Hospitals and Clinics
Iowa City, Iowa

Kenneth B. Simon, MD, MBA
Chief of Staff
Gulf Coast Veterans Healthcare System
Biloxi, Mississippi

Amir F. Sleiman, MD
Department of General Surgery
American University of Beirut Medical Center
Beirut, Lebanon

Jessica K. Smith
Clinical Assistant Professor
Department of Surgery
University of Iowa
Iowa City, Iowa

Raphael C. Sun, MD
Resident in General Surgery
Department of Surgery
University of Iowa Roy J. and Lucille A. Carver
    College of Medicine
Iowa City, Iowa

Jose E. Torres, MD, MSc
Visiting Associate
Department of Cardiothoracic Surgery
University of Iowa Roy J. and Lucille A. Carver
   College of Medicine
Iowa City, Iowa

Christine J. Waller, MD
Resident in General Surgery
Department of Surgery
University of Iowa Roy J. and Lucille A. Carver
   College of Medicine
Iowa City, Iowa

Jarrett E. Walsh, MD, PhD
Resident in Otolaryngology
Department of Otolaryngology
University of Iowa Roy J. and Lucille A. Carver
   College of Medicine
Iowa City, Iowa

Steven D. Wexner, MD, PhD (Hon)
Director, Digestive Disease Center
Chair, Department of Colorectal Surgery
Emeritus Chief of Staff, Cleveland Clinic Florida
Affiliate Professor and Associate Dean for Academic Affairs
Florida Atlantic University College of Medicine
Clinical Professor and Affiliate Dean for Clinical Education
Florida International University College of Medicine
Weston, Florida

Neal Wilkinson, MD
Associate Professor of Surgery & Oncology
Roswell Park Cancer Institute
Buffalo, New York

Foreword to the First Edition

It is a privilege to introduce this fine and literary volume. It comes at a time when the hours of instruction in gross anatomy that medical students receive have been gradually but drastically reduced in many, if not most, medical schools, often by at least one-half that of thirty years ago. Formal instruction in embryology virtually disappeared from some curricula but has recently been partially restored.

To be sure, different medical specialists have different needs for precise anatomical knowledge. Thus, a significant reduction in gross anatomy hours and detail for the majority of medical students was doubtless justified, as the rise in other disciplines such as genetics, molecular biology, psychiatry, and still others laid claim to increased classroom attention. The surgeon's need for precise anatomical knowledge, however, has not decreased. In fact, it has increased, as mini-invasive surgery, in which the first author has special expertise, has exploded worldwide. Incomplete or imprecise knowledge of the regional anatomy involved in a given operation can result in severe injuries and devastating complications. Hence, the need for this operative anatomy atlas by a practicing academic surgeon, Dr. Carol Scott-Conner, and a professional anatomist, Dr. David L. Dawson, is clear. Their intimate collaboration over a period of some years during and after which Dr. Scott-Conner took her second doctorate degree, in anatomy, has culminated in a volume practical not only for medical students and residents but also for practicing surgeons who may need to refresh their knowledge of regional anatomy.

But, while operative anatomy remains the central focus, this book conveys much additional information and guidance and many admonitions—all of great value. Operative techniques for over 101 procedures, involving six regions of the body, are detailed. With each operation, the discussion is divided into "anatomic points" and "technical points." Operative safeguards and potential errors are stressed. Up-to-date references appear at the end of each section. Normal organ function and its preservation or restoration after surgery are emphasized throughout.

The major strength of the work is represented by the line drawings developed with Michael P. Schenk, James Goodman, Myriam E. Kirkman, Steven H. Oh, Charles Boyter, David J. Mascaro, and Mary K. Shirazi, medical illustrators.

This writer is confident that *Operative Anatomy* will be received enthusiastically and will quickly become a standard source in its field.

James D. Hardy
Professor of Surgery Emeritus
Department of Surgery
University of Mississippi Medical Center
Jackson, Mississippi

Preface

What is new with this edition? A lot. The entire book has been structured around SCORE™, the Surgical Council on Resident Education, Curriculum Outline (2012–2013). Procedures in the print version concentrate on the "Essential Common" and "Essential Uncommon" categories, and many "Complex" procedures have been moved to the web version. New procedures have been added. Color photographs have been added. The chapters still begin with three tables—"Steps in Procedure," "Hallmark Anatomic Complications," and "List of Structures." These tables are intended for quick review before performing an operation, or before taking the boards. "Steps in Procedure" is simply a quick list of the order in which various steps are done. "Hallmark Anatomic Complications" lists those problems unique to the procedure, as opposed to more generic complications such as bleeding or infection that may follow any operation. For example, bile duct injury is a hallmark anatomic complication of cholecystectomy (laparoscopic or open), ureteral injury is a hallmark anatomic complication of hysterectomy or colon resection.

The challenge in revising a text like Operative Anatomy lies not in deciding which procedures to add, but rather in choosing those to delete. Can the author assume, for example, that vagotomy is an obsolete operation? Not yet. What about lumbar sympathectomy? Safest to include these procedures and hope for the clemency of the publisher.

Because we were able to move material to the web version (accessible to registered users), little has been deleted. Some material has been condensed, some has been changed, and much has been added. The first edition had 72 chapters; this edition has 134. The number of contributing authors has grown and we have added a significant number of new color images.

Sadly, during our work on this revision, my friend and colleague David L Dawson died. He remained an active clinical anatomist and gifted teacher to the end. Virtually all of the "Anatomic Points" were written by him. Thus, this revision was enriched by his previous contributions and I deeply regret that I will not be able to consult him in the future.

As with prior editions, the goal has been to provide the surgeon—whether trainee or experienced—with a reference for both the surgical technique and the relevant anatomy. Emphasis has been placed on proven, mainstream techniques rather than "how I do it," and references are included for alternative or infrequently employed maneuvers.

Carol E. H. Scott-Conner, MD, PhD, MBA
Iowa City, Iowa

Preface to the First Edition

To paraphrase the familiar proverb "necessity is the mother of invention," *frustration is the genesis of books.* As a surgical resident, the first author was often frustrated because the regional gross anatomy studied as a freshman in medical school had too often been forgotten or was inadequate or inappropriate for the procedures to be done the next day. Various surgical atlases and descriptions were of some help with complex procedures, but these often ignored the anatomy relevant to common procedures that all residents must perform.

The second author, trained as a traditional gross anatomist, also became frustrated when attempting to develop surgical anatomy programs based upon procedures which, although commonplace to surgical residents, had not been included in his training. Moreover, he discovered that dissection in the gross anatomy lab was vastly different, both in technique and in concept, from that practiced by surgeons. Also daunting was the realization that the anatomy taught in such anatomy courses was often inappropriate for a single medical discipline, such as surgery. Finally, he, like most traditional anatomists, was only vaguely familiar with the technical aspects of the many procedures required of developing surgeons.

In light of these frustrations, this book was developed to provide a concise reference to the relevant operative anatomy of procedures encountered by most general surgery residents. We also expect that this text will be useful to medical students rotating through surgery. Finally, we hope that this book will be of value to anatomy instructors and to surgeons who would like a quick review of the anatomy germane to common procedures.

The volume is divided into sections based on anatomic regions, permitting the curious user a rapid review of the relevant operative anatomy of a given region. In each section, individual chapters present technical anatomic considerations for specific operative procedures. The illustrations are designed to show both the topographic and regional anatomy, as well as to focus on the anatomy visualized as the procedure progresses. The text is divided into technical and anatomic points, for successful surgery depends on a knowledge of both. At the end of each section, selected references are provided for the reader who is interested in learning more. These carefully selected entries are, in our opinion, benchmark articles. Lastly, appreciating the frustrations inherent in learning the technical aspects of general surgery, we have included an appendix that describes common surgical instruments and their use. Because this text is intended for surgeons-in-training and for practicing surgeons, we have used terminology consistent with current surgical usage. In some cases this corresponds to *Nomina Anatomica,* but in many cases it does not.

This work is not intended to be all-inclusive, either anatomically or surgically. Rather, our aim is to enable the reader to review the anatomy necessary to perform successfully those procedures that form the core of most general surgery residency programs—procedures that comprise the "bread and butter" of a general surgeon's practice.

Carol E. H. Scott-Conner, MD, PhD, MBA
David L. Dawson, PhD

Acknowledgments

The authors once again wish to thank Dr. James D. Hardy, now deceased, and Dr. Robert S. Rhodes for their enthusiasm and advice during the preparation of the first edition.

We have been blessed with patient and wise editors at Lippincott Williams & Wilkins—Lisa McAllister, who shepherded this book through the first two editions, followed by Brian Brown and Keith Donnellan, who have seen this one through to completion. An expert developmental editor, Brendan Huffman, expedited the process of bringing the book together.

Finally, we thank our students, residents, and co-workers for their patience. The editor gives special thanks to her husband, Dr. Harry F. Conner, whose love and support makes all of this possible.

Contents

SECTION I   The Head and Neck

e = web only chapter

SECTION II   The Pectoral Region and Chest

e = web only chapter

SECTION III The Upper Extremity

SECTION IV The Abdominal Region

e = web only chapter

ℰ = web only chapter

@ = web only chapter

ⓔ = web only chapter

e = web only chapter

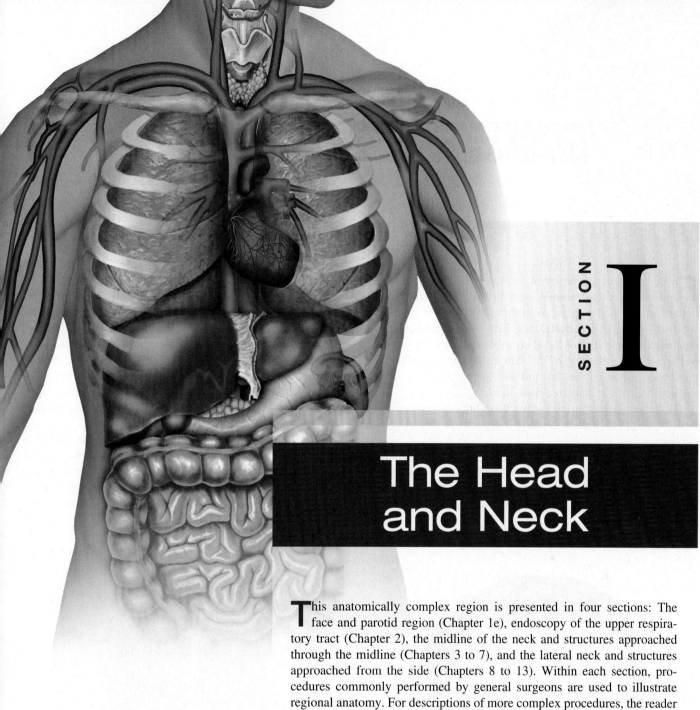

SECTION

I

The Head and Neck

This anatomically complex region is presented in four sections: The face and parotid region (Chapter 1e), endoscopy of the upper respiratory tract (Chapter 2), the midline of the neck and structures approached through the midline (Chapters 3 to 7), and the lateral neck and structures approached from the side (Chapters 8 to 13). Within each section, procedures commonly performed by general surgeons are used to illustrate regional anatomy. For descriptions of more complex procedures, the reader should consult an atlas of plastic surgery or surgery of the head and neck (see references listed below).

REFERENCES

1. Lore JM, Medina JM. *An Atlas of Head and Neck Surgery.* Philadelphia: Saunders; 2004. (This classic text provides detailed information on specialized surgical techniques.)
2. Thorne CH, Beasley RW, Aston SJ, et al., eds. *Grabb and Smith's Plastic Surgery.* 6th ed. Philadelphia: Lippincott Williams & Wilkins; 2007. (A brief but comprehensive overview of plastic surgery, this book includes extremely useful information on suturing facial lacerations and local flaps.)

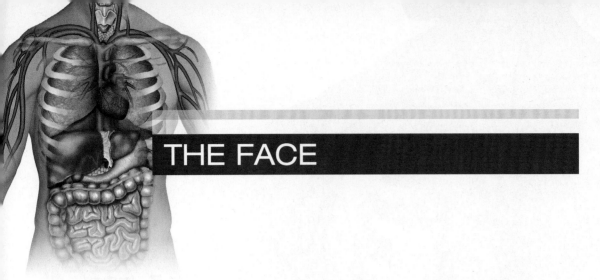

THE FACE

Facial incisions are designed to preserve facial symmetry and motion and to minimize scarring. To remove small skin tumors, make elective incisions in natural skin "wrinkle lines," if possible (Fig. 1). Generally, these lines run perpendicular to the underlying muscles of facial expression, as they are formed by the repetitive pleating of the skin caused by the action of these muscles. Scars that fall in these lines will be less conspicuous than those that cross these lines.

Traumatic lacerations that cross these lines can sometimes be debrided or modified by Z-plasty to conform to natural wrinkle lines.

Approximate the eyebrow and vermilion border of the lip with special precision because even a small degree of malalignment will be permanently obvious. Never shave the eyebrow as regrowth of eyebrow hair is unpredictable.

The muscles of facial expression (Fig. 2) are innervated by the seventh cranial nerve, aptly named the facial nerve. The anatomy of the facial nerve and parotid region are illustrated in Chapter 1.

Deep lacerations of the cheek may divide branches of the facial nerve or the parotid (Stensen's) duct. Evaluate nerve function by asking the patient to raise and lower the eyebrows (temporal branches of the facial nerve), close the eyes tightly (zygomatic branches), and smile (zygomatic and buccal branches). If a nerve injury is diagnosed, attempt primary repair.

Look inside the mouth, gently retracting the cheek with a tongue blade, and identify the internal opening of the parotid duct as a small punctum opposite the maxillary second molar. Cannulate this with a fine Silastic tube. The appearance of the tube within the wound confirms injury to the duct. Identify both

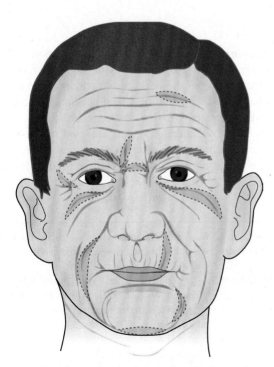

Figure 1 Incisions and excision sites that are chosen to lie along natural skin crease heal with minimal scarring and are generally hidden within normal facial wrinkles.

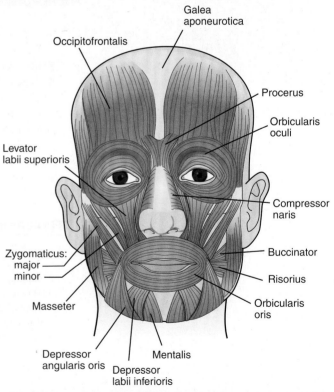

Figure 2 The muscles of facial expression create wrinkles in the skin through natural skin movement.

ends of the duct, repairing it with fine, interrupted sutures of an absorbable material. Use the Silastic tube to stent the repair.

Close deep lacerations in layers, carefully approximating muscle, fascia, and skin. Complex injuries involving muscle, nerve, or the parotid duct are best repaired in the operating room.

REFERENCES

1. Armstrong BD. Lacerations of the mouth. *Emerg Med Clin North Am.* 2000;18:471–480.
2. Brown DJ, Jaffee JE, Henson JK. Advanced laceration management. *Emerg Med Clin North Am.* 2007;25:83–99.
3. Hollier L Jr, Kelley P. Soft tissue and skeletal injuries of the face. In: Thorne CH, Beasley RW, Aston SJ, et al., eds. *Grabb and Smith's Plastic Surgery.* 6th ed. Philadelphia: Lippincott Williams & Wilkins; 2007:315–332.
4. Kreissl CJ. The selection of appropriate lines for elective surgical incisions. *Plast Reconstr Surg.* 1951;8:1. (This brief classic paper discusses the rationale for choosing various incisions to minimize scarring.)
5. Thomas JR, Somenek M. Scar revision review. *Arch Facial Plast Surg.* 2012;14:162.

e1 Parotidectomy

This chapter can be accessed online at www.lww.com/eChapter1.

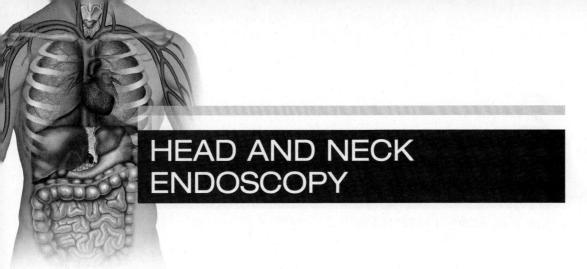

HEAD AND NECK ENDOSCOPY

Although not strictly operative procedures, laryngoscopy and endotracheal intubation are frequently performed by surgeons. Endotracheal intubation is considered an ESSENTIAL COMMON technique by SCORE, the Surgical Committee on Resident Education. Mirror laryngoscopy is essentially unchanged since Czermark's description in 1865 and Kirstein's technique for direct laryngoscopy in 1895. Newer video technology has improved the safety of endotracheal intubation; nevertheless, both techniques continue to demand respect for the complex anatomy of this region and the ability to obtain a secure airway.

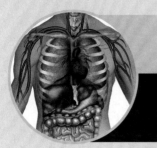

2

Laryngoscopy and Endotracheal Intubation

Laura A. Adam and Kent Choi

Laryngoscopy, or visualization of the larynx, is performed for both diagnostic and therapeutic purposes. In this chapter, indirect (or mirror) laryngoscopy and the direct laryngoscopy for the purpose of endotracheal intubation are discussed. The use of the fiberoptic laryngoscope is described as part of fiberoptic bronchoscopy (see Chapter 25).

SCORE™, the Surgical Council on Resident Education, classified endotracheal intubation as an "ESSENTIAL COMMON" procedure.

STEPS IN INDIRECT LARYNGOSCOPY

Obtain adequate topical anesthesia
Warm the mirror to avoid fogging

Introduce the mirror into back of oropharynx

STEPS IN ENDOTRACHEAL INTUBATION

Positioning the patient
  Placing the patient in the sniffing position
    when possible
  Providing cervical spine stabilization
    when necessary
Inducing appropriate sedation and relaxation
Introducing the laryngoscope blade
  Advancing a straight (Miller) blade over
    the epiglottis
  Advancing a curved (Macintosh) blade in
    front of the epiglottis

Lifting the larynx gently in the anterior
  caudal direction
Visualizing the laryngeal aperture
Passing the endotracheal tube through cords
  Confirming endotracheal placement of
    tube
Securing in place
Obtaining a chest x-ray to verify appropriate
  positioning

ANATOMIC COMPLICATIONS

Oral trauma
Tracheal stenosis

Esophageal intubation
Right mainstem bronchial intubation

LIST OF STRUCTURES

Tongue
Uvula
Pharynx
  Nasopharynx
  Oropharynx
  Laryngopharynx (hypopharynx)
Palatoglossal arch
Hyoid bone
Hyoepiglottic ligament
Larynx
  Laryngeal inlet
  Epiglottis

True vocal cords
Vestibular folds (false vocal cords)
Rima glottidis, glottis
Arytenoid cartilages
Cuneiform and corniculate cartilages
Interarytenoid notch
Hyoepiglottic ligament
Trachea
  Cricoid cartilage
  Thyroid cartilage
  Carina

Indirect Laryngoscopy

Mirror Laryngoscopy (Fig. 2.1)

Technical Points

The patient should be seated facing the examiner for this procedure. Adequate topical anesthesia of the posterior pharynx is essential. Ask the patient to open the mouth and stick out the tongue. Spray a topical anesthetic over the tongue, soft palate, uvula, and posterior pharynx. Gently grasp the tongue with a dry sponge or deflect it down with a tongue blade to improve visibility. Use a headlamp to provide illumination. Warm a dental mirror by holding it under hot running water so that it does not fog when placed in the warm, moist environment of the posterior pharynx. Use your nondominant hand to apply posterior pressure to the thyroid cartilage to increase visualization.

Place the mirror in the oropharynx, just anterior to the uvula. Push back gently on the uvula and visualize the larynx by adjusting the angle of the mirror slightly (Fig. 2.1). Observe the vocal cords for color, symmetry, abnormal growths, and mobility during phonation. The mirror can also be used to inspect the lateral pharyngeal wall and can be reversed to view the posterior nasopharynx.

Recognize that the mirror produces an apparent reversal of anterior and posterior regions. Visualization of the anterior commissure and base of the epiglottis and the subglottic regions is limited by overhanging structures.

Anatomic Points

The upper aerodigestive tract is divided into the oral cavity proper and the pharynx on the basis of embryologic origin.

The oral cavity is lined by epithelium of ectodermal origin. It ends at about the level of the palatoglossal arch. The pharynx is lined with epithelium that is endodermally derived. It is divided into the nasopharynx, the oropharynx, and the laryngopharynx. The nasopharynx is posterior to the nose and superior to the soft palate. The oropharynx extends from the soft palate to the hyoid bone. The laryngopharynx extends from the hyoid bone to the cricoid cartilage and is also known as the hypopharynx.

The larynx is made of a combination of skeletal structures, muscles, and connective tissues, and is responsible for phonation, assistance with respiration, and protection against aspiration. At the superior aspect of the larynx is the hyoid bone which during swallowing elevates the larynx via the hyoepiglottic ligament to prevent aspiration. The epiglottis along with the thyroid, cricoid, and arytenoid cartilages make up the skeletal portion of the larynx. The thyroid cartilage is attached to the epiglottis and forms the externally prominent Adam's apple. The cricoid cartilage is also a single cartilage and is the only complete cartilage. The posterior cartilages are paired and consistent of the arytenoid, the cuneiform, and corniculate cartilages. During laryngoscopy, the vocal cords are encircled posteriorly from lateral to medial by the paired structures of the aryepiglottic folds, cuneiform cartilages, and corniculate cartilages where they fuse at the interarytenoid notch. This is the most posterior portion of the laryngeal inlet and must be viewed for endotracheal intubation. The lateral mucosal folds known as the vestibular folds (false vocal cords) are covered by respiratory epithelium and are responsible for resonance. The true vocal cords via posterior attachments to the arytenoids and anterior attachments to the thyroid and cricoid cartilages are

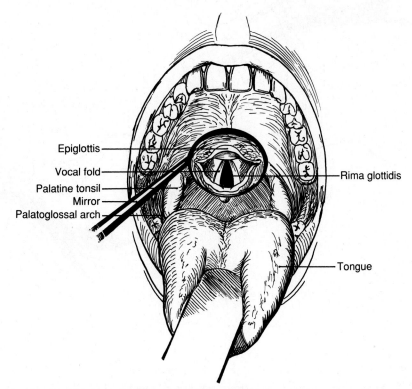

Epiglottis
Vocal fold
Palatine tonsil
Mirror
Palatoglossal arch
Rima glottidis
Tongue

Figure 2.1 Mirror laryngoscopy

responsible for phonation. The opening that is viewed between them is known as the rima glottidis whereas the glottis is the vocal cords and the space between them.

Endotracheal Intubation

Positioning the Patient (Fig. 2.2)

Technical Points

Position the patient supine with the neck slightly flexed and a small roll under the head. Stand at the head of the operating table or bed. If you are intubating a patient in bed, remove the headboard whenever possible to gain better access to the patient.

The "sniffing position" (Fig. 2.2A) decreases the distance from the teeth to the larynx and facilitates visualization of the larynx. Hyperextension of the neck (Fig. 2.2B) increases the distance from the teeth to the larynx and makes intubation more difficult. Flexion of the head on the neck compresses the airway, again making intubation more difficult. Achieve the correct position by placing a small pillow or folded sheet under the head.

Do not manipulate the head and neck in a patient with a known or possible cervical spine injury. Displacement of vertebrae can cause irreversible damage to the spinal cord. In the situation of known or suspected injury to the cervical spine, fiberoptic laryngoscopy, blind nasotracheal intubation (generally only successful in breathing patients), or cricothyroidotomy is safer than orotracheal intubation. These difficult airway problems are discussed in the references.

Anatomic Points

Note the relative orientation of the structures involved in endotracheal intubation. In the anatomic position, the orientation of the horizontally displaced oral cavity is about 90 degrees with respect to the vertical laryngeal pharynx. The laryngeal inlet forms the anterior wall of the cranial portion of the laryngeal pharynx. The rima glottidis is again approximately horizontal, but the infraglottic cavity and trachea are oblique, coursing from superoanterior to inferoposterior. With the neck gently flexed and the atlanto-occipital joint extended, the involved pathway has gentle curves rather than acute angles. Straightening the

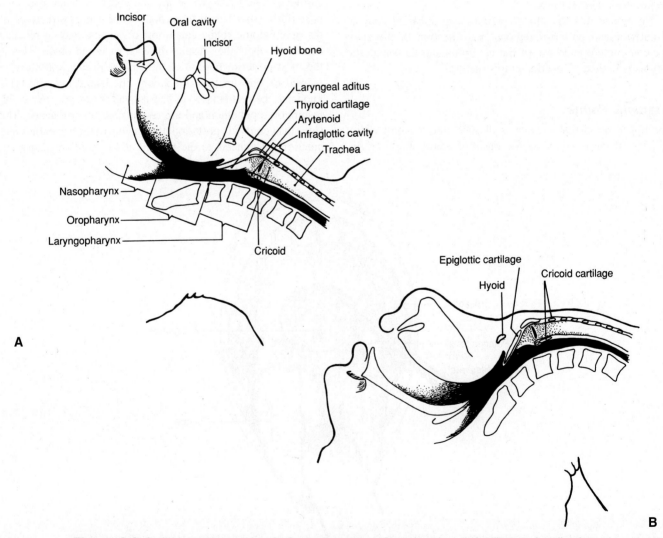

Figure 2.2 Positioning the patient. **A:** Correct position of head and neck facilitates visualization of glottis. **B:** Incorrect position makes it harder to see the glottis.

airway in this manner also shortens the distance from the teeth to the trachea. Allow for this when tube length is estimated before intubation.

Introducing the Laryngoscope (Fig. 2.3)

Technical Points

Preoxygenate the patient by bag and mask ventilation with 100% oxygen before attempting intubation. This allows intubation to progress in an orderly, unhurried fashion. Check all the equipments carefully. Verify that the laryngoscope light works, the proper size of endotracheal tube is available, and check the cuff on the endotracheal tube. One needs to have a working suction available and have at hand an assortment of laryngoscope blade types and lengths, endotracheal tubes, and a stylet. Probably, the most important part of intubation is establishing additional alternatives should direct laryngoscopy be unsuccessful. Alternatives include video laryngoscopy, optical laryngoscopy, fiberoptic intubation, optical stylet, alternative tubes such as an intubating laryngeal mask airway (LMA), and surgical airways.

After administration of appropriate sedation and relaxation, use the fingers of your gloved right hand to open the jaws by spreading apart the upper and lower incisors. Use your thumb to push the lower incisors down and your third finger to elevate the upper incisors in a "scissor technique." Hold the laryngoscope by its handle in your left hand and gently introduce the blade, sliding it over the tongue toward the oropharynx. When opening the jaw and inserting the laryngoscope, be very careful to avoid chipping the teeth or using them as a fulcrum to lever the laryngoscope blade. Think of the laryngoscope as a lighted tongue blade with a handle that is used to elevate the tongue, mandible, and epiglottis to expose the larynx. The initial angle of the scope should be toward the toes to divert the tongue and jaw downward. Once the blade is fully around the base of the tongue, the handle can be elevated more paralell to the patient's body for improved visualization.

Two types of laryngoscope blades (straight and curved) are commonly used. To some extent, personal preference dictates which blade is used. Many people prefer the curved blade for routine intubation, using the straight blade only when exposure is difficult.

When using a curved blade, insert the blade fully into the vallecula. Once the tip is fully within the vallecula, the blade can be retracted to a 40-degree angle to visualize the epiglottis. Insert the curved (Macintosh) blade to a point just in front of the epiglottis (Fig. 2.3A). The curve of the blade tends to follow the curve of the tongue and is advanced downward until the tip of the blade rests against the hyoepiglottic ligament. Gentle upward and forward pressure elevates the epiglottis. Visualization should progressively include from posterior to anterior, the interarytenoid notch, the glottis, and the vocal cords.

Alternatively, insert the straight (Miller) blade just past the epiglottis (Fig. 2.3B). Elevate the epiglottis by direct pressure to expose the vocal cords. Careful positioning of the patient to align the airway before insertion of the blade will help to ensure success. Note that the view obtained is slightly different because the straight blade covers and obscures the view of the epiglottis, but visualization of the interarytenoid notch, the rima glottidis, and the vocal cords should progress in the same manner.

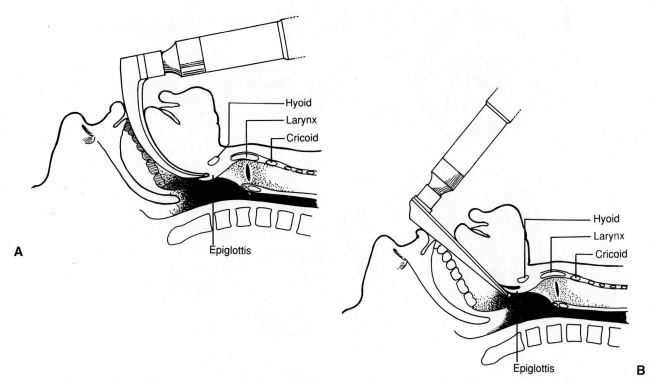

Figure 2.3 Introducing the laryngoscope. **A:** Curved blade is positioned in front of epiglottis. **B:** Straight blade is passed beyond epiglottis.

Anatomic Points

Note that the base of the tongue and the anterior surface of the epiglottis are apposed. Both have attachments to the hyoid bone (the tongue via the hyoglossus muscle, the epiglottis via the hyoepiglottic ligament). Elevating the tongue and mandible will reduce tension on the hyoid bone and epiglottis and will allow increased mobility of the epiglottis. Moving the epiglottis anteriorly is accomplished with a straight blade by applying gentle pressure on the epiglottic cartilage itself. The curved blade presses on the hyoepiglottic ligament to pull the epiglottis anteriorly.

Visualizing the Laryngeal Aperture (Fig. 2.4)

Technical Points

Ideally the entire larynx including both the anterior and posterior vocal cords should be visible (Fig. 2.4). A Grade I view of the larynx is similar to that seen in Figure 2.1. Although one is now looking at the larynx directly, rather than using a mirror, the examiner's position relative to the airway has changed, and thus the view obtained has the same orientation. If the cords cannot be visualized, provide anterior pressure of the thyroid cartilage to increase visualization of the larynx. Airway visualization is graded from I to IV. A Grade I view includes visualization of the entire laryngeal aperture, Grade II only the posterior commissure of the laryngeal aperture, Grade III only the epiglottis, and

Grade IV only the soft palate. Grade III and Grade IV views not surprisingly are predictive of difficult intubations.

In rapid sequence intubation, the Sellick maneuver is used to prevent regurgitation from the stomach by occluding the esophagus. An assistant provides cricoid pressure in order to use the rigid back wall of cricoid cartilage (remember it is the only completely ringed cartilage) to compress the esophagus against the vertebral column. The assistant must be instructed not to release the pressure until the cuff of the endotracheal tube is inflated in the trachea and position confirmed.

Anatomic Points

The true vocal cords appear whitish. The more cephalad vestibular folds (false vocal cords) are pink and are not as prominent. Gentle downward pressure on the thyroid cartilage will compress the esophagus and other soft tissues posterior to the larynx, thus enhancing the alignment of the laryngeal cavity with the passageway from mouth to vocal cords.

Passing of the Endotracheal Tube Through the Cords (Fig. 2.5)

Technical Points

Once visualization is optimal, one can pass the tube under direct vision through the vocal cords (Fig. 2.5A). If a Grade I

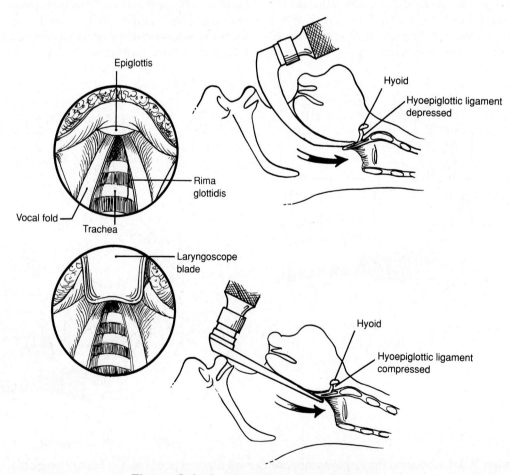

Figure 2.4 Visualizing the laryngeal aperatus

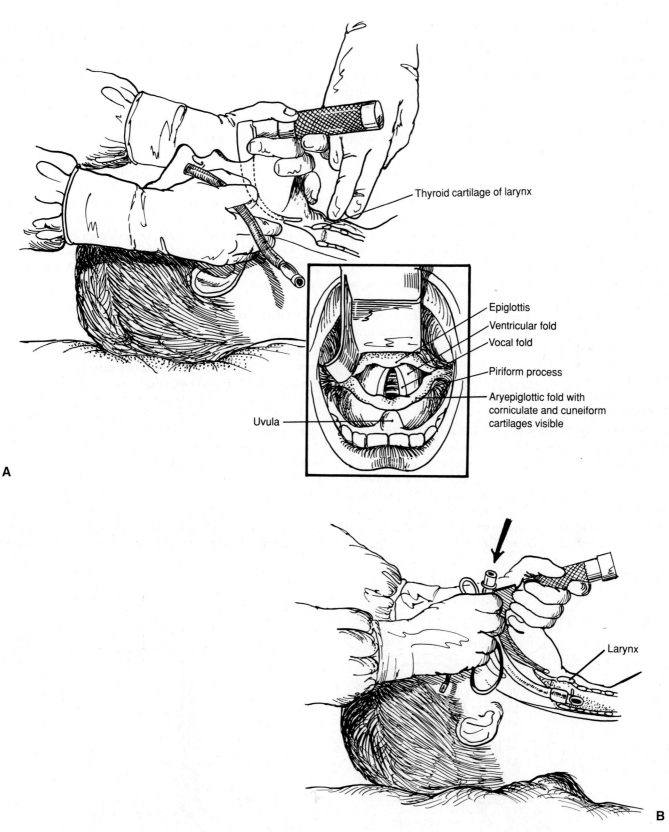

Figure 2.5 Passing the endotracheal tube through the cords. **A:** Visualizing glottis.
B: Passing tube.

or Grade II view cannot be obtained, consider an alternative intubation strategy as previously described.

The endotracheal tube is constructed with a gentle curve, which aids in passage through the cords (Fig. 2.5B). If a greater curvature is needed because of a very anterior larynx, use a stylet. Many practitioners routinely use a stylet; this stiffens the tube but increases the risk for laryngeal damage if the tube is forced. The tube should pass easily. Once the tip of the tube has passed through the cords have an assistance pull out the stylet.

Anatomic Points

As previously stated, visualization of the entire laryngeal aperture should include progressive visualization from posterior to anterior, the interarytenoid notch, the rimi glottidis, and the vocal cords. (Fig. 2.5A, inset). In inserting the tube, guide it through the rima glottidis to inflict as little trauma as possible to the laryngeal mucosa. Such trauma can denude regions of the larynx and elicit involuntary reflexes carried by sensory fibers of the internal branch of the superior laryngeal nerve cephalad to the vocal cords and fibers of the recurrent laryngeal nerve inferior to the vocal cords.

Positioning the Tube (Fig. 2.6)

Technical Points

Advance the cuff past the cords and inflate until no air leak is detected while maintaining the cuff pressure below 25 mm Hg. This ensures that the cuff pressure is lower than the tracheal capillary perfusion pressure, thereby minimizing pressure necrosis of the trachea and long-term risk of tracheal stenosis. The esophagus lies directly posterior to the trachea; blind passage of the tube, particularly when the larynx is more anterior than usual, may result in esophageal intubation. Guard against this by always passing

the tube under direct vision when possible. Additional procedures should be performed to confirm appropriate position including CO_2 detection with colorimetric change and/or capnometry and presence of bilateral breath sounds with lack of gastric resonance. A disposable colorimetric CO_2 detector is often readily available and demonstrates a change of color when CO_2 is detected. In the operating room or intensive care unit, capnometry can help to confirm adequacy of ventilatory exchange.

The tip of the tube should lie approximately 2.5 cm above the carina to allow downward migration with increasing neck flexion (Fig. 2.6B). Confirm the position of the tube by auscultation. Breath sounds should be heard clearly over both lung fields. If the tube is inserted too far, it will enter one of the principal bronchi, usually the right. Overinflation of one lung and collapse of the contralateral lung will result. When this occurs, deflate the cuff and reposition the tube. Confirm the position of the tube by obtaining a chest radiograph.

Anatomic Points

The blood supply to the trachea, derived from branches of the inferior thyroid arteries, is not particularly rich. In addition, the tracheal cartilages provide a relatively rigid framework. Thus overinflation of the cuff can easily compromise the blood supply to the mucosa—in particular, that covering the cartilages.

Estimate the distance from the incisor teeth to the carina in order to ensure that the tip of the tube is properly placed. The distance from incisors to vocal cords and then to the carina increases with age. Further, there is a disproportionate increase in the length of the trachea. The length of the trachea (cords to carina) essentially triples from birth to age 65 years, whereas the length of the oropharyngeal cavity (incisors to vocal cords) essentially doubles. The approximate length of tube needed can be determined before intubation by placing the tube alongside

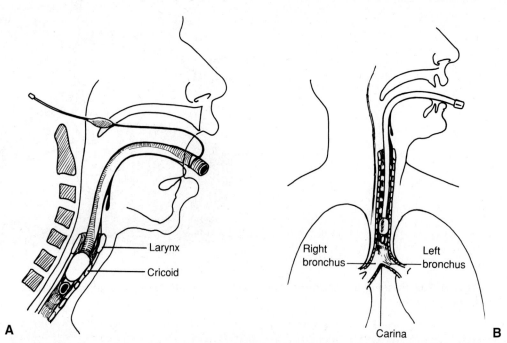

Larynx

Cricoid

Right bronchus

Left bronchus

Carina

A   **B**

Figure 2.6 Positioning the tube. **A:** Balloon at cricoid cartilage, tube is a bit too high. **B:** Tube in good position above carina.

the face and neck, and extending it to the sternal angle (of Louis), which approximates the level of the carina. The tube should be 2 to 3 cm shorter than this distance.

At the carina, the trachea divides into left and right principal bronchi. The left mainstem bronchus is smaller in diameter than the right and takes off at a more acute angle. This explains why endotracheal tubes, if inserted too far, typically enter the right mainstem bronchus.

REFERENCES

1. Applebaum EL, Bruce DL. *Tracheal Intubation.* Philadelphia: WB Saunders; 1976. (This monograph describes basic intubation techniques including tracheostomy.)
2. Blanc VF, Tremblay NA. The complications of tracheal intubation. *Anesth Analg.* 1974;53:202–213.
3. Dripps RD, Eckenhoff JE, Van Dam LD. Intubation of the trachea. In: Dripps RD, Eckenhoff JE, Van Dam LD, eds. *Anesthesia: The Principles of Safe Practice.* 6th ed. Philadelphia: WB Saunders; 1982.
4. Mahajan R, Ahmed P, Shafi F, et al. Dual bougie technique for nasotracheal intubation. *Anesth Prog.* 2012;59:85–86.
5. McGovern FH, Fitz-Hugh GS, Edgeman LJ. The hazards of endotracheal intubation. *Ann Otol Rhinol Laryngol.* 1971;80: 556–564.
6. Orringer MB. Endotracheal intubation and tracheostomy: Indications, techniques, and complications. *Surg Clin North Am.* 1980; 60:1447–1464. (Provides a clear description of blind nasotracheal intubation, as well as of other techniques; also discusses what to do if intubation is not possible after induction of anesthesia.)
7. Rothfield KP, Russo SG. Videolaryngoscopy: Should it replace direct laryngoscopy? A pro-con debate. *J Clin Anesth.* 2012;24: 593–597.
8. Thierbach AR, Lipp MD. Airway management in trauma patients. *Anesth Clin North Am.* 1999;17:63–81. (Discusses options when possible cervical spine injury complicates management.)
9. Wilson WC, Benumof JL. Pathophysiology, evaluation, and treatment of the difficult airway. *Anesth Clin North Am.* 1998; 16:29–75.

THE MIDLINE AND STRUCTURES APPROACHED THROUGH THE MIDLINE

General surgical procedures involving the neck can be divided into those that are performed through a midline approach and those that are performed through a lateral incision. Accordingly, the anatomy of the neck is explored in this section first through structures approached through the midline (trachea, thyroid, parathyroid) and then through structures approached laterally (lymph nodes, major vessels, cervical esophagus).

Important structures approached from the midline of the neck include the thyroid and parathyroid glands and the trachea. Although the esophagus is a midline structure, it is often approached laterally because it lies deep to the trachea. *The anatomy of the neck is separated by multiple fascial planes and commonly oriented by "triangle" groupings. Understanding these boundaries is* essential to good surgical technique in the neck. For simplicity, visualize the multiple fascial layers as a set of "tubes within tubes" (Fig. 1).

After incising through skin and subcutaneous fat through the midline, the platysma muscle is exposed. This thin muscular layer is innervated by a branch of facial nerve, cranial nerve VII. The first encountered cervical fascial layer—forming the outer tube—invests all cervical structures and is just deep to the platysma. This layer, called the deep cervical fascia, splits to encompass the sternocleidomastoid muscle, the trapezius muscle, the corresponding spinal accessory nerve (cranial nerve XI), and the paired strap muscles (sternothyroid, sternohyoid, thyrohyoid, and omohyoid). This fascial layer attaches posteriorly to the ligamentum nuchae, which is the supraspinous ligament. At the root of the neck, the fascia splits to attach to both the anterior and posterior surfaces of the manubrium. The intervening suprasternal space (of Burns) contains the lower portion of the anterior jugular veins and their connecting branch, the jugular venous arch.

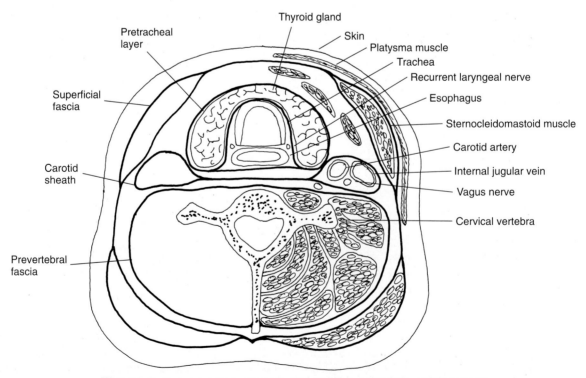

Figure 1 Cross-section of neck showing fascial "tubes within tubes"

Triangles of the Neck

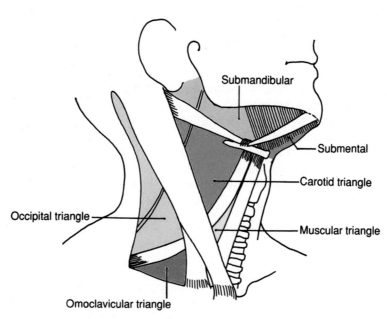

Figure 2 Triangles of the neck as defined by muscle boundaries

Within the deep cervical fascia are *four more tubes.* Two of these tubes, the *carotid sheaths,* are paired. Each carotid sheath contains the vagus nerve, common carotid artery and its internal carotid branch, the internal jugular vein, and the associated lymph nodes. Another tube, the *prevertebral fascia,* encompasses the cervical vertebrae and their associated muscles, the emerging cervical spinal nerve roots and branches thereof (including the phrenic nerve), the cervical portion of the sympathetic chain, and the cervical part of the subclavian artery. The fourth and final tube is the *pretracheal fascia.* This fascial layer surrounds the larynx, esophagus, thyroid and parathyroid glands, and recurrent laryngeal nerve. In the vicinity of the thyroid gland, the pretracheal fascia splits to entirely invest the thyroid and parathyroid glands, forming the false capsule of the thyroid gland. Between the deep surface of the thyroid gland and the upper two or three tracheal rings, this fascia is strongly adherent to the gland and trachea, forming the so-called "adherent zone" or lateral suspensory ligament (ligament of Berry). The recurrent laryngeal nerve is located laterodorsal to this ligament. This is verified in a review of 486 thyroid surgery cases and 25 autopsy cases, which demonstrated that the recurrent laryngeal nerves was identified laterodorsal to the ligament without any examples of recurrent laryngeal nerve passing through the ligament. Parathyroid glands are typically located within the false capsule derived from pretracheal fascia, but outside the true capsule of the thyroid gland.

Off of midline the superficial neck is divided into triangles for convenience (Fig. 2). These triangles are bounded by bony or muscular fixed landmarks and provide important guides to the location of nerves and other critical structures. Two major triangles, both of which are roofed by the deep cervical fascia on each side of the neck, are based on the location of the sternocleidomastoid muscle (Fig. 3). The *anterior triangle* is bounded

posteriorly by the sternocleidomastoid muscle, superiorly by the body of the mandible, and anteriorly by the midline. The *posterior triangle* is bounded anteriorly by the sternocleidomastoid muscle, inferiorly by the clavicle, and posteriorly by the trapezius muscle.

Each triangle can be further subdivided. The *anterior triangle* can be divided into four lesser triangles. The *submental triangle* is bounded by the hyoid bone, the midline of the neck, and the anterior belly of the digastric muscle. The *submandibular triangle* lies between the body of the mandible and the two bellies of the digastric muscle. The *carotid triangle* is delimited by the sternocleidomastoid muscle, the superior belly of the omohyoid muscle, and the posterior belly of the digastric muscle. The *muscular triangle* is bounded by the sternocleidomastoid muscle, the superior belly of the omohyoid muscle, and the midline.

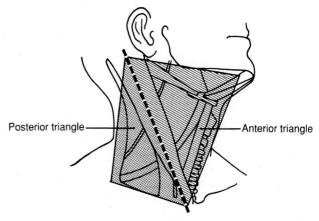

Figure 3 The sternocleidomastoid muscle divides the neck into anterior and posterior triangles.

The *posterior triangle* is only divided into two lesser triangles. The larger of these is the *occipital triangle,* which is bounded by the trapezius muscle, the sternocleidomastoid muscle, and the inferior belly of the omohyoid muscle. The smaller *omoclavicular triangle* is delimited by the inferior belly of the omohyoid muscle, the clavicle, and the sternocleidomastoid muscle. It is quite important to realize that several important structures of the neck are not, in the strictest sense, located in either the anterior or posterior triangle or their subdivisions but, rather, are located deep to the sternocleidomastoid muscle itself. Examples include the carotid sheath and the vertebral vessels. These structures are typically rendered accessible either by lateral retraction of the sternocleidomastoid muscle or, immediately superior to the clavicle, by dissecting in the interval between the sternal and clavicular heads of the sternocleidomastoid muscle, a space known as the minor supraclavicular fossa or *scalene triangle.*

REFERENCES

1. Demetriades D, Salim A, Brown C, et al. The neck with complex anatomic features and dense concentration of numerous vital structures. *Curr Probl Surg.* 2007;44(1):6–10.
2. Sasou S, Nakamura S, Kurihara H. Suspensory ligament of Berry: Its relationship to recurrent laryngeal nerve and anatomical examination of 24 autopsies. *Head Neck.* 1998;20(8):695–698.

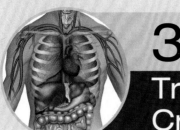

3
Tracheostomy and Cricothyroidotomy

Grant O. Lee and Kent Choi

Tracheostomy is necessary when long-term access to the airway for ventilatory support or respiratory toilet is required. It may also be indicated during emergency situation when surgical airway is needed. This chapter describes open tracheostomy and open cricothyroidotomy; percutaneous tracheostomy (Chapter 4) is an alternative in selected patients. Open tracheostomy is best performed in a controlled setting with a fully equipped operating room where adequate lighting, electrocautery, suction, and airway control. Percutaneous tracheostomy may be performed at the bedside, generally in the intensive care unit, but requires the same attention to airway control as formal tracheostomy (see Chapter 4).

SCORE™, the Surgical Council on Resident Education, classified Tracheostomy as an "ESSENTIAL COMMON" procedure.

SCORE™, the Surgical Council on Resident Education, classified Cricothyrodotomy as an "ESSENTIAL UNCOMMON" procedure.

STEPS IN PROCEDURE (TRACHEOSTOMY)

Position patient, check equipment, test balloon of tracheostomy tube

Identify five midline landmarks

Transverse or vertical incision at midline, one finger breadth above the suprasterna notch

Divide tissues in midline

Retract or divide thyroid isthmus

Expose trachea and count rings down from cricoid

Incision between second and third ring

Pull back endotracheal tube slowly until it is just above the tracheal opening

Spread incision and insert tube

Confirm position of tube by passage of suction catheter; secure tube

STEPS IN PROCEDURE (CRICOTHYROIDOTOMY)

Position patient, check equipment, check balloon of tracheostomy tube

Transverse incision over cricothyroid membrane

Control bleeding by manual pressure

Stab into membrane

Spread and insert tube, secure tube, pack wound to control bleeding

HALLMARK ANATOMIC COMPLICATIONS

Supraglottic tracheostomy

Tracheoinnominate arterial fistula (delayed complication)

LIST OF STRUCTURES

Larynx

Thyroid cartilage

Cricoid cartilage

Median cricothyroid ligament

Cricothyroid artery

Trachea

Landmarks

Mental protuberance

Hyoid bone

Laryngeal prominence

Manubrium sterni

Jugular (suprasternal) notch

Associated Structures

Thyroid gland

Isthmus

Pyramidal lobe

Anterior jugular vein

External jugular vein

Platysma muscle

Brachiocephalic (innominate) trunk

Brachiocephalic (innominate) vein

Jugular venous arch

Brachial plexus

surgical airway may be required in an emergency when the patient cannot be intubated in the normal fashion (e.g., when massive facial trauma or edema precludes safe intubation). In this situation, cricothyroidotomy (see Fig. 3.8) can be performed more quickly and more safely than formal tracheostomy.

Positioning the Patient (Fig. 3.1)

Technical Points

Slightly hyperextend the neck by placing a small roll under the patient's shoulders (Fig. 3.1A). Do not hyperextend the neck in a patient with a known or suspected cervical spine injury, because the resulting vertebral motion may cause irreversible damage to the spinal cord.

Select a tracheostomy tube appropriate to the size of the patient; for an average-sized adult, a number 7 or 8 tube will work well. Test the balloon and then deflate and lubricate it with sterile lubricant. Place the obturator inside the tube. Be sure that a soft rubber suction catheter is available on the sterile field for suctioning the tracheostomy after the tube is inserted. Sterilize the skin and drape the patient while allowing access to the endotracheal tube.

Whereas tracheostomy can be performed in infants younger than 1 month of age with acceptable procedure-related morbidity, cricothyroidotomy should be avoided in patients younger than 12 years of age due to increased incidence of subglottic stenosis. Endotracheal intubation over a flexible bronchoscope is the procedure of choice as an alternative.

Anatomic Points

Landmark structures of this region are shown in Fig. 3.1B. The thyroid gland, often with a pyramidal lobe, overlies the trachea. The thyroid cartilage and cricoid cartilage are easily palpable above the thyroid gland. The hyoid bone can be palpated above the thyroid cartilage. The paired sternocleidomastoid muscles are located laterally to it.

The phrenic nerve arises from spinal cord levels C3 to C5 and the brachial plexus is derived from C5 to T1. Spinal cord damage at or above C3 will result in death secondary to paralysis of all respiratory muscles. Damage of the cord at levels involving the brachial plexus can result in quadriplegia. Hyperextension of the neck stretches the cord and may compress the cord against a damaged cervical vertebra; such a maneuver may also result in complete transection as the cord is caught between broken fragments of cervical vertebrae.

Identification of Landmarks (Fig. 3.2)

Technical and Anatomic Points

Palpate five midline landmarks, including the mental protuberance, or tip of the chin; the body of the hyoid bone; the laryngeal prominence of the thyroid cartilage (Adam's apple); the cricoid cartilage; and the suprasternal notch of the manubrium sterni. All of these constant bony or cartilaginous landmarks should be identified with certainty to avoid inadvertent supraglottic incision. Repeated palpation of these readily identifiable

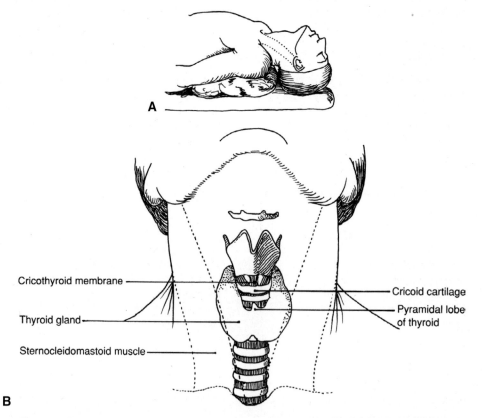

A

B

Figure 3.1 Positioning the patient. **A:** Patient position. **B:** Regional anatomy.

Cricothyroid membrane

Thyroid gland

Sternocleidomastoid muscle

Cricoid cartilage

Pyramidal lobe of thyroid

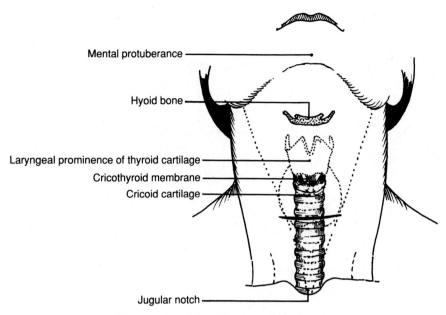

Figure 3.2 Identification of landmarks

midline structures will help ensure that the dissection remains in the midline.

Skin Incision for Tracheostomy (Fig. 3.3)

Technical Points

A vertical incision at midline one finger breadth above the suprasternal notch provides the best exposure and is preferred in emergency situations. With this incision, there is less bleeding and less risk for damage to nerves and vessels. The incision shown is slightly larger than usually required. Do not hesitate to make a generous incision if exposure is difficult.

A transverse incision, made at the same level, yields a somewhat better cosmetic result; however, the advantage is marginal because scarring occurs around the tracheal stoma. Open tracheostomy is performed between the second and third tracheal rings. If a transverse incision is used, it should be planned to lie directly over the appropriate level, confirmed by palpation of the anatomic landmarks.

Anatomic Points

The theoretic cosmetic advantage of a transverse incision is that it follows the direction of Langer's lines (resulting from the predominant orientation of dermal collagen bundles and elastic fibers in the skin) and also parallels the natural wrinkle lines of the area.

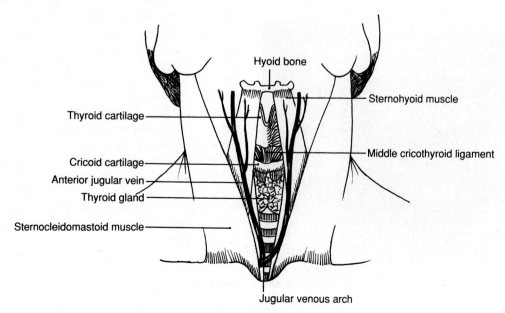

Figure 3.3 Skin incision

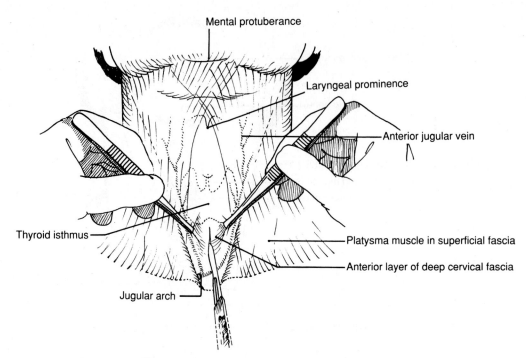

Figure 3.4 Dissection down to the trachea

Dissection Down to the Trachea (Figs. 3.4 and 3.5)

Technical Points

Proceed with sharp and blunt dissection in the midline, confirming correct placement by repeated palpation of anatomic landmarks.

Anatomic Points

The platysma muscle, which should be identified and retracted, is deficient in the median plane. The superficial veins in this region (anterior and external jugulars and their tributaries) run in a predominantly vertical direction deep to the platysma. With the exception of the jugular venous arch, these superficial veins do not cross or occupy the median plane. No motor nerves, and only the terminal branches of sensory nerves, cross or occupy the median plane.

Isthmus of Thyroid Gland (Fig. 3.6)

Technical Points

The next important structure to identify is the isthmus of the thyroid gland. The isthmus may be retracted cephalad or caudad, or divided, to obtain access to the appropriate segment of the trachea. To facilitate retraction of the isthmus, spread the tissues with a blunt-tipped hemostat (such as a small Kelly clamp) in the plane between the thyroid and the trachea. Then place a vein retractor on the isthmus to retract it away from the second and third tracheal rings. Decide whether to divide the isthmus according to the amount of dissection necessary to expose the second and third tracheal rings and the space in between. Generally, it is possible to achieve this exposure by retraction.

If it is necessary to divide the isthmus of the thyroid partially or completely, first confirm that the plane between the thyroid and the trachea has been developed adequately. Then double clamp and oversew or suture ligate the highly vascular thyroid tissue before proceeding.

Anatomic Points

The thyroid begins its development as a diverticulum in the region of the incipient tongue and migrates from its site of

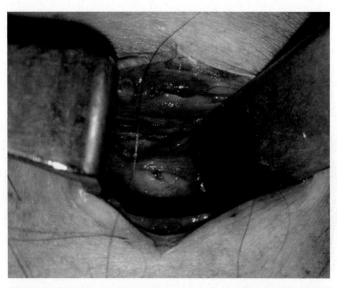

Figure 3.5 Neck dissection down to the trachea. The second tracheal ring is visible.

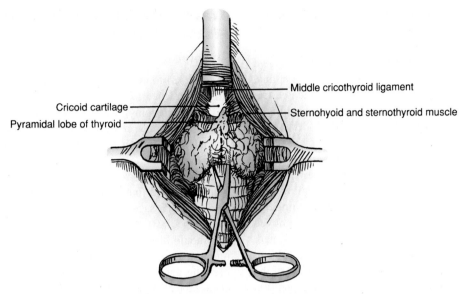

Figure 3.6 Isthmus of thyroid gland

origin (marked by the foramen cecum) to its definitive location. Although the large lobes are paratracheal, the isthmus is in the median plane and typically covers the second and third tracheal rings. Furthermore, its developmental route is frequently indicated by the presence of a pyramidal lobe, the result of "residual" thyroid tissue being deposited along the path of descent. This lobe is usually slightly to the left of the midline, but it may be in the midline or on the right.

Exposure of Pretracheal Fascia and Tube Insertion (Fig. 3.7)

Technical Points

Dissect the pretracheal fascia (which invests the thyroid gland) from the trachea to provide a clear view of the trachea. To perform a formal tracheostomy, count the rings down from the cricoid cartilage. Incise and spread the tissue between the second and third rings (Fig. 3.7A). A simple transverse incision is generally all that is required; however, some prefer to make an H-shaped or T-shaped cut. It is rarely necessary to excise any cartilage.

A tracheostomy hook—a small, sharp, hooked device—may be used to pull the trachea cephalad and anterior into the field and maintain visibility when the incision is deep. However, care must be taken to avoid puncture of the cuff of the tracheostomy tube when using the hook. An alternative method is to place a 2–0 monofilament suture through the third tracheal cartilage and use that for retraction. The suture can be left long and brought out through the skin incision to aid in replacing the tube if it becomes dislodged. The trachea is opened between the second and third tracheal ring space. A "T" shape incision with

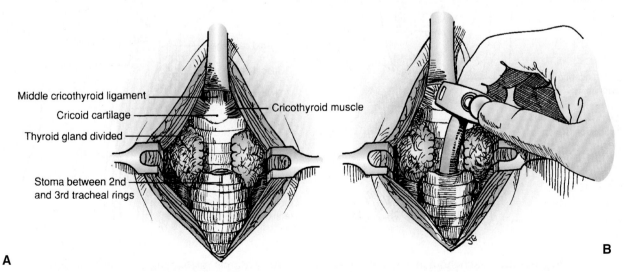

Figure 3.7 Exposure of pretracheal fascia. **A:** Incision between tracheal rings. **B:** Insertion of tube.

the third tracheal ring cut at midline will help accommodate the tracheostomy tube insertion.

Have an assistant at the head of the table deflate the cuff of the endotracheal tube and withdraw it slowly until it is just inferior to the vocal cords but superior to the tracheal stoma. With the stoma spread, insert the pretested and lubricated tracheostomy tube, with the obturator in place, by pushing it straight in and then downward (Fig. 3.7B). Push downward only after feeling the tube pop into the tracheal lumen; otherwise, it is possible to place the tube in the pretracheal space. Inflate the cuff, and connect the tracheostomy to the ventilator or to oxygen. The tracheostomy tube placement shall always be confirmed by either end-tidal detection or listening for bilateral breath sound. The endotracheal tube may be removed after the placement of tracheostomy tube has been confirmed. Pass a soft-suction catheter down the tracheostomy tube to remove blood and mucus from the airway. Free passage of the catheter into the bronchial tree also helps confirming position of the tracheostomy tube within the airway.

Anatomic Points

It is critical that the incision *not* be made through the cricoid cartilage. This is the only totally circumferential cartilage in the airway and provides important stability. Repeated identification of anatomic landmarks and careful dissection in a bloodless field will prevent such an error as well as the equally unfortunate circumstance of entering the airway above the glottis.

Tracheobrachiocephalic Artery Fistula (Fig. 3.8)

Technical and Anatomic Points

If a tracheostomy is performed below the level of the fourth ring, the tracheostomy tube may tilt upward, resulting in the tip of the tracheostomy tube kicking forward. The tip of the tracheostomy tube may erode into the brachiocephalic (innominate) arterial trunk, which runs obliquely across the thoracic outlet immediately anterior to the trachea (Fig. 3.8A). This will result in delayed presentation of massive bleeding into the airway. The left brachiocephalic (innominate) vein often lies in the suprasternal notch in its passage from the root of the neck to the superior vena cava (Fig. 3.8B). A very low incision could injure this vessel.

Should bleeding from either of these vessels occur, obtain temporary control by placing a finger in the tracheal stoma and pressing anteriorly or by inflating the balloon of an endotracheal tube. This will compress the vessel against the undersurface of the manubrium, allowing time to transport the patient to the operating room for open or endovascular repair. Definitive management of this difficult problem is detailed in the surgical references at the end of this chapter.

Cricothyroidotomy (Fig. 3.9)

Technical Points

Cricothyroidotomy is performed through the median cricothyroid ligament, which is the most superficial part of the trachea and hence affords the easiest approach during emergency

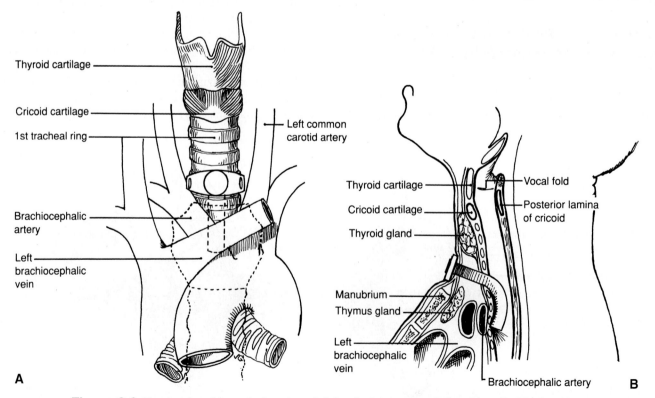

Figure 3.8 Tracheobrachiocephalic artery fistula. **A:** Anatomic relationships. **B:** Mechanism of injury.

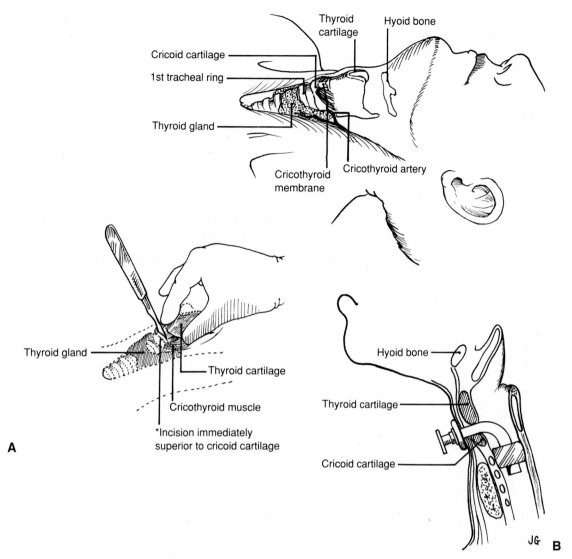

Figure 3.9 Cricothyroidotomy. **A:** Incision into cricothyroid membrane. **B:** Position of tube.

situations. During an emergency, percutaneous needle cannulation with 14- or 16-gauge catheter of this ligament may be lifesaving, allowing time for subsequent, more orderly control of the airway. The landmarks for this procedure are the thyroid cartilage, the cricoid cartilage, and the hyoid bone (Fig. 3.9A).

To perform an emergency cricothyroidotomy, first stabilize the larynx with the fingers of the nondominant hand and palpate the space between the larynx and the cricoid. (Fig. 3.9B). A secure grasp is essential to prevent skiving during incision. Stab into the median cricothyroid ligament transversely with a scalpel. Spread the hole with a hemostat or clamp and insert a tracheostomy tube. In patients who are obese or have a short neck, the treacheal may be deep. A needle access followed by wire-guided cricothyroidotomy tube insertion using the Seldinger technique can be helpful and safer. Be careful to avoid injury to the cricoid cartilage! Most bleeding will be venous; control it by direct pressure with the fingers of the nondominant hand until the tube is in and the patient is successfully ventilated. Then expose and ligate individual bleeders.

If time permits, cricothyroidotomy may be performed by dissection in a manner similar to that described for tracheostomy. Visualize the median cricothyroid ligament and incise it transversely, then spread the tissues and insert the tracheostomy tube as discussed previously.

Anatomic Points

The cricoid cartilage is the narrowest part of the trachea. Concern about subglottic stenosis in children under 12 years limits the application of this approach.

A branch of the superior thyroid artery—the cricothyroid artery (and its accompanying vein)—runs transversely across the median cricothyroid ligament. This artery occasionally has a branch that penetrates the median cricothyroid ligament to anastomose with the laryngeal arteries. It is typically closer to the thyroid cartilage than to the cricoid cartilage. Thus, to avoid injury to these vessels, and to avoid damage to the closely situated vocal cords, cricothyroidotomy should be performed by making a transverse incision along the superior border of the cricoid cartilage, rather than along the inferior border of the thyroid cartilage.

SURGICAL REFERENCES

1. Chew JW, Cantrell RW. Tracheostomy: Complications and their management. *Arch Otolaryngol.* 1972;96:538. (Provides an excellent review of complications, including tracheoinnominate artery fistula.)
2. Dulguerov P, Gysin C, Perneger TV, et al. Percutaneous or surgical tracheostomy: A meta-analysis. *Crit Care Med.* 1999;27:1617. (Compares complications as reported in literature.)
3. Eliachar I, Zohar S, Golz A, et al. Permanent tracheostomy. *Head Neck Surg.* 1984;7:99. (Describes construction of a permanent stoma.)
4. Gysin C, Dulguerov P, Guyot JP, et al. Percutaneous versus surgical tracheostomy: A double-blind randomized trial. *Ann Surg.* 1999;230:708. (Details complications associated with both techniques.)
5. Hamaekers AE, Henderson JJ. Equipment and strategies for emergency tracheal access in the adult patient. *Anaesthesia.* 2011; 66(suppl 2):65.
6. Heffner JE, Miller KS. Tracheostomy in the intensive care unit. I. Indications, techniques, management. *Chest.* 1986;90:269. (Offers a good description of the management of a patient with a tracheostomy.)
7. Higgins KM, Punthakee X. Meta-analysis comparison of open versus percutaneous tracheostomy. *Laryngoscope.* 2007;117:447–454. (Trend in favor of percutaneous techniques.)
8. Hsaiao J, Pacheco-Fowler V. Videos in clinical medicine. Cricothyroidotomy. *N Engl J Med.* 2008;29:e25.
9. Van-Hasselt EJ, Bruining HA. Elective cricothyroidotomy. *Intensive Care Med.* 1985;11:207. (Provides reviews of clinical experience.)

ANATOMIC REFERENCES

1. American Association of Clinical Anatomists, Educational Affairs Committee. The clinical anatomy of several invasive procedures. *Clin Anat.* 1999;12:43.
2. Ger R, Evans JT. Tracheostomy: An anatomico-clinical review. *Clin Anat.* 1993;6:337.
3. Salassa JR, Pearson BW, Payne WS. Gross and microscopical blood supply of the trachea. *Ann Thorac Surg.* 1977;24:100.

TECHNICAL COMPLICATIONS: MANAGEMENT OF TRACHEOINNOMINATE ARTERY FISTULA REFERENCES

1. Allan JS, Wright CD. Tracheoinnominate fistula: Diagnosis and management. *Chest Surg Clin N Am.* 2003;13:331–341.
2. Cohen JE, Klimov A, Rajz G, et al. Exsanguinating tracheoinnominate artery fistula repaired with endovascular stent-graft. *Surg Neurol.* 2008;69:306–309.
3. Marone EM, Esposito G, Kahlberg A, et al. Surgical treatment of tracheoinnominate fistula after stent-graft implantation. *J Thorac Cardiovasc Surg.* 2007;113:1641–1643.
4. Palchik E, Bakkien AM, Saad N, et al. Endovascular treatment of tracheoinnominate artery fistula: A case report. *Vasc Endovascular Surg.* 2007;41:258–261.
5. Ridley RW, Zwischenberger JB. Tracheoinnominate fistula: Surgical management of an iatrogenic disaster. *J Laryngol Otol.* 2006;120:676–680.

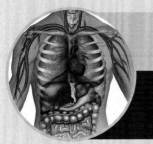

4

Percutaneous Dilatational Tracheostomy

Carlos A. Pelaez

Percutaneous dilatational tracheostomy is now the standard operative technique for long-term airway access at many institutions around the world. There are two slightly different technical approaches to this procedure, which differ primarily in the use or omission of bronchoscopic guidance. Both are discussed in this chapter.

SCORE™, the Surgical Council on Resident Education, classified tracheostomy as an ESSENTIAL COMMON procedure.

STEPS IN PROCEDURE

Check equipment including balloon of tracheostomy tube

Hyperextend the neck if no cervical spine injury

Bronchoscopic visualization of proximal trachea (optional)

Vertical incision (or horizontal) extending 2 cm inferiorly from cricoid cartilage

Palpate/visualize second and third tracheal rings

Insert needle into trachea and aspirate air

Advance catheter and pass guidewire (bronchoscopic control)

Pass lubricated dilator

Using dilator as obturator, pass lubricated tracheostomy tube and secure

Confirm placement, achieve hemostasis and secure the tube

COMPLICATIONS

Bleeding

Injury to posterior wall of trachea

Improper placement

Erosion into innominate artery/ tracheoinnominate artery fistula

Tracheal stenosis

Percutaneous dilatational tracheostomy is generally not recommended for achieving emergency airway control or access. Endotracheal intubation or cricothyrotomy is the most appropriate emergency technique to achieve adequate airway control and ventilation. Percutaneous dilatational tracheostomy is a safe and appropriate technique for use in the intubated patient who requires elective tracheostomy. It may be done at the bedside in the intensive care unit, with direct visualization of the trachea or under bronchoscopic guidance.

Absolute contraindications to percutaneous dilatational tracheostomy include the following:

1. Patient younger than 8 years of age
2. Emergency airway due to acute airway compromise
3. Gross distortion of neck anatomy due to hematoma, tumor, large thyromegaly, or high innominate artery

Relative contraindications include the following:

1. Obese patient with short neck that obscures landmarks
2. Coagulopathy with prothrombin time or activated partial thromboplastin time more than 1.5 times the reference range, platelet count less than 50,000, or bleeding time longer than 10 minutes
3. Positive end-expiratory pressure (PEEP) of more than 20 cm of water
4. Infection of the soft tissues of the neck

Appropriate positioning and preparation of the patient are essential to achieving good operative results. Therefore, in both techniques, the following preparations must be made. Place the intubated patient in a supine position. Continuous monitoring should include electrocardiographic monitoring of heart rate, blood pressure, pulse oximetry, inspired title volume, and ventilator pressures. Increase the inspired oxygen fraction to 100% and ensure adequate ventilation. Extend the cervical spine by placing a rolled towel between the shoulder blades. In patient with cervical spine injury, the neck is kept in neutral position. This procedure is not considered sterile but one should always prep and drape the anterior neck with the solution of choice and sterile towels. The procedure is done with a preliminary cutdown and then a Seldinger technique, as summarized in Figure 4.1.

Percutaneous Dilatational Tracheostomy Without Bronchoscopic Guidance

Technical and Anatomic Points

Identify the anterior neck landmarks, including the thyroid and cricoid cartilages. Infiltrate the skin and subcutaneous tissues with 1% lidocaine solution with epinephrine before making the skin incision. Make the skin incision starting at the inferior edge of the cricoid cartilage and extending vertically 1.5 to 2 cm. Divide the subcutaneous tissues bluntly with hemostats at the level of the second and third tracheal rings until the trachea is visualized and its cartilage rings are palpable (Fig. 4.2). This allows for a clear visual delineation of tracheal anatomy, including the location of the tracheal midline, and obviates the need for concomitant bronchoscopy.

Achieve hemostasis with absorbable suture or electrocautery as necessary. Under laryngoscopic guidance, partially deflate the cuff of the endotracheal tube and slowly withdraw it until the cuff is seen just below the vocal cords. Stabilize the trachea in the midline and insert the needle and catheter this into the trachea between the second and third cartilage rings under direct vision. Confirm entry into the trachea by free aspiration of air. Advance the overlying catheter into the trachea and withdraw the needle. Again confirm the position of the catheter within the trachea by aspirating air. Advance the J-tipped guidewire through the catheter into the trachea (Fig. 4.3) and remove the catheter. Next, place a dilator guide over the guidewire, followed by a lubricated, tapered dilator up to its external 38 French mark (Fig. 4.4A,B). Perform this dilation carefully and without excessive force. Remove the dilator, leaving the dilator guide and guidewire in place. Pass a size 6 or 8 cuffed Shiley tracheostomy tube over the appropriate dilator, which will function as an obturator. Lubricate the tracheostomy tube and dilator and pass these into the trachea (Fig. 4.5). When the tracheostomy tube is seated in its final position, remove the dilator, dilator guide, and guidewire as a unit. Inflate the tracheostomy balloon until the air leak is sealed. Leave the endotracheal tube in place, but disconnect it from the ventilator. Connect the tracheostomy tube to the ventilator tubing with a flexible adaptor. Initiate ventilation. Confirm satisfactory oxygenation and minute ventilation before withdrawing the endotracheal tube. Apply the CO_2 detector to ensure proper endotracheal position of the tracheostomy tube. Secure the tracheostomy tube by four-point fixation using sutures and a tracheostomy tape. Chest x-ray is not routinely necessary.

Percutaneous Dilatational Tracheostomy with Bronchoscopic Guidance

Technical and Anatomic Points

For this procedure, you will need an extra operator to navigate the bronchoscope during the procedure. After preparing the

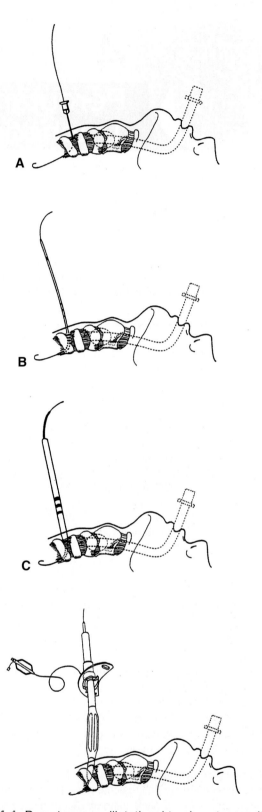

Figure 4.1 Percutaneous dilatational tracheostomy without bronchoscopic guidance. **A:** Guidewire passed through needle into trachea. **B:** Needle removed and dilator guide placed. **C:** Tapered dilator passed. **D:** Dilator removed and tracheostomy tube passed (from Singh RK. Timing and type of tracheostomy. *Probl Gen Surg.* 2000;17:101–109, with permission).

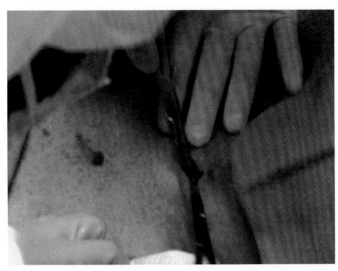

Figure 4.2 Blunt dissection with hemostats at the level of the second and third tracheal rings until the trachea is visualized and its cartilage rings are palpable.

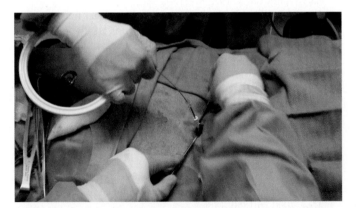

Figure 4.3 The J-tipped guidewire is advanced through the catheter into the trachea.

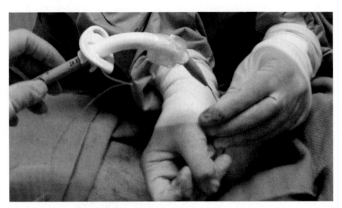

Figure 4.5 Lubricated tracheostomy tube and dilator are passed into the trachea over the guidewire.

patient as described previously, attach a bronchoscopy adapter between the endotracheal tube and the ventilator tubes. Perform a bronchoscopic inspection of the airway. Withdraw the endotracheal tube to immediately below the vocal folds. Reinflate the cuff of the endotracheal tube to ensure adequate ventilation, and identified the anterior neck landmarks, including the thyroid and cricoid cartilages. Infiltrate the skin and subcutaneous tissues with 1% lidocaine solution with epinephrine before making the skin incision. Make the skin incision starting at the inferior edge of the cricoid cartilage and extending vertically 1.5 to 2 cm. Bronchoscopic transillumination of the anterior trachea is a useful guide, but does not absolutely guarantee an initial midline tracheal puncture. Palpate and define the cricoid and tracheal rings. Infiltrate the skin and subcutaneous tissue over the second and third tracheal rings with 1% lidocaine solution with epinephrine. Insert the needle and catheter percutaneously between the first and third tracheal rings into the trachea under direct bronchoscopic guidance. To prevent damage to the bronchoscope, leave it within the endotracheal tube while advancing the needle. Confirm that the needle entry is in the midline between the 11- and the 1-o'clock positions (Fig. 4.6A). Withdraw the needle, leaving the catheter in place as previously described. Pass the J wire under bronchoscopic observation, confirming that the

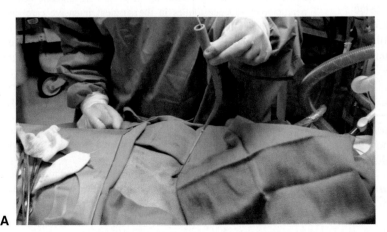

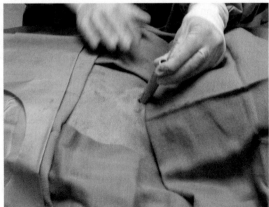

A   **B**

Figure 4.4 The dilator is advanced over the guidewire up to its external 38-French mark.
A: Dilator passed over guidewire. **B:** Dilator passed to appropriate mark.

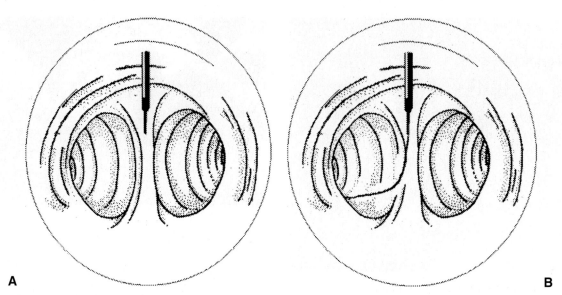

Figure 4.6 Percutaneous dilatational tracheostomy with bronchoscopic guidance. **A:** Needle and tip of guidewire visualized. **B:** Guidewire seen to pass distally in tracheobronchial tree.

J wire passes toward the carina (Fig. 4.6B). Insert the dilator guide over the guidewire into the trachea. Dilate the trachea using the tapered flexible dilator up to its external 38 French mark (Fig. 4.4A,B). Perform the dilatation carefully and without excessive force. Remove the tapered dilator. Place a size 6 or 8 Shiley tracheostomy tube snugly over the appropriate dilator. Lubricate the tracheostomy tube and dilator and pass them over the guidewire and into the trachea (Fig. 4.5). Withdraw the dilator, dilator guide, and guidewire as a single unit. Insert the inner cannula of the tracheostomy tube, inflate the cuff of the tube, and attach the ventilator.

Insert the bronchoscope into the tracheostomy tube to confirm the intratracheal position of the tracheostomy tube and to inspect for bleeding. Withdraw the oral endotracheal tube only after the confirmation of appropriate positioning of the tracheostomy tube. Secure the tracheostomy tube using four-point fixation sutures and the tracheostomy tape. Chest x-ray is not routinely necessary.

The key to successful percutaneous dilatation tracheostomy is careful surgical technique preceded by appropriate positioning of an intubated patient. Bronchoscopically directed guidewire insertion into the trachea ensures anterior midline placement of the tracheostomy tube and eliminates the anterior dissection of the neck structures and paratracheal tissues.

REFERENCES

1. Byhahn C, Wilke HJ, Halbig S, et al. Percutaneous tracheostomy: Ciaglia blue rhino versus the basic Ciaglia technique of percutaneous dilatational tracheostomy. *Anesth Analg.* 2000;91:882–886.
2. Cheng E, Fee WE Jr. Dilatational versus standard tracheostomy: A meta-analysis. *Ann Otol Rhinol Laryngol.* 2000;109:803–807.
3. Ciaglia P, Firsching R, Syniec C. Elective percutaneous dilatational tracheostomy: A new simple bedside procedure, preliminary report. *Chest.* 1985;87:715–719.
4. Ciaglia P, Graniero K. Percutaneous dilatational tracheostomy: Results and long-term follow-up. *Chest.* 1992;101:464–467.
5. Delaney A, Bagshaw SM, Nalos M. Percutaneous dilatational tracheostomy versus surgical tracheostomy in critically ill patients: A systematic review and meta-analysis. *Crit Care.* 2006;10:1–13.
6. Fernadez L, Norwood S, Roettger R, et al. Bedside percutaneous tracheostomy with bronchoscopic guidance in critically ill patients. *Arch Surg.* 1996;131:129–132.
7. Higgins KM, Punthakee X. Meta-analysis comparison of open versus percutaneous tracheostomy. *Laryngoscope.* 2007;117:447–454.
8. Hinerman R, Alvarez F, Keller CA. Outcome of bedside percutaneous tracheostomy with bronchoscopic guidance. *Intensive Care Med.* 2000;26:1850–1856.
9. Kilic D, Findikcioglu A, Akin S, et al. When is surgical tracheostomy indicated? Surgical "U-shape" versus percutaneous tracheostomy. *Ann Thorac Cardiovasc Surg.* 2011;17:29–32.
10. Kornblith LZ, Burlew CC, Moore EE, et al. One thousand bedside percutaneous tracheostomies in the surgical intensive care unit: Time to change the gold standard. *J Am Coll Surg.* 2011;212:163–170.
11. Moe KS, Schmid S, Stoeckli SJ, et al. Percutaneous tracheostomy: A comprehensive evaluation. *Ann Otol Rhinol Laryngol.* 1999;108:384–391.
12. Norwood S, Valina VL, Short K, et al. Incidence of tracheal stenosis and other late complications after percutaneous tracheostomy. *Ann Surg.* 2000;232:233–241.
13. Rosenbower TJ, Morris JA Jr, Eddy VA, et al. The long-term complications of percutaneous dilatational tracheostomy. *Am Surg.* 1998;64:82–87.
14. Van Natta TL, Morris JA Jr, Eddy VA, et al. Elective bedside surgery in critically injured patients is safe and cost-effective. *Ann Surg.* 1998;227:618–626.

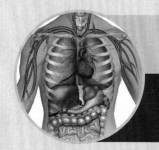

5

Thyroglossal Duct Cyst

In this section, the anatomy of the upper midline of the neck is explored, and the embryology of the thyroid gland and associated anomalies is discussed through the operation of removal of thyroglossal duct cyst.

Thyroglossal duct cysts form along the path of descent of the thyroid gland. They present as upper midline neck masses. Often, these cysts become infected and present as abscesses. Incision and drainage or simple excision of the cyst results in a high recurrence rate. Complete removal of the cyst and its associated tract is necessary for cure.

SCORE™, the Surgical Council on Resident Education, has classified surgery for thyroglossal duct cyst as a "COMPLEX" Pediatric Surgical procedure.

STEPS IN PROCEDURE

Position patient: Neck hyperextended, lower face, and mouth draped into field

Transverse incision (include sinus tract if present)

Retract sternohyoid muscles and expose cysts

Dissect cyst free of surrounding tissues medially, laterally, cephalad, and caudad

Seek and dissect fibrous tract leading to hyoid bone

Trace to hyoid and resect midportion of hyoid bone in continuity with tract

Follow tract to base of tongue, using pressure on foramen cecum if necessary; ligate termination

HALLMARK ANATOMIC COMPLICATION

Recurrence resulting from inadequate dissection

LIST OF STRUCTURES

Embryologic Structures and Terms
Thyroid anlagen
Pharyngeal arches
Tuberculum impar (pharyngeal arch I)
Copula (pharyngeal arches II through IV)
Thyroglossal duct

Adult Structures
Tongue
Foramen cecum
Hyoid bone
Suprahyoid muscles

Mylohyoid muscle
Geniohyoid muscle
Sternohyoid muscle
Genioglossus muscle
Hypoglossal nerve (XII)
Mandibular division of trigeminal nerve (V)
Mylohyoid nerve
Lingual nerve
Thyroid gland
Pyramidal lobe
Thyroid cartilage

Positioning the Patient and Incising the Skin (Fig. 5.1)

Technical Points

Position the patient supine with the neck hyperextended and the chin directly anterior. Include the lower face and lips in the surgical field. (Access to the mouth may facilitate subsequent dissection.)

Make a transverse skin incision over the cyst (Fig. 5.1A). If previous drainage of the cyst resulted in an external sinus tract or scar, excise this in transverse elliptical fashion with the skin incision. Plan the incision to lie parallel to, or within, the natural skin lines. Elevate flaps in the plane deep to the platysma muscle to expose the deep cervical fascia and paired sternohyoid muscles overlying the cyst. Incise this fascia in the midline.

Anatomic Points

Thyroid anlagen begin as an epithelial thickening of endodermal origin during the fourth intrauterine week. This thickening

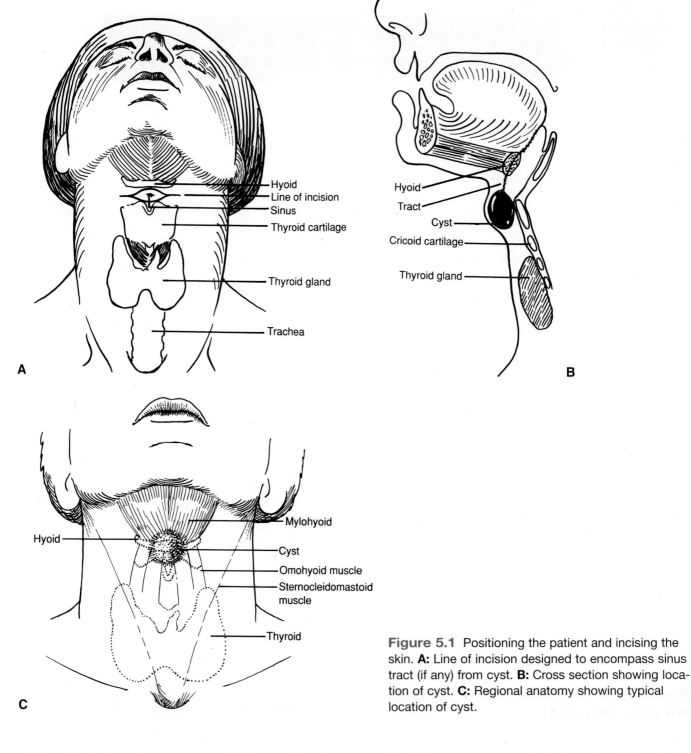

Figure 5.1 Positioning the patient and incising the skin. **A:** Line of incision designed to encompass sinus tract (if any) from cyst. **B:** Cross section showing location of cyst. **C:** Regional anatomy showing typical location of cyst.

is located in the floor of pharyngeal arch II, between the tuberculum impar (pharyngeal arch I) and copula (arches II through IV) that participate in the formation of the tongue. The anlage rapidly evaginates, coming into contact with the aortic sac of the developing heart. Owing to differential growth, the thyroid migrates from its point of origin, marked by the foramen

cecum of the mature tongue (at the junction of the anterior two-thirds and posterior one-third), to its definitive location. During this migration, the gland is connected to the tongue by the thyroglossal duct (Fig. 5.1B). The path of migration passes anterior to the developing hyoid bone, whose paired anlagen, from pharyngeal arch II, fuse in the ventral midline and also undergo some rotation. Because of the relationship of the thyroglossal duct to the developing hyoid bone, the duct can be drawn posterocranially with respect to the hyoid, be enveloped in hyoid periosteum or hyoid bone proper, or pass posterior to the hyoid. Typically, the duct degenerates, leaving a short diverticulum at the foramen cecum proximally, a longer cord distally that develops into the pyramidal lobe of the thyroid gland (typically displaced slightly to the left of the median plane), and an intervening fibrous cord. If the discontinuous epithelial cells present in the fibrous remnant differentiate and subsequently assume a secretory function, a thyroglossal duct cyst results.

A thyroglossal duct cyst should be suspected in any person presenting with a median or paramedian lump in the neck, especially if the lump is superior to the level of the cricoid cartilage and if it moves with the excursion of the hyoid bone during swallowing or tongue protrusion (Fig. 5.1C). A lingual thyroid, usually the result of maldescent of the thyroid, has to be considered if the lump is located intralingually. In this case, preoperative evaluation with a radioisotope scan is essential because 65% to 75% of patients with this condition lack other thyroid tissues.

Dissection of the Cyst (Fig. 5.2)

Technical Points

Retract the paired sternohyoid muscles laterally to expose the cyst. Carefully dissect the cyst from the surrounding soft tissues on all sides. Often, the inferior border can be delineated most easily. Start the dissection here and divide any attachments to the pyramidal lobe of the thyroid that may be present (Fig. 5.2A). Search for and identify the tract leading up to the hyoid bone. This will be palpable as a firm, cord-like structure passing superiorly and deep in a relatively straight path to

the midportion of the hyoid (Fig. 5.2B). If the cyst is densely adherent to the hyoid and the tract cannot be identified, simply proceed to excise the cyst and midportion of the hyoid *en bloc*.

Anatomic Points

The tract typically is to the left of midline, juxtaposed to the thyroid cartilage. If a pyramidal lobe is present, the dissection should start at its apex and proceed superiorly to the body of the hyoid bone. Although the tract typically ascends posterior to the body of the hyoid and then is recurved to pass superficial to the anterior surface of the hyoid, it must be emphasized that the tract can lie within the hyoid periosteum or within the bone, or it can continue its ascent to the foramen cecum posterior to the hyoid.

Dissection Through the Hyoid to the Base of the Tongue (Fig. 5.3)

Technical Points

Detach the mylohyoid and deeper geniohyoid muscles from the hyoid superiorly and the sternohyoid muscles inferiorly. Divide the hyoid laterally with a small, heavy scissor. Excise a block of the midportion of the hyoid bone in continuity with the cyst and its tract (Fig. 5.3A). Continue the dissection proximally. Excise a core of tissue surrounding the fibrous tract (Fig. 5.3B).

Anatomic Points

Because of the variability of the path of the thyroglossal duct with respect to the hyoid, resect a portion of the body of the hyoid bone in continuity with soft tissues to ensure that no part of the duct remains.

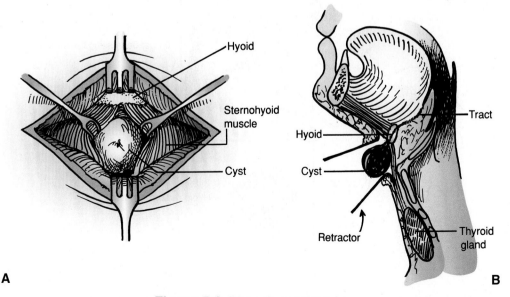

A　　　　　　　　　　　　　　　　　　　　　　　　　　**B**

Figure 5.2 Dissection of the cyst

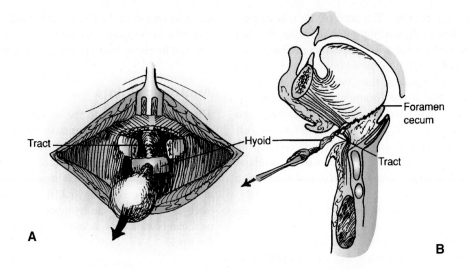

Figure 5.3 Dissection through the hyoid to the base of the tongue. **A:** Cyst visualized in operative field. **B:** Cross section showing resection of portion of hyoid bone to remove tract.

Tract Followed to the Foramen Cecum (Fig. 5.4)

Technical Points

Place a second surgical glove (one-half size larger than the size normally worn) over the glove of your nondominant hand or have an assistant do this. Insert the index and second finger of this hand into the mouth and press downward in the vicinity of the foramen cecum. Then continue the dissection up toward the foramen cecum, using the hand within the mouth as a guide. Excise the tract. Do not excise the foramen cecum through the cervical incision. Suture–ligate the base of the tract just below the foramen cecum.

Check hemostasis in the operated field. If only a small portion of the hyoid bone has been resected, reapproximate it with a monofilament nonabsorbable suture. When a large cyst necessitates removal of a large portion of the hyoid bone, close the defect by suturing the sternohyoid muscle inferiorly to the mylohyoid muscle superiorly. Then close the cervical fascia and skin.

Anatomic Points

As the tract is followed to the foramen cecum, the surrounding soft tissues are "cored out" along with the tract. This includes the median portions of the mylohyoid muscle and its raphe, the

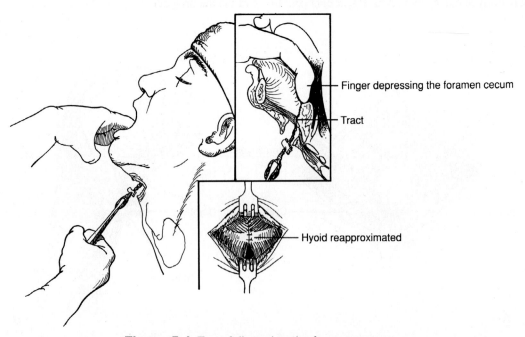

Figure 5.4 Tract followed to the foramen cecum

geniohyoid muscle, and the genioglossus muscles. Removing this median core should not endanger the nerves of this region, the hypoglossal nerve (cranial nerve XII) or the mylohyoid and lingual branches of the mandibular division of the trigeminal nerve (cranial nerve V), because these arise posterolaterally, course anterolaterally, and remain lateral to the anterior midline.

Because the foramen cecum lies posterosuperior to the hyoid, digital pressure in the vicinity of the foramen cecum not only stabilizes the soft tissues, but also forces these tissues anteriorly, enhancing their excision.

SURGICAL REFERENCES

1. Acierno SP, Waldhausen JH. Congenital cervical cysts, sinuses and fistulae. *Otolaryngol Clin North Am.* 2007;40:161–176.

2. Bennett KG, Organ CH, Williams GR. Is the treatment for thyroglossal duct cysts too extensive? *Am J Surg.* 1986;152:602. (This clinical review confirms the need for excision of the midportion of the hyoid.)

3. Chon SH, Shinn SH, Lee CB, et al. Thyroglossal duct cyst within the mediastinum: An extremely unusual location. *J Thorac Cardiovasc Surg.* 2007;133:1671–1672.

4. Gupta P, Maddalozzo J. Preoperative sonography in presumed thyroglossal duct cysts. *Arch Otolaryngol Head Neck Surg.* 2001;127:200–202. (Discusses the use of preoperative ultrasound to confirm the existence of normally placed thyroid.)

5. Joseph J, Lim K, Ramsden J. Investigation prior to thyroglossal duct cyst excision. *Ann R Coll Surg Engl.* 2012;94:181.

6. LaRiviere CA, Waldhausen JH. Congenital cervical cysts, sinuses, and fistulae in pediatric surgery. *Surg Clin North Am.* 2012;92:583.

7. Maddalozzo J, Venkatesan TK, Gupta P. Complications associated with the Sistrunk procedure. *Laryngoscope.* 2001;111:119–123. (Wound complications dominate.)

8. Mussak EN, Kacker A. Surgical and medical management of midline ectopic thyroid. *Otolaryngol Head Neck Surg.* 2007;136:870–872.

9. Organ GM, Organ CH Jr. Thyroid gland and surgery of the thyroglossal duct: Exercise in applied embryology. *World J Surg.* 2000;24:886–890. (Reviews surgery and associated embryology.)

10. Sistrunk WE. The surgical treatment of cysts of the thyroglossal tract. *Ann Surg.* 1920;71:121. (Provides an original description of the classic procedure.)

11. Sistrunk WE. Technique of removal of cysts and sinuses of the thyroglossal duct. *Surg Gynecol Obstet.* 1928;46:109.

GENERAL REFERENCES

1. Brown RL, Azizkhan RG. Pediatric head and neck lesions. *Pediatr Clin North Am.* 1998;45:889–905. (Discusses this and other common lesions.)

2. Marshall SF. Thyroglossal cysts and sinuses. *Surg Clin North Am.* 1953;33:633. (Reviews the results of extensive experience with the Sistrunk technique.)

3. McClintock JC, Mahaffey DE. Thyroglossal tract lesions. *J Clin Endocrinol.* 1950;10:1108. (Discusses embryology with particular reference to development of the hyoid bone.)

4. Nichollas R, Girelfucci B, Roman S, et al. Congenital cysts and fistulas of the neck. *Int J Pediatr Otorhinolaryngol.* 2000;55:117–124. (Good review of branchial cleft and thyroglossal duct cysts.)

5. Sprinzl GM, Koebke J, Wimmers-Klick J, et al. Morphology of the human thyroglossal tract: A histologic and macroscopic study in infants and children. *Ann Otol Rhinol Laryngol.* 2000;109:1135–1139. (Reaffirms the need to excise part of the hyoid bone.)

EMBRYOLOGY REFERENCES

1. Albers GD. Branchial anomalies. *JAMA.* 1963;183:399.

2. Boyd JD. Development of the thyroid and parathyroid glands and the thymus. *Ann R Coll Surg Engl.* 1950;7:455.

3. Gilmour JR. The embryology of the parathyroid glands, the thymus and certain associated rudiments. *J Pathol Bacteriol.* 1937;45:507.

4. Sgalitzer KE. Contribution to the study of the morphogenesis of the thyroid gland. *J Anat.* 1941;75:389.

5. Weller GL. Development of the thyroid, parathyroid and thymus glands in man. *Contrib Embryol.* 1933;24:93.

6. Wilson CP. Lateral cysts and fistulas of the neck of developmental origin. *Ann R Coll Surg Engl.* 1955;17:1.

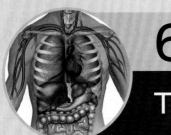

6

Thyroid Lobectomy

Anuradha R. Bhama and Geeta Lal

The thyroid gland, the largest endocrine gland in the body, is located in the midline of the neck and is composed of two lobes connected by a midline isthmus and a variable pyramidal lobe. It is purple-pink in color and normally weighs approximately 20 g. The isthmus lies inferior to the cricoid cartilage and the lobes extend superiorly over the lateral aspects of the thyroid cartilage. In relation to the spine, the thyroid gland extends from approximately C5 to T1. It is closely associated with the external branch of the superior laryngeal nerve, the recurrent laryngeal nerve, and the parathyroid glands. Success in thyroid surgery requires careful and meticulous dissection and hemostasis, which aids in the identification and preservation of these vital structures.

SCORE™, the Surgical Council on Resident Education, has classified Partial or Total Thyroidectomy as "ESSENTIAL COMMON" procedures.

STEPS IN PROCEDURE

Beach chair position, with neck extended and roll between scapulae

Incision 1 cm caudal to cricoid cartilage

Raise flaps in subplatysmal plane

Incise midline and mobilize strap muscles

Mobilize thyroid gland medially and divide middle thyroid vein

Mobilize superior pole and divide vessels on thyroid

Ligate inferior pole structures, working from medial to lateral

Identify recurrent laryngeal nerve

Identify and mobilize parathyroid glands

Skeletonize and divide branches of inferior thyroid artery directly on thyroid

Divide ligament of Berry

Mobilize pyramidal lobe, if present

For lobectomy, clamp and ligate isthmus on contralateral side

For total thyroidectomy, mobilize contralateral lobe as previously described

For subtotal lobectomy, leave approximately 4 g remnant posteriorly

Reapproximate strap muscles and platysma

Close incision without drainage

HALLMARK ANATOMIC COMPLICATIONS

Injury to recurrent laryngeal nerve

Injury to superior laryngeal nerve

Hypoparathyroidism

LIST OF STRUCTURES

Thyroid Gland and Associated Structures

Thyroid gland
    Left and right lobes
    Isthmus
    Pyramidal lobe
Parathyroid glands
    Superior parathyroid glands
    Inferior parathyroid glands

Nerves

Vagus nerve (CN X)
Facial nerve (CN VII)
Spinal accessory nerve (CN XI)
Recurrent laryngeal nerve
Superior laryngeal nerve
    External branch

    Internal branch
Ansa cervicalis

Muscles

Platysma
Strap muscles
    Sternohyoid muscle
    Sternothyroid muscle
    Thyrohyoid muscle
    Omohyoid muscle
Sternocleidomastoid muscle

Vessels

External jugular vein
Anterior jugular vein
Jugular venous arch
Internal jugular vein

Common carotid artery	**Landmarks**
External carotid artery	Trachea
Internal carotid artery	Thyroid cartilage
Superior thyroid vein	Cricoid cartilage
Middle thyroid vein	Sternal notch
Inferior thyroid vein	Esophagus
Thyrocervical trunk	Pretracheal fascia
Superior thyroid artery	Ligament of Berry
Inferior thyroid artery	Hyoid bone
Thyroid ima artery	Tubercle of Zuckerkandl

Preoperative Preparation (Fig. 6.1)

Technical Points

Patients requiring thyroid surgery should undergo careful preoperative preparation. This may include measurement of thyroid function tests, ultrasonography, fine needle aspiration, and radionucleotide scanning. To avoid thyroid storm, hyperthyroid patients should be treated with antithyroid medications, beta-blockers, and Lugol's iodine or supersaturated potassium iodide solution, and occasionally steroids. Patients with medullary thyroid cancer should be screened for pheochromocytoma and primary hyperparathyroidism, as these conditions are associated with multiple endocrine neoplasia syndromes. Patients who have undergone prior neck surgery or those with suspected pre-existing vocal cord dysfunction should undergo documentation of vocal cord function by direct or indirect laryngoscopy.

Anatomic Points

Recurrent laryngeal nerve injury generally results in the ipsilateral vocal cord lying in a paramedian position. Injury to both the external branch of the superior laryngeal nerve and the recurrent laryngeal nerve causes the vocal cord to lie in an intermediate position, as shown in Figure 6.1.

Patient Positioning (Fig. 6.2)

Technical Points

The patient should be positioned supine on the operating room table in a modified "beach chair" position, that is, with a moderate reverse Trendelenburg and with the knees flexed. This will help reduce venous pressure. Place a sandbag or roll between the scapulae allowing the shoulders to fall backward. Extend the neck and place the head on a donut cushion.

Anatomic Points

Proper positioning displaces the thyroid anteriorly and superiorly, allowing for an easier dissection. Suboptimal positioning

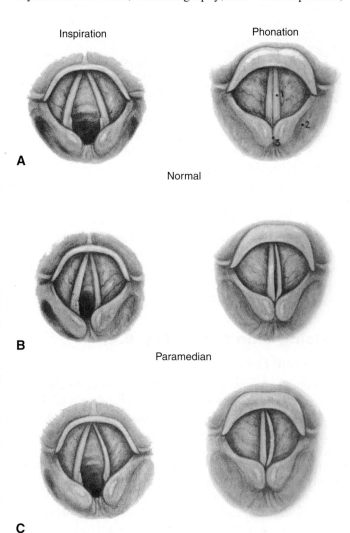

Figure 6.1 Preoperative preparation (from Dedo HH. The paralyzed larynx: An electromyographic study in dogs and humans. *Laryngoscope.* 1970;80:1455–1517. Wolters Kluwer/Lippincott Williams & Wilkins, with permission).

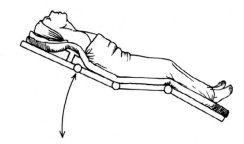

Figure 6.2 Patient positioning

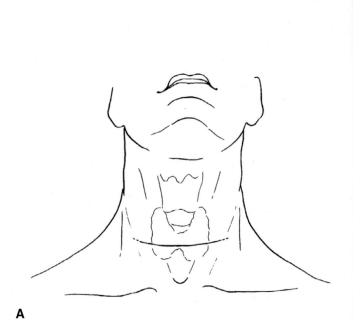

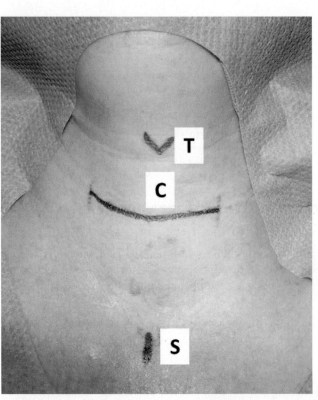

A

B

Figure 6.3 A: Choice of skin incision (from Clark OH, Caron. NR Fine-needle aspiration of the thyroid: Thyroid lobectomy and subtotal thyroidectomy. In: Baker RJ, Fischer JE, eds. *Mastery of Surgery.* 4th ed. Philadelphia: Lippincott Williams & Wilkins; 2001, with permission). **B:** Operative photo showing anatomic landmarks for placing the incision (T, thyroid cartilage notch; C, cricoid cartilage; S, sternal notch). The incision is generally placed in a pre-existing skin crease, if feasible.

translates into inadequate exposure and may result in a larger incision.

Choice of Skin Incision (Fig. 6.3)

Technical Points

Make a slightly curved transverse collar incision in a natural skin crease approximately 1 cm below the cricoid cartilage. A 2-0 silk suture may be pressed against the skin to mark out the planned course of the incision. Take care to measure the distance on each side of the midline to ensure symmetry. A 4- to 5-cm incision is generally adequate; however, patients with a short neck, large thyroid gland, or limited neck extension may require a longer incision. Carry this incision through the skin, the subcutaneous tissues, and the platysma. It is generally easier to identify the fibers of the platysma along the lateral aspect of the incision.

Anatomic Points

An incision 1 cm caudal to the cricoid cartilage generally places the incision over the thyroid isthmus. The platysma arises in the superficial fascia of the neck and is continuous with the fascia that covers the pectoralis major and deltoid muscles. It is a

sheet-like muscle that extends from the mandible or the subcutaneous tissues of the face to the clavicles. Its fibers decussate over the chin and become continuous with the facial musculature. As a muscle of facial expression, it is innervated by the seventh cranial nerve.

Raising Skin Flaps (Fig. 6.4)

Technical Points

Raise the flaps in the subplatysmal plane. Place straight Kelly clamps, skin hooks, or rake retractors on the dermis to elevate the flaps anteriorly. Provide countertraction with a finger, Kitner, or gauze as the flaps are elevated, starting medially and carrying the dissection laterally, with electrocautery and/or a scalpel. Sometimes, portions of this dissection can be accomplished bluntly with a Kitner. Extend this elevation superiorly to the level of the thyroid cartilage and inferiorly to the level of the suprasternal notch. Take care not to injure the superficial network of veins that lie deep to the platysma. This potentially extensive collection of veins, including the paired anterior jugular veins, external jugular veins, and communicating veins, lies beneath the platysma muscle, overlying the sternocleidomastoid and midline strap muscles. Place towels along the skin edges to protect them and use a self-retaining retractor to aid in exposure.

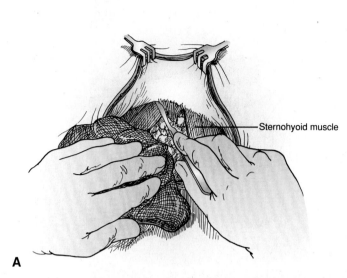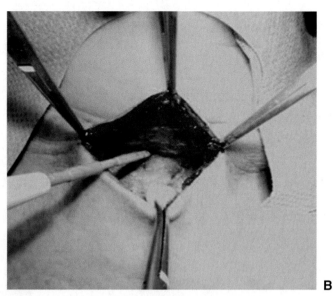

—Sternohyoid muscle

A   **B**

Figure 6.4 Raising skin flaps in the subplatysmal plane can be accomplished as shown in **(A)** sharply using a scalpel or **(B)** using electrocautery, as shown in this operative photo. A Sponge or Kitner is useful to provide countertraction.

Anatomic Points

Elevating subplatysmal flaps takes advantage of an avascular plane that lies between the platysma and the underlying superficial veins and strap muscles. The muscles encountered during thyroid surgery become apparent after the mobilization of subplatysmal flaps. These include the sternocleidomastoid muscles and the paired strap muscles (sternohyoid, sternothyroid, thyrohyoid, and omohyoid muscles). The sternocleidomastoid muscles mark the lateral boundaries of the dissection. The sternocleidomastoid muscle has two muscle bellies, both inserting onto the mastoid process with dual origins, on the sternum and the proximal clavicle. The sternocleidomastoid muscle is innervated by the spinal accessory nerve (CN XI). The omohyoid muscle inserts on the hyoid bone and originates from the scapula. Only the superior belly is generally encountered. The sternohyoid muscles lie in the midline overlying the sternothyroid and thyrohyoid muscles. The sternohyoid originates from the sternum and inserts on the hyoid bone. The sternothyroid extends from the sternum to the thyroid cartilage, and the thyrohyoid muscle extends from the thyroid cartilage to the hyoid bone.

The superficial jugular veins lie just beneath the platysma. The paired external jugular veins lie laterally and over the sternocleidomastoid muscles. The paired anterior jugular veins directly overlie the sternohyoid muscles. There is often an extensive network of communicating veins connecting the anterior jugular veins and the external jugular veins. The jugular venous arch, a communication between the right and left anterior jugular veins, is often seen in the lower part of the neck and may have to be ligated and divided to provide optimal exposure and separation of the strap muscles. Although ligation of these veins is of little clinical consequence, identification and avoidance of these vessels is often possible.

Division/Mobilization of Strap Muscles (Fig. 6.5)

Technical Points

Identify the midline raphe between the paired strap muscles. Using electrocautery, separate the paired sternohyoid and sternothyroid muscles in the midline from the sternal notch to the thyroid cartilage to expose the underlying thyroid gland. On the side to be approached first, bluntly dissect the sternohyoid muscle from the deeper sternothyroid muscle lying just beneath it. This step often assists with exposure, particularly when working via smaller incisions. Identify and preserve the ansa cervicalis as it courses over the lateral aspect of the sternothyroid, if possible. Then dissect the sternothyroid muscle off the thyroid bluntly. Identify the internal jugular vein by gently retracting laterally on the sternocleidomastoid muscle.

The strap muscles may occasionally require division to gain exposure to the thyroid gland, particularly in large goiters. In the rare occasion that division is necessary, divide the muscles as high as possible to preserve the strap muscles' innervation by the ansa cervicalis. These muscles can then be sutured together at the end of the operation. If a tumor directly invades into the strap muscles, resect the strap muscle en bloc with the underlying thyroid tissue.

Anatomic Points

The thyroid gland lies deep to the strap muscles. Dividing the midline raphe between the left and right sternohyoid and sternothyroid muscles and retracting the muscles laterally allows visualization of the thyroid gland. The midline raphe between the strap muscles represents a condensation

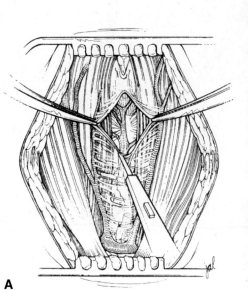

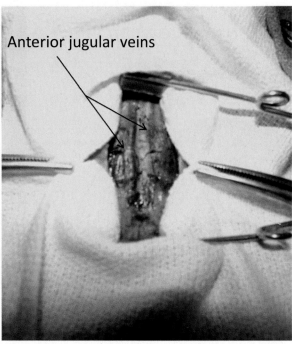

Anterior jugular veins

Figure 6.5 **A:** Separation/mobilization of strap muscles (from Moore FH, Jr, Gawande AA. Parathyroidectomy for hyperplasia and secondary hyperparathyroidism. In: Baker RJ, Fischer JE, eds. *Mastery of Surgery.* 4th ed. Philadelphia: Lippincott Williams & Wilkins; 2001, with permission). **B:** The anterior jugular veins are easily identified on either side of the midline raphe.

of the superficial layer of deep cervical fascia. The strap muscles are farthest apart just above the suprasternal notch, making this the ideal spot to start the dissection. The thyrohyoid muscle is innervated by a branch of the first cervical nerve, and the remaining strap muscles are innervated by the ansa cervicalis (C1 to C3). Although denervation of the strap muscles is of little clinical significance, it may lead to subtle changes in swallowing and cosmesis. Preservation of the ansa cervicalis is therefore desired. Motor branches of the ansa cervicalis usually enter the muscles at two points, near the level of the thyroid cartilage and just cephalad to the sternal notch. The underlying thyroid is purple-pink in color and its surrounding capsule represents the division of the deep pretracheal fascia of the neck into the anterior and posterior divisions.

Identification and Division of the Middle Thyroid Vein (Fig. 6.6)

Technical Points

Mobilization of the thyroid gland requires division of the middle thyroid vein or veins. Retract the thyroid medially and anteriorly as you sweep the lateral tissues posterolaterally with a Kitner. This should expose the middle thyroid vein, which can then be ligated. Sometimes, several branches, rather than one middle vein, are encountered. Divide and ligate these as close to the thyroid as possible.

Anatomic Points

The middle thyroid vein is variable; it has been reported to exist in approximately 50% of patients, and often, multiple veins are encountered. The middle thyroid vein extends from the lateral border of the gland and passes superficial to the common carotid artery to drain into the ipsilateral internal jugular vein. The recurrent laryngeal nerve and inferior thyroid artery lie posterior and in close proximity to the middle thyroid vein. Division of the middle thyroid vein allows mobilization of the thyroid gland anteriorly and medially, assisting in the exposure of the lateral compartment containing the inferior thyroid artery, recurrent laryngeal nerve, and parathyroid glands. In large goiters, the internal jugular vein and the middle thyroid vein may be pushed against the thyroid capsule, making the plane between the internal jugular vein and the thyroid gland difficult to define.

The thyroid is also drained by superior and inferior thyroid veins that parallel its arterial supply. The superior veins also drain into the internal jugular veins; however, the inferior veins drain into the brachiocephalic veins.

Mobilization of the Superior Pole (Fig. 6.7)

Technical Points

Next, identify the midline pyramidal lobe and the Delphian group of lymph nodes. Identify the superior pole by retracting

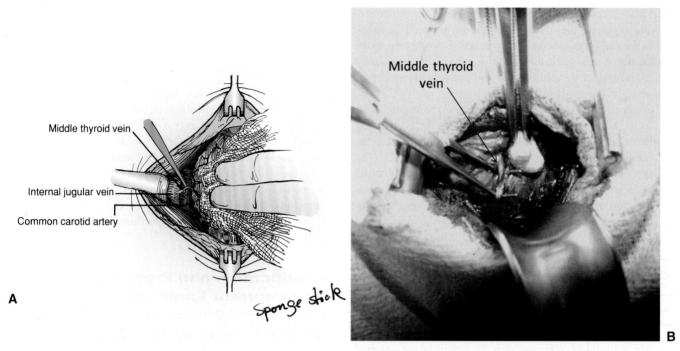

Figure 6.6 Identification and division of the middle thyroid vein. **A:** Anatomic diagram. **B:** Operative photograph.

the strap muscles laterally and cephalad, and the thyroid lobe inferiomedially. Next, retract the upper pole caudally and laterally; this puts tension on the superior pole vessels and allows for their easier identification. Keep the plane of dissection as close to the thyroid as possible. Individually identify, skeletonize, and ligate the superior pole vessels low on the thyroid gland. A clamp may be placed around the superior pole to provide downward traction and exposure of the superior pole vessels and is especially useful when dissecting large goiters. Caution is necessary to avoid injury to the external branch of the superior laryngeal nerve. After the vessels are divided, the tissues posterior and lateral to the superior pole can be swept away from the gland to avoid injuring the vascular supply to the

superior parathyroid gland. The superior pole vessels can also be divided after delivering the lower thyroid pole into the incision and identifying the recurrent laryngeal nerve, as described in the following sections.

Anatomic Points

The superior thyroid artery and vein and the external branch of the superior laryngeal nerve lie in close proximity to the superior pole of the thyroid. The relationship of the nerve and vessels is variable. Cernea classified the location of the external branch of the superior laryngeal nerve into three types. In type 1, the nerve crosses the superior pole vessels 1 cm or more above the upper

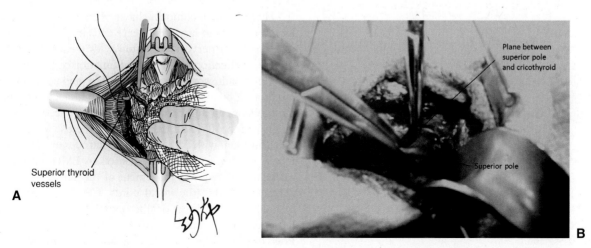

Figure 6.7 Mobilization of the superior pole. **A:** Anatomic diagram. **B:** Operative photograph.

pole. In type 2a, the nerve crosses within 1 cm of the upper border of the superior pole. The type 2b variant, in which the nerve crosses the vessels below the upper border of the superior pole, puts the nerve at a particular risk of iatrogenic injury. Safety requires staying close to the gland and individually skeletonizing and dividing each vessel.

The superior laryngeal nerve is a branch of the vagus nerve. It arises high in the neck, near the skull base. It travels along the internal carotid artery and then tracks medially. Near the hyoid cornu, it divides into an internal and external branch. The internal branch pierces the thyrohyoid membrane and receives sensory input from the pharynx. It may anastomose with sensory branches of the recurrent laryngeal nerve forming the loop of Galen. The external branch descends along the lateral edge of the pharyngeal constrictor muscles and inserts onto the cricothyroid muscle. The external branch is a motor nerve to the cricothyroid muscle and plays a role in tensing the vocal cords. Injury to the external branch of the superior laryngeal nerve leads to difficulty in reaching high notes and may lead to voice fatigue.

The superior thyroid artery is the first branch of the external carotid artery. It originates near the origin of the external carotid from the common carotid artery. The superior thyroid vein drains into the internal jugular vein and its course closely approximates that of the superior artery.

Ligation of Inferior Pole Structures (Fig. 6.8)

Technical Points

The inferior thyroid vessels can now be ligated. Again, the dissection is kept close to the thyroid gland and proceeds medial to lateral. Avoid ligating too much tissue en bloc to avoid injury to the recurrent laryngeal nerve, which has not been identified yet. Although not always present, the thyroid

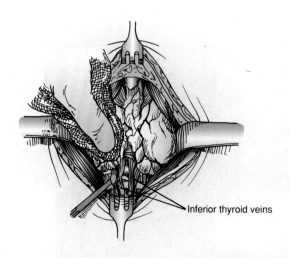

Figure 6.8 Ligation of inferior pole structures

ima artery may enter the inferior pole. This vessel can be ligated and divided.

Anatomic Points

The inferior thyroid veins, which emerge from the thyroid gland near the lower pole, drain into the brachiocephalic veins. These veins usually arise as two trunks on the medial aspect of the thyroid lobes and pass inferiorly to drain into the ipsilateral brachiocephalic veins. A thyroid ima artery is variably present and arises from the brachiocephalic artery, aortic arch, right common carotid artery, internal thoracic artery, or the subclavian artery. Occasionally, the right and left inferior thyroid veins join to form a thyroidea ima vein, which drains into the left brachiocephalic vein.

Identification and Preservation of the Recurrent Laryngeal Nerve and Parathyroid Glands and Ligation of Inferior Thyroid Artery (Fig. 6.9)

Technical Points

Next, identify the recurrent laryngeal nerve; this step can also be performed before mobilizing the inferior pole. A bloodless operative field is imperative at this juncture. Mobilize the thyroid gland medially, up and into the operative field. The recurrent laryngeal nerve is most consistently identified at the level of the cricoid cartilage near the ligament of Berry. Begin the dissection lateral to the tubercle of Zuckerkandl with a fine hemostat or right angle clamp. The recurrent laryngeal nerve often lies close to the tubercle of Zuckerkandl near the tracheoesophageal groove. The inferior thyroid artery is also a helpful landmark; the recurrent laryngeal nerve almost always makes contact with the vessel, passing directly above, under, or between the branches of the vessel. If the recurrent laryngeal nerve is not readily identified, it may be uncovered by dissecting the loose fibrous tissue just caudal to the inferior thyroid artery with a fine hemostat. Use of a neurostimulator, as described below, may also be helpful.

Three main techniques have been used to functionally monitor recurrent laryngeal nerve activity: Intermittent recurrent laryngeal nerve stimulation with postcricoid palpation, direct visualization of vocal cord function by laryngoscopy or fiberoptic endoscopy during dissection, and continuous nerve monitoring by electromyography (EMG) electrodes placed in the larynx or in an endotracheal tube. Of these, nerve stimulation with postcricoid palpation and the use of endotracheal tubes outfitted with EMG surface electrodes are the most commonly used modalities. The use of an EMG-outfitted endotracheal tube requires placement of the surface electrodes in contact with the true vocal cords. Correct positioning may be confirmed by direct or fiberoptic laryngoscopy. Recurrent laryngeal nerve function may be tested with a monopolar Prass or Montgomery nerve stimulator, typically with currents of 1 to 2 mA, while monitoring evoked potential on a monitor

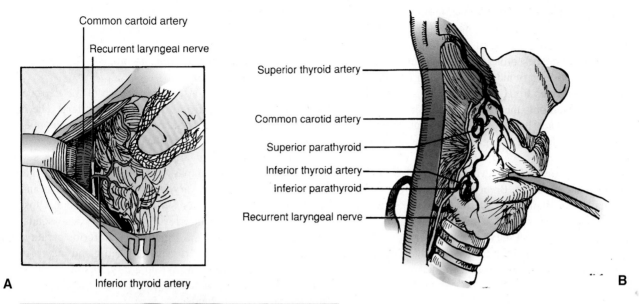

Common cartoid artery

Recurrent laryngeal nerve

Inferior thyroid artery

A

Superior thyroid artery

Common carotid artery

Superior parathyroid

Inferior thyroid artery

Inferior parathyroid

Recurrent laryngeal nerve

B

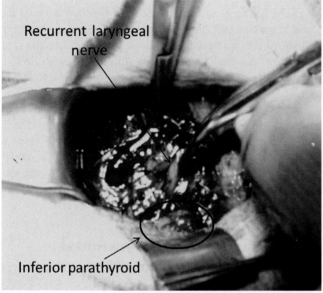

Recurrent laryngeal nerve

Inferior parathyroid

C

Figure 6.9 A: Identification and preservation of the recurrent laryngeal nerve and parathyroid glands and ligation of the inferior thyroid artery. **B:** Lateral view showing the relationships of the inferior thyroid artery, the recurrent laryngeal nerve, and the parathyroid glands. **C:** Operative photo showing the relationship between the inferior parathyroid and the recurrent laryngeal nerve.

screen. As opposed to observing evoked potentials, postcricoid palpation of a laryngeal twitch provides a direct assessment of recurrent laryngeal nerve activity. Laryngeal palpation after recurrent laryngeal nerve stimulation is a simple and readily available technique. Mere visual inspection after nerve stimulation does not suffice. Recurrent laryngeal nerve motor branches may supply inferior constrictor and esophageal musculature, the contraction of which can be confused with true laryngeal contractions. A finger inserted deep to the posterior lamina of the cricoid cartilage allows palpation of the posterior cricoarytenoid muscle contraction through the wall of the hypopharynx.

After successful identification, carry the dissection superficially along the course of the nerve to its final insertion on the larynx. The recurrent laryngeal nerve is closely associated with the ligament of Berry, traversing it in 25% of patients, before entering the cricothyroid membrane, between the cricoid

cartilage and the inferior cornu of the thyroid cartilage. Next, identify the parathyroid glands, which can generally be identified within 1 cm of the intersection of the recurrent laryngeal nerve with the inferior thyroid artery. The superior parathyroid gland lies superior and posterior, whereas the inferior parathyroid lies anterior and caudal. Mobilize the parathyroid glands and reflect them posterolaterally along with their vascular pedicle, if technically feasible. If a parathyroid gland is inadvertently devascularized, confirm its identity by a frozen section of a tiny fragment, and prepare the gland for autotransplantation. Section the gland into 1-mm fragments, create a pocket in the sternocleidomastoid muscle, and autotransplant these fragments into the pocket. Mark the pocket with a Prolene stitch and a metal clip to allow easy identification in the future, if necessary.

Next, individually dissect, skeletonize, and ligate branches of the inferior thyroid artery on the surface of the gland, using caution not to injure the recurrent laryngeal nerve or vascular branches to the parathyroid glands. Identification of the parathyroid glands and the recurrent laryngeal nerve followed by dissection close to the thyroid best protects these structures. Lateral retraction on the carotid artery aids in identifying the inferior thyroid artery as it emerges from behind the carotid artery and travels medially to insert onto the thyroid gland. Maintaining a bloodless field is important; however, avoid blind placement of hemostats and control bleeding with gentle pressure rather than electrocautery.

At this point, the thyroid is elevated off the trachea by ligating the ligament of Berry. Branches of the inferior thyroid artery, small veins draining the thyroid, and the recurrent laryngeal nerve are intimately associated with the ligament of Berry. The recurrent laryngeal nerve is injured most often at this location; ligate vessels with care, ensuring that the recurrent laryngeal nerve has been positively identified.

Anatomic Points

The right recurrent laryngeal nerve branches off the vagus and crosses anterior to the subclavian artery, whereas the left recurrent laryngeal nerve loops around the ligamentum arteriosum and then passes anterior to the aortic arch. They both ascend near the tracheoesophageal groove to enter the larynx near the caudal aspect of the cricothyroid muscle. The right recurrent laryngeal nerve generally follows a more oblique course than the left. In approximately 0.5% to 1% of individuals, a nonrecurrent right laryngeal nerve exists. A nonrecurrent left laryngeal nerve is rare, but has been described in patients with a right-sided aortic arch or a retroesophageal left subclavian artery.

The recurrent laryngeal nerve provides motor input to the laryngeal musculature, except for the cricothyroid muscle, which is innervated by the external laryngeal nerve. Unilateral injury leads to paralysis of the ipsilateral vocal cord, causing it to lie in the paramedian or abducted position. The paramedian position results in a normal, but weak voice; whereas, the abducted position leads to hoarseness and an ineffective cough. Bilateral injury may lead to airway obstruction or loss of voice. If both cords lie in an abducted position, air movement may occur, but the patient has an ineffective cough and is at an increased risk of aspiration. The recurrent laryngeal nerve is closely associated with the inferior thyroid artery, which may cross it anteriorly, posteriorly, or between its branches. The recurrent laryngeal nerve and its intersection with the inferior thyroid artery are most consistently identified near the cricoid cartilage in the vicinity of the ligament of Berry. The nerve is also intimately associated with the tubercle of Zuckerkandl, a lateral projection of the middle third of the thyroid, which represents the embryologic fusion between the ultimobranchial bodies and the median thyroid process. When enlarged, it may develop into a nodular process with the recurrent laryngeal nerve most often running medial to it in a fissure. As described by Dedo, only one branch of the recurrent laryngeal nerve

supplies the laryngeal musculature; the other branches are sensory. One branch may anastomose with a branch of the internal laryngeal nerve forming the loop of Galen (as described previously). Interrupting the sensory branches to the pharynx may lead to aspiration.

The inferior thyroid artery is a branch of the thyrocervical trunk, which arises from the subclavian artery. The inferior thyroid artery ascends over the anterior scalenus muscle. It then crosses medially behind the carotid sheath and emerges from behind the carotid artery to pass medially to supply the thyroid gland. As it passes medially toward the gland, it crosses the recurrent laryngeal nerve, with its branches posterior to, anterior to, or surrounding the nerve. Close to the thyroid gland, the inferior thyroid artery also sends off small branches to both the superior and inferior parathyroid glands. Although the superior parathyroid gland may receive branches from the superior thyroid artery, the inferior thyroid artery is the primary blood supply to both the superior and inferior parathyroid glands.

The ligament of Berry is derived from pretracheal fascia and represents the lateral fascial attachment of the thyroid gland to the trachea. It is located just caudal to the cricoid cartilage. A small branch of the inferior thyroid artery and small venous branches from the thyroid traverse the ligament, as does the recurrent laryngeal nerve. The tubercle of Zuckerkandl, a lateral projection of the thyroid tissue, often obscures or points to the recurrent laryngeal nerve at the level of the ligament of Berry. The recurrent laryngeal nerve may lie anterior to, posterior to, or in the substance of the ligament of Berry. Any bleeding encountered in this area should be controlled by gentle pressure, rather than blindly placing clamps.

Mobilization of the Pyramidal Lobe and Resection of the Thyroid (Fig. 6.10)

Technical Points

Attention is again turned to the midline. If a pyramidal lobe is identified, retract it caudally. Then dissect alongside the pyramidal lobe in a cephalad direction. Ligate and divide small vessels along the lobe.

After the parathyroid glands are swept posteriorly off the thyroid and the ligament of Berry is divided, the thyroid gland can be resected. If a lobectomy is to be performed, clamp the isthmus on the contralateral side and divide it flush with the trachea. The remaining side is then suture ligated with 2-0 silk sutures. Some surgeons prefer to divide the isthmus early in the course of the procedure (i.e., before mobilization of the superior pole, particularly if a lobectomy is planned). This allows enhanced mobility and exposure, particularly when working through a small incision. Devices such as the harmonic scalpel or vessel-sealing devices are often used in place of suture ligature to divide the isthmus and throughout the procedure.

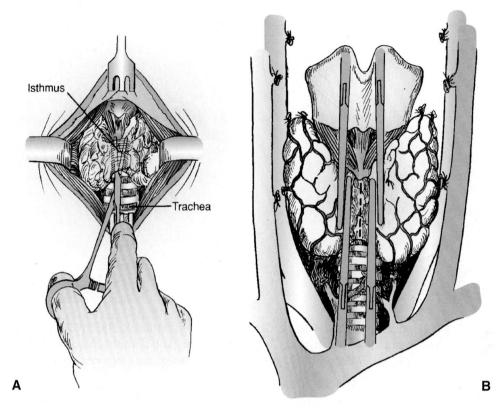

A   B

Figure 6.10 A: Mobilization of the isthmus. **B:** Transection of the isthmus can be accomplished by a sharp division between clamps.

Anatomic Points

A pyramidal lobe is present in about 60% of individuals. It represents a remnant of the thyroglossal duct and its caudal course to the neck from the foramen cecum.

Total and Subtotal Thyroidectomy

Technical Points

If a total thyroidectomy is indicated, repeat the lobectomy procedure on the opposite side.

In order to perform a subtotal thyroidectomy, first dissect and ligate the superior pole vessels and then clamp the remaining gland and transect it, leaving approximately 4 g of tissue posteriorly. Divide the remnant, taking care not to injure the recurrent laryngeal nerve.

Conclusion of Operation and Skin Closure (Fig. 6.11)

Technical Points

Use of a drain is rarely necessary. After obtaining adequate hemostasis, reapproximate the strap muscles in the midline with interrupted or running absorbable sutures. If the strap muscles were divided, approximate these with horizontal mattress sutures. Approximate the platysma using interrupted

absorbable suture. Finally, close the skin with a running subcuticular stitch or clips.

Minimally Invasive Thyroidectomy (Fig. 6.12)

Minimally invasive thyroidectomy encompasses a variety of operations that includes open operations via small incisions, video-assisted dissections, and completely endoscopic dissections. The size of the incision needed to remove the thyroid specimen appears to be one major limitation to these techniques. Thyroid cancers, thyroid nodules greater than 3 cm, thyroid volume greater than 30 mL, thyroiditis, and previous neck operations have generally been considered contraindications to minimally invasive techniques. Applications to other patient populations remain to be determined.

Endoscopic techniques can be broadly divided into two categories: Cervical and noncervical approaches. Of the cervical approaches, the minimally invasive video-assisted technique, an endoscopically assisted technique using a small transverse central neck incision, is the most commonly used. It uses the same landmarks as the standard open approach, reduces incision length, allows bilateral dissection, and allows for conversion to an open technique by merely expanding the incision. Some surgeons have also advocated an endoscopic lateral approach, whereby the incision is located in the lateral neck. Total endoscopic thyroidectomies using small incisions in the

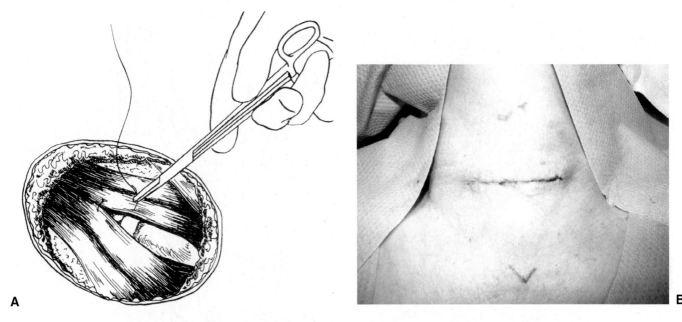

Figure 6.11 Conclusion of operation. **A:** Closure of the strap muscles (from Clark OH, Caron NR. Fine-needle aspiration of the thyroid: Thyroid lobectomy and subtotal thyroidectomy. In: Baker RJ, Fischer JE, eds. *Mastery of Surgery.* 4th ed. Philadelphia: Lippincott Williams & Wilkins; 2001). **B:** Skin closure.

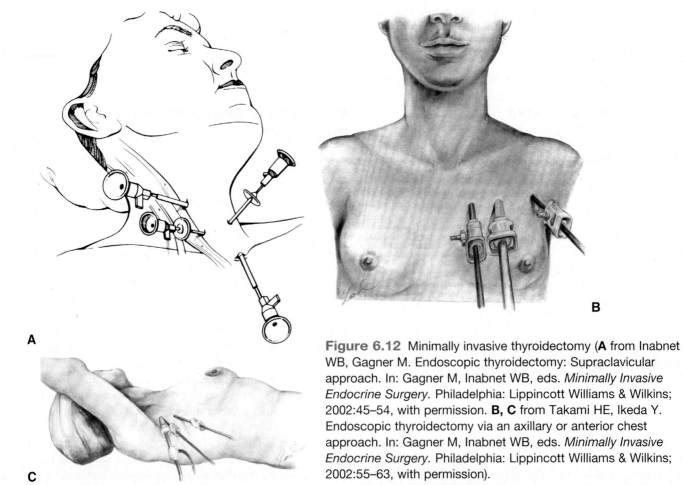

Figure 6.12 Minimally invasive thyroidectomy (**A** from Inabnet WB, Gagner M. Endoscopic thyroidectomy: Supraclavicular approach. In: Gagner M, Inabnet WB, eds. *Minimally Invasive Endocrine Surgery.* Philadelphia: Lippincott Williams & Wilkins; 2002:45–54, with permission. **B, C** from Takami HE, Ikeda Y. Endoscopic thyroidectomy via an axillary or anterior chest approach. In: Gagner M, Inabnet WB, eds. *Minimally Invasive Endocrine Surgery.* Philadelphia: Lippincott Williams & Wilkins; 2002:55–63, with permission).

suprasternal notch and along the sternocleidomastoid muscle have also been described (Fig. 6.12A). The noncervical approaches move the incisions to the chest, axilla, or breast (Fig. 6.12B, C). Although these minimize visible scars, all of the total endoscopic approaches require dissection of additional tissue planes. Some centers have explored the use of robotic-assisted thyroid surgery with encouraging results. Long-term outcome data will ultimately determine the role of these techniques in the management of patients with thyroid disease.

REFERENCES

1. Bliss RD, Gauger PG, Delbridge LW. Surgeon's approach to the thyroid gland: Surgical anatomy and the importance of technique. *World J Surg.* 2000;24:891–897.
2. Cernea CR, Ferraz AR, Nishio S, et al. Surgical anatomy of the external branch of the superior laryngeal nerve. *Head Neck.* 1992; 14:380–383.
3. Clark OH. Surgical treatment. In: Clark OH, ed. *Endocrine Surgery of the Thyroid and Parathyroid Glands.* St. Louis: C.V. Mosby; 1985:256–292.
4. Dhiman SV, Inabnet WB. Minimally invasive surgery for thyroid disease and thyroid cancer. *J Surg Oncol.* 2008;97:665–668.
5. Dozois RR, Beahrs OH. Surgical anatomy and technique of thyroid and parathyroid surgery. *Surg Clin North Am.* 1977;57:647–661.
6. Droulias C, Tzinas S, Harlaftis N, et al. The superior laryngeal nerve. *Am Surg.* 1976;42:635–638.
7. Duh QY. Presidential Address: Minimally invasive endocrine surgery—standard of treatment or hype? *Surgery.* 2003;134:849–857.
8. Friedman M, Vidyasagar R, Bliznikas D, et al. Intraoperative intact parathyroid hormone level monitoring as a guide to parathyroid reimplantation after thyroidectomy. *Laryngoscope.* 2005;115:34–38.
9. Gauger PG, Delbridge LW, Thompson NW, et al. Incidence and importance of the tubercle of Zuckerkandl in thyroid surgery. *Eur J Surg.* 2001;167:249–254.
10. Harness JK, Fung L, Thompson NW, et al. Total thyroidectomy: Complications and technique. *World J Surg.* 1986;10:781–786.
11. Henry JF, Audiffret J, Denizot A, et al. The nonrecurrent inferior laryngeal nerve: Review of 33 cases, including two on the left side. *Surgery.* 1988;104:977–984.
12. Hisham AN, Lukman MR. Recurrent laryngeal nerve in thyroid surgery: A critical appraisal. *ANZ J Surg.* 2002;72:887–889.
13. Hunt PS, Poole M, Reeve TS. A reappraisal of the surgical anatomy of the thyroid and parathyroid glands. *Br J Surg.* 1968;55:63–66.
14. Kandil EH, Noureldine SI, Yao L, et al. Robotic transaxillary thyroidectomy: An examination of the first one hundred cases. *J Am Coll Surg.* 2012;214:558–564.
15. Katz AD. Extralaryngeal division of the recurrent laryngeal nerve. Report on 400 patients and the 721 nerves measured. *Am J Surg.* 1986;152:407–410.
16. Lal G, Clark OH. Thyroid, parathyroid, and adrenal. In: Brunicardi FC, ed. *Schwartz's Principles of Surgery.* 8th ed. Chicago: McGraw-Hill; 2005:1395–1470.
17. Lennquist S, Cahlin C, Smeds S. The superior laryngeal nerve in thyroid surgery. *Surgery.* 1987;102:999–1008.
18. Mamais C, Charaklias N, Pothula VB, et al. Introduction of a new surgical technique: Minimally invasive video-assisted thyroid surgery. *Clin Otolaryngol.* 2011;36:51–56.
19. Nemiroff PM, Katz AD. Extralaryngeal divisions of the recurrent laryngeal nerve. Surgical and clinical significance. *Am J Surg.* 1982;144:466–469.
20. Pagedar NA, Freeman JL. Identification of the external branch of the superior laryngeal nerve during thyroidectomy. *Arch Otolaryngol Head Neck Surg.* 2009;135(4):360–362.
21. Pelizzo MR, Toniato A, Gemo G. Zuckerkandl's tuberculum: An arrow pointing to the recurrent laryngeal nerve (constant anatomical landmark). *J Am Coll Surg.* 1998;187:333–336.
22. Randolph GW, Kobler JB, Wilkins J. Recurrent laryngeal nerve identification and assessment during thyroid surgery: Laryngeal palpation. *World J Surg.* 2004;28:755–760.
23. Robertson ML, Steward DL, Gluckman JL, et al. Continuous laryngeal nerve integrity monitoring: Does it reduce risk of injury? *Otolaryngol Head Neck Surg.* 2004;131:596–600.
24. Rossi RL, Cady B. Surgical anatomy. In: Cady B, Rossi RL, eds. *Surgery of the Thyroid and Parathyroid Glands.* 3rd ed. Philadelphia: W.B. Saunders Company; 1991:13–30.
25. Ruggieri M, Straniero A, Genderini M, et al. The size criteria in minimally invasive video-assisted thyroidectomy. *BMC Surg.* 2007;25:2.
26. Schwartz AE, Friedman EW. Preservation of the parathyroid glands in total thyroidectomy. *Surg Gynecol Obstet.* 1987;165:327–332.
27. Sebag F, Palazzo FF, Harding J, et al. Endoscopic lateral approach thyroid lobectomy: Safe evolution from endoscopic parathyroidectomy. *World J Surg.* 2006;30:802–805.
28. Skandalakis JE, Droulias C, Harlaftis N, et al. The recurrent laryngeal nerve. *Am Surg.* 1976;42:629–634.
29. Thompson NW, Olsen WR, Hoffman GL. The continuing development of the technique of thyroidectomy. *Surgery.* 1973;73:913–927.
30. Tzinas S, Droulias C, Harlaftis N, et al. Vascular patterns of the thyroid gland. *Am Surg.* 1976;42:639–644.
31. Yeung GH. Endoscopic thyroid surgery today: A diversity of surgical strategies. *Thyroid.* 2002;12:703–706.

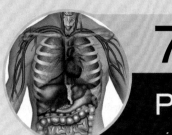

7

Parathyroidectomy

Jarrett E. Walsh and Geeta Lal

In experienced hands, parathyroidectomy is >95% successful in curing hyperparathyroidism. Hyperparathyroidism may result from the overactivity of one gland, as in the case of a parathyroid adenoma or rarely a parathyroid carcinoma, or it may result from the overactivity of multiple glands, as in the case of diffuse hyperplasia or multiple adenomas. The goal of parathyroidectomy is to remove all hyperfunctioning parathyroid tissues.

The gold standard operation for hyperparathyroidism is a bilateral neck exploration, which entails identification of all parathyroid glands. Advances including localization studies, use of intraoperative parathyroid hormone (PTH) assays, and endoscopic techniques have allowed for less invasive and more focused explorations. This chapter will focus on the standard, formal four-gland exploration. Various minimally invasive techniques in use will also be briefly discussed.

SCORE™, the Surgical Council on Resident Education, classified parathyroidectomy as an "ESSENTIAL COMMON" procedure.

STEPS IN PROCEDURE

Initial positioning and exposure are similar as those for thyroidectomy (see Chapter 6)

Standard Four-gland Exploration
Ligate middle thyroid vein and retract gland medially
Identify and preserve recurrent laryngeal nerve
Identify all parathyroid glands bilaterally before biopsy or resection
Superior parathyroid glands commonly found dorsal to recurrent laryngeal nerve and posterior to the upper thyroid capsule

Inferior parathyroid glands commonly found anterior to recurrent laryngeal nerve near lower thyroid pole and thyrothymic ligament
If single adenoma—resect
If multiglandular disease—subtotal parathyroidectomy or total parathyroidectomy and autotransplantation

Focused Exploration or Reoperation
Consider lateral incision for re-exploration
Proceed as guided by ultrasound, radioisotope studies, or intraoperative PTH levels
Close without drains

HALLMARK COMPLICATIONS

Hypoparathyroidism
Recurrent or persistent hyperparathyroidism

Injury to recurrent laryngeal nerve
Bleeding

LIST OF STRUCTURES

Adult Structures
Parathyroid glands
    Superior parathyroid glands
    Inferior parathyroid glands
Thyroid gland
Middle thyroid vein
Inferior thyroid artery
Superior thyroid artery
Recurrent laryngeal nerve
Thymus
Thyrothymic ligament
Mediastinum

Cricoid cartilage
Thyroid cartilage
Esophagus
Tracheoesophageal groove

Embryologic Structures
Pharyngeal pouch III
    Ventral wing
    Dorsal wing
Pharyngeal pouch IV
    Ventral wing
    Dorsal wing

Patients requiring parathyroidectomy should be suitable candidates for general anesthesia. Special attention should be given to preoperative planning in those patients with significant hypercalcemia (i.e., calcium levels higher than 12.5 mg/dL) or marginal renal function. Specifically, this patient population may benefit from the administration of furosemide, bisphosphonates, or calcitonin to address their significant hypercalcemia, and adequate hydration is essential. Document vocal cord function by direct or indirect laryngoscopy in those already suspected of having vocal cord dysfunction (i.e., those with prior neck surgery or altered phonation), because bilateral injury may lead to airway obstruction.

Initial Exposure of Parathyroid Glands

Technical Points

Position the patient with adequate neck exposure in mind. The neck should be dorsally extended on a donut cushion with a bean bag beneath the shoulders in a modified "beach chair" position. Consider additional reverse Trendelenburg positioning of the patient to facilitate venous outflow from the cervical region during the procedure. Make an incision approximately 1 cm below the cricoid cartilage (Fig. 7.1) and carry this through the subcutaneous tissues and platysma. Develop subplatysmal flaps superiorly to the thyroid cartilage notch and inferiorly to the suprasternal notch using electrocautery. After placing a self-retaining retractor, divide the strap muscles through the midline raphe (Fig. 7.2A) and mobilize them laterally off the thyroid gland.

Dissect the sternothyroid muscle off the thyroid and prethyroidal fascia by blunt and sharp dissection, with careful attention to hemostasis. Then retract the strap muscles laterally

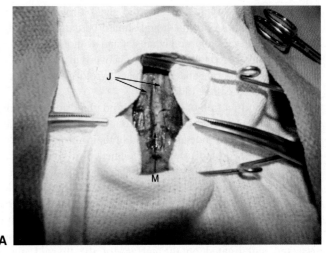

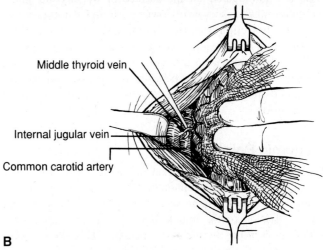

Figure 7.2 A: Operative photo showing the midline raphe (*M*) flanked by the anterior jugular veins (*J*). **B:** Identification and division of the middle thyroid vein.

to expose the middle thyroid vein. Ligate and divide this vein (Fig. 7.2B) and retract the thyroid lobe medially. Sometimes, several branches, rather than one middle thyroid vein, are encountered. These branches may be similarly ligated and divided. A Kitner or 2-0 silk suture placed in the surface of the thyroid gland may be used to help retract the thyroid gland medially. Develop the space between the thyroid gland and the carotid sheath bluntly or with gentle sharp dissection. Identify and protect the recurrent laryngeal nerve using a neurostimulator, if desired.

Most parathyroid glands are found within 1 cm of the junction of the inferior thyroid artery and the recurrent laryngeal nerve. The superior parathyroid glands are usually found dorsal to the recurrent laryngeal nerve and posterior to the upper thyroid capsule. The inferior parathyroid glands are usually located anterior to the recurrent laryngeal nerve near the lower thyroid pole and thyrothymic ligament. Location of glands can vary widely, reflecting differences in the degree of embryologic migration and the extent of displacement as glands enlarge.

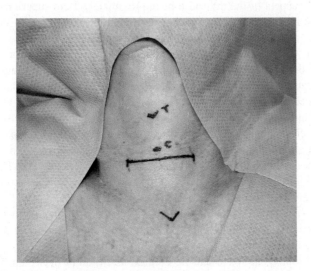

Figure 7.1 Operative photo showing anatomic landmarks and placement of the incision approximately 1 cm inferior to the cricoid cartilage (*C*). The thyroid cartilage is also Identified (*T*).

Any fat lobule at a typical parathyroid gland location could be harboring a parathyroid gland and should be carefully evaluated. A fine, curved Jacobson hemostat and a tenotomy scissors or scalpel can be used to incise the fascia overlying a suspicious fat lobule allowing an underlying parathyroid gland to come into view, the so-called "float sign."

After identification of the parathyroid glands on one side, the exploration should be continued on the contralateral side. When glands on one side are located in their normal position, the contralateral gland is usually located in a similar position. Contralateral symmetry is observed 80% of the time with superior parathyroid glands and 70% of the time with inferior parathyroid glands. Ideally in a four-gland exploration, all parathyroid glands are identified before removing any parathyroid tissue. During thyroidectomy, vessels are dissected and ligated on the surface of the thyroid gland (extrathyroidal dissection). However, during parathyroidectomy, the dissection is carried out more laterally to facilitate identification of the parathyroid glands and avoid inadvertent devascularization. As in the case of thyroidectomy, careful dissection and meticulous hemostasis are essential to prevent blood-stained tissues that can obscure parathyroid gland identification.

Anatomic Points

The middle thyroid vein is varied and is present in only about half of the patients. The vein drains into the ipsilateral internal jugular vein after traveling superficial to the common carotid artery. Division of the middle thyroid vein or veins allows mobilization of the thyroid gland medially. This allows exposure of the space between the thyroid gland and the carotid sheath (containing the carotid artery, internal jugular vein, and vagus nerve). This space contains the recurrent laryngeal nerve, the inferior thyroid artery, and the parathyroid glands.

Normal parathyroid glands are golden yellow to light brown in color. The color does vary depending on the fat and oxyphil cell content of the gland and on the gland's vascularity. Each gland generally weighs between 40 and 50 mg and is 3 to 7 mm in size. Although the parathyroid glands usually derive their blood supply from branches of the inferior thyroid artery, branches of the superior thyroid artery supply approximately 20% of superior glands.

Most individuals (approximately 84%) have four glands, 13% to 20% have more than four glands, and 3% have fewer than four glands. The superior parathyroid glands are generally superior and dorsal to the intersection of the inferior thyroid artery and the recurrent laryngeal nerve. The inferior parathyroid glands are usually inferior and ventral to the intersection (Fig. 7.3).

Parathyroid glands are generally soft and molded by their anatomic position. Distinguishing between a normal and hypercellular gland is often difficult. Generally, hypercellular glands are larger in size (i.e., >7 mm) and darker, firmer, and more vascular. An intraoperative density test may prove useful. Hypercellular glands tend to sink when submersed in a

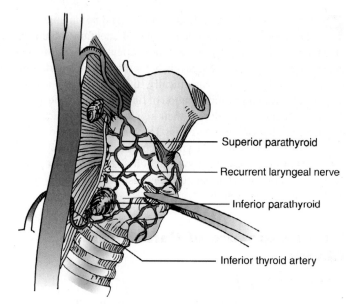

Figure 7.3 The anatomic relationships between the inferior thyroid artery, the recurrent laryngeal nerve, and the parathyroid glands.

Labels:
- Superior parathyroid
- Recurrent laryngeal nerve
- Inferior parathyroid
- Inferior thyroid artery

saline solution, whereas normal glands usually float. No single characteristic is 100% reliable in distinguishing normal from hypercellular glands. The surgeon must therefore rely on a combination of factors; this gestalt recognition favors the well-trained and experienced eye.

Identification of the Superior Parathyroid Glands

Technical Points

The superior parathyroid gland generally resides at the posterior aspect of the thyroid lobe approximately 1 cm superior to the intersection of the inferior thyroid artery and the recurrent laryngeal nerve. The gland is often found within a globule of fat. Careful dissection with a Jacobson or right angle clamp of the fascial layers covering the gland usually aids in identification. Gentle probing with a Kitner often causes the gland to come into view. If differentiation between a fat lobule and gland is still in question, a fine scissors or scalpel can be used to cut a small piece from the nonhilar aspect of the gland. A parathyroid gland diffusely oozes from its cut surface where fat generally bleeds from distinct small blood vessels. The sample of tissue obtained can also be sent for frozen section analysis if there is still a question.

If after an extensive search, a superior gland has not been located, dissection should proceed posteriorly, examining the tracheoesophageal groove and retroesophageal space. The retroesophageal space can be entered and bluntly dissected by passing a finger between the esophagus and vertebral column. The operative field should be first explored visually, and then using a finger, this space should be palpated from the larynx down to the posterior mediastinum. The dissection plane

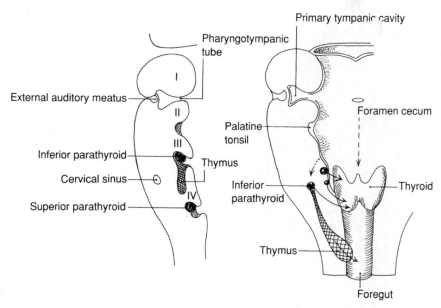

Figure 7.4 Embryology of the parathyroid glands

is generally posterior to the recurrent laryngeal nerve. The inferior thyroid artery can generally be preserved by carefully dissecting around it. Tracing the course of the inferior thyroid artery, which usually supplies the superior gland, may also aid in its identification. Open the carotid sheath and explore this space both visually and by palpation. If a superior gland is still not found, it may be present under the thyroid capsule or within the substance of the thyroid gland. Incise the capsule of the upper thyroid pole sharply with fine scissors, and seek a subcapsular gland. Intraoperative ultrasound of the thyroid may help in identifying an intrathyroidal parathyroid gland, particularly if an ultrasound was not obtained preoperatively. In a hyperparathyroid patient in whom all other glands have been confirmed as normocellular by frozen section, an ipsilateral thyroid lobectomy may be performed and the lobe "bread-loafed" or cut into fine sections to reveal an intrathyroidal gland. Of note, this maneuver is not necessary if a preoperative ultrasound has ruled out intrathyroid nodules.

Anatomic Points

The superior parathyroid gland is derived embryologically from the dorsal wing of the fourth pharyngeal pouch (Fig. 7.4). The ventral wing gives rise to the ultimobranchial body, which contributes to the lateral thyroid tissues and the parafollicular cells. Its descent to its final location in the neck generally follows a shorter course than the inferior gland; therefore, its location is less variable. Approximately 80% of the time, the superior parathyroid gland is located near the cricothyroid junction, about 1 cm superior to where the inferior thyroid artery crosses the recurrent laryngeal nerve. It is usually located at the posterior aspect of the upper thyroid lobe covered by the fascial sheath connecting the upper thyroid pole to the pharynx or is evident more anteriorly beneath the thyroid capsule.

Occasionally, the superior parathyroid lies in an ectopic location (Fig. 7.5A). Knowledge of the glands' embryologic pathway and an understanding that enlarged glands move along areolar planes are invaluable tools when looking for missing glands. When the superior glands enlarge, they usually remain posterior and track caudally in the tracheoesophageal groove, retroesophageal space, or posterior to the carotid sheath. The superior gland may even descend to a position inferior, albeit posterior, to the inferior parathyroid (Fig. 7.5B). On rare occasions, an ectopic superior parathyroid may come to lie in the aortopulmonary window or posterior mediastinum. The occurrence of an intrathyroidal superior gland is rare and occurs in less than 0.5% of cases. The presence of a gland in this location may be explained by the superior gland's close embryologic proximity to the ultimobranchial bodies, which also arise from the fourth pharyngeal pouch and contribute to the lateral thyroid complex.

Identification of the Inferior Parathyroid Glands

Technical Points

The search for an inferior gland should commence with a thorough dissection of the lower thyroid pole. A Jacobson or fine right angle clamp can be used to gently spread the surrounding areolar and fatty tissues near the lower thyroid pole. Often, the gland may be found in the fatty tissue in between branches of the inferior thyroid veins. When the inferior gland is not identified, the junction of the lower pole and the thyrothymic ligament should be carefully dissected. Dissection should then proceed along the posterior aspect of the lower thyroid lobe. One should visually inspect along the tracheoesophageal grove and then, with a finger, palpate down into the superior mediastinum. Next, the thin sheath covering the thymus should be incised. If a gland

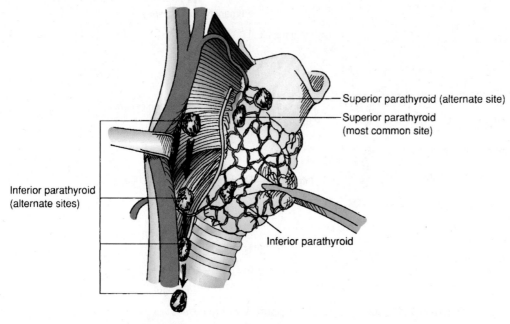

Superior parathyroid (alternate site)

Superior parathyroid (most common site)

Inferior parathyroid (alternate sites)

Inferior parathyroid

A

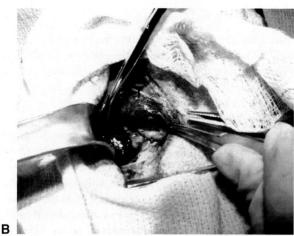

B

Figure 7.5 A: Ectopic locations of the upper parathyroid gland. **B:** Operative photo showing an upper gland adenoma (*P*) in an ectopic (paraesophageal location). This gland was present in the inferior location, posterior to the plane of the thyroid (*T*).

still eludes identification, the thymus can be pulled cranially up into the neck by "walking down" on the thymus with sequential right angle clamps. The upper thymus can then be excised and inspected. The carotid sheath should then be opened and this space should be visually inspected and palpated. If an inferior gland is still not identified and the other glands appear normal, a thyroid lobectomy can be performed. The thyroid lobe can then be "bread-loafed" and inspected for an ectopic gland. As for superior glands, this maneuver is not necessary if a preoperative ultrasound has ruled out thyroid nodules.

Anatomic Points

The inferior parathyroid gland is derived embryologically from the dorsal wing of the third pharyngeal pouch and courses caudally to its final location near the inferior pole of the thyroid (Fig. 7.4B). The ventral wing gives rise to the thymus, which descends into the superior mediastinum. Because of the longer course of migration of the inferior parathyroid gland compared

with the superior gland, its location tends to be more variable. Nonetheless, more than 50% of inferior parathyroid glands are located around the lower pole of the thyroid. Twenty-eight percent of the time, the inferior parathyroid glands are found in the thymus or in the thyrothymic ligament (Fig. 7.6). Both the inferior parathyroid gland and the thymus originate from the third pharyngeal pouch, providing an embryologic explanation for this close relationship. Rarely, in cases where the inferior gland fails to migrate caudally, it may be found higher in the neck near the carotid bifurcation. When inferior glands enlarge, they tend to migrate along areolar planes into the anterior mediastinum.

Excision of Abnormal Glands

Technical Points

If a single large gland is identified, dissect it free from the surrounding thyroid tissue using a sharp dissection and deliver it into the field (Fig. 7.5). The surrounding connective tissue

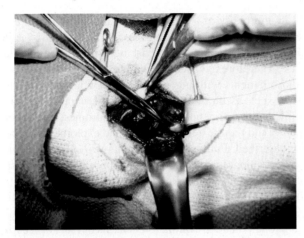

Figure 7.6 Operative photo showing a normal lower parathyroid gland (*P*) located in the thyrothymic ligament, inferior to the thyroid gland (*T*).

can be carefully lysed with electrocautery until just a vascular pedicle remains. This pedicle is then clamped with a right angle clamp and tied with a 3-0 silk suture. Alternatively, small hemoclips may be used. The parathyroid gland is then excised and sent to pathology.

If several glands are enlarged, they are removed in a similar fashion. If there is a question as to whether a gland is normal or not, a biopsy of the gland may be taken and sent for frozen section analysis. The surrounding connective tissue is gently teased off the gland, using care to preserve the gland's vascular supply. A small clip is placed across the edge of the gland and a biopsy is obtained with a fine scissors or scalpel.

When all four glands are enlarged, the surgeon may choose between a subtotal parathyroidectomy and a total parathyroidectomy with autotransplantation. For a subtotal parathyroidectomy, the most normal appearing gland is identified. A clip is placed across the gland and the nonhilar aspect is resected with a fine scissors or scalpel, leaving a 40 to 50 mg remnant behind. If this remnant remains viable, then the remaining glands are removed. If the remnant has been inadvertently devascularized, then the next most normal appearing gland is selected and the process is repeated.

For autotransplantation, all parathyroid glands are removed. A remnant of a gland is then minced into approximately 15 pieces of tissue measuring 1 mm each. These fragments are then implanted into two or three separate pockets in the brachioradialis muscle of the nondominant hand (Fig. 7.7A). Make a horizontal or vertical skin incision over the brachioradialis muscle a few centimeters below the antecubital fossa. Create pockets by gently spreading the muscle fibers with a curved hemostat. Place the remnants into the muscle belly and close the pockets with a 3-0 Prolene stitch and mark them with a clip.

We prefer subtotal parathyroidectomy because total parathyroidectomy with autotransplantation commits the patient to a period of hypoparathyroidism. Failure of autotransplanted tissues has been reported in up to 5% of cases. Rates of recurrent hyperparathyroidism; however, are similar between these two methods. Proponents of total parathyroidectomy argue that in cases of recurrent hyperparathyroidism, it is easier to

remove autotransplanted tissue from the forearm than to reoperate in a scarred neck.

In cases of hyperplasia, we also prefer to perform an upper cervical thymectomy because supernumerary glands occur in up to 20% of patients. Grasp the thyrothymic ligament with a right angle clamp (Fig. 7.7B). With gentle traction, sequentially use right angle clamps to bring the cervical thymus up into the neck incision. Take care to identify and avoid injury to the

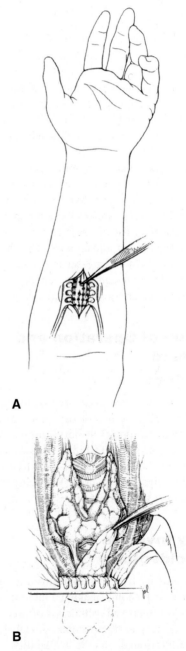

A

B

Figure 7.7 A: Parathyroid autotransplantation. **B:** Mobilization of thymus (from Moore FD Jr, Gawande AA. Parathyroidectomy for hyperplasia and secondary hyperparathyroidism. In: Baker RJ, Fischer JE, eds. *Mastery of Surgery*. 4th ed. Philadelphia: Lippincott Williams & Wilkins; 2001, with permission).

recurrent laryngeal nerves. A Kitner or finger may be used to bluntly and gently dissect the thymus out of the mediastinum. Because of the close proximity to the great vessels, avoid sharp dissection. Ligate thymic veins on the gland's medial and lateral aspects with 3-0 silk sutures or with hemoclips. When no further thymus can be easily delivered, resect the upper thymus and ligate the distal tissue with a 2-0 silk.

Anatomic Points

The brachioradialis muscle is commonly used as a reservoir for autotransplanted parathyroid remnants. The muscle originates from the lateral supracondylar ridge of the humerus and inserts on the base of the styloid process of the radius. It is easily accessible and identifiable. It starts as a rounded elevation above the lateral epicondyle and forms a prominent mass on the radial side of the upper forearm. An incision on the radial side of the forearm, a few centimeters below the antecubital fossa, will allow access to its muscle belly.

The thymus is a common location of ectopic inferior parathyroid glands and supernumerary glands. The common origin of the thymus and inferior parathyroid glands from the third pharyngeal pouches likely explains these findings. The thymus is a bilobed organ that usually resides in the superoanterior mediastinum, although variations exist. The thymus is most prominent in childhood and regresses into adulthood, except in pathologic states. The dominant arterial supply to the thymus is via the inferior thyroid arteries and internal mammary arteries.

Conclusion of Operation and Skin Closure

Technical Points

Use of a drain is rarely necessary. After obtaining adequate hemostasis, the midline raphe of the strap muscles is reapproximated with interrupted 3-0 Vicryl sutures. The platysma is approximated in a similar fashion. The skin is then closed with a running subcuticular stitch of 4-0 Monocryl, or alternatively, Michel clips may be used. Skin glue or Steri-strips may be placed over the incision. Dressings are then placed.

Minimally Invasive Parathyroidectomy

Most cases of primary hyperparathyroidism are secondary to a single parathyroid adenoma, making a more limited exploration feasible. With improved techniques of preoperative noninvasive imaging, such as 99m-technetium–labeled sestamibi, high-resolution ultrasound, and the availability of rapid intraoperative PTH assays, which can objectively assess the adequacy of resection, many centers favor limited or "minimally invasive" explorations instead of a formal bilateral exploration. Proponents cite decreased operative time, length of stay, and cost and improved cosmesis. Opponents argue that a focused exploration is unlikely to improve on the >95% success rate

and low morbidity of a formal, bilateral exploration in experienced hands. Furthermore, a focused exploration is associated with an inherent increased risk of missing multiple gland disease. Therefore, great care should be exercised in screening for those patients with higher risks of having multiple gland disease, such as those with familial hyperparathyroidism or multiple endocrine neoplasia (MEN) syndromes. These populations would require a formal four-gland exploration as previously described. Further, those patients with limited, equivocal, or no radiographic localization of abnormal glands despite biochemical abnormalities or those with discordant findings among imaging techniques necessitate four-gland exploration.

Although some studies show no difference between unilateral and bilateral neck exploration in terms of rates of recurrent or persistent disease, a limited number of studies with various methods and endpoints have only perpetuated debate on this issue. More long-term follow-up data will be needed to identify the optimal use of "minimally invasive" techniques in the general population. That being said, the minimally invasive techniques are widely used. The most common ones are described briefly in the following sections.

Focused Parathyroidectomy

This approach is what is most commonly referred to as a "minimally invasive" parathyroidectomy. A focused approach commences by drawing a blood sample for PTH before making an incision. The sample may be drawn from a peripheral vein or from the jugular vein, once it has been exposed. It is our preference to draw the PTH from an intravenous catheter placed in the antecubital vein. A 2.5- to 3-cm skin crease incision is then made 1 cm caudal to the cricoid cartilage as described previously. Dissection proceeds on the affected side (as determined by preoperative imaging) in a fashion similar to that described above for a bilateral exploration. After the parathyroid adenoma is identified, it is dissected from the surrounding tissues and removed. A PTH level is drawn immediately before excision and 10 minutes postexcision. A fall in PTH level ≥50% from the highest pre-excision level is considered adequate and the procedure is terminated. Some patients may require 20 to 30 minutes for the PTH level to fall secondary to gland manipulation during dissection. In these patients, an additional blood sample may be sent.

Ultrasound and sestamibi scans have 65% and 80% sensitivity, respectively, for identifying an abnormal gland. When both studies identify the same abnormal gland, the sensitivity increases to more than 95% (Fig. 7.8). Discordant imaging results are often due to thyroid nodules that may complicate results. It is these authors' practice to perform a focused exploration when both studies are concordant. In patients with secondary hyperparathyroidism or with a family history suggestive of inherited primary hyperparathyroidism, we perform a bilateral exploration, because these patients are likely to have multigland disease. Although our preference is to perform focused explorations under general anesthesia, using a local anesthetic and sedation is also feasible.

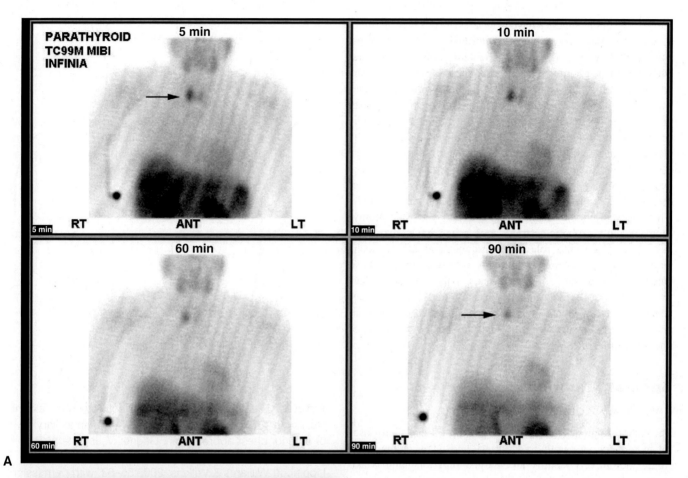

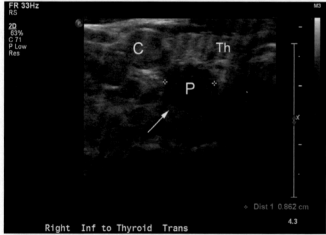

Figure 7.8 A: Sestamibi scan showing right parathyroid uptake. **B:** Ultrasound showing concordance for a right parathyroid adenoma, which is typically hypoechoic when compared to the thyroid gland. C, carotid; Th, thyroid; P, parathyroid adenoma.

Radio-Guided Parathyroidectomy

The technique involves using a hand-held gamma probe to identify parathyroid adenomas in patients with positive sestamibi scans. The radionuclide is administered within 2 hours of surgery. The patient is then explored through a 2- to 3-cm incision, and the dissection is directed toward areas with the highest counts. Ex vivo counts of excised adenomas are generally 20% above background counts. Reported advantages include easier localization, particularly in reoperative cases, and the ability to perform the procedure under local anesthetic or seda-

tion using smaller incisions. Although feasible, this approach has not been widely used as it is often difficult to differentiate a "hot" parathyroid adenoma from background activity in the thyroid gland, which also takes up the tracer. Moreover, it has little advantage over a good preoperative sestamibi scan.

Endoscopic Parathyroidectomy

Purely videoscopic and video-assisted parathyroidectomies have proven both feasible and safe in experienced hands.

Many different techniques have been described. Early attempts at parathyroidectomy using conventional insufflation were complicated by hypercarbia and subcutaneous emphysema, but since then, groups have reported success with both conventional and gasless approaches. The parathyroids have been approached via the central neck, laterally, and even via ports in the axilla and anterior chest (Fig. 7.9). Relative contraindication for videoscopic or video-assisted means include multiglandular disease and large goiters or concurrent thyroid disease. Absolute contraindications include parathyroid cancer and reoperative necks. Endoscopic techniques have also been described to remove ectopic mediastinal parathyroid glands, where they provide a less invasive alternative to sternotomy. More recently, robotic-assisted approaches have also been described. The future role of endoscopic and robotic techniques in parathyroid surgery remains to be determined. These techniques have been shown by many to be safe and effective, but the benefit in terms of decreasing incision length may be exaggerated compared to a conventional open exploration, and endoscopic techniques are usually associated with longer operative times.

Special Situations

Lateral Approach

The lateral approach to parathyroidectomy is especially useful in reoperative parathyroid surgery and when preoperative studies definitively identify an enlarged superior gland. Make an incision as previously described or alternatively, centered along the anterior border of the sternocleidomastoid muscle. Develop the plane between the sternocleidomastoid and strap muscles with a sharp and blunt dissection. Retract the common carotid artery and internal jugular vein laterally and the thyroid gland medially. Identify the recurrent laryngeal nerve and

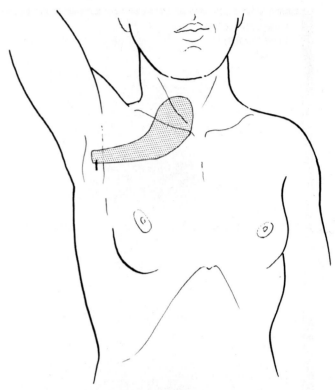

Figure 7.9 Endoscopic parathyroidectomy (from Takami HE, Ikeda Y. Endoscopic thyroidectomy via an axillary or anterior chest approach. In: Gagner M, Inabnet WB, eds. *Minimally Invasive Endocrine Surgery.* Philadelphia: Lippincott Williams & Wilkins; 2002:55–63, with permission).

the enlarged gland. Remove the gland as previously described (Fig. 7.10). One obvious disadvantage of a lateral approach is the requirement for two neck incisions if multiglandular disease is encountered.

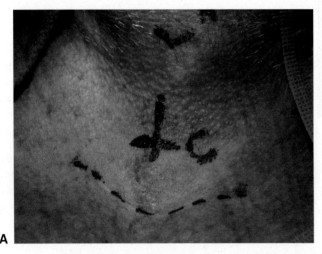
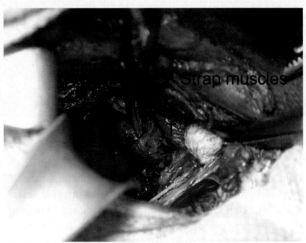

Figure 7.10 Operative photos showing the lateral approach in a patient with persistent hyperparathyroidism. The neck was approached via the previous scar **(A)** and the dissection was carried out in the plane between the straps and sternocleidomastoid muscle **(B).** SCM, sternocleidomastoid; T, thyroid; P, parathyroid adenoma.

Sternotomy

Sternotomy should only be performed after a thorough exploration of the neck. Generally, sternotomy is not performed at the time of original neck exploration and is only considered after preoperative imaging modalities (e.g., sestamibi scanning, computed tomography, magnetic resonance imaging, or occasionally angiography) have demonstrated a mediastinal tumor. The anterior mediastinum can generally be explored via a neck incision, but, when necessary, a vertical incision from the suprasternal notch to the second or third intercostal space can be made along with a partial sternal split. Care should be taken not to injure the internal thoracic arteries laterally and the left innominate vein posteriorly. Ectopic parathyroid glands in the posterior mediastinum usually require a complete sternotomy or thoracoscopic approach.

REFERENCES

1. Akerstrom G, Rudberg C, Grimelius L, et al. Causes of failed primary exploration and technical aspects of re-operation in primary hyperparathyroidism. *World J Surg.* 1992;16:562–568.
2. Arici C, Cheah WK, Ituarte PH, et al. Can localization studies be used to direct focused parathyroid operations? *Surgery.* 2001;129:720–729.
3. Bilezikian JP, Khan AA, Potts JT Jr, et al. Guidelines for the management of asymptomatic primary hyperparathyroidism: Summary statement from the third international workshop. *J Clin Endocrinol Metab.* 2009;94:335–339.
4. Duh QY. Presidential Address: Minimally invasive endocrine surgery–standard of treatment or hype? *Surgery.* 2003;134:849–857.
5. Duh QY, Uden P, Clark OH. Unilateral neck exploration for primary hyperparathyroidism: Analysis of a controversy using a mathematical model. *World J Surg.* 1992;16:654–661.
6. Edis AJ. Surgical anatomy and technique of neck exploration for primary hyperparathyroidism. *Surg Clin North Am.* 1977;57:495–504.
7. Edis AJ, Purnell DC, van Heerden JA. The undescended "parathymus": An occasional cause of failed neck exploration for hyperparathyroidism. *Ann Surg.* 1979;190:64–68.
8. Esselstyn CB Jr, Levin HS. A technique for parathyroid surgery. *Surg Clin North Am.* 1975;55:1047–1063.
9. Fraker DL, Doppman JL, Shawker TH, et al. Undescended parathyroid adenoma: An important etiology for failed operations for primary hyperparathyroidism. *World J Surg.* 1990;14:342–348.
10. Freeman JB, Sherman BM, Mason EE. Transcervical thymectomy: An integral part of neck exploration for hyperparathyroidism. *Arch Surg.* 1976;111:359–364.
11. Gagner M. Endoscopic subtotal parathyroidectomy in patients with primary hyperparathyroidism. *Br J Surg.* 1996;83:875.
12. Gilmour JR. The gross anatomy of the parathyroid glands. *J Pathol.* 1938;46:133–149.
13. Gilmour JR, Martin WJ. The weight of the parathyroid glands. *J Pathol Bacteriol.* 1937;44:431–462.
14. Inabnet WB 3rd, Kim CK, Haber RS, et al. Radioguidance is not necessary during parathyroidectomy. *Arch Surg.* 2002;137:967–970.
15. Irvin GL 3rd, Dembrow VD, Prudhomme DL. Clinical usefulness of an intraoperative "quick parathyroid hormone" assay. *Surgery.* 1993;114:1019–1022.
16. Kebebew E, Clark OH. Parathyroid adenoma, hyperplasia, and carcinoma: Localization, technical details of primary neck exploration, and treatment of hypercalcemic crisis. *Surg Oncol Clin N Am.* 1998;7:721–748.
17. Lee NC, Norton JA. Multiple-gland disease in primary hyperparathyroidism: A function of operative approach? *Arch Surg.* 2002;137:896–899.
18. Levin K, Clark OH. The reasons for failure in parathyroid operations. *Arch Surg.* 1989;124:911–914.
19. Liechty RD, Weil R 3rd. Parathyroid anatomy in hyperplasia. *Arch Surg.* 1992;127:813–815.
20. Moley JF, Lairmore TC, Doherty GM, et al. Preservation of the recurrent laryngeal nerves in thyroid and parathyroid reoperations. *Surgery.* 1999;126:673–677.
21. Nathaniels EK, Nathaniels AM, Wang CA. Mediastinal parathyroid tumors: A clinical and pathological study of 84 cases. *Ann Surg.* 1970;171:165–170.
22. Okamoto T, Obara T. Parathyroid: Bilateral neck exploration. In: Hubbard JG, Inabnet WB, Lo CY, eds. *Endocrine Surgery: Principles and Practice.* 1st ed. London: Springer-Verlag; 2009:279–289.
23. Pollock WF. Surgical anatomy of the thyroid and parathyroid glands. *Surg Clin North Am.* 1964;44:1161–1173.
24. Prinz RA, Lonchyna V, Carnaille B, et al. Thoracoscopic excision of enlarged mediastinal parathyroid glands. *Surgery.* 1994;116:999–1004.
25. Rossi RL, Cady B. Surgical anatomy. In: Cady B, Rossi RL, eds. 3rd ed. Philadelphia: W.B. Saunders Company; 1991:13–30.
26. Thompson NW, Eckhauser FE, Harness JK. The anatomy of primary hyperparathyroidism. *Surgery.* 1982;92:814–821.
27. Tolley N, Arora A, Palazzo F, et al. Robotic-assisted parathyroidectomy: A feasibility study. *Otolaryngol Head Neck Surg.* 2011;144(6):859–866.
28. Udelsman R. Six hundred fifty-six consecutive explorations for primary hyperparathyroidism. *Ann Surg.* 2002;235:665–670.
29. Wang CA. Surgical management of primary hyperparathyroidism. *Curr Probl Surg.* 1985;22:1–50.
30. Wang C. The anatomic basis of parathyroid surgery. *Ann Surg.* 1976;183:271–275.
31. Wang CA, Rieder SV. A density test for the intraoperative differentiation of parathyroid hyperplasia from neoplasia. *Ann Surg.* 1978;187:63–67.
32. Wells SA Jr, Farndon JR, Dale JK, et al. Long-term evaluation of patients with primary parathyroid hyperplasia managed by total parathyroidectomy and heterotopic autotransplantation. *Ann Surg.* 1980;192:451–458.

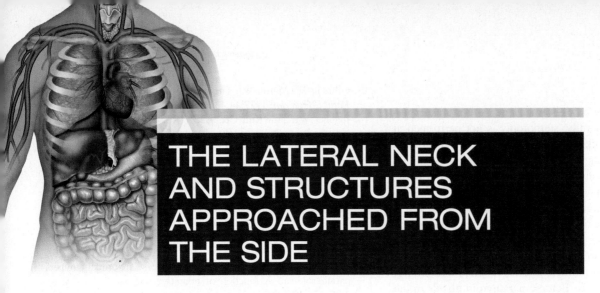

THE LATERAL NECK AND STRUCTURES APPROACHED FROM THE SIDE

Structures of significance in the lateral neck are primarily vascular. The internal and external jugular veins and the common, internal, and external carotid arteries are all approached from the side. The internal and external jugular veins are primarily used for vascular access (Chapter 8), either by percutaneous puncture or by cutdown. This chapter also discussed how to place long-term access devices such as ports and tunneled catheters. Surgery for stroke prevention is performed on the carotid artery in the region of its bifurcation (Chapter 9).

As are all major vessels, the carotid arteries and jugular veins are accompanied by lymph nodes. Lymph node biopsy (Chapter 10) introduces the anatomy of the cervical lymph node groups. The anatomy of the major lymph node groups is related to major vascular structures and nerves by the meticulous operation undertaken for cancer (termed *radical neck dissection*) (Chapter 11).

Although the esophagus is a midline structure, it lies so deep in the neck that it is easier to approach from the side. Therefore, exposure of the cervical esophagus and the anatomic relationships of this portion of the gastrointestinal tract are included in this section (Chapter 12).

Neck exploration for trauma (Chapter 13)—a systematic inspection of the major vascular and visceral compartments of the neck—completes the procedures commonly performed in this area.

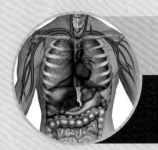

8

Venous Access: External and Internal Jugular Veins

The external and internal jugular veins are frequently used for access to the central venous circulation. In this chapter, external jugular venous cutdown, internal jugular venous cutdown, and percutaneous internal jugular venous cannulation are presented. Because the most common method is percutaneous internal jugular venous cannulation, several approaches (posterior, anterior, and ultrasound-guided) are discussed.

This chapter also discusses placement of two types of implantable venous access devices: Ports and tunneled venous catheters.

Special considerations referable to placement of large-diameter venous access devices for hemodialysis are discussed in Chapter 38.

The anatomy of the carotid sheath is introduced. The carotid artery and the anatomy of the carotid region are discussed in greater detail in Chapter 9.

SCORE™, the Surgical Council on Resident Education, classified central venous line placement, ultrasound use for intravascular access, insertion of implantable venous access devices, and pulmonary artery catheter placement as "ESSENTIAL COMMON" procedures.

Pulmonary artery catheter placement is not explicitly described in this text; critical care references at the end explain this procedure, which begins with the access procedures described in this chapter and in Chapter 14.

STEPS IN PROCEDURE—EXTERNAL JUGULAR VEIN CUTDOWN

Position patient with head turned to one side, slight Trendelenburg positioning
Identify external jugular vein
Small transverse incision in midneck
Identify vein and dissect proximally and distally
Tunnel catheter
Ligate vein cephalad and cannulate vein, directing it centrally
Confirm central location
Tie vein around catheter
Close skin incision and secure catheter

HALLMARK ANATOMIC COMPLICATIONS

Carotid artery puncture
Pneumothorax
Failure of catheter to pass centrally

LIST OF STRUCTURES

External jugular vein
Internal jugular vein
Common facial vein
Common carotid artery
Platysma muscle
Sternocleidomastoid muscle

External Jugular Venous Cutdown

The external jugular vein, because of its superficial location, is an easy site for venous cutdown or percutaneous cannulation. Difficulty is often encountered in passing a catheter centrally from this location. In addition, the vein is often thrombosed in patients in whom the procedure has been attempted before. For these reasons, the more difficult internal jugular approaches may be preferred.

Venous Anatomy of the Neck and External Jugular Venous Cutdown (Fig. 8.1)

Technical Points

Position the patient with the head turned to one side. A slight Trendelenburg position will increase venous pressure in the neck, facilitating identification of the vein and decreasing the chance of venous air embolism. Apply pressure to the platysma muscle just above the clavicle and identify the external jugular

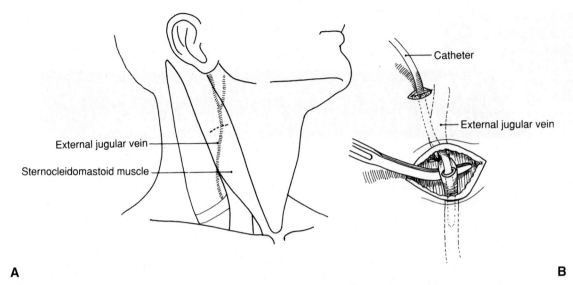

A   **B**

Figure 8.1 Venous anatomy of the neck and external jugular venous cutdown. **A:** Venous anatomy of the neck. **B:** External jugular venous cutdown.

vein as it distends with blood. Infiltrate the area overlying the vein with local anesthetic and make a small transverse skin incision over the vein in the midneck. Make the incision with care to avoid injury to the vein, which lies very superficially. Identify the vein and dissect parallel to the vein proximally and distally for a length of about 1 cm. Elevate the vein into the wound with a hemostat. Ligate the vein proximally (cephalad) and place a ligature around the distal vein.

The catheter should enter the skin at a separate site, rather than through the cutdown incision. Make a small incision about 2 cm above the skin incision and tunnel the catheter under the skin to the incision. A Broviac- or Hickman-type catheter is tunneled under the skin of the chest wall to an exit site located at a flat, stable location (see subsequent sections of this chapter). Generally, the parasternal region, about 10 cm below the clavicle, is selected as the exit site.

Use a number 11 blade for performing a small anterior venotomy, then introduce the catheter. Because of angulation at the juncture of the external jugular vein and the subclavian vein, there may be a tendency for the catheter to "hang up" or to pass out toward the arm rather than centrally. If this occurs, turn the patient's head back toward the side of cannulation and reattempt to pass the catheter centrally. If necessary, use a floppy-tipped guidewire, under fluoroscopic control, to guide the catheter into the superior vena cava. Tie the catheter in place distally.

Secure the catheter in position and close the incision with interrupted absorbable sutures. If the external jugular vein cannot be cannulated or the central venous circulation cannot be accessed using this approach, extend the incision medially and proceed to the internal jugular vein (Fig. 8.2).

Anatomic Points

The external jugular vein begins in the vicinity of the angle of the mandible, within or just inferior to the parotid gland. It runs just deep to the platysma muscle. Its course is approximated by a line connecting the mandibular angle and the middle of the clavicle. It crosses the sternocleidomastoid muscle and pierces the superficial lamina of the deep cervical fascia roofing the omoclavicular triangle. It continues its vertical course to end in either the subclavian or, about one-third of the time, the internal jugular vein. When it pierces the superficial lamina, its wall adheres to the fascia. This tends to hold a laceration of the vein open and predisposes the patient to air entrance if the vein is severed at this site. The vein can be occluded by pressure just superior to the middle of the clavicle, a point slightly posterior to the clavicular origin of the sternocleidomastoid muscle. The diameter of the external jugular vein is quite variable and appears to have an inverse relation to the diameter of the internal jugular veins. The right external jugular vein is typically larger in diameter than the

---

STEPS IN PROCEDURE—INTERNAL JUGULAR CUTDOWN

Choose right side if possible, turn head to left, slight Trendelenburg position

Transverse incision centered over division of sternocleidomastoid

Deepen incision through platysma and spread two heads of sternocleidomastoid

Identify internal jugular vein

Dissect in anterior adventitial plane to free several centimeters of vein

Place purse-string suture

Tunnel catheter

Cannulate vein

Tie purse-string suture around vein

Confirm position of catheter

Close incision

left, partly because it is more closely aligned with the superior vena cava and thus the right atrium.

At midneck, the external jugular vein is covered only by the platysma muscle and minor branches of the transverse cervical nerve. This branch of the cervical plexus, carrying sensory fibers of C2 and C3, pierces the superficial lamina of the cervical fascia at the posterior edge of the middle of the sternocleidomastoid, then crosses the sternocleidomastoid muscle, passing deep to the external jugular vein to innervate the skin of the anterior triangle of the neck.

Internal Jugular Venous Cutdown

Dissection to the Internal Jugular Vein (Fig. 8.2)

Technical Points

Choose the right internal jugular vein whenever possible. Position the patient supine with the head turned to the contralateral side. The table should be flat or in a slight Trendelenburg position to distend the veins of the neck and minimize the chances of venous air embolism. Infiltrate the skin of a planned transverse skin incision about 2 cm above the clavicle. Make an incision about 3 cm in length, centered over the triangle formed by the division of the sternocleidomastoid muscle into its medial and lateral heads.

Deepen the incision through the platysma until the sternocleidomastoid muscle is encountered, then spread the tissue between the two heads of the muscle to expose the underlying internal jugular vein.

If approaching the internal jugular vein after a failed external jugular vein cutdown, the incision may be high enough to access the common facial vein as it empties into the internal jugular vein. Extend the incision medially across the medial border of the sternocleidomastoid muscle. Retract the sternocleidomastoid muscle and identify the internal jugular vein just deep to the muscle and lying within the carotid sheath. Search along the anterior and upper aspect of the vein for a large common facial vein. If this can be identified, it can often be cannulated and ligated. This is a simpler way to access the internal jugular vein than is the purse-string suture method (Fig. 8.3).

Anatomic Points

The right internal jugular vein takes a relatively straight course to the central venous circulation, unlike the left, which first enters the brachiocephalic vein. For this reason, it is the preferred site of cannulation.

The minor supraclavicular fossa is the triangle bounded by the clavicle and the sternal and clavicular heads of the sternocleidomastoid muscle. This fossa is covered by skin, superficial fascia (in which there may be branches of the medial supraclavicular nerve), fibers of the platysma muscle, and the superficial lamina of the cervical fascia.

The internal jugular vein is the dominant structure within the fossa itself. Its exposure may be somewhat tedious owing to the presence of deep cervical lymph nodes. It is located in its own compartment in the carotid sheath and tends to diverge anteriorly from the common carotid artery. This facilitates circumferential dissection of the vein. Because the vein is completely surrounded by the connective tissue elements of the carotid sheath, it does not collapse completely. This can lead to air embolus. Remember that the common carotid artery is posterior to the internal jugular vein at this level and that the apex of the lung is posterior to the common carotid artery. Slightly more inferior, the termination of the internal jugular vein and the beginning of the brachiocephalic vein are in contact with the parietal pleura and the apex of the lung.

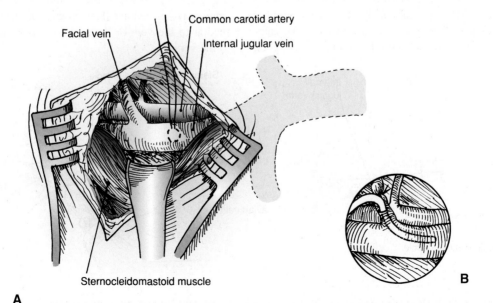

Facial vein

Common carotid artery

Internal jugular vein

Sternocleidomastoid muscle

A

B

Figure 8.2 Dissection to the internal jugular vein. **A:** Location of purse-string suture on internal jugular vein. **B:** Alternative placement into facial vein.

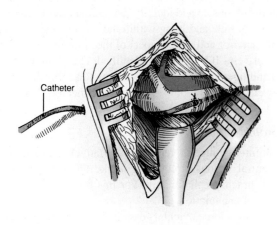

Figure 8.3 Placement of purse-string suture and cannulation of the internal jugular vein

Placement of Purse-String Suture and Cannulation of the Internal Jugular Vein (Fig. 8.3)

Technical and Anatomic Points

Carefully dissect the anterior adventitial plane of the vein to free several centimeters of vein proximally and distally. Pass a right-angle clamp under the vein and place silastic loops proximal and distal to the vein. Lift up on the vein gently with DeBakey pickups, if necessary, to facilitate passage of the right-angle clamp. The internal jugular vein can be ligated if necessary. If injury to the vein occurs, ligation and division of the vein is the safest course.

Place a 4-0 Prolene purse-string suture on the anterior surface of the vein. Place this suture in four bites, drawing a small square on the vein. Make a small incision, using a number 11 blade, in the center of the purse-string and insert the catheter. Confirm passage into the central circulation and good position of the catheter tip. Tie the purse-string suture and close the incision in layers with interrupted absorbable suture.

Percutaneous Cannulation of the Internal Jugular Vein by Posterior Approach

Posterior Approach to the Internal Jugular Vein by Anatomic Landmarks (Fig. 8.4)

Technical Points

Position the patient supine, in a moderate Trendelenburg position, with the head turned to the contralateral side. Palpate the lateral border of the sternocleidomastoid muscle about two fingerbreadths above the clavicle (Fig. 8.4A). Use the thumb of the nondominant hand to stabilize and elevate the sternocleidomastoid muscle by hooking the tip of the thumb under the edge of the muscle and lifting slightly. Place the index finger of the same hand in the sternal notch for orientation. Visualize an imaginary line passing just deep to the thumb of that hand and aiming at the index finger (Fig. 8.4B). Infiltrate the skin with local anesthetic, then infiltrate the deeper tissues, aspirating carefully as the needle is advanced. Use this small-gauge needle to identify the internal jugular vein by aspirating venous blood about 1- to 2-cm deep to the skin. If no blood is obtained, vary the depth below the sternocleidomastoid muscle, but not the angle of the needle, until blood is obtained.

Anatomic Points

At the entrance site of the needle, no major anatomic structures should be located. Remember that the internal jugular vein is immediately deep to the sternocleidomastoid muscle and anterolateral to the common carotid artery. The apex of the lung is protected by the anterior scalene muscle and its fascia, but it can be entered if the needle is directed too deeply. An improperly placed needle can enter the common carotid artery medial to the vein or damage the vagus nerve posteromedial to the vein.

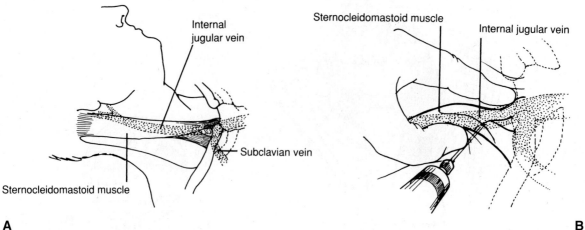

A

B

Figure 8.4 Posterior approach to the internal jugular vein by anatomic landmarks. **A:** Anatomic landmarks. **B:** Passage of needle.

STEPS IN PROCEDURE—PERCUTANEOUS CANNULATION OF THE INTERNAL JUGULAR VEIN

Position Patient Supine, Moderate
Trendelenburg position, head turned to contralateral side

Posterior Approach by Landmarks
Stand at the patient's side
Lateral border of sternocleidomastoid muscle, two fingerbreadths above the clavicle
Hook the thumb of your nondominant hand under this muscle and elevate it
Place the index finger of nondominant hand in sternal notch
Visualize a line passing just deep to the thumb, aiming at the index finger
Infiltrate with local anesthetic, pass needle into deep tissues while aspirating to find vein
Use larger needle to access vein along same trajectory
Pass guidewire, dilator, and sheath, followed by catheter
Obtain chest x-ray to confirm position of catheter and absence of pneumothorax

Anterior Approach by Landmarks
Stand at the head of the patient
Identify triangle formed by sternal and clavicular heads of sternocleidomastoid muscle

Inject local anesthesia and pass needle deeper, directing it inferiorly and very slightly laterally, aspirating to find vein
Proceed with larger needle, guidewire, dilator and sheath, followed by catheter
Obtain chest x-ray to check position of catheter and absence of pneumothorax

Anterior Approach, Ultrasound-Guidance
Stand at head of patient
Use ultrasound to localize vein and optimize head position
Entry site of catheter will be cephalad to that previously described when landmarks are used
Transverse orientation of transducer
Visualize cross section of vein in middle of field
Needle will appear as bright spot in lumen of vein
Longitudinal orientation of transducer
Visualize vein in longitudinal orientation
Hold transducer parallel to vein; maintain critical orientation of transducer, vein, and needle in same plane
Needle will appear to enter from side and slant into lumen of vein

Anterior Approach to the Internal Jugular Vein (Fig. 8.5) and Seldinger Technique (Fig. 8.6)

Technical Points

Identify the triangle formed by the sternal and clavicular heads of the sternocleidomastoid muscle (Sedillot's triangle) (Fig. 8.5). Introduce the small-caliber finder needle at the apex of this triangle, directing it inferiorly and very slightly laterally as you progress deeper through the tissues. Aspirate continuously until free flow of blood is obtained. The anterior approach to the right internal jugular vein is often used to place catheters using the Seldinger technique because it provides a straight pathway to the superior vena cava.

The *Seldinger technique* is a versatile maneuver in which a guidewire is used to exchange the initial cannulating needle for a cannulating device. It is applied in a variety of circumstances ranging from venous access through percutaneous cystostomy. To introduce a catheter with the Seldinger technique, first familiarize yourself thoroughly with the particular kit that you have at hand and all of its components. Ensure that everything is there and laid out easily to hand.

After identifying the vein with a small-caliber needle, use a slightly larger needle to cannulate the vein, then introduce the floppy end of a guidewire into the vein (Fig. 8.6A). Note that it is important to withdraw the curved end of the guidewire fully into the plastic introducer that has been supplied with the kit. The guidewire should pass very easily. Fluoroscopy, if available,

helps confirm central passage of the guidewire. Remove the cannulating needle. Ensure that the skin opening is large enough to accommodate the dilator and sheath easily; if the skin opening is too small, the sheath will not pass. Frequently, this attempted failed passage will damage the smooth leading edge of the sheath so that it cannot be used again.

Next, pass a vessel dilator and sheath of the desired size over the guidewire (Fig. 8.6B) and withdraw the guidewire. Put your gloved finger over the end of the sheath to prevent significant loss of blood, but do visually confirm that dark venous rather than pulsatile arterial blood is obtained. If bright red blood is obtained when the vessel is cannulated, the carotid artery may have been entered. Before making another attempt, withdraw the needle and apply firm but gentle pressure to the site for 10 minutes. If attempting a new venipuncture on the opposite internal jugular vein, it is always safest to obtain a chest radiograph before proceeding any further. Although rare, a bilateral pneumothorax can occur and is a potentially serious, if not lethal, complication if it is not recognized.

Pass the catheter into the sheath (Fig. 8.6C). To avoid buckling of thin flexible catheters, push straight into the sheath in small increments with a DeBakey forceps as shown. Next, snap the sheath to break the rigid plastic and begin pulling back both parts while continuing to pull the sheath apart where it has been scored. Visually confirm complete removal of both parts of the sheath (Fig. 8.6D). Note that the catheter is not seen in this

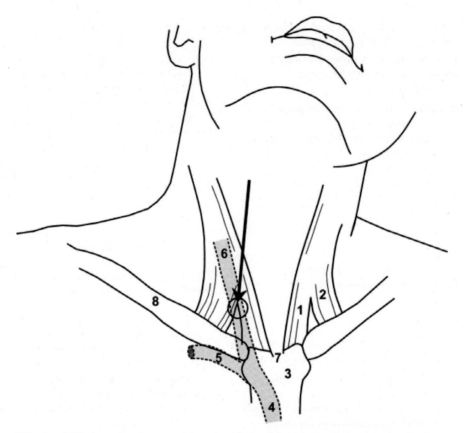

Figure 8.5 Anterior approach to the internal jugular vein by anatomic landmarks. *Arrow* shows direction of needle as vein is accessed from anterior approach.

photograph because a completely subcutaneous "port" type device has been placed (as described later in this chapter).

After the catheter is successfully positioned, confirm its location by chest radiography and check carefully for the presence of a pneumothorax.

Note that this access route is frequently used to place very large diameter venous cannulae for hemodialysis access. See Chapter 38, Figures 38.5A,B for additional considerations in this circumstance.

Anatomic Points

The carotid artery lies immediately medial to the internal jugular vein. Palpation of this landmark at the beginning of the procedure assists in identification of the, probably, tract of the vein. The apex of the pleura extends for a variable amount into the path of the needle and pneumothorax may result if the needle is passed too deeply.

Ultrasound-Guided Cannulation of the Internal Jugular Vein (Anterior Approach) (Figs. 8.7 and 8.8)

Scan the neck on the proposed side before preparing a sterile field; use the information gained to optimize position of the head and neck. The jugular vein will be larger, more superficial, and more compressible than the artery. Doppler, if available, will show arterial flow in the carotid artery and not in the vein. Move the head into a more neutral position, if necessary, to allow the carotid artery to move medially away from the vein, thus diminishing the chance of carotid artery puncture. Next, create the sterile field, including a drape and sterile conducting jelly for the ultrasound probe.

There are two ways to use ultrasound to visualize the vein during cannulation. The ultrasound probe may be held transverse to the long axis of the vein, so that the vein is seen in cross section. The operator then watches for the needle to appear in the lumen of the vein. This method is simpler because precise alignment of the needle, vein, and ultrasound probe axis are not required.

In the second method, the ultrasound transducer is aligned parallel with the long axis of the vein (Fig. 8.7). The needle is visualized as a long, slender hyperechoic object entering the vein. Precise alignment of three objects—vein, needle, and ultrasound transducer—is required. Recall that the typical high-resolution ultrasound beam is about the thinness of a credit card, and you will appreciate the inherent difficulty of this approach. References at the end of the chapter give further details on this alternative method, which is preferred by some and may be easier in some special situations.

With either approach, the entry site will be cephalad to the location of the transducer; this results in a more cephalad puncture site than when anatomic landmarks are used.

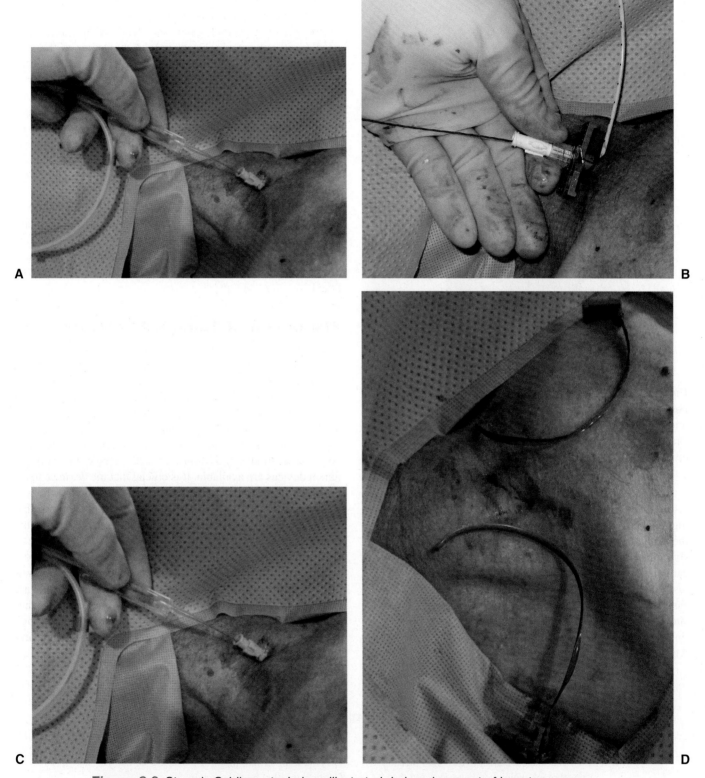

Figure 8.6 Steps in Seldinger technique illustrated during placement of long-term access device through anterior approach to the right internal jugular vein. **A:** Guidewire is placed into the vein. **B:** Needle is removed, and dilator and sheath are passed into the vein over the guidewire. **C:** Catheter is passed into sheath after removal of dilator. **D:** Catheter is now in place (unseen, under the skin) and both pieces of the sheath have been removed intact. Photographs courtesy of Drs Ryan Conway and Scott Sherman, University of Iowa Carver College of Medicine.

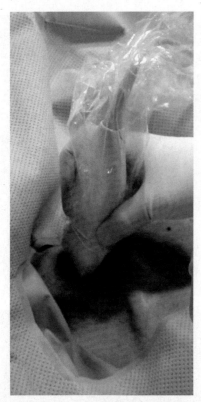

Figure 8.7 Ultrasound probe is draped into sterile field and used to identify the internal jugular vein and associated structures. Photograph courtesy of Drs Ryan Conway and Scott Sherman, University of Iowa Carver College of Medicine.

Stand at the head of the patient. Hold the ultrasound probe in your nondominant hand. Visualize the internal jugular vein with the ultrasound probe (Fig. 8.8A,B). Place the probe transverse to the axis of the vein. Note that excessive pressure with the probe will compress the vein, making cannulation more difficult; therefore, be careful to maintain just enough pressure to get a good image. Note and, if necessary, measure the depth of the vein. Choose a skin entry site just cephalad to the ultrasound probe and directly in line with the vein. Inject local anesthetic. The advancing wheal of local anesthetic may be visible in the surrounding tissues and the injecting needle may be seen. Then pass the introducer needle into the vein, using a visual estimate of the likely trajectory given the depth of the vein. The needle will appear as a bright spot in the center of the vein (Fig. 8.8C–E). Insertion guides, pieces of plastic that limit the path of the needle, are available, but most surgeons prefer to freehand the needle entry. After the entry of the needle into the vein is confirmed both by ultrasound and by free aspiration of venous blood, set the transducer down on the sterile field, and then pass a guidewire. Use ultrasound confirmation that the guidewire has passed intraluminally and then proceed with Seldinger technique cannulation as previously described. Obtain a chest x-ray at the end.

If the longitudinal approach is chosen, the procedure is quite similar except that the vein will appear in longitudinal section and the needle will be visualized passing through soft tissues and into the vein at an angle. Precise alignment of the transducer, vein, and needle are required as previously noted.

Placement of Tunneled Catheter

When patients require long-term indwelling central venous access for nutritional support, hemodialysis, chemotherapy, or administration of other drugs, there are two basic options. The first is a cuffed tunneled catheter, often referred to as a Broviac or Hickman catheter, and the second is a completely implanted device with a subcutaneous reservoir called a port. There are advantages and disadvantages to both. Catheters and ports are available in a variety of sizes. Single and multiple lumen devices are available. It is crucial that the device chosen fit the needs of the patient. If you are *not* the physician who will be directing the long-term needs of the patient, it is crucial that you speak with the appropriate physician in charge, so that the appropriate device is placed.

Tunneled catheters, as a general rule, are used when more or less continuous access or rapid infusion of large volumes of blood (e.g., in a bone marrow transplant or dialysis unit) are required. Ports are used when intermittent use (e.g., for chemotherapy for breast cancer patients) is needed. Ports provide convenience for the patient because the device is completely subcutaneous and needs little care.

STEPS IN PROCEDURE—PLACEMENT OF TUNNELED CATHETER

Access the vein as above

Choose an exit site for the catheter several centimeters caudal to the small incision through which you have accessed the vein

Use the tunneler to create a subcutaneous tunnel between the two incisions

Estimate the length of the catheter needed and cut it to length

Affix the end of the catheter to the passer

Pass the catheter end from the exit site incision into the vein access site incision

Pass the catheter into the vein

Confirm position by fluoroscopy

Confirm ease of aspiration of venous blood and flush the catheter with heparinized saline

Ensure that the cuff on the tunneled catheter is under the skin

Close incisions

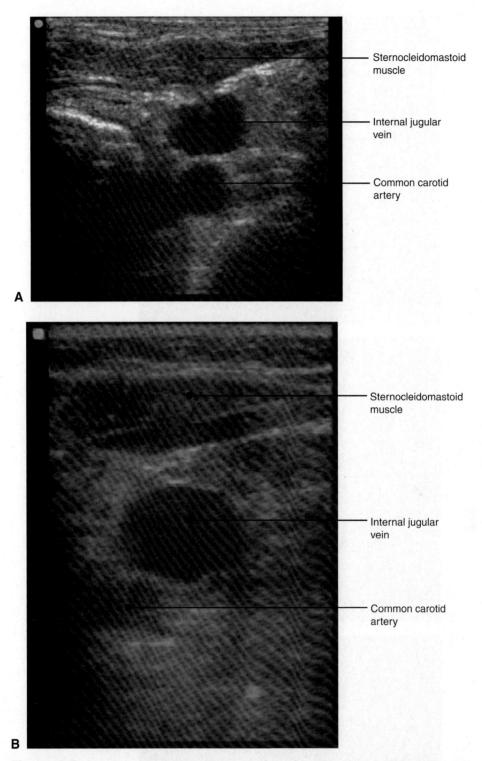

Figure 8.8 Anterior approach to the internal jugular vein—ultrasound guidance. **A:** Normal anatomic relations in transverse ultrasound view. **B:** Vein expanded by Trendelenburg positioning. (*continued*)

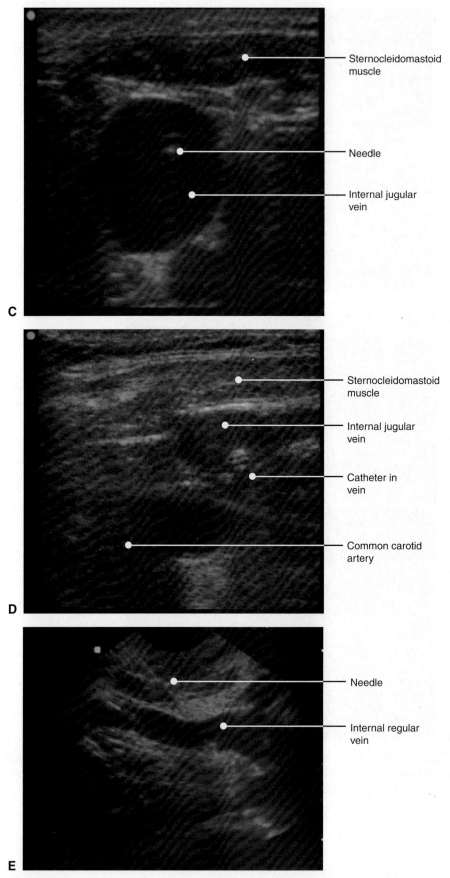

Sternocleidomastoid
muscle

Needle

Internal jugular
vein

C

Sternocleidomastoid
muscle

Internal jugular
vein

Catheter in
vein

Common carotid
artery

D

Needle

Internal regular
vein

E

Figure 8.8 *Continued*. **C:** Needle in internal jugular vein-transverse view.
D: Catheter in vein. Note common carotid artery. **E:** Longitudinal internal
jugular vein.

In addition to device selection, location may be important. To take an obvious example, do *not* put the device on the side of the breast cancer.

Route of access is also a consideration. The large-bore catheters placed for temporary dialysis access are often placed through the right internal jugular vein.

To place a tunneled catheter, prep and drape the entire neck and chest. Choose an exit site on a stable area of the chest wall, several centimeters from the vein access site. A relatively medial parasternal location is popular for that reason. Lower catheter exit sites make it easier for the patient to conceal the catheter or scar with clothes. In female patients, particularly those with large breasts, do *not* place the exit site on the breast itself if at all possible, lest motion of the breast lead to catheter displacement over time.

Make a small transverse incision at the exit site. This incision should be a little under 1 cm in length. Make a second incision at the likely venous access site. Use the subcutaneous tunneler supplied with the catheter to create a tunnel for the catheter. The appropriate plane is usually about 0.5 to 1 cm deep.

If you anticipate difficulty in accessing the vein, you may wish to create a catheter exit site and tunnel *after* you access the vein. This avoids the embarrassing situation where you find you must go to the contralateral side to gain venous access. In patients who have had multiple vascular access procedures, this scenario can certainly occur.

Access the vein as previously described. If you have used a percutaneous technique, you will want to have the guidewire in place at this point, but do not proceed to pass the dilator or sheath.

Estimate the appropriate length of the catheter and cut it cleanly across (i.e., at right angles, rather than at a bevel). Beveling the catheter does not make it any easier to pass and may cause the catheter to "suck up" against the vessel wall when blood withdrawal is attempted.

Secure the catheter to the passer. Pull it through from the skin exit site. The cuff should lie comfortably in the subcutaneous tissues fairly close to the exit site.

Detach the catheter from the passer and pass it into the vein as you would any other central venous catheter.

Use fluoroscopy to confirm good placement of the catheter tip in the superior vena cava. Confirm that the cuff is in good position. Ideally, the cuff should be close to the skin exit site, but not immediately under the incision. If the cuff is too far from the skin exit site, it may be more difficult to remove both the catheter and the cuff when the catheter is no longer needed. If the cuff is too close to the skin entry site, it may extrude from the skin before it is fully incorporated. Adjust the curve of the catheter in the vein access incision so that it lies comfortably without kinking. Raise a small flap to allow this, if necessary.

Close the skin entry and vein access incisions. Obtain a chest x-ray to document position.

When the catheter is no longer needed, remove it by prepping the skin exit site and injecting some local anesthesia. Palpate the catheter track by placing it on a slight stretch and identify the location of the cuff by palpation or by noting where the catheter seems to be tethered. Generally, the cuff will be close to the skin exit site. Dilate the skin exit site with a hemostat and spread gently in the plane between the cuff and the surrounding tissues. Maintain a gentle but firm pull on the catheter. The goal is to detach the cuff from the surrounding scar tissue and remove it intact. Enlarge the skin exit site if necessary to do this safely. Confirm complete removal of the catheter and cuff. Maintain pressure on the vein entry site incision to minimize back-bleeding after catheter removal. Slight reverse Trendelenburg position may also be used at this point, in stark contrast to removal of uncuffed nontunneled catheters, because the long tunnel will prevent venous air embolism.

Figure 8.9—Placement of Venous Port

As previously discussed, it is crucial that you choose the proper device for the patient. A port is a good choice for a patient who needs intermittent access for chemotherapy; for example, for breast cancer. Put the device on the opposite side from the cancer.

Prep both the chest and neck. Access the vein as previously described. Plan the placement of the port in the infraclavicular fossa not distant from the vein entry site (if the subclavian or cephalic vein were used) or at least on the same side. Check the port and determine how long an incision you will need in order to place it. Make an incision at the cephalad aspect of the

---

STEPS IN PROCEDURE—PLACEMENT OF VENOUS PORT

Access the vein

Choose a place for the port in the infraclavicular fossa

Raise the flaps to create a pocket

Trim the catheter to length as above

If the port site is distant from the vein entry site (as may be the case if the internal jugular vein has been used), create a tunnel for the catheter

Pass the catheter into the vein and confirm the position by fluoroscopy

Access the port with a Huber needle and confirm free aspiration of venous blood; fill the port with heparinized saline

Tack the port in place with several sutures of nonabsorbable material

Close the incisions

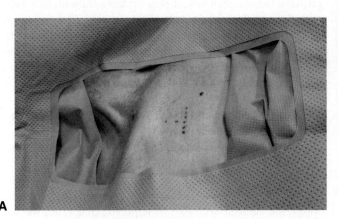
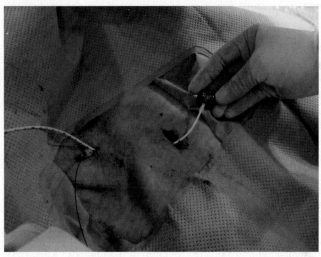

A   **B**

Figure 8.9 A: Incision is marked for port placement and tract for catheter to entry site into internal jugular vein. **B:** Catheter is passed through tunnel and brought out through vein access site. Photographs courtesy of Drs. Ryan Conway and Scott Sherman, University of Iowa Carver College of Medicine.

proposed pocket and create a subcutaneous pocket caudal to this, with a smaller pocket cephalad (Fig. 8.9A). The large caudal pocket will accommodate the device and the smaller cephalad pocket provides room for the catheter course to be adjusted so as to avoid kinks, if necessary. Avoid placing the incision directly over the device. The goal is to allow the device to be accessed ("needled") through intact skin rather than through the surgical incision.

Obtain meticulous hemostasis in the pocket. Use a noncoring (Huber-type) needle to access the port and fill it with heparinized saline. Pass the catheter through the tunnel (Fig. 8.9B). Cut the catheter to length as previously described and place it in the vein. Confirm easy aspiration of blood and flush the device with heparinized saline. If desired, secure the catheter to the subcutaneous tissues with an absorbable suture. Tack the device in place in the pocket with several simple sutures of nonabsorbable material to prevent rotation or displacement. Close the incisions.

When the device is no longer needed, remove it. Prep and drape the skin around the pocket and anesthetize the skin incision with local anesthesia. Dissect down to the device with care. The goal is to enter the pseudocapsule that has formed around the port. Apply gentle pressure to the device to displace it up (cranial) in the incision, if necessary, to avoid transecting the catheter. Use a piercing towel clip to grasp the suture ring of the device and pull it up and partially out of the incision, leaving the catheter in situ. Sequentially cut and remove the tacking sutures and deliver the port completely out of the incision. Applying pressure to the vein entry site, gently pull the catheter out.

Use precautions to avoid venous air embolism. This means, apply pressure to the vein entry site and if necessary place a single suture of absorbable material to close it. Generally backbleeding ceases with pressure. Close the incision in layers (do not try to strip out the pseudocapsule).

REFERENCES

1. American Association of Clinical Anatomists, Educational Affairs Committee. The clinical anatomy of invasive procedures. *Clin Anat.* 1999;12:43–54.
2. Boon JM, van Schoor AN, Abrahams PH, et al. Central venous catheterization—an anatomical review of a clinical skill. Part 2. Internal jugular vein via the supraclavicular approach. *Clin Anat.* 2008;21:15–22.
3. Cavatorta F, Zollo A, Galli S, et al. Real-time ultrasound and endocavitary electrocardiography for venous catheter placement. *J Vasc Access.* 2001;2:40–44. (Describes use of electrocardiogram to confirm central venous placement.)
4. Dolla D, Cavatorta F, Galli S, et al. Anatomical variations of the internal jugular vein in non-uremic outpatients. *J Vasc Access.* 2001;2:60–63.
5. Edwards Corporation. Video on Swan Ganz Catheter Placement. Available at: http://www.edwards.com/Products/PACatheters/Pages/placementvideo.aspx (accessed November 25, 2012).
6. Feller-Kopman D. Ultrasound-guided internal jugular access: A proposed standardized approach and implications for training and practice. *Chest.* 2007;132:302–309.
7. Harvey S, Young D, Brampton W, et al. Pulmonary artery catheters for adult patients in intensive care. *Cochrane Database Syst Rev.* 2006;19:CD003408. (PA catheterization did not affect outcome in critically ill surgical patients.)
8. Irwin RS, Rippe JM, Lisbon A, Heard SO (eds.). *Irwin & Rippe's Procedures, Techniques and Minimally Invasive Monitoring in Intensive Care Medicine.* Philadelphia, PA: Wolters Kluwer Lippincott Williams & Wilkins; 2011. (Excellent source of detailed information on procedures required in the critical care setting, including pulmonary artery catheterization.)
9. Kaushik S, Dubey PK, Ambesh SP. Internal jugular vein cannulation in neurosurgical patients: A new approach. *J Neurosurg Anesthesiol.* 1999;11:185–187. (Describes a modified technique that is useful when head and neck must be maintained in neutral position.)

10. Koroglu M, Demir M, Koroglu BK, et al. Percutaneous placement of central venous catheters: Comparing the anatomical landmark method with the radiologically guided technique for central venous catheterization through the internal jugular vein in emergent hemodialysis patients. *Acta Radiol.* 2006;47:43–47. (Advocates for ultrasound and real-time fluoroscopic guidance to minimize complications.)

11. Krausz MM, Berlatzky Y, Ayalon A, et al. Percutaneous cannulation of the internal jugular vein in infants and children. *Surg Gynecol Obstet.* 1979;148:591–594. (Describes variations in anatomy in young children.)

12. Leung J, Duffy M, Finckh A. Real-time ultrasonographically-guided internal jugular vein catheterization in the emergency department increases success rates and reduces complications: A randomized, prospective study. *Ann Emerg Med.* 2006;48:540–547.

13. Lowell JA, Bothe A Jr. Venous access. Preoperative, operative, and postoperative dilemmas. *Surg Clin North Am.* 1991;71:1231–1246.

14. Marik PE, Flemmer M, Harrison W. The risk of catheter-related bloodstream infection with femoral venous catheters as compared to subclavian and internal jugular venous catheters: A systematic review of the literature and meta-analysis. *Crit Care Med.* 2012;40:2479–2485.

15. Recht MP, Burke DR, Meranze SG, et al. Simple technique for redirecting malpositioned central venous catheters. *AJR Am J Roentgenol.* 1990;154:183–184. (Describes a useful technique when the catheter is misdirected.)

16. Silberzweig JE, Mitty HA. Central venous access: Low internal jugular vein approach using imaging guidance. *AJR Am J Roentgenol.* 1998;170:1617–1620. (Explains rationale for low approach; advocates adjunctive use of ultrasound.)

17. Wang R, Snoey ER, Clements RC, et al. Effect of head rotation on vascular anatomy of the neck: An ultrasound study. *J Emerg Med.* 2006;31:283–286. (Important for patients in whom the neck cannot be manipulated.)

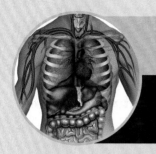

9

Carotid Endarterectomy

Parth B. Amin and Timothy F. Kresowik

The carotid bifurcation in the neck is a frequent site of atherosclerosis. Thromboembolic events originating from atherosclerotic plaque at this location are a common cause of ischemic stroke. Fortunately, the disease is most often limited to the region of the bifurcation and is surgically accessible. Randomized clinical trials have established the efficacy of carotid endarterectomy (surgical plaque removal) for stroke prevention in patients who have high-grade stenosis of the proximal internal carotid artery.

SCORE™, the Surgical Council on Resident Education, has classified this as an "ESSENTIAL COMMON" procedure.

STEPS IN PROCEDURE

Identify mastoid process and sternal notch

Incision parallels anterior border of sternocleidomastoid and curves medially at the inferior aspect toward the sternal notch

Mobilize medial border of sternocleidomastoid

Preserve great auricular nerve if possible

Expose medial border of internal jugular vein

Identify and ligate the facial vein

Expose common carotid artery and dissect lateral border of the internal carotid artery

Protect vagus nerve and identify hypoglossal nerve; divide branch from occipital artery if needed

Administer systemic heparin

Clamp the internal carotid artery, common carotid artery, and external carotid artery

Place arteriotomy on middle portion of common carotid and extend toward carotid bifurcation

Transect internal carotid artery off of the common carotid

Eversion endarterectomy of internal carotid artery

Feather to good endpoint; transect plaque at appropriate endpoint if needed

Separate and evert plaque from orifice of external carotid artery

Anastomosis from internal carotid artery to carotid bifurcation

Flush debris before completing suture line by opening each clamp

Restore circulation to external carotid artery first

Close wound in two layers

HALLMARK ANATOMIC COMPLICATIONS

Embolic stroke

Injury to marginal mandibular nerve

Injury to hypoglossal nerve

Injury to spinal accessory nerve

Injury to vagus nerve

LIST OF STRUCTURES

Sternocleidomastoid muscle

Mandible

Mastoid process

Clavicular head

Langer's lines

Platysma muscle

Parotid gland

Sternocleidomastoid muscle

Mastoid process

Clavicular head

Langer's lines

Platysma muscle

Parotid gland

External jugular vein

Great auricular nerve

Marginal mandibular branch of facial nerve

Internal jugular vein

Facial vein

Digastric muscle

Hypoglossal nerve (XII)

Sternocleidomastoid branch of occipital artery

Ansa cervicalis

Vagus nerve

Glossopharyngeal nerve (IX)

Omohyoid muscle

Common carotid artery

Internal carotid artery

External carotid artery

Superior thyroid artery

Superior laryngeal nerve

Regional Anatomy and Skin Incision (Fig. 9.1)

Technical Points

Preoperative determination of extent of disease and location of the carotid bifurcation, through either duplex ultrasound imaging or angiography, allows the skin incision to be planned for optimal access. The description that follows would apply to patients whose carotid bifurcation is in the typical position in the mid-neck and in whom the disease does not extend unusually far distally or proximally.

Position the patient with the neck extended and the head rotated to the side opposite the procedure. It is also helpful to have the head of the bed elevated about 30 degrees to decrease venous pressure and bleeding. The most important landmark for planning the incision is the anterior border of the sternocleidomastoid muscle, which can be visualized or palpated. Initiate the distal end of the incision along this border at the level of the angle of the mandible or 2 to 3 cm from the mastoid process. The upper portion of the incision should follow the border of the sternocleidomastoid muscle. At a point two-thirds of the distance between the mastoid process and the head of the clavicle, curve the incision into a more transverse direction to produce a better cosmetic result than the traditional straight incision.

Anatomic Points

The incision described previously allows the best balance between exposure and cosmesis. Langer's lines in the neck are predominately horizontal, and making the inferior portion of the incision more transverse results in a better scar that follows the normal skin creases.

Exposure of the Sternocleidomastoid Muscle (Fig. 9.2)

Technical Points

Deepen the skin incision through the subcutaneous tissue and platysmal layer. Mobilize the medial border of the sternocleidomastoid muscle along the entire length of the incision. If the incision is extended superiorly, the tail of the parotid gland is encountered. If necessary for exposure, this portion of the parotid can be mobilized along the inferior and posterior aspects of the gland. The external jugular vein and great auricular nerve may be encountered at this level. The external jugular vein may be ligated. Preserve the great auricular nerve if possible. The dissection plane should remain over the medial border of the sternocleidomastoid muscle and not drift anteriorly toward the mandible because injury to the marginal mandibular branch of the facial nerve could result. Near the upper end of the incision, an arterial branch from the occipital artery going to the sternocleidomastoid muscle may be encountered and should be divided. This arterial branch usually loops over the hypoglossal nerve in its course from the occipital artery, and division allows the hypoglossal nerve to retract medially away from the dissection plane.

If more proximal exposure of the common carotid is necessary, develop a subplatysmal flap at the inferior end of the

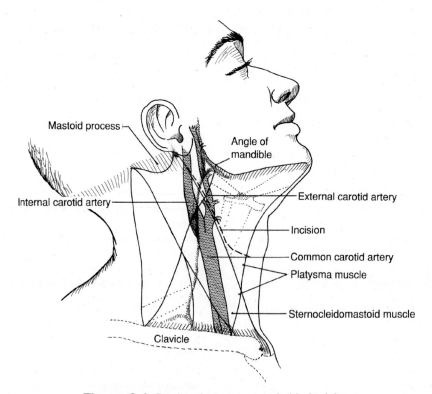

Figure 9.1 Regional anatomy and skin incision

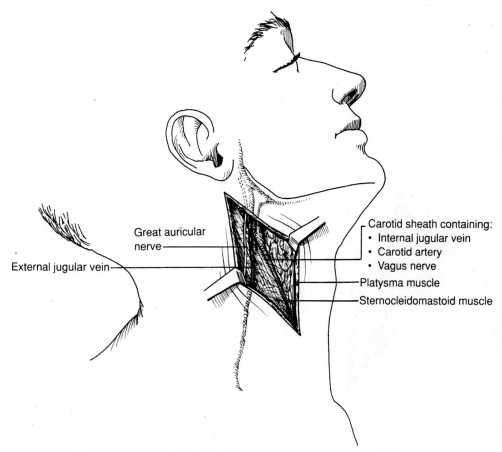

Figure 9.2 Exposure of the sternocleidomastoid muscle

incision to allow continued mobilization of the medial border of the sternocleidomastoid muscle to its clavicular insertion despite the transverse course of the skin incision.

Anatomic Points

The platysma muscle has little functional importance but is the division between a plane superficial to the muscle, which is devoid of significant neurovascular structures, and the plane deep to the muscle that contains nerves that should be preserved if possible. The great auricular nerve is a sensory branch of C2 and C3 that parallels the external jugular vein. Sacrifice or injury to the great auricular nerve leads to numbness or paresthesia of the ear. The marginal mandibular branch of the facial nerve normally parallels the ramus of the mandible but can extend as much as 2.5 cm inferior to the mandible. The nerve is a motor branch to the muscles of the corner of the mouth. Injury to this nerve can lead to a significant cosmetic and functional impairment, with ipsilateral drooping of the corner of the mouth and drooling. Keeping the dissection plane along or posterior to the border of the sternocleidomastoid muscle will usually avoid direct injury to this nerve. This nerve can also be injured by injudicious placement of mechanical retractors against the mandible.

Exposure of the Carotid Sheath and Internal Jugular Vein (Fig. 9.3)

Technical Points

The next portion of the dissection involves mobilizing the medial border of the internal jugular vein. It is important to perform the dissection using this anatomic landmark rather than proceeding directly to dissecting out the carotid artery. Take care to stay along the border of the vein to minimize the chance of cranial nerve injury. As the medial border of the vein is mobilized, the common facial vein is encountered. Division of the facial vein can be performed after exposure of the internal jugular vein proximal and distal to it. As the dissection progresses superiorly, additional small draining veins may be encountered and may need to be ligated. If very distal exposure of the internal carotid is necessary, the posterior belly of the digastric muscle can be divided, but dissection at this level is not necessary in most carotid endarterectomy procedures.

In performing the superior portion of the dissection, avoid drifting laterally in the plane between the posterior aspect of the sternocleidomastoid muscle and the internal jugular vein. The eleventh cranial nerve (spinal accessory) may be encountered in this area.

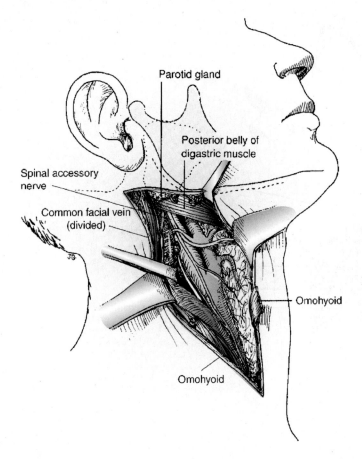

Figure 9.3 Exposure of the carotid sheath and internal jugular vein

At the inferior end of the dissection, the omohyoid muscle is encountered looping across the field. The muscle may be divided, but adequate exposure is often obtained by mobilizing and retracting the muscle inferiorly.

Anatomic Points

The common facial vein is the largest vein draining into the internal jugular vein. It is formed from the confluence of the retromandibular vein and facial vein. The junction of the common facial and internal jugular veins is usually a good marker of the level of the carotid bifurcation. The accessory nerve is found deep to the sternocleidomastoid muscle lateral to the internal jugular vein. Injury to this nerve, which supplies the trapezius muscle, can lead to a shoulder drop and difficulty in arm abduction.

Exposure of the Carotid Bifurcation (Fig. 9.4)

Technical Points

Exposure and mobilization of the carotid is normally begun along the lateral aspect of the common carotid artery and then extended distally. Gently mobilize the vagus nerve from the

lateral aspect of the carotid. Take care not to inadvertently create a crush injury of the nerve by injudicious use of the forceps during dissection. Continue the dissection distally along the lateral aspect of the internal carotid. Locate the hypoglossal nerve as it runs between the internal carotid and external carotid and then courses anteriorly. If the previously mentioned arterial branch looping over the nerve from the occipital artery to the sternocleidomastoid muscle has been divided, mobilizing the nerve along the posterior and inferior aspects will generally cause it to fall medially and out of danger.

The superior (descending) branch of the ansa cervicalis will also usually retract medially, but it may be occasionally necessary to divide this branch or the inferior branch arising from the cervical plexus to obtain adequate exposure.

Completely mobilize the internal carotid artery to allow clamping well distal to the most distal aspect of the carotid plaque. Minimize manipulation of the bifurcation to decrease the likelihood of dislodging atherothrombotic debris by gently dissecting the tissues away from the artery. In addition, avoid dissecting the internal carotid on its medial aspect (i.e., at the bifurcation between the internal and external carotid) to minimize trauma to the carotid baroreceptors and carotid sinus nerve.

Mobilize the proximal portion of the external carotid and its first branch, the superior thyroid artery, for clamping. In a similar fashion, completely mobilize the common carotid artery proximally and identify a minimally diseased section for clamping.

Anatomic Points

The vagus nerve is within the carotid sheath and, in the superior portion of the dissection, is posterior to the internal carotid and then courses lateral to the common carotid. The nerve may course anterior to the carotid, especially proximally in the neck. The major disability associated with injury to the vagus in the neck is vocal cord paresis because of the recurrent laryngeal nerve fibers that are traveling with the vagus in the neck. The hypoglossal nerve emerges between the internal jugular vein and the internal carotid. The nerve loops anterior to the branches of the external carotid artery superficial to the carotid sheath, usually just superior to the carotid bifurcation. The hypoglossal nerve is a motor nerve to the intrinsic muscles of the tongue, and injury to this nerve can cause significant disability owing to speech and eating difficulties. Traveling with the hypoglossal nerve are fibers from C1 that form the superior root of the ansa cervicalis. The ansa fibers normally diverge from the hypoglossal nerve as it crosses the internal carotid and descend superficial to the internal and common carotid arteries. The superior root is joined by the inferior root, which comprises fibers originating from C2 and C3 and emerges from between the internal jugular vein and common carotid. The ansa cervicalis innervates the strap muscles. Although the nerve is spared if possible, division of the inferior or superior root is sometimes necessary to obtain adequate mobilization of

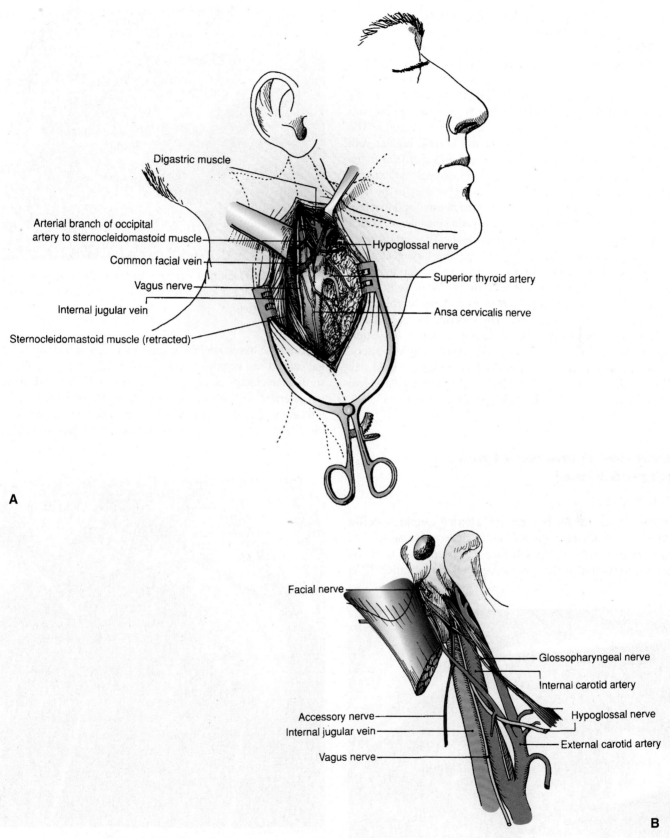

Figure 9.4 Exposure of the carotid bifurcation. **A:** Exposure. **B:** Regional anatomy.

the hypoglossal nerve or exposure of the carotid and does not result in significant disability.

There are other nerves in the vicinity that are not encountered in the usual carotid endarterectomy procedure. The glossopharyngeal nerve parallels the course of the hypoglossal nerve but is much more superior; its inferior extent is rarely below the angle of the mandible. It may, however, be encountered in very high dissections of the internal carotid. The nerve is superiorly located between the internal jugular vein and the internal carotid artery. It then passes superficial to the internal carotid and courses between the internal and external carotid arteries to enter the base of the tongue deep to the hyoglossus muscle. As it passes between the internal and external carotid arteries, it gives rise to the carotid sinus nerve, which supplies the carotid sinus and carotid body. The carotid body also receives vagal innervation. The superior laryngeal nerve is sensory (through the internal branch) to the laryngopharynx and laryngeal mucosa superior to the vocal cords and is motor (through its external branch) to the cricothyroid muscle, a tensor of the vocal cords. The superior laryngeal nerve is usually medial to the carotid sheath, although the external branch comes in proximity to the superior thyroid artery. Dissection of the external carotid and its branches should stay close to the vessels to avoid injury to the superior laryngeal nerve. Injury to the superior laryngeal nerve may cause voice fatigue.

Eversion Endarterectomy (Figs. 9.5–9.8)

Technical Points

In most cases, the internal carotid, external carotid, superior thyroid, and common carotid are occluded separately. The internal carotid is clamped before the external or common carotid to minimize the risk for cerebral embolization. It is

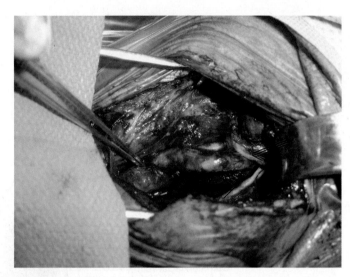

Figure 9.6 Thick black arrow points to the vagus nerve. The ansa cervicalis can help identify the hypoglossal nerve (*triple-line arrow*).

important to have created adequate exposure of both the internal carotid and common carotid beyond the diseased portions so that the clamps can be safely applied in locations that will not interfere with obtaining adequate endpoints of the endarterectomy. The arteriotomy should be initiated on the common carotid and extended toward the carotid bifurcation. Care

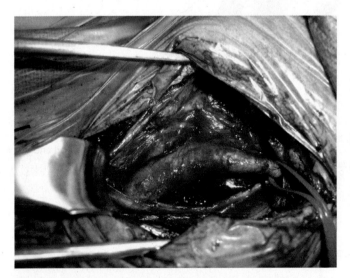

Figure 9.5 A red silastic loop has been placed around the internal carotid artery.

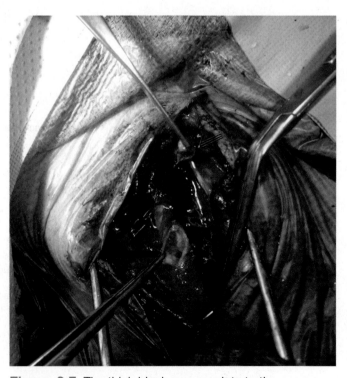

Figure 9.7 The thick black arrow points to the endarterectomized common carotid artery. The triple-line arrow points to the endarterectomized internal carotid artery.

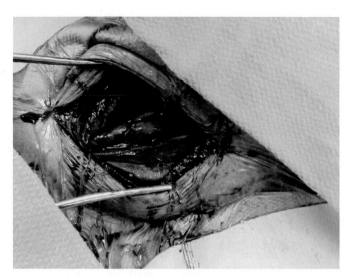

Figure 9.8 The internal carotid artery is sewn back onto the bifurcation.

should be taken to stay on the lateral aspect of the bifurcation so as not cut into the external carotid artery. Using the anterior aspect of the arteriotomy (toward the carotid bifurcation) as a guide, the internal carotid should then be transected off the bifurcation. The correct endarterectomy plane is in the outer media, leaving only undiseased circular muscle fibers and the adventitia.

Some surgeons routinely place an indwelling shunt to maintain cerebral perfusion during the endarterectomy. Only 5% to 10% of patients actually have inadequate collateral flow and experience significant ischemia during the period of clamping. Since placing an indwelling shunt interferes with the endarterectomy and adds a small risk for intimal damage proximal or distal to the endarterectomy site, many surgeons prefer to shunt selectively. Selective shunting requires some form of cerebral perfusion or collateral flow monitoring. The most common forms of monitoring include performing the procedure under regional or local anesthesia so that neurologic testing of the awake patient can be performed, using intraoperative electroencephalogram monitoring, or measuring internal carotid back pressure (with the common and external carotid clamped) as an indicator of adequate collateral flow. I prefer to perform the procedure under a cervical block and insert a shunt only if the patient develops a neurologic deficit with clamping.

Begin the endarterectomy in the proximal internal carotid and completely separate the plaque from the vessel wall. Maintain steady traction on the internal carotid plaque while an assistant everts the internal carotid. This is done until an area of distal feathering is identified. Often, the best way to achieve a good endpoint is to pull the plaque in a proximal direction, allowing the diseased portion to separate. We have found that sharply transecting the plaque at an area where the plaque becomes thin and adherent may preclude the creation of distal intimal flaps. After completing the endarterectomy, remove any loose intimal fronds and check the endpoints for adherence.

Create the common carotid endpoint by elevating the plaque proximally, stopping at a point beyond the most severe disease. The common carotid usually has thickened intima, and the disease does not "feather out" as it does in the internal carotid. Sharply divide the plaque proximally. Ascertain that the remaining proximal intima is adherent. Although it seems counterintuitive, the proximal endpoint can elevate despite the apparent direction of blood flow. This lifting of a proximal endpoint intimal flap has been observed on ultrasound evaluation and is a potential source of thromboembolism or recurrent stenosis.

Closure is then performing by, in a sense, reimplanting the internal carotid artery onto the bifurcation. The benefit of this approach is that anastamotic stenoses at the level of the internal carotid are far less likely than patch closure. Furthermore, there is the additional benefit of not requiring prosthetic material. A closure is generally performed with a running continuous anastomosis using 5-0 or 6-0 polypropylene suture. Before completing closure, temporarily release each clamp individually to "flush out" any residual debris. Restore flow into the external carotid circulation first (removing the internal carotid clamp last) to minimize the possibility of cerebral embolization of any residual debris or air. Close the wound in two layers with continuous absorbable suture. The only deep layer that needs to be approximated is the platysmal layer. A continuous subcuticular skin closure with absorbable suture provides an excellent cosmetic result in most patients.

Endarterectomy with Patch Angioplasty (Fig. 9.9A–G)

Another technique employed for carotid endarterectomy proceeds with the same exposure of the internal carotid, common carotid, superior thyroidal, and external carotid arteries. Once systemic heparin has been administered, the internal carotid artery, common carotid artery, and external carotid artery are clamped. A longitudinal arteriotomy is then made, beginning on the distal common carotid and extending beyond the area of palpable disease on the internal carotid artery (Fig. 9.9A). Shunting can then be performed either routinely, or selectively based on EEG monitoring or patient responsiveness (Fig. 9.9B).

The outer media should then be removed leaving only undiseased circular muscle fibers and the adventitia. One key principle in this maneuver is to push the vessel wall away from the plaque using a Freer elevator. If an incorrect plan is entered, attempt to start the endarterectomy at another site (Fig. 9.9C–E). The proximal portion of the plaque can be sharply divided and the distal endpoint should be aimed at creating a smooth, feathered endpoint (Fig. 9.9F). At this point, heparinized saline irrigation is used to remove any loose debris and examine the distal endpoint for any potential intimal flaps. Once the endarterectomy has been completed, a standard Dacron patch is sewn with a standard 6-0 polypropylene continuous anastomosis. The remainder of the procedure continues in the fashion previously described.

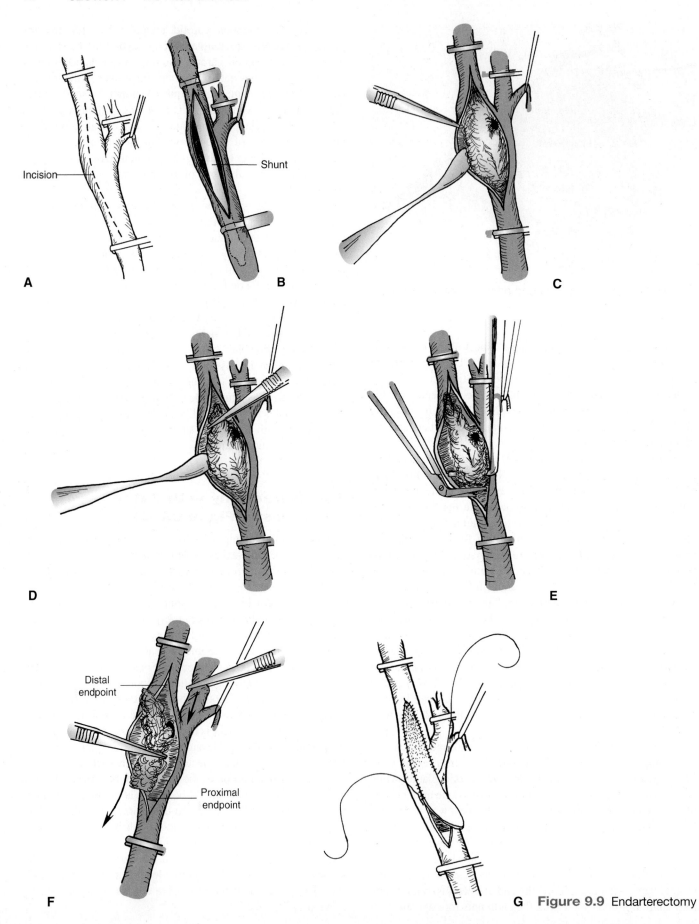

A

Incision

B

Shunt

C

D

E

F

Distal
endpoint

Proximal
endpoint

G   **Figure 9.9** Endarterectomy

REFERENCES

1. Byrne J, Feustel P, Darling RC 3rd. Primary closure, routine patching, and eversion endarterectomy: What is the current state of the literature supporting use of these techniques? *Semin Vasc Surg.* 2007;20(4):226–235. Review.

2. European Carotid Surgery Trialists' Collaborative Group. Randomised trial of endarterectomy for recently symptomatic carotid stenosis: Final results of the MRC European Carotid Surgery Trial (ECST). *Lancet.* 1998;351:1379–1387.

3. Executive Committee for the Asymptomatic Carotid Atherosclerosis Study. Endarterectomy for asymptomatic carotid artery stenosis. *JAMA.* 1995;273:1421–1428.

4. Jackson MR, Clagett GP. Use of vein or synthetic patches in carotid endartectomy. In: Loftus CM, Kresowik TF, eds. *Carotid Artery Surgery.* New York, NY: Thieme Medical Publishers; 2000:281.

5. Kresowik TF, Bratzler D, Karp HR, et al. Multistate utilization, processes, and outcomes of carotid endarterectomy. *J Vasc Surg.* 2001;33:227–235.

6. Kresowik TF, Hoballah JJ, Sharp WJ, et al. Intraoperative B-mode ultrasonography is a useful adjunct to peripheral arterial reconstruction. *Ann Vasc Surg.* 1993;7:33–38.

7. Mayberg MR, Wilson SE, Yatsu F, et al. Carotid endarterectomy and prevention of cerebral ischemia in symptomatic carotid stenosis. Veterans Affairs Cooperative Studies Program 309 Trialist Group. *JAMA.* 1991;273:1421–1428.

8. North American Symptomatic Carotid Endarterectomy Trial Collaborators. Beneficial effect of carotid endarterectomy in symptomatic patients with high-grade carotid stenosis. *N Engl J Med.* 1991;325:445–453.

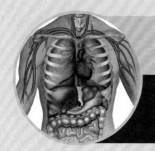

10

Cervical Lymph Node Biopsy and Scalene Node Biopsy

Lymph node biopsy is only very rarely performed now for diagnostic purposes. Cervical lymph node biopsy should only be performed when a careful examination of the aerodigestive tract has failed to demonstrate a primary carcinoma and other means of diagnosis have failed. Biopsy of a cervical lymph node that is found to contain metastatic carcinoma from a head and neck primary tumor is a grave error because such biopsy contaminates the field should subsequent radical neck dissection be contemplated. For this reason, open surgical biopsy has largely been supplanted by fine-needle aspiration cytology. Open surgical biopsy is rarely indicated.

For optimum histologic classification of lymphomas, an entire lymph node with its capsule may be needed. Thus, the goal of diagnostic lymph node biopsy is to remove the node intact with minimal trauma.

Scalene node biopsy is performed by removing the fatty node-bearing tissue in the scalene triangle. Formerly performed for diagnosis and staging of lung cancer, it is now occasionally used for other malignancies.

Cervical lymph node biopsy and the closely related scalene node biopsy are discussed in this section, and the major cervical lymph node groups are presented. The anatomy of this region is described in greater detail in Chapter 11.

SCORE™, the Surgical Council on Resident Education, does not list cervical or scalene node biopsy; it does, however, classify excisional and incisional biopsy of soft tissue lesions as an "ESSENTIAL COMMON" procedure. That procedure requires the skills described in the current chapter.

STEPS IN PROCEDURE

Transverse skin crease incision over node of interest

Deepen through platysma

Retract sternocleidomastoid muscle if necessary to expose node

Remove node, ligating hilum

HALLMARK ANATOMIC COMPLICATIONS

Compromise future radical neck dissection field

Injury to thoracic duct (left side)

LIST OF STRUCTURES

Platysma muscle

Sternocleidomastoid muscle

Omohyoid muscle

Anterior scalene muscle

Carotid sheath

Thoracic duct

Phrenic nerve

Thyrocervical trunk

Cervical lymph nodes

Scalene lymph nodes

Major Lymph Node Groups of the Neck (Fig. 10.1)

Technical Points

Lymph nodes are clustered in regions where major vessels converge. In the head and neck, the nodes most commonly selected for biopsy follow the internal jugular vein.

Anatomic Points

Although the position of lymph nodes and the groups of lymph nodes in the neck are relatively constant, the terminology applied to these nodes is not. Here, we follow the terminology of *Terminologia Anatomica* (Fig. 10.1A) and compare it with that used for cancer staging as described in the American Joint Committee on Cancer Staging Manual (Fig. 10.1B).

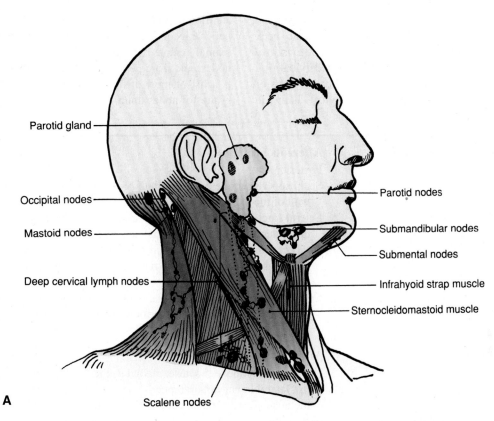

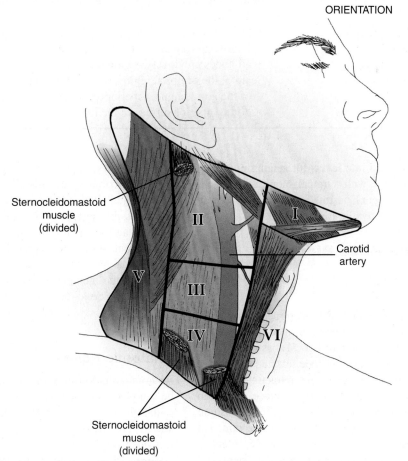

Figure 10.1 Major lymph node groups of the neck. **A:** Terminologia anatomica; **B:** Cervical lymph node biopsy.

In general, lymph node groups in the neck can be considered to form a *pericraniocervical ring* (essentially at the head–neck junction), superficial and deep *vertical chains,* and *perivisceral deep nodes.* Lymph node groups in the pericraniocervical ring receive afferent lymph vessels from adjacent head regions or from other groups in the ring. The vertical cervical chains, in addition to receiving afferent lymph vessels from nodes in the pericraniocervical ring, also receive afferents directly from the cranial regions (lymph thus "skips" the immediate regional nodes) and from perivisceral nodes in the neck. The following is a list of most of the regional lymph nodes and what these groups of nodes drain.

Pericraniocervical Node Groups	Afferents From
1. Occipital	Posterior scalp
2. Mastoid (posterior auricular)	Scalp superior to the ear, upper half of the inner aspect of the auricle, posterior wall of the external acoustic meatus
3. Parotid, superficial, and deep	Lateral forehead, temporal region, upper half of the lateral aspect of the auricle, anterior wall of the external acoustic meatus, lateral eyelids, skin over the zygomatic arch, middle ear and mastoid antrum, all the conjunctiva, lateral cheek and skin on the root of the nose, posterior nasal floor, parotid gland, infratemporal region
4. Submental	Central portion of the lower lip, central portion and floor of the mouth, apex of the tongue and frenulum, anterior triangle of the neck superior to the hyoid bone

Cervical Node Groups	Afferents From
5. Submandibular	Frontal region above the nose, medial eyelids, external nose, cheeks and upper lip, lateral lower lip, oral mucosa, anterior nasal cavity, skin of the root of the nose, gingiva, palate, lateral floor of the mouth, submental nodes
6. Anterior cervical, superficial	Skin of the neck inferior to the hyoid, and deep lower larynx, thyroid gland, cervical trachea
7. Superior deep cervical (including jugulodigastric nodes)	Scalp of the occipital region, auricle, back of the neck, most of the tongue, larynx, thyroid gland, trachea, nasopharynx and nasal cavity, esophagus, and all nodes previously mentioned
8. Inferior deep cervical (including jugulo-omohyoid nodules)	Scalp of the occipital region, back of the neck, superficial pectoral region, part of the arm, tongue, superior deep cervical nodes, and sometimes, a portion of the superior surface of the liver

These nodes are grouped into levels for staging purposes. Since these levels correlate with surgical biopsies, they are easily identified during surgery on this anatomic area. These correspond to the regions shown in Figure 10.1B.

Cervical Lymph Node Biopsy (Fig. 10.2)

Technical Points

Position the patient supine with the head turned away from the side on which the biopsy is to be performed. Infiltrate the region of the proposed skin incision with local anesthetic. Make a transverse incision over the palpable node selected for biopsy. Deepen the incision through the platysma, retracting the sternocleidomastoid muscle to expose the node. Place a traction suture of 2-0 silk through the node in a figure-of-eight fashion to facilitate mobilization. This allows the node to be removed intact, with minimal trauma. As dissection progresses, identify the hilum of the lymph node (containing a small artery and vein). Clamp and ligate the hilum.

Sometimes, a matted group of nodes, extending much farther proximally and distally than previously expected, is encountered. If this happens, remove an adequate portion of the accessible surface of the mass rather than attempting complete removal. Attempt to shell out an entire node from the matted, but often still lobulated, mass. Achieve hemostasis in the residual nodal mass by electrocautery or suture ligature.

Close the incision in layers with fine interrupted absorbable sutures. Send the lymph node specimen to the laboratory fresh.

Anatomic Points

Anatomic relationships vary depending on which nodes are to be sampled. Anterior cervical nodes are closely related to terminal filaments of the cervical branch of the facial nerve (VII) and to the anterior jugular vein and its tributaries. The superior deep cervical lymph nodes, including the jugulodigastric node, are closely related to the hypoglossal nerve (XII), accessory nerve (XI), and vagus nerve (X) and its superior laryngeal

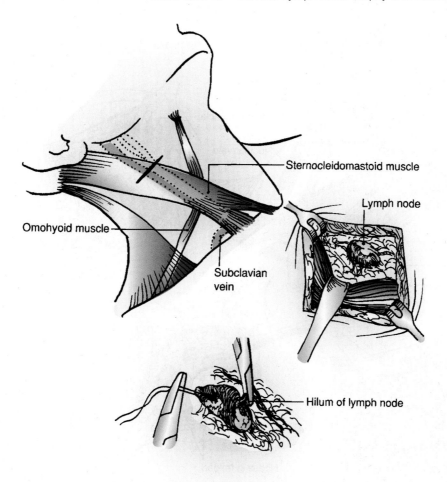

Figure 10.2 Cervical lymph node biopsy

branch; the cervical, and sometimes marginal mandibular branch of the facial nerve (VII); the superior root of the ansa cervicalis; the external carotid artery and its superior thyroid, occipital, and facial branches; the internal carotid artery; the termination of the common carotid artery; the carotid body and its nerve supply (a branch of the glossopharyngeal nerve); and the internal jugular vein. The inferior deep cervical nodes are most closely related to the internal jugular vein, the common carotid and subclavian arteries, the vagus nerve (X), the thyrocervical trunk and its branches (inferior thyroid, suprascapular, and transverse cervical arteries), the phrenic nerve (C3, C4, and C5), the recurrent laryngeal nerve, the thyroid gland, the inferior root of the ansa cervicalis, parts of the sympathetic trunk, and, sometimes, the brachial plexus (C5 to TI).

The occipital nodes are closely related to the occipital artery and to the greater (C2, dorsal ramus) and lesser (C2, ventral ramus) occipital nerves. Mastoid lymph nodes are most closely related to the lesser occipital (C2), posterior auricular (cranial nerve VII), and great auricular (C2 and C3) nerves and to the posterior auricular artery.

Nodes in the posterior triangle lie in relation to the spinal accessory nerve.

Submental nodes are not closely related to neurovascular structures of any consequence. By contrast, submandibular nodes are closely related to the submandibular gland, hypoglossal nerve, marginal mandibular and cervical branches of the facial nerve, and the facial artery and its submental branch.

Scalene Node Biopsy (Fig. 10.3)

Technical Points

In the absence of palpable nodes, do the procedure on the right side to avoid injury to the thoracic duct. Make a transverse incision about one fingerbreadth above the clavicle over the space between the sternal and clavicular heads of the sternocleidomastoid muscle. Place retractors to spread and develop the space between the two heads of the sternocleidomastoid muscle, exposing the omohyoid muscle and internal jugular vein. Identify a pad of fatty node-bearing tissue overlying the anterior scalene muscle (which is palpable but not visible), free it up by sharp and blunt dissection, and excise it. Identify and remove any enlarged or palpable nodes. Be

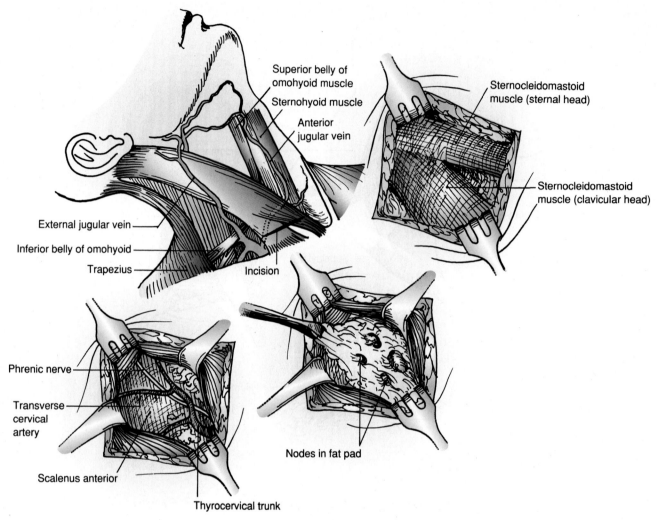

Figure 10.3 Scalene node biopsy

careful to avoid the phrenic nerve (running along the anterior scalene muscle deep to the fat pad) and transverse cervical artery.

On the left side, avoid the thoracic duct. If the thoracic duct is injured, milky or opalescent fluid will appear in the operative field. The duct should then be identified and ligated.

Close the incision in layers with interrupted absorbable sutures. Send the fat pad and associated nodes to the laboratory fresh.

Anatomic Points

The scalene triangle, as described, is bounded inferiorly by the clavicle, medially by the sternal head of the sternocleidomastoid muscle, and laterally by the clavicular head of that muscle. Opening this triangle exposes a lymph node-bearing fat pad immediately lateral to the carotid sheath and superficial to the prevertebral fascia, here investing the anterior scalene muscle, phrenic nerve, and lateral branches of the thyrocervical trunk. Gentle retraction of the carotid sheath and its contents medi-

ally protects the internal jugular vein, common carotid artery, and vagus nerves. If the dissection is limited posteriorly by the scalene fascia, the phrenic nerve, which closely approximates the direction of the anterior scalene muscle fibers, as well as the lateral branches of the thyrocervical trunk (transverse cervical and suprascapular arteries), should be avoided. On the left side, the thoracic duct enters the neck posteromedial to the common carotid artery. It then arches laterally, passing posterior to the common carotid artery and internal jugular vein, but anterior to the thyrocervical trunk (and its branches) and phrenic nerve to enter the venous system near the junction of the internal jugular and subclavian veins. Again, gentle medial retraction of the carotid sheath and cautious dissection lateral to the sheath should allow this biopsy to be performed with minimal complications.

REFERENCES

1. American Joint Committee on Cancer. Introduction to head and neck sites. *AJCC Cancer Staging Atlas.* Chicago: Springer Verlag; 2006:13–18.

2. Edge SB, Byrd DR, Compton CC, et al., eds. *AJCC Cancer Staging Manual.* 7th ed. New York, NY: Springer Verlag; 2010.

3. Hood RM. *Techniques in General Thoracic Surgery.* Philadelphia, PA: WB Saunders; 1985:145. (Provides an excellent description of scalene node biopsy.)

4. Horowitz NS, Tamimi HK, Goff BA, et al. Pretreatment scalene node biopsy in gynecologic malignancy: Prudent or passe? *Gynecol Oncol.* 1999;75:238–241. (Reviews current indications and complications in gynecologic practice.)

5. Kierner AC, Zelenka I, Heller S, et al. Surgical anatomy of the spinal accessory nerve and the trapezius branches of the cervical plexus. *Arch Surg.* 2000;135:1428–1431.

6. Nason RW, Abdulrauf BM, Stranc MF. The anatomy of the accessory nerve and cervical lymph node biopsy. *Am J Surg.* 2000;180:241–243. (Specific tactics for posterior cervical triangle biopsy.)

7. Skandalakis JE, Skandalakis LJ, Skandalakis PN. Anatomy of the lymphatics. *Surg Oncol Clin N Am.* 2007;16:1–16. (Excellent description of location of thoracic duct.)

8. Talmi YP, Hoffman HT, Horowitz Z, et al. Patterns of metastases to the upper jugular lymph nodes (the "submuscular recess"). *Head Neck.* 1998;20:682–686.

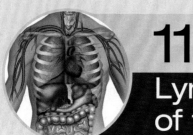

11

Lymph Node Dissections of the Neck

Anuradha R. Bhama and Geeta Lal

Neck dissections encompass a wide variety of terminology and procedures. Each operation is tailored to the illness and the suspected degree of metastasis. It is essential to have an understanding of the levels of the lymph nodes in the neck to grasp the surgical variations. The classic radical neck dissection entails en bloc resection of all soft tissues bordered superiorly by the inferior aspect of the mandible, inferiorly by the clavicle, medially by the midline of the neck, and posteriorly by the trapezius muscle.

A modified radical neck dissection differs from a radical neck dissection in that it preserves one or more structures, namely the sternocleidomastoid (SCM) muscle, the spinal accessory nerve, and the internal jugular vein. The modified radical neck dissection has largely replaced radical neck dissections because of improved cosmetic and functional results with minimal morbidity and less than 1% risk of mortality.

Selective neck dissection and "berry picking" respectively refer to operations in which the surgeon has chosen to remove an isolated compartment or only those nodes that are clinically positive. Berry picking is generally not recommended at an initial operation because of the high rate of compartment recurrence. A central neck dissection refers to a neck dissection of level VI nodes in the paratracheal, paraesophageal, and upper mediastinal regions. It is typically performed for carcinoma of the thyroid and may include resection of level VII or upper mediastinal nodes.

Complications after neck dissection primarily include nerve injury, hypoparathyroidism, and wound complications including seroma, hematoma, infection, and chyloma. A rare complication of bilateral neck dissection is the syndrome of inappropriate antidiuretic hormone.

This chapter begins with the standard radical neck dissection and then presents the common types of modified radical neck dissection and central neck dissection. Selective node dissection is also briefly discussed.

SCORE™, the Surgical Council on Resident Education, classified modified neck dissection as a "COMPLEX" procedure.

STEPS IN PROCEDURE

Standard or Modified Radical Neck Dissection

Position patient with head turned to contralateral side and elevate head of table slightly

Avoid placing incision in a line directly over carotid artery

Elevate flaps at level just deep to platysma

Identify and ligate facial artery and facial vein

Identify and protect marginal mandibular branch of facial nerve

Begin at inferior margin of field

Ligate and divide external jugular vein

If standard neck dissection:

Divide and elevate sternocleidomastoid muscle (may preserve for modified)

Identify, ligate, and divide internal jugular vein (may preserve for modified)

Elevate all surrounding fatty tissues with the divided structures, preserving underlying nerves

Terminate dissection at cephalad aspect, including submandibular gland with specimen

Meticulous closure, with closed-suction drains if desired

Selective Node Dissection

Generally, smaller incision—tailored to node group to be removed

En bloc selective removal of one or more groups of lymph nodes

Generally surrounding structures are preserved

Central Node Dissection

Generally done through a collar (thyroid) incision

Elevate subplatysmal flaps

Divide strap muscles in midline

Begin dissection at inferior aspect of field, resecting thymus

Skeletonize trachea and fatty tissues along esophageal groove to hyoid

Preserve recurrent laryngeal nerves

Preserve superior parathyroid glands

HALLMARK ANATOMIC COMPLICATIONS

Injury to Regional Nerves

Ansa cervicalis

Spinal accessory nerve

Hypogastric nerve

Vagus nerve

Recurrent laryngeal nerve

Injury to parathyroid glands (central neck dissection)

Blowout of carotid artery (delayed)

LIST OF STRUCTURES

Cricoid cartilage

Strap Muscles

Sternothyroid muscle

Omohyoid muscle

Sternohyoid muscle

Anterior jugular veins

Sternocleidomastoid muscle

Ansa cervicalis

Carotid Sheath

Carotid artery

Vagus nerve

Internal jugular vein

Digastric muscle

Spinal accessory nerve

Hypogastric nerve

Parotid Gland

Facial nerve

Innominate artery and vein

Thoracic inlet

Thymus

Thyrothymic ligament

Parathyroid glands, superior and inferior

Introduction

A critical understanding of the zones of the neck and tissue planes is necessary before performing a neck dissection. Lymph node classifications can be either by anatomic description or by levels of the neck. The named nodal groups include submental (level IA), submandibular (level IB), upper jugular (includes sublevels IIA and IIB), middle jugular (level III), lower jugular (level IV), posterior triangle group (includes sublevels VA and VB), and anterior compartment group (level VI). Level IA nodes lie within the boundaries of the anterior belly of the digastric and the hyoid bone. Level IB nodes lie within the boundaries of the anterior belly of the digastric, the stylohyoid muscle, and the body of the mandible. Levels II, III and IV are defined by the upper, middle, and lower third of the sternocleidomastoid (SCM). Level II is subdivided into IIA and IIB, based upon a vertical plane defined by the spinal accessory nerve. IIA nodes lie anteromedial to the plane, while IIB nodes lie posterolateral to the plane. Level V is subdivided into VA and VB by a plane defined by the level of the cricoid cartilage. VA lies superior to this horizontal plane, while VB lies inferior. Finally, level VI nodes are bound superiorly by the hyoid bone, inferiorly by the suprasternal notch, and laterally by the common carotid arteries. Level VI includes the pretracheal, precricoid (Delphian), and perithyroidal nodes (Fig. 11.1).

Standard Radical Neck Dissection

Incision and Development of Flaps (Fig. 11.2)

Technical Points

Position the patient supine with the neck in slight extension and the head turned slightly to the contralateral side. Prepare and drape a surgical field that includes the neck, lower face, and upper chest. Elevate the head of the table slightly to reduce venous bleeding.

A variety of incisions have been used for radical neck dissection. All involve elevation of flaps so that the entire area illustrated can be removed en bloc. Because many of these

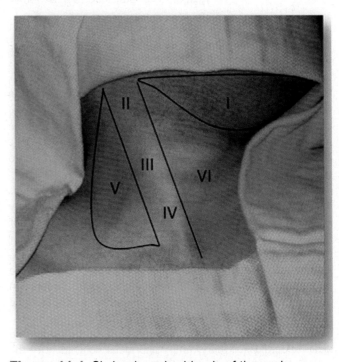

Figure 11.1 Six levels and sublevels of the neck

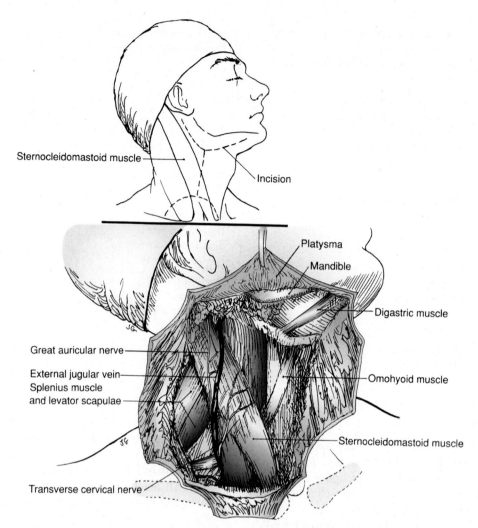

Sternocleidomastoid muscle

Incision

Platysma

Mandible

Digastric muscle

Great auricular nerve

External jugular vein
Splenius muscle
and levator scapulae

Omohyoid muscle

Sternocleidomastoid muscle

Transverse cervical nerve

Figure 11.2 Standard radical neck dissection—incision and development of flaps

patients have received radiation therapy, or may in the future undergo irradiation, viability of skin flaps is especially important. The H-shaped or double Y-shaped incision shown allows complete lymphadenectomy while preserving good, viable skin flaps. Alternative incisions are also illustrated.

Make an H-shaped incision, placing the vertical arm of the incision so that it does not lie directly over the carotid vessels. Make this limb of the incision vertical, rather than oblique, to place it away from the carotid sheath.

Identify the platysma and include it with the skin flaps as this improves blood supply to the skin flaps and greatly enhances the chances for their survival. Elevate the posterior flaps to the anterior border of the trapezius muscle, the superior flap to the mandible, the medial flap to the midline of the neck, and the inferior flap to the clavicle. The external jugular vein should be visible as it courses obliquely across the midportion of the SCM. As the flaps are raised, be careful to dissect in the adventitial plane of this vein.

At the superior border of the field, divide and ligate the facial (external maxillary) artery and facial vein. Identify the marginal mandibular branch of the facial nerve, which may

be injured during the elevation of flaps. It generally is located parallel to and 1 to 2 cm below the lower border of the mandible, crossing superficial to the facial artery and facial vein. Gentle upward traction on the divided stumps of these vessels will retract the marginal mandibular branch safely up out of the field.

Anatomic Points

The platysma is innervated by the cervical branch of the facial nerve, which courses inferiorly deep to the platysma, with anterior branches supplying the platysma. The skin incision and the subsequent elevation of myocutaneous flaps will, of necessity, denervate all or part of the platysma.

The marginal mandibular branch of the facial nerve is important for cosmetic and functional reasons. This nerve innervates the muscles of the lower lip and chin and can lie as much as 2.5 cm inferior to the ramus of the mandible. It is at risk during the development of the upper flap. Begin the incision to raise the superior myocutaneous flap at the mastoid process and then follow a gentle curve inferiorly, about 3 cm inferior to the posterior third of the ramus of the mandible.

Then gently curve the incision superiorly and anteriorly to the mental protuberance of the chin.

Branches of the great auricular nerve, a sensory branch of the cervical plexus bearing fibers from C2 and C3, will be severed during exposure of the upper attachment of the SCM. The vertical limb of the incision almost approximates the course of the external jugular vein, lying immediately deep to the platysma muscle. Be careful to identify this vein and keep the incision superficial to it. The incision also divides branches of the transverse cervical nerve, a sensory branch of the cervical plexus that also carries fibers of C2 and C3. The inferior limb of the incision is relatively risk-free. The supraclavicular nerves (sensory divisions of the cervical plexus carrying fibers of C3 and C4) that supply the skin of the lower neck and extend onto the upper thorax will be encountered and must be divided. The sensory branches of the cervical plexus all emerge from under the middle of the SCM and fan out from this point. Those that supply regions anterior to the SCM cross the superficial surface of that muscle. Several superficial veins will also be encountered deep to the platysma and should be controlled.

Dividing the Sternocleidomastoid Muscle and Beginning the Posterior and Inferior Dissection (Fig. 11.3)

Technical Points

Incise the fascia overlying the anterior border of the trapezius muscle to enter the posterior triangle of the neck. Ligate and divide the transverse cervical artery and vein at the lateral margin of the dissection. Sweep fatty and areolar tissues upward and medially. Identify the spinal accessory nerve, which may be sacrificed or preserved depending on individual preference and the degree of nodal involvement. This nerve is sacrificed in the classic radical neck dissection, but in practice, most surgeons preserve it.

Advance the incision medially, just above the clavicle, and, by sharp and blunt dissection, expose the external jugular vein. Ligate and divide this vein about 1 cm above the clavicle. Begin to sweep fatty and areolar tissues upward as the dissection progresses medially. Divide the posterior belly of the omohyoid muscle and the medial ends of the transverse cervical artery and vein, which run deep to the omohyoid muscle.

Incise the fascia medial to the SCM and gently elevate it, freeing the muscle from the underlying internal jugular vein. Divide the SCM from its attachments to the clavicle and sternum. Place a clamp on the divided stump of the SCM and use it to provide upward traction.

The brachial plexus, phrenic nerve, anterior scalene muscle, and internal jugular vein should be visible in the floor of the dissection.

Anatomic Points

The fascia investing the SCM, or the investing layer of the deep cervical fascia, also invests the trapezius muscle and the section of the spinal accessory nerve that passes from the SCM to the trapezius muscle. This nerve crosses the posterior triangle along a line running from slightly superior to the middle of the SCM to the anterior border of the trapezius muscle about 5 cm

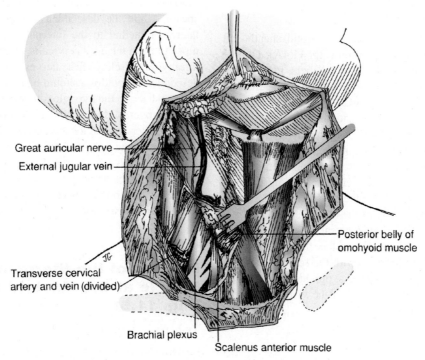

Great auricular nerve

External jugular vein

Posterior belly of omohyoid muscle

Transverse cervical artery and vein (divided)

Brachial plexus

Scalenus anterior muscle

Figure 11.3 Standard radical neck dissection—dividing the sternocleidomastoid muscle and beginning the posterior and inferior dissection

superior to the clavicle. Some surgeons routinely sacrifice this nerve, while others sacrifice it only if it is directly invaded by tumor. Division of this nerve causes significant disability, as this potentially results in diminished trapezius muscle mass and partial paralysis of the trapezius and SCM.

The external jugular vein crosses the superficial surface of the SCM, passing inferiorly from its beginning in the parotid gland to its junction with the subclavian vein, just lateral to the clavicular attachment of the SCM. The termination of the subclavian veins and the internal jugular veins is immediately deep to the SCM, as is the end of the thoracic duct on the left and its counterparts—the right lymphatic ducts—on the right.

The omohyoid muscle has two bellies. The inferior belly originates from the superior border of the scapula and passes medially to join the superior belly through an intermediate tendon. The superior belly then courses vertically and inserts into the hyoid bone. The inferior belly lies immediately superficial to the supraclavicular part of the brachial plexus, suprascapular and transverse cervical vessels, and phrenic nerve, which lies on the anterior scalene muscle. As the specimen is reflected craniad, the transverse cervical vessels are carefully ligated and divided. The phrenic nerve, which lies posterior to these vessels, must be identified and preserved. It lies deep to the lateral branches of the thyrocervical trunk and superficial to the anterior scalene muscle and is the only longitudinal structure coursing superolaterally to inferomedially in the lower neck.

Dissection in the Carotid Sheath and Ligation of the Internal Jugular Vein (Fig. 11.4)

Technical Points

By sharp and blunt dissection, open the carotid sheath and identify the internal jugular vein within (Fig. 11.4A). Double ligate and divide this vein just above the clavicle. Identify the vagus nerve and carotid artery lying posterior to the internal jugular vein. Sweep the internal jugular vein upward with the specimen protecting the vagus nerve and underlying carotid.

Dissection may then proceed relatively rapidly up along the carotid sheath until the carotid bifurcation is reached (Fig. 11.4B). Proceed slowly past the carotid bifurcation and identify and protect the hypoglossal nerve. This crosses the internal and external carotid arteries just above their bifurcation and then passes deep to the posterior belly of the digastric muscle.

The bed of the dissection should reveal the medial border of the trapezius muscle, the middle scalene muscle, and the levator scapulae muscle posteriorly (with the spinal accessory nerve, if preserved). The brachial plexus, phrenic nerve, vagus nerve, and common carotid artery should be visible and preserved in the floor of the dissection.

Anatomic Points

Within the carotid sheath, just above the medial end of the clavicle, the internal jugular vein lies anterolateral, the common carotid artery lies anteromedial, and the vagus nerve is posterior in the groove between these two vessels. As the internal jugular vein is exposed, the middle thyroid vein should be identified, ligated, and divided; this vein, which is present in about half of cases, will be encountered at about the level of the lower and middle third of the thyroid gland. It passes anterior to the common carotid artery.

On the left, the thoracic duct enters the neck by passing along the left side of the esophagus. It arches (as much as 3 to 4 cm superior to the clavicle) anterior to the thyrocervical trunk, phrenic nerve, and medial border of the anterior scalene muscle and posterior to the left common carotid artery, vagus nerve, and internal jugular vein. From the apex of this arch, the duct descends anterior to the left subclavian artery. It may empty into the junction of the subclavian vein and internal jugular vein or into either of these great veins near their junction, or it may divide into smaller vessels before terminating. On the right, typically three major lymphatic trunks (right subclavian, right jugular, and right bronchomediastinal trunks) terminate independently on the anterior aspect of the jugulosubclavian junction, the internal jugular vein, the subclavian vein, or any combination of these. If these lymphatic vessels are injured, they should be ligated to prevent the development of a chylous fistula.

The sympathetic chain lies immediately posterior to the carotid sheath. As with the phrenic nerve, it lies deep to prevertebral fascia and should be protected. Other than the vagus nerve, which is of substantial size and must be preserved, the only other nerves that should be encountered while dissecting the carotid sheath from its contents are the descendens hypoglossi and the descendens cervicalis. The descendens hypoglossi is typically located on the anterior surface of the carotid sheath, while the descendens cervicalis is generally located lateral or medial to the internal jugular vein. These anastomose to form the ansa cervicalis, which innervates the strap or infrahyoid muscles. These nerves have to be sacrificed, but the descendens hypoglossi should be identified because it leads the surgeon back to the hypoglossal nerve. Other nerves that might be encountered during this dissection include the recurrent laryngeal nerve—the location of which is more variable on the right than on the left—and the internal and external branches of the superior laryngeal nerve. Both the superior and the inferior laryngeal nerves lie deep to fascial layers that normally would not be included in the specimen, but their presence is the cause for the surgeon to proceed cautiously.

Division of the Sternocleidomastoid Muscle at the Mastoid Process (Fig. 11.5)

Technical Points

Posteriorly, dissect the specimen from the levator scapulae muscle and the splenius capitis muscle. Divide the SCM at its insertion on the mastoid process.

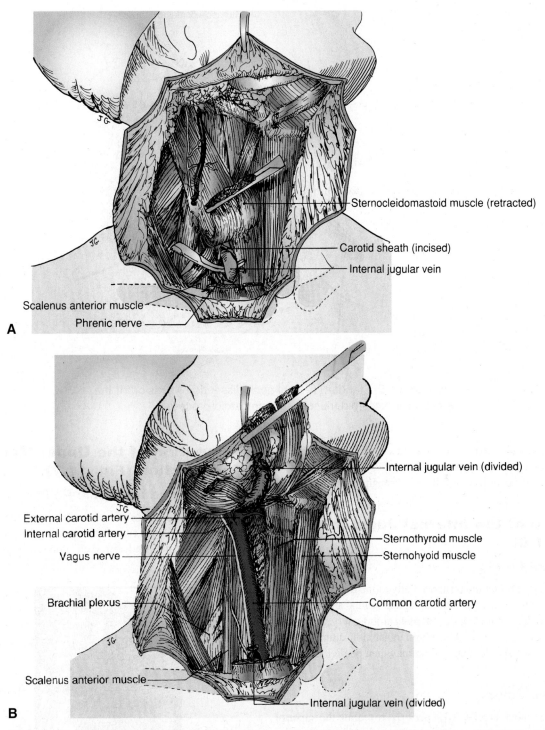

Figure 11.4 Standard radical neck dissection—dissection in the carotid sheath and ligation of the internal jugular vein. **A:** Begin by dividing the sternocleidomastoid muscle and retracting it cephalad. **B:** Field near completion of dissection, showing skeletonized residual structures.

The spinal accessory nerve passes through the part of the SCM several centimeters below the mastoid. Gently tease this nerve out from beneath the cut muscle fibers. Divide the small motor branch to the SCM. Allow the main trunk of the nerve to retract back onto the floor of the dissection. Reflect the specimen medially.

Anatomic Points

As the spinal accessory nerve passes posteriorly, it usually crosses superficial to the internal jugular vein, although it may instead pass deep to the jugular vein. It innervates the SCM approximately 4 cm inferior to the tip of the mastoid and then either pierces or passes deep to that muscle to innervate the trapezius muscle. To

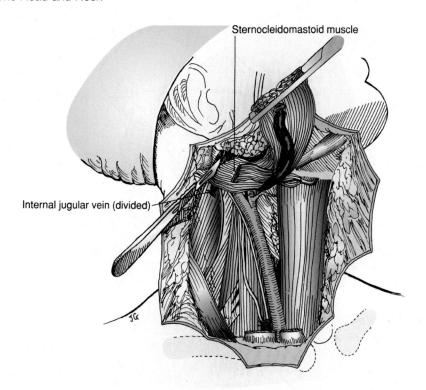

Figure 11.5 Standard radical neck dissection—division of the sternocleidomastoid muscle at the mastoid process

spare the innervation to the trapezius muscle, carefully detach the SCM from the mastoid process and carefully dissect the nerve free from the deep surface or follow it through the muscle.

Division of the Internal Jugular Vein (Fig. 11.6)

Technical Points

Place a retractor under the posterior belly of the digastric muscle and elevate it to expose the internal jugular vein. Carefully clean the vein to delineate it from the internal carotid artery, hypoglossal nerve, and vagus nerve. Use a high transfixion suture ligature to secure the internal jugular vein; it may then be divided.

Anatomic Points

As the tissue block is reflected superiorly, revealing the superior extent of the internal jugular vein and its tributaries, care must again be taken to ligate these veins. Branches of the facial nerve, especially the marginal mandibular, should be preserved. In the lateral groove between the internal jugular vein and the internal carotid artery, care should be taken to avoid the descending segment of the hypoglossal nerve, which will curve anteriorly immediately inferior to the occipital artery. In the medial groove between the jugular and the carotid, the vagus nerve should be avoided. Again, the key to avoiding these nerves when ligating and dividing is to skeletonize the vein gently, making sure to include only the vein in the clamp or ligature.

Delineation of the Upper Margin of Dissection (Fig. 11.7)

Technical and Anatomic Points

Allow the specimen to fall back down into the bed of the dissection. Identify the marginal mandibular nerve, which was previously located and retracted along with the facial artery

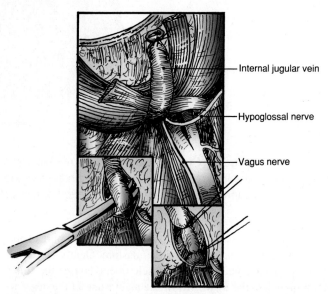

Figure 11.6 Standard radical neck dissection—division of the internal jugular vein

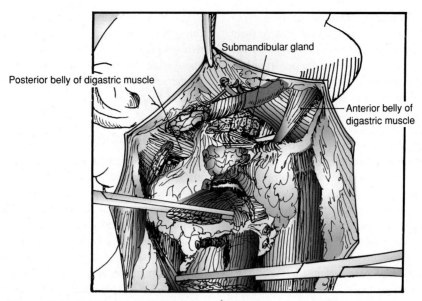

Figure 11.7 Standard radical neck dissection—delineation of the upper margin of dissection

and facial vein. Preserve the nerve by tracing it along the angle of the mandible. Divide the soft tissues from the mental process out along the ramus of the mandible.

Superior Aspect of the Dissection and Completion of Procedure (Fig. 11.8)

Technical Points

Reflect the fatty and areolar tissues medially, exposing the anterior belly of the digastric muscle. The submandibular gland is then identified and should be taken with the specimen. Identify and ligate the duct of the submandibular gland, preserving the lingual nerve. Retract the mylohyoid muscle medially to facilitate exposure of the salivary duct. In the depths, identify and preserve the hypoglossal nerve. Check the field for hemostasis. Place closed-suction drains under both the medial and lateral flaps and approximate the platysma and then the skin with care.

Anatomic Points

This part of the dissection can be challenging because many structures are present in a relatively small space. Excision of

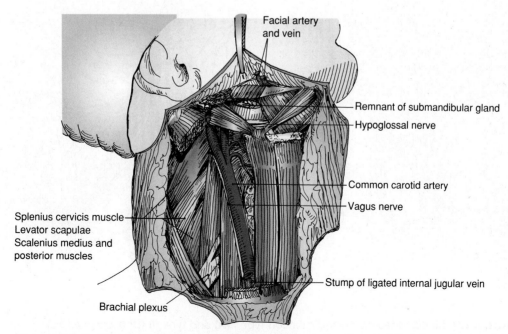

Figure 11.8 Standard radical neck dissection—superior aspect of the dissection and completion of procedure

the submandibular gland necessitates ligation and division of its duct (Wharton's duct). This duct extends anteriorly from the deep surface of the gland, in the interval between the more superficial mylohyoid muscle and the deeper hyoglossus muscle. Here, it lies between the more inferior hypoglossal nerve and the lingual nerve. As the lingual nerve passes forward deep to the mylohyoid muscle, it passes lateral to the duct, gently curves inferiorly, and finally terminates on the medial aspect of the duct by giving off terminal branches. Close to the posterior border of the mylohyoid muscle, preganglionic parasympathetic secretomotor fibers diverge from the lingual nerve to synapse with postganglionic fibers in the submandibular ganglion. Postganglionic fibers provide parasympathetic innervation to the submandibular gland. Traction on the gland can stretch the lingual nerve; because of these anatomic relations, it is necessary to skeletonize the submandibular gland gently before ligating and dividing it to ensure that these important nerves are preserved.

Modified Radical Neck Dissection

The definition of a modified radical neck dissection (MRND) varies by authors. However, the procedure typically involves excision of all the lymph nodes typically removed in a radical neck dissection (levels I–V) with preservation of one or more of the following nonlymphatic structures—the internal jugular vein, the SCM muscle, or the spinal accessory nerve. The spared structure is specifically named. The Type I MRND involves preservation of the spinal accessory nerve (Fig. 11.9A), whereas the Type II MRND preserves the nerve and the internal jugular vein. The Type III MRND spares all the three structures (Fig. 11.9B).

Technical Points

Position the patient as for a radical neck dissection. If a previous scar is present, as is often the case in patients who have undergone thyroidectomy for thyroid cancer, use this incision and extend it several centimeters to the ipsilateral side. Extend the incision vertically along the border of the trapezius muscle to create a hockey stick incision. Some surgeons prefer an apron flap design (Fig. 11.10A) that extends from the mastoid tip to the mandibular symphysis. A variety of alternative incision options exist including making a counter incision along the angle of the mandible (MacFee) (Fig. 11.10) or making an incision along the angle of the mandible and continuing inferiorly with or without extension along the clavicle (Crile and Martin incisions).

The remainder of the dissection is as described in the preceding sections. If the spinal accessory nerve is to be preserved, it should be dissected atraumatically to the trapezius muscle, using a small hemostat. If the SCM muscle is being preserved, it is imperative to identify and dissect the spinal accessory nerve

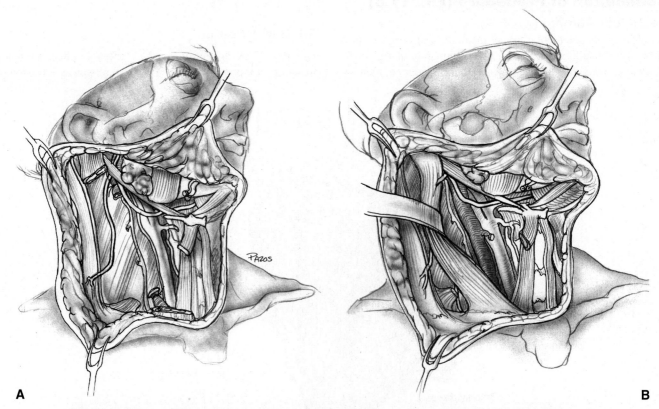

A   **B**

Figure 11.9 Modified radical neck dissection type I **(A)** and type III **(B)** (from Bailey BJ, Johnson JT, eds. *Head & Neck Surgery—Otolaryngology.* 4th ed. Philadelphia, PA: Lippincott Williams & Wilkins; 2006:1594–1595, with permission).

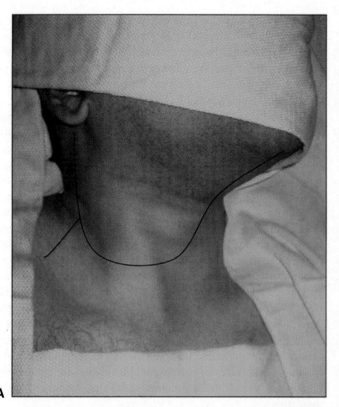

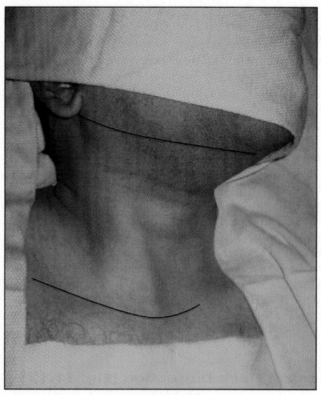

A

B

Figure 11.10 Incisions for MRND include apron-type **(A)** and MacFee **(B)**

both anterior and posterior to the SCM. To accomplish this, the spinal accessory nerve is dissected free from the tissues in the posterior triangle and carefully retracted with a vessel loop. The contents of the posterior triangle superior and posterior to the nerve are then passed under the nerve and the dissection is continued to the posterior border and undersurface of the SCM. If the SCM is to be sacrificed, it is bisected at this juncture and elevated in continuity with the specimen. Lymph node tissues in level IIB will also need to be rotated under the nerve and dissected to the lateral aspect of the internal jugular vein. The muscle can then be transected at the mastoid tip superiorly and just above the clavicle inferiorly. If the muscle is preserved, the nodal contents can be passed anterior to the mobilized muscle. If the internal jugular vein is being preserved, the nodal tissues immediately adjacent and posterior to the vein are removed en bloc with the remainder of the dissection and dissected off the vein sharply.

Selective Neck Dissection (Fig. 11.11)

Technical and Anatomic Points

A selective lymph node dissection of the neck refers to isolated resection of lymph node levels or the removal of retained nodal tissue seen on repeat imaging (e.g., metastatic lymph node visualized on Iodine 131 scanning). The technique can involve either reincising a previous incisional scar and extending it laterally or creating a new longitudinal scar on the ipsilateral side over the enlarged nodes. The illustration shows one example

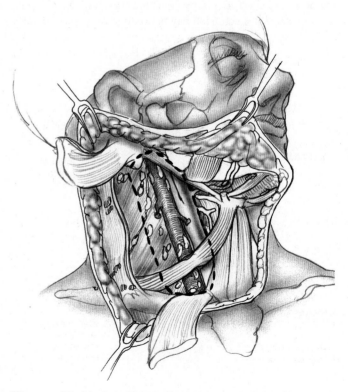

Figure 11.11 Selective radical neck dissection (from Bailey BJ, Johnson JT, eds. *Head & Neck Surgery—Otolaryngology*. 4th ed. Philadelphia, PA: Lippincott Williams & Wilkins; 2006:1597, with permission).

of a selective node dissection, in which lateral nodes (levels II–IV) are removed.

In this procedure, separate the entire SCM off of the strap muscles with either cautious electrocautery or a combination of sharp and blunt dissection. When the sternal border of the SCM has been fully mobilized, retract the SCM laterally and the strap muscles medially. Identify the omohyoid muscle and retract it laterally. Alternatively, some surgeons divide the omohyoid muscle to obtain adequate exposure. Place retractors as needed. As the sternal border of the SCM is mobilized laterally, the internal jugular vein will come into view. Start in the lowest visualized portion of the neck (level IV) and begin dissecting the fibrofatty tissues off of the internal jugular vein. Carry the dissection inferiorly to the level of the clavicle and then return superiorly to dissect to the level of the mandible (level II). Be cautious to identify internal jugular branches and lymphatic channels as the dissection is continued, because these will need to be ligated. As the dissection progresses superiorly, the spinal accessory nerve will come into view and will need to be carefully preserved.

Central Neck Dissection (Fig. 11.12)

This refers to the removal of level VI nodes. Place the patient in a semi-Fowler (modified beach chair) position after appropriately inducing general anesthesia and prepping and draping the neck and chest. Begin by palpating the tip of the chin and the suprasternal notch. Halfway between these points, identify the cricoid cartilage and the cricothyroid membrane. Create a transverse incision equidistant from the midline at the nearest skin crease by the cricoid cartilage or approximately two fingerbreadths above the suprasternal notch. Carry the incision through the platysma and create superior and inferior subplatysmal flaps (see Figs. 6.2–6.4).

Divide the strap muscles in the midline with electrocautery and bluntly dissect them free of the thyroid. Carry this dissection laterally each way to the carotid sheath. Perform total thyroidectomy if appropriate. Inferior to the sternothyroid muscles, expose the thoracic inlet at the level of the innominate artery and vein, resecting the inferior sternohyoid and sternothyroid muscles as necessary. The thymus will be easily evident in this area. Using a combination of electrocautery and blunt dissection, mobilize the thyrothymic ligament to allow for complete resection of the thymic fat pad. Removal of these upper mediastinal nodes (inferior to the sternal notch) constitutes a level VII dissection and is often included in central neck clearance for thyroid cancers. Continue by mobilizing the specimen superiorly. Skeletonize the trachea and fatty tissues along the esophageal groove to the level of the hyoid, being cautious of the recurrent laryngeal nerves. In addition, be wary of injury to the superior parathyroid glands because the inferior parathyroid glands usually cannot be separated from the lower dissection.

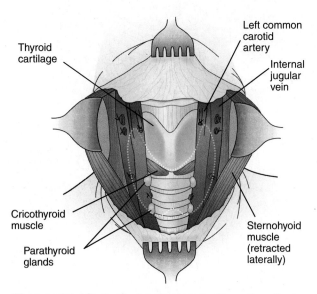

Figure 11.12 Central radical neck dissection (from Donohue JH, van Heerden JA, Monson JRT. *Atlas of Surgical Oncology*. Cambridge, MA: Blackwell Science; 1995:75, Fig. 7.21, with permission).

SURGICAL REFERENCES

1. Attie JN. Modified neck dissection in treatment of thyroid cancer: A safe procedure. *Eur J Cancer Clin Oncol.* 1988;24: 315–324.
2. Day TA, Hornig JD, Sharma AK, et al. Melanoma of the head and neck. *Curr Treat Options Oncol.* 2005;6:19–30.
3. DeCamp MM Jr, Ercan S. Chapter 38: Transsternal, transcervical, and thoracoscopic thymectomy for benign and malignant disease including radical mediastinal dissection. In: Fischer JE, Bland KI, eds. *Mastery of Surgery*. 5th ed. Philadelphia, PA: Lippincott Williams & Wilkins; 2007:445–455.
4. Fleming JB, Lee JE, Bouvet M, et al. Surgical strategy for the treatment of medullary thyroid carcinoma. *Ann Surg.* 1999;230: 697–707.
5. Grant CS. Chapter 33: Surgical anatomy of the thyroid, parathyroid, and adrenal glands. In: Fischer JE, Bland KI, eds. *Mastery of Surgery*. 5th ed. Philadelphia, PA: Lippincott Williams & Wilkins; 2007:388–397.
6. Karakousis CP. Therapeutic node dissections in malignant melanoma. *Ann Surg Oncol.* 1998;5:473–482.
7. Mack LA, McKinnon JG. Controversies in the management of metastatic melanoma to regional lymphatic basins. *J Surg Oncol.* 2004;86:189–199.
8. O'Brien CJ, Petersen-Schaefer K, Ruark D, et al. Radical, modified, and selective neck dissection for cutaneous malignant melanoma. *Head Neck.* 1995;17:232–241.
9. Robbins KT. Indications for selective neck dissection: When, how, and why. *Oncology.* 2000;14:1455–1464.
10. Shaha AR. Management of the neck in thyroid cancer. *Otolaryngol Clin North Am.* 1998;31:823–831.

Figure labels:
Thyroid cartilage
Left common carotid artery
Internal jugular vein
Cricothyroid muscle
Sternohyoid muscle (retracted laterally)
Parathyroid glands

11. Wells SA Jr. Chapter 35: Total thyroidectomy, lymph node dissection for cancer. In: Fischer JE, Bland KI, eds. *Mastery of Surgery.* 5th ed. Philadelphia, PA: Lippincott Williams & Wilkins; 2007:411–422.

SPECIAL PROBLEM REFERENCES

1. Bocca E, Pignataro O, Sasaki CT. Functional neck dissection: A description of operative technique. *Arch Otolaryngol.* 1980;106:524. (Describes a technique for modified node dissection that spares the spinal accessory nerve, sternocleidomastoid muscle, and internal jugular vein.)
2. Roses DF, Harris MN, Ackerman AB, eds. *Diagnosis and Management of Cutaneous Malignant Melanoma.* Philadelphia, PA: WB Saunders; 1983:159. (Describes the modification of radical neck dissection for melanomas of the head and neck, including superficial parotidectomy when appropriate.)
3. Rossi RL, Cady B. Surgery of the thyroid gland. In: Cady B, Rossi RL, eds. *Surgery of the Thyroid and Parathyroid Glands.* 3rd ed. Philadelphia, PA: WB Saunders; 1991:187. (Clearly describes the role and extent of radical neck dissection in the treatment of well-differentiated thyroid carcinoma.)
4. Stack BC Jr, Ferris RL, American Thyroid Association Surgical Affairs Committee, et al. American Thyroid Association consensus review and statement regarding the anatomy, terminology, and rationale for lateral neck dissection in differentiated thyroid cancer. *Thyroid.* 2012;22:501–508.

ANATOMIC REFERENCES

1. Beahrs OH, Gossel JD, Hollinshead WH. Techniques and surgical anatomy of radical neck dissection. *Am J Surg.* 1955;90:490. (Presents an original detailed description of anatomy.)
2. Branstetter BF 4th, Weissman JL. Normal anatomy of the neck with CT and MR imaging correlation. *Radiol Clin North Am.* 2000; 38:925–929.
3. Coleman JJ. Complications in head and neck surgery. *Surg Clin North Am.* 1986;66:149. (Briefly enumerates the technical complications that can arise, emphasizing anatomy.)
4. Nason RW, Abdulrauf BM, Stranc MF. The anatomy of the spinal accessory nerve and cervical lymph node biopsy. *Am J Surg.* 2000; 180:241–243.
5. Robbins KT, Clayman G, American Head and Neck Society, et al. Neck dissection classification update: Revisions proposed by the American Head and Neck Society and the American Academy of Otolaryngology-Head and Neck Surgery. *Arch Otolaryngol Head Neck Surg.* 2002;128(7):751–758.

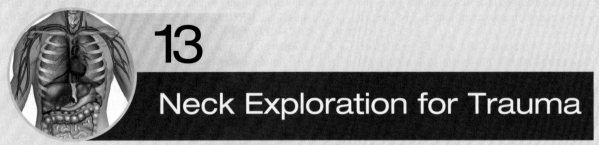

12 Operations for Zenker's Diverticulum

This chapter can be accessed online at www.lww.com/eChapter12.

13

Neck Exploration for Trauma

Kevin D. Helling and Carlos A. Pelaez

Traumatic injuries to the neck can be complicated and difficult to treat as they threaten both life and function. Due to the close proximity of multiple important structures, a systematic approach to exploration and repair must be employed. In order to accomplish this, the neck is divided into three zones numbered in a caudocranial fashion (Fig. 13.1).

Zone I lies between the cricoid cartilage superiorly and the thoracic inlet (clavicles and sternal notch) inferiorly. Injuries in this area of the neck can also extent into the chest and mediastinum. Therefore, the surgeon must have high index of suspicion for injuries at this level and also be prepared to explore the chest and mediastinum. Hemodynamically

ORIENTATION

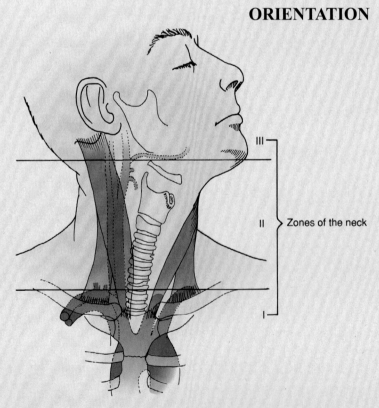

Figure 13.1 Zones of the neck as defined for purposes of trauma

unstable patients are taken directly to the operating room, whereas stable patients should first undergo further evaluation to characterize their injuries. Computed tomography with angiography (CTA) is a useful method to evaluate for vascular injuries. Angiography is also diagnostic and provides therapeutic options. Chest radiography is done to look for associated hemopneumothorax. Esophageal contrast studies with or without endoscopy, as well as bronchoscopy, are necessary to complete the nonoperative evaluation. These studies may be selectively omitted if the CTA reveals the path of penetration to be remote from the aerodigestive tract. Positive findings direct operative repair. If operative intervention is required, exposure can be difficult and usually requires a combination of incisions to gain access to the neck and mediastinum. Most injuries can be managed by a median sternotomy with extension to the neck over the anterior aspect of the sternocleidomastoid muscle. A supraclavicular incision, removal of the clavicle or a trapdoor thoracotomy (where an incision is made from midclavicular to the sternal notch, then carried along the midline onto the sternum to the fourth intercostal space, and out along the fourth interspace to the midaxillary line) are sometimes required. These approaches are described at the end of the chapter.

Zone II extends from the angle of the mandible superiorly to the cricoid cartilage inferiorly. Injuries to this zone that penetrate the platysma generally warrant exploration, and prompt surgery is required in unstable patients. Injuries superficial to the platysma require only local exploration and irrigation. Massive hemorrhage possible as a result from injury to the common carotid artery or its branches, vertebral artery, jugular vein, or a combination of them. Initial control of bleeding can be accomplished by manual pressure; blind clamp application for hemorrhage control is to be condemned. Stable patients may undergo further preoperative evaluation by duplex ultrasonography, CTA or angiography, followed by radiographic or endoscopic hypopharyngeal and esophageal evaluation. The larynx and trachea must be examined by fiberoptic or rigid endoscopy if appropriate signs or symptoms are present, such as cervical subcutaneous emphysema, stridor, respiratory difficulties, hemoptysis, or hoarseness. A selective approach to exploration may be appropriate if diagnostic studies yield negative results. Zone II injuries are explored through a neck incision over the anterior border of the sternocleidomastoid muscle.

Zone III extends from the skull base superiorly to the angle of the mandible inferiorly. Operative exposure can be difficult. If possible, patients with injuries in zone III should undergo preoperative imaging to allow better operative strategy and planning. Unstable patients should be taken expeditiously to the operating room. A Fogarty or Foley catheter may be gently inserted into the wound and its balloon inflated to the point of hemorrhage control. If this results in hemodynamic improvement, diagnostic and therapeutic arteriography may then be possible. In the case of profound bleeding, operative management is focused on obtaining proximal and distal control of the bleeding vessel. Obtaining distal control near the skull base or vertebrae may be exceedingly difficult if not impossible. Placement of bone wax into the bleeding orifice can accomplish distal control in injuries in which the distal end of the vessel cannot be reached to ligate or repair the vessel. When nonoperative evaluation is pursued, fiberoptic endoscopic evaluation of the pharyngeal area should be conducted as well.

SCORE™, the Surgical Council on Resident Education, classified neck exploration for trauma as a "COMPLEX" procedure.

STEPS IN PROCEDURE

Position the patient with neck extended and the head turned laterally

Place a roll under the shoulders for better support

Prepare and drape the neck and chest in case sternotomy or thoracotomy is required

Perform an oblique incision through the skin and platysma, along anterior border of sternocleidomastoid muscle, curving posteriorly as the incision approaches the angle of the mandible to avoid injury to the marginal mandibular nerve

Retract sternocleidomastoid muscle laterally to expose carotid sheath

Explore carotid sheath if hematoma is encountered

Retract thyroid medially after dividing middle thyroid vein

Expose and inspect esophagus and trachea by retracting the carotid sheath laterally

Close incision in layers

Obtain hemostasis of all small muscles and subcutaneous bleeders

Place drain if contaminated wound or any concern for possible esophageal injury

LIST OF STRUCTURES

Platysma
Sternocleidomastoid muscle
Trachea
Esophagus
Thyroid gland
Carotid sheath

Carotid artery (common, internal, and external)
Internal jugular vein
Facial vein
Vagus nerve
Recurrent laryngeal nerve

Neck exploration can be thought of as a means of systematically inspecting two main compartments in the neck. The vascular compartment includes the common carotid, internal carotid, external carotid, and vertebral arteries, as well as the internal jugular vein and its branches. The visceral compartment includes the pharynx and esophagus, larynx and trachea, thyroid, parathyroids, and associated structures. Even when preoperative clinical findings or diagnostic studies point to injury of a specific structure, a complete and systematic examination of all structures should be performed.

Positioning of the Patient and Skin Incision (Fig. 13.2)

Technical and Anatomic Points

Position the patient supine with the head turned slightly away from the injury or neutral if cervical spine injury is possible. Recently, the routine use of cervical spine collar in isolated penetrating neck trauma has been called into question due to the propensity of the collar to obscure injuries, and the surgeon must evaluate the entire circumference of the neck to avoid missing wounds, hematomas, tracheal abnormalities, or spinal

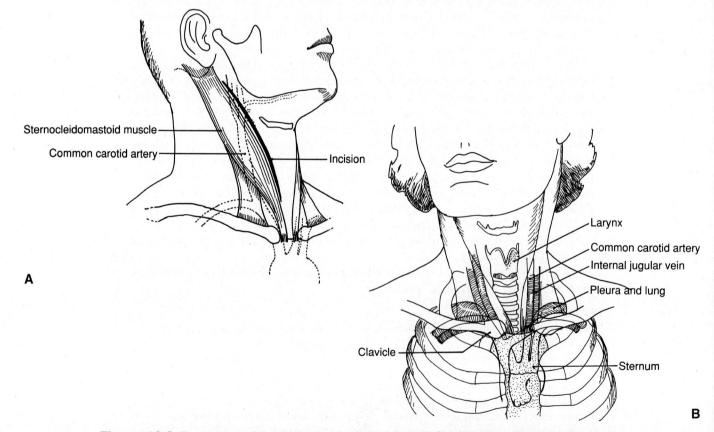

Figure 13.2 Positioning of the patient and skin incision. **A:** Skin incision along anterior border of sternocleidomastoid muscle. **B:** Regional anatomy.

defects. Once the head is positioned appropriately, prepare and drape both sides of the neck and the entire chest, as exploration of the mediastinum through partial or complete median sternotomy or anterolateral thoracotomy may be necessary. Prepare and drape both groins to allow vascular access and harvest of the saphenous veins in the event they are needed for vessel repair.

Make a long incision along the anterior border of the sternocleidomastoid muscle on the side of injury. Curve the incision posteriorly near the angle of the mandible in order to prevent injury to the marginal mandibular branch of the facial nerve. Bilateral neck exploration can be accomplished through bilateral incisions. Alternatively, a collar-type incision can be used. However, this incision requires that flaps be raised and thus takes longer than lateral neck incisions. The slightly better cosmetic result achieved with this technique rarely justifies the extra operative time. Control major bleeding by direct digital pressure until proximal and distal control can be achieved. If difficulty obtaining vascular control is encountered, a Fogarty catheter or Foley balloon can be used to tamponade the vessel. Always attempt to obtain proximal and distal vascular control before opening any hematoma.

Exploration of the Vascular Structures (Fig. 13.3)

Technical and Anatomic Points

Ligate any superficial bleeding vessels. Retract the sternocleidomastoid muscle laterally to expose the carotid sheath. A hematoma involving the carotid sheath requires exploration. Achieve sufficient exposure for proximal and distal control before opening the sheath. This may require extension of the incision to expose uninjured vessel.

Persistent arterial hemorrhage not originating from the common carotid artery or its branches indicates possible injury to the vertebral artery. Such bleeding can be copious. In zone I of the neck, gentle retraction of the carotid sheath contents allows exposure of the more posterior vertebral artery. After proximal and distal control is obtained, arterial repair can be performed. If necessary, the vertebral artery can be ligated with low risk for stroke. In zone III and the cephalad aspect of zone II, vertebral artery exposure is much more difficult, generally requiring removal of the anterior aspect of the vertebral transverse process, a maneuver that can produce additional hemorrhage. Alternatively, bone wax can be placed over the opening to temporarily control hemorrhage until further, more definitive therapy can occur. An alternative to direct operative exposure is wound packing followed by therapeutic angiography.

Hemorrhage from within the carotid sheath is often from the internal jugular vein or a large branch thereof. Simple lacerations of the internal jugular vein may be repaired by simple closure with a running monofilament suture (lateral venorrhaphy). Venous repair has high risk of thrombosis and anticoagulation should be considered. For more significant injuries, the vein may be ligated. Air embolism may occur, particularly in patients who are breathing spontaneously. Avoid bilateral internal jugular vein ligation, if possible, to avert adverse neurologic complications from venous congestion.

For injuries to the common, external, and internal carotid arteries, proximal and distal control must be obtained before exposing the vessel. Debride the injury. Repair injuries of the common or internal carotid artery by simple suture (permanent monofilament), vein patch angioplasty, or interposition saphenous vein grafting. Consider using an intraluminal shunt if common or internal carotid artery repair is necessary. As an alternative to interposition vein grafting for proximal internal carotid artery injuries, the uninjured external carotid artery may

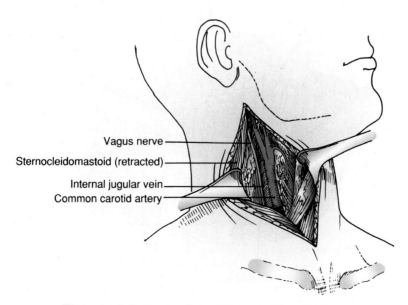

Vagus nerve
Sternocleidomastoid (retracted)
Internal jugular vein
Common carotid artery

Figure 13.3 Exploration of the vascular structures

be transposed, making an anastomosis between it and the distal internal carotid. An injured external carotid artery itself can be ligated with impunity. Ligation of the common and internal carotid arteries is reserved for patients who are obtunded and comatose, or when there is uncontrollable hemorrhage and a temporary shunt is not possible. Inspect the vagus nerve, but handle it minimally to avoid injury to its medially located recurrent laryngeal nerve fibers.

Exploration and Repair of Midline Structures (Fig. 13.4)

Technical and Anatomic Points

Control bleeding from the thyroid gland by direct suture ligation as such bleeding usually does not respond to cautery. Visualize the recurrent laryngeal nerve if the injury lies close to its position in the tracheoesophageal groove. Expose the trachea from an anterior approach. Close simple tracheal lacerations with one-layer interrupted absorbable suture material, tying knots externally to avoid intraluminal granuloma formation. When adjacent injuries to the trachea and esophagus are present, a well-vascularized muscle flap should be interposed between the tracheal and esophageal repairs. Laryngeal injuries are similarly repaired but also require endoscopic evaluation of internal laryngeal structures.

The pharynx and esophagus are located slightly left of the midline, and are ideally approached from the left side. Full exposure of the cervical esophagus and distal pharynx requires ligation and division of the middle thyroid vein and inferior thyroid artery. The thyroid can then be rotated anteromedially with the trachea as the sternocleidomastoid muscle and carotid sheath are retracted posterolaterally. After appropriate debridement, repair pharyngeal and esophageal

injuries using a standard two-layer suture technique. Esophageal repair over a 40- to 46-French bougie prevents clinically significant esophageal narrowing. Place a small drain in proximity to the suture line.

Close the wound in layers, approximating the anterior border of the sternocleidomastoid muscle to the divided cervical fascia with absorbable sutures. Bring the drain out through a separate stab wound. Care should be taken to control any small muscular bleeders to prevent hematoma formation within the wound.

Additional Exposure for Injuries Involving the Thoracic Inlet (Fig. 13.5)

Technical and Anatomic Points

When the exact extent of injury is not known in the unstable patient, median sternotomy provides the best exposure. This incision can be extended superiorly along the anterior border of either sternocleidomastoid muscle as necessary to expose the carotid sheath. Median sternotomy with cervical extension allows excellent exposure and proximal control of the brachiocephalic, proximal right subclavian and proximal common carotid arteries. A contiguous incision along the right supraclavicular region exposes the more distal right subclavian artery. The very proximal left subclavian artery can be controlled through median sternotomy, but a high left anterolateral thoracotomy (third or fourth interspace) usually provides better proximal exposure.

Coupled with a left supraclavicular incision, access to most of the left subclavian artery can be achieved. Rarely, left clavicular division, partial excision, or both may be required. Alternatively, combining upper sternotomy from sternal notch to fourth intercostal space with dual left lateral incisions

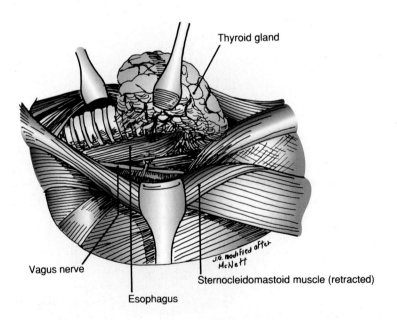

Thyroid gland

Vagus nerve

J.G. modified after McNett

Sternocleidomastoid muscle (retracted)

Esophagus

Figure 13.4 Exploration and repair of midline structures

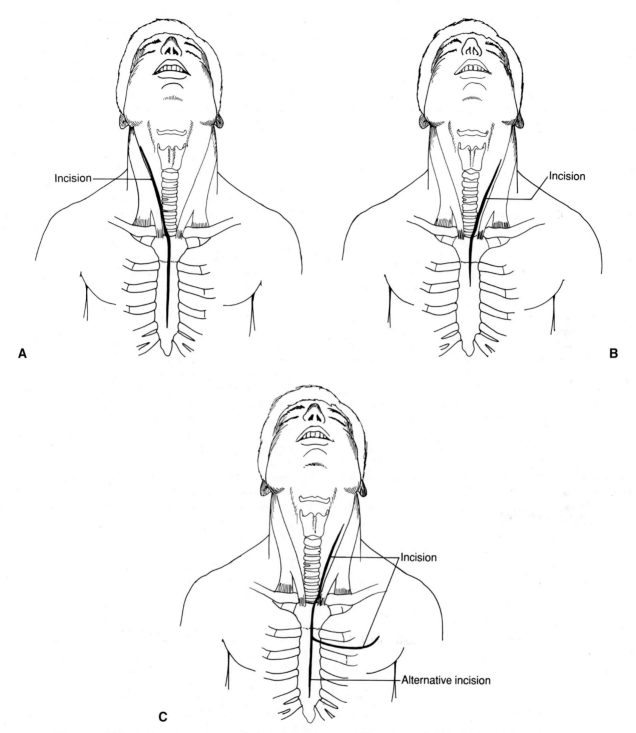

Figure 13.5 Additional exposure for injuries involving the thoracic inlet. **A:** Combination of median sternotomy and right neck exploration incisions. **B:** Combination of median sternotomy and left neck exploration incisions. **C:** Trapdoor incision to allow better proximal exposure on the left.

(supraclavicular and fourth interspace anterolateral thoracotomy)—the so-called "trapdoor" incision—allows left subclavian artery exposure from origin to terminus. The latter two options are justified if vascular control cannot be obtained by other means, but these maneuvers are associated with significant morbidity because of resultant brachial plexopathy and complex regional pain syndrome.

REFERENCES

1. Bishara RA, Pasch AR, Douglas DD, et al. The necessity of mandatory exploration of penetrating zone II neck injuries. *Surgery.* 1986;100:655–660.
2. Brywczynski JJ, Barrett TW, Lyon JA, et al. Management of penetrating neck injury in the emergency department: A structured literature review. *Emerg Med J.* 2008;25(11):711–715.

3. Cox MW, Whittaker DR, Martinez C, et al. Traumatic pseudo-aneurysms of the head and neck: Early endovascular intervention. *J Vasc Surg.* 2007;46:1227–1233.

4. Demetriades D, Asensio JA, Velmahos G, et al. Complex problems in penetrating neck trauma. *Surg Clin North Am.* 1996;76:661–683.

5. Demetriades D, Chahwan S, Gomez H, et al. Penetrating injuries to the subclavian and axillary vessels. *J Am Coll Surg.* 1999; 188:290–295. (Contains a wealth of information about dealing with these difficult injuries.)

6. Dichtel WJ, Miller RH, Woodson GE, et al. Lateral mandibu-lotomy: A technique of exposure for penetrating injuries of the internal carotid artery at the base of the skull. *Laryngoscope.* 1984;94:1140–1144. (Describes division of the mandible to allow significant upward extension of exposure.)

7. Eddy VA. Is routine arteriography mandatory for penetrating injuries to zone 1 of the neck? Zone I penetrating neck injury study group. *J Trauma.* 2000;48:208–214.

8. Gaspert MG, Lorelli DR, Kralovich KA, et al. Physical examination plus chest radiography in penetrating periclavicular trauma: The appropriate trigger for angiography. *J Trauma.* 2000;49:1029–1033.

9. Gilroy D, Lakhoo M, Charalambides D, et al. Control of life-threatening hemorrhage from the neck: A new indication for balloon tamponade. *Injury.* 1992;23:557–559.

10. Graham JM, Mattox KL, Feliciano DV, et al. Vascular injuries of the axilla. *Ann Surg.* 1982;195:232–238. (Describes exposure of axillary and sub-clavian vessels.)

11. Grewal H, Rao PM, Mukerji S, et al. Management of penetrating laryngotracheal injuries. *Head Neck.* 1995;17:494–502.

12. Hirshberg A, Mattox KL. The neck: Safari in tiger country. In: Allen MK, ed. *Top Knife: The Art and Craft of Trauma Surgery.* UK: tfm; 2005:199–214.

13. Landrenau RJ, Weigelt JA, Megison SM, et al. Combined carotid-vertebral arterial trauma. *Arch Surg.* 1992;127:301–304.

14. Lustenberger T, Talving P, Lam L, et al. Unstable cervical spine fracture after penetrating neck injury: A rare entity in an analysis of 1,069 patients. *J Trauma.* 2011;70(4):870–872.

15. McIntyre WB, Ballard JL. Cervicothoracic vascular injuries. *Semin Vasc Surg.* 1998;11:232–242.

16. Noyes LD, McSwain NE, Markowitz IP. Panendoscopy with arte-riography versus mandatory exploration of penetrating wounds of the neck. *Ann Surg.* 1986;204:21–31. (Presents alternative to neck exploration.)

17. Patel AV, Marin ML, Veith FJ, et al. Endovascular graft repair of penetrating subclavian artery injuries. *J Endovasc Surg.* 1996;3:382–388. (An alternative to operative management in highly selected cases.)

18. Peitzman A, Rhodes M, Schwab CW, et al. Penetrating neck trauma. In: Schermer CR, Boffard K, eds. *The Trauma Manual: Trauma and Acute Care Surgery.* 3rd ed. Philadelphia: Lippincott Williams and Wilkins; 1998:197–202.

19. Richardson JD, Martin LF, Borzotta AP, et al. Unifying concepts in treatment of esophageal leaks. *Am J Surg.* 1985;149:157–162.

20. Schenk WG. Neck injuries. In: Moylan JA, ed. *Trauma Surgery.* Philadelphia: JB Lippincott; 1988:417. (Describes the management of blunt and penetrating neck injuries.)

21. Shaha A, Phillips T, Scalea T, et al. Exposure of the internal carotid artery near the skull base: The posterolateral anatomic approach. *J Vasc Surg.* 1988;8:618–622. (Provides an excellent description of the exposure obtained through a radical neck–type approach.)

22. Stuke LE, Pons PT, Guy JS, et al. Prehospital spine immobiliza-tion for penetrating trauma-review and recommendations from the prehospital trauma life support executive committee. *J Trauma.* 2011;71(3):763–770.

23. Thoma M, Navsaria PH, Edu S, et al. Analysis of 203 patients with penetrating neck injuries. *World J Surg.* 2008;32(12):2716–2723.

24. Van Waes OJ, Cheriex KCAL, Navsaria PH, et al. Management of penetrating neck injuries. *Br J Surg.* 2012;99(S1):149–154.

25. Yee LF, Olcott EW, Knudson M, et al. Extraluminal, transluminal, and observational treatment for vertebral artery injuries. *J Trauma.* 1995;39:480–486.

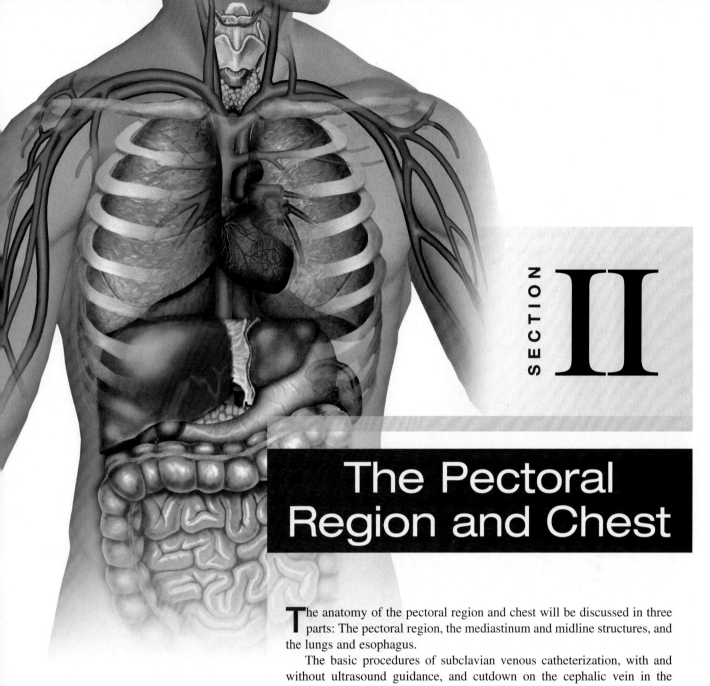

The Pectoral Region and Chest

The anatomy of the pectoral region and chest will be discussed in three parts: The pectoral region, the mediastinum and midline structures, and the lungs and esophagus.

The basic procedures of subclavian venous catheterization, with and without ultrasound guidance, and cutdown on the cephalic vein in the deltopectoral groove will be used to illustrate the anatomy of the subclavian region (Chapter 14). A series of breast procedures beginning with the ultrasound-guided percutaneous breast biopsy (Chapter 15) and progressing through modified radical and classic radical mastectomy (Chapter 18) illustrate the anatomy of the breast, pectoral region, and axilla. Sentinel lymph node biopsy for breast cancer and axillary dissection (Chapters 20 and 21) conclude this section.

The structures of the chest are first discussed by presenting the anatomy of the mediastinum (the "space between"). A rare procedure now, Mediastinoscopy (Chapter 22e) is included in the electronic text because it is a useful introduction to the topography of the region. A discussion of median sternotomy and thymectomy (Chapter 23e) completes the introduction to the anterior mediastinum.

Chapter 25 introduces pulmonary anatomy endobronchially, through fiber-optic and rigid bronchoscopy. Thoracostomy and thoracotomy (Chapter 26) illustrate the anatomy of an intercostal space and the muscles of the chest wall. This is complemented by Chapter 27, which presents the thoraco-scopic view. Pulmonary resections—both pneumonectomies (Chapter 28e) and lobectomies (Chapters 29e and 30e)—complete the discussion of the anatomy of the lungs. Because these are infrequently performed by general surgeons, they have been moved to the electronic text.

The thoracic outlet is the opening through which major neurovascular structures enter and leave the chest for the neck and upper extremity. The anatomy of this complex space is illustrated in Chapter 31e, where surgery for thoracic outlet compression syndromes is considered.

The esophagus, although it is a midline structure, is approached through a thoracotomy incision and hence is discussed with other structures accessed through that approach (Chapters 32e and 33e). It provides an introduction to the abdominal region (Section IV).

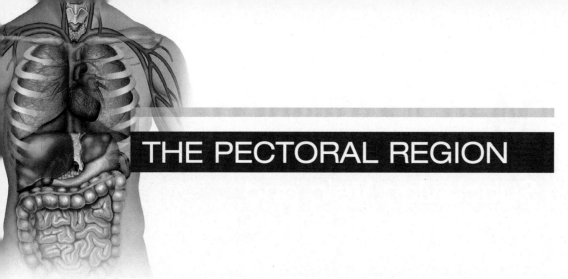

THE PECTORAL REGION

The pectoral region is described in this section. Structures of importance for venous access include the subclavian and cephalic veins. The approach to the axillary artery is described in Section III (The Upper Extremity), Chapter 36e (Axillobifemoral Bypass). The breast and axilla are included in this section, along with operative descriptions of a large number of breast procedures including axillary node dissection and sentinel node biopsy for breast cancer.

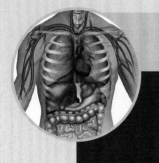

14

Venous Access: The Subclavian Vein and the Cephalic Vein in the Deltopectoral Groove

Percutaneous cannulation of the subclavian vein is frequently used for rapid access to the central venous circulation and for the placement of long-term intravascular access devices such as tunneled catheters and ports. Because the vein follows a relatively constant course that is easily estimated by readily palpable bony landmarks, this is a convenient site for cannulation. However, this vein's proximity to other major vascular structures and to the apex of the lung necessitates a thorough understanding of the anatomy so that complications may be avoided when performing this routine procedure. Two approaches to this procedure are described—first, cannulation by anatomic landmarks; second, cannulation under ultrasound guidance. Details on the Seldinger technique are illustrated and described in Chapter 8 (Figure 8.6) and will not be repeated here.

Performing a cutdown on the cephalic vein in the deltopectoral groove is an alternative mean of achieving access to the central circulation. In selected patients, it may be easier or safer than percutaneous methods.

The subclavian and deltopectoral groove approaches may also be used for the placement of implantable venous access devices. Details on these devices and how to place them are included in Chapter 8 (Figures 8.9 and 8.10) and are not repeated here.

SCORE™, the Surgical Council on Resident Education, classified Central venous line placement, Ultrasound use for intravascular access, and Insertion of implantable venous access devices as "ESSENTIAL COMMON" procedures.

LIST OF STRUCTURES

Superior vena cava

Brachiocephalic (Innominate) Vein
Internal jugular vein
Subclavian vein
Vertebral vein
Inferior thyroid vein
Internal thoracic vein
Thymic vein
Left superior intercostal vein
Axillary vein
Cephalic vein

Aorta
Brachiocephalic artery
Subclavian artery

Thoracic Duct
Arch of thoracic duct
Cervical portion of thoracic duct
Thoracic portion of thoracic duct

Acromion process
Sternal notch
Clavicle
Sternoclavicular joints
Anterior scalene muscle
Sternohyoid muscle
Sternothyroid muscle
Pectoralis major muscle
Pectoralis minor muscle
Clavipectoral fascia
Prevertebral fascia
Deltopectoral groove
Deltopectoral triangle
Pleura
Thymus
Trachea
Phrenic nerve
Vagus nerve

ORIENTATION

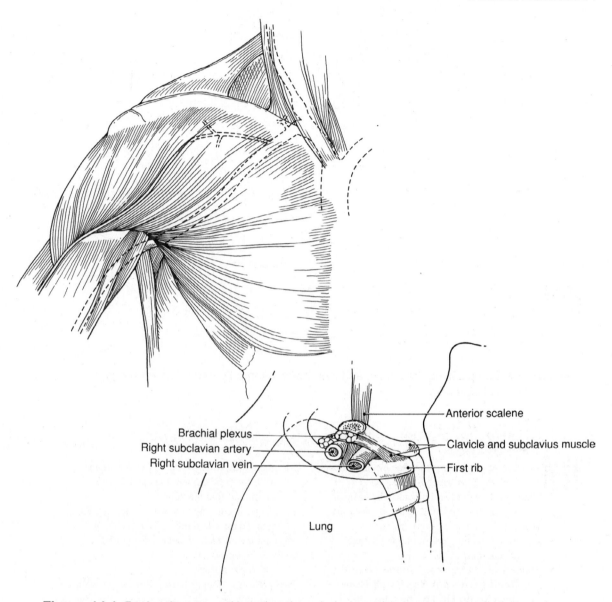

Figure 14.1 Regional anatomy. Note that the subclavian vein passes anterior to the subclavian artery and anterior scalene muscle.

Orientation (Fig. 14.1)

Percutaneous Cannulation of the Subclavian Vein by Landmarks

Cannulation by Landmarks—Positioning the Patient and Identifying Landmarks (Fig. 14.2)

Technical Points

Position the patient supine with arms at the side. Elevate the foot of the bed to a 5- or 10-degree Trendelenburg position.

This will increase venous pressure in the central veins, distending the subclavian vein and rendering the possibility of venous air embolus less likely. Place a vertical roll under the thoracic spine to allow the shoulders to "fall back" slightly, thus opening the angle between the clavicle and the ribs. Inspect both infraclavicular regions for evidence of previous cannulation or local infections. In general, the left subclavian vein is somewhat easier to cannulate and will more reliably provide access to the central circulation than the right subclavian vein. Both, however, are usable.

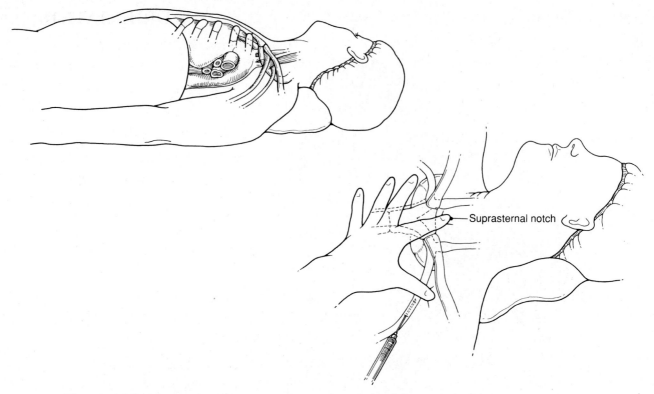

Figure 14.2 Positioning the patient and identifying landmarks—subclavian venous cannulation by landmarks

Suprasternal notch

STEPS IN PROCEDURE—PERCUTANEOUS SUBCLAVIAN VENOUS CANNULATION

Position patient with ipsilateral arm at side and in slight Trendelenburg position

Place a roll under the thoracic spine to open up the infraclavicular space, if necessary

Identify the following bony landmarks: Acromion process, sternal notch, and medial third of the clavicle

Place Index Finger of Nondominant Hand in Sternal Notch and Hook the Thumb Under the Clavicle

Usually one-third of the distance from the acromion to the sternal notch

Infiltrate skin and subcutaneous tissues

Maintaining needle parallel to plane of floor, walk the needle under the clavicle and aspirate to find the vein

Pass larger needle supplied with the kit into the vein; confirm free flow of venous blood

Pass guidewire under fluoroscopic guidance

Make skin incision

Pass dilator and sheath

Pass catheter through sheath, peel away sheath and remove

Confirm catheter position

Secure catheter

HALLMARK ANATOMIC COMPLICATIONS—PERCUTANEOUS SUBCLAVIAN CANNULATION

Pneumothorax
Subclavian artery cannulation
Mediastinal perforation

Catheter placed too far medial; pinched off by clavicle

Identify the constant bony landmarks before cannulation. These include the acromion process, the sternal notch, and the medial third of the clavicle. Prepare and drape a field that includes the medial half of the clavicle. Using your nondominant hand, place the index finger in the sternal notch and the thumb under the clavicle. Identify the place where the curvature of the clavicle begins to change (remember that the clavicle is S-shaped). This should be about one-third of the distance from the sternal notch to the acromion and medial to the pulse of the subclavian artery if it is palpable. Use a fine-gauge needle to infiltrate the area with lidocaine without epinephrine. Aspirate as the skin, subcutaneous tissues, and periosteum are infiltrated. "Walk" the needle under the periosteum of the clavicle and aspirate. Free aspiration of venous blood with this fine-gauge needle will help to identify where the subclavian vein lies. Do not inject local anesthesia into the subclavian vein.

After identifying the probable location of the subclavian vein, place an 18-gauge needle on a Luer slip syringe. Maintaining the orientation of the bony landmarks previously described, "walk" the tip of the needle under the clavicle. The point of the needle should be aimed at the sternal notch. The shaft of the needle should remain parallel to the floor at all times. Never point the needle toward the chest wall. You should feel the needle strike the periosteum of the underside of the clavicle and slip under the clavicle; aspirate until free return of venous blood is obtained.

After free return of venous blood, use a hemostat to grasp the needle and maintain it in position as the Luer slip syringe is gently removed. Conscious, cooperative patients should then be asked to perform a Valsalva maneuver before the syringe is disconnected to avoid producing a venous air embolus. Immediately place a gloved finger over the hub of the needle so that no air can enter the vein. Introduce the floppy end of the guidewire through the needle as shown in Figure 8.6. It should pass freely and easily, indicating a central position. Remove the needle, taking care not to lose contact with the guidewire at any time. If resistance is encountered while introducing the wire through the needle, withdraw the needle and guidewire as a unit. Otherwise, withdrawal of the wire through the needle may result in cutting of the wire, which can then embolize to the heart.

If fluoroscopy is available, check the position of the guidewire at this time. Demonstrate by fluoroscopy that the guidewire is centrally located. Use a number 11 blade to enlarge the skin hole around the guidewire and pass a venous dilator and sheath over the guidewire coaxially into the subclavian vein. These should pass easily, although some resistance will be felt as the tissue is dilated. Injuries to mediastinal structures can occur during this phase, and many prefer to use fluoroscopy and only pass the dilator and sheath as far as needed (rather than "up to the hub"). Remove the dilator and wire, leaving the sheath in place. Again, place a gloved finger over the hub of the needle as the wire and dilator are removed to avoid venous air embolus. Introduce the catheter through the sheath; break and peel away the sheath. Confirm the final position of the catheter using fluoroscopy and document, by upright chest radiographic studies, that pneumothorax has not occurred. Secure the catheter in position and place a sterile dressing over the device.

Anatomic Points

The subclavian veins, which represent continuations of the axillary veins, begin at the outer border of the first rib. Posterior to the sternoclavicular joint on each side, the subclavian vein joins the internal jugular vein to form either the right or left brachiocephalic (innominate) vein. The two brachiocephalic veins join posterior to the right side of the sternum, at the level of the first intercostal space, to form the superior vena cava. Both subclavian veins lie more or less posterior to the clavicle and the subclavius muscle (although the relationship of the clavicle varies as one progresses from lateral to medial), anterior and slightly inferior to the subclavian artery, and anterior to the anterior scalene muscle. The anterior scalene muscle lies between the subclavian vein (which lies anterior) and the subclavian artery (posterior). Medial to the anterior scalene muscles, both left and right veins lie on the superior surface of the first rib and then on the dome of the pleura. The fascial relations of the subclavian veins make the threat of an air embolus more than theoretical. Laterally, the vein is firmly attached to the clavipectoral fascia, whereas more medially, it is attached to prevertebral fascia. These attachments prevent collapse of the vein, and during certain movements, such as during inspiration or raising of the arm, they can increase the diameter of the subclavian veins.

The two brachiocephalic veins are quite different in length, orientation, significant tributaries, and relations. Both begin posterior to their respective sternoclavicular joints. The right brachiocephalic vein is usually about 2.5 cm long and is essentially vertical; thus, its axis lies at an angle of almost 90 degrees with respect to the axis of the subclavian vein. Because the left brachiocephalic vein joins the right at a point posterior to the right edge of the sternum and superior to the second sternocostal articulation, it is, of necessity, longer (about 6 cm), and its oblique course approaches the horizontal. As a consequence, the axis of the subclavian and brachiocephalic veins is obtuse, approaching 180 degrees. It is the orientation of subclavian and brachiocephalic veins that makes cannulation of the left side easier than cannulation of the right.

In addition to the subclavian and internal jugular veins, tributaries of both brachiocephalic veins typically include vertebral, inferior thyroid, and internal thoracic veins. The left brachiocephalic vein typically also receives the left superior intercostal vein, the thymic veins, and an inferior thyroid vein when the latter is present.

On the right, typically (80% of cases), three lymphatic trunks (right bronchomediastinal, subclavian, and jugular) join the venous system at or near the beginning of the brachiocephalic vein. In about 20% of cases, these trunks join to form a short right lymphatic duct. On the left, these trunks typically join the thoracic duct, which then drains into the venous system as a single vessel at or near the beginning of the brachiocephalic vein.

The anatomic relationships of the brachiocephalic veins are a prime source of morbidity. The right brachiocephalic vein is related anteriorly to the sternohyoid and sternothyroid attachments on the deep aspect of the sternum and, more inferiorly, to the first costal cartilage. Posteriorly, it is related to the pleura and brachiocephalic artery. Medial to it are the brachiocephalic artery and vagus nerve, whereas the pleura and phrenic nerve lie lateral to it. Anterior to the left brachiocephalic vein, the thymus or its remnant separates the vein from the sternum and its related muscles. Posterior to the vein are the arch of the aorta, the roots of all three great arteries, the trachea, the vagus, and the phrenic nerves. Remember that, frequently, a part of the left brachiocephalic vein is superior to the top of the manubrium and, thus can be palpated in the jugular notch.

STEPS IN PROCEDURE—ULTRASOUND-GUIDED SUBCLAVIAN VENOUS CANNULATION

Scan infraclavicular region with ultrasound and use this information to optimize patient position

Drape transducer into sterile field

Scan infraclavicular region and visualize subclavian vein

Holding transducer with your nondominant hand, anesthetize skin and subcutaneous tissues

Aspirate as You Walk the Needle Under the Clavicle to Find the Vein

(Maintain Needle in a Plane Parallel to the Floor)

Maintain transducer in plane of vein and plane of needle, visualize needle as it enters vein

Noting trajectory, remove smaller gauge needle and pass large-gauge needle under ultrasound guidance

Needle will first tent the vein, then pierce it

When intraluminal position is confirmed by free aspiration of blood, proceed as outlined in Section 14.1

Ultrasound-Guided Approach to the Subclavian Vein

Landmarks and Incision (Fig. 14.3)

Technical and Anatomic Points

Perform an initial scan of the infraclavicular region with a 3-cm linear 5-MHz ultrasound transducer and identify the subclavian vein. The clavicle and the subclavian artery may also be seen. Use this information to optimize patient positioning to maximize the lumen and accessibility of the vein.

Then prepare the sterile field as usual, but in addition drape the ultrasound transducer so it is accessible. Place the transducer slightly inferior to the midportion of the clavicle. Find the vein by angling the transduced superiorly. Color Doppler may be helpful, but is not essential. The vein will be seen to be compressible, and the lumen will change with respiratory phase. The subclavian artery will not be compressible, will generally be slightly smaller than the vein, and will not vary with respiratory phase.

Holding the transducer in your nondominant hand, choose a skin entry site lateral to the transducer and anesthetize the skin and subcutaneous tissues. Find the subclavian vein with the small caliber anesthetizing needle. Then pass the larger needle along the same trajectory, watching it first tent the vein and then pierce and enter the lumen of the vein. After venous access is confirmed by free flow of venous blood, proceed as previously described.

STEPS IN PROCEDURE—CUTDOWN ON THE CEPHALIC VEIN IN THE DELTOPECTORAL GROOVE

Identify the deltopectoral groove by palpating head of humerus and muscular heads of deltoid muscle and pectoralis major muscle

Transverse skin crease incision about two fingerbreadths below lateral aspect of clavicle, just medial to head of humerus

Dissect to fascia overlying pectoralis major muscle

Follow this muscle laterally and identify a slight change in muscle fiber direction

where the deltoid adjoins the pectoral muscle

Work in the fatty tissues in this groove to identify the cephalic vein

Elevate the vein and encircle it with two loops of 2-0 silk

Create a venotomy and pass the catheter

Confirm adequate position by fluoroscopy and tie silks

Close incision in layers

Secure catheter

Cutdown on the Cephalic Vein in the Deltopectoral Groove

Landmarks and Incision (Fig. 14.4)

Technical Points

The cephalic vein runs in a fairly constant position in the deltopectoral groove. Identify the deltopectoral groove by palpating the head of the humerus and the muscular heads of the deltoid muscle and the pectoralis major muscle. Prep and drape the field, which includes the lateral half of the pectoralis major muscle, the inferior border of the clavicle, and the medial portion of the head of the humerus. Make a transverse skin incision about two fingerbreadths below the clavicle, just medial to the head of the humerus.

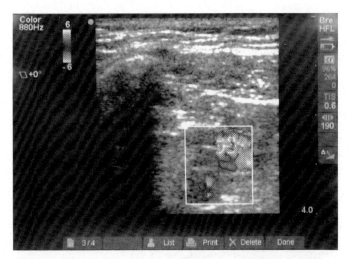

Figure 14.3 Percutaneous subclavian venous cannulation using ultrasound guidance

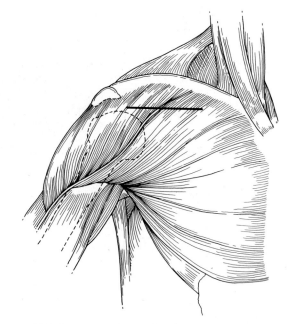

Figure 14.4 Landmarks and incision

HALLMARK ANATOMIC COMPLICATIONS—CUTDOWN ON THE CEPHALIC VEIN IN THE DELTOPECTORAL GROOVE
Inability to find the vein
Inability to pass catheter because of angulation
    at entry site into axillary vein

Anatomic Points

The cephalic vein begins on the radial side of the dorsum of the hand and then ascends in the superficial fascia to the deltopectoral triangle, where it pierces the deep fascia, ultimately ending in the axillary vein. In the arm, it is typically located in the groove lateral to the biceps brachii muscle; in the upper arm, this groove and the vein are medial to the anterior edge of the deltoid muscle.

Location of the Vein and Cannulation (Fig. 14.5)

Technical Points

By sharp and blunt dissection, carry the dissection down to the fascia overlying the pectoralis major muscle. Follow this muscle and identify where it lies separate from the adjacent deltoid muscle. This site is identifiable by a slight change in muscle fiber direction. Often, a distinct groove can be found. Spread with a hemostat in the fatty tissue of the groove and identify the cephalic vein. Elevate it into the field and secure it with two loops of 2-0 silk. Make a venotomy on the anterior surface of the vein and introduce the catheter through the venotomy.

The catheter should place easily. Occasionally, the catheter will "hang up" at the angulation between the cephalic vein and the axillary vein. If this happens, move the arm slightly or apply digital pressure in the field to guide the catheter around the bend. Confirm adequate positioning of the catheter by fluoroscopy and tie it in position in the vein. Ligate the distal end of the vein. Close the incision in layers with absorbable suture material.

Anatomic Points

When the cephalic vein reaches the deltopectoral triangle, it pierces the investing fascia covering the pectoralis major and deltoid muscles, continues for a short distance in the plane just deep to that fascia, and then pierces the clavipectoral fascia, just inferior to the clavicle, ending in the axillary vein. Difficulty in locating the vein in the deltopectoral triangle may be attributable to a developmental variation (e.g., absence, hypoplasia) or failure to divide the investing fascia, which will result in looking for the vein in an inappropriate tissue plane. Another variant—a branch that passes anterior to the clavicle and ends in the external jugular vein—could also present problems.

A final point to remember is that, when the cephalic vein ends, its junction with the axillary vein is almost 90 degrees with respect to the latter vein. Further, it tends to terminate on the superior aspect of the axillary vein, so that elevation of the arm may make the angle between the cephalic and axillary veins sharper, thereby making passage of the catheter into the subclavian vein more difficult than need be.

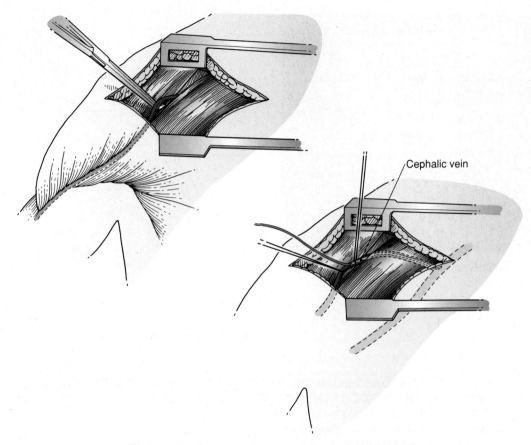

Figure 14.5 Location of the vein and cannulation

REFERENCES

1. Abboud PA, Kendall JL. Ultrasound guidance for vascular access. *Emerg Med Clin North Am.* 2004;22:749–773.
2. Au FC. The anatomy of the cephalic vein. *Am Surg.* 1989;55:638–639.
3. Brooks AJ, Alfredson M, Pettigrew B, et al. Ultrasound-guided insertion of subclavian venous access ports. *Ann R Coll Surg Engl.* 2005;87:25–27.
4. Hawkins J, Nelson EW. Percutaneous placement of Hickman catheters for prolonged venous access. *Am J Surg.* 1982;144:624–626.
5. Heimbach DM, Ivey TD. Technique for placement of a permanent home hyperalimentation catheter. *Surg Gynecol Obstet.* 1976;143:634–636. (This original technique of placement by cutdown includes a description of catheter placement in the cephalic or internal jugular vein, a procedure that is still applicable when percutaneous subclavian access is contraindicated.)
6. Holland AJ, Ford WD. Improved percutaneous insertion of long-term central venous catheters in children: The 'shrug' manoeuvre. *Aust N Z J Surg.* 1999;69:231–233.
7. Jensen MO. Anatomical basis of central venous catheter fracture. *Clin Anat.* 2008;21:106–110.
8. Karanlik H, Kurul S, Saip P, et al. The role of antibiotic prophylaxis in totally implantable venous access device placement: Results of a single-center prospective randomized trial. *Am J Surg.* 2011;202:10–15.
9. Lefrant JY, Cuvillon P, Benezet JF, et al. Pulsed Doppler ultrasonography guidance for catheterization of the subclavian vein: A randomized study. *Anesthesiology.* 1998;88:1195–1201.
10. Muhm M, Sunder-Plassmann G, Apsner R, et al. Supraclavicular approach to the subclavian/innominate vein for large-bore central venous catheters. *Am J Kidney Dis.* 1997;30:802–808. (Describes an alternative approach to the infraclavicular method described in this chapter.)
11. Narducci F, Jean-Laurent M, Boulanger L, et al. Totally implantable venous access port systems and risk factors for complications: A one-year prospective study in a cancer centre. *Eur J Surg Oncol.* 2011;37:913–918.
12. Orsi F, Grasso RF, Arnaldi P, et al. Ultrasound guided versus direct vein puncture in central venous port placement. *J Vasc Access.* 2000;1:73–77.
13. Sterchi JM, Fulks D, Cruz J, et al. Operative technique for insertion of a totally implantable system for venous access. *Surg Gynecol Obstet.* 1986;163:381–382. (Describes the modification needed for placement of totally implantable devices.)
14. Tan BK, Hong SW, Huang MH, et al. Anatomic basis of safe percutaneous subclavian venous catheterization. *J Trauma.* 2000;48:82–86.
15. Tercan F, Ozkan U, Oguzkurt L. US-guided placement of central vein catheters in patients with disorders of hemostasis. *Eur J Radiol.* 2008;65:253–256.
16. Walser EM. Venous access ports: Indications, implantation technique, follow-up, and complications. *Cardiovasc Intervent Radiol.* 2012;35:751–764.
17. Wilson SE, Stabile BE, Williams RA, et al. Current status of vascular access techniques. *Surg Clin North Am.* 1982;62:531–551.

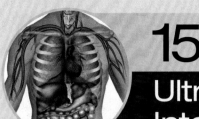

15

Ultrasound-Guided Breast Interventions

This chapter introduces the ultrasound anatomy of the breast and how to use ultrasound to guide various interventions including cyst aspiration, core needle biopsy, and lumpectomy.

SCORE™, the Surgical Council on Resident Education, classified Aspiration of breast cyst as an "ESSENTIAL COMMON" procedure.

STEPS IN PROCEDURE

Ultrasound-Guided Aspiration

Visualize lesion and establish ergonomically sound and safe approach for needle

Prepare sterile field and anesthetize skin

Introduce needle under ultrasound guidance and record image

Aspirate fluid until structure collapses and record image

If cyst is complex or there is suspicion of malignancy, submit fluid for cytology and place marking clip

Ultrasound-Guided Core Biopsy

Visualize lesion and prepare as noted above

Create skin nick with number 11 blade

Introduce spring-loaded core biopsy needle so that it is just touching lesion (ultrasound guidance) and record image

Fire device and record image

Remove needle and retrieve core

Obtain six cores in this fashion

Place clip into biopsy site

Ultrasound-Guided Lumpectomy

Use ultrasound to image lesion or biopsy cavity and clip (having previously confirmed ability to visualize in clinic)

Mark skin overlying lesion

Perform lumpectomy in usual fashion

Confirm presence of target lesion and adequacy of margins by ultrasound of specimen, x-ray of specimen, or immediate pathologic examination

HALLMARK ANATOMIC COMPLICATIONS

Puncture of chest cavity (needle passed too deep)   Missed lesion

LIST OF STRUCTURES

Areola

Internal thoracic (mammary) vessels

Pectoral fascia

Cooper's ligaments

Ribs

Ultrasound Landmarks (Fig. 15.1)

Technical and Anatomic Points

This section covers the basic ultrasound anatomy of the normal breast and describes how ultrasound may be used to guide various percutaneous interventions ranging from aspiration of breast cysts through core biopsy of lesions and drainage of seromas. References at the end of this chapter give additional information. Hands-on courses such as those offered by the American College of Surgeons or the American Society of Breast Surgeons are essential to the process of learning how to use ultrasound in this area.

The transducer generally used for breast ultrasound is a 7.5-MHz linear array transducer. Two standard orientations (transverse and vertical) are used and indicated on a diagram or pictogram on the image. A radial orientation for the transducer may be preferred, particularly when ducts near the nipple are scanned; in this case, the second image is taken at right angles to the first. Surgeons typically perform focused (as apposed to screening) ultrasound examinations. A focused examination places the transducer over a specific region of concern, such as a palpable abnormality.

The normal ultrasound anatomy of the breast (Fig. 15.1A) includes skin, subcutaneous fat, Cooper's ligament, pectoralis major muscle and/or ribs, and pleura.

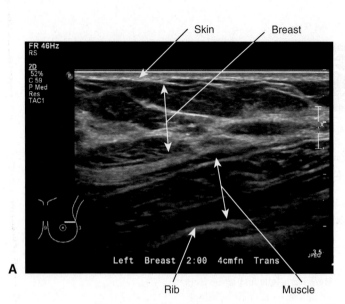

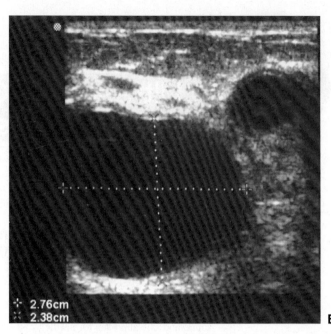

Figure 15.1 Ultrasound landmarks. **A:** Ultrasound landmarks. **B:** Breast cysts showing approximate measurements of larger cyst.

Place the transducer over the region of interest and scan slowly over the area. Realize that the transducer may slip rapidly off the surface of a mobile lesion such as a fibroadenoma, making it difficult to image the mass. In this case, "trap" the lesion between the fingers of your nondominant hand as you guide the transducer with your dominant hand.

After the abnormality is imaged, optimize the image using the time-gain, resolution, and depth controls. Record two orthogonal views for the medical record. For each view, place calipers to measure the lesion. By convention, the first caliper is placed along the greatest dimension and the second caliper is placed at right angles to the first.

Note the characteristics of the mass. Fluid-filled structures such as cysts or seromas are hypoechoic (black), clearly demarcated, and show posterior enhancement and some degree of edge enhancement (Fig. 15.1B). They are usually compressible and often wider than they are tall. Benign lesions in general tend to be very well demarcated and to displace rather than invade adjacent structures. In contrast, malignancies are irregular, sometimes speculated, and invade adjacent structures. They are frequently hypoechoic and exhibit posterior shadowing. An increase in vasculature may be seen with Doppler. They are generally not compressible and are frequently taller than they are wide. Note: *Do not rely on your interpretation of the appearance of a lesion to determine that it is benign—you are not a radiologist!* Rather use the ultrasound to guide a diagnostic intervention such as aspiration or core biopsy.

Ultrasound-Guided Aspiration (Fig. 15.2)

Technical and Anatomic Points

If an ultrasound-guided intervention is planned, take care to find an optimum transducer location and skin entry site. Take

a few minutes to establish an ergonomically satisfactory layout. You should be able to stand or sit comfortably facing the screen. An assistant will manipulate the controls.

Prep a sterile field including a sterile cover for the ultrasound transducer. Anesthetize the area. Introduce a long needle at a shallow angle under ultrasound visualization. A spinal needle works well for this purpose. The shallower your angle of entry, the brighter the reflection will appear on the screen.

Watch the needle enter the fluid-filled structure (Fig. 15.2A). Record an image. Be aware that the ultrasound beam is only about the thickness of a credit card. The beam and needle must be in the same plane for the ultrasound to "see" the needle. A needle guide is available, but most surgeons prefer to free hand the needle.

Aspirate fluid and record an image with the needle in the collapsed cyst or seroma (Fig. 15.2B).

If you are sufficiently concerned about possible malignancy to send the fluid for cytology, place a clip (see below). Otherwise, you may not be able to identify the location of the (now completely collapsed) cyst for excision.

Core Biopsy of Lesions (Fig. 15.3)

Technical and Anatomic Points

A variety of spring-loaded and vacuum-driven biopsy devices are available. This section describes the use of the spring-loaded devices.

Know the characteristics of the biopsy device you will be using. Practice firing it so that the patient will become accustomed to the sound (and so that you will be facile with the use of the device). Most devices are designed to be placed touching the mass. Firing the device triggers a spring-loaded release that shoots the needle forward for a fixed distance and cutting the core. The distance that the needle shoots forward is termed

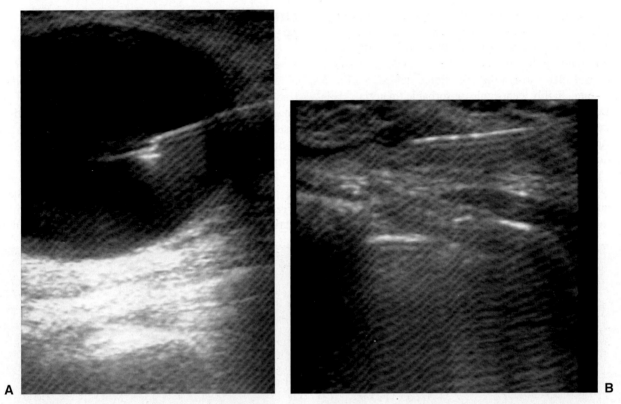

Figure 15.2 Ultrasound-guided aspiration. **A:** Needle in good position in cyst. **B:** Cyst almost completely collapsed after aspiration.

throw. It is essential to know the throw of the device you are using.

Identify the lesion of concern and find a transducer position that allows easy access to the mass. Prep and anesthetize the skin, taking care to use sufficient local anesthesia to flood the subcutaneous tissues. Generally 10 to 20 mL will be required to infiltrate the skin and entire proposed track.

Make a nick in the skin using a number 11 blade. Take the precocked device in your dominant hand in such a way that a finger or thumb is positioned right over the trigger button. Introduce the needle under ultrasound guidance so that it is just touching the lesion (Fig. 15.3A). Record an image.

Warn the patient to expect a loud click. Fire the needle. Record a second image with the needle in the lesion (Fig. 15.3B). Remove the device and harvest the core. Tumor tissue tends to be very white or gray (as apposed to yellow fat) and to sink when put into formalin (fatty tissue will float). Try to obtain six good "sinker" cores.

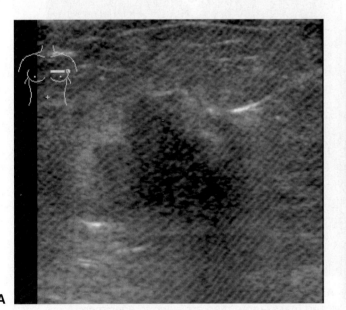
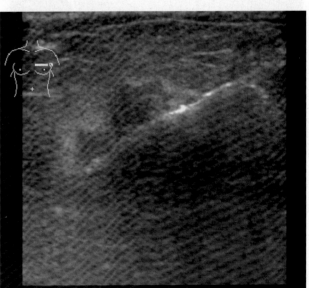

Figure 15.3 Ultrasound-guided core biopsy. **A:** Needle in pre-fire position. **B:** Needle in post-fire position.

Place a clip into the center of the region that was sampled. As with biopsy devices, there are several clip appliers available. All work in a similar way. Place the hollow needle containing the clip into the biopsy cavity under ultrasound guidance and then extrude the clip. Some devices will also extrude some highly echogenic absorbable material. This enhances the ability to find the cavity again under ultrasound guidance.

Compare the pathology report with the ultrasound findings for concordance. If the biopsy was done for presumed cancer, and the pathology does not reveal carcinoma or yield a satisfactory alternative diagnosis such as fibroadenoma, then the biopsy must be repeated. Often the safest course in this situation is to excise the abnormality.

Ultrasound-Guided Lumpectomy (Fig. 15.4)

When excision of a nonpalpable mass is required, operative ultrasound provides an alternative to preoperative needle localization (Chapter 16). First determine in the clinic that you can image the target lesion. If you are unable to image the target lesion with certainty in the clinic, do not attempt to localize it this way in the operating room; perform needle-localized biopsy as previously described.

In the operating room, use the ultrasound before the sterile prep is initiated to determine the location of the lesion (Fig. 15.4A). Mark the location in two dimensions with a skin marker. Make the incision and excise the lesion in the usual

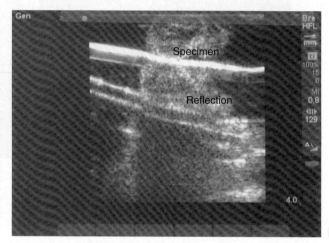

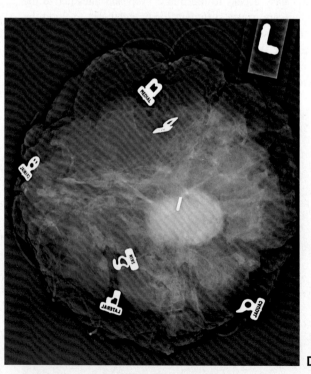

Figure 15.4 Ultrasound-guided lumpectomy. **A:** Ultrasound showing mass. **B:** Ultrasound of specimen. **C:** Specimen radiograph showing clip and mass—note markers sewn to specimen for orientation. **D:** Another view of a specimen radiograph.

fashion. Confirm adequacy of excision by one of the following methods: Ultrasound of excised lesion (Fig. 15.4B), specimen radiograph (Fig. 15.4C,D), or immediate gross examination in the pathology laboratory. Note the use of six metallic markers which provide specimen orientation. These help in assessing potentially close margins on specimen radiograph, and assure accurate orientation in the pathology laboratory. It is crucial to ensure adequate excision of the target at the time of surgery, just as it is with needle-localized biopsy.

Some surgeons prefer to drape the ultrasound probe into the sterile field and use it to guide excision, in the hope that this will improve margin control. Studies are ongoing to determine which technique will work best.

REFERENCES

1. American Society of Breast Surgeons. Ultrasound certification program. Available online at: http://www.breastsurgeons.org/certification.shtml. (This site also gives information about courses in breast ultrasound.)
2. Arentz C, Baxter K, Boneti C, et al. Ten-year experience with hematoma-directed ultrasound-guided (HUG) breast lumpectomy. *Ann Surg Oncol.* 2010;17:378–383.
3. Cardenosa G. *The Core Curriculum: Breast Imaging.* Philadelphia, PA: Lippincott Williams & Wilkins; 2003.
4. Hernanz F, Regano S, Vega A, et al. Needle-wire-guided breast tumor excision. *J Surg Oncol.* 2006;94:165–166.
5. Kass RB, Lind DS, Souba WW. Chapter 5. Breast procedures. In: Souba WW, Fink MP, Jurkovich GJ, Kaiser LP et al., eds. *ACS Surgery: Principles and Practice.* 6th ed. Section 5. Breast Procedures. New York, NY: WebMD Professional Publishing; 2005.
6. Kopans DB. Breast ultrasound. In: Kopans DB, ed. *Breast Imaging.* 3rd ed. Philadelphia, PA: Lippincott Williams & Wilkins; 1998:555–606.
7. Larrieux G, Cupp JA, Liao J, et al. Effect of introducing hematoma ultrasound-guided lumpectomy in a surgical practice. *J Am Coll Surg.* 2012;215:237–243.

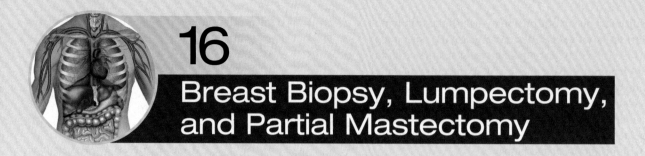

16

Breast Biopsy, Lumpectomy, and Partial Mastectomy

This chapter describes how palpable and nonpalpable masses are excised. Every effort should be made before surgery to determine whether the mass is benign or malignant, because this determines the width of margins necessary. With the wealth of image-guided percutaneous biopsy techniques available, as well as fine needle aspiration for cytology, it is rarely necessary to excise a mass simply to get a diagnosis.

When the lesion is not palpable, or when resection is needed after core biopsy, the lesion must be localized by hookwire placement under radiographic or ultrasound guidance (see Fig. 16.3). Ultrasound-guided localization is an alternative described in Chapter 15.

The chapter also describes how lumpectomy and partial mastectomy are performed for the treatment of breast cancer or ductal carcinoma in situ (DCIS).

SCORE™, the Surgical Council on Resident Education, classified breast biopsy with or without needle localization, and partial mastectomy, as "ESSENTIAL COMMON" procedures.

STEPS IN PROCEDURE

Palpable Mass
Circumareolar incision where feasible
Incision directly over mass if necessary
Raise flaps
Transfix mass with traction suture
Excise with appropriate margin, orient specimen

Nonpalpable Mass with Needle Localization
Inspect localization radiographs and trajectory of needle, estimate position of lesion
Make incision over likely location of mass
Circumareolar incision may be used for lesion close to areolar margin

Deliver wire into wound
Transfix tissue around wire with traction suture
Excise tissue around wire, leaving tip of wire to final part of dissection
Orient specimen
Radiograph specimen to determine adequacy of excision
    Larger margin and more careful excision of all abnormal tissue needed for DCIS or breast cancer (partial mastectomy)
Obtain hemostasis
Close incision in layers without a drain

HALLMARK ANATOMIC COMPLICATIONS

Missed lesion or failure of localization (needle localized)

Broken wire, necessitating retrieval with metal detector
Hematoma

LIST OF STRUCTURES

Breast
Nipple areola
Axillary tail of Spence

Choice of Incision (Fig. 16.1)

Technical Points

For most easily palpable lesions that lie within several centimeters of the areola, a circumareolar incision is appropriate for obtaining a biopsy specimen. However, biopsy of ill-defined masses that are not easily reached using this approach should be accomplished through an incision placed directly over the mass. In such cases, the incision should be gently curved in the upper or lower parts of the breast, and should be transverse, or nearly so, in the medial or lateral aspects. This allows the scar to be hidden by clothing or readily incorporated into a mastectomy incision should that procedure be indicated.

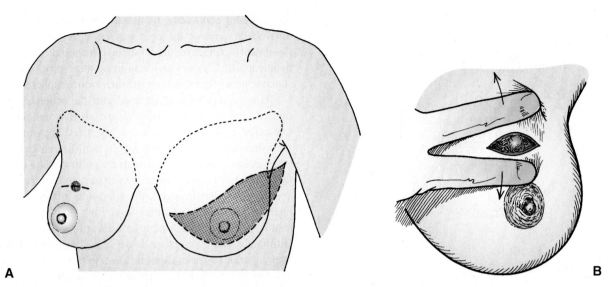

Figure 16.1 Choice of incision. **A:** Incision made as low as possible in natural skin crease. **B:** Incision in skin crease directly over palpable mass.

Radial incisions, once advocated because they parallel the underlying duct structure of the breast, yield poor cosmetic results and should be used only for very medial or lateral lesions. When planning the incision, remember that the biopsy site will have to be excised with a skin margin should subsequent mastectomy be required. For this reason, inframammary incisions, although cosmetically appealing, are generally avoided.

Choose a site for incision and infiltrate the area with local anesthetic. If the mass becomes difficult to palpate after the skin preparation has been done, wash the skin of the breast with sterile saline and palpate by sliding gloved fingers over the wet skin.

Anatomic Points

The breast, which is wholly contained within superficial fascia, extends from the second rib superiorly to the sixth rib inferiorly and from the sternum to the midaxillary line. The axillary tail of Spence is an extension of breast tissue into the axilla. The breast is composed of 15 to 20 glandular lobes and adipose tissue arranged radially around the nipple-areolar complex. These are separated by fibrous septa, fibers of which attach to the deep surface of the skin and to the deep layer of the superficial fascia (suspensory ligaments of Spence). The glandular tissue of the lobes, each based on a lactiferous duct that drains at the apex of the nipple, tends to be located more centrally, whereas the adipose tissue tends to be located more peripherally.

A circumareolar incision produces a scar that is almost hidden in the abrupt change in skin pigmentation at the areolar margin. If the location of the lesion makes this impossible, the incision should approximate the direction of the skin cleavage lines. These lines are concentrically arranged around the nipple, although in pendulous breasts, the effects of gravity are superimposed on this pattern. The surgeon should be aware of the underlying radial breast architecture and should restrict the initial incision to the skin.

Biopsy of a Palpable Mass (Fig. 16.2)

Technical Points

Make a circumareolar incision and raise a flap (generally, 0.5 cm in thickness) in the cleavage plane between the subcutaneous tissue and the breast. This is the same plane in which mastectomies are performed. Place retractors to pull the incision closer to the mass. Identify the mass by palpation. If necessary, cut through the overlying breast tissue to expose the mass. Place a traction suture of 2-0 silk in a figure-of-eight fashion through the mass. (Use a curved cutting needle because the tough, fibrous breast tissue will bend a tapered-point needle.) Pull up on the traction suture to elevate the mass into the field. Excise the mass by sharp dissection using a knife or Mayo scissors. Avoid overzealous use of electrocautery on the biopsy specimen because this can render assessment of margins difficult, particularly in borderline lesions. Take care not to violate the pectoral fascia by cutting too deeply because this fascia provides a natural barrier that will help to prevent contamination of the mastectomy field with spilled tumor cells if subsequent mastectomy is performed.

Feel both the excised mass and the residual breast cavity to ascertain that the palpable lesion has been removed. Request that receptor and tumor markers be done if the biopsy is positive for carcinoma. Some laboratories may require that fresh tissue be submitted; know the requirements of your pathologist.

If the mass is ill-defined or is located at some distance from the areola, it is safest to make the incision directly over the mass. In such cases, cosmetic considerations should be set aside because the first priority is an accurate diagnosis. Stabilize the mass with the fingers of the nondominant hand and infiltrate the overlying skin with anesthetic. Continue to hold the mass firmly anchored as you make the skin incision. Place retractors to visualize the underlying breast tissue. Place a traction suture in the mass. The traction suture can then be used to manipulate the mass as it is excised.

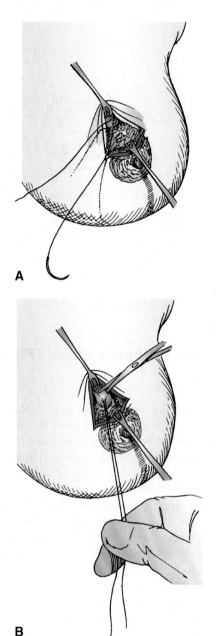

A

B

Figure 16.2 Biopsy of a palpable mass. **A:** Traction suture placed to deliver benign mass into low incision. **B:** Excision of retracted mass.

Perform local excision (lumpectomy) of early breast carcinomas as an excisional biopsy, taking care not to contaminate the biopsy field by cutting into tumor. Remove the lesion along with a generous rim of the surrounding, grossly normal breast tissue, and have the pathologist ink the specimen and check the margins for adequacy of excision. Orient the specimen for the pathologist.

Anatomic Points

In raising a skin flap, one gets the impression that the breast is surrounded by an adipose "capsule" that is prominent everywhere except deep to the nipple and the areola. However, throughout this capsule, connective tissue strands connect interlobar and interlobular septa to the deep surface of the dermis. The more prominent connective tissue strands constitute the suspensory ligaments (of Cooper) and tend to be more pronounced on the superior hemisphere than on the inferior hemisphere.

After a skin flap is elevated and the adipose capsule is opened, the breast parenchyma and stroma will be encountered. The glandular parenchyma, organized in pyramidal lobes with their apices toward the nipple, will be recognized by its white color, which contrasts with the yellow-white color of the fat. Although fibrous connective tissue tends to be interlobar and thus radially arranged, the continuity of these septa with interlobular fibers and fibers separating adipose tissue loculi results in an irregular, spongy distribution of this tissue type. Ultimately, the connective tissue septa connect to the fibrous deep layer of superficial fascia. Deep to this fascial layer, a thin layer of loose connective tissue with a small amount of retromammary fat separates the breast from the pectoral fascia, the deep or investing fascia of the muscles of the pectoral region. This loose areolar tissue should warn you of impending exposure of pectoral fascia.

Needle-Localized Breast Biopsy (Fig. 16.3)

Technical and Anatomic Points

Close communication between the mammographer or the ultrasonographer and surgeon is essential. Review the prelocalization and postlocalization radiographic films with the radiologist and be certain that you understand the three-dimensional relationship between the skin entry site, the shaft of the wire, the thickened portion of the shaft, the hooked tip of the wire, and the target lesion.

Standard hookwires are used for mammographic and ultrasound localization. These are fairly robust. The hookwires used for MRI localization are significantly less robust and are easily transected by electrocautery.

Remove the dressing from the breast with care because the wire can become dislodged if pulled too hard. Prepare the entire breast and the wire. Gently tug on the exposed wire while feeling the underlying breast along the projected course of the needle. Often, the site of the target lesion can be identified by noting the region of the breast that moves slightly as the wire is tugged. Plan an incision that is cosmetically acceptable yet close to the tip of the wire. It may be possible to use a circumareolar incision; however, most of the time, it is preferable to make the incision as close as possible to the terminal 2 to 3 cm of wire. Generally, the incision should not be made over the skin entry site of the wire, which is commonly at some distance from the areola and also far from the target lesion.

Elevate a flap toward the wire and expose it. If dissection becomes difficult, use a knife because scissors can cut the wire. Identify the wire by the tactile sensation of the steel on steel and by noting motion of the exposed wire as you probe. Anchor

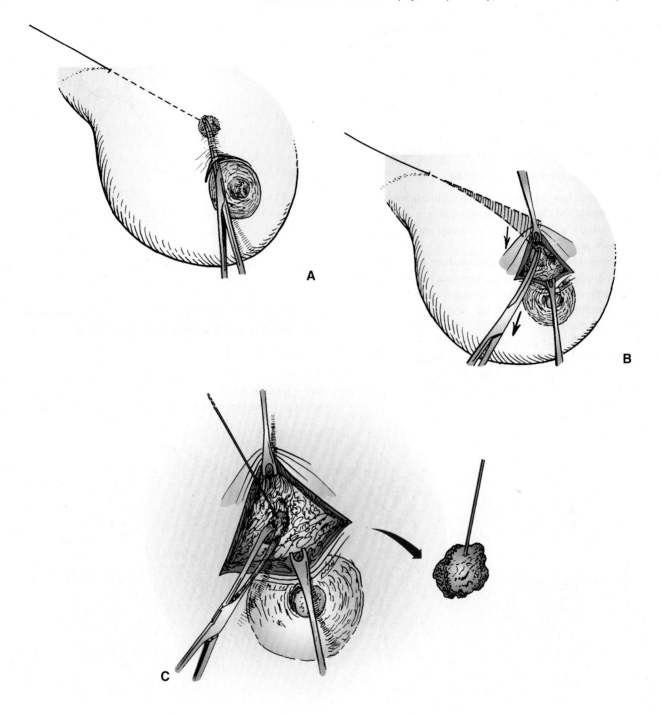

Figure 16.3 Needle-localized breast biopsy. **A:** Incision made over mass. **B:** Dissection to mass and wire. **C:** Removal of mass and wire.

the distal wire with a hemostat so that it is not inadvertently pulled out, and then deliver the proximal end of the wire into the wound by pulling it back through the skin. Periodically verify, by gentle traction on the wire, the probable location of the tip. Dissect down parallel to, but 1 to 2 cm distant from, the wire. Start the dissection behind the wire and work toward the tip. Often, a previously nonpalpable target lesion becomes palpable as dissection progresses.

Terminate the dissection by cutting well past the tip of the wire. Remember that the best chance to excise the target lesion is at the first pass. After the wire has been removed, orientation is lost. Submit the wire and specimen for radiographic study, returning the mammograms with the specimen for comparison. Feel the cavity for any residual abnormal tissue. Excise and submit for specimen radiography any palpably abnormal residual tissue in the biopsy cavity.

Close the incision after receiving confirmation that the target area was included in the specimen. If the lesion was missed, a review of localization films and specimen radiographs will frequently provide a clue as to which portion of the cavity wall undergoing biopsy is likely to contain the area of interest.

Closure of the Incision (Fig. 16.4)

Technical and Anatomic Points

Achieve complete hemostasis in the biopsy incision by irrigating it to remove blood clots and then sequentially grasping portions of the cavity wall with an Allis clamp and pulling them up for inspection.

Most surgeons do not place sutures deep in the breast to close the cavity or to attempt to "reconstruct" the breast, especially for minor excisions such as fibroadenomas. Such sutures create a deformity by tethering the normally mobile, fluid breast tissue. Place several interrupted fine absorbable sutures to approximate the subcutaneous fat just under the skin and close the skin incision with a subcuticular suture. Drains are rarely used. Either a pressure dressing or, preferably, a light dressing held by a snugly fitting brassiere will help to prevent hematoma formation.

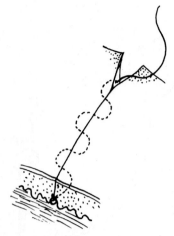

Figure 16.4 Closure of the incision

Partial Mastectomy or Lumpectomy for DCIS or Cancer (Fig. 16.5)

Technical and Anatomic Points

Lumpectomy (partial mastectomy) is performed for cancer using most of the same techniques already described. However, several important differences warrant special consideration.

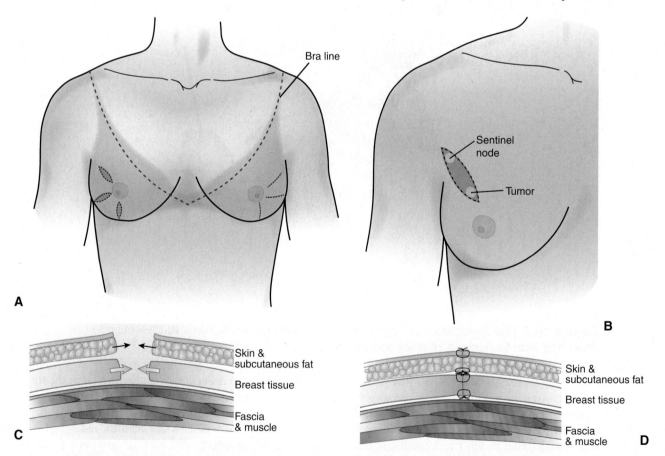

Figure 16.5 Partial mastectomy for cancer or DCIS. **A:** Radial incisions allow resection of some skin, if necessary, without distorting shape. **B:** Long radial incision with skin excision for lumpectomy and sentinel node biopsy. **C:** Undermining layers to facilitate closure. **D:** Oncoplastic closure to eliminate dead space and maximize cosmetic appearance.

First, it is extremely important to plan the incision with care. Generally the incision is made directly over the malignancy. If the tumor is close to the skin, it may be necessary to excise an ellipse of skin to get an adequate superficial margin. This is best accomplished with a radial incision (Fig. 16.5A) as an incision parallel to the areola is likely to pull the nipple-areolar complex toward the incision.

Many cancers occur in the upper outer quadrant, simply because this is where the largest amount of breast tissue is located. A long radially oriented incision in this area may also be used to access the sentinel node, if sentinel node biopsy is planned (Fig. 16.5B). Alternatively, sentinel node biopsy can be done through a separate incision (see Chapter 20).

If at all possible, keep the incision below an imaginary "bra line" running from the acromioclavicular joint lateral to the xiphoid medially, so that the scar will be concealed by clothing. Incisions under this line are also easier to incorporate into a mastectomy if subsequent mastectomy is required.

Generally the excision of breast tissue is taken down to the fascia. It may be necessary to excise a disk of fascia or even underlying muscle to get a clear margin.

The amount of clean margin required for adequate treatment continues to be a matter of some contention, and failure to attain an adequate margin is a major cause of return to the operating room for additional surgery. Generally, this will require excision of a greater amount of tissue than described for breast biopsy or excision of a benign mass. This results in a larger cavity. Some surgeons will close this cavity by mobilizing the breast tissue off the underlying fascia to mobilize the remaining breast tissue (Fig. 16.5C) and placing deep sutures (Fig. 16.5D), with the goal of remodeling the breast to a slightly smaller size which is; however, normal in conformation. Excising a lens-shaped segment of overlying skin actually helps this process by eliminating dead space under the skin. Oncoplastic resection techniques described in Chapter 19 combine the excision of large amounts of breast tissue with remodeling of the shape of the breast.

Postoperative radiation therapy is an important part of breast conservation for the majority of patients. Intraoperative radiation therapy is described in references at the end of this chapter.

For decades, it was necessary to place clips to mark the boundaries of the lumpectomy cavity to help the radiation oncologist plan postoperative treatment. This is rarely needed with current treatment planning techniques; however, it is always good to communicate closely with your radiation oncologist and learn local preferences. If oncoplastic techniques will result in tissue rearrangement, clip placement is helpful.

Clip placement, if desired, is simple. Use medium hemo-clips to mark the medial, lateral, cephalad, caudad, and deep sides of the cavity. Simply pinch some tissue up with forceps and apply the clip. It is usually not necessary to mark the superficial boundary of the cavity. Place your clips before mobilizing breast tissue for closure.

Close the partial mastectomy incision without drains, even when sentinel lymph node biopsy is performed through the same incision.

REFERENCES

1. Arentz C, Baxter K, Boneti C, et al. Ten-year experience with hematoma-directed ultrasound-guided (HUG) breast lumpectomy. *Ann Surg Oncol.* 2010;17(suppl 3):378–383.
2. Baynosa J, Horst K, Dirbas FM. Chapter 72. Accelerated partial breast irradiation with intraoperative radiotherapy. In: Direbas FM, Scott-Conner CEH, eds. *Breast Surgical Techniques and Interdisciplinary Management.* New York, NY: Springer Verlag; 2011:883–897.
3. Biggers BD, Lamont JP, Etufugh CN, et al. Inframammary approach for removal of giant juvenile fibroadenomas. *J Am Coll Surg.* 2009;208:e1–e4.
4. Clough KB, Kaufman GJ, Nos C, et al. Improving breast cancer surgery: A classification and quadrant per quadrant atlas for oncoplastic surgery. *Ann Surg Oncol.* 2010;17:1375–1391. (Excellent description and careful explanation of oncoplastic techniques.)
5. Gainer SM, Lucci A. Oncoplastics: Techniques for reconstruction of partial breast defects based on tumor location. *J Surg Oncol.* 2011;103:341–347.
6. Henry-Tillman R, Johnson AT, Smith LF, et al. Intraoperative ultrasound and other techniques to achieve negative margins. *Semin Surg Oncol.* 2001;20:206–213.
7. Kaufman CS, Littrup PJ, Freeman-Gibb LA, et al. Office-based cryoablation of breast fibroadenomas with long-term follow-up. *Breast J.* 2005;11:344–350. (An alternative for biopsy-proven fibroadenomas that require intervention.)
8. Margenthaler JA. Optimizing conservative breast surgery. *J Surg Oncol.* 2011;103:306–312.
9. Nurko J, Mabry CD, Whitworth P, et al. Interim results from the Fibroadenoma Cryoablation Treatment Registry. *Am J Surg.* 2005; 190:647–651.
10. Silverstein MJ, Recht A, Lagios MD, et al. Special report: Consensus conference III. Image-detected breast cancer: State-of-the-art diagnosis and treatment. *J Am Coll Surg.* 2009;209:504–520.
11. Thompson M, Henry-Tillman R, Margulies A, et al. Hematoma-directed ultrasound-guided (HUG) breast lumpectomy. *Ann Surg Oncol.* 2007;14:148–156.

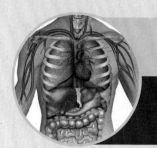

17

Surgery for Subareolar Abscess; Duct Excision

James P. De Andrade and Jesse L. Dirksen

An acute subareolar abscess can initially be treated with antibiotics and needle aspiration or incision and drainage as appropriate. However, these abscesses generally are associated with underlying duct pathology that predisposes to recurrence of abscess or formation of a mammary duct fistula. Thus, it is often necessary to excise the diseased subareolar ducts to prevent recurrence. Duct excision is also used to diagnose and treat nipple discharge. This chapter describes the management of subareolar abscesses as well as definitive surgical ductal excision for nipple discharge or chronic subareolar abscess.

SCORE™, the Surgical Council on Resident Education, classified incision, drainage, debridement for soft tissue infections, and duct excision as "ESSENTIAL COMMON" procedures.

STEPS IN PROCEDURE

Surgery for Subareolar Abscess
Inspect, palpate, and perform ultrasound imaging (if needed) of the abscess and overlying skin
Aspirate if small and liquid
Incise if complex
    Small, radially oriented incision at areolar border
Send fluid for culture

Duct Excision (Microdochectomy and Central Duct Excision)
Place lacrimal duct in offending duct

Incision
Circumareolar for nipple discharge
Radial ellipse for chronic subareolar abscess/ mammary fistula
Elevate flaps
Ligate duct(s) at undersurface of the nipple and do a wedge resection proximally
Orient the specimen
Obtain hemostasis
Close incision in two layers

HALLMARK ANATOMIC COMPLICATIONS

Subareolar Abscess
Recurrence or fistula formation
Incomplete evacuation of necrotic or purulent material
Undiagnosed inflammatory breast carcinoma

Duct Excision (Microdochectomy and Central Duct Excision)
Inverted nipple
Insensate nipple
Nipple necrosis

LIST OF STRUCTURES

Nipple
Areola
Subareolar ducts

Intercostal nerves 4 to 6
Lateral cutaneous branch
Anterior cutaneous branch

Subareolar Abscess

Technical and Anatomic Points

Examine the patient in the supine position with the ipsilateral arm extended above the patient's head. Suspect a subareolar abscess by location and setting (generally seen in nonlactating women). First, visually inspect the breast for the degree of erythema and the integrity of the skin overlying the abscess (Fig. 17.1). Second, palpate the area to determine the amount of induration and fluctuance. Finally, use an ultrasound machine to visualize if an abscess cavity is present and to determine if other adjacent loculated collections exist (please refer to breast ultrasound techniques described in Chapter 15). If the skin is not overly thinned or necrotic and an abscess cavity containing liquid contents and without loculations is visualized with ultrasound, the subareolar abscess is amenable to needle aspiration, either under direct palpation or with ultrasound guidance.

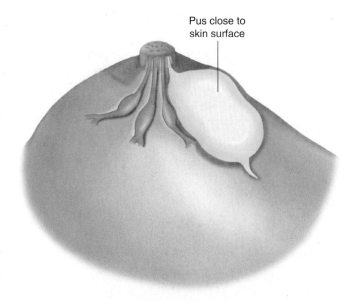

Pus close to
skin surface

Figure 17.1 Subareolar abscess shown in cross-section. Incision and drainage is best performed at areolar margin, where purulence is closest to skin surface (from Bland KI, Klimberg VS. *Master Techniques in General Surgery: Breast Surgery.* Philadelphia, PA: Lippincott Williams & Wilkins; 2011, with permission).

Aspiration is performed in a manner similar to cyst aspiration (see Chapter 15). Prep and drape the area in a sterile fashion. Most often, aspiration can be performed under palpation. If ultrasound is needed, drape the ultrasound transducer with a sterile cover. Anesthetize the area with local anesthetic using a 22- or 25-gauge needle. Using an 18-gauge needle, aspirate the abscess cavity under ultrasound guidance and then culture the fluid to tailor antibiotic therapy. The abscess cavity will collapse on ultrasound imaging if an adequate aspiration has been achieved. Ultrasound-guided aspiration may need to be

repeated every 2 to 3 days as the abscess cavity slowly collapses and heals in conjunction with antibiotics.

If the skin is significantly thinned or necrotic, the abscess should be managed with incision and drainage. Prep and drape the area and anesthetize with local anesthetic. A number 15 blade is used to make a stab incision into the abscess cavity and the purulent fluid is evacuated and cultured (Fig. 17.2A). The incision should be made along the areolar border, if possible, as this lends to a better cosmetic result. A small radially oriented incision facilitates subsequent ductal excision should this be required. Avoid using a long circumareolar incision as this may complicate subsequent excision. Use local anesthetic or sterile saline to irrigate the abscess cavity. Debride grossly nonviable tissue and send cultures. A small drain may be placed. Packing is not routinely utilized in the management of a subareolar abscess.

These abscesses are generally caused by ductal ectasia or other problem in the distal ducts such as stricture from nipple piercing (Fig. 17.2B). This underlying problem is not cured by aspiration or incision and drainage. Always warn the patient that recurrence is common. Recurrence may take the form of another abscess, or a chronic draining fistula at the areolar margin. This chronic draining fistula is termed a mammary duct fistula or mammary fistula. Definitive management requires duct excision.

Duct Excision (Microdochectomy and Central Duct Excision) for Nipple Discharge

Technical Points

If the offending duct(s) can be localized, a selective duct excision (microdochectomy) can be performed. If duct(s) cannot be identified, or in the case of a recurrent subareolar abscess with multiple diseased ducts, a central (or complete) duct excision should be completed.

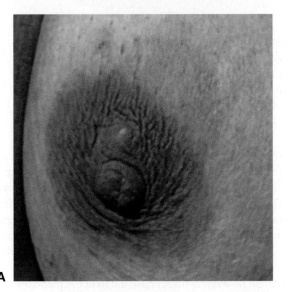

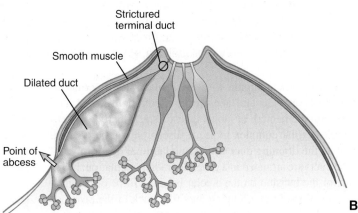

Strictured
terminal duct

Smooth muscle

Dilated duct

Point of
abcess

A   **B**

Figure 17.2 A: Chronic mammary fistula resulting from drainage of subareolar abscess. (Courtesy of Ingrid Lizarraga, MD.) **B:** Distal stricture in ducts leads to stagnation and abscess formation at areolar border.

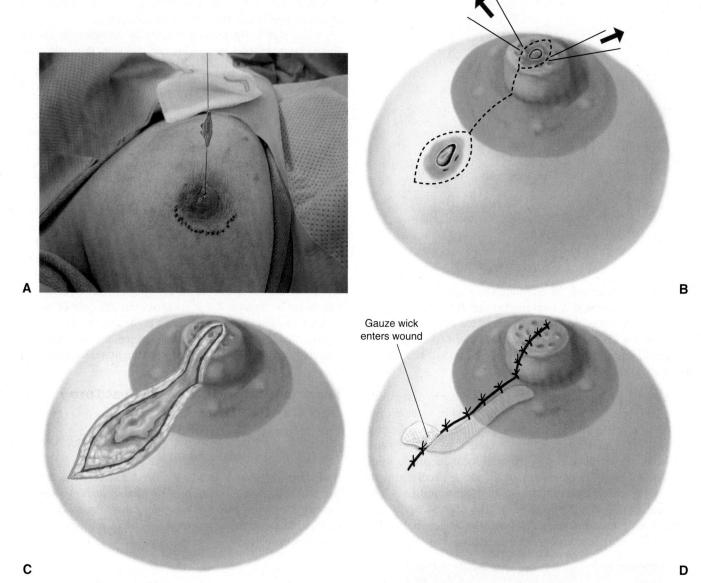

Figure 17.3 A: A circumareolar incision has been outlined and a lacrimal duct probe has been used to cannulate the offending duct. **B,C,D:** Alternative radial incision used primarily for the treatment of chronic mammary fistula (sinus tract and duct exit onto nipple surface, as well as entire duct, removed). A gauze wick or small diameter Penrose drain may be left in if purulence is encountered (from Bland KI, Klimberg VS. *Master Techniques in General Surgery: Breast Surgery.* Philadelphia, PA: Lippincott Williams & Wilkins; 2011, with permission).

Place the patient supine with the ipsilateral arm extended on an arm board. General anesthesia is commonly used, and may be supplemented by local anesthesia. Gently squeeze the nipple-areolar complex to see if discharge can be elicited. Cannulate the draining duct with a fine lacrimal duct probe.

The ducts are arranged in a generally radial orientation; hence the site of the incision on the areolar border will be determined by the direction of the offending duct (the track of the probe) if doing a selective duct excision. If performing a complete duct excision, the inferior areolar border is the preferred incision site, incorporating any previous scars when possible. A circumareolar incision provides the best cosmetic result as the scar is not easily visualized in the change in pigmentation at the areolar border.

Do not make an incision greater than 50% of the entire circumference of the areola, in order to avoid the risk of devascularization of the nipple and areola and to provide the best opportunity at maintaining sensation to the area. Of note, it might be helpful to outline the areolar border with a marking pen before prepping the patient, especially in those patients with a lightly pigmented areola, as a distinct areolar border might become difficult to visualize after prepping the patient (Fig. 17.3).

Once the incision is made, raise a flap in the plane between the subcutaneous tissue and the breast parenchyma on the side of the incision away from the nipple. On the areolar side of the incision, create a plane between the undersurface of the areolar and the central ducts (Fig. 17.4). This is often accomplished

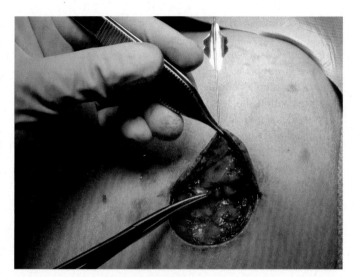

Figure 17.4 A plane of dissection is being developed on the undersurface of the areola.

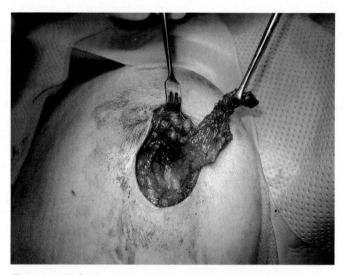

Figure 17.6 Excision of the offending duct and a wedge-shaped portion of proximal tissue.

with Metzenbaum scissors or a scalpel. Take care during this step to avoid back-walling instruments into the skin of the areola, especially common when the nipple is inverted (Fig. 17.5).

If doing a selective duct excision, use the lacrimal probe as a guide and ligate the duct from its termination under the nipple using fine absorbable suture. Dissect out and remove a wedge-shaped portion of proximal breast tissue (Fig. 17.6). It is important to ligate the remaining distal portion of the duct to prevent leakage of blood or fluid from the operative site through the transected duct.

For complete duct excision, use a curved hemostat to develop a plane on either side of the central ducts and subsequently connect the two planes to completely encircle the terminal ducts (Fig. 17.7). The terminal end under the nipple is ligated and excise a wedge-shaped portion of proximal breast tissue for 3 to 5 cm with electrocautery.

Orient the specimen before sending to pathology. If the nipple is inverted at the end of the case, place an absorbable

purse-string suture at the nipple base to keep the nipple everted. Hemostasis is achieved and the incision is closed in two layers with absorbable suture (Fig. 17.8). Take care when applying dressings to create a little "nest" within which the nipple can remain in an everted position. The goal is to allow the nipple-areolar complex to remain in a natural position during healing.

Anatomic Points

There is a layer of smooth muscle immediately under the areolar skin. Dissection deep to this plane allows easy access to the ductal and glandular structures with the least disturbance of nerves and blood supply, and can be performed in a relatively avascular plane.

The terminal ducts converge on the underside of the nipple as multiple small openings, arranged in a roughly radial orientation. Thus, a duct opening at the periphery of the nipple will generally drain a duct that tracks radially outward in a predictable direction.

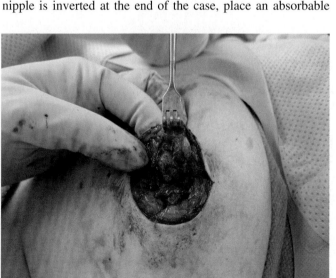

Figure 17.5 Undersurface of the nipple after the terminal ducts have been ligated.

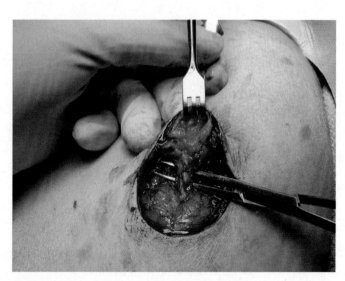

Figure 17.7 Encircling the terminal ducts

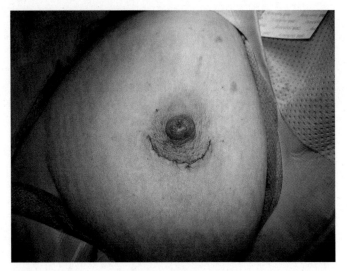

Figure 17.8 Final closure with incision disguised in the areolar border.

There is a slight narrowing at the skin opening, and then the duct opens into a slightly larger ampulla. Thus, when passing the lacrimal duct probe, you may feel a "popping" sense as the lacrimal duct probe falls into the ampulla. Never use force, as this may produce a false passage. Rather, a gentle twisting motion and steady light pressure in the anticipated direction that the duct is likely to take will generally result in successful passage.

The nipple-areolar complex is innervated by lateral and anterior cutaneous branches of the third, fourth, and fifth intercostal nerves. The fourth intercostal nerve is the most constant source of innervation. The lateral cutaneous branch approaches from lateral to medial, and the anterior cutaneous branch from medial to lateral. As with many segmental sensory innervation patterns, overlap of territories may allow recovery of sensation if only one nerve branch is divided.

Long circumareolar incisions at the lateral or medial aspect may divide these superficial branches, causing transient or permanent sensory deficit in a very sensitive area. This may be more common with medial (as opposed to other locations around the areola) circumareolar incisions. Radially oriented incisions within the areolar skin avoid this problem but may not provide as good exposure.

The blood supply to the nipple-areolar complex is highly variable and usually derives from several sources. In the most common pattern, branches of the internal mammary (internal thoracic) artery come from medial to anastomose with branches of the intercostal perforators which approach from lateral. Devascularization of part of the areolar skin may occur with long circumareolar incisions, and this is another reason to avoid creating any such incision longer than one-third of the circumference.

Duct Excision for Chronic Subareolar Abscess or Mammary Fistula

Technical and Anatomic Points

Generally it will be necessary to excise at least the ducts of the involved quadrant. This is done in women who desire to retain the ability to breast feed. If the woman does not wish to breast feed in the future, complete duct excision is the best way to prevent recurrence.

Plan a lens-shaped radially oriented incision that encompasses the skin over the previous incision and drainage site, or includes the chronic fistula tract (Fig. 17.2A). If partial duct excision is desired, cannulate the fistula with a lacrimal duct probe and seek a tract to the nipple. If this can be identified, subsequent excision of all indurated tissue around the probe should remove the responsible duct (Fig. 17.9A).

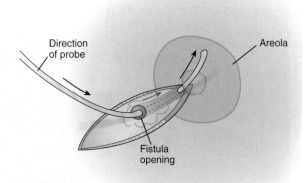
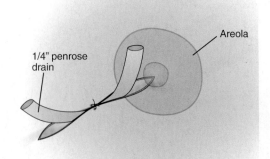

Figure 17.9 A: Excision of tissue for chronic subareolar abscess. **B:** Closure over Penrose drain in cases of frank purulence.

If you encounter frank purulence, close the midportion of the incision with a single interrupted fine nylon suture to approximate the areolar margin and pass a ¼″ Penrose drain under the suture, allowing the two ends to exit medially and laterally (Fig. 19.9B). This is a much less desired closure; hence it is best to spend sufficient time allowing the acute infectious process to subside.

Despite this excision, recurrence may occur and it is important to counsel the patient. These problems appear to be more prevalent in smokers; smoking cessation should be advised. Contralateral involvement may also occur in the future and the patient should be so counseled.

REFERENCES

1. Dixon JM, Bundred NJ. Management of disorders of the ductal system and infections. In: Harris JR, Lippman ME, Morrow M, et al., eds. *Diseases of the Breast,* 4th ed. Philadelphia, PA: Lippincott Williams & Wilkins; 2010:42–51.
2. Dixon JM, Hardy RG. Breast infection. In: Dirbas FM, Scott-Conner CE. *Breast Surgical Techniques and Interdisciplinary Management.* New York, NY: Springer; 2011:161–177.
3. Elder EE, Brennan M. Nonsurgical management should be first-line therapy for breast abscess. *World J Surg.* 2010;34:2257–2258.
4. Gollapalli V, Liao J, Dudakovic A, et al. Risk factors for development and recurrence of primary breast abscesses. *J Am Coll Surg.* 2010;211:41. (Draws attention to nipple piercing as a cause of subareolar abscess.)
5. Morrogh M, Park A, Elkin EB, et al. Lessons learned from 416 cases of nipple discharge of the breast. *Am J Surg.* 2010;200: 73–80.
6. Nakajima H, Imanishi N, Aiso S. Arterial anatomy of the nipple-areola complex. *Plast Reconstr Surg.* 1995;96:843–845.
7. O'Dey D, Prescher A, Pallua N. Vascular reliability of nipple-areola complex pedicles: An anatomical microdissection study. *Plast Reconstr Surg.* 2007;119:1167.
8. Sabel MS, Helvie MA, Breslin T, et al. Is duct excision still necessary for all cases of suspicious nipple discharge? *Breast J.* 2011;10:1524.
9. Sarhadi NS, Shaw Dunn J, Lee FD, et al. An anatomical study of the nerve supply of the breast, including the nipple and areola. *Br J Plast Surg.* 1996;49:156.
10. Sarhadi NS, Shaw-Dunn J, Soutar DS. Nerve supply of the breast with special reference to the nipple and areola: Sir Astley Cooper revisited. *Clin Anat.* 1997;10:283.
11. Schlenz I, Kuzbari R, Gruber H, et al. The sensitivity of the nipple-areola complex: An anatomic study. *Plast Reconstr Surg.* 2000; 105:905.
12. Schwarz RJ, Shrestha R. Needle aspiration of breast abscesses. *Am J Surg.* 2001;182(2):117–119.
13. Sharma R, Dietz J, Wright H, et al. Comparative analysis of minimally invasive microductectomy versus major duct excision in patients with pathologic nipple discharge. *Surgery.* 2005;138:591.

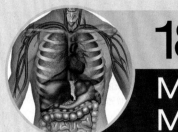

18
Mastectomy: Total (Simple), Modified, and Classic Radical

Total (sometimes called *simple*) mastectomy removes all the glandular tissue of the breast. It is sometimes required for the treatment of extensive ductal carcinoma in situ. In combination with reconstructive surgery, bilateral total mastectomy is sometimes used for breast cancer prophylaxis in carefully selected patients.

Modified radical mastectomy adds the removal of the node-bearing tissue of the axilla while preserving the muscular contours of the upper chest wall. The operation was modified from the original or classic radical mastectomy to enhance the cosmetic result without compromising the control of the disease. Many modifications of the original classic radical mastectomy have been described. They differ in the extent of tissue removed and the completeness of axillary dissection. The modification described here combines a thorough axillary dissection with the preservation of muscle contour. Other modified radical mastectomy techniques are detailed in the references.

Classic radical mastectomy is still used in those rare circumstances in which wider excision of the pectoral muscles might enhance local control. This is increasingly rare as better neoadjuvant chemotherapy has become available.

When mastectomy is performed for risk reduction (sometimes termed *cancer prophylaxis*) or for early disease, skin-sparing mastectomy with immediate reconstruction is generally appropriate. Nipple-areolar–sparing mastectomy may be employed in suitable patients. Technical considerations referable to these procedures are mentioned throughout. These procedures are also briefly discussed in Chapter 19.

Sentinel lymph node biopsy (see Chapter 20) is frequently combined with mastectomy. It may be performed through the lateral aspect of the incision or, if a skin-sparing technique is employed, through a separate axillary incision.

SCORE™, the Surgical Council on Resident Education, classified total mastectomy and modified radical mastectomy as "ESSENTIAL COMMON" procedures. SCORE™ classified radical mastectomy as an "ESSENTIAL UNCOMMON" procedure.

STEPS IN PROCEDURE

Total Mastectomy
Position patient with arm out; may drape arm free if desired
Ellipse of skin including nipple-areolar complex and skin over tumor
   Nipple-areolar complex may be spared in selected patients
Develop flaps at the level of fusion plane between subcutaneous fat and fatty envelop of breast to sternum medially, clavicle superiorly, rectus inferiorly, latissimus laterally
Elevate breast from pectoralis major muscle from superior medial to inferior lateral
Take pectoral fascia for cancer
Leave pectoral fascia for immediate reconstruction with implant
Identify and ligate (if necessary) perforating branches of internal thoracic (mammary) vessels

Sweep all fatty tissue downward and terminate dissection
Obtain hemostasis and lymph stasis and close over two closed suction drains

Dog Ear Correction by V-Y Flap Advancement
Close middle of incision
Elevate apex of dog ears to define pyramids of tissue
Excise triangles of redundant tissue
Suture the resulting reverse arrowheads in place
Record length of dog ear in operating note

Modified Radical Mastectomy
Develop flaps and dissect breast from pectoralis major muscle as described above
Leave breast attached at lateral aspect and use weight of breast to enhance retraction
Incise pectoral fascia at lateral edge of pectoralis major and elevate muscle

Dissect under pectoralis major muscle, removing all fatty node-bearing tissues

Preserve median pectoral nerve

Sweep fatty tissue laterally and expose and protect long thoracic nerve

Identify axillary vein and sweep fatty tissue downward

Sweep all fatty tissues downward and terminate dissection

Obtain hemostasis and lymph stasis and close over two closed suction drains

Radical Mastectomy

Position patient as noted, prep abdomen or thigh for possible skin graft

Develop flaps as previously outlined

Shave pectoralis major muscle (with overlying breast tissue) off chest wall from medial to lateral

Ligate perforating branches of internal thoracic (mammary) vessels as encountered

Similarly excise pectoralis minor muscle when exposed

Axillary dissection proceeds as previously outlined but includes level III nodes

Close as previously described, placing skin graft in midportion if required

HALLMARK ANATOMIC COMPLICATIONS

Injury to long thoracic nerve

Injury to thoracodorsal nerve

Injury to intercostobrachial nerves

Injury to axillary vein

Seroma formation

LIST OF STRUCTURES

Pectoralis major muscle

Pectoralis minor muscle

Subclavius muscle

Clavipectoral fascia

Coracoid process

Lateral pectoral nerve

Medial pectoral nerve

Thoracodorsal nerve

Long thoracic nerve

Axillary artery

Axillary vein

Thoracoacromial artery

Thoracodorsal vein

Internal thoracic (mammary) artery

Internal thoracic (mammary) vein

Axillary lymph nodes

Landmarks

Clavicle

Anterior rectus sheath

Latissimus dorsi muscle

Sternum

Total and Modified Radical Mastectomy

Position of the Patient and Choice of Skin Incision (Fig. 18.1)

Technical and Anatomic Points

The operation is performed under general anesthesia. After the initial intubation, muscle relaxants are avoided so that nerve function can be assessed. Position the patient supine with the ipsilateral arm extended on an arm board (Fig. 18.1A). If necessary, place a small, folded sheet under the shoulder to improve exposure. Avoid hyperextending the shoulder because this can cause neurapraxia. Some surgeons routinely drape the arm free so that it can be moved during the course of the dissection.

The choice of incision depends on several factors, including the location of the lesion, any prior biopsy incisions, and planned reconstruction. When immediate reconstruction is to be performed, design the skin incision in consultation with the plastic surgeon who will scrub in to do the reconstruction. In many cases, skin-sparing flaps can be created in such a manner as to be oncologically correct and yet provide an aesthetically pleasing outcome. See Chapter 19 for skin-sparing and nipple-areolar–sparing incisions and further details on these more complex procedures.

When delayed reconstruction is a possibility, a generally transverse incision is favored as it facilitates reconstruction. When reconstruction will not be performed, a generally oblique incision that is high at the axillary end and low medially provides excellent access. Flaps generally heal very well with this incision and the end result is a flat chest wall to which prostheses can easily be adapted.

For a standard mastectomy, the skin incision should include the nipple-areolar complex and the skin overlying the tumor, biopsy cavity, and any prior biopsy incision (Fig. 18.1B). The biopsy cavity is considered to be contaminated by the tumor cells and frequently contains gross residual disease. It must be excised in its entirety as dissection progresses. Therefore, if the biopsy is performed through an incision located at some distance from the mass, a correspondingly larger amount of skin should be sacrificed. Alternatively, an ellipse of skin around the biopsy incision may be excised separately. Do not compromise the skin incision because of the fear of difficulty in closure. A skin graft will heal well over the underlying muscle and may be used if necessary. This is rarely necessary if flaps are designed properly.

Figure 18.1C and D shows how a "lazy S" type incision provides flaps that can accommodate a variety of lesion locations, yet slide together to afford primary closure with minimal

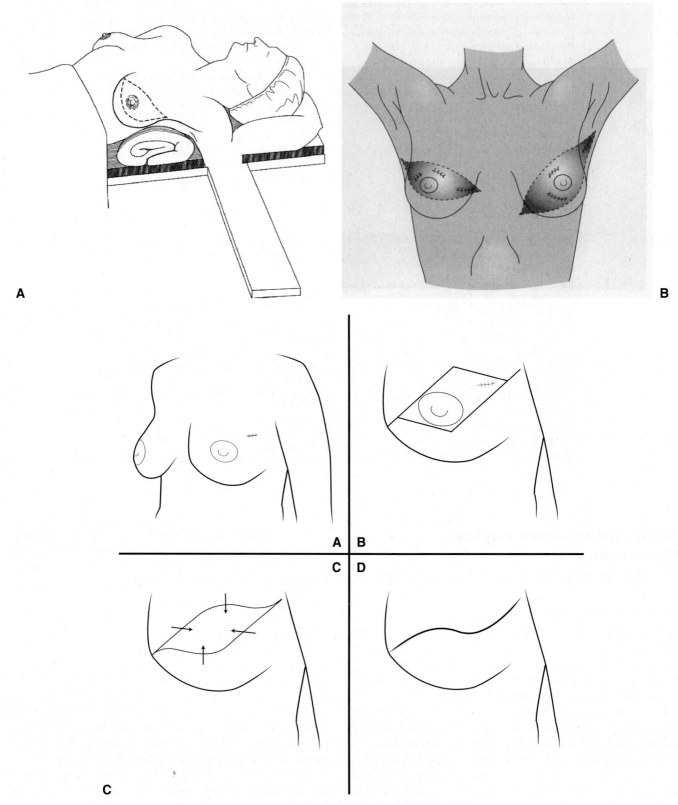

Figure 18.1 Position of the patient and skin incision. **A:** Patient position. **B:** Standard oval incisions. **C:** Construction of lazy-S skin incision from trapezoid (sub-figures A–D show how this can be accomplished for a relatively high lesion—A. Site of lesion B. Trapezoid outlined C. Edges of trapezoid are smoothed and skin brought together from four directions to close flaps D. Incision after closure of flaps).

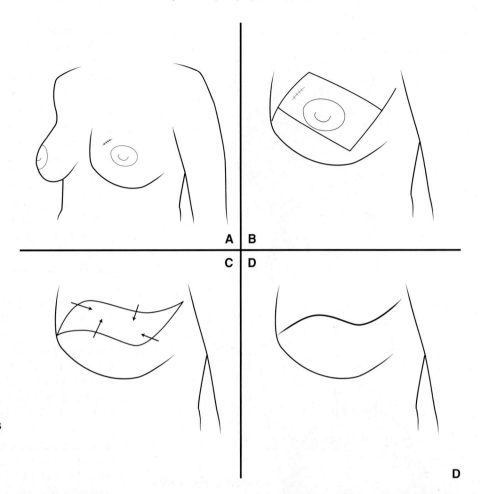

Figure 18.1 *Continued.* **D:** Construction of lazy-S skin incision for high medial lesion (Sub-figure A. Site of lesion. B. Trapezoid outlined. C. Edges of trapezoid smoothed and edges approximated. D. Incision after flap closure).

tension. The easiest way to create the lazy S is to first outline a diamond shape around the nipple areola and tumor location, then round the corners a bit. Remember, whenever possible, to keep the skin incision low medially and high laterally. This will make it easier for the patient to conceal the scar under her clothes and will also facilitate your access to the axillary tail of the breast and any axillary nodal tissue as needed.

As the incision is closed, flaps are allowed to slide from side to side and from top to bottom as shown. The result is a flat scar that may be hidden under clothing even for some upper inner quadrant lesions.

Development of Flaps (Fig. 18.2)

Technical Points

Incise the skin and subcutaneous tissue. Visualize the breast as lying encapsulated in a separate layer of subcutaneous fat that lies 0.5 to 1 cm below the skin. Often, this layer can be defined as the skin incision is made. Place Lahey clamps on the dermal side of the upper flap and have an assistant place these under strong upward traction (Fig. 18.2A). Apply countertraction by pulling the breast tissue down and toward you strongly with a lap sponge. Avoid manipulating the breast overlying the biopsy site. Develop flaps by sharp dissection using a shaving motion with a sharp knife or electrocautery. If a knife is used, change the blades frequently. Dissection in the proper plane is surpris-

ingly bloodless. A network of large subcutaneous veins is often visible on the underside of the flap and will be preserved if dissection progresses in the proper plane. Ligate occasional bleeders on the underside of the flap. (Use electrocautery with caution on the flap because it can burn through the thin flap to damage the overlying skin surface.) Confirm the thickness of the flap by palpation as the dissection progresses.

An alternative technique uses slightly opened Mayo scissors to develop the flaps by a push-cut technique. This is particularly useful when the skin incision is small as during skin-sparing mastectomy.

In the axilla, the skin flap will be crossed by hair follicles and apocrine glands. Divide these sharply or pass into a very slightly deeper plane to avoid these. Raise the flaps to the level of the clavicle superiorly, the midline medially, the anterior rectus sheath inferiorly, and the anterior border of the latissimus dorsi muscle laterally (Fig. 18.2B). Of these, the lateral border of the latissimus dorsi is generally the most difficult to find.

Identify this muscle by palpation of a longitudinal ridge of muscle tissue. Dissect sharply down to confirm its identity by visualizing longitudinal muscle fibers. Trace the muscle up toward the axilla. Check the upper flap for hemostasis and place a moist laparotomy pad under the flap. Place the Lahey clamps on the inferior skin incision and develop the inferior flap by the same technique. The plane between the breast and the subcutaneous tissue is frequently less well-defined inferiorly, and unless care

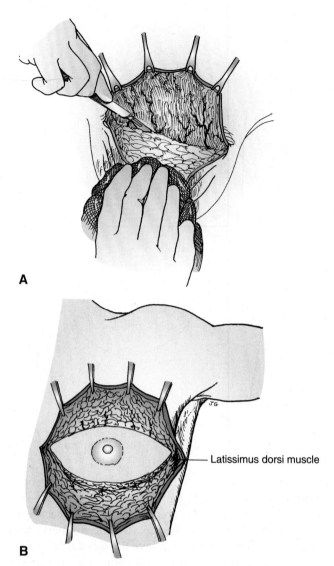

A

B

Latissimus dorsi muscle

Figure 18.2 Development of flaps. **A:** Flaps developed in subcutaneous plane. **B:** Lateral border of dissection is latissimus dorsi muscle.

is taken, the inferior flap may be cut too thick. Guard against this by constant palpation of the thickness of the flap. If white fibrous tissue (breast or suspensory ligaments of the breast [Cooper ligaments]) is seen the flap is too thick and must be cut thinner.

Draw a line around the margins of the dissection by incising the fascia at the perimeter of the field with electrocautery. This will prevent your dissecting too far in any direction. Recheck both flaps for hemostasis and place warm moist lap pads under them. Take care throughout the operation not to allow the subcutaneous fat of the underside of the flaps to become exposed and desiccated.

Anatomic Points

The breast is a conical ectodermal derivative limited to superficial fascia. The base of the breast overlies the chest wall from the second rib to the sixth and from the edge of the sternum to the midaxillary line. A lateral tongue of breast tissue—the axillary tail of Spence—extends into each axilla from the otherwise

conical breast. This tail sometimes passes through the deep fascia of the axilla and approaches the pectoral group of axillary lymph nodes. Superficial to the breast is the superficial layer of the superficial fascia, whereas deep into the breast is the deep layer of superficial fascia. The subcutaneous fat lobules are small and easy to differentiate from the larger fat lobules of the breast itself.

As the skin flaps are developed, the suspensory ligaments (of Cooper) must be severed. These ligamentous bands traverse the fat of the gland and attach to the deep layer of superficial fascia and dermis. They are especially well developed in the upper portion of the breast.

Because the extent of the skin flaps can be related to musculoskeletal structures, the anatomy of these structures should be reviewed. The clavicle extends laterally from the superolateral corner of the manubrium to the acromion process of the scapula. Those muscles that attach to the clavicle and are palpable include a part of the pectoralis major muscle (medial half), the deltoid muscle (lateral third), and the sternocleidomastoid muscle (medial third). Most of the breast lies on the pectoralis major muscle. This muscle forms the anterior wall of the axilla. Its free lower edge is the muscular framework for the anterior axillary fold. In addition to its clavicular part, it also has a sternocostal part and an abdominal part. The sternocostal part originates from the anterior surface (essentially to the midline) of the sternum (manubrium and body) and from the cartilage of all true ribs. The abdominal part arises from the aponeurosis of the external abdominal oblique muscle. From this wide origin, the fibers converge on a flat tendon inserted into the lateral lip of the intertubercular sulcus of the humerus. Thus fibers of the clavicular part pass obliquely inferiorly and laterally, those of the sternocostal part pass horizontally or superolaterally and those of the abdominal part ascend almost vertically.

The rectus abdominis attaches to the costal cartilage of ribs five to seven. It is covered superficially by the anterior rectus sheath, here composed only of external oblique aponeurosis. The lateral edge of the upper rectus (and hence, the rectus sheath) lies at the midclavicular line.

The latissimus dorsi forms the muscular basis for the posterior axillary fold. It originates either directly or through an aponeurosis from all vertebrae between T5 and the coccyx, the lower three to four ribs, the inferior angle of the scapula, and the iliac crest. From this origin, fibers pass laterally to converge on a tendon that inserts on the medial wall and floor of the intertubercular groove of the humerus. The most superior fibers pass almost horizontally and the lower fibers ascend at an increasingly oblique angle toward the humerus. Thus fibers originating from the iliac crest, especially the more anterior ones, have an almost vertical course. The latter fibers contribute to the posterior axillary fold. The direction of the muscle fibers is the key to their identification during surgery.

Removal of Breast from the Pectoralis Major Muscle (Fig. 18.3)

Technical Points

Place retractors in the medial aspect of the upper and lower flaps to expose the midline. Place Allis clamps on the pectoral fascia

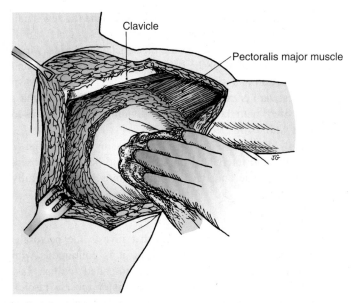

Figure 18.3 Removal of breast from the pectoralis major muscle

as breast and pectoral fascia are removed medially to laterally. Look for, and either preserve or carefully ligate and divide, a series of perforating branches of the internal thoracic (mammary) artery and vein; these will be encountered as dissection progresses past the sternum. Generally, these are located within 1 to 2 cm of the edge of the sternum, one at each interspace.

Be aware that some free flap reconstructive techniques will anastomose to one of these vessels deep in the intercostal space.

Use a knife to remove pectoral fascia cleanly with the breast. Only the exposed fibers of the pectoralis major muscle should remain. If tumor is locally fixed to the pectoralis major muscle, excise a portion of the muscle with the specimen. Progress from medial to lateral until the lateral border of the pectoralis major muscle is seen. Clean this lateral border allowing the attached breast to fall laterally.

As dissection progresses inferior and lateral to the pectoralis major muscle, take care to preserve a thin layer of areolar tissue investing the underlying muscles. This will put you in the proper plane to preserve the long thoracic nerve if axillary dissection is planned.

If the operation is planned as a total mastectomy, the breast is then excised from the underlying axillary tissues with electrocautery. Axillary node dissection is not performed.

Anatomic Points

The blood supply of the breast is derived from axillary, internal thoracic (mammary), and intercostal arteries. The branches of the axillary artery that supply the breast include the thoracoacromial, lateral thoracic, and subscapular branches. The internal thoracic (mammary) artery, a branch of the subclavian, usually supplies the breast through comparatively large perforating arteries in the second, third, and fourth intercostal spaces; of these, the one in the second space is typically the largest. Finally, the anterior intercostal arteries provide small perforators that are distributed to the deep aspect of the breast. Thus the principal

blood supply of the breast enters the gland superolaterally (axillary branches) and superomedially (internal thoracic branches).

Pectoral fascia is the deep fascia associated with the pectoralis major muscle. Although it is typically quite thin, it increases in thickness laterally, where it forms the floor of the axilla; it then becomes continuous with the latissimus dorsi fascia and fascia of the arm. The fascial layer, of which the pectoral fascia is one regional expression, is distinct and superficial to the clavipectoral fascia. The latter fascial layer is associated with the pectoralis minor muscle.

Modified Radical Mastectomy—Dissection Under the Pectoralis Major Muscle and Optional Removal of the Pectoralis Minor Muscle (Fig. 18.4)

Technical Points

This procedure begins as outlined in Figures 18.1 to 18.3. Subsequent complete axillary dissection is greatly facilitated by relaxing the pectoral muscles by elevating the arm. Have an assistant lift the arm and hold it up and over the chest wall. Place Allis clamps on the lateral edge of the pectoralis major muscle and have the assistant elevate it. Clean the underside of the pectoralis major muscle by removing fatty, areolar, node-bearing tissue and exposing the underlying pectoralis minor muscle.

Identify and preserve the medial and lateral pectoral nerves that innervate the pectoralis major and minor muscles. The lateral pectoral nerve pierces the clavipectoral fascia, whereas the medial pectoral nerve pierces the pectoralis minor muscle to enter the pectoralis major muscle relatively medially. Sacrifice of these nerves causes atrophy of the pectoralis major muscle. The muscle then becomes a fibrous cord, at which point it is both a cosmetic and a functional liability.

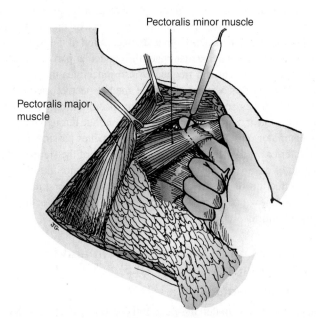

Figure 18.4 Modified radical mastectomy—dissection under the pectoralis major muscle and removal of the pectoralis minor muscle

If access to level III nodes is required, it may be necessary to resect the pectoralis minor muscle. This is not done in common practice, but may be required in exceptional circumstances. Incise the clavipectoral fascia on both sides of the pectoralis minor muscle in the superior portion of the field. Pass a finger behind this muscle. Look underneath to confirm that the underlying fascia is intact and that no major structures were inadvertently raised with the muscle. If visualization under the muscle is difficult, divide the muscle using electrocautery, thus detaching it from the coracoid process.

Anatomic Points

Innervation of the pectoralis major muscle is provided by the lateral and medial pectoral nerves. These nerves are named according to their respective origins from the lateral and medial cords of the brachial plexus, not on the basis of their relative location on the anterior thoracic wall. They carry fibers of spinal cord levels C5 to C7 and C5 to T1, respectively. The lateral pectoral nerve crosses anterior to the first part of the axillary artery and vein (that segment proximal to the pectoralis minor muscle), and there sends an anastomotic branch to join the medial pectoral nerve. The main ramus pierces the clavipectoral fascia with the thoracoacromial artery and is distributed to the pectoralis major and minor muscles along with the pectoral branches of this artery. The medial pectoral nerve arises from the medial cord somewhat more distally than the lateral pectoral nerve— that is, at the level of the second part of the axillary artery (that segment posterior to the pectoralis minor muscle). Typically, this nerve pierces the pectoralis minor muscle (providing innervation to the muscle) and then ramifies on the deep surface of the pectoralis major muscle. In addition, it usually gives off two or three branches that accompany the lateral pectoral artery along with the inferior border of the pectoralis minor muscle and that ultimately are distributed to the pectoralis major muscle.

In addition to the variably developed natural separation between the clavicular and sternocostal parts of the pectoralis major muscle, there is a difference in innervation of the two parts. The lateral pectoral nerve innervates the clavicular part of the pectoralis major muscle and frequently also innervates the superior part of the sternocostal portion. The medial pectoral nerve has several branches, some of which enter the pectoralis minor muscle and innervate it. Some of these branches continue through the pectoralis minor muscle and, in addition to branches passing around the inferior border of this muscle, supply most of the sternocostal and all of the abdominal parts of the pectoralis major muscle.

Reflection or retraction of the pectoralis major muscle is done to allow access to lymph nodes that lie posterior to this muscle, ultimately including all axillary nodes.

Identification of the Axillary Vein and Initial Axillary Dissection (Fig. 18.5)

Technical Points

Incise the fascia under the pectoralis minor muscle and look carefully for the underlying axillary vein. It is often lower than expected, particularly if the pectoralis major muscle has been divided. Dissect medially in the anterior adventitial plane of

the vein to the surgical apex of the axilla. Divide the few small vessels that cross over the vein.

The highest axillary nodes are the subclavian nodes, which lie in the medial apex of the field. Remove them by sharp and blunt dissection and sweep all fatty node-bearing tissue down as the chest wall is exposed. Remove the pectoralis minor muscle (if desired) with the specimen by dividing its attachments to the chest wall using electrocautery.

Cleanly dissect the chest wall, progressing from medial to lateral. Ribs and intercostal muscles should be well exposed. Sweep fatty tissue and the pectoralis minor muscle laterally with the breast.

Anatomic Points

Clavipectoral fascia is that fascia that invests the pectoralis minor muscle. Inferior to the muscle, it is continuous with serratus anterior fascia and with the so-called axillary fascia (primarily derived from pectoralis major muscle fascia). Superomedially, it blends with intercostal fascia, whereas superolaterally, it continues as a dense sheet, splitting to invest the subclavius muscle. When splitting this fascia, care should be taken not to damage either the thoracoacromial artery or the lateral pectoral nerve, both of which pierce the fascia superior to the pectoralis minor muscle.

Division of the pectoralis minor muscle allows exposure of all the three parts of the axillary artery and vein. The axillary vein is the most inferior (or medial) of the major neurovascular structures in the axilla. Components of the brachial plexus are closely associated with the axillary artery; thus nerves will lie in the interval between the vein and the artery, where appropriate. The axillary sheath, in continuity with scalene fascia, surrounds the artery and nerves but not the vein.

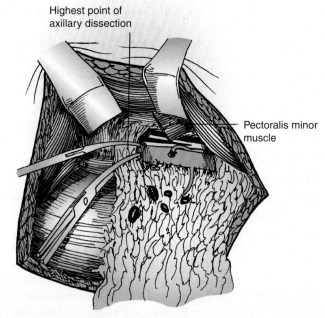

Highest point of axillary dissection

Pectoralis minor muscle

Figure 18.5 Modified radical mastectomy—identification of the axillary vein and initial axillary dissection

Exposure of the axillary vessels provides complete access to axillary lymph nodes (chiefly those of the central and apical group), which are located adjacent to the second and first part of these vessels, respectively.

On average, there are 35 axillary lymph nodes, which are loosely arranged in groups associated with the major arteries and veins. Although major anatomy texts frequently list five groups, perhaps the best classification system is that of Haagensen, who maintains that there are six groups, as follows:

1. *External mammary nodes:* An average of 1.7 nodes lying deep to the lateral edge of the pectoralis major muscle and associated with the lateral thoracic artery. Lymphatic drainage from these nodes passes to the central or subclavicular nodes.

2. *Interpectoral (Rotter's) nodes:* An average of 1.4 nodes associated with the pectoral branches of the thoracoacromial artery. These nodes are located in the areolar tissue between the pectoralis major muscle and the clavipectoral fascia that envelops the pectoralis minor muscle. Lymphatic drainage from these nodes passes to the central or subclavicular nodes.

3. *Scapular nodes:* An average of 5.8 nodes associated with the subscapular vessels and their thoracodorsal branches. Because the intercostobrachial and thoracodorsal nerves pass through this group of nodes, these nerves may have to be sacrificed to allow removal of the nodes. Lymphatic drainage from these nodes passes to the central nodes.

4. *Central nodes:* An average of 12.1 nodes lying in fat in the central axilla, about halfway between the anterior and posterior axillary folds. Frequently, one or more of these nodes is located between the skin and the superficial fascia. Lymphatic drainage from these nodes passes to the axillary nodes.

5. *Axillary nodes:* An average of 10.7 nodes closely associated with the axillary vein from the tendon of the latissimus dorsi muscle to the termination of the thoracoacromial vein. Lymphatic drainage from these nodes passes to the subclavicular nodes.

6. *Subclavicular nodes:* An average of 3.5 nodes associated with the axillary vein proximal to the termination of the thoracoacromial vein. These nodes, then, are located in the apex of the axilla and are primarily posterior to the subclavius muscle, which is enveloped by the clavipectoral fascia. Access to the nodes is facilitated by the division of the pectoralis minor muscle and its enveloping clavipectoral fascia. This group of nodes receives lymphatics from all other axillary nodes. Lymphatic drainage from these nodes passes into the inferior deep cervical nodes or directly into the venous system in the vicinity of the jugulosubclavian junction. These nodes are considered to be the highest, or apical, lymph nodes, at least from the standpoint of the breast surgeon.

Modified Radical Mastectomy—Dissection of the Axillary Vein and Identification of Nerves (Fig. 18.6)

Technical Points

Follow the axillary vein laterally, dividing any small vessels that cross over it and any venous tributaries that pass inferiorly.

As the chest wall starts to curve down away from you, look for the long thoracic nerve just under the fascia. Identify it as a long, straight nerve. Incise the fascia and confirm the identity of the nerve by gentle mechanical stimulation with a forceps or with an electrical nerve stimulator. Extend the incision of the overlying fascia inferiorly and gently push the nerve down against the chest wall and posterior axilla.

Continue dissecting laterally in the anterior adventitial plane of the axillary vein. Look for a large venous tributary, the thoracodorsal vein. Ligate and divide this vein. It is a landmark for the second important nerve in the region, the thoracodorsal nerve. The thoracodorsal artery and nerve pass about 1 cm deep to the plane of the axillary vein. The thoracodorsal nerve lies in close proximity to, and generally just deep to, the thoracodorsal artery. Confirm the identity of this nerve by gentle stimulation.

Sweep the axillary contents downward, keeping both nerves in view and preserving them. The thoracodorsal artery can be ligated, and the thoracodorsal nerve can be sacrificed, if necessary, if it is involved by tumor. The long thoracic nerve should be preserved; however, significant functional and cosmetic liabilities accompany its sacrifice.

Remove the specimen by rapidly dividing the remaining attachments inferiorly.

Anatomic Points

A triangular surgical field, which almost corresponds to the anatomic axilla, is accessible when the pectoral muscles are retracted or divided. This surgical field is limited superolaterally by the axillary vein, inferolaterally by the latissimus dorsi muscle, medially by the serratus anterior muscle, and posteriorly by the subscapular, teres major, and latissimus dorsi muscles. The apex of this triangle is superomedial, deep to the clavicle. Here, the dominant feature of immediate concern is the axillary vein.

The long thoracic nerve is formed in the posterior triangle of the neck by anastomosis of the branches of brachial plexus roots C5 to C7. It enters the field deep to the vein and parallels the curvature of the thoracic wall, being on the axillary surface of the serratus anterior muscle. It descends into the axilla posterior to the brachial plexus, the first part of the axillary vessels, and all other neurovascular structures. It then continues its descent along the superficial (axillary) surface of the serratus anterior muscle, supplying each digitation of this muscle in its course. The long thoracic nerve can be located at the point where the axillary vein passes over the second rib. Injury of the nerve impairs the serratus anterior muscle, whose prime function is to protract the scapula, especially its inferior angle. Without rotation of the scapula, it is impossible to raise the arm above the level of the shoulder. In addition, the serratus muscle holds the vertebral border of the scapula to the trunk; therefore, loss of function of the serratus muscle results in "winging" of the scapula. Thus injury to this nerve can be both disabling and disfiguring.

The thoracodorsal or middle subscapular nerve carries fibers from C6 to C8. It originates from the posterior cord of the brachial plexus posterior to the second part of the axillary vessels and accompanies the thoracodorsal branch of the subscapular artery along the posterior axillary wall to supply the latissimus

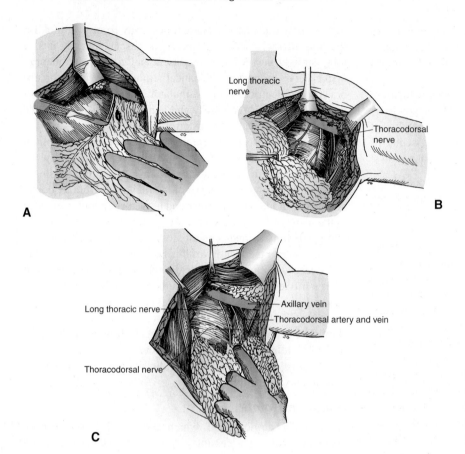

A

B

C

Long thoracic nerve

Thoracodorsal nerve

Long thoracic nerve

Axillary vein

Thoracodorsal artery and vein

Thoracodorsal nerve

Figure 18.6 Modified radical mastectomy—dissection of the axillary vein and identification of nerves. **A:** Dissection of node-bearing tissue from long thoracic nerve. **B** and **C:** Dissection from axillary vein and thoracodorsal trunk.

dorsi muscle. The nerve lies on the subscapular and teres major muscles. Damage to this nerve that is sufficient to paralyze the latissimus dorsi muscle weakens adduction, inward rotation, and extension of the arm (as in a swimming stroke). It also hinders the ability to depress the scapula, a function that is important when using crutches to support the weight of the body.

Modified Radical Mastectomy—Closure of the Wound and Correction of Dog Ears (if Needed) (Fig. 18.7)

Technical and Anatomic Points

Achieve careful hemostasis and irrigate the field to remove debris and loose bits of fat. Place a skin hook in each end of the incision and pull these in opposite directions to judge how the incision will come together and determine if dog ears, redundant flaps of skin, will be created.

Place closed suction drains under upper and lower flaps (Fig. 18.7A). Excise any redundant skin and dog ears, but remember that extra skin may be an asset to the plastic surgeon if postmastectomy reconstruction is planned. Dog ears are common at the medial and lateral aspects, particularly if a generous skin ellipse has been taken, and they can cause great annoyance to patients.

If primary closure will result in dog ears (Fig. 18.7B), a V-Y advancement flap technique can be used to flatten the ends. First, close the midportion of the wound (Fig. 18.7C).

Take the apex of the incision medially or laterally and pull it upward, creating a small pyramid (Fig. 18.7D). Experiment with laying this apex down flat along the line of the incision and determine the skin that needs to be excised (triangles from the upper and lower aspects as shown). Excise these triangles (Fig. 18.7E) and then sew the resulting inverted arrowhead into place. The result should be an incision that is flat and smooth (Fig. 18.7F). Record the length of the limbs in the operative note. Other correction techniques are described in the references at the end of the chapter.

Close the skin with multiple fine interrupted sutures, skin clips, or a subcuticular suture. Deep dermal sutures of absorbable material are helpful in avoiding closure under tension.

Classic Radical Mastectomy

Surgical Technique (Fig. 18.8)

Technical and Anatomic Points

Make the incision and raise the flaps exactly as described previously. Because classic radical mastectomy is generally used for more advanced lesions, a larger amount of breast skin may need to be sacrificed. Prepare and drape a thigh in case a skin graft is needed.

Place retractors in the medial aspect of both flaps and shave the pectoralis major muscle off the chest wall from medial to lateral. Take care to identify and ligate the perforating branches

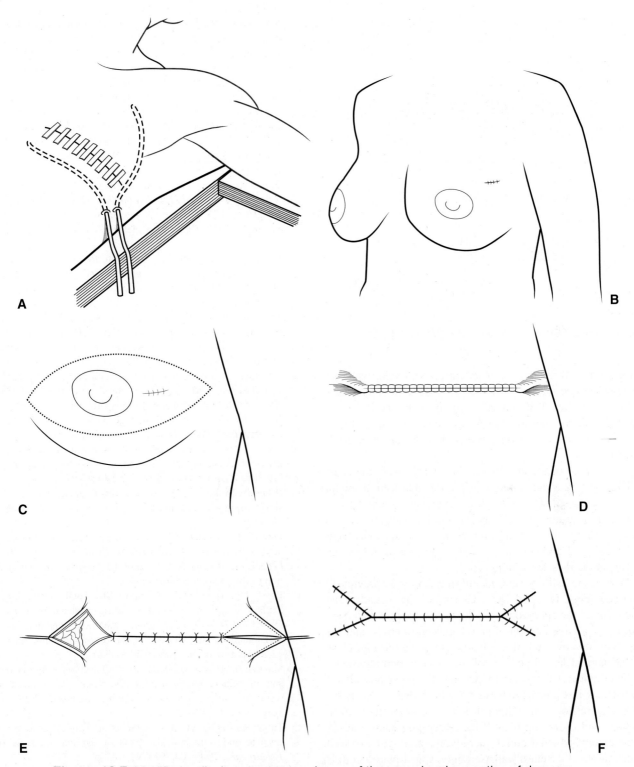

Figure 18.7 Modified radical mastectomy—closure of the wound and correction of dog ears. **A:** Incision closed with drains in place. **B:** Typical carcinoma of lateral breast that might be approached through a transverse incision. **C:** Outline of transverse incision. **D:** Simple closure yields dog-ears at both ends. **E:** To avoid this, excise a diamond-shaped piece of tissue at each end as shown. **F:** Complete the closure by folding it back onto the chest wall and suturing the two legs as shown. (Technique courtesy of Mark A. Gittelman, MD.)

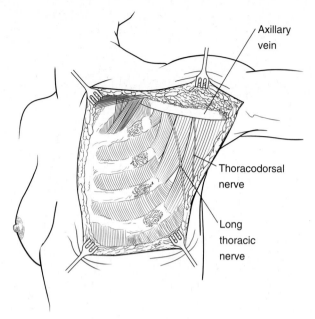

Figure 18.8 Classic radical mastectomy—surgical technique

of the internal thoracic (mammary) artery and vein, which at this point will be seen to emerge directly from the interspaces. Secure any vessels that "retract" into an interspace by suture ligature. Take care not to poke the tips of a hemostat into the interspace because it is extremely easy to enter the chest inadvertently.

As the pectoralis major muscle is elevated from the chest wall, the pectoralis minor muscle will be encountered. It should likewise be shaved off. Divide the attachments of the pectoralis major muscle to the clavicle and the humerus superiorly and laterally. Divide the pectoralis minor muscle at its attachment to the coracoid process, as previously described. Allow the breast and the muscles to fall laterally.

Dissect the axillary vein, identifying nerves as previously described (Figs. 18.5 and 18.6). Closure of the wound at the conclusion of the operation is similar to that for modified mastectomy. If a large amount of skin has been removed and the flaps will not come together without excessive tension, close the medial and lateral portions of the incision partially, leaving an elliptical defect centrally. Change the gown and gloves and use new instruments to harvest a split-thickness skin graft. Place the graft over the elliptical defect, suturing the graft to the flaps and anchoring both to the underlying chest wall. A tie-over stent is often useful. Generally, the graft will take well to the muscle of the chest wall. Certainly, a well-placed graft is preferable to closure of flaps under tension, with the attendant risk for subsequent flap necrosis.

REFERENCES

1. Bland KI, O'Neal B, Weiner LJ, et al. One-stage simple mastectomy with immediate reconstruction for high-risk patients. An improved technique: The biologic basis for ductal-glandular mastectomy. *Arch Surg.* 1986;121:221–225. (Provides a clear and concise description of a cosmetic yet biologically sound prophylactic mastectomy.)

2. Carlson GW, Bostwick J 3rd, Styblo TM, et al. Skin-sparing mastectomy. Oncologic and reconstructive considerations. *Ann Surg.* 1997;225:570–575. (Provides an excellent description of an increasingly popular alternative, particularly for early lesions.)

3. Ching-Wei DT, Howard H, Bland KI. Chapter 35. Mastectomy. In: Dirbas FM, Scott-Conner CEH, eds. *Breast Surgical Techniques and Interdisciplinary Management.* New York, NY: Springer Verlag; 2011:409–422.

4. Edlich RF, Winters KL, Faulkner BC, et al. Risk-reducing mastectomy. *J Long Term Eff Med Implants.* 2006;16:301–314.

5. Haagenson CD. *Diseases of the Breast.* Philadelphia, PA: WB Saunders; 1986. (Presents a clear description of classic radical mastectomy.)

6. Hoffman GW, Elliott LF. The anatomy of the pectoral nerves and its significance to the general and plastic surgeon. *Ann Surg.* 1987;205:504–507. (Presents a brief review of relevant anatomy.)

7. Kato M, Simmons R. Chapter 36. Nipple and areola-sparing mastectomy. In: Dirbas FM, Scott-Conner CEH, eds. *Breast Surgical Techniques and Interdisciplinary Management.* New York, NY: Springer Verlag; 2011:423–430.

8. Moosman DA. Anatomy of the pectoral nerves and their preservation in modified mastectomy. *Am J Surg.* 1980;139:883–886. (Reviews the variant anatomy of pectoral nerves.)

9. Nava MB, Cortinovis U, Ottolenghi J, et al. Skin-reducing mastectomy. *Plast Reconstr Surg.* 2006;118:603–610.

10. Patani N, Devalia H, Anderson A, et al. Oncological safety and patient satisfaction with skin-sparing mastectomy and immediate breast reconstruction. *Surg Oncol.* 2008;17:97–105.

11. Patani N, Mokbel K. Oncological and aesthetic considerations of skin-sparing mastectomy. *Breast Cancer Res Treat.* 2008;111: 391–403.

12. Patey DH. A review of 146 cases of carcinoma of the breast operated on between 1930 and 1943. *Br J Cancer.* 1967;21:260–269. (This is the original description of the Patey technique with resection of the pectoralis minor muscle.)

13. Roses DF, Harris MN, Gumport SL. Total mastectomy with axillary dissection: A modified radical mastectomy. *Am J Surg.* 1977;134:674–677. (Describes a modified technique involving division of the sternal head of the pectoralis major muscle for wide exposure of the apex of the axilla.)

14. Slavin SA, Schnitt SJ, Duda RB, et al. Skin-sparing mastectomy and immediate reconstruction: Oncologic risks and aesthetic results in patients with early-stage breast cancer. *Plast Reconstr Surg.* 1998;102:49–62.

15. Tubbs RS, Salter EG, Custis JW, et al. Surgical anatomy of the cervical and infraclavicular parts of the long thoracic nerve. *J Neurosurg.* 2006;104:792–795.

16. Weisberg NK, Nehal KS, Zide BM. Dog-ears: A review. *Dermatol Surg.* 2000;26:363–370. (Describes alternative methods for treatment of dog ear deformities.)

17. Wijayanayagam A, Kumar AS, Foster RD, et al. Optimizing the total skin-sparing mastectomy. *Arch Surg.* 2008;143:38–45.

18. Yano K, Hosokawa K, Masuoka T, et al. Options for immediate breast reconstruction following skin-sparing mastectomy. *Breast Cancer.* 2007;14:406–413.

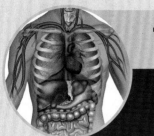

19

Oncoplastic Techniques in Breast Surgery

Oncoplastics is a term used to describe the application of plastic surgical techniques to cancer surgery of the breast. This chapter describes the use of two oncoplastic techniques to resect large areas of the upper or lower aspect of the breast with subsequent re-creation of the breast shape. Often a corresponding procedure must be done on the other side to achieve symmetry.

This chapter also describes some considerations for skin and nipple-areolar complex sparing mastectomy.

SCORE™, the Resident Council on Surgical Education, does not classify these procedures.

STEPS IN PROCEDURE

Oncoplastic Resection Through Batwing Incision
Outline incision along upper aspect of areola
Draw medial and lateral transverse extensions
Create upper incision in similar fashion so that "batwing" of skin is excised with specimen
Raise flaps and excise specimen in usual fashion
Confirm adequacy of excision by specimen radiography or other means
Optional—mobilize remaining breast tissue at the level of pectoral fascia and reapproximate to eliminate dead space
Close incision in usual fashion

Oncoplastic Resection Through Education Mastopexy Incision
Outline incision with the assistance of plastic surgeon
Resect area of involvement and confirm adequacy of resection

Mark edges of the cavity with clips
Closure generally done by plastic surgeon

Skin-Sparing Mastectomy
Incision may be circumareolar, have a keyhole extension, or be modified to incorporate prior biopsy site
Develop cone of skin and subcutaneous tissue by dissecting circumferentially
Mobilize breast from underlying pectoral fascia
Obtain hemostasis and allow plastic surgeon to complete the procedure

Nipple-Areolar–Sparing Mastectomy
Incision may be lateral or inframammary (hockey stick)
Ducts are dissected off the nipple
Biopsy terminal ducts
Finish mastectomy as above

HALLMARK ANATOMIC COMPLICATIONS
Skin-flap necrosis (skin-sparing mastectomy)
Nipple necrosis (nipple-areolar–sparing mastectomy)

LIST OF STRUCTURES
Areola
Internal thoracic (mammary) vessels
Pectoral fascia

Cooper's ligaments
Ribs

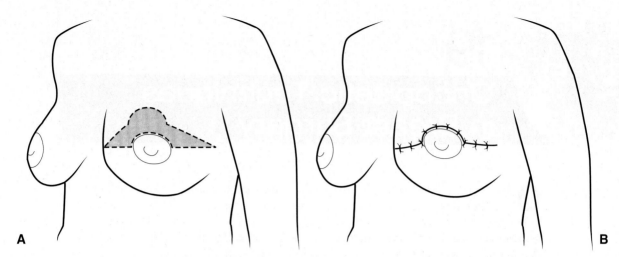

A

B

Figure 19.1 Oncoplastic resection—batwing incision. **A:** Incision. Note extent of skin resection. **B:** Result after resection and closure of incision. Note this will lift the operated breast; hence, a corresponding lift may be needed on the opposite side for symmetry.

Oncoplastic Lumpectomy—Batwing Incision (Fig. 19.1)

Technical and Anatomic Points

This incision allows removal of a significant amount of tissue from the upper aspect of the breast. It is useful for excising large regions of ductal carcinoma in situ (DCIS) or for removal of large benign tumors such as giant fibroadenomas. When the incision is closed, the result is a breast that is slightly smaller and less ptotic than it was before surgery. Sometimes a similar re-excision will be performed on the opposite side to achieve symmetry.

Outline the incision by first defining the area of the tissue to be removed. Outline the upper aspect of the areolar boundary. Then draw medial and lateral extensions. Create the upper part

of the incision in a similar fashion, outlining a contour that will naturally mate to the inferior aspect (Fig. 19.1A).

Elevate flaps and remove tissue as described for lumpectomy. Some surgeons will mobilize the breast tissue from the pectoral fascia and approximate it to eliminate the dead space. Close without drains (Fig. 19.1B).

Oncoplastic Resection—Reduction Mastopexy Incision (Fig. 19.2)

Technical and Anatomic Points

For a woman with relatively large, ptotic breasts, resection of large lesions in the inferior half of the breast may be combined with reduction mastopexy. Reduction mastopexy is usually done on the contralateral breast to re-establish symmetry.

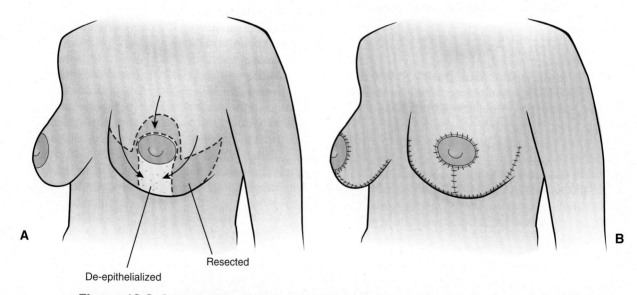

A

B

De-epithelialized

Resected

Figure 19.2 Oncoplastic resection—reduction mastopexy approach. **A:** Incision. **B:** Closure—note reduction on contralateral side for symmetry.

The incision is shown in Figure 19.2A. Generally, the cancer surgeon performs the resection and assures adequacy of the excision. This may require needle localization, ultrasound, specimen radiograph, or any of the techniques in current use to maximize the chance of a negative margin. The plastic surgeon then reconstructs the shape of the breast by bringing the tissue together. This may require resection of additional tissue (which should be oriented and submitted for pathologic examination), elevation of flaps, and/or transposition of some tissue. For that reason, it is prudent to place marking clips in the excision bed before the reconstructive phase of this operation is performed.

The final result is shown in Figure 19.2B. Surgery on the opposite breast may be performed at the same setting or deferred until all cancer-directed treatment is accomplished.

Skin-Sparing Mastectomy Incision (Fig. 19.3)

Technical and Anatomic Points

There are two key points to successful performance of this operation. First, choice of incision; second, careful development of the flaps with preservation of good blood supply. If the operation is being performed for DCIS, generally a circumare-

olar incision will be made (Fig. 19.3A). If the areolae are small and the breast mounds large, a lateral incision can be made to enhance visibility (Fig.19.3B). When a prior biopsy has been done for early breast cancer, some creativity may be needed to maximize skin harvest yet excise nipple-areolar skin and skin around biopsy site (Fig. 19.3C).

Skin-Sparing Mastectomy— Development of Flaps and Completion of Mastectomy (Fig. 19.4)

Technical and Anatomic Points

Flaps are developed in the plane between the subcutaneous tissues and fatty capsule of the breast as during conventional mastectomy, but rather than delineating an upper and lower flap, it is better to conceptualize a conical single envelope of tissue that is being dissected. Work circumferentially, moving from region to region as one area becomes difficult. Often a push-cut technique with almost closed Mayo scissors will enable dissection better than conventional dissection with electrocautery or knife (Fig. 19.4A). Place retractors as the dissection becomes deeper.

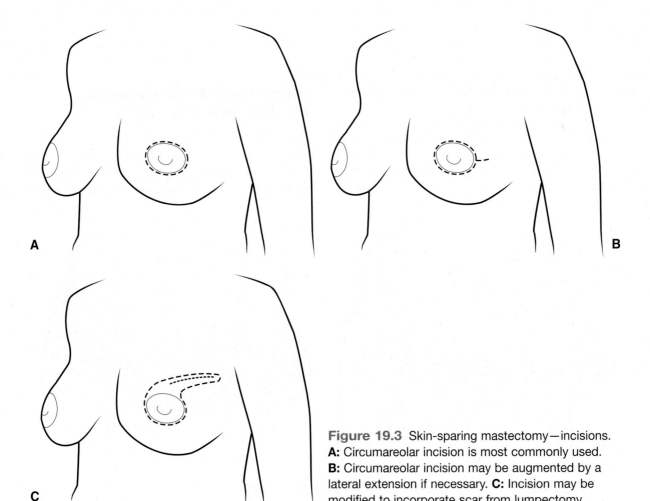

Figure 19.3 Skin-sparing mastectomy—incisions. **A:** Circumareolar incision is most commonly used. **B:** Circumareolar incision may be augmented by a lateral extension if necessary. **C:** Incision may be modified to incorporate scar from lumpectomy.

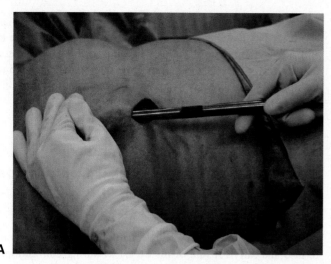
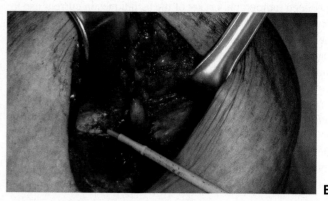

Figure 19.4 Skin-sparing mastectomy—removal of breast. **A:** Development of flaps by blunt dissection with Hegar dilators or closed curved Mayo scissors (from Bland KI, Klimberg VS. *Master Techniques in General Surgery: Breast Surgery*. Philadelphia, PA: Lippincott Williams & Wilkins; 2011, with permission). **B:** Development of inframammary plane (from Bland KI, Klimberg VS. *Master Techniques in General Surgery: Breast Surgery*. Philadelphia, PA: Lippincott Williams & Wilkins; 2011, with permission).

After the flaps have been developed, initiate dissection of the breast from the underlying muscles and fascia at a place where the interface is easily visualized. Often this will be the inferior aspect of the field, rather than superior as during conventional mastectomy. Take care not to inadvertently go deep to pectoralis major muscle as you work cephalad. This risk can be minimized by starting at the medial aspect of the field, where the pectoralis major muscle is easier to find.

The plane deep to the breast and superficial to the pectoralis major muscle is essentially avascular and can be developed by blunt dissection with a finger. Developing this plane early allows greater mobility of the breast, facilitating dissection (Fig. 19.4B).

At some point, it will become possible to deliver the specimen out through the incision and complete dissection by working on the everted skin edge. Take care not to buttonhole the skin.

Obtain hemostasis and allow the plastic surgeon to complete the initial phase of reconstruction and wound closure.

Nipple- and Areola-Sparing Mastectomy (Fig. 19.5)

Technical and Anatomic Points

This approach is used primarily for risk-reducing mastectomy or for small cancers distant from the nipple-areolar complex. There are two basic kinds of incisions in common use. The first

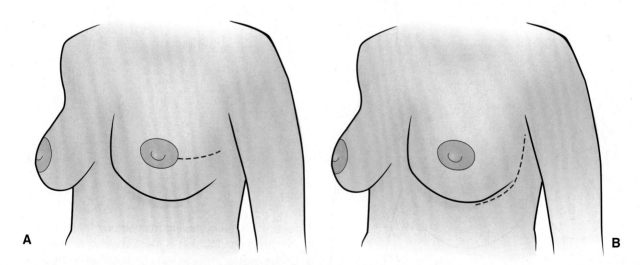

Figure 19.5 Nipple- and areola-sparing mastectomy. **A:** Lateral transverse incision. **B:** Inframammary and lateral (hockey-stick) incision.

is a lateral transverse incision (Fig. 19.5A). This incision can be extended along the areolar border to get greater visibility. The second is a hockey-stick incision that combines an inframammary incision with a lateral vertical component (Fig. 19.5B). This incision gives an excellent cosmetic result and is easily extended, if necessary, without compromising the cosmetic result.

Choice of reconstruction may influence incision location. For this reason, it is wise to discuss the planned approach with the plastic surgeon who will do the reconstruction. Microvascular free flap reconstruction usually requires access to a parasternal intercostal space.

Create the incision and then develop flaps in the usual fashion until the subareolar region is reached. Carefully dissect the ducts to their termination in the nipple as shown for duct excision (Chapter 17). Combine strong downward traction on the duct bundle (easily achieved by grasping the bundle with a right angle clamp and pulling down) with digital pressure on the nipple skin, essentially everting the nipple. Scrape the terminal ducts from the underside of the nipple with a scalpel. Send a biopsy of the terminal ducts for biopsy and mark the termination of the ducts on the breast specimen with a silk suture. Dissection then progresses in the normal fashion.

REFERENCES

1. Clough KB, Ihrai T, Oden S, et al. Oncoplastic surgery for breast cancer based on tumour location and a quadrant-per-quadrant atlas. *Br J Surg.* 2012;99:1389–1395. (Excellent summary of a wide variety of techniques and their application to resections.)
2. Cunnick GH, Mokbet K. Skin-sparing mastectomy. *Br J Surg.* 2006; 93:276–281.
3. Cunnick GH, Mokbel K. Oncological considerations of skin-sparing mastectomy. *Int Semin Surg Oncol.* 2006;3:14.
4. Cutress RI, Simoes T, Gill J, et al. Modification of the Wise pattern breast reduction for oncological mammoplasty of upper outer and upper inner quadrant breast tumours: A technical note and case series. *J Plast Reconstr Aesthet Surg.* 2013;66:e31–e36.
5. Gainer SM, Lucci A. Oncoplastics: Techniques for reconstruction of partial breast defects based on tumor location. *J Surg Oncol.* 2011;103:341–347.
6. Garwood ER, Moore D, Ewing C, et al. Total skin-sparing mastectomy: Complications and local recurrence rates in 2 cohorts of patients. *Ann Surg.* 2009;249:26–32.
7. Greenway RM, Schlossberg L, Dooley WC. Fifteen-year series of skin-sparing mastectomy for stage 0 to 2 breast cancer. *Am J Surg.* 2005:190:918–922.
8. Hernanz F, Regano S, Redondo-Figuero C, et al. Oncoplastic breast-conserving surgery: Analysis of quadrantectomy and immediate reconstruction with latissimus dorsi flap. *World J Surg.* 2007;31:1934–1940. (Another approach; rather than transposing the tissue and creating a smaller breast, the defect is filled with latissimus dorsi.)
9. Huemer GM, Schrenk P, Moser F, et al. Oncoplastic techniques allow breast-conserving treatment in centrally located breast cancers. *Plast Reconstr Surg.* 2007;120:390–398.
10. Jones JA, Pu LL. Oncoplastic approach to early breast cancer in women with macromastia. *Ann Plast Surg.* 2007;58:34–38.
11. Kato M, Simmons R. Chapter 36. Nipple and Areola-Sparing Mastectomy. In: Dirbas FM, Scott-Conner CEH, eds. *Breast Surgical Techniques and Interdisciplinary Management.* New York, NY: Springer Verlag; 2011:423–430.
12. Malata CM, Hodgson EL, Chikwe J, et al. An application of the LeJour vertical mammaplasty pattern for skin-sparing mastectomy: A preliminary report. *Ann Plast Surg.* 2003;51:345–350.
13. Margenthaler JA. Optimizing conservation breast surgery. *J Surg Oncol.* 2011;103:306–312.
14. Masetti R, Di Leone A, Franceschini G, et al. Oncoplastic techniques in the conservative surgical treatment of breast cancer: An overview. *Breast J.* 2006;12(5 suppl 2):S174–S180.
15. Munhoz AM, Aldrighi CM, Ferreira MC. Paradigms in oncoplastic breast surgery: A careful assessment of the oncological need and esthetic objective. *Breast J.* 2007;13:326–327.
16. Nava MB, Cortinovis U, Ottolenghi J, et al. Skin-reducing mastectomy. *Plast Reconstr Surg.* 2006;118:603–610.
17. Rainsburgy RM. Skin-sparing mastectomy. *Br J Surg.* 2006;93: 276–281.
18. Rietjens M, Urban CA, Rey PC, et al. Long-term oncological result of breast conservative treatment with oncoplastic surgery. *Breast.* 2007;16:387–395.
19. Wijayanayagam A, Kumar AS, Foster RD, et al. Optimizing the total skin-sparing mastectomy. *Arch Surg.* 2008;143:38–45.

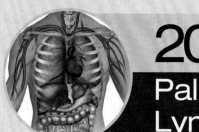

20

Palpable and Sentinel Axillary Lymph Node Biopsies

Laura A. Adam

Simple node excisions are utilized for excision of palpable nodes and in conjunction with sentinel lymph node injections for cancer staging. Although the technique remains essentially the same, anatomy is, of course, variable based on the location of the nodal excision. Most commonly, simple node excisions are performed in the groin or the axilla; however, suspicious palpable nodes can be excised from any nodal basin including the cervical chain, supraclavicular region, preauricular region, and others. The surgical anatomy of the axilla and groin are detailed in Chapters 21 and 119, respectively.

SCORE™, the Surgical Council on Resident Education, classified sentinel lymph node biopsy for melanoma as an "ESSENTIAL UNCOMMON" procedure. SCORE™ has not classified sentinel lymph node biopsy for breast.

STEPS IN PROCEDURE

Palpable Node
Make incision over node
Incise axillary fascia
Elevate node into incision
Clip or ligate hilar pedicle and remove node
Obtain hemostasis and lymph stasis and close incision in layers

Sentinel Lymph Node Biopsy
Lymphoscintigraphy with a radiocolloid is performed preoperatively
Inject blue dye in operating room, if desired
Prep and drape breast and axilla in the usual fashion
If a large breast hangs over and compromises exposure of the axilla, use a sterile adhesive drape to retract it medially and cephalad, improving access
Use a sterile gamma probe to identify location for incision based upon greatest activity and obtain baseline Geiger count

Open axillary fat and enter axillary fascia
Use sterile gamma probe to identify hot spots
Seek blue lymphatics which will lead to blue nodes (if blue dye is used)
Excise any blue, radioactive, or abnormally palpable nodes
Elevate fat surrounding target node into incision
Clip and divide lymphatics and hilar pedicle
Obtain ex vivo count
Check base of incision for radiation—base should be less than 10% of counts of hottest node
Repeat procedure until all blue, radioactive, or abnormal nodes have been removed—but consider terminating after six nodes have been excised
Obtain hemostasis and lymph stasis and close incision without drains

HALLMARK ANATOMIC COMPLICATIONS
Lymphocele
Injury to intercostobrachial or other nerves

False negative biopsy

LIST OF STRUCTURES
Langer's Lines
Tension lines of Kraissl

Axillary Fascia
Pectoralis major
Latissimus dorsi
Serratus anterior
Suspensory ligament of the axilla
Clavipectoral fascia

Axillary Nodes (Haagensen's System)
Lateral group (axillary)
Subscapular (scapular)

Pectoral (external mammary)
Central (central)
Apical (subclavian)
Superficial fascia of the groin
Fascia lata of the thigh

Inguinal Nodes
Superficial inguinal nodes
Deep inguinal nodes
Iliac nodes
Inguinal ligament
Saphenous, femoral, and iliac vessels

Selective sentinel lymphadenectomy refers to excision of a single node or small number of lymph nodes identified by dye staining or lymphoscintigraphy technology. Sentinel lymph node resection is based on the idea that metastasis occurs in a systematic fashion. Because a negative sentinel lymph node strongly predicts a negative nodal basis, patients can have a more extensive lymphadenectomy averted. Sentinel lymph node technology is primarily used in cutaneous malignancies and breast cancers, but has been employed in other cancers, including colorectal, gastroesophageal, lung, urologic, gynecologic, and head and neck. This chapter discusses the technical modifications surrounding palpable and sentinel lymph node biopsies (SLNBs) in the axilla primarily related to breast cancer.

Excisional biopsy of a palpable node is rarely required and should be done only upon careful consideration. Fine needle aspiration for cytology or core needle biopsy (with ultrasound assistance, if necessary) will generally be used first, with excision reserved for difficult cases in which these modalities fail.

Accuracy of sentinel lymph node rates is found to be 97% with a 9.8% false negative rate with multiple trials validating SLNB. In addition, SLNB has been evaluated in other previously controversial breast cancer conditions. High rates of accuracy have been found in multicentric and multifocal breast cancer patients and can be utilized for ductal carcinoma in situ when a mastectomy is being performed. Also SLNB can be used in pregnancy after 30 weeks' gestation when utilizing only a radiocolloid (not blue dye). Controversy still remains as to which patients receive benefit from axillary lymph node dissection after a positive SLNB.

Palpable Node Biopsy (Fig. 20.1)

Technical Points

Position the patient supine with the appropriate extremity exposed. For an axillary node excision, the ipsilateral arm should be extended on an armboard. If necessary, place a small folded sheet under the shoulder to improve exposure. The anatomy of the axilla and location of node groups significant for breast cancer are shown in Figure 20.1A.

Palpate and mark the node before prepping because it may become difficult to palpate the node after infiltration of local anesthetic. In most cases, plan a transverse incision over the area of the palpable node, keeping in mind that the incision may need to be included in a future lymph node dissection. In the case of an axillary node excision, plan to make the incision below the hair-bearing region of the axilla and raise a flap, if necessary, to avoid this area.

Infiltrate the area with local anesthetic and incise the skin. As you begin to dissect, keep in mind that lymph nodes often feel deceptively superficial. To assist in exposure, raise flaps as necessary to expose the node and place a fixed retractor to expose the node (Fig. 20.1B). A traction suture through the node may be used to help elevate it out the wound. Excise the node by dissecting investing tissues off the node circumferentially

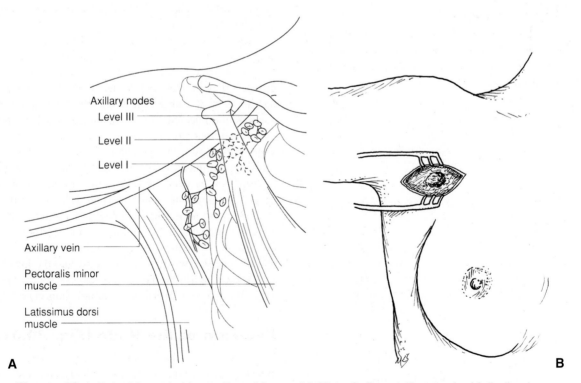

Axillary nodes
Level III
Level II
Level I

Axillary vein

Pectoralis minor muscle

Latissimus dorsi muscle

A

B

Figure 20.1 Palpable node biopsy (from Morrow M, Khan S. Breast disease. In: Mulholland MW, Lillemoe KD, Doherty GM, et al., eds. *Greenfield's Surgery: Scientific Principles and Practice.* 4th ed. Philadelphia, PA: Lippincott Williams & Wilkins; 2006:1252, with permission).

coming around the node. A vascular and lymphatic channel pedicle will be present that should be ligated with a hemoclip or suture before excision. After assuring hemostasis, close the incision in two layers with absorbable suture.

Anatomic Points

The incision should be made as close as possible to the palpable node. For cosmetic reasons, here as elsewhere, Langer's lines should be followed. In the region of the axilla and the groin, these lines are approximately transverse. Corresponding to the relaxed skin tension lines, they are perpendicular to the line of action of the underlying muscle fibers. Avoid the hair-bearing area of the axilla—not for cosmetic reasons, but rather to avoid the morbidity associated with its moist and bacteria-laden environment. This is more difficult to do in the groin region, especially in an overweight individual, so it is best advised to place the incision directly over the palpable node.

Briefly, axillary lymph nodes are located on the medial side of the axillary, but surgeons typically use topographic terminology for axillary lymph nodes. Level I nodes are the most inferior and lie below the pectoralis minor muscle. Level II nodes lie deep to the pectoralis minor muscle and Level III nodes lie medial to this muscle above the axillary vein. A more detailed description of axillary nodes is described in Chapter 19.

Sentinel Node Biopsy—Injection (Fig. 20.2)

Technical Points

First, decision should be made about what identification method will be used: Blue dye, radioactive tracer, or both. Greatest accuracy is achieved when both are used, and that is the method described here.

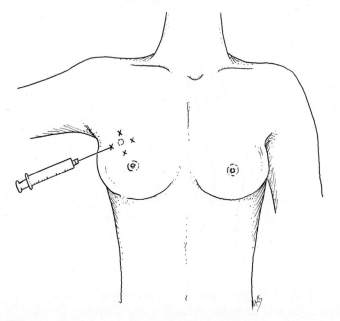

Figure 20.2 Sentinel node biopsy—injection

Lymphazurin 1% (isosulfan blue) dye is readily available at most facilities. It has been associated with a 0.7% risk of anaphylaxis. Methylene blue dye is less expensive and does not carry the risk of anaphylaxis, but it should be diluted to avoid skin necrosis and sterile abscess formation. Either works well for localization purposes.

Radioactive tracer requires a nuclear medicine team and preoperative injection. The radiocolloid used is either 99mTc-antimony sulfide or 99mTc-sulfur colloid and may thus result in allergic reactions in patients with pre-existing sulfa allergies. The operative technique for the excision of lymph nodes is no different than that of a palpable node as long as the techniques for identification of the sentinel node are adhered to.

If the patient is undergoing lymphoscintigraphy mapping, this should be done before bringing the patient to the operating room. Radiocolloids are trapped and retained by sentinel lymph nodes because of the inability of the nodes to filter them. This process occurs about 2 hours after injection and remains present for up to 24 hours after injection.

Consider performing the SLNB before excising the primary tumor so that the blue dye will be excised with the specimen, resulting in improved cosmesis. In addition, a touch preparation (if desired) can be performed while resecting the primary tumor. This allows for a single anesthesia without operative delay; that is, if the sentinel lymph node is positive for metastasis, it can be immediately followed by a lymphadenectomy. If performing a mastectomy for breast cancer at the same time, consider using the lateral aspect of the mastectomy incision to access the axilla for a single surgical incision. If a skin-sparing mastectomy is being performed, a small separate axillary incision may be required.

After positioning the patient and induction of anesthesia, prep with alcohol or chlorhexidine over the skin over the tumor site or the lateral areolar border. Inject a total of 1.5 to 5 mL intradermally into the four corners of the tumor or into the four quadrants of the subareolar tissue. Keep the patient warm and massage the injected area to encourage lymphatic flow. Avoid excess external pressure while massaging because this may slow or even stop the lymphatic flow. Lymph flow rates vary based on the injection site and should therefore result in varying times of incision. Average flow rates are as follows: Head/neck 1.5 cm/minute, anterior trunk 2.8 cm/minute, posterior trunk 3.9 cm/minute, arm/shoulder 2 cm/minute, forearm/hand 5.5 cm/minute, thigh 4.2 cm/minute, and leg/foot 10.2 cm/minute. The faster the flow rate, greater the chance of involving second tier nodes. Thus blue dye injected into the lower extremity sites should be followed relatively soon by sentinel lymph node excision to prevent excision of multiple unnecessary nodes.

Excision of the Node (Fig. 20.3)

If access to the axilla is compromised by a large overhanging breast, gently retract the breast medially and inferiorly with a sterile adhesive drape. Generally, the easiest path to the sentinel node in a large patient is along a curvilinear line where the axillary fat pad meets the fat of the lateral breast (Fig. 20.3A).

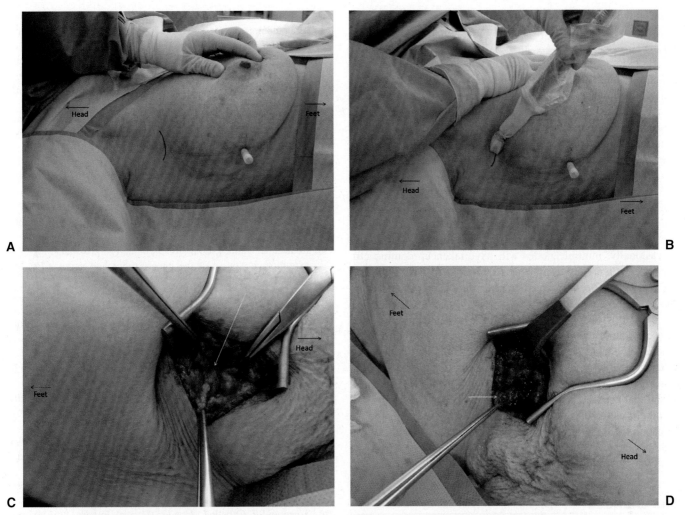

Figure 20.3 Excision of the sentinel node. **A:** Incision in natural skin crease (from Bland KI, Klimberg VS. *Master Techniques in General Surgery: Breast Surgery.* Philadelphia, PA: Lippincott Williams & Wilkins; 2011, with permission). **B:** Identification of hot spot with sterile gamma probe (from Bland KI, Klimberg VS. *Master Techniques in General Surgery: Breast Surgery.* Philadelphia, PA: Lippincott Williams & Wilkins; 2011, with permission). **C:** Blue lymphatics lead to the blue-stained sentinel lymph node (from Bland KI, Klimberg VS. *Master Techniques in General Surgery: Breast Surgery.* Philadelphia, PA: Lippincott Williams & Wilkins; 2011, with permission). **D:** The blue node is excised (from Bland KI, Klimberg VS. *Master Techniques in General Surgery: Breast Surgery.* Philadelphia, PA: Lippincott Williams & Wilkins; 2011, with permission).

The exact site along this line is determined by localization with the gamma probe.

Begin by exposing the site as if for a palpable node. Use a gamma probe to identify the area of highest radioactivity. This is best accomplished by determining the greatest activity along both the x- and y-axes and planning the incision over their intersection (Fig. 20.3B). The operative gamma probe is collimated so that it detects activity along a narrow cone projecting from the end of the device. Take advantage of this collimation by angling the probe away from the primary injection site as shown. Many nuclear medicine centers mark the area of greatest activity; however, this can be misleading as the patient

may not be in the same position as during operation. Perform a transverse incision as described earlier in this chapter.

Occasionally, a node will be located under the lateral edge of the pectoralis major muscle, and in this case an oblique incision along the edge of this muscle may facilitate identification, particularly in a slender individual. Be mindful that a positive sentinel lymph node may require completion axillary dissection with a corresponding extension of the incision.

Expose and incise the axillary fascia and identify the fat around the nodes by a change in texture. Subcutaneous fat is usually lumpy and bumpy, whereas axillary fat is much smoother in texture, similar to visceral fat. Although an occasional sentinel node will be found in the subcutaneous fat (or even in the axillary tail of the breast), most are contained in the axillary fat.

Follow the gamma probe activity deep while looking for any blue-laden lymphatic channels (Fig. 20.3C). Remember that the sentinel lymph node is defined as "any lymph node that receives lymph drainage directly from the tumor site" and may not be the first node encountered. Any node that avidly stains blue or is radioactive should be included within the specimen until a 90% drop in total radioactive counts is obtained.

Isolate and dissect the node or nodes of interest (Fig. 20.3D). Remember that a node that is totally replaced by tumor may not take up either tracer. Hence it is important to remove any palpably abnormal node encountered during dissection. Occasionally, multiple nodes will have taken up contrast. In this case, it is common practice to terminate dissection when six nodes have been removed or when dissection progresses to the level of the axillary vein.

Use clips and/or ties to secure any lymphatics and the hilar pedicle of the node in order to help prevent lymphoceles. Check the background activity and seek additional nodes if it is unacceptably high (>10% of the baseline reading). Keep in mind, The American College of Surgeons Oncology Group has found that age ≥70 years and having ≥5 lymph nodes removed results in increased rates of axillary seromas. Additional complications include an 8.6% risk of axillary paresthesias, 3.8% risk of decreased arm range of motion, and 6.9% risk of proximal upper extremity lymphedema.

REFERENCES

1. Cox CE, Salud CJ, Harrinton MA. The role of selective sentinel lymph node dissection in breast cancer. *Surg Clin North Am.* 2000;80:1759–1777. (The appendix lists technical "pearls" which are particularly valuable.)
2. Cunnick GH, Upponi S, Wishart GC. Anatomical variants of the intercostobrachial nerve encountered during axillary dissection. *Breast.* 2001;10:160–162.
3. Freeman SR, Washington SJ, Pritchard T, et al. Long term results of a randomised prospective study of preservation of the intercostobrachial nerve. *Eur J Surg Oncol.* 2003;29:213–215.
4. Giuliano AE, Hunt KK, Ballman KV, et al. Axillary dissection vs no axillary dissection in women with invasive breast cancer and sentinel node metastasis. A randomized clinical trial. *JAMA.* 2011;305:569–575.
5. Leong SP, Kitagawa Y, Kitajima M. *Selective Sentinel Lymphadenectomy for Human Solid Cancer.* New York, NY: Springer Science+Business Media, Inc; 2005.
6. Lopchinsky RA. Locating the axillary vein and preserving the medial pectoral nerve. *Am J Surg.* 2004;188:193–194. (Describes some tricks useful when operating through a very small incision.)
7. Loukas M, Louis RG Jr, Fogg QA, et al. An unusual innervation of pectoralis minor and major muscles from a branch of the intercostobrachial nerve. *Clin Anat.* 2006;19:347–349.
8. Loukas M, Hullet J, Louis RG Jr, et al. The gross anatomy of the extrathoracic course of the intercostobrachial nerve. *Clin Anat.* 2006;19:106–111.
9. Lyman GH, Giuliano AE, Somerfield MR, et al. American Society of Clinical Oncology guideline recommendations for sentinel lymph node biopsy in early-stage breast cancer. *J Clin Oncol.* 2005; 20:7703–7720.
10. O'Rourke MG, Tang TS, Allison SI, et al. The anatomy of the extrathoracic intercostobrachial nerve. *Aust N Z J Surg.* 1999;69: 860–864.
11. Pandelidis SM, Peters KL, Walusimbi MS, et al. The role of axillary dissection in mammographically detected carcinoma. *J Am Coll Surg.* 1997;184:341–345.
12. Pavlista D, Eliska O, Duskova M, et al. Localization of the sentinel node of the upper outer breast quadrant in the axillary quadrants. *Ann Surg Oncol.* 2007;14:633–637.
13. Taylor KO. Morbidity associated with axillary surgery for breast cancer. *ANZ J Surg.* 2004;74:314–347.
14. Torresan RZ, Cabello C, Conde DM, et al. Impact of the preservation of the intercostobrachial nerve in axillary lymphadenectomy due to breast cancer. *Breast J.* 2003;9:389–392.
15. Van Zee KJ, Manasseh DM, Bevilacqua JL, et al. A nomogram for predicting the likelihood of additional nodal metastases in breast cancer patients with a positive sentinel node biopsy. *Ann Surg Oncol.* 2003;10:1140–1151. (One of several predictive models for likelihood of additional positive nodes.)

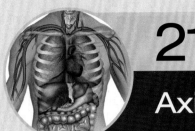

21

Axillary Node Dissection

Laura A. Adam and Neal Wilkinson

Axillary lymph node dissection typically refers to the more limited resection of topographic group I and group II axillary lymph nodes (Fig. 21.1). It is most commonly performed for breast cancer, but can be used for treatment of other malignancies like melanoma. When performed in conjunction with mastectomy it is termed as modified radical mastectomy (see Chapter 18), but it is often performed as an isolated axillary node dissection with lumpectomy. Often a sentinel lymph node biopsy will have been performed prior to axillary lymph node dissection, either as a separate surgical procedure or during the initial phase of the same operation.

This chapter first discusses the technical modifications required when axillary node dissection is done alone followed by description of a more limited axillary node sampling procedure previously used in staging of breast carcinomas. This procedure is now rarely performed following the widespread use of sentinel lymph node biopsy.

SCORE™, the Surgical Council on Resident Education, did not specifically classify Axillary node dissection.

STEPS IN PROCEDURE

Position patient supine, with arm extended on arm board

Transverse incision below hair-bearing area or oblique incision just behind lateral edge of pectoralis major muscle

Raise flaps

Identify lateral edge of pectoralis major muscle

Dissect under pectoralis major muscle, preserving median pectoral neurovascular bundle

Identify pectoralis minor muscle and dissect under it (sometimes, it may be divided or excised to facilitate dissection)

Identify axillary vein and trace it laterally

Identify long thoracic nerve and incise fascia lateral to it; mobilize the nerve medially

Identify thoracodorsal neurovascular bundle and preserve it

Sweep all fatty node-bearing tissue inferiorly and laterally, preserving nerves and axillary vein

Orient specimen

Obtain hemostasis and place closed suction drains

Close incision in layers

Axillary Sampling

Shorter but similar incision

Dissection is limited to level I and some level II nodes

Preserve nerves as noted above

HALLMARK ANATOMIC COMPLICATIONS

Injury to median pectoral nerve

Injury to long thoracic nerve (winged scapula)

Injury to thoracodorsal nerve

Injury to axillary vein

Division or injury to intercostobrachial nerve

LIST OF STRUCTURES

Pectoralis major muscle

Pectoralis minor muscle

Clavipectoral fascia

Lateral pectoral nerve

Medial pectoral nerve

Thoracodorsal nerve

Long thoracic nerve

Axillary artery

Axillary vein

Thoracoacromial artery

Thoracodorsal vein

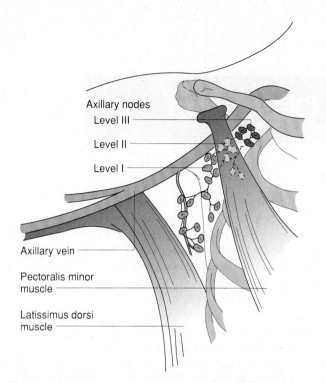

Figure 21.1 Regional anatomy, showing axillary vein and pectoralis minor muscle, and their relationship to nodes in levels I to III (from Morrow M, Khan S. Breast disease. In: Mulholland MW, Lillemoe KD, Doherty GM, et al., eds. *Greenfield's Surgery: Scientific Principles and Practice*. Philadelphia, PA: Lippincott Williams & Wilkins; 2006, with permission).

Axillary Node Dissection

Choice of Incision and Elevation of Flaps (Fig. 21.2)

Technical Points

Position the patient with the arm extended on an arm board with a bump under the shoulder (see Chapter 18). If sentinel node biopsy has been performed at an earlier time, plan an incision that excises and extends the previous scar. It will, in general, be easiest to stay wide of the sentinel lymph node dissection field and dissect in fresh tissue around that field. Excising the old scar may help avoid going back into a scarred area. If sentinel node biopsy was done during the same operative procedure and returned positive, then simply extend the sentinel node incision in both directions. Again, allowing subsequent dissection to progress through fresh undissected planes is generally the safest strategy.

An oblique incision just lateral to the pectoralis major muscle provides excellent access to the axilla, and this lateral location allows the scar to fall behind the muscle, where it is less noticeable. A more cosmetically appealing transverse or U-shaped incision may also be used. A transverse incision should be planned to lie below the hair-bearing portion of the axilla. Patient habitus and location of sentinel lymph node often determine incision preference. As with sentinel node biopsy, in corpulent patients an incision in the line between the axillary fat pat and the breast fat may provide the easiest access to the axilla (see Chapter 20).

After incising the skin, create skin flaps to expose the subcutaneous tissues.

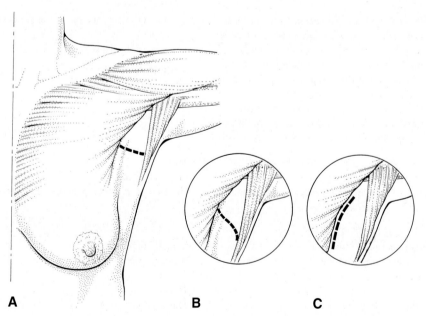

A   B   C

Figure 21.2 Choice of incision and elevation of flaps. **A,B,** and **C:** Show several alternatives incisions (from Dixon JM, Soon PSH. Breast-conserving surgery. In: Fischer JE, Bland KI, eds. *Mastery of Surgery*. 5th ed. Philadelphia, PA: Lippincott Williams & Wilkins; 2007).

Anatomic Points

Discrete superficial and deep fascia is not encountered in the axilla. Instead, the axillary fascia (derived from the fascia of the pectoralis major, latissimus dorsi, serratus anterior muscles, and investing the muscles of the arm) is adherent to the superficial fascia and is, in the hollow of the armpit, along with the suspensory ligament of the axilla, a continuation of the clavipectoral fascia.

The axillary lymph nodes are predominantly located on the medial side of the axillary neurovascular bundle, and along the medial axillary wall. Terminology is complicated by multiple nomenclature systems including the anatomic system, Haagensen's system (explained later in this chapter), and the surgeon's topographic levels I to III (as shown in Fig. 21.1). The anatomic *lateral group* on the third part of the axillary neurovascular bundle drains the upper limb. The *subscapular group* located around the subscapular artery and vein drains the shoulder and posterior thorax. The *pectoral* group associated with the lateral thoracic vessels along the inferolateral border of the pectoralis major muscle drains the anterior thoracic wall including the lateral breast. These three groups drain into the *central group* lymph nodes located on the second part of the axillary neurovascular bundle which then further joins with the upper outer quadrant of the breast to drain into the *apical group*.

Surgeons commonly use a different terminology (topographic) for axillary lymph nodes. Topographic group I nodes include the pectoral, subscapular, and lateral nodes. These are the nodes lateral to the pectoralis minor muscle. Topographic group II nodes are under the pectoralis minor muscle and correspond to the central nodes, whereas topographic group III nodes are medial to the pectoralis minor muscle and correspond to the apical nodes (see Fig. 21.1).

Exposure of Nerves and Axillary Vein (Fig. 21.3)

Technical Points

If a sentinel node biopsy has been done, avoid the temptation to re-enter the sentinel node cavity. Instead, work through clean tissue planes and excise this cavity with the specimen. First, identify the lateral border of the pectoralis major muscle and clean the fatty tissue from the underside of the muscle (Fig. 21.3A,B). Take care to preserve the neurovascular bundle to the pectoralis major muscle. This bundle originates superiorly and will generally retract medially and cephalad out of the field when gently pushed in that direction with a finger or Kittner dissector. Place a retractor under pectoralis major muscle. Identify the pectoralis minor muscle and incise the clavipectoral fascia on each side of this muscle. If necessary, divide the pectoralis minor muscle to gain access to the axillary vein. Dissect medially in the anterior adventitial plane of the vein to the surgical apex of the axilla. Follow the axillary vein laterally, dividing any small vessels that cross over the vein. The general rule is that any structure that crosses over or

terminates within the axillary vein is safe to take because motor nerves pass deep to the vein.

Sensory nerves arise from the intercostal spaces and pass through the surgical field from the chest wall toward the upper arm. These include the intercostobrachial nerve, which generally arises from the second intercostal space and several smaller nerves that similarly arise from intercostal nerves. These were previously commonly divided resulting in numbness of the inner aspect of the arm. Preservation probably does not increase rates of local recurrence and results in improved sensory outcomes.

Follow the axillary vein laterally, dividing any small vessels that cross over it and any venous tributaries that pass inferiorly. As the chest wall starts to curve down away from you, look for the long thoracic nerve just under the fascia. Identify it as a long, straight nerve. Incise the fascia and confirm the identity of the nerve by gentle mechanical stimulation with a forceps or with an electrical nerve stimulator. Extend the incision of the overlying fascia inferiorly and gently push the nerve down against the chest wall and posterior axilla away from your specimen.

Continue dissecting laterally in the anterior adventitial plane of the axillary vein looking for the thoracodorsal vein, a relatively large venous tributary passing about a centimeter deep to the axillary vein. It serves as an important landmark for the thoracodorsal nerve and, for safety, the vein may need to be ligated at this point. The thoracodorsal nerve lies in close proximity to, and in general just deep to the thoracodorsal artery. Confirm the identity of this nerve. Look for any small tributaries that can often pass from this neurovascular bundle to the specimen and ligate or clip as needed.

Anatomic Points

Figure 21.3C shows the major structures that are preserved during dissection including the intercostobrachial nerve. The innervation of the pectoralis major muscle is provided by the lateral and medial pectoral nerves. These nerves, named according to their origin on the lateral and medial cords of the brachial plexus (not on the basis of their relative location on the anterior thoracic wall), carry fibers of spinal cord levels C5 to C7 and C8 to T1, respectively. The lateral pectoral nerve crosses anterior to the first part of the axillary artery and vein and the medial pectoral nerve arises at the level of the second part of the axillary artery. Both have several rami which innervate both the pectoralis minor and major muscles.

Clavipectoral fascia is that fascia that invests the pectoralis minor muscle. Inferior to the muscle, it is continuous with the serratus anterior fascia and with the so-called axillary fascia (primarily derived from the pectoralis major fascia), whereas superomedially, it blends with intercostal fascia, and superolaterally, it continues as a dense sheet, splitting to invest the subclavius muscle. When splitting this fascia, care should be taken not to damage either the thoracoacromial artery or the lateral pectoral nerve, both of which pierce the fascia superior to the pectoralis minor muscle.

When performed, division of the pectoralis minor muscle allows exposure of all the three parts of the axillary artery

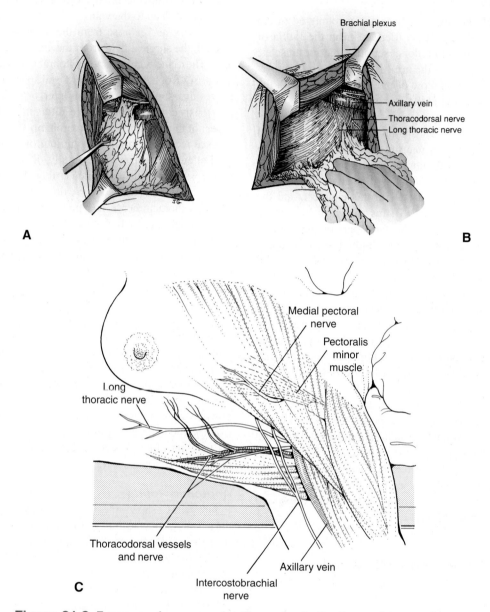

A

B

Brachial plexus

Axillary vein
Thoracodorsal nerve
Long thoracic nerve

Medial pectoral
nerve

Pectoralis
minor
muscle

Long
thoracic nerve

Thoracodorsal vessels
and nerve

Axillary vein

Intercostobrachial
nerve

C

Figure 21.3 Exposure of nerves and axillary vein. **A:** Gentle caudal retraction on fat pad exposes axillary vein. **B:** Once axillary vein has been cleared, lateral retraction exposes nerves. **C:** Regional anatomy (**C** from Dixon JM, Soon PSH. Breast-conserving surgery. In: Fischer JE, Bland KI, eds. *Mastery of Surgery.* 5th ed. Philadelphia, PA: Lippincott Williams & Wilkins; 2007).

and vein. This improves access to the axillary lymph nodes (chiefly those of the central and apical groups) located adjacent to the second and first part of these vessels, respectively. When removing the node-bearing axillary tissue, one should remember that the long thoracic nerve, formed in the posterior triangle of the neck by anastomosis of branches of brachial plexus roots C5 to C7, descends into the axilla posterior to the brachial plexus and the first part of the axillary vessels. It continues its descent along the superficial (axillary) surface of the serratus anterior muscle, supplying each digitation of this muscle in its course. Damage to this nerve that is sufficient to cause paralysis of the serratus anterior muscle is manifested by "winging"

of the scapula and an inability to elevate the arm above the horizontal level.

The thoracodorsal nerve, which carries fibers from C6 to C8, originates from the posterior cord of the brachial plexus posterior to the second part of the axillary vessels, accompanying the thoracodorsal branch of the subscapular artery along the posterior axillary wall to supply the latissimus dorsi muscle. Damage to the thoracodorsal nerve results in paralysis of the latissimus dorsi muscle weakening adduction, inward rotation, and extension of the arm (as in a swimming stroke), and aids in depression of the scapula a function necessary to support the weight of the body when using crutches.

Completion of Dissection (Fig. 21.4)

Sweep the axillary contents downward, keeping both nerves in view and preserving them. If there is malignant invasion, the thoracodorsal artery and nerve can be sacrificed, but this is rare. Terminate the dissection at the latissimus dorsi muscle. When dissection is performed properly, ribs and intercostal muscles will be well exposed. Amputate and orient the specimen. Check for hemostasis and place closed-suction drains under the flaps. Close the wound in two layers with absorbable suture.

Anatomic Points

The anatomic axilla, is a triangular field accessible when the pectoral muscles are retracted or when necessary divided bounded superolaterally by the axillary vein, inferolaterally by the latissimus dorsi muscle, medially by the serratus anterior muscle, and posteriorly by the subscapular, teres major, and latissimus dorsi muscles (Fig. 21.4A). The apex of this triangle is superomedial, deep to the clavicle. Here, the dominant feature of immediate concern is the axillary vein.

On average, there are 35 axillary lymph nodes, which are loosely arranged in groups associated with the major arteries

and veins (Fig. 21.4B). As reviewed earlier in this chapter, multiple classifications exist for axillary nodes. Although major anatomy texts frequently list five groups, perhaps the best classification system is that of Haagensen, who maintains that there are six groups, as follows:

1. *External mammary nodes:* An average of 1.7 nodes lying deep to the lateral edge of the pectoralis major muscle and being associated with the lateral thoracic artery. Lymphatic drainage from these nodes passes to the central or subclavicular nodes.

2. *Interpectoral (Rotter's) nodes:* An average of 1.4 nodes are associated with the pectoral branches of the thoracoacromial artery. These nodes are located in the areolar tissue between the pectoralis major muscle and the clavipectoral fascia that envelops the pectoralis minor muscle. Lymphatic drainage from these nodes passes to the central or subclavicular nodes.

3. *Scapular nodes:* An average of 5.8 nodes are associated with the subscapular vessels and their thoracodorsal branches. Because the intercostobrachial and thoracodorsal nerves pass through this group of nodes, these nerves may have to

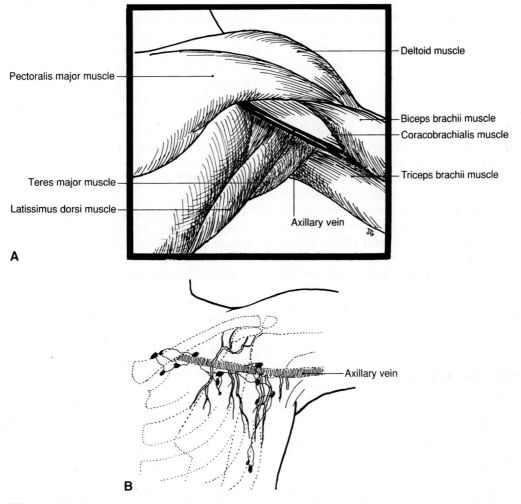

Figure 21.4 Completion of dissection. **A:** Relationships of axillary vein to muscles in the region. **B:** Lymphatics of region, removed during dissection.

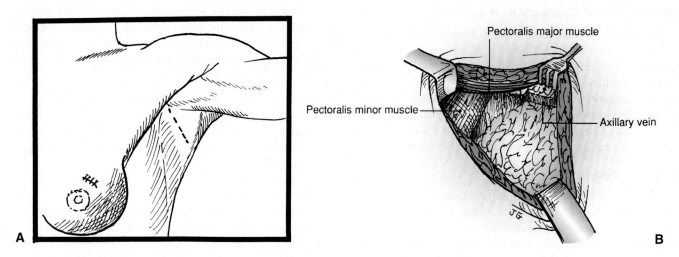

Figure 21.5 Incision and extent of dissection. **A:** Incision **B:** Exposure of level I and level II nodes.

be sacrificed to allow the removal of the nodes. Lymphatic drainage from these nodes passes to the central nodes.

4. *Central nodes:* An average of 12.1 nodes lying in fat in the central axilla, about halfway between the anterior and posterior axillary folds. Frequently, one or more of these nodes is located between the skin and the superficial fascia. Lymphatic drainage from these nodes passes to the axillary nodes.

5. *Axillary nodes:* An average of 10.7 nodes are closely associated with the axillary vein from the tendon of the latissimus dorsi muscle to the termination of the thoracoacromial vein. Lymphatic drainage from these nodes passes to the subclavicular nodes.

6. *Subclavicular nodes:* An average of 3.5 nodes are associated with the axillary vein proximal to the termination of the thoracoacromial vein. These nodes, then, are located in the apex of the axilla, and are primarily posterior to the subclavius muscle, which is enveloped by the clavipectoral fascia. Access to the nodes is facilitated by the division of the pectoralis minor muscle and its enveloping clavipectoral fascia. This group of nodes receives lymphatics from all other axillary nodes. Lymphatic drainage from these nodes passes into the inferior deep cervical nodes or directly into the venous system in the vicinity of the jugulosubclavian junction. These nodes are considered to be the highest, or apical, lymph nodes, at least from the standpoint of the breast surgeon.

Axillary Node Sampling

Incision and Extent of Dissection (Fig. 21.5)

Technical and Anatomic Points

This low axillary dissection may be used when sentinel node localization fails. It is designed to remove only the lowest nodes. Make an incision similar to that described for complete axillary dissection, but shorter in length (Fig. 21.5A). Raise skin flaps to expose the area indicated. Begin at the lateral border of the pectoralis major muscle to sweep fatty tissue later-

ally and out of the axilla. Place a retractor under the pectoralis major muscle to aid in exposure of the pectoralis minor muscle. The aim of the dissection is to remove a representative sampling of group I and a few group II axillary nodes (Fig. 21.5B). These nodes lie lateral to the breast up to, but not beyond, the medial border of the pectoralis minor muscle. Remove fatty tissue down to the level of the pectoralis minor muscle, but do not dissect under this muscle. Sweep the fatty node-bearing tissue laterally out of the axilla. Do not carry the dissection as far posteriorly as would be appropriate for a formal node dissection. Nerves are generally not formally identified; hence, the dissection must remain relatively superficial. Check hemostasis and place a small closed-suction drain under the flaps. Close the incision with a single subcuticular layer.

REFERENCES

1. Cunnick GH, Upponi S, Wishart GC. Anatomical variants of the intercostobrachial nerve encountered during axillary dissection. *Breast.* 2001;10:160–162.

2. Freeman SR, Washington SJ, Pritchard T, et al. Long term results of a randomized prospective study of preservation of the intercostobrachial nerve. *Eur J Surg Oncol.* 2003;29:213–215. (Preservation of this nerve provided a modest improvement in long-term symptoms.)

3. Gobardhan PD, Wijsman JH, van Dalen T, et al. ARM: Axillary reverse mapping – the need for selection of patients. *Eur J Surg Oncol.* 2012;38:657–661. (Use of tracer to identify and preserve lymphatics draining the arm, potentially minimizing lymphedema.)

4. Harris MN, Gumport SL, Maiwandi H. Axillary lymph node dissection for melanoma. *Surg Gynecol Obstet.* 1972;135:936–940. (Describes division of the sternal head of the greater pectoral muscle for wide exposure of the apex of the axilla; also discusses incontinuity wide excision of melanoma.)

5. Hoffman GW, Elliott LF. The anatomy of the pectoral nerves and its significance to the general and plastic surgeon. *Ann Surg.* 1987;205:504–507. (Presents a brief review of relevant anatomy.)

6. Khan A, Chakravorty A, Gui GP. In vivo study of the surgical anatomy of the axilla. *Br J Surg.* 2012;99:871–877. (excellent discussion of common anatomic variants.)

7. Luini A, Zurrida S, Galimberti V, et al. Axillary dissection in breast cancer. *Crit Rev Oncol Hematol.* 1999;30:63–70.

8. Margolese R, Poisson R, Shibata H, et al. The technique of segmental mastectomy (lumpectomy) and axillary dissection: A syllabus from the National Surgical Adjuvant Breast Project workshops. *Surgery.* 1987;102:828–834. (Describes axillary dissection through a small, separate incision when done as part of breast conservation surgery.)

9. McNeil C. Endoscopy removal of axillary nodes gains ground abroad, toehold in US. *J Natl Cancer Inst.* 1999;91:582–583. (Presents an alternative technique that is under development.)

10. Nos C, Kaufmann G, Clough KB, et al. Combined axillary reverse mapping (ARM) technique for breast cancer patients requiring axillary dissection. *Ann Surg Oncol.* 2008;15:2550–2555.

11. O'Rourke MG, Tang TS, Allison SI, et al. The anatomy of the extrathoracic intercostobrachial nerve. *Aust NZJ Surg.* 1999;69:860–864.

12. Pavlista D, Eliska O. Relationship between the lymphatic drainage of the breast and the upper extremity: A postmortem study. *Ann Surg Oncol.* 2012;19:3410–3415.

13. Temple WJ, Ketcham AS. Preservation of the intercostobrachial nerve during axillary dissection for breast cancer. *Am J Surg.* 1985;150:585–588.

14. Torresan RZ, Cabello C, Conde DM, et al. Impact of the preservation of the intercostobrachial nerve in axillary lymphadenectomy due to breast cancer. *Breast J.* 2003;9:389–392.

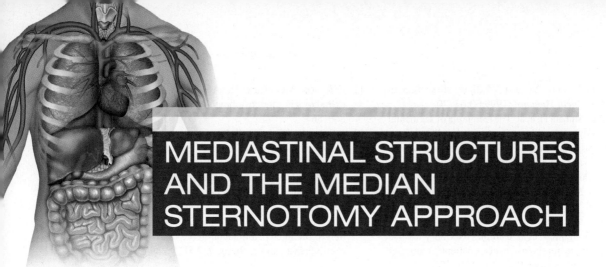

MEDIASTINAL STRUCTURES AND THE MEDIAN STERNOTOMY APPROACH

The mediastinum is the "thoracic space" between the two pleural sacs, the root word originally meaning septum. The mediastinum extends from the thoracic inlet cephalad to the superior surface of the diaphragm. The undersurface of the mediastinum is bounded posteriorly by the anterior longitudinal spinal ligament (dorsal) and the posterior mantel of the sternum anteriorly (ventral). Although lesions of the paravertebral region (costovertebral sulci) are traditionally classified as mediastinal in nature, this area is not formally within the mediastinum.

Multiple surgical and radiologic subdivisions within the mediastinum have been described in the literature. Most commonly, the mediastinum has been divided either into four compartments (superior, anterior, middle, and posterior) or three compartments (anterosuperior, middle or visceral, and posterior).

The anterior mediastinum can be defined as the area bounded by the thoracic inlet superiorly, the sternum anteriorly, and the pericardium and vertebral column inferiorly (see Figure 1). Each compartment extends to the diaphragm inferiorly and is bounded laterally by the mediastinal surface of the respective parietal pleura.

Within the subdivisions of the mediastinum are numerous structures that are of frequent surgical interest. The anterosuperior compartment contains multiple lymph node stations and the thymus. In addition, it can be the site of displaced parathyroid tissue, ectopic thyroid tissue, and other benign and malignant tumors.

The regional lymph nodes can give rise to primary tumors or pathologic processes or, more commonly, can be regionally (or systemically) involved with malignant lesions. Additional structures within this compartment include the trachea, great vessels, and their proximal tributaries. The middle, or visceral, compartment contains the heart, proximal great vessels, proximal pulmonary arteries and veins, lymph nodes, and the pericardium. The posterior mediastinum contains the azygos and hemiazygos veins, sympathetic trunks, esophagus, thoracic duct, lymph nodes, and the descending aorta.

In this chapter, the anatomy of the mediastinum is explored through a series of operative procedures. Cervical mediastinoscopy, anterior mediastinoscopy, and mediastinotomy (Chamberlain's procedure) (Chapter 22e) are diagnostic maneuvers used to gain access to mediastinal lymph nodes. These invasive procedures are rarely used in current practice, having been largely supplanted by ultrasound-guided transbronchial biopsy, and a variety of imaging studies. They are included in the web version of this text because they illustrate the anatomy well and because they still have occasional application when other techniques fail.

Median sternotomy (Chapter 23e) provides wide access to the anterior mediastinum and heart. It is used for major cardiac surgery, some pulmonary surgery, exposure of the thymus gland, great vessel and proximal upper vascular exposure, and, occasionally, improved hepatic exposure. The posterior mediastinum is most easily approached laterally through a thoracotomy incision because the heart, lungs, and great vessels form a barrier limiting adequate access from the front.

The esophagus is a mediastinal structure. However, because of its posterior location, it is approached either through a thoracotomy incision or through combined cervical and abdominal approaches. Hence the thoracic esophagus can be included in the next part of this text (The Lungs and Structures Approached Through a Thoracotomy Incision).

ORIENTATION

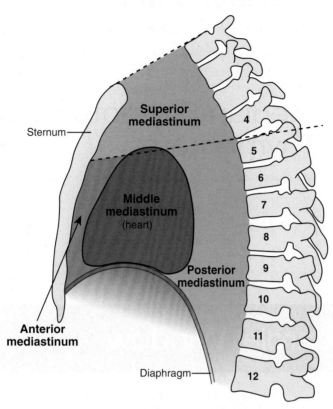

Figure 1 Orientation

22 Mediastinoscopy and Mediastinotomy

This chapter can be accessed online at www.lww.com/eChapter22.

23 Median Sternotomy and Thymectomy

This chapter can be accessed online at www.lww.com/eChapter23.

24

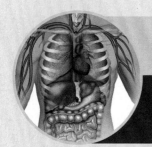

Pericardial Window

This procedure is performed for the treatment of pericardial effusions. The most common indication is malignancy. Two approaches are described here—the open subxiphoid approach and the thoracoscopic approach. Rarely, subxiphoid exploration is performed during trauma resuscitations when pericardial tamponade is suspected. This has largely been superseded by echocardiography.

Subxiphoid pericardial window is an easy way to decompress the pericardium if cardiac tamponade is diagnosed during trauma laparotomy.

The open subxiphoid approach provides only limited drainage but can be performed rapidly under local anesthesia, if the patient is in extreme distress.

SCORE™, the Surgical Council on Resident Education, classified pericardial window for drainage as an "ESSENTIAL UNCOMMON" procedure.

STEPS IN PROCEDURE

Subxiphoid Approach
Short midline incision from just above xiphoid extending approximately 5 cm inferiorly

Resect xiphoid process

Suture ligate small branches of inferior phrenic artery if encountered

Sweep diaphragm and preperitoneal fat inferiorly to expose pericardium

Elevate pericardium from heart and incise it (do not use cautery)

Excise pericardium to create an approximately 2 cm circular defect; send to pathology (if cancer)

Gently explore pericardium and break down any soft loculations

Suture edges of defect to surrounding tissues

Place one or two small diameter chest tubes or closed suction drains

Close incision in layers

Thoracoscopic Approach
Three ports

Divide inferior pulmonary ligament and retract lung cephalad

Visualize phrenic nerve

Create anterior window by elevating pericardium and incising it, then excising a rectangular window anterior to phrenic nerve (do not use cautery)

On the left side, space may allow creation of a similar window inferior to the phrenic nerve

Place chest tubes

Close trocar sites

HALLMARK ANATOMIC COMPLICATIONS

Injury to phrenic nerve

Bleeding from inferior phrenic artery

Cardiac herniation through lateral window

LIST OF STRUCTURES

Pericardium

Mediastinal pleura

Sternum

Manubrium

Body

Xiphoid process

Inferior pericardiosternal ligament

Diaphragm

Peritoneal cavity

Inferior phrenic artery

Phrenic nerve

Inferior pulmonary ligament

Subxiphoid Approach (Fig. 24.1)

Technical Points

This is the quickest and simplest approach. It is easily performed under local anesthesia, or, with minor modification, during trauma laparotomy. When the pericardium is simply entered and drained, the term *drainage* is used. The term *window* is used if a connection is established between the pericardium and the peritoneal cavity.

Make a short midline incision from just above the xiphoid extending inferiorly for several centimeters. Deepen this incision through subcutaneous tissues to expose the xiphoid cartilage. Surround this and resect it at its junction with the sternum (Fig. 24.1A). Small branches of the inferior phrenic arteries commonly run on each side of the xiphoid process and must be suture ligated if encountered. Deep to the xiphoid process some preperitoneal fat and muscular slips of the diaphragm will be encountered. Sweep these inferiorly to expose the pericardium (Fig. 24.1B).

Assess the pericardium for the presence of fluid, tumor nodules, or blood. Elevate the pericardium with forceps and make a small incision. Aspirate fluid and culture it if indicated. With scissors, excise a disc of pericardium approximately 2 cm in diameter and send it for pathologic examination (in cases of malignancy). Do not use cautery, because the current may cause the heart to fibrillate. Gently explore the pericardium with your finger and break down any soft loculations.

If a permanent window is desired, suture the edges of the pericardial defect to the surrounding tissues and drain the pericardial space with tubes as shown (Fig. 24.1C). If desired, a permanent opening into the peritoneal space may be created by excising a small portion of the dome of the diaphragm as the pericardium is entered. This may provide a better mechanism for long-term drainage.

Note that the diaphragmatic pericardium is easily seen during laparotomy. Generally, the motion of the heart can be seen with sufficient clarity to determine visually if blood is present. If tamponade is suspected during trauma laparotomy, it is sim-

ply a matter to place two traction sutures and aspirate blood to gain time in an emergency situation.

Anatomic Points

The xiphoid process is the third of three parts of the sternum. The other two are the manubrium and the body. In adolescence, the xiphoid is cartilaginous, but as one ages, it becomes ossified. It varies in size and shape. Most commonly, it has the form of an inverted triangle, with the point directed inferiorly. Loss of the xiphoid causes no morbidity.

The fibrous pericardial sac forms a tough sac in which the heart moves freely, covered by the serous pericardium (a much thinner membrane). If fluid accumulates slowly within the pericardial sac, it can distend and stretch to a considerable extent, but it does not accommodate rapid increase in volume well. The fibrous pericardium is attached inferiorly to the xiphoid process by the inferior pericardiosternal ligament which is divided during the resection of the xiphoid. Inferiorly, the pericardial sac attaches to and lies upon the dome of the diaphragm. Laterally, it is apposed to the pleural sacs.

Thoracoscopic Pericardial Window (Fig. 24.2)

Technical Points

Either side of the chest (or both) may be used. This procedure takes advantage of the fact that the fibrous pericardium is fused to the mediastinal pleura and is easily entered via a thoracoscopic approach. The phrenic nerve is protected by creating windows anterior and (on the left side) posterior to this structure.

Typically, three ports are placed (Fig. 24.2A). Divide the inferior pulmonary ligament and sweep the lung cephalad. Identify the phrenic nerve. Grasp the pericardium and elevate it from the heart. Use scissors to excise a rectangular window above the phrenic nerve, preserving a strip of pericardium on

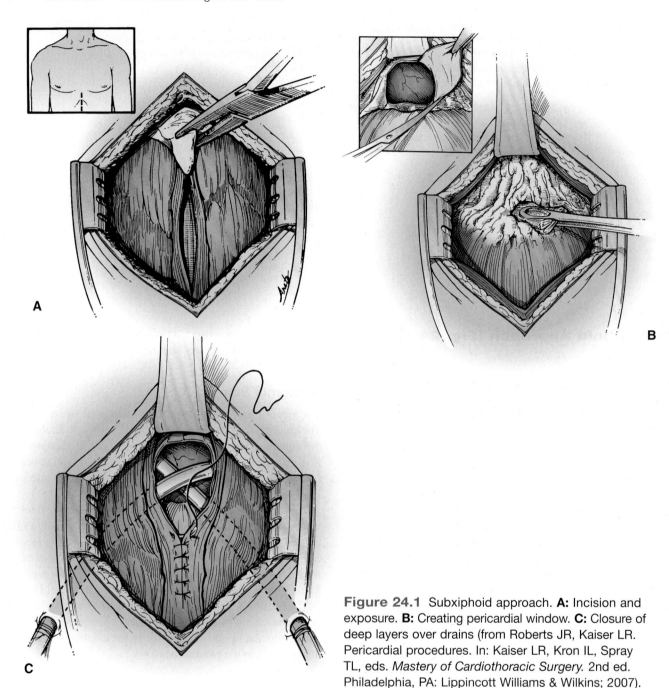

Figure 24.1 Subxiphoid approach. **A:** Incision and exposure. **B:** Creating pericardial window. **C:** Closure of deep layers over drains (from Roberts JR, Kaiser LR. Pericardial procedures. In: Kaiser LR, Kron IL, Spray TL, eds. *Mastery of Cardiothoracic Surgery.* 2nd ed. Philadelphia, PA: Lippincott Williams & Wilkins; 2007).

which the nerve runs. On the left side, it may be possible to create a second window inferior to the phrenic nerve (Fig. 24.2B). On the right side, the nerve runs relatively more posterior and only an anterior window is usually feasible (Fig. 24.2C). Submit the excised pericardium for pathologic examination as noted before. Place two chest tubes; one in the pleural space and a second in the pericardium (Fig. 24.2D).

Anatomic Points

The phrenic nerve is both sensory and motor. It originates from the fourth cervical nerve, with contributions from the third and

fifth nerves. It is the primary motor nerve to the diaphragm, and division of this nerve results in paralysis of the hemidiaphragm on the side of the injury.

The left phrenic nerve is slightly longer (to accommodate the increased size of the heart on the left side) and has a more anterior course on the pericardium than the right phrenic nerve. Delicate branches of both nerves enter the upper portion of the pericardium to provide sensory innervation; these are not encountered during the present dissection.

The phrenic nerves give branches to the diaphragm, and also contribute terminal fibers to the phrenic plexus and phrenic ganglion (on the right) and the celiac plexus (on the left).

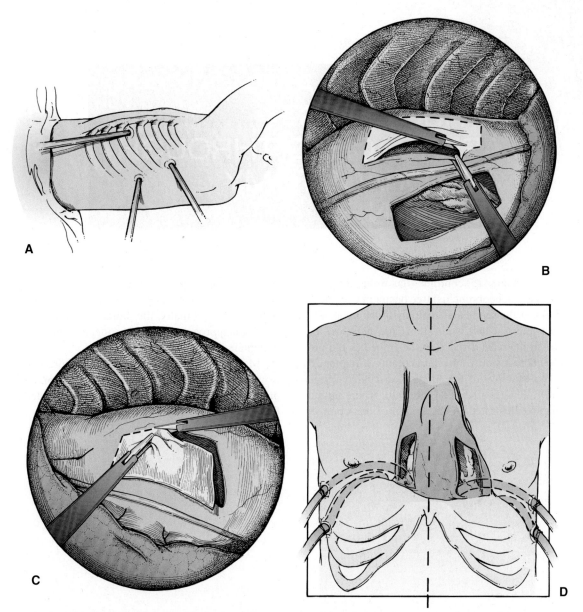

Figure 24.2 Thoracoscopic pericardial window. **A:** Patient position and location of trocars. **B:** Creation of anterior window (posterior window has been made). **C:** Completion of anterior window. **D:** Placement of drains (from Roberts JR, Kaiser LR. Pericardial procedures. In: Kaiser LR, Kron IL, Spray TL, eds. *Mastery of Cardiothoracic Surgery.* 2nd ed. Philadelphia, PA: Lippincott Williams & Wilkins; 2007).

REFERENCES

1. Arom KV, Franz JL, Grover FL, et al. Subxiphoid anterior mediastinal exploration. *Ann Thorac Surg.* 1977;24:289–290. (A similar approach to the anterior mediastinum for mediastinoscopy.)
2. Becit N, Unlu Y, Ceviz M, et al. Subxiphoid pericardiostomy in the management of pericardial effusions: Case series analysis of 368 patients. *Heart.* 2005;91:785–790.
3. Gross JL, Younes RN, Deheinzelin D, et al. Surgical management of symptomatic pericardial effusion in patients with solid malignancies. *Ann Surg Oncol.* 2006;13:1732–1738.
4. Jimenez E, Martin M, Krukenkamp I, et al. Subxiphoid pericardiotomy versus echocardiography: A prospective evaluation of the diagnosis of occult penetrating cardiac injury. *Surgery.* 1990;108:676–679.

5. O'Brien PK, Kucharczuk JC, Marshall MB, et al. Comparative study of subxiphoid versus video-thoracoscopic pericardial "window." *Ann Thorac Surg.* 2005;80:2013–2019. (More morbidity with thoracoscopic approach, but better long-term patency.)
6. Roberts JR, Kaiser LR. Pericardial procedures. In: Kaiser LR, Kron IL, Spray TL, eds. *Mastery of Cardiothoracic Surgery.* 2nd ed. Philadelphia, PA: Lippincott Williams & Wilkins; 2007: 254–261.
7. Smith CA, Galante JM, Pierce JL, et al. Laparoscopic transdiaphragmatic pericardial window: Getting to the heart of the matter. *J Am Coll Surg.* 2011;213:736.
8. Yonemori K, Kunitoh H, Tsuta K, et al. Prognostic factors for malignant pericardial effusion treated by pericardial drainage in solid-malignancy patients. *Med Oncol.* 2007;24:425–430.

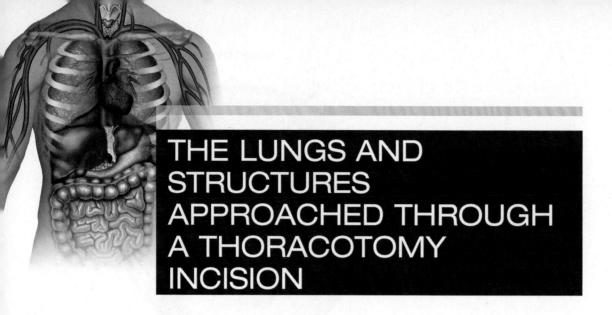

THE LUNGS AND STRUCTURES APPROACHED THROUGH A THORACOTOMY INCISION

Bronchoscopy (Chapter 25) continues the discussion of the anatomy of the tracheobronchial tree begun in Chapters 2 and 3 and introduces the segmental anatomy of the lungs. Following this, the lateral chest wall, associated muscles, and the anatomy of an intercostal space are described as the procedures of tube thoracostomy and thoracotomy (Chapter 26) are detailed. The anatomy of the lungs is discussed further in chapters that follow (available on the web), where pulmonary resections are illustrated. A discussion of one common operative approach to the thoracic outlet syndrome presents additional anatomy relevant to both the chest and the neck (Chapter 31e). Finally, the thoracic esophagus, a mediastinal structure approached from the side, is included in this section (Chapters 32e and 33e).

Major thoracic vascular operations, thoracoscopy, resection of posterior mediastinal tumors, and less common esophageal procedures are described in the references listed at the end of this section.

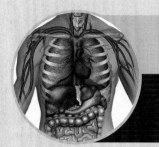

25

Bronchoscopy

M. Victoria Gerken and Phillip C. Camp, Jr.

Fiberoptic bronchoscopy is frequently performed for diagnosis and for management of secretions. This chapter describes how to access various segments of the bronchial tree with both the fiberoptic and the rigid bronchoscope. References at the end detail special additional procedures such as endobronchial ultrasound (used to stage lung cancer) and bronchoalveolar lavage for pneumonia.

SCORE™, the Surgical Council on Resident Education, has classified bronchoscopy as an "ESSENTIAL COMMON" procedure.

STEPS IN PROCEDURE

Flexible Fiberoptic Bronchoscopy
Provide adequate topical anesthesia and
    sedation, and ensure adequate monitoring
Introduce fiberoptic bronchoscope through
    anesthetized naris
Identify larynx and vocal cords
Pass scope through cord into proximal trachea
Look first where the lesion is suspected on the
    basis of imaging studies; obtain biopsies
    or brushings if desired
Then examine remainder of tracheobronchial
    tree in systematic fashion

Rigid bronchoscopy
General anesthesia, patient positioned with
    neck in slight hyperextension
Ventilation port is used by anesthesiologist
    to maintain ventilation during
    procedure
Introduce scope through mouth, elevate
    epiglottis and pass through cords
Continuously support the rigid bronchoscopy
    and avoid sudden movements
Advance scope along tracheobronchial tree to
    desired location

HALLMARK ANATOMIC COMPLICATIONS
Incomplete examination or inability to
    cannulate selected segmental bronchus
Bleeding from biopsy

LIST OF STRUCTURES
Inferior nasal meatus
Nasopharynx
Oropharynx
Pharynx
Laryngeal aditus
Larynx
Vocal cords
Cricoid cartilage
Aryepiglottic folds
Trachea
Carina

Right Main Stem Bronchus
Bronchus intermedius (intermediate bronchus)

Left Main Stem Bronchus

Right Lung
Right upper lobe
Right middle lobe
Right lower lobe

Left Lung
Left upper lobe
Lingula
Left lower lobe
Bronchopulmonary segments
Left and right vagus nerves
Stomach
Cardioesophageal junction
Spleen
Gastrosplenic (lienogastric) ligament

Fiberoptic Bronchoscopy

Introduction of the Bronchoscope
(Fig. 25.1)

Technical Points

Anesthesia is crucial for successful fiberoptic bronchoscopy. There are certain situations in which it is expedient to perform this procedure under general anesthesia (i.e., when the patient cannot tolerate topical anesthesia, when the patient is anesthetized for another reason, or before a thoracotomy that is being performed to resect a small, peripheral nodule). Although general anesthesia does allow the endoscopist to examine the periphery closely without having to deal with coughing, the proximal trachea and the cords cannot be examined in an intubated patient. This is especially pertinent when one is evaluating central lung lesions and when there is a possibility of involvement of the recurrent laryngeal nerve. However, more than half of the life-threatening complications stemming from bronchoscopy are related to hypoxemia, hypercapnia, respiratory depression (oversedation), and medication side effects. Each clinical scenario should be carefully considered.

Most diagnostic bronchoscopy procedures are performed using topical anesthesia. However, all too often, the inexperienced endoscopist fails to achieve adequate anesthesia and ends up with an incomplete bronchoscopy because the patient is coughing and is clearly dyspneic. With an adequate balance of sedation (i.e., with diazepam or midazolam hydrochloride), adequate analgesia and antitussive management (meperidine, morphine), and adequate topical anesthesia of the naris, the posterior pharynx, the aryepiglottic folds, and the cords, the average patient will be able to tolerate the procedure with little or no coughing, dyspnea, or agitation.

Place viscous lidocaine jelly on a series of cotton-tipped applicators and use these to anesthetize the naris, progressing slowly to the back of the nasopharynx as an anesthetic effect is achieved. Anesthetize the rest of the airway by connecting an atomizer filled with 4% lidocaine to a high-flow oxygen system with a Y connector. The anesthetic can then be sprayed gently over the mucous membranes with good control.

The use of intravenous sedation, careful monitoring of pulse oximetry, adequate topical anesthesia, and antisialogogues (atropine, glycopyrrolate) when indicated will allow careful and systematic examination of the proximal tracheobronchial tree. With the fiberoptic bronchoscope, you should be able to reach, without difficulty, the orifices of the third order of bronchi in all lobes.

Introduce the fiberoptic bronchoscope through the anesthetized naris. Pass the instrument into the back of the oropharynx and identify the larynx and vocal cords. Ask the awake patient to speak to confirm equal and full movement of the true cords. You may wish to inject additional topical anesthetic at this point to ensure its direct application to the cords. Under direct visualization, pass the fiberoptic bronchoscope through the cords into the proximal trachea. Inspect the area for neoplasms (both tumors and granulomas), excessive collapse of the trachea (tracheomalacia), points of external compression, and injuries (erosions, trauma, hematoma, disruption). The U shape of the tracheal cartilages and the comparatively flat, softer, membranous posterior wall make easy landmarks for maintaining proper orientation. The carina should appear to have a very acute angle with a sharp edge. Blunting of this angle can be seen with disease involving the subcarinal lymph nodes.

Anatomic Points

The fiberoptic bronchoscope should be advanced through the nose by way of the inferior nasal meatus (below the inferior nasal concha) because this is the widest passageway. As the bronchoscope is advanced into the nasopharynx, the tip should be directed 60 to 90 degrees caudally because this is the angle of the pharyngeal cavity with respect to the nasal cavity.

An alternative approach is to pass the flexible bronchoscope orally through an oral (bite block) specifically designed to allow passage of a scope. The advantage of this approach allows easier removal and reinsertion than when cleaning or unplugging of the scope's channels is required.

After the bronchoscope is advanced through the laryngeal aditus, the trachea should be clearly visible. This part of the

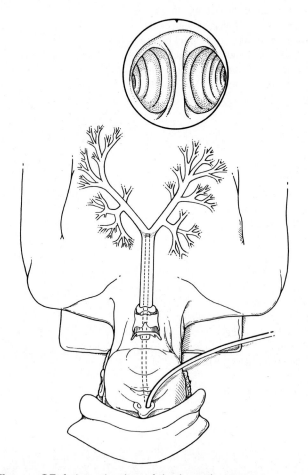

Figure 25.1 Introduction of the bronchoscope

airway is about 11 cm long and 2 to 2.5 cm wide. It is narrowest at its beginning, where the only complete cartilaginous ring, the cricoid cartilage, is located. From there on, it assumes an inverted U shape owing to the signet ring-shaped cartilages. The mucosa of the posterior wall, which widens as the carina is approached, has distinct longitudinal corrugations. The endoscopist should note that, during inspiration, the posterior membrane in the thorax moves posteriorly, whereas during expiration, it moves anteriorly in response to interairway pressure changes.

The carina, located at the end of the trachea and between the left and right main bronchi, is normally vertical, sharp, and narrow at its center, widening as its anterior and posterior limits are approached (normally, it is widest anteriorly). Although the normal orientation of the carina is vertical, it can vary from the perpendicular by as much as 45 degrees.

Examination of the Bronchial Tree (Fig. 25.2)

Technical Points

It is always advisable to "go where the money is" first. If chest radiographic studies show a mass on the left, examine that side first in case the patient develops dyspnea and the procedure needs to be terminated before a complete examination can be performed.

If the patient's condition allows, proceed to examine the entire tracheobronchial tree systematically. Develop a routine so that, in the excitement of identifying pathologic changes, you do not forget to examine the entire tree. The routine described here examines the right side first, then the left.

When looking down the right main stem bronchus, the orifice to the upper lobe usually will be seen to be in a very lateral location. However, there is some variability to this finding (in contrast to the anatomy of the rest of the right lung). Occasionally, the orifice will lie directly opposite the carina, but usually it lies 2 to 3 cm distally. Herein lies one of the strong advantages of fiberoptic bronchoscopy over rigid bronchoscopy: The tip of the scope must be flexed fairly sharply to be able to look into the right upper lobe bronchus (clearly not possible with a rigid instrument). When looking up the right upper lobe bronchus, the three segmental bronchial orifices can easily be identified.

Just past the takeoff of the right upper lobe, you enter the bronchus intermedius. The anatomy here rarely varies. Anteriorly, a bronchial orifice will be seen that leads to the middle lobe. Down this orifice, the two segmental orifices that quickly branch further can usually be identified without difficulty. Directly posterior (and typically directly opposite the middle lobe orifice) is the orifice of the superior segment of the lower lobe. Between these two orifices is the bronchus leading to the four basilar segments of the right lower lobe.

The left main stem bronchus branches much less acutely, with division into the upper and lower lobes. The upper lobe orifice lies superior to and slightly lateral to the lower lobe orifice. The upper lobe bronchus quickly bifurcates to go to the upper lobe and the lingula. The superior segment bronchial orifice is clearly seen posterior to the bronchus to the basal segments of the lower lobe.

One caveat pertains to the excessive use of suction. The ability to suction blood or mucus is critical to adequate visualization. However, the inexperienced endoscopist can unwittingly leave a finger on the suction port throughout the entire procedure. This virtually guarantees hypoxia and should be avoided.

Anatomic Points

Successful fiberoptic bronchoscopy demands knowledge of the bronchopulmonary segments. These segments, supported by third-order (segmental) bronchi, are the surgical units of the lung because there is little or no communication between segments. Each segment is based on the ramifications of a segmental bronchus and the accompanying ramifications of the pulmonary and bronchial arteries. Tributaries of the pulmonary vein, on the other hand, are intersegmental.

The right lung has 10 segments, whereas the left lung has 8 (although in the British literature, 10 segments are recognized on the left). As seen endoscopically, the 10 segments of the right lung and the relative positions (related to a clock face) of the orifices of their bronchi are as follows:

Upper Lobe Apical segment (B I)—orifice at 4 o'clock Anterior segment (B II)—orifice at 12 o'clock Posterior segment (B III)—orifice at 8 o'clock **Middle Lobe** Lateral segment (B IV)—orifice at 3 o'clock to 6 o'clock Medial segment (B V)—orifice at 9 o'clock to 12 o'clock	**Lower Lobe** Superior segment (B VI)—orifice at 5 o'clock, immediately past the middle lobe bronchus Medial basal segment (B VII)—orifice at 9 o'clock, usually more proximal than other basal segments Anterior basal segment (B VIII)—orifice at 1 o'clock Lateral basal segment (B IX)—orifice at 3 o'clock Posterior basal segment (B X)—orifice at 6 o'clock

It should be noted that, in more than half of the patients, there is a subapical segment in the lower lobe, the bronchus of which is posterior. This tertiary bronchus can arise anywhere along the lower lobe bronchus from the opening of the superior segment to the final division of the lobar bronchus.

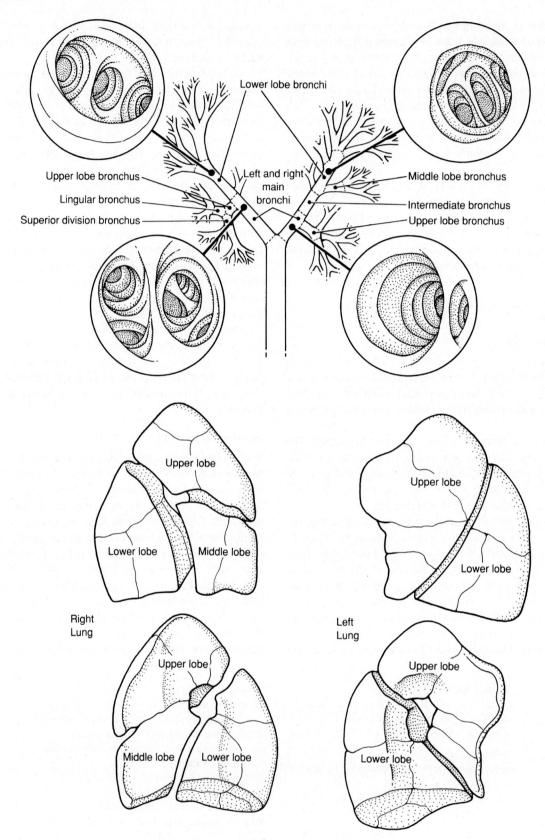

Figure 25.2 Examination of the bronchial tree

In a similar fashion, the bronchopulmonary segments of the left lung, and the relative location of the openings of their bronchi, are as follows:

Upper Lobe

Upper division—orifice at 8 o'clock
Apicoposterior segment (B I + III)

Anterior Segment (B II)

Lingular division—orifice at 2 o'clock
Superior segment (B IV)—orifice at 10 o'clock
Inferior segment (B V)—orifice at 2 o'clock

Lower Lobe

Superior segment (B VI)—orifice at 6 o'clock, shortly past the origin of the lower lobe
Anteromedial basal segment (B VIII + VII)— orifice at 12 o'clock
Lateral basal segment (B IX)—orifice at 9 o'clock
Posterior basal segment (B X)—orifice at 5 o'clock

Rigid Bronchoscopy

Rigid bronchoscopy, the only technique available before the development of the fiberoptics that have revolutionized endoscopy, still has much to offer. True, fiberoptic bronchoscopy does allow manipulation within the bronchial tree, permitting much improved visualization of the distal tree (especially the right upper lobe), and it is well tolerated by the awake patient. However, rigid bronchoscopy is preferable for the retrieval of foreign bodies, for severe hemoptysis, and for suctioning and hyperexpansion of an atelectatic lung. In addition, rigid bronchoscopes are designed to allow concurrent ventilation, accept Hopkins telescopes, accommodate large biopsy forceps without obstructing the view, and allow passage of flexible bronchoscope.

Positioning the Patient and Manipulating the Scope (Fig. 25.3)

Technical and Anatomic Points

This procedure is usually done using general anesthesia, providing concurrent ventilation through the scope's side port.

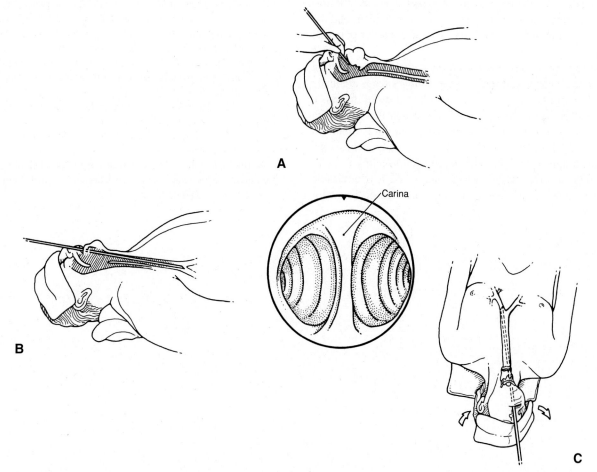

Figure 25.3 Positioning the patient and manipulating the scope. **A:** Initial insertion of scope. **B:** Deeper insertion of scope should allow visualization of carina. **C:** Move the patient's head to access the left or right bronchus.

Much of the technique is a matter of personal preference. Just as there are anesthesiologists with varying ideas as to how the head of a patient should be positioned for intubation, so, too, do thoracic surgeons vary in their bronchoscopic techniques. A single, rolled towel under the patient's shoulders creates a very slight hyperextension of the neck and chin extension, facilitating exposure. Marked hyperextension will make exposure much more difficult.

Introduce the scope through the mouth, elevating the epiglottis with the tip of the lubricated scope and passing the instrument through the glottis and the cords and into the upper trachea. Alternatively, a laryngoscope can be used to expose the posterior oropharynx and vocal cords. Always place the scope through the cords under direct visualization. Care must be taken to continuously support the rigid bronchoscope and to prevent sudden or jarring motions. The rigid scope can cause significant trauma when not manipulated in a coordinated fashion.

Give the ventilation port to the anesthesiologist for continued ventilation of the patient during the procedure. While viewing through the glass-covered eyepiece, advance the scope along the tracheobronchial tree until the desired area is reached.

It is extremely important to communicate and work well with the anesthesiologist. Wedging the scope into a lobar bronchus (especially if it is obstructed by a foreign body) may not allow adequate ventilation. Having an experienced anesthesiologist monitoring the ventilator bag, the pulse oximeter, and the carbon dioxide monitor will ensure early detection of potential problems.

Extraction of foreign bodies, although challenging, is often an interesting endeavor. A variety of grasping forceps are made for this purpose. Occasionally, one will find it useful to pass a Fogarty catheter past the offending object and then, with the Fogarty balloon inflated, to draw back on it until it is impacted in the end of the bronchoscope. At this time, the bronchoscope, with the entrapped foreign body, is removed to allow for adequate ventilation through the anesthesia mask. It is advisable in this circumstance to then reintroduce the cleaned broncho-scope to check for any remaining remnants of the foreign body. (Peanuts are notorious for fracturing during removal.)

When performing this procedure on children, many endoscopists administer racemic epinephrine (by nebulizer), dexamethasone (Decadron), or both, in an attempt to reduce further swelling of the small airway.

In cases of severe hemoptysis, examination of the tracheobronchial tree can be performed better with the rigid scope because it permits much better suctioning through larger suction catheters. In the setting of airway hemorrhage, an obstructing balloon catheter can be purposefully directed and inflated quickly, protecting the remainder of the airway. If the hemorrhage is massive, the rigid bronchoscope can then be introduced into the main stem bronchus of the unaffected side to allow ventilation through it during a subsequent thoracotomy. However, this is rarely done any more because the fit is seldom tight enough to rule out spillage of blood into the "good" side around the bronchoscope. Use of a Robert-Shaw or Carlens tube tends to be much more satisfactory.

REFERENCES

1. Krinzman SJ, Oliveria PJ, Irwin RS. Chapter 9. Bronchoscopy. In: Irwin RS, Rippe JM, Lisbon A, et al, eds. *Irwin & Rippe's Procedures, Techniques and Minimally Invasive Monitoring in Intensive Care Medicine.* 5th ed. Philadelphia, PA: Wolters Kluwer Lippincott Williams & Wilkins; 2012:89–95. (Excellent description of critical care applications including bronchoalveolar lavage for pneumonia, and management of hemoptysis.)
2. McField D, Bauer T. A review of noninvasive staging of the mediastinum for non-small cell lung carcinoma. *Surg Oncol Clin N Am.* 2011;20:681.
3. Meyer KC. The role of bronchoalveolar lavage in interstitial lung disease. *Clin Chest Med.* 2004;25:637.
4. Oho K, Amemiya R. *Practical Fiberoptic Bronchoscopy.* Tokyo: Igaku-Shoin; 1980.
5. Yasufuku K, Chiyo M, Koh E, et al. Endobronchial ultrasound guided transbronchial needle aspiration for staging of lung cancer. *Lung Cancer.* 2005;50:347.

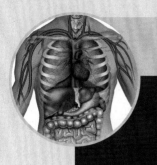

26

Tube Thoracostomy, Thoracotomy, Partial Pulmonary (Wedge) Resection, and Pleural Abrasion

M. Victoria Gerken and Phillip C. Camp, Jr.

In this chapter, the basic procedure of tube thoracostomy (chest tube placement) is used to introduce chest wall anatomy. A fundamental thoracic surgery incision—posterolateral thoracotomy—is described in detail, as is a less-painful muscle-sparing approach. Two common, simple, open thoracic surgery procedures—wedge resection and pleural abrasion—are then described.

SCORE™, the Surgical Council on Resident Education, classified chest tube placement as an "ESSENTIAL COMMON" procedure. SCORE™ classified exploratory thoracotomy as an "ESSENTIAL UNCOMMON" procedure, and partial pulmonary resection as a "COMPLEX" procedure.

STEPS IN PROCEDURE

Tube Thoracostomy

Location (interspace) is determined by nature of material to be drained

Obtain adequate local anesthesia and widely prep and drape the area

Check equipment, including drainage device, to ensure everything is ready

Make an incision one interspace below the desired interspace

Gently spread the tissues cephalad until the top of the next rib is encountered

Spread the intercostal muscles just above the rib and control the clamp as you pop into the pleural space

Spread the opening until it is large enough to admit your finger

Digitally explore the space, break down any loculations or adhesions, and confirm intrathoracic placement by palpating diaphragm

Insert the chest tube into this interspace, passing it just far enough to place the last hole within the pleural space

Connect to the tubing of the drainage device and secure tube in position

Standard Posterolateral Thoracotomy

Carefully position patient in full lateral decubitus position, padding and securing patient with care

Prepare hemithorax and drape widely

Standing at patient's back, draw an incision from anterior axillary line (inframammary fold, for a sixth interspace thoracotomy) to a point 2 to 3 cm inferior to the inferior angle of scapula, then angled gently cephalad to end midway between spine of scapula and thoracic vertebral column

Divide subcutaneous tissues to and through muscles, preserving the paraspinal muscles

Enter the chest through third, fourth, or fifth interspace depending on operation to be performed

Divide intercostals muscles and enter pleura

Extend intercostal incision and place rib spreader

At conclusion of procedure, check for air leaks and place chest tubes under direct vision

Remove rib spreader and approximate ribs with six to eight figure-of-eight pericostal sutures

Approximate muscles over chest wall

Close subcutaneous tissues and skin, secure chest tubes in place

Muscle-Sparing Thoracotomy

Same incision as above, but not so long posteriorly

Divide subcutaneous tissue and free it from fascia of latissimus dorsi muscle

Mobilize latissimus dorsi muscle and serratus anterior to allow retraction of both muscles

Enter pleural space

Use two small rib spreaders placed at right angles

Partial Pulmonary (Wedge) Resection

Identify the region to be resected

Tent up the lesion by elevating it with lung clamps

Fire stapler across region to be resected
(generally two firings will be needed, at
right angles to each other)

Pleural Abrasion

Resect blebs if present, using wedge resection
technique, and check for air leaks

Abrade pleural surfaces briskly with dry
laparotomy sponge

HALLMARK ANATOMIC COMPLICATIONS

Injury to lung or diaphragm (during tube
thoracostomy)

Injury to intercostal neurovascular bundle

Creation of devitalized or nonaerated remnant
during wedge resection

LIST OF STRUCTURES

Pleura

Pleural space

Intercostal space

External intercostal muscles

Internal intercostal muscles

Innermost intercostal muscles

Intercostal Neurovascular Bundle

Intercostal vein

Intercostal artery

Intercostal nerve

Diaphragm

Costal margin

Xiphoid process

Serratus anterior muscle

Endothoracic fascia

Latissimus dorsi muscle

Scapula

Trapezius muscle

Triangle of auscultation

Rhomboideus major muscle

Erector spinae muscles (paraspinous muscles)

Long thoracic nerve

Orientation (Fig. 26.1)

Tube Thoracostomy

Placement of a Tube Thoracostomy (Fig. 26.2)

Technical Points

The relatively simple procedure of tube thoracostomy demands careful attention to detail. Poor performance will cause patient discomfort and underlying lung injury, and may even necessitate open thoracotomy or laparotomy for correction.

In the past, chest tubes placed for pneumothoraces were inserted in the anterior chest, causing much unnecessary discomfort for the patient and substantially increasing the risk for hemorrhage from the anterior chest wall. Current practice dictates that chest tubes for uncomplicated pleural effusions, hemothoraces, or pneumothoraces be placed between the anterior axillary line and the midaxillary line, resulting in best results and minimum pain to the patient. Loculated collections of fluid or air may often require variations in technique that will not be discussed in this chapter.

Adequate analgesia is the key to successful, uncomplicated tube thoracostomy. Create a 2- to 3-cm skin wheal with 0.5% to 1% lidocaine about one interspace width below the planned thoracic entrance site. Subsequent or serial injections of lidocaine (5 mg/kg maximum dose), including the rib periosteum, intercostal muscles, and chest wall pleura, will greatly improve the ease of the procedure and patient comfort.

Prepare the skin widely and drape the area. For most purposes, chest tube insertion at the sixth interspace is adequate and safe. To prevent pneumothorax at the time of tube removal, plan to make the skin incision a full interspace lower than where you intend to enter the chest. In this way, the tube will pass through a subcutaneous tunnel measuring 2 to 3 cm in length between the skin and the entry site between the ribs. Thus the skin incision should be made at the seventh interspace.

Incise the skin with the scalpel and then create the subcutaneous tunnel with a long curved clamp. Repetitive, gentle spreading to a width equal to your finger and the chest tube will allow adequate access. Identify the top of the rib with the clamp and spread the intercostal muscle just over it, carefully hugging the superior surface. Control the clamp carefully so that when you "pop" through the pleura, the tip of the clamp does not injure underlying tissue. While the clamp is still in, spread the tips to widen the intercostal defect. Place your index finger through this incision into the chest and "sweep" down any adhesions, feeling for rind on the lung, pleural implants, and blood clots. Confirm the intrathoracic placement of a low chest tube by palpating the superior surface of the diaphragm.

Grasp the tip of the chest tube with the tip of a curved clamp and introduce it into the chest as shown (Fig. 26.2A). Inset the tube just far enough so that the last drainage hole is well within the chest cavity. An alternative method is to leave your finger

ORIENTATION

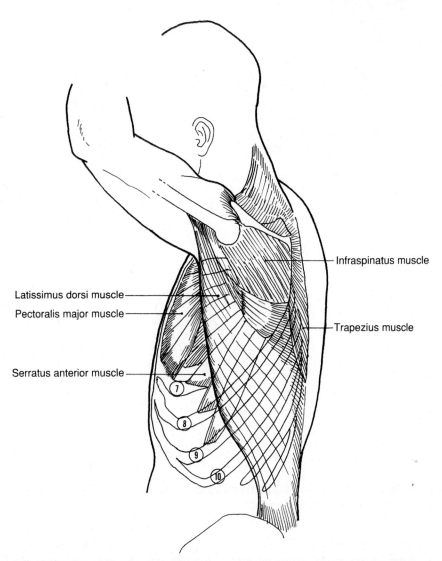

Latissimus dorsi muscle

Pectoralis major muscle

Serratus anterior muscle

Infraspinatus muscle

Trapezius muscle

Figure 26.1 Regional anatomy, showing ribs 7–10 and the muscles of the lateral chest wall, as encountered from a lateral approach such as that used for chest tube placement and thoracotomy.

in the tunnel and feed the tube next to it. The fingertip is blunt and allows the tube to be directed in a more specific direction. Either way, spinning the tube in a counterclockwise direction while advancing will help keep the tube from kinking and being misplaced into a fissure.

Secure the tube at the skin level with a heavy silk suture. The suture should be a U stitch or a single horizontal mattress stitch, which will allow skin approximation at the time of closure (Fig. 26.2B). Connect it to a chest drainage and suction device, such as a Pleurovac. Dress the site appropriately.

Chest tube management is described in the references at the end, which also describe placement of small-bore catheters in lieu of chest tube in selected cases.

Removal of the tube is best accomplished by two people. Prepare an occlusive dressing by placing a petroleum jelly

gauze on 4 × 4's. Expose the chest tube site and mobilize the stitch. Ask the patient to hold his or her breath in full inspiration. Place the dressing over the site with petroleum jelly apposing the incision. Quickly withdraw the tube, secure the suture, and tape the dressing tightly down while holding it firmly to the chest wall.

Anatomic Points

One of the potential hazards of tube thoracostomy—inadvertent placement of the tube below the diaphragm—can be avoided by analyzing the structure and morphology of the diaphragm. This muscle has a circumferential origin and divides the thoracic cavity from the abdominal cavity. Posteriorly, the diaphragm takes its origin from the anterolateral surfaces of the upper two or three lumbar vertebrae. It has a costal origin

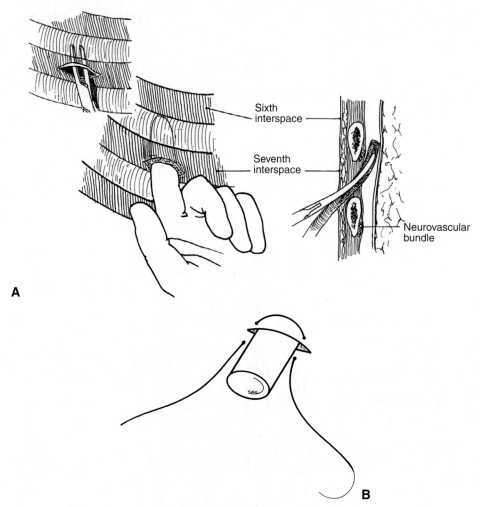

A

B

Figurè 26.2 Placement of a tube thoracostomy. **A:** Insertion of thoracostomy tube. **B:** One method of securing tube.

from the internal surfaces of the lower six ribs and costal cartilages at the costal margin; hence, as one progresses anteriorly, the origin of the diaphragm becomes progressively more cranial. Anteriorly, it has two small slips of origin from the deep surface of the xiphoid process. From this origin, the muscular fibers insert on the expansive, aponeurotic central tendon.

The upper limits of the diaphragm are at the level of the nipple, or fourth intercostal space, so that it is dome shaped. As a consequence, the peripheral part of the thoracic cavity becomes progressively attenuated inferiorly, resulting in a sharp, narrow costophrenic recess. In the midclavicular line, the reflection of parietal pleura from body wall to diaphragm is at the level of the eighth rib, whereas in the midaxillary line, this reflection is at the level of the tenth rib. Because of this reflection and the dome shape of the diaphragm, incisions below the level of the eighth rib may not enter the pleural cavity and can easily pass through the diaphragm into the abdominal cavity. The sharp costophrenic recess is precisely why excellent clamp control when popping into the chest is mandatory. Overly aggressive entry can easily continue on

through the adjacent diaphragm and into the abdomen. The slippery dome has been known to be confused with the diaphragm. Digitally palpating the diaphragm and lung wall helps confirm accurate location.

The other main hazard is injury to the intercostal neurovascular bundle. Each major intercostal neurovascular bundle is located in the costal groove (on the inferior surface of the rib), which helps to protect it. From superior to inferior, the arrangement of neurovascular structures is *vein–artery–nerve*. The nerve, lying lowest, is most susceptible to iatrogenic injury. To avoid this neurovascular bundle, make the intercostal incision close to the superior margin of the lower rib, rather than along the inferior margin of the upper rib.

In the midaxillary line, muscle fibers that must be divided before entering the intercostal neurovascular plane include those of the serratus anterior, external intercostal, and internal intercostal muscles. The neurovascular bundle lies in the plane between the deep innermost intercostal muscle layer and the more superficial internal intercostal layer. Deep to the innermost intercostal layer is the endothoracic fascia, a thin layer to which the costal pleura is adherent.

Standard Posterolateral Thoracotomy

Position of Patient and Incision (Fig. 26.3)

Technical Points

Correct patient positioning is mandatory for the safe performance of this procedure. To have the patient roll slightly forward or backward during the procedure is, at best, extremely frustrating, and, at worst, dangerous.

Place the patient in the lateral decubitus position with a roll under the dependent axilla to protect the shoulder and the axillary contents. In general, the diameter of the roll should approximate the diameter of the upper arm. The roll remains parallel to and just caudal to the dependent arm, which is flexed 90 degrees at the shoulder. The roll should prop up the chest wall, allowing the shoulder to drop down, thus relieving pressure on the brachial plexus. A common misperception is that the roll is tucked into the axilla, which is incorrect. Fold a soft pillow double and place it over this arm. Drape the superior arm over the pillow or onto a sling cephalad to the dependent arm.

A vacuum-activated "beanbag," previously placed under the patient, should be molded to the patient's dependent half of the torso and hips and aspirated until rigid. Alternatively, place a 4.5-kg (10-lb) sandbag just anterior to the patient's abdomen, supporting any panniculus. Leave the lower, dependent leg straight. Flex the upper leg 90 degrees at both the hip and the knee. Support the calf with two pillows. A strip of wide tape will help stabilize the patient in this position. The tape should extend from the table edge over the buttocks and hip and down the length of the flexed thigh to the table edge on the opposite side. Take care not to place the tape over the fibular head on the upper leg, where it may press on the common peroneal nerve. In addition, avoid undue force in applying the tape because this may cause a counter-pressure point.

After the patient has been securely positioned, prepare the hemithorax extending across the midline both anteriorly and posteriorly. The prep should extend up to the prominent spine of the seventh cervical vertebra and over the exposed shoulder and should include the nipple on the operative side. Extend the prep down to the iliac crest inferiorly.

Stand at the patient's back. Draw an incision beginning at the anterior axillary line at the level of the inframammary fold in a woman, or at a point about 6 cm inferior to the nipple in a man. Extend the incision laterally so that it passes 2 to 3 cm inferior to the inferior angle of the scapula and then curves gently cephalad, ending midway between the spine of the scapula and the thoracic vertebral column. Incise the skin.

Use electrocautery to divide the subcutaneous tissue down to the level of the muscles. Expose and divide the latissimus dorsi muscle with electrocautery. Posteriorly, expose the lateral edge of the trapezius muscle and divide it in the same way. Identify the auscultatory triangle, which is just inferior and posterior to the inferior angle of the scapula, and divide its thin connective tissue. Slip your hand under the posterior edge of the serratus anterior muscle.

Divide the serratus anterior muscle with electrocautery or identify and divide its attachments to the chest wall, exposing these attachments by retracting the inferior edge of the divided latissimus dorsi muscle with a sharp-pronged rake retractor.

Posteriorly, divide the lateral edge of the rhomboideus major muscle with cautery. Slide your hand up under the

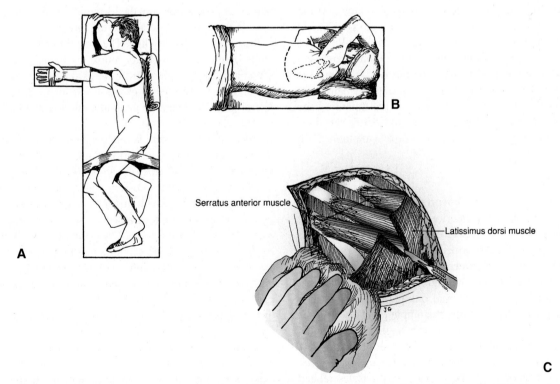

Serratus anterior muscle

Latissimus dorsi muscle

Figure 26.3 Position of patient and incision. **A:** Patient position. **B:** Skin incision. **C:** Division of muscle.

scapula to identify the ribs. The first rib can seldom be felt; hence, the identification process usually begins with the second rib, the outer aspect of which has a characteristic, flattened surface. A helpful marker of the second rib is the insertion of the subclavius and anterior scalene muscles.

In general, enter the chest in the third, fourth, or fifth interspace depending on the operation being performed. Very seldom is it necessary to resect a rib; this is done almost exclusively when there is dense pleural disease or when the rib is needed for a bone graft.

Divide the external and internal intercostal muscles, staying just superior to the lower rib in order to avoid the neurovascular bundle. As you approach the parietal pleura, ask the anesthesiologist to "drop the lung," or to deflate the lung to reduce the risk for injury to the underlying pulmonary parenchyma. Using the tip of a hemostat or careful, delicate strokes with a scalpel, pop into the pleura. Place an index finger or a plastic Yankauer suction catheter into the pleural cavity and advance the intercostal incision anteriorly, keeping the cautery on your finger (or suction catheter) to protect the underlying lung. Stay directly on the superior edge of the lower rib. If the intercostal space is so narrow as to be uncomfortable on your finger, place the blade of the smallest available Richardson retractor in the intercostal space and use it to widen the space. Posteriorly, extend the intercostal incision, using cautery, to the anterior border of the paraspinous muscles. *Do not divide the paraspinous muscles;* these define the posterior extent of your soft-tissue dissection. Identify and score the anterior margin of these muscles with electrocautery. Using a large periosteal elevator, elevate the muscle off the outer surface of the ribs and slide a small Army–Navy elevator in to keep this outer surface exposed.

Place the rib spreader in such a way as to "catch" or trap the tip of the scapula to prevent its protruding into your line of vision. Open the intercostal space along its length, taking care not to divide the internal mammary artery about 1 to 2 cm from the most anteromedial aspect of the rib. Dividing the intercostal muscles under direct vision (through the spreader) without dividing the overlying muscles of the thoracic cage allows excellent exposure, typically avoids deliberate division of the rib for exposure, and minimizes unplanned rib fractures.

Anatomic Points

Here, as elsewhere, knowledge of surface anatomy is important in planning the incision. The anterior axillary fold is formed by the inferolateral border of the pectoralis major muscle, whereas the posterior axillary fold is formed by the lateral margin of the latissimus dorsi muscle. Between these two muscles, the thoracic wall is covered by the interdigitating costal attachments of the serratus anterior and external oblique muscles. In men and in women with small breasts, the nipple typically overlies the fourth intercostal space. The inferior angle of the scapula usually overlies the eighth rib, whereas the root of the spine of the scapula is located at about the third intercostal space.

After skin incisions have been made, the muscles related to the posterior thoracic wall and scapula are identified next.

Adjacent to the posterior midline and for a variable distance laterally, the most superficial muscle fibers, directed superolaterally, are those of the inferior border of the trapezius, a muscle that originates from the superior nuchal line of the occipital bone and the spinous processes of all cervical and thoracic vertebrae and that inserts on the spine of the scapula and lateral clavicle. The lower trapezius fibers overlie the essentially horizontal upper fibers of the latissimus dorsi, a muscle whose broad origin includes the lower six thoracic vertebral spines, all lumbar and sacral spines, and the posterior iliac crest by way of its attachment to the thoracolumbar fascia, and the iliac crest lateral to the erector spinae muscles. The latissimus dorsi fibers converge to form a flat tendon of insertion onto the lateral floor of the humeral intertubercular sulcus.

Division of the lower trapezius fibers and upper latissimus dorsi fibers effectively increases the size of the triangle of auscultation, a triangle bounded by the upper border of the latissimus dorsi muscle, the lower lateral border of the trapezius muscle, and the vertebral border of the scapula. Division of the trapezius and latissimus dorsi fibers allows increased mobility of the lower part of the scapula. A margin of 2 to 3 cm inferior to the inferior angle of the scapula should be maintained to allow adequate closure and to not disrupt the local capsule.

The anatomic relationships of the serratus anterior muscle are potentially confusing. This muscle arises from muscular digitations of the anterolateral aspect of the upper eight to ten ribs, and then passes posteriorly between the thoracic wall and the scapula to insert along the entire length of the vertebral border of the scapula. It is innervated by the long thoracic nerve, which originates from the roots (C5 to C7) of the brachial plexus and descends on the external surface of the serratus muscle deep to the fascia covering this muscle, approximately in the posterior axillary line. The long thoracic nerve is accompanied, especially low in its course, by branches from the subscapular artery. Higher up in the axilla, behind the pectoralis minor muscle, the nerve passes posterior to the origin of the lateral thoracic artery, an anatomic relation that can be used to identify this nerve.

Some difficulty may be encountered in counting ribs deep to the scapula. Here, as anteriorly, it is easiest to start counting with the second rib. This rib can be identified by palpating the insertion of the serratus posterior superior muscle because this is the highest rib to which this muscle is attached.

The term *paraspinous muscles,* as used here, refers to the erector muscles of the spine. These muscles are divisible into a medial spinalis muscle column adjacent to spinous processes, an intermediate longissimus column occupying the interval between the spinalis muscle column and the angles of the lower ribs, and a lateral iliocostalis column, attached to the angles of ribs. Division of iliocostal or longissimus fibers should not affect the function of these muscular columns because their innervation, through branches from the posterior primary divisions of spinal nerves, is segmental. However, division of these muscle groups is rarely required and should be avoided if possible.

Closure of Thoracotomy (Fig. 26.4)

Technical Points

At the completion of the procedure, ask the anesthesiologist to inflate the lung fully. This is the best time to expand any lung that may have become atelectatic intraoperatively; atelectasis is difficult enough to treat postoperatively without starting the problem in the operating room.

At this time, instill bupivacaine hydrochloride into the posterior intercostal spaces for two or three spaces above and below the incision. This strategy helps to control postoperative pain if regional anesthesia or analgesia is not being used.

At the completion of the case, place one or two chest tubes into the hemithorax; these should exit caudal on the chest wall, anterior to the midaxillary line, for greatest patient comfort. If two tubes are used, place a right-angled tube in the posterior position to promote batter basilar fluid drainage. Place the anterior chest tube with the tip in the apex of the pleural space. Secure the tubes to the skin with heavy silk.

Use six to eight figure-of-eight "pericostal" stitches of heavy absorbable suture material to approximate the ribs. A nice method to minimize accidental punctures is to use a large "liver" needle (blunted tip, large 180-degree curve) to place the intercostal sutures. We have found this to be quick and rather safe. After placing the sutures, fully inflate the lung and approximate the ribs. Again, take care to avoid the intercostal neurovascular bundles. Although some surgeons prefer to use the Bailey rib approximator to appose the ribs while tying these

sutures, a slipknot permits snug approximation of the ribs without endangering the intercostal vessels. Individually reapproximate the serratus anterior, rhomboideus, latissimus dorsi, and trapezius muscles anatomically with heavy absorbable suture material.

Approximate the subcutaneous tissue with absorbable suture, after which the skin edges should be approximated, either with skin staples or a subcuticular running monofilament suture.

Anatomic Points

The use of a local analgesic injected two to three spaces above and below the incision is partially based on the anatomic principles of segmental innervation. Seemingly, only the interspace of the incision should require analgesia because it should be wholly within a dermatome. However, there is overlap of dermatomes, which means that about half of a segment is at least partially innervated by the nerve preceding that for the given segment and about half is at least partially innervated by the nerve succeeding the segment.

When the anterior chest tube is placed, the tube should be in the apex, about 2.5 cm cephalad to the medial third of the clavicle. The lower chest tube is placed just anterior to the posterior axillary line. If this is placed as low as possible, it will be in the eighth or ninth intercostal space. Again, caution should be exercised to prevent trauma to the diaphragm or the abdominal contents.

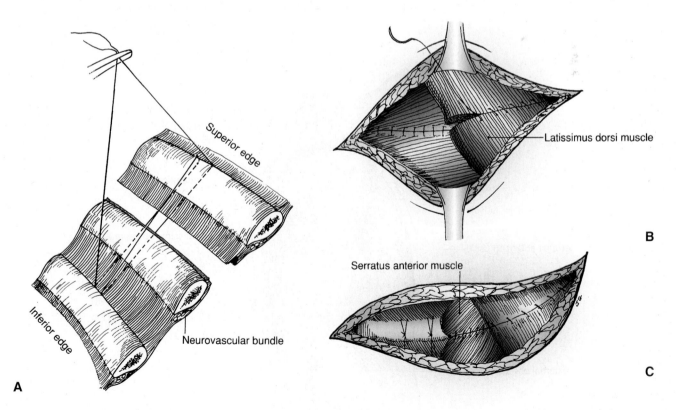

Figure 26.4 Closure of thoracotomy. **A:** Closure of ribs. **B:** Suture of muscle layers. **C:** Completed deep closure.

Muscle-Sparing Thoracotomy
(Fig. 26.5)

Technical Points

The division of the latissimus dorsi muscle causes severe post-operative pain, which often leads to splinting of the chest wall and a long recovery period and can hinder good pulmonary function and toilet in the postoperative period. For intrathoracic operations not requiring maximal exposure (pleural abrasions, wedge resections, biopsies), a procedure associated with less morbidity—a muscle-sparing thoracotomy—can be performed in many cases.

Use the same skin incision as for the standard thoracotomy, but do not make it as long posteriorly. Divide the subcutaneous tissue and free it up from the fascia of the latissimus dorsi muscle superiorly to the scapula and inferiorly to the iliac crest. Mobilize the anterior edge of the latissimus dorsi muscle and free the undersurface. Free the serratus muscle in a similar fashion so that the latissimus dorsi can be freely retracted posteriorly and the serratus anteriorly to expose the ribs.

Enter the chest in the intercostal space as described previously. Use two smaller rib-spreader retractors: The first for separating the free edges of the latissimus dorsi and serratus muscles, and the second for placement in the usual intercostal space. This creates a window through which the procedure can be performed.

At the completion of the procedure, place the chest tubes and the pericostal stitches as described previously. Place a flat suction drain under the muscle flaps, bringing it out through a separate stab wound. Approximate the subcutaneous tissue and close the skin.

Anatomic Points

Again, be aware that the intercostal bundle, containing the intercostal vein, artery, and nerve, runs medial and inferior to the lower edge of the corresponding rib. This unfortunately makes it a structure that is easy to injure during chest closure.

Partial Pulmonary (Wedge) Resection (Fig. 26.6)

Technical Points

Many procedures are easily approached by thoracoscopy, but often the nature of the lesion, the stability of the patient, or the tolerance of single-lung ventilation may favor open approaches. Pulmonary procedures generally begin with exploration of the hemithorax. Just as the peritoneal cavity should be explored before proceeding with a formal hemicolectomy, so, too, should an examination of the hilum of the lung, the entire lung, the pleural surfaces, and the anterior and posterior mediastina be performed before proceeding with lobectomy, segmentectomy, or wedge resection. Wedge resections of lung tissue for diagnostic purposes (e.g., diffuse infiltrative disease, acute respiratory distress syndrome) allow for a minimal incision but will, by their size, limit complete thoracic exploration. This approach will help to determine the appropriateness of curative versus palliative resection, compared with a simple biopsy.

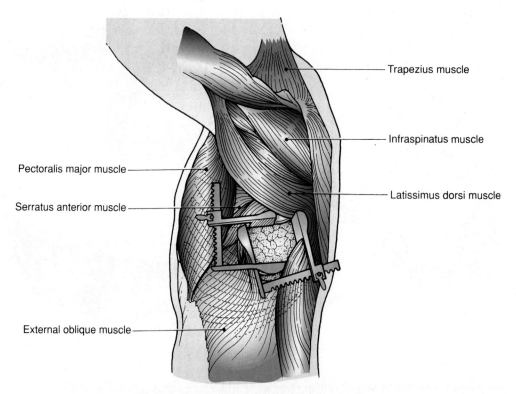

Figure 26.5 Muscle-sparing thoracotomy

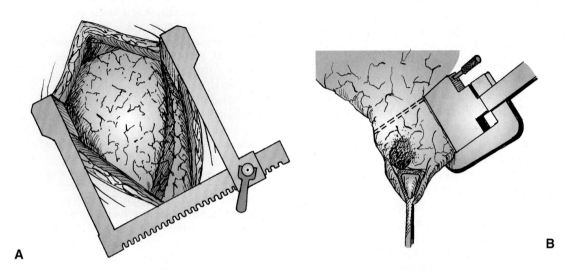

A   **B**

Figure 26.6 Wedge resection. **A:** Exposure of area. **B:** Stapled wedge resection of nodule.

For small subpleural (peripheral) masses, grasp the lung on either side with lung clamps. Elevate these regions to "tent up" the lesion. Use a stapling device to divide under the lesion. Bolstering stapled margins with bovine pericardium can be advantageous and minimize postoperative air leaks.

Air leak. This approach also can be somewhat stronger when wedging out thicker portions of tissue. For lesions that are large or that lie deep within the parenchyma, it may be necessary to fire the stapler twice to "wedge out" the lesion. In such cases, it is extremely important to remember the segmental anatomy of the lung. It is possible, and quite disastrous, to resect a wedge in such a fashion that the bronchial or vascular communication of the remaining lung is compromised. This leaves nonaerated, nonperfused lung behind to serve as a septic source. After performing a wedge resection, deflate the remaining lung and then have the anesthesiologist reinflate it to confirm the adequate function of all remaining lung.

Anatomic Points

The segmental anatomy of the lung is of crucial importance. It is discussed in detail in the chapters devoted to bronchoscopy (Chapter 26) and lobectomy (Chapter 28). Because a nonanatomic wedge resection crosses subsegmental boundaries, aeration of the adjacent pulmonary parenchyma must be confirmed at operation.

Pleural Abrasion (Fig. 26.7)

Technical and Anatomic Points

Recurring spontaneous pneumothoraces usually occur in otherwise healthy young people. After the second occurrence, most surgeons recommend thoracostomy or thoracotomy. This chapter discusses the open approach.

This is an ideal situation for muscle-sparing thoracotomy. Open the chest in the fifth or sixth intercostal space and exam-

ine the lung parenchyma carefully for subpleural blebs. These occur at the apex of the upper lobe, along the apical edge of the superior segment of the lower lobe, and rarely, along the fissures. If any are visualized, exclude them with the stapling device. It is not necessary to resect much tissue if a minimal amount of parenchyma is involved. Fill the hemithorax with sterile saline and inflate the lung to a pressure of 30- to 40-cm H_2O. Anything more than minimal air leaks should be addressed by oversewing the staple line or restapling.

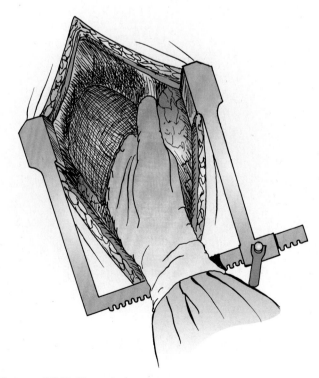

Figure 26.7 Pleural abrasion

Suction all saline from the chest. Abrade the parietal pleura by rubbing briskly with a dry laparotomy sponge. As the sponge becomes moistened with serous fluid, replace it with a dry one. An alternative approach is to use an abrasive pad (we use the disposable pad designed for electrocautery cleaning) to cause numerous microlacerations in the pleural surface. The key to successful pleural abrasion is causing significant inflammation between the two pleural surfaces, thus obliterating the potential space.

In the setting of apical blebs causing the recurrent pneumothorax, we will physically excise the apical pleural cap from within the thorax. This is a more aggressive maneuver and will definitely scar in the problematic portion of the lung. It is important that all pleura be abraded to the point of mild hemorrhage to ensure success. Include the diaphragm and the apex of the chest. Just before closing, 5-g talc poudrage should be evenly applied to the inner thoracic surface.

Place two chest tubes in the usual positions and close the chest. It is imperative that the chest tubes be kept patent and suctioned; the visceral and parietal pleural surfaces must be kept in direct apposition if adhesions are to form as desired.

TUBE THORACOSTOMY REFERENCES

1. Cooke DT, David EA. Large-bore and small-bore chest tubes: Types, function, and placement. *Thorac Surg Clin.* 2013;23:17.

2. Millikan JS, Moore EE, Steiner E, et al. Complications of tube thoracostomy for acute trauma. *Am J Surg.* 1980;140:738.

3. Peters J, Kubitschek KR. Clinical evaluation of a percutaneous pneumothorax catheter. *Chest.* 1984;86:714. (Describes the "dart" percutaneous technique for simple pneumothoraces.)

4. Silver M, Bone RC. The technique of chest tube insertion. *J Crit Illness.* 1986;1:45.

5. Torres U, Lancy RA. Chapter 8. Chest tube insertion and care. In: Irwin RS, Rippe JM, Lisbon A, et al., eds. *Irwin & Rippe's Procedures, Techniques and Minimally Invasive Monitoring in Intensive Care Medicine.* 5th ed. Philadelphia, PA: Wolters Kluwer Lippincott Williams & Wilkins; 2012:83–89.

THORACOTOMY REFERENCES

1. Bayram AS, Ozcan M, Kaya FN, et al. Rib approximation without intercostal nerve compression reduces post-thoracotomy pain: A prospective randomized study. *Eur J Cardiothorac Surg.* 2011;39:570.

2. Burlew CC, Moore EE, Moore FA, et al. Western trauma association critical decisions in trauma: Resuscitative thoracotomy. *J Trauma Acute Care Surg.* 2012;73:1357.

3. Seamon MJ, Chovanes J, Fox N, et al. The use of emergency department thoracotomy for traumatic cardiopulmonary arrest. *Injury.* 2012;43:1355.

4. Ziyade S, Baskent A, Tanju S, et al. Isokinetic muscle strength after thoracotomy: Standard vs. muscle-sparing posterolateral thoracotomy. *Thorac Cardiovasc Surg.* 2010;58:295.

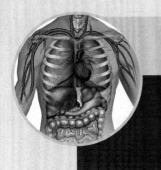

27
Thoracoscopy, Thoracoscopic Wedge Resection

Kemp H. Kernstine, Sr.

A thoracotomy incision is traumatic and painful and frequently leaves the patient with a cosmetically unappealing scar. Two percent of thoracotomy patients have incapacitating pain that lasts for more than a year, 4% have upper extremity disability, and 40% have persistent mild-to-moderate discomfort. Reducing the incision size and avoiding the use of a rib retractor appears to reduce the trauma, pain, and disability. Endoscopic thoracic surgery appears to accomplish these goals. This chapter discusses the basic principles of thoracoscopy as applied to two common problems.

SCORE™, the Surgical Council on Resident Education, classified thoracoscopy with or without biopsy and thoracoscopic pleurodesis as "COMPLEX" procedures.

STEPS IN PROCEDURE

Single lung ventilation is preferred, if feasible

Most procedures are performed in lateral decubitus position; some procedures require prone or supine position to access lesions

Have radiographs available in OR

Initial port placement is generally in anterior axillary line at fifth to seventh intercostal space

Place additional ports as required

To achieve the highest pathological yield in a lung biopsy, identify region of interest by radiographic studies, fluoroscopy, palpation, hook wire, or other method

The lung biopsy should be performed in the most cephalad region and near an edge to minimize the risk of prolonged air leak and

Check for air leaks

Close incisions with small chest tube or fluted drain to bulb suction in place

For spontaneous pneumothorax:
Resect blebs with stapler
Abrade pleural surfaces or remove parietal pleura from fourth rib to apex
Place chest tube into apical region and leave in place for 2 to 3 days

HALLMARK ANATOMIC COMPLICATIONS

Inability to localize target lesion
Air leak

Three types of thoracic endoscopic procedures can be performed:

Pleuroscopy usually involves a single puncture wound and portal for visualization, biopsy, and dissection. Visualization is either directly through an open scope, such as a Pilling or Storz mediastinoscope, or indirectly with a digital scope. The direct scope gives a limited view, but is very efficient in that it allows visualization and manipulation through the same port. Pleuroscopy is ideally suited to evaluate and treat pleural effusions or pleural masses. It may also assist in placement of pleural drains. Although pleuroscopy is done most frequently under general anesthesia, it may also be performed using fairly mild sedation with local anesthesia, if the planned procedure is brief with minimal manipulation.

Thoracoscopy involves two or more portals through which the visualization, dissection, and resection are performed.

Video-assisted thoracoscopic surgery (VATS) employs multiple ports or ports plus a small access incision. All the dissection that would be performed through an open thoracotomy is performed by endoscopic visualization. A nonrib-spreading incision may be necessary to dissect and extract the surgical specimen. To minimize pain, retractors are not used. Thoracoscopy and VATS are used for a wider variety of procedures: Lung biopsies; wedge resections; resections of thoracic masses; intrapleural, extrapleural, hilar, and mediastinal masses; and resection of lesions within the esophageal wall, portions of the esophagus, and myotomies.

It is essential to obtain a chest computed tomography (CT) scan before performing any form of endoscopic thoracic surgery. This allows three-dimensional operative planning and appropriate positioning of the surgical ports. The most appropriate patients for the thoracoscopic or video-assisted procedure are those who have had no prior thoracotomy, have a large thoracic cavity, are not ventilator dependent, and are not obese. Lesions most suitable for access through this approach are smaller than 3 cm and are peripherally located, although with more advanced techniques selected cases involving larger lesions and those more centrally located can be resected. Preoperative pulmonary function testing is very helpful in assisting intraoperative and postoperative management.

Anesthetic intubation management is dependent on the procedure planned. All three procedures may be performed using (a) single-lumen intubation with apnea or CO_2 insufflation, (b) double-lumen intubation, or (c) bronchial blocker. For brief, pleurally based procedures, apnea may be appropriate. Ventilator-dependent patients may require CO_2 insufflation taking care to avoid excess intrapleural pressure and hypotension. Single-lung ventilation by either double-lumen tube technique or bronchial blocker is desirable because it improves intrathoracic visibility, minimizes respiratory motion, reduces pulmonary parenchymal bleeding, and decreases the damage to the lung and the pulmonary vasculature. The greater the complexity of the intended endoscopic procedure, the greater these factors must be realized.

Patient Position and Port Placement (Fig. 27.1)

Technical Points

Patients are typically placed in the lateral decubitus position, although the supine or prone position may be necessary. Always have radiologic studies available for intraoperative review.

Incisions of 5 mm to 1 cm are then placed. In the case of pleuroscopy, especially in those situations where malignant mesothelioma or other locally recurrent tumors are likely, a single port should be placed in the fifth to seventh intercostal space at the anterior axillary line. The port site must be planned in anticipation of an extrapleural pneumectomy or pleural decortication resection, which would include the chest wall area where the port site is placed. Use the chest wall topical anatomy, such as the tip of the scapula, the manubriosternal junction, and the xiphoid process in comparison to these chest wall landmarks on the chest computed tomography (CT) scan to place the ports as they relate to the intended surgical target. For particularly small pulmonary masses, those smaller than 5 mm and deeper than 1 to 2 cm from the pleural surface, preoperative, CT-guided wire localization may prove useful to identify lesions that are less likely palpable at the time of thoracoscopy or VATS.

When more than one port is used, we usually place the first port in the low anterior chest wall in the anterior axillary line and pass a straight or 30-degree angled thoracoscope. For single ports, an open direct visualization scope, such as is used for mediastinoscopy, may be used when there is a limited view, as described earlier. Further ports may be placed as

necessary, especially when performing complex procedures. For thoracoscopy, portal arrangement is placed as a baseball diamond, with the video port placed at home plate, grasping and biopsy portals at first and third bases, and the region of interest at second base.

The instrumentation is dependent on the planned procedure. Plastic and rubber portals can be used when instrumentation must be repeatedly changed to prevent injury to the chest wall

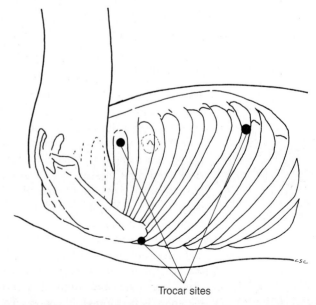

Trocar sites

Figure 27.1 Patient position and port placement

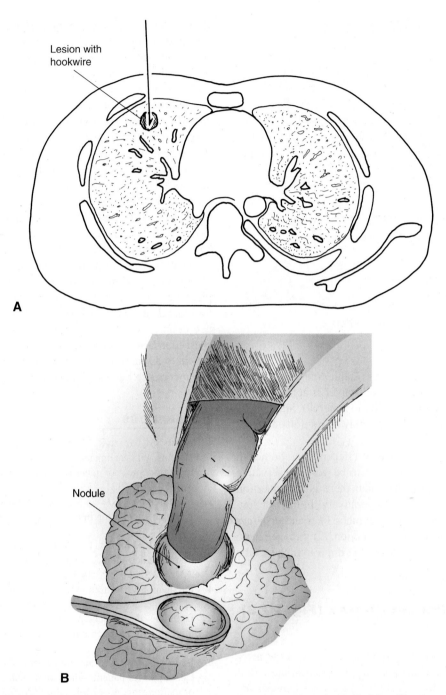

Lesion with
hookwire

Nodule

A

B

Figure 27.2 Lung biopsy. **A:** Hookwire in lesion (cross-section view). **B:** Identification of
lesion by direct palpation.

and intercostal nerves. Grasping, retracting, dissecting, suturing, and clip applying equipment are all available. We prefer
to grasp the lung with ring clamps. Endoscopic stapling equipment is very beneficial to seal the lung after resection.

Lung Biopsy (Fig. 27.2)

Technical Points

The chest CT scan is used to identify the most diseased portion
of the lung. Ports are placed to reach the diseased lung. It is
essential that the lesion be either palpable or easily visualized.

If this is not likely, perform preoperative CT-guided wire localization and resection with fluoroscopic assistance (Fig. 27.2A).

Enlarge the axillary port and insert a finger to palpate the
lung, using an opposing operative grasping clamp to bring the
lung into range (Fig. 27.2B). Take all adhesions down bluntly,
or use electrocautery if the adhesions are dense. Biopsy may be
performed with a forceps or by performing a wedge resection
using a standard stapling device. If possible, biopsy the most
cephalad portion of the lung or a portion adjacent to an edge
in order to obtain an adequate sample and reduce the likelihood for postoperative air leak. Typically, there is no need to

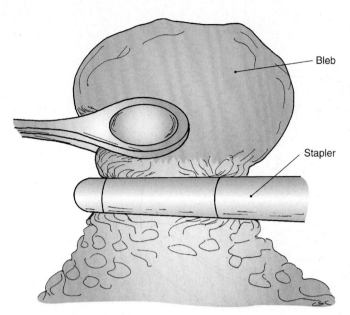

Figure 27.3 Spontaneous pneumothorax

cauterize any bleeding sites along the staple line. For particularly friable lung, we use a reinforced stapler (staplers may be reinforced with pericardium or synthetic material). Staple lines that appear weak or that are bleeding may be reinforced with a knife-lacking stapler.

Chest tube drainage is optional and depends on the health of the lung and the patient. We tend to be very conservative and leave a chest tube in place when there is any question rather than place a chest tube postoperatively. In the last several years, we have been placing a number 19 round or larger fluted drain that is connected to bulb suction. If by chance there is an air leak, we can easily connect the drain to a chest tube suction apparatus.

Spontaneous Pneumothorax (Fig. 27.3)

Technical Points

Three ports are placed in the following locations: Low anterior axillary line for the video port, third to fourth intercostal space in the midaxillary line, and high middle back between the scapula and the posterior spinous process. Thoroughly inspect the pulmonary space for bullous disease, because missed bullae represent one of the most common causes of recurrence.

Bullous disease is most common at the apex of the upper lobe, followed by the superior segment of the lower lobe, the tail of the right middle lobe, and the base of the lower lobe adjacent to the inferior pulmonary ligament. The diseased lung must be treated as well as the pleural space to achieve optimal results.

After all bullous disease has been identified, judicious resection (using the stapling device) is performed. In most young patients, the apex of the lung is all that is necessary to be resected, although we have been referred recurrent pneumothorax patients with disease in the other locations who were successfully treated with repeat thoracoscopy.

After resecting all bullous disease, remove or abrade the apical parietal pleural. We prefer to remove the parietal pleura from the fourth rib level to the apex making certain that we have removed the very apical pleura.

Place a chest tube to the apex. Leave this tube on suction for 48 hours for maximal adherence of the lung to the exposed intrapleural chest wall. Patients rarely require chest tube suctioning for more than 3 days. In the last few years, we have been placing two drains, a chest tube and a fluted drain to bulb suction, the chest tube being removed within the first 24 hours, leaving the patient to discharged home with the fluted drain within 24 hours. The recurrence rate should be less than 2% to 3%.

REFERENCES

1. Basso SM, Mazza R, Marzano B, et al. Improved quality of life in patients with malignant pleural effusion following videoassisted thoracoscopic talc pleurodesis. Preliminary results. *Anticancer Res.* 2012;32:5131–5134.
2. Deshmukh SP, Krasna MJ, McLauglin JS. Video assisted thoracoscopic biopsy for interstitial lung disease. *Int Surg.* 1996;81:330–332.
3. Kakuda J, Omari B, Renslo R, et al. CT guided needle localization for video-thoracoscopic resection of pulmonary nodules. *Eur J Med Res.* 1997;2:340–342.
4. Pursnani SK, Rausen AR, Contractor S, et al. Combined use of preoperative methylene blue dye and microcoil localization facilitates thoracoscopic wedge resection of indeterminate pulmonary nodules in children. *J Laparoscendosc Adv Surg Tech A.* 2006;16:184–187.
5. Sortini D, Feo CV, Carcoforo P, et al. Thoracoscopic localization techniques for patients with solitary pulmonary nodule and history of malignancy. *Ann Thorac Surg.* 2005;79:258–262.
6. Yim AP, Liu HP. Video assisted thoracoscopic management of primary spontaneous pneumothorax. *Surg Laparosc Endosc.* 1997;7:236–240.

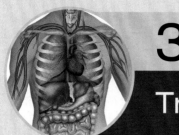

34

Transhiatal Esophagectomy

In this procedure, the mediastinal dissection of the esophagus is done from below (through the esophageal hiatus during the laparotomy phase) and from above (through a left neck incision). When successful, thoracotomy (or thoracoscopy) and the associated morbidity are avoided. The surgeon should be prepared to perform a thoracotomy if difficulties, including bleeding, occur.

The operation may be performed for benign disease or for selected patients with esophageal carcinoma. Accurate preoperative staging is essential. Tumors of the upper and middle third of the esophagus must be shown not to be adherent to adjacent structures. Variations of the procedure including laparoscopic and robotic dissection are given in references at the end.

SCORE™, the Surgical Council on Resident Education, classified esophageal resection as a "COMPLEX" procedure.

STEPS IN PROCEDURE

Supine position, head turned slightly to the right

Upper Midline Incision, Thorough Abdominal Exploration
Mobilize the stomach, preserving vascular arcades
Incise phrenoesophageal membrane
Encircle distal esophagus with Penrose drain
Gently circumferentially mobilize distal esophagus
Wide Kocher maneuver
Pyloromyotomy
Feeding jejunostomy (if desired)

Incision Along Anterior Border of Sternocleidomastoid Muscle
Divide omohyoid muscle
Retract carotid sheath laterally and trachea and esophagus medially
Divide middle thyroid vein
Circumferentially mobilize esophagus and encircle with Penrose drain

Mediastinal Dissection
Posterior mobilization by passing a sponge stick down from above, hand up from below
Similar anterior mobilization
Lateral mobilization performed last
Pull several centimeters of esophagus into cervical wound
Divide with GIA
Pull stomach and esophagus down into abdomen
Divide proximal stomach with GIA
Check hemostasis in mediastinal tunnel and ensure that it is large enough
Pass stomach up into neck
GIA anastomosis of stomach with esophagus
Hand sew rest of anastomosis
Close incisions without drainage
Check chest x-ray, place chest tubes if pneumothorax or hemothorax present

HALLMARK ANATOMIC COMPLICATIONS

Injury to recurrent laryngeal nerve
Injury to azygos vein
Injury to posterior (membranous) portion of trachea

Anastomotic leak
Pneumothorax

ANATOMIC STRUCTURES

Esophagus

Stomach
Pylorus
Gastroepiploic arteries and veins
Lesser curvature
Short gastric arteries

Left gastric artery
Azygos vein
Trachea
Carotid sheath
Sternocleidomastoid muscle
Omohyoid muscle
Middle thyroid vein

Although the operation was, in the past, termed *blind* or *blunt* esophagectomy, in reality, only a very small part of the dissection is performed without visual control. This chapter gives the basic steps in the procedure. More detailed accounts are given in the references at the end.

Patient Position and Initial Abdominal Dissection (Fig. 34.1)

Technical Points

Position the patient supine, with the head turned slightly to the right and the neck slightly extended by a roll under the shoulders (Fig. 34.1A). In addition to the usual monitoring devices, place an indwelling arterial line so that blood pressure can accurately be measured on a beat-to-beat basis. Compression on the heart and vena cava during the mediastinal dissection may cause hemodynamic compromise, and accurate blood pressure monitoring and communication between the surgeon and the anesthesiologist are crucial during this operation.

Begin with an upper midline incision and thorough abdominal exploration, including palpation of liver and regional nodes, to confirm that resection is appropriate. Take down the triangular ligament of the liver and fold it to the right, placing a padded retractor over it (Fig. 34.1B) to provide wide exposure of the gastroesophageal hiatus and distal esophagus.

Mobilize the stomach as described in Chapter 30, taking care to preserve the vascular arcades along the lesser and greater curvature.

Next, incise the peritoneum overlying the esophageal hiatus and divide the phrenoesophageal membrane. Encircle the distal esophagus with a Penrose drain (Fig. 34.2) and place gentle downward traction on it. Place a heart-shaped retractor on the esophageal hiatus and elevate it, providing direct exposure into the lower mediastinum. Enter the mediastinum, gently displacing the pleura to each side of the esophagus and taking care not to enter the pleura. Progress upward, gently assessing the mobility of the esophagus and circumferentially mobilizing it by sequentially dividing fibrous attachments and small vessels with electrocautery under direct vision. Take periesophageal soft tissues with this dissection and slowly proceed to the level of the carina.

Place a pack in the mediastinum. Perform a wide Kocher maneuver (if not already done) and a pyloromyotomy. If desired, a feeding jejunostomy can be done at this stage to complete the abdominal phase of the operation.

Anatomic Points

The stomach has a rich anastomotic blood supply that must be preserved during this dissection. The left gastric artery, a major branch of the celiac artery, is the single most important artery supplying the stomach. The right gastric artery is much shorter and smaller than the left. It arises from the common hepatic artery above the duodenum. The right and left gastroepiploic arteries form an arcade that supplies the greater curvature.

The right gastroepiploic artery arises from the gastroduodenal artery. The left arises from the splenic artery or one of its derivatives. Anastomosis between left and right gastroepiploic arteries occurs in the omentum. Several short gastric arteries run in the gastrosplenic ligament between the spleen and the stomach to supply the proximal greater curvature and sometimes distal esophagus. These are divided during the dissection described.

The esophageal hiatus is formed from muscle fibers of the right and left crura of the diaphragm. The only structures that traverse this hiatus are the esophagus and the vagus nerves. Division of the vagal trunks during this dissection necessitates pyloromyotomy, as delayed gastric emptying is a frequent result of bilateral truncal vagotomy.

The phrenoesophageal ligament (or membrane) is formed from the fusion of the layers of endoabdominal fascia closing the gap between hiatus and esophagus. It thus separates the retroperitoneum from the mediastinum. It covers the muscular arch of the hiatus and the lower part of the esophagus.

In the lower mediastinum, the left side of the esophagus is in close contact with the left and right pleura. The thoracic duct enters the mediastinum through the aortic hiatus but comes to lie posterior and to the right of the esophagus where it is vulnerable to injury during esophagectomy.

The distal esophagus derives its blood supply from the ascending (esophageal) branches of the left gastric artery with frequent contribution from the branch of the inferior phrenic artery. These vessels enter the esophagus beneath the phrenoesophageal membrane. They anastomose with descending esophageal branches of the thoracic aorta.

Cervical Dissection (Fig. 34.2)

Technical Points

Make an incision along the anterior border of the sternocleidomastoid muscle. Divide the overlying platysma muscle with electrocautery and identify the border of the sternocleidomastoid muscle. Retract this muscle laterally to expose the omohyoid muscle. Divide the central tendon of the omohyoid with electrocautery and incise the fascia superiorly and inferiorly to expose the carotid sheath.

Gently retract the carotid sheath and contents laterally and the trachea and esophagus (with associated recurrent laryngeal nerve) medially. Seek the middle thyroid vein, which generally crosses the field at approximately the level of the cricoid cartilage or slightly inferiorly, coursing from the thyroid to the internal jugular vein. Doubly ligate and divide it.

Have your assistant provide gentle upward traction on the esophagus as you carefully clear the esophagus of surrounding tissue and mobilize it circumferentially. Encircle it with a Penrose drain.

Anatomic Points

The omohyoid muscle is the only substantial structure crossing the field of this oblique incision. Division of the muscle

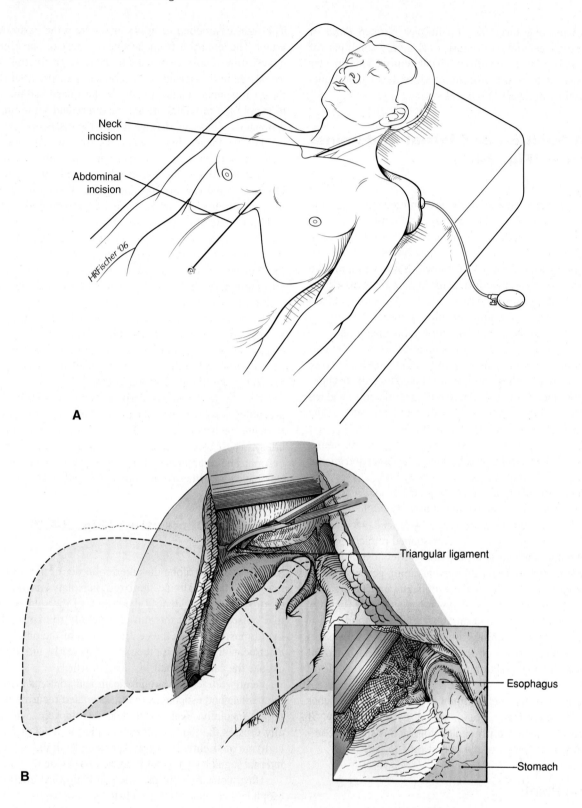

Figure 34.1 A: Patient position and initial abdominal dissection (from Ashrafi AS, Sundaresan RS. Transhiatal esophagectomy. In: Kaiser LR, Kron IL, Spray TL, eds. *Mastery of Cardiothoracic Surgery.* 2nd ed. Philadelphia, PA: Lippincott Williams & Wilkins; 2008:131–138, with permission). **B:** Exposure of esophageal hiatus.

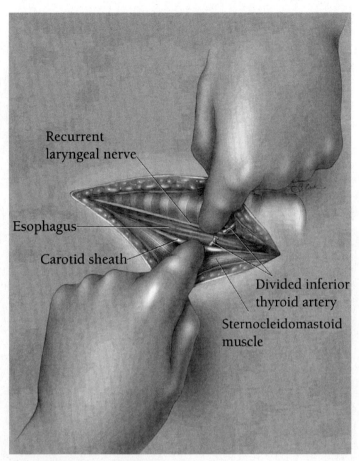

Figure 34.2 Cervical dissection (from Orringer MB. Transhiatal esophagectomy without thoracotomy. *Oper Tech Thorac Cardiovasc Surg.* 2005;10:63, with permission).

provides access to the deeper compartments. The anatomy of this region is illustrated in the chapters that describe carotid endarterectomy (Chapter 9) and operations for Zenker's diverticulum (Chapter 12).

In this region, the esophagus begins at the inferior border of the cricoid cartilage, just below the cricopharyngeus muscle, where circular fibers attain a longitudinal muscular coat. Anterior to the esophagus lies the trachea and posteriorly the vertebral column and longus colli muscles are found. Laterally, the carotid sheath and lobes of the thyroid gland are encountered. Thus the exposure described retracts the carotid sheath laterally and the thyroid medially, exposing the space within which the aerodigestive tract (trachea and esophagus) is found. Mobilization of the esophagus is easy in this region because it is surrounded only by loose areolar tissue. The blood supply of this portion of the esophagus is from branches of the inferior thyroid branch of the thyrocervical trunk. As it passes into the upper mediastinum, the esophagus gains branches derived from the descending portion of the thoracic aorta and the bronchial arteries.

The recurrent laryngeal nerve is at risk during this dissection. This nerve most commonly runs in the tracheoesophageal groove but may be encountered anterior (closer to the trachea) or posterior (closer to the esophagus).

Mediastinal Dissection (Fig. 34.3)

Technical Points

Dissection now proceeds from above and below with traction on the two Penrose drains (Fig. 34.3A). Perform as much as possible under direct vision, but inevitably a part comes that can only be done by feel. Pass a sponge stick from above and use this to gently mobilize the esophagus off the vertebral bodies posteriorly, as a hand passed from below gently displaces the esophagus and heart anteriorly (Fig. 34.3B). Constant monitoring of arterial pressure is essential during this phase as the resulting cardiac displacement can result in significant hypotension. When the sponge stick meets the hand, this phase of the dissection is complete.

Progress in a similar fashion to perform the anterior dissection, but take extreme care to avoid injury to the azygos vein or the posterior membranous portion of the trachea. Throughout, periodically assess mobility (and therefore resectability) of the tumor until it is fully mobilized.

Divide the lateral attachments in a similar manner.

When the esophagus is completely mobilized, pull several centimeters of the esophagus up into the cervical wound, pull back the nasogastric tube, and divide the esophagus with the GIA

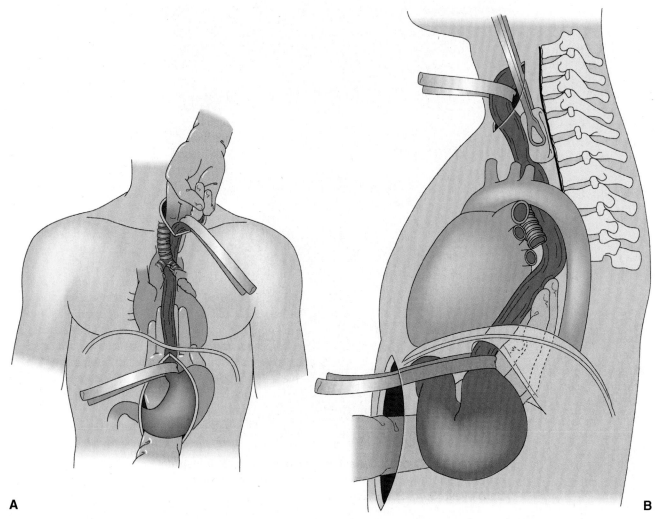

A   B

Figure 34.3 Mediastinal dissection (from Kucharczuk JC, Kaiser LR. Esophageal injury, diverticula, and neoplasms. In: Mulholland MW, Lillemoe KD, Doherty GM, et al., eds. *Greenfield's Surgery: Scientific Principles and Practice.* 4th ed. Philadelphia, PA: Lippincott Williams & Wilkins; 2006:691–708, with permission).

stapler. This line of transection should be oblique from anterior to posterior, so that the anterior part is slightly longer than the posterior, and should leave a generous length of cervical esophagus for anastomosis. Draw the esophagus out through the abdomen. Inspect the mediastinal tunnel for hemostasis and pack it, taking care not to produce hemodynamic compromise.

Lay the stomach out on the anterior chest wall and identify that portion of greater curvature that will reach with least tension toward the neck. Create an opening in the lesser omentum and divide the stomach from mid lesser curvature up toward greater curvature with several applications of the GIA stapler. Oversew this staple line with a running Lembert suture.

Remove the packs from the mediastinum and recheck hemostasis. Pass your hand and forearm up through this tunnel until two to three fingers emerge from the neck, ensuring adequate room for the stomach.

Gently pass the stomach up through the mediastinal tunnel to exit from the cervical wound.

Reconstruction and Anastomosis (Fig. 34.4)

Technical and Anatomic Points

Align the cervical esophagus and stomach (with the gastric staple line to the patient's right). Place stay sutures and create an opening in the esophagus and stomach through which you can pass the GIA stapler. Fire the stapler (Fig. 34.4A). Inspect the staple line for hemostasis.

Guide the nasogastric tube down into the stomach under direct vision.

Complete the anastomosis by hand-sewing the esophagus to stomach along the lateral and anterior sides of the anastomosis (Fig. 34.4B–D).

The completed reconstruction is shown in Figure 34.4E. Confirm that the anastomosis rests comfortably without tension.

Close the cervical incision without drainage.

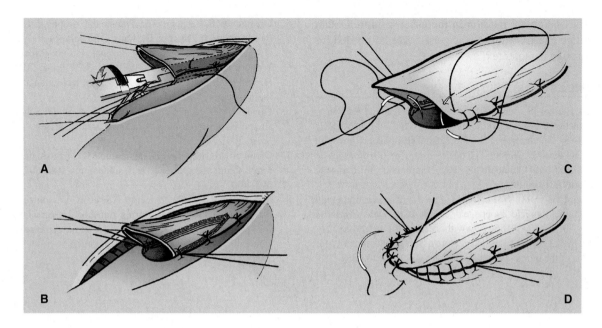

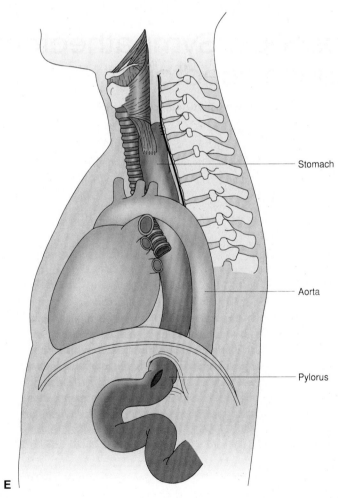

Stomach

Aorta

Pylorus

Figure 34.4 Reconstruction and anastomosis (**A–D** from Orringer MB, Marshall B, Iannettoni MD. Eliminating the cervical esophagogastric anastomotic leak with a side-to-side stapled anastomosis. *J Thorac Cardiovasc Surg.* 2000;119:277–288. **E** from Kucharczuk JC, Kaiser LR. Esophageal injury, diverticula, and neoplasms. In: Mulholland MW, Lillemoe KD, Doherty GM, et al., eds. *Greenfield's Surgery: Scientific Principles and Practice.* 4th ed. Philadelphia, PA: Lippincott Williams & Wilkins; 2006:691–708, with permission).

Close the abdominal incision in the usual fashion. Obtain a postoperative chest x-ray and place chest tubes if needed for pneumothorax or hemothorax.

REFERENCES

1. Ajani JA, Barthel JS, Bentrem DJ, et al. Esophageal and esophago-gastric junction cancers. *J Natl Compr Canc Netw.* 2011;9:830–887.
2. Ashrafi AS, Sundaresan RS. Transhiatal esophagectomy. In: Kaiser LR, Kron IL, Spray TL, eds. *Mastery of Cardiothoracic Surgery.* 2nd ed. Philadelphia, PA: Lippincott Williams & Wilkins; 2008:131–138.
3. Malthaner RA, Collin S, Fenlon D. Preoperative chemotherapy for resectable thoracic esophageal cancer. *Cochrane Database Syst Rev.* 2006;3:CD001556 (www.thecochranelibrary.com).
4. Orringer MB. Transhiatal esophagectomy without thoracotomy for carcinoma of the thoracic esophagus. *Ann Surg.* 1984;200:282–288.
5. Orringer MB. Chapter 75: Transhiatal esophagectomy without thoracotomy. In: Fischer JE, Jones DB, Pomposelli FB, Upchurch GR, eds. *Fisher's Mastery of Surgery.* 6th ed. Philadelphia, PA: Wolters Kluwer Lippincott Williams & Wilkins; 2012:903–918. (Excellent, highly detailed description of technique and pitfalls by the major developer of the operation.)
6. Orringer MB, Marshall B, Chang AC, et al. Two thousand transhiatal esophagectomies: Changing trends, lessons learned. *Ann Surg.* 2007;246:363–372.
7. Orringer MB, Marshall B, Iannettoni MD. Transhiatal esophagectomy: Clinical experience and refinements. *Ann Surg.* 1999;230: 392–400.
8. Pop D, Venissac N, Nadeemy AS, et al. Lesson to be learned: Beware of lusoria artery during transhiatal esophagectomy. *Ann Thorac Surg.* 2012;94:1010–1011. (Anatomic anomaly of significance during performance of this operation.)

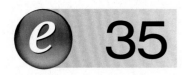

Thoracoscopic Sympathectomy and Splanchnicectomy

This chapter can be accessed online at www.lww.com/eChapter35.

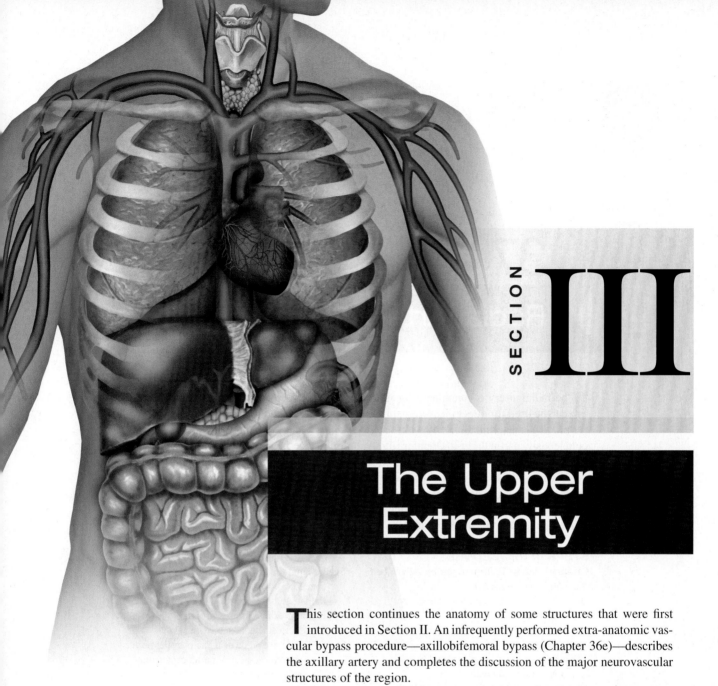

The Upper Extremity

This section continues the anatomy of some structures that were first introduced in Section II. An infrequently performed extra-anatomic vascular bypass procedure—axillobifemoral bypass (Chapter 36e)—describes the axillary artery and completes the discussion of the major neurovascular structures of the region.

The remaining sections describe those areas of upper extremity anatomy that are likely to be encountered in the operating room by the general surgeon or surgery resident on specialty rotations. References at the end include texts of hand and orthopedic surgery that give greater detail on these procedures as well as information about other operations.

Vascular anatomy of the arm and hand is explored further in Chapters 38, 39 and 40e, in which the nerves of the hand, radial artery, ulnar artery, brachial artery, and associated veins are described. Two specialized procedures—tendon repair (Chapter 40e) and carpal tunnel release (Chapter 41e)—are included because they are commonly performed or observed and because they illustrate well the regional anatomy of the tendons and nerves of the hand.

e **36** Axillobifemoral Bypass

This chapter can be accessed online at www.lww.com/eChapter36.

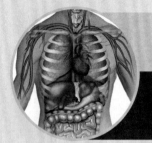

37

Radial Artery Cannulation

The radial artery is cannulated for monitoring purposes. A catheter in the radial artery can be used for direct measurement of arterial pressure and for sampling arterial blood for blood gas determinations. It is almost always possible to cannulate the radial artery percutaneously, particularly if Doppler ultrasound guidance is used in difficult cases. Under rare circumstances, a patient with significant vascular disease or shock may require direct cutdown on the artery, with subsequent introduction of the catheter under direct vision. Both procedures are described in this chapter.

SCORE™, the Surgical Council on Resident Education, classified arterial line placement as an "Essential Common" procedure.

STEPS IN PROCEDURE

Confirm Patent Palmar Arch by Allen Test
Ask patient to clench fist
Occlude both radial and ulnar arteries by
    direct pressure
Have patient open hand, which should be
    blanched
Release ulnar artery—hand should become
    pink within 3 seconds
Alternatively, use Doppler ultrasound

Secure hand on arm board with wrist slightly
    cocked
Palpate radial artery
Inject lidocaine around artery
Introduce catheter at approximately
        45-degree angle using an over-the-needle
        system or a special arterial cannulation
        system incorporating a guidewire

If Cutdown is Necessary:
Transverse incision over radial artery
Isolate and elevate radial artery
Cannulate under direct vision

HALLMARK ANATOMIC COMPLICATION
Ischemia of digits or hand due to lack of
    adequate collateral circulation

LIST OF STRUCTURES
Radial Artery
Superficial palmar branch of radial artery
Principal artery of the thumb
Radial artery of the index finger

Deep Palmar Arch
Palmar metacarpal arteries

Ulnar Artery
Deep palmar artery
Superficial palmar arch
Common palmar digital arteries

Radius
Radial styloid process
Ulna
Palmaris longus tendon
Brachioradialis tendon
Tendon of the flexor carpi radialis
Tendons of the flexor digitorum superficialis
Tendon of the flexor carpi ulnaris
Median nerve
Ulnar nerve

Position of the Extremity, Identification of Landmarks, and Cannulation of Artery (Fig. 37.1)

Technical Points

Before inserting an indwelling radial artery catheter, perform an Allen test to assess the adequacy of collateral circulation of the ulnar artery across the palmar arch. Because the arch is variable, the adequacy of circulation must be checked in each individual and in each extremity. Instruct the patient to clench the fist tightly. Use both of your hands to occlude both the radial and ulnar arteries. Then have the patient open the fist, which should be blanched. Release pressure on the ulnar artery and note the time required for the hand to become pink. The hand should become pink within 3 seconds after the release of occlusion. Alternatively, a Doppler ultrasound stethoscope may be used as a more objective means of determining the adequacy of circulation. Place the Doppler stethoscope over the palmar arch and do the test as previously described. In this case, use the appearance of Doppler flow in the palmar arch as evidence of collateral flow by the ulnar artery.

Place the patient's hand on an arm board with a roll under the wrist and secure the hand in a slightly wrist-cocked position. Palpate the radial pulse. Prepare the area over the radial pulse with povidone–iodine (Betadine) about 1 to 2 cm proximal to the crease in the wrist. Infiltrate the area with 1% lidocaine (Xylocaine).

Several systems are available for cannulation. They differ in whether or not a guidewire is used as an intermediary in catheter placement. The simplest system uses a small gauge (20G for the average adult) over-the-needle catheter similar to those used for intravenous access. The advantage of this system is that the equipment is readily available in all hospital settings.

Take care to identify the spot where the pulse is most prominent and feels closest to the skin. Then palpate the patient's pulse just proximal to this site with the fingers of your nondominant hand while gently introducing the needle–catheter assembly at an angle of about 45 degrees. The goal is to pierce the anterior wall of the artery and then have nearly tangential access to the artery to advance the catheter (Fig. 37.1B). Pass the needle–catheter assembly into the artery under palpation guidance. As soon as pulsating arterial blood is obtained from the needle, slide the catheter over the needle into the artery. The catheter should pass easily and pulsating blood should exit the catheter freely after the needle is removed. To stop the flow, simply occlude the radial artery proximal to the catheter entry site. If you encounter difficulty passing the catheter or accessing the artery, try moving proximal a centimeter or two. The artery will be generally larger, but may be deeper and more mobile. If necessary, ultrasound can be used as an aid or

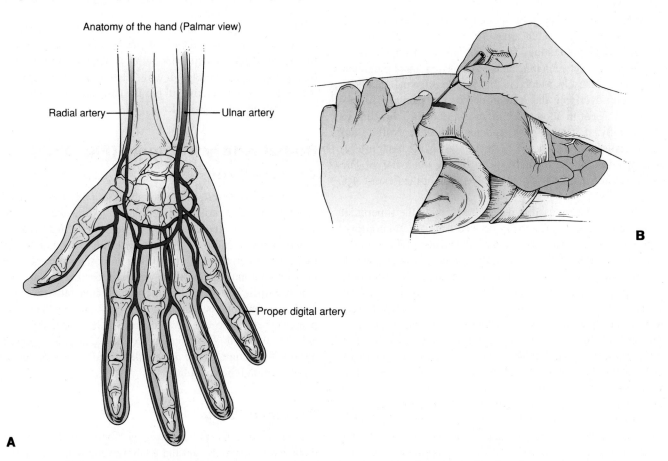

Anatomy of the hand (Palmar view)

Radial artery —   — Ulnar artery

— Proper digital artery

A

B

Figure 37.1 Position of the extremity and identification of landmarks. **A:** Regional anatomy. **B:** Position of hand and insertion of needle.

a cutdown can be performed. Secure the catheter in place and secure the extremity.

An alternative specialized assembly using a guidewire is described next.

Anatomic Points

To perform radial artery cannulation and cutdown successfully and safely, it is necessary to understand the relationships of skin creases, bony landmarks, and neurovascular structures at the wrist and to ascertain the blood supply and collateral circulation in the hand.

Typically, the flexor surface of the wrist has a proximal, middle, and distal skin crease. The proximal wrist crease does not correspond to any palpable landmarks. The middle wrist crease corresponds approximately to the radial styloid processes of both the radius and ulna as well as to the proximal extent of the common flexor synovial sheath. The consistent distal wrist crease is the most important of the three. From the radial to ulnar sides of the wrist, it overlies the tip of the radial styloid process, is just proximal to the tuberosity of the scaphoid, crosses the distal part of the lunate, and terminates just proximal to the pisiform. Furthermore, it marks the proximal border of the flexor retinaculum. The palmaris longus tendon bisects the distal skin crease and overlies the median nerve.

Identification of palpable structures at the wrist enables identification of the radial artery. The most lateral tendon is the brachioradialis tendon. The radial artery, identified by its pulsations, lies between this tendon and the tendon of the flexor carpi radialis muscle. Medial to this muscle is the palmaris longus tendon overlying the median nerve. The palmaris longus tendon is absent in about 10% of cases. Medial to this tendon (or centrally, if it is absent), tendons of the flexor digitorum superficialis can be palpated. Medial to this is the ulnar artery, accompanied (on its medial aspect) by the ulnar nerve. The most medial palpable structure is the tendon of the flexor carpi ulnaris.

The Allen test is used to determine whether the superficial palmar arterial arch, principally derived from the ulnar artery, is complete. The ulnar artery, always located superficial to the flexor retinaculum, gives off a small deep palmar artery, which passes deeply between the hypothenar muscles to contribute to the deep palmar arterial arch. The continuation of the ulnar artery past this point is the superficial palmar arterial arch, lying just deep to the palmar aponeurosis and curving laterally. The apex of this arch is located approximately at the level of the distal base of the extended thumb, or close to the proximal palmar skin crease. In about 88% of hands examined, it anastomoses with an artery derived from the radial artery, such as the small superficial radial artery (35%), the principal artery of the thumb, or the radial artery of the index finger. In its course through the hand, the superficial arch gives off four common digital arteries; typically, these digital arteries are joined by a palmar metacarpal artery derived from the deep palmar arterial arch.

The deep palmar arterial arch is the major continuation of the radial artery. After the radial artery gives off its small superficial palmar branch, it wraps around the lateral aspect of the wrist, passing through the anatomic snuffbox, to lie on the dorsum of the hand. At the base of the first intermetacarpal space, this artery dives between the muscles of this space to enter the hand and becomes known as the *deep palmar arterial arch*. This arch runs medially across the palm of the hand in the interval between the long flexor tendons and the metacarpal bones with their attached interosseous muscles and usually is completed by anastomosing with a small derivative of the ulnar artery. Branches of the distal radial artery/deep palmar arterial arch include the principal artery of the thumb, the radial artery of the index finger (in 13%, this was found to arise solely from the superficial arch), the carpal arteries, and the metacarpal arteries.

Cannulation of Radial Artery with Guidewire System (Fig. 37.2)

Kits are available which incorporate a needle (for entry), a small gauge guidewire, and a catheter in a single unit. These are designed to minimize splash of blood, by providing a chamber to contain the blood. The guidewire may facilitate atraumatic passage into the lumen of the artery, particularly if the artery is at all tortuous.

Position the hand and perform the Allen's test as previously described. Insert the needle–catheter–guidewire apparatus into the artery. When pulsatile blood flow is obtained into the chamber, gently advance the guidewire. Then pass the catheter over the guidewire and remove all but the catheter. Secure the catheter as previously described.

Radial Artery Cutdown (Fig. 37.3)

Technical Points

Perform the Allen test, as previously described, to confirm adequacy of the ulnar collateral circulation. A transverse incision that is parallel to the wrist crease and 1 to 2 cm proximal to it may be used. Infiltrate the area with lidocaine and make an incision through the skin only. Use a hemostat to spread gently in a longitudinal direction as you look for the radial artery, which will lie just medial to the radius. Generally, it is identifiable by pulsations that, although they may not have been palpable before the wrist was open, will be palpable once the artery is exposed. The artery is exposed and then cannulated by direct puncture, as previously described. Close the incision loosely around the cannula.

Anatomic Points

Remember that the radial artery lies between the brachioradialis tendon laterally and the tendon of the flexor carpi radialis medially. It is worthwhile to note that the superficial radial nerve, which accompanies the radial artery proximally, is lateral

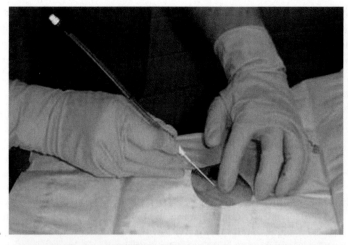

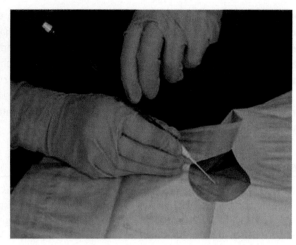

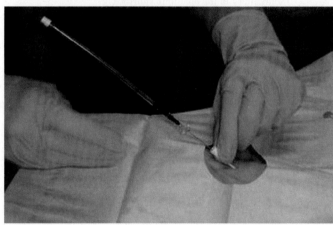

Figure 37.2 Cannulation of the radial artery with a needle–guidewire apparatus. **A:** The catheter–needle–guidewire apparatus is inserted into the skin at a 30- to 60-degree angle. **B:** The guidewire is advanced into the artery after pulsatile blood flow is obtained. **C:** The catheter is advanced over the guidewire into the artery (from Irwin RS, Rippe JM. *Manual of Intensive Care Medicine.* 4th ed. Philadelphia, PA: Lippincott Williams & Wilkins, 2006:17, with permission).

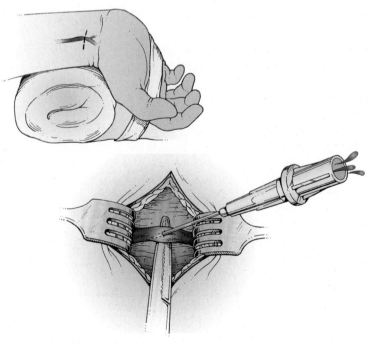

Figure 37.3 Radial artery cutdown

(dorsal) to the brachioradialis tendon at the wrist. Likewise, the median nerve is medial to the tendon of the flexor carpi radialis muscle. Consequently, there is no nerve accompanying the radial artery at the wrist, although branches of the lateral antebrachial cutaneous nerve (a continuation of the musculocutaneous nerve) are located in the superficial fascia over the radial artery. Because no nerves actually accompany the radial artery at this level, iatrogenic nerve injuries are virtually nonexistent.

REFERENCES

1. Allen EV. Thromboangiitis obliterans: Methods of diagnosis of chronic occlusive arterial lesions distal to the wrist with illustrative cases. *Am J Med Sci.* 1929;178:237–244. (This is the original description of the test that bears the author's name.)
2. Brodsky JB. A simple method to determine patency of the ulnar artery intraoperatively prior to radial artery cannulation. *Anesthesiology.* 1975;42:626.
3. Cronin KD. Radial artery cannulation: The influence of method on blood flow after decannulation. *Anaesth Intens Care.* 1986;14:400.
4. Durbin CG Jr. Radial arterial lines and sticks: What are the risks? *Respir Care.* 2001;46:229–231. (Presents review of complications.)
5. Ejrup B, Fischer B, Wright IS. Clinical evaluation of blood flow to the hand: The false positive Allen test. *Circulation.* 1966;33:778.
6. Gellman H, Botte MJ, Shankwiler J, et al. Arterial patterns of the deep and superficial palmar arches. *Clin Orthop Relat Res.* 2001;383: 41–46. (Provides thorough review of anatomy and anomalies.)
7. Kamienski RW, Barnes RW. Critique of the Allen test for continuity of the palmar arch assessed by Doppler ultrasound. *Surg Gynecol Obstet.* 1976;142:861.
8. Lee-Llacer J, Seneff M. Chapter 3. Arterial Line Placement and Care. In: Irwin RS, Rippe JM, Lisbon A, Heard SO, eds. *Irwin & Rippe's Procedures, Techniques and Minimally Invasive Monitoring in Intensive Care Medicine.* 5th ed. Philadelphia, PA: Wolters Kluwer Lippincott Williams & Wilkins; 2012:36–45. (Describes cannulation of other arteries as alternative to radial. Excellent description of use of ultrasound to guide cannulation in difficult circumstances.)
9. Pyles ST. Cannulation of the dorsal radial artery: A new technique. *Anesth Analg.* 1982;61:876. (Describes cannulation of the radial artery in the anatomic snuffbox.)
10. Scheer BV, Perel A, Pfeiffer UJ. Clinical review: Complications and risk factors of peripheral arterial catheters used for haemodynamic monitoring in anesthesia and intensive care medicine. *Critical Care.* 2002;6:199–204.
11. Tegtmeyer K, Brady G, Lai S, et al. Videos in clinical medicine. Placement of an arterial line. *N Engl J Med.* 2006;354:e13.
12. Valentine RJ, Modrall JG, Clagett GP. Hand ischemia after radial artery cannulation. *J Am Coll Surg.* 2005;201:18.

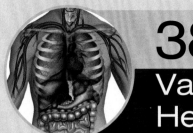

38

Vascular Access for Hemodialysis

Courtney L. Olmsted and Rachael Nicholson

The creation of an arteriovenous fistula is a common procedure for surgeons involved in dialysis programs. The goal of this procedure is to create an accessible, high-flow (500 mL/minute) conduit that can withstand repeated puncture by large-bore needles and yet remain patent and uninfected. The most common access procedures are performed in the forearm, although upper arm and even lower extremity arteriovenous fistulas may be used if options in both upper limbs have been exhausted. The native arteriovenous fistula is the preferred form of access because it is constructed from the patient's own tissue, making it durable and resistant to infection. When a fistula cannot be constructed, an arteriovenous hemodialysis graft using polytetrafluoroethylene (PTFE) is then created.

If the patient's disease process develops rapidly, a dialysis appropriate central venous catheter may need to be placed for weeks to months until a more permanent option such as an arteriovenous fistula can be placed and mature. However, in patients with multiple failed arteriovenous fistulas, placement of a large diameter tunneled catheter may be the final option. Placement of such a catheter is described in the final part of this chapter (which should be read in conjunction with Chapter 8).

STEPS IN PROCEDURE

Arteriovenous Fistula
Preoperative venous marking with Doppler ultrasound—optional
Brescia–Cimino
Create longitudinal incision lateral to radial artery at wrist
Identify and mobilize vein, ligating collaterals—vein should be at least 2.5 mm in diameter
Divide forearm fascia to expose radial artery
Mobilize sufficient length for proximal and distal control and 5- to 7-mm anastomosis
Divide vein and ligate distal end
Spatulate proximal end of vein
Create end vein to side artery anastomosis with running 6-0 polypropylene

Brachiocephalic AVF Access with Prosthetic Graft
Transverse incision one fingerbreadth below the antecubital joint crease
Expose brachial artery, medial antebrachial vein, median basilic vein, and median cephalic vein

Mobilize brachial artery
Choose a large vein from among those encountered
Create subcutaneous tunnel for graft
Anastomose spatulated ends of graft to artery and vein

Tunneled Catheter Placement
Use ultrasound to assess the right internal jugular (or central vein of choice)
Perform ultrasound-guided venipuncture using micropuncture needle (21-gauge)
Exchange over 0.018-inch wire for micropuncture sheath (4- or 5-French) using Seldinger technique
Create a subcutaneous tunnel
Determine length of catheter needed and cut to length
Exchange micropuncture sheath for larger peel-away sheath
Insert catheter and remove sheath
Check catheter tip location (with fluoroscopy)
Test function of catheter and secure in place

HALLMARK ANATOMIC COMPLICATIONS

Arteriovenous Fistula
Steal syndrome from excess flow through fistula
Sore thumb syndrome from venous hypertension
Injury to median nerve in antecubital fossa

Tunneled Catheter Placement
Pneumothorax

Hemothorax
Possible arterial canalization
Air embolization

LIST OF STRUCTURES

Radial artery
Cephalic vein
Basilic vein
Superficial fascia
Median basilic vein
Median cephalic vein
Median antebrachial vein
Brachial artery
Median nerve
Biceps brachii tendon
Bicipital aponeurosis
Brachioradialis tendon

Supinator muscle
Radial nerve
Superficial radial nerve
Lateral antebrachial cutaneous nerve
Medial antebrachial cutaneous nerve
Musculocutaneous nerve
Anatomic snuffbox
Internal jugular vein
Carotid artery
Clavicle
Superior vena cava
Right atrium

Arteriovenous Fistula

Incision and Identification of a Suitable Vein (Fig. 38.1)

Technical Points

The radial artery and the cephalic vein may be exposed through a single incision placed 1 cm lateral to the longitudinal axis of the radial artery. The nondominant upper extremity is preferred for dialysis access, presuming the vessels are of good quality because this allows freedom of movement for the dominant hand during the considerable hours spent undergoing hemodialysis. The nondominant upper extremity should be used only if both arms have equal access opportunities; otherwise the side with the better veins will take precedence. In diabetic patients with calcified radial arteries at the wrist that are seen to be inadequate on preoperative Doppler study, it may be prudent to consider more proximal access sites in the arm.

Establish the position of the wrist joint crease by inspecting the skin folds of the flexed wrist. If needed, place a tourniquet above the elbow to facilitate inspection of the distended veins of the forearm. Phlebitic, occluded, or stenotic veins, whether at the forearm, brachial, or axillosubclavian level, will mandate selection of an alternate site. Large side branch tributaries of the cephalic vein may be identified on ultrasound; these should be ligated to promote fistula maturation. A straight vein that is confined to the anterior surface of the arm and has few tributaries is ideal for the creation of a fistula.

Place the incision proximal to the mobile areas of the wrist to prevent normal joint motion from affecting the anastomosis. A longitudinal incision, placed parallel to the vessels, allows the vein to be dissected far enough distally to reach the artery easily. Sharp dissection will minimize adventitial loss and destruction of the vasa vasorum when dissecting the vein. Bathing the vein in papaverine minimizes vasospasm and allows more accurate assessment of conduit quality and size.

Anatomic Points

The goal of this procedure is to anastomose the cephalic vein, located in the superficial fascia lateral (or dorsal) to the brachioradialis tendon, to the radial artery, located deep to the deep fascia and medial to the brachioradialis tendon. An incision 1 cm lateral to the axis of the radial artery, or directly over the brachioradialis tendon, generally provides access to both of the radial artery and the cephalic vein. A longitudinal incision carries less risk of dividing the sensory nerves in this area, which are branches of the superficial branch of the radial nerve. These branches frequently communicate with branches of the lateral antebrachial cutaneous nerve, a sensory branch of the musculocutaneous nerve. This incision can also easily be extended. The cephalic vein begins on the dorsum of the hand over the anatomic snuffbox, draining the lateral aspect of the dorsal venous arch. At approximately the junction of the distal and medial thirds of the forearm, it courses from the lateral aspect of the forearm to lie on its anterolateral surface. Distal to the cubital fossa, it has a wide communication with the median cubital vein, which is an oblique communication with the basilic vein. In the cubital region, there is typically

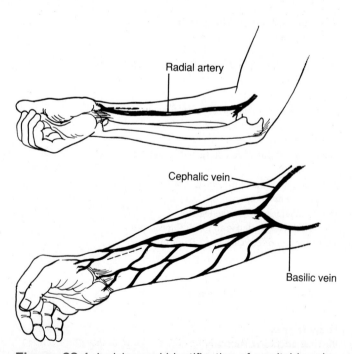

Radial artery

Cephalic vein

Basilic vein

Figure 38.1 Incision and identification of a suitable vein

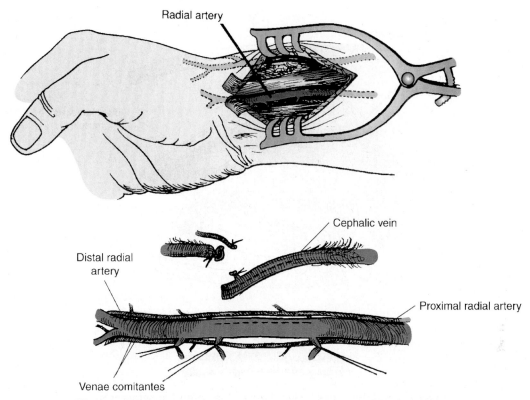

Figure 38.2 Exposure of the radial artery and its venae comitantes

a large communication between the superficial cephalic or median cubital vein and the deep venous drainage in the cubital fossa. The cephalic vein usually is accompanied by branches of the superficial radial nerve.

Exposure of the Radial Artery and its Venae Comitantes (Fig. 38.2)

Technical Points

Expose the radial artery by division of the forearm fascia. Mobilize a sufficient length of artery to allow proximal and distal control as well as construction of an anastomosis that is 6- to 10-mm long. Sharply dissect the venae comitantes from the artery to maintain a bloodless field for anastomotic control. Avoid ligating branches of the radial artery. Place a Silastic tourniquet or small atraumatic vascular clamp around these vessels, removing them at the end of the procedure.

Anatomic Points

The deep fascia of the forearm is continuous with the deep fascia of the arm and cubital fossa proximally, and also with the subcutaneous fascia of the hand. It is thicker proximally, where muscle fibers are seen to originate from it, and is attached to the epicondyles of the humerus and the olecranon process. Distally, it is thin except where it thickens to form the superficial and deep divisions of the flexor retinaculum; here, it is attached to the distal portions of the radius and ulna. Division of this fascia over the brachioradialis tendon, with reflection anteromedially, will expose the radial artery, which at this location emerges from under cover of the belly of the brachioradialis muscle and lies immediately deep to the deep fascia. Several branches of the radial artery may be seen near the wrist. Because most of these communicate with branches derived directly or indirectly from the ulnar artery, these branches should be controlled for hemostasis.

Again, remember that this artery, which in the proximal forearm is accompanied by the radial nerve, in the distal forearm at the wrist has no nerve accompanying it. Lateral to the cubital fossa, the radial nerve divides into deep and superficial branches. The deep branch pierces fibers of the supinator muscle to gain access to the posterior forearm, where it continues distally in the plane between superficial and deep extensors. The superficial branch, which is all sensory, leaves the company of the radial artery in the distal third of the forearm, passes dorsally deep to the tendon of the brachioradialis muscle and becomes superficial (i.e., piercing the deep fascia) near the dorsum of the wrist. This course places the main trunk of the superficial radial nerve out of the dissection field.

Brescia–Cimino Fistula (Side-to-end Anastomosis) (Fig 38.3)

Technical and Anatomic Points

Spatulate the divided vein end to create a patulous anastomosis. Within the general guidelines of 5 to 7 mm, the actual length

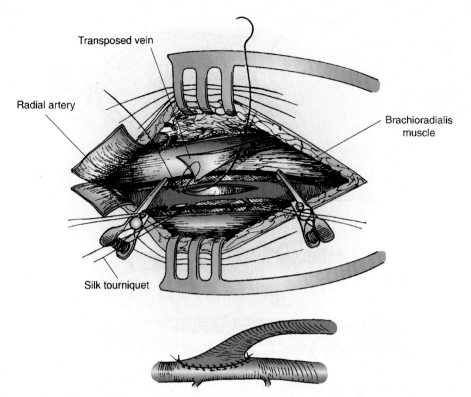

Figure 38.3 Brescia–Cimino fistula (side-to-end anastomosis)

of the anastomosis is individually tailored. A vein 2.5 mm in diameter or greater is sufficiently large to promote successful fistula maturation. Avoid inserting dilators into the vein to minimize intimal injury. Carefully align the vein so that when it is distended with blood it will not be twisted or kinked because either may limit flow. Take note of the orientation of any branches which have been ligated as another guide to maintain proper alignment. Use a running 6-0 or 7-0 monofilament suture for the anastomosis. Sew the anastomosis from the lumen to the adventitia side of the artery and the vein from the adventitia-side to the lumen-side.

Arteriovenous Hemodialysis Access with Prosthetic Graft (Fig. 38.4)

Technical Points

A graft of prosthetic material is used when the veins of the distal forearm are not adequate for creation of an arteriovenous fistula. Create a transverse incision one fingerbreadth below the antecubital joint crease. Expose the brachial artery, median antebrachial vein, median basilic vein, and median cephalic vein (Fig. 38.4A). Expose the artery by retracting the bicipital aponeurosis, the fibrous expansion of the biceps brachii tendon, laterally. If necessary, divide a few of the aponeurosis fibers. Any of the veins may be used, depending on its position and quality. The veins in the antecubital region are relatively variable, but generally one of them is of sufficient caliber to serve as the venous outflow for the dialysis graft. Avoid dividing communicating venous branches because

their patency will enhance graft venous outflow and graft patency.

Create a subcutaneous tunnel for the graft to lie in an ovoid or loop shape. The loop should be gently curved distally and about 10- to 12-cm long and 5- to 6-cm wide. A counterincision at the distal forearm will facilitate tunneling. Position a prestretched 6-mm, nonringed PTFE graft in the tunnel. Use care to avoid twisting or kinking of the graft, especially at the distal forearm. The counterincision will aid in graft positioning. Systemically heparinize the patient. Perform the arterial anastomosis first. Create a longitudinal arteriotomy 6- to 8-mm long after clamping the artery. Minimally spatulate the arterial end of the PTFE graft. Create the anastomosis with a running 6-0 monofilament suture.

Perform the venous anastomosis second. Carefully position the venotomy on the vein so that when the vein is distended with blood, it is neither twisted nor kinked. Spatulate the venous end of the graft to create an anastomosis of 6 to 10 mm. Use 6-0 or 7-0 monofilament suture for the anastomosis. Refrain from inserting dilators into the vein to avoid intimal injury.

Anatomic Points

There may be variability in the superficial veins of the forearm (Fig. 38.4B). In many instances, there is a median antebrachial vein that drains into the origins of the medial basilic and median cephalic veins. In other situations, it can drain into either. Recognizing anatomic variability is helpful so that a vein of appropriate quality and caliber can be identified for use.

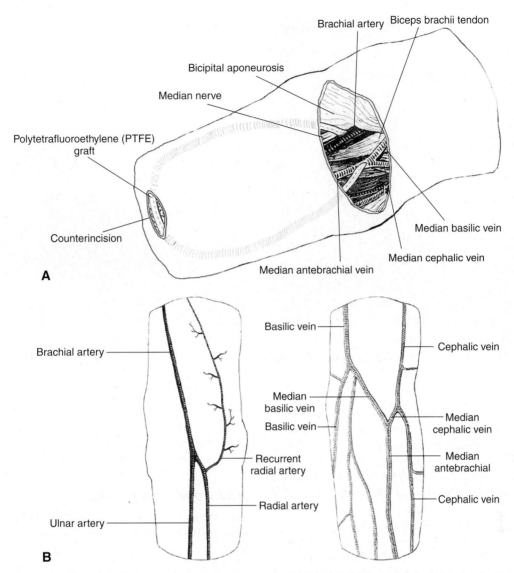

Figure 38.4 Arteriovenous hemodialysis access with prosthetic graft. **A:** Placement of graft. **B:** Regional arterial and venous anatomy.

Exposure of the median cephalic and median basilic veins should be done carefully to avoid injury to adjacent cutaneous nerves. Although these veins lie in the superficial fascia of the forearm, they are in close proximity to the medial and lateral antebrachial cutaneous nerves. These veins may cross superficially over these nerves. The median nerve enters the forearm medial to the brachial artery and should be carefully protected during arterial dissection.

Tunneled Catheter Placement (Fig. 38.5)

Technical Points

When dialysis access is needed and sufficient time is not available for creation of an arteriovenous fistula or if arteriovenous fistula fails, then a large bore tunneled catheter may be placed. These can be used immediately. As with all central access procedures, follow a standardized protocol for best results. Although there are several options for access, the right internal jugular vein is preferred as it offers a straight course in comparison to the left and is not as prone to stenosis and catheter fracture as the subclavian veins (see also Chapter 8). Identify the right internal jugular vein with ultrasound, confirming patency (see Fig. 8.8). Anesthetize the skin overlying the vein with lidocaine. Create a larger opening with blunt spread to minimize subcutaneous tissues from causing catheter kinking at this point. With the ultrasound probe resting on the cephalad portion of the clavicle and a micropuncture (21-gauge) needle adjacent to the cephalad portion of the ultrasound probe as shown in Figure 38.5B, access the internal jugular vein under ultrasound guidance (see Fig. 8.8 for actual ultrasound images). Observe the tip of the needle entering the vein. Aspirate to verify intraluminal positioning. Place a guidewire into the superior vena cava under ultrasound guidance and use it to exchange the needle for the micropuncture sheath with Seldinger technique (see Fig. 8.6). Confirm guidewire position with fluoroscopy.

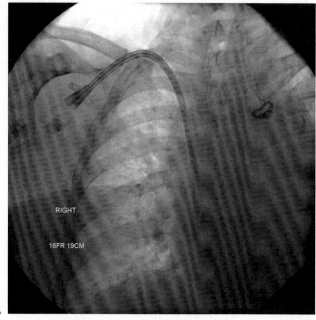

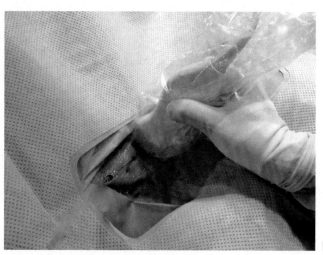

Figure 38.5 A: Ultrasound-guided puncture of right internal jugular vein. **B:** Fluoroscopic image of final placement of hemodialysis catheter.

Choose a site on the chest wall 3 to 4 fingerbreadths below the clavicle along the midclavicular line for the exit of the catheter. Generously anesthetize the site and a tract to the neck incision and make one transverse incision. Pass a tunneler from the chest wall incision to the access site at the neck and pull the catheter through the tunneled area until the cuff is positioned 1 cm from the exit site (see Chapter 8, Figs. 8.6 and 8.9 for additional details in tunneled catheter placement).

Measure the length needed for the tunneled catheter with fluoroscopy by advancing a wire through the sheath to caval–atrial junction and placing the clamp on the wire at the hub of the sheath. Withdraw the wire and the distance from the tip of the wire to the clamp minus the length of the hub is the length necessary for tunneled catheter. Under fluoroscopy, position a 0.035-inch J-wire with the tip in the inferior vena cava. Cut the catheter to the appropriate length.

Over the J-wire, exchange the micropuncture sheath for the peel away sheath and dilator under fluoroscopy. Remove the dilator and wire. If the sheath is not equipped with a valve, place a finger over the sheath opening to avoid air entry. Place the catheter into the sheath and peel away the sheath. Using fluoroscopy, check the catheter tip position as well as the course of the catheter. (Fig. 38.5B) Aspirate and flush the catheter with heparinized saline.

Anatomic Points

Entry with a micropuncture set and ultrasound guidance greatly minimizes access complications. Low puncture of the internal jugular vein just above the clavicle minimizes kinking of the catheter at the turning point. Access through the subclavian vein can be performed, but carries a higher complication rate and it may also compromise future arteriovenous fistulas in the ipsilateral arm. The catheter tip should be positioned at or just above the caval–atrial junction. See also Chapter 8 for more detailed anatomical discussion of the internal jugular vein.

Acknowledgments

The authors of this revised chapter would like to acknowledge Beth A. Ballinger for her significant previous contribution to this chapter.

REFERENCES

1. Ash SR. Advances in tunneled central venous catheters for dialysis: Design and performance. *Semin Dial.* 2008;21(6):504–515.
2. Barama AA. Evaluating the impact of an aggressive strategy to create wrist arterio-venous fistula in patients on hemodialysis. *J Vasc Access.* 2003;4:140–145.
3. Bonalumi V, Civalleri D, Rovidas S, et al. Nine years' experience with end-to-end arteriovenous fistula at the anatomical snuffbox for maintenance hemodialysis. *Br J Surg.* 1982;69:486. (Discusses most distal arteriovenous fistula.)
4. Brescia MJ, Cimino JE, Appel K, et al. Chronic hemodialysis using venipuncture and a surgically created arteriovenous fistula. *N Engl J Med.* 1966;275:1089. (This is the original description of this technique.)
5. Hakim NS. Chapter 8: Arteriovenous Fistulas. In: JA Akoh and Hakim NS, eds. *Dialysis Access: Current Practice.* Singapore: World Scientific Publishing Company; 2001;169–180.
6. Heberlein W. Principles of tunneled cuffed catheter placement. *Tech Vasc Interv Radiol.* 2011;14(4):192–197.
7. Humphries AL, Nesbit RR, Caruana RJ, et al. Thirty-six recommendations for vascular access operations: Lessons learned from our first thousand operations. *Am Surg.* 1981;47:145.

8. Kapala A, Szczesny W, Stankiewicz W, et al. Vascular access for chronic dialysis using the superficial femoral vein. *J Vasc Access.* 2003;4:150–153. (An alternative when other access is used up.)

9. Koontz PG, Helling TS. Subcutaneous brachial vein arteriovenous fistula for chronic hemodialysis. *World J Surg.* 1983;7:672. (Describes technique using autologous tissue.)

10. Leblanc M, Saint-Sauveur E, Pichette V. Native arterio-venous fistula for hemodialysis: What to expect early after creation? *J Vasc Access.* 2003;4:39–44.

11. Matsumoto T, Simonian S, Kholoussy AM. *Manual of Vascular Access Procedures.* Norwalk, CT: Appleton Century Crofts; 1987. (Provides concise, portable guide to a variety of access procedures for chronic renal failure and chemotherapy.)

12. McCormack LJ, Cauldwell EW, Anson BJ. Brachial and antebrachial arterial patterns; a study of 750 extremities. *Surg Gynecol Obstet.* 1953;96:43–54.

13. Moosa HH, Peitzman AB, Thompson BR, et al. Salvage of exposed arteriovenous hemodialysis fistulas. *Surgery.* 1985;2: 610.

14. Morsy AH, Kulbaski M, Chen C, et al. Incidence and characteristics of patients with ischemia after hemodialysis access procedure. *J Surg Res.* 1998;187:421–426.

15. Robbin ML, Chamberlain NE, Lockhart ME, et al. Hemodialysis arteriovenous fistula maturity: US evaluation. *Radiology.* 2002; 225(1):59–64.

16. Shemesh D, Mabjeesh NJ, Abramowitz HB. Management of dialysis access-associated steal syndrome: Use of intraoperative duplex ultrasound scanning for optimal flow reduction. *J Vasc Surg.* 1999;30:193–195.

17. So SKS. Arteriovenous communication: Internal fistulas. Arteriovenous communication: Bridge grafts. In: Simmons RL, Finch ME, Ascher NL, et al., eds. *Manual of Vascular Access, Organ Donation, and Transplantation.* New York, NY: Springer-Verlag; 1984;47:60.

18. Srivastava A, Sharma S. Hemodialysis vascular access aptions after failed Brescia-Cimino arteriovenous fistula. *Indian J Urol.* 2011;27(2):163–168.

19. Wixon CL, Hughes JD, Mills JL. Understanding strategies for the treatment of ischemic steal syndrome after hemodialysis access. *J Am Coll Surg.* 2000;191:301–310.

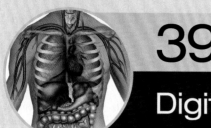

39

Digital Nerve Block

Digital nerve block is used to provide quick, reliable anesthesia of a finger or toe. Nerve block avoids injection of anesthetic into injured or more sensitive distal tissues, while providing sufficient anesthesia to allow nail removal, drainage of paronychia, reduction of minor dislocations, and other emergent and urgent procedures. This chapter describes the use of the basic web-space block in both the upper and lower extremities. Alternative techniques are described in references at the end.

SCORE™, the Surgical Council on Resident Education, classified digital nerve block as an "ESSENTIAL UNCOMMON" procedure.

STEPS IN PROCEDURE

Finger Block

Position the hand with the palm down on a padded well-supported surface

Prep the web spaces on each side of the digit to be anesthetized

For the thumb:

  Prep the web space between thumb and index finger

  Prep lateral aspect of thumb

Prepare a 5- to 10-mL syringe with local anesthetic *without epinephrine* and a 15- to 30-gauge needle

Enter the web space in the loose skin overlying the dorsum of the hand (or lateral aspect of the thumb, for thumb block)

Gently inject 2- to 4-mL of local anesthetic while advancing the needle toward the palmar aspect

Take care not to pierce the skin of the palm

Repeat the procedure on the other side

Gently massage the anesthetic into the tissues

Allow several minutes to achieve an effective block

Toe Block

Position the patient with easy access to the web spaces and great toe

Prep the web spaces and inject as noted above

For the great toe:

  Inject the web space between the great toe and the next digit as described above

  Inject soft tissues medial to great toe

  It may be necessary to use a third injection across the dorsum of the toe to achieve adequate anesthesia

HALLMARK ANATOMIC COMPLICATIONS

Digital ischemia

LIST OF STRUCTURES

Ulnar nerve
  Dorsal digital branches
Median nerve
  Dorsal digital branches
Radial nerve
  Dorsal digital branches

Proper palmar digital nerve, artery, and vein
Superficial fibular (peroneal) nerve
  Dorsal digital branches
Lateral dorsal cutaneous nerve of foot
Deep fibular (peroneal) nerve
Digital arteries

The cutaneous innervation of the hand is shown in Figure 39.1A. Note how branches of the ulnar, median, and radial nerves bifurcate in complex patterns but in general local anesthesia injected along the medial and lateral aspects of each digit will produce a nerve block for the distal portion. These dorsal digital branches course in close proximity to the proper palmar digital arteries and veins as shown in Figure 39.1B. It is this close proximity to the proper palmar digital artery that creates the potential for ischemic complications when injections are made in this region. *Do not use epinephrine-containing anesthetics because these may induce arterial spasm and ischemia.*

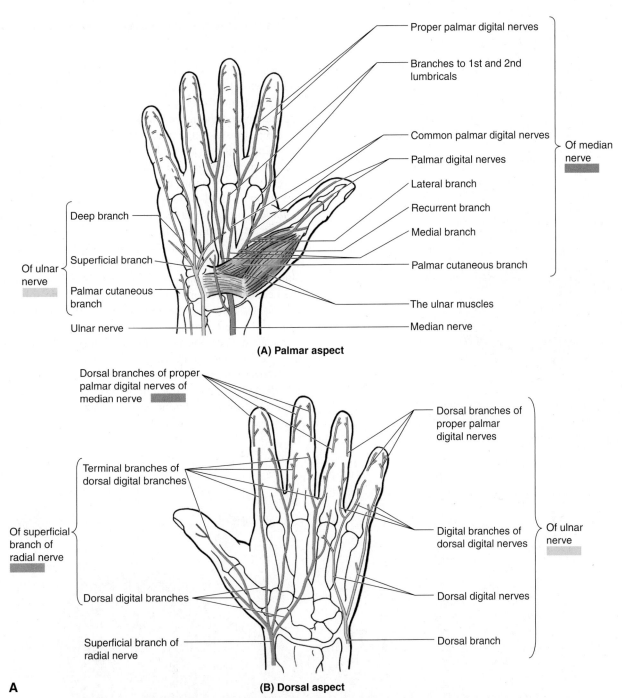

Figure 39.1 A: Cutaneous innervation of the hand (from Moore KL, Dalley AF, Agur AMR. *Clinically Oriented Anatomy.* 6th ed. Philadelphia, PA: Lippincott Williams & Wilkins; 2010, with permission). **B:** Transverse section through proximal phalanx showing neurovascular bundles. Note that palmar surface is up in this illustration. (*continued*)

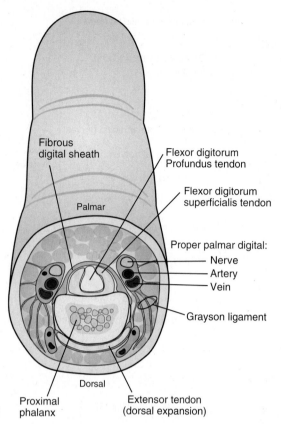

Fibrous
digital sheath

Flexor digitorum
Profundus tendon

Flexor digitorum
superficialis tendon

Palmar

Proper palmar digital:

Nerve
Artery
Vein

Grayson ligament

Dorsal

Proximal
phalanx

Extensor tendon
(dorsal expansion)

B

Figure 39.1 *Continued*

Digital Block of Finger (Fig. 39.2)

Technical points

Position the patient with the hand on a stable, padded surface, palm down. Prep the web spaces on both sides of the affected digit. If a thumb block is required, prep the web space between the thumb and the index finger, and the medial aspect of the thumb just distal to the metacarpophalangeal joint.

Gently insert a needle into the loose tissue of the web space, aiming to remain in the subcutaneous tissues (Fig. 39.2A). Aspirate before injection, to confirm that you are not in a vessel. Slowly inject 1 to 2 mL of local anesthetic (*without epinephrine*) as you advance the needle (continue to aspirate as you go). The trajectory of the needle should be approximately perpendicular to the long axis of the fingers (i.e., directly toward the palm). Take care not to pierce the skin of the palmar surface. Continue to inject as you withdraw the needle. Gently massage the local anesthetic solution into the tissues. Note that the goal is to enter the soft tissues adjacent to the neurovascular bundle as shown in Figure 39.2B. The massage promotes diffusion and entry of the solution into the space around the nerve.

Repeat the process on the other side of the finger. If you are blocking a thumb, inject tissues on the medial side of the thumb just distal to the metacarpophalangeal joint and gently massage.

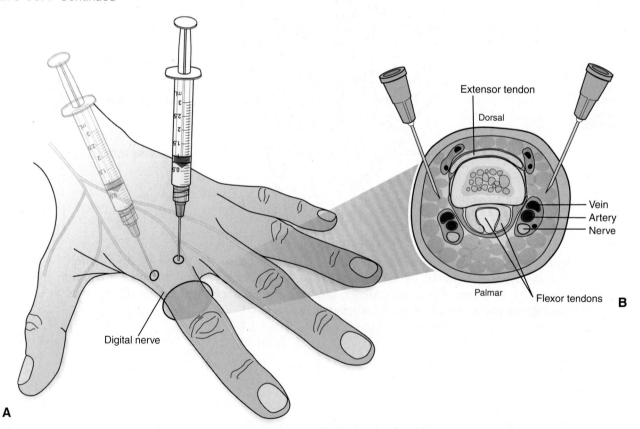

Extensor tendon

Dorsal

Vein
Artery
Nerve

Palmar

Flexor tendons   **B**

Digital nerve

A

Figure 39.2 A: Injection is made into the loose tissues of the web space on the medial and lateral aspects of the digit. Introduce the needle at nearly right angles to the long axis of the digit. **B:** Injection sites shown in transverse section of proximal phalanx.

Allow sufficient time for the block to take effect, and always test adequacy of the block before proceeding.

If the block is not adequate, inject a small amount of local anesthetic in the soft tissues over the dorsal surface of the digit, massage, and give time for the block to work.

Anatomic Points

The sensory nerves which supply the fingers and thumb derive from branches of the radial, ulnar, and median nerves. While the pattern of branching is variable, in general the ulnar nerve provides sensory innervation of lateral aspect of the middle finger, as well as the ring and the little finger. The thumb, index finger, and medial aspect of the middle finger are supplied by the medial and radial nerves. In each digit, the nerve travels on the medial and lateral aspects. There is also frequently a dorsal digital branch; thus, when block fails, injection along the dorsum of the digit (to block this branch) may be required.

It bears repeating that these nerves travel in close proximity to the arteries. The goal is to place the local anesthesia into the soft tissues around the neurovascular bundle, rather than to enter the neurovascular bundle and risk injury.

In the lower extremity, the sensory nerves derive primarily from the terminal branches of the lateral dorsal cutaneous nerve of foot and the deep fibular (peroneal) nerve. Again, the exact pattern of innervation and branching is variable, but in general the nerves travel along the medial and lateral aspects of each digit in close proximity to the arteries.

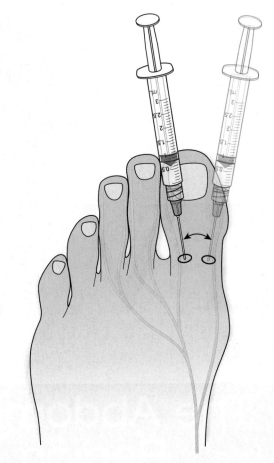

Figure 39.3 Injection sites for great toe

Digital Block of Great Toe (Fig. 39.3)

Technical and Anatomic Points

In the lower extremity, digital block is commonly used for procedures on the great toe. Perform the block in a similar manner to that already described. It is common to require a third injection across the dorsal aspect of the great toe to produce adequate anesthesia. If so, inject from medial to lateral into the loose subcutaneous tissues over the dorsum of the toe.

REFERENCES

1. Maga JM, Cooper L, Gebhard RE. Outpatient regional anesthesia for upper extremity surgery update (2005 to present) distal to shoulder. *Int Anesthesiol Clin.* 2012;50:47.
2. Tzeng YS, Chen SG. Tumescent technique in digits: A subcutaneous single-injection digital block. *Am J Emerg Med.* 2012;30:592. (Nice description of alternative techniques.)
3. Volfson D. Anesthesia, Regional, Digital Block. Medscape Reference. http://emedicine.medscape.com/article/80887-overview#a15 (accessed December 13, 2012). (Includes a video of the procedure.)

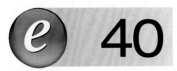 **40** Tendon Repair

This chapter can be accessed online at www.lww.com/eChapter40.

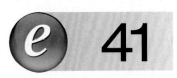 **41** Carpal Tunnel Release

This chapter can be accessed online at www.lww.com/eChapter41.

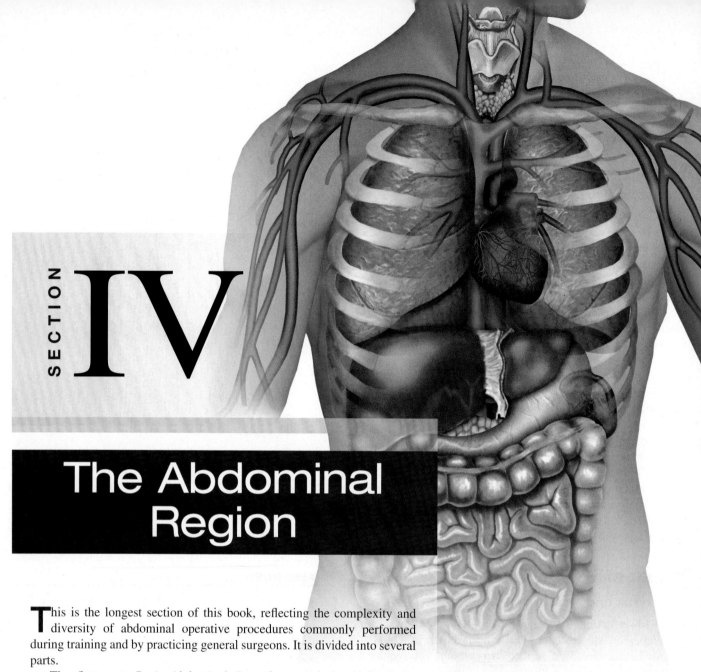

SECTION IV

The Abdominal Region

This is the longest section of this book, reflecting the complexity and diversity of abdominal operative procedures commonly performed during training and by practicing general surgeons. It is divided into several parts.

The first part, *Basic Abdominal Procedures and the Abdomen in General* (Chapters 42 to 49), deals with the anatomy of the anterior abdominal wall and peritoneal recesses. The general layout of the peritoneal cavity is described.

The next part, *The Upper Gastrointestinal Tract and Structures of the Left Upper Quadrant* (Chapters 50 to 71), continues the anatomy first introduced in Chapters 32e to 34. The distal esophagus, stomach, duodenum, and spleen are described.

Next, the right upper quadrant is addressed in the part on *The Liver, Biliary Tract, and Pancreas* (Chapters 72 to 87), including a description of the operative procedures performed on the extrahepatic biliary tree and liver. The pancreas, which strictly speaking is a retroperitoneal structure, is included here because of tradition and because operations involving the pancreas and biliary tree often overlap.

The next part, devoted to *The Small and Large Intestine* (Chapters 88 to 100), continues the discussion of the alimentary tract, presenting the anatomy of the small and large intestine. Both operative and endoscopic procedures are discussed as a means of describing these organs. A vascular procedure, superior mesenteric artery embolectomy (Chapter 89) is included here. The anatomy of *The Pelvis* is described through the operations of abdominoperineal and low anterior resection of the rectum (Chapters 101 and 102e) as well as total abdominal hysterectomy and oophorectomy (Chapters 103 and 104).

The next part, *The Retroperitoneum* (Chapters 105 to 114), explores renal and adrenal (suprarenal) surgery and aortic surgery. Finally, the part entitled *The Inguinal Region* (Chapters 115 to 120) provides a transition to the next section of the text, *The Sacral Region and Perineum.*

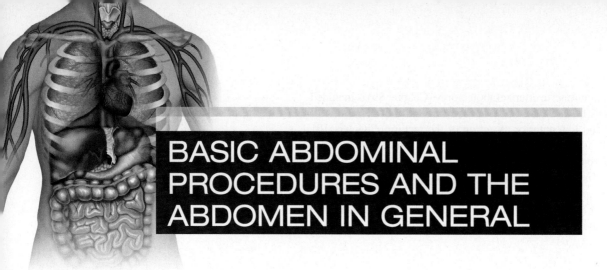

BASIC ABDOMINAL PROCEDURES AND THE ABDOMEN IN GENERAL

The detailed anatomy of the muscles and fascial layers of the anterior abdominal wall is described in Chapters 42 to 46. Peritoneal lavage is the first procedure illustrated in this section because it is often the first "laparotomy" performed by the junior resident or student. The general topography of the abdominal cavity is introduced in Chapter 42. The relationships of the viscera and a method for systematic exploration of the abdominal cavity, with considerations for trauma laparotomy, are described in Chapters 44 to 46. Additional information on the lateral abdominal wall may be found in chapters on specific procedures, such as appendectomy (Chapter 94), in which special abdominal incisions are described.

Weakness in the anterior abdominal wall may lead to hernia formation. Congenital weakness in the region of the umbilicus causes the formation of umbilical hernias, and imperfect healing of laparotomy incisions can result in incisional (ventral) hernia formation. The repair of these defects is described in Chapters 47 to 49. Other, less common, abdominal wall hernias and their repair are described in references at the end of these chapters.

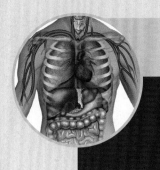

42

Peritoneal Lavage: Insertion of a Peritoneal Dialysis Catheter

Peritoneal lavage is a diagnostic maneuver in which a catheter is inserted into the peritoneal cavity and fluid is aspirated. The character of the fluid (presence of blood, bile, or food particles, and its odor) is noted. If no fluid is obtained, 1 L of Ringer's lactate solution is instilled, allowed to equilibrate with any fluid in the peritoneal cavity, and then aspirated. Although peritoneal lavage has largely been superseded by other diagnostic modalities such as FAST (focused abdominal ultrasound for trauma; see Chapter 40) or computed tomography scan, the procedure is still indicated under special circumstances.

A temporary or permanent peritoneal dialysis catheter is placed for peritoneal dialysis in patients with acute or chronic renal failure.

In this chapter, placement of a catheter for diagnostic peritoneal lavage is discussed first, followed by a description of the modifications necessary for placement of a permanent catheter. This procedure is used to introduce the anatomy of the anterior abdominal wall and the topography of the peritoneal recesses.

SCORE™, the Surgical Council on Resident Education, classified insertion of peritoneal dialysis catheter as an "ESSENTIAL COMMON" procedure.

STEPS IN PROCEDURE—DIAGNOSTIC PERITONEAL LAVAGE

Lower midline incision (modified if previous scars)

Careful hemostasis as fascia is identified

Identify and lift up peritoneum

Create small incision and insert catheter, directing it toward the pelvis

Place purse-string suture if desired

Confirm entry into peritoneum by free flow of intravenous fluid through catheter

Aspirate—free blood or succus indicates positive tap

Otherwise, instill 1-L Ringer's lactate or normal saline and allow to dwell

Place bag on floor and submit effluent for laboratory analysis

STEPS IN PROCEDURE—PLACEMENT OF TENCKHOFF CATHETER

Access peritoneal cavity through small paramedian incision

Place small purse-string suture in peritoneum

Insert catheter, using guidewire if necessary to direct it to the pelvis

Position with one cuff in subcutaneous tissues, second cuff just superficial to the peritoneum

Tie purse-string suture and close incision

HALLMARK ANATOMIC COMPLICATIONS

Preperitoneal catheter placement

Injury to bowel during access of peritoneum or placement of catheter

LIST OF STRUCTURES

Linea alba

Umbilicus

Rectovesical pouch

Rectouterine pouch (of Douglas)

Pyramidalis muscle

Rectus Abdominis Muscle

Rectus sheath

Pubis

ORIENTATION

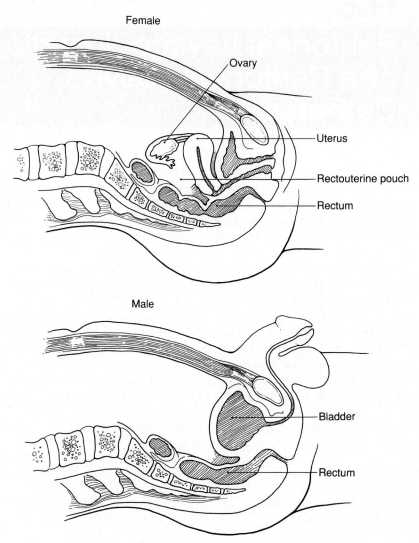

Female

Ovary

Uterus

Rectouterine pouch

Rectum

Male

Bladder

Rectum

Figure 42.1 Cross sections of female and male pelvis

Placement of a peritoneal dialysis catheter takes advantage of the deep recesses of the pelvis. The cross-sectional anatomy of the female and male pelvis is shown in Figure 42.1. Note that the deepest recess of the female pelvis is posterior to the uterus, tubes, and ovaries.

Diagnostic Peritoneal Lavage: Choice of Site (Fig. 42.2)

Technical Points

Note any scars from prior abdominal surgery. Because intraperitoneal adhesions form most densely on the underside of old scars, avoid such areas. In the absence of old scars or pelvic fractures, the preferred site is the lower midline, about 4 to 5 cm below the umbilicus. Alternative sites include the upper midline (for patients with pelvic fractures) and right lower

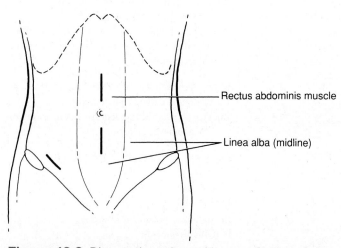

Rectus abdominis muscle

Linea alba (midline)

Figure 42.2 Diagnostic peritoneal lavage: Choice of site

quadrant. Ensure that the patient's bladder is empty by having the conscious, cooperative patient void or by placing an indwelling Foley catheter. Shave, prepare, and infiltrate the area of the proposed skin incision. The use of lidocaine with epinephrine minimizes bleeding into the incision and may decrease the chance of a false-positive result. Careful hemostasis throughout the procedure is important.

Make an incision about 5 cm long in the midline. Place a self-retaining retractor and deepen the incision until the linea alba is seen.

Anatomic Points

The linea alba changes as one progresses from the pubic crest to the costal margin. Inferior to the umbilicus, it is quite thin, because the rectus abdominis muscles attach immediately adjacent to the pubic symphysis. Medial fibers of the recti can originate from the linea alba, or quite inferiorly, tendinous fibers of one side can interdigitate with fibers of the contralateral rectus. The pyramidalis muscles lie in the rectus sheath immediately anterior to the rectus. These paired muscles originate from the anterior surface of the pubis and from the pubic ligament and insert into the linea alba. Fibers of this muscle are attached to the linea alba midway between the umbilicus and pubis. Above the umbilicus, the rectus muscles widen (but become thinner), diverging from the midline to attach to the costal cartilages of the fifth to seventh ribs. Here, the linea alba is about 1.5 to 2 cm wide.

The topographic anatomy of the abdomen in the sagittal plane provides a rationale for making an incision 4 to 5 cm below the umbilicus. At this location, you should be directly anterior to the fifth lumbar vertebral body or L5 or S1 disk. Because the aorta bifurcates superiorly and the right common iliac artery crosses the midline superiorly, no major arteries are at risk for injury. The left common iliac vein; however, does cross the midline somewhat lower than the major arteries and thus can be susceptible to injury. If the bladder is empty, the only structures between the retroperitoneum and the anterior parietal peritoneum should be mesenteric (greater omentum) or suspended by mesentery (loops of small bowel or redundant transverse or sigmoid colon).

Placement of Catheter (Fig. 42.3)

Technical Points

If the tap is to be done completely open, make a longitudinal incision 1 to 2 cm in length in the linea alba. Infiltrate the preperitoneal fat with local anesthetic. Spread the fatty preperitoneal tissues with a hemostat until the peritoneum is identified. Grasp it with two hemostats and incise between them with a knife. Place the catheter in the incision thus made and slide it in gently until all its holes are within the abdomen.

Perform a semiclosed tap (as shown in the figure) using a peritoneal dialysis catheter with a central trocar. Make a nick in the linea alba and pop the catheter–trocar assembly through

the peritoneum and slide the catheter down into the pelvis. Withdraw the trocar.

The catheter should slip in easily, without resistance. Direct the catheter downward into the dependent recesses of the pelvis. Aspirate fluid. If blood, bile, or fecal material is obtained, the test is positive, and the procedure can be terminated at this point.

If no fluid is obtained, instill Ringer's lactate solution and proceed with a formal peritoneal lavage. Place a purse-string suture in the peritoneum around the catheter and tie it tightly. Place a gauze sponge in the wound both to decrease the chance of any blood from the incision contaminating the lavage and to cover the incision.

Connect the dialysis catheter to an intravenous infusion setup equipped with a macrodrip chamber. Instill 1-L Ringer's lactate solution. It should flow in "wide open" by gravity alone. If the solution does not run in easily, the catheter may be in preperitoneal fat rather than in the peritoneal cavity. In this case, stop the infusion, cut the purse string, and remove the catheter. Wash it clean of any blood. Check the incision into the peritoneum and confirm the location by visualizing omentum or bowel. Replace and resuture the catheter.

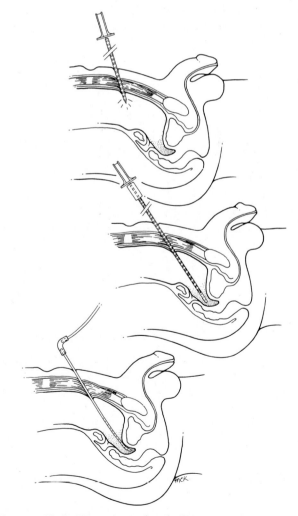

Figure 42.3 Placement of catheter

Allow the fluid to equilibrate for 5 minutes. Then place the bag of solution on the floor, allowing drainage from the peritoneum by gravity. If the intravenous infusion setup has a one-way valve in the tubing, it will not drain. In this case, cut the tubing and allow the lavage fluid to flow into a basin on the floor. Send the lavage fluid for amylase determination and cell count.

Close the incision in layers. If the lavage is clearly positive and laparotomy will be required, closure is not necessary.

Anatomic Points

The objective of catheter placement is to place the catheter in the lowest point possible in the peritoneal cavity. Ideally, this is the rectovesical pouch in the male, or the rectouterine pouch (of Douglas) in the female.

Insertion of a Tenckhoff Catheter for Dialysis in Patients with Chronic Renal Failure (Fig. 42.4)

Technical Points

When a permanent catheter is placed, special care must be taken (as with the implantation of any foreign device) to ensure

asepsis. A paramedian incision is preferred by many surgeons because this approach permits better sealing of the tract.

Alternatively, place the catheter under laparoscopic guidance (see references at the end of this chapter).

The procedure may be done using local or general anesthesia.

The Tenckhoff chronic peritoneal dialysis catheter is designed for long-term peritoneal dialysis. It has two Dacron cuffs that encourage tissue ingrowth and provide a barrier against bacterial migration along the catheter. These cuffs must be positioned properly at the time of implantation. The deep cuff should lie just superficial to the peritoneum, whereas the superficial cuff should be located in the subcutaneous tissue below the skin.

Make a short paramedian incision and place a 4-0 Dexon purse-string suture on the peritoneum. Guide the Tenckhoff catheter into the pelvis and the rectovesical pouch (in males) or the rectouterine pouch of Douglas (in females) using a guidewire, if necessary. Position the first cuff just superficial to the fascia.

Instill fluid and confirm that there is no leakage of fluid when the purse-string suture is tied. If fluid leaks, place additional sutures to ensure a watertight closure. Close the fascia around the catheter and position the second cuff just superficial to the fascia in a subcutaneous position. Tunnel the exit site of the catheter a short distance from the surgical incision. Secure the catheter in place.

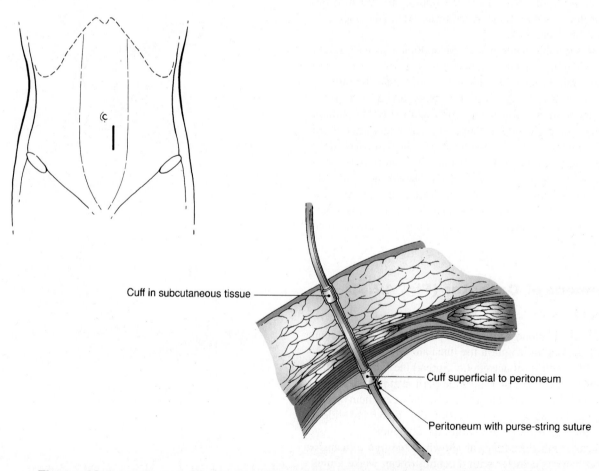

Figure 42.4 Insertion of a Tenckhoff catheter for dialysis in patients with chronic renal failure

REFERENCES

1. Asif A, Gadalean F, Vieira CF, et al. Salvage of problematic peritoneal dialysis catheters. *Semin Dial.* 2006;19:180–183.
2. Borazan A, Comert M, Ucan BH, et al. The comparison in terms of early complications of a new technique and percutaneous method for the placement of CAPD catheters. *Ren Fail.* 2006;28:37–42.
3. Crabtree JH. Selected best demonstrated practices in peritoneal dialysis access. *Kidney Int Suppl.* 2006;103:S27–S37.
4. Crabtree JH, Burchette RJ, Siddiqi NA. Optimal peritoneal dialysis catheter type and exit site location: An anthropometric analysis. *ASAIO J.* 2005;51:743–747.
5. Frost JH, Bagul A. A brief recap of tips and surgical manoeuvres to enhance optimal outcome of surgically placed peritoneal dialysis catheters. *Int J Nephrol.* 2012;2012:251584.
6. Gajjar AH, Rhoden DH, Kathuria P, et al. Peritoneal dialysis catheters: Laparoscopic versus traditional placement techniques and outcomes. *Am J Surg.* 2007;194:872–875.
7. Harissis HV, Katsios CS, Koliousi EL, et al. A new simplified one port laparoscopic technique of peritoneal dialysis catheter placement with intra-abdominal fixation. *Am J Surg.* 2006;192:125–129.
8. Hodgson NF, Stewart TC, Girotti MJ. Open or closed diagnostic peritoneal lavage for abdominal trauma? A meta-analysis. *J Trauma.* 2000;48:1091–1095. (Results show no difference between open and closed technique.)
9. Jwo SC, Chen KS, Lee CC, et al. Prospective randomized study for comparison of open surgery with laparoscopic-assisted placement of Tenckhoff peritoneal dialysis catheter – a single center experience and literature review. *J Surg Res.* 2010;159:489–496.
10. Numanoglu A, McCulloch MI, Van Der Pool A, et al. Laparoscopic salvage of malfunctioning Tenckhoff catheters. *J Laparoendosc Adv Surg Tech A.* 2007;17:128–130.
11. Tenckhoff H, Schechter H. A bacteriologically safe peritoneal access device. *Trans Am Soc Artif Intern Organs.* 1968;14:181–187. (This is the original description of device that bears Tenckhoff's name.)

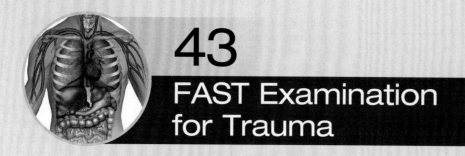

43

FAST Examination for Trauma

Focused assessment with sonography for trauma (FAST) examination has largely replaced diagnostic peritoneal lavage for initial evaluation of the patient with multiple trauma. The examination is performed in the trauma room by trauma surgeons. An accurate knowledge of the ultrasound anatomy of the regions examined is crucial for accurate interpretation. The key finding on FAST is the presence of fluid in one of the four areas examined; that finding is indicative of some internal injury requiring further investigation or exploratory laparotomy. If FAST is negative at initial evaluation, repeat examination in 30 minutes may be warranted.

SCORE™, The Surgical Council on Resident Education, classified Focused assessment with sonography (FAST scan) as an "ESSENTIAL UNCOMMON" procedure.

STEPS IN PROCEDURE

3- to 5-MHz transducer
Patient supine, clamp Foley catheter

Subxiphoid Examination

Transducer placed in epigastric region, just under the xiphoid process
Firm downward pressure to allow sound wave to go under xiphoid process
Direct transducer cephalad and toward patient's left shoulder

Right Upper Quadrant View

Transducer placed at midaxillary line just below right costal margin
Identify right kidney, then angle transducer upward to find liver

If difficulty is encountered, try a more posterior location

Left Upper Quadrant View

Transducer placed at midaxillary line just below costal margin
Angle transducer slightly downward to identify left kidney
Then slowly angle transducer upward to find spleen

Suprapubic View

Make sure that bladder is full
Place transducer in suprapubic region
Identify the two fossae on each side of bladder

HALLMARK ANATOMIC COMPLICATIONS

False-negative examination
Inability to access window because of overlying bowel gas

Inability to access window because of overlying bone or lung

LIST OF STRUCTURES

Xiphoid process
Pericardium
Liver

Right and left kidneys
Bladder
Paravesicular fossae

Transducer Placement Locations for Performing FAST (Fig. 43.1)

Technical Points

FAST is performed with a 3- to 5-MHz transducer placed sequentially in the following locations: Subxiphoid (to image the pericardium), right upper quadrant, left upper quadrant, suprapubic. In preparation for the examination, make sure that

the patient has a full bladder by clamping the Foley catheter, if present. The purpose of the examination is simply to determine if fluid is, or is not, present in the locations examined. Fluid may be blood, gastric contents, bile, or succus. The examination is not designed to yield a definitive diagnosis. Interpretation of the FAST examination must be done in conjunction with clinical picture and other imaging studies. In some circumstances, a

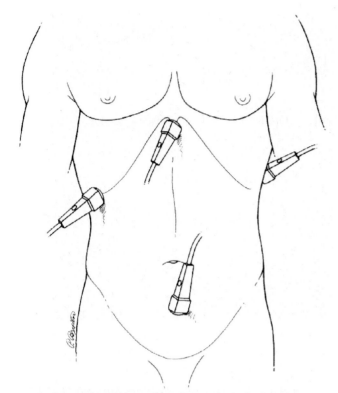

Figure 43.1 Transducer placement locations for performing focused abdominal sonography for trauma (from Rozycki GS, Ballard RB, Feliciano DV, et al. Surgeon-performed ultrasound for the assessment of truncal injuries. Lessons learned from 1,540 patients. *Ann Surg.* 228;4: 557–567, with permission).

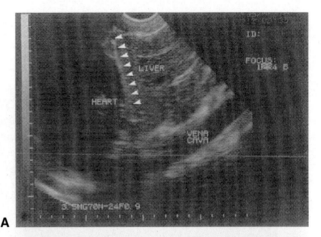

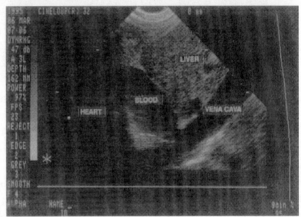

Figure 43.2 Subxiphoid examination **A:** Normal anatomy. **B:** Blood in pericardium is visible between heart and liver (from Rozycki GS, Ballard RB, Feliciano DV, et al. Surgeon-performed ultrasound for the assessment of truncal injuries. Lessons learned from 1,540 patients. *Ann Surg.* 228;4:557–567, with permission).

repeat FAST examination may be helpful, because it takes time for blood or fluid to accumulate in these locations.

Anatomic Points

These four locations are chosen for two reasons: First of all, they provide good ultrasound "windows" into the peritoneal cavity; second, they are regions were fluid accumulation is likely to occur in trauma.

The concept of an acoustic window is quite simple. Ultrasound is strongly reflected by interfaces between liquid/tissue and air (i.e., the lungs) or bone, and this reflection obscures the visualization of deeper structures. A good window avoids these interfaces. Thus the subxiphoid approach to the pericardium avoids potential overlap of ribs or lung and takes advantage of the anatomy illustrated in Chapter 20.

Free fluid most commonly results from bleeding from the spleen or liver. Initially this blood may accumulate under these organs, where it is detectable by examination of Morrison's pouch or in the splenorenal space. Blood also tends to pool in the pelvis, where it may be picked up on suprapubic examination. Although it is true that blood will also be found around loops of small bowel or in the paracolic gutters, these regions are more difficult for the nonradiologist to interpret.

Subxiphoid Examination (Fig. 43.2)

Technical and Anatomic Points

Place the transducer in the subxiphoid region and angle it cephalad and very slightly toward the patient's left shoulder. Firm downward pressure is required to allow the sound beam to pass under the xiphoid and into the pericardium. A four-chamber view of the beating heart should result (Fig. 43.2A). Often the liver will be seen between transducer and pericardium. Fluid in the pericardium produces a dark shadow between the heart and the pericardium (Fig. 43.2B), and suggests impending pericardial tamponade in the trauma setting.

Right Upper Quadrant View (Fig. 43.3)

Technical Points

Place the transducer just under the right costal margin at the midaxillary line and angle it slightly cephalad. It may be helpful to first identify the right kidney, seen in cross-section as an oval structure with internal echoes corresponding to the renal

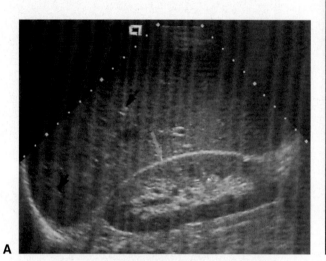

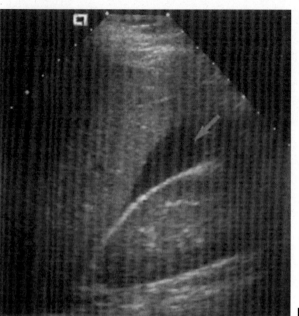

Figure 43.3 Right upper quadrant examination **A:** Normal anatomy showing liver above and kidney below. **B:** Blood between liver and kidney (*gray arrow*) (from Brant WE. *Ultrasound: The Core Curriculum.* Philadelphia, PA: Lippincott Williams & Wilkins; 2001, with permission).

pelvis. After the kidney is confidently identified, angle the transducer cephalad to seek the liver. It is essential to image the interface between the underside of the liver and the upper surface of the right kidney. A thin bright line should be seen (Fig. 43.3A) between the kidney and the liver. A black crescent indicates fluid (Fig. 43.3B). This is the easiest view to obtain in most patients, because the liver and right kidney can be accessed below the costal margin.

Anatomic Points

Posteriorly, the right lobe of the liver overlies the right kidney. This is the region that is imaged for this view. Anteriorly, hepatic flexure and descending colon obscure the view. The key to a good view in this region is to place the transducer sufficiently posteriorly. If it proves difficult to image the kidney, place the transducer in a more posterior location to avoid overlying colon gas.

Left Upper Quadrant View (Fig. 43.4)

Technical Points

This is often the most difficult view to obtain. Place the transducer at the left costal margin, midaxillary line, and angle it slightly downward. Identify the left kidney and work upward from the left kidney to find the spleen. As with the right upper quadrant view, a bright line between the kidney and the spleen is normal (Fig. 43.4A). A black crescent indicates the presence of fluid (Fig. 43.4B).

Anatomic Points

As with the subhepatic space, the key to obtaining this image is to place the transducer sufficiently far posteriorly. This allows

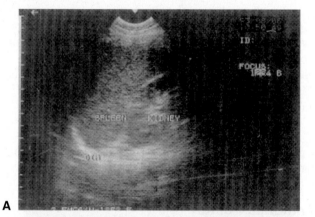

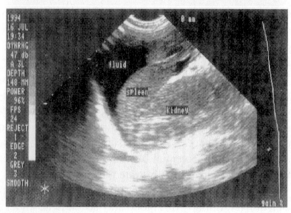

Figure 43.4 Left upper quadrant examination **A:** Normal anatomy showing liver and spleen. **B:** Blood above spleen and under liver (not visible, at upper left of image) (from Rozycki GS, Ballard RB, Feliciano DV, et al. Surgeon-performed ultrasound for the assessment of truncal injuries. Lessons learned from 1,540 patients. *Ann Surg.* 228;4: 557–567, with permission).

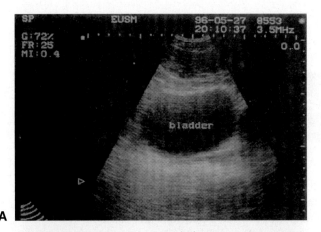

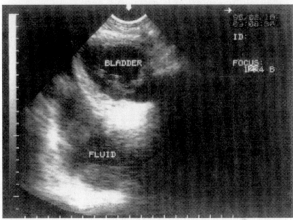

Figure 43.5 Suprapubic examination **A:** Normal view of bladder. **B:** Blood or fluid posterior to bladder (from Rozycki GS, Ballard RB, Feliciano DV, et al. Surgeon-performed ultrasound for the assessment of truncal injuries. Lessons learned from 1,540 patients. *Ann Surg.* 228;4:557–567, with permission).

the sound waves to pass unimpeded by overlying splenic flexure of colon and left colon.

Suprapubic View (Fig. 43.5)

Technical and Anatomic Points

Place the transducer in the suprapubic region and image the bladder, which should be a large black (i.e., fluid-filled) structure. Next image the two fossae on each side of the bladder (Fig. 43.5A). It may be necessary to angle the probe slightly downward to see these fossae. As before, the presence of anechoic material (black on ultrasound) suggests fluid (Fig. 43.5A,B).

REFERENCES

1. Brooks AJ, Price V, Simms M. FAST on operational military deployment. *Emerg Med J.* 2005;22:263–265.
2. Jang T, Kryder G, Sineff S, et al. The technical errors of physicians learning to perform focused assessment with sonography in trauma. *Acad Emerg Med.* 2012;19:98–101.
3. McKenney KL, Nunez DB Jr, McKenney MG, et al. Sonography as the primary screening technique for blunt abdominal trauma: Experience with 899 patients. *AJR Am J Roentgenol.* 1998;170:979–985.
4. Nagdev A, Racht J. The "gastric fluid" sign: An unrecognized false-positive finding during focused assessment for trauma examinations. *Am J Emerg Med.* 2008;26:630.
5. Quinn AC, Sinert R. What is the utility of the focused assessment with sonography in trauma (FAST) exam in penetrating torso trauma? *Injury.* 2011;42:482–487.
6. Rozycki GS, Ballard RB, Feliciano DV, et al. Surgeon-performed ultrasound for the assessment of truncal injuries: Lessons learned from 1,540 patients. *Ann Surg.* 1998;228:557–567.
7. Rozycki GS, Newman PG. Surgeon-performed ultrasound for the assessment of abdominal injuries. *Adv Surg.* 1999;33:243–259.

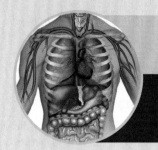

44

Exploratory Laparotomy

The choice of incision for laparotomy is influenced by the operation planned, the location of the probable pathology, the body habitus of the patient, and the presence or absence of previous scars. Choose an incision that will provide good exposure, can be extended if necessary, and will heal well. The vertical midline incision is discussed here as the prototype for an abdominal incision. The McBurney and Rockey-Davis incisions, Kocher incision, paramedian incision, and transverse and oblique incisions are discussed in conjunction with the operative procedures for which they are most frequently used. This chapter also describes the general principles for adhesiolysis and trauma laparotomy.

SCORE™, the Surgical Council on Resident Education, classified open exploratory laparotomy and open adhesiolysis as "ESSENTIAL COMMON" procedures.

STEPS IN PROCEDURE

Vertical midline incision provides best access

Lift up abdominal wall when entering peritoneum, watch for bowel

Lyse any adhesions with care, use sharp dissection

Thorough exploration is mandatory

In trauma situation, consider damage control laparotomy

Place omentum under incision and around any anastomoses

Close fascia; consider retention sutures

When heavy contamination is encountered, pack skin open or use vacuum dressing

HALLMARK ANATOMIC COMPLICATIONS

Missed pathology or injury

Injury to bowel during entry into peritoneal cavity

LIST OF STRUCTURES

External oblique muscle and aponeurosis

Internal oblique muscle and aponeurosis

Transversus abdominis muscle

Preperitoneal fat

Peritoneum

Linea alba

Median umbilical fold (urachus)

Bladder

Orientation

The vertical midline incision is versatile, rapidly made, and affords equal access to all quadrants of the abdomen. Few vessels are encountered in the midline, and no nerves are sacrificed (Fig. 44.1). It is the preferred incision in cases of traumatic injury in situations in which access to multiple areas is required and in any situation in which the nature of the pathology is in doubt. The potential disadvantages of the incision are that only one layer of fascia is present to be closed and that contraction of the abdominal wall muscles tends to pull the incision apart (in contrast to transverse or muscle-splitting incisions, in which the pull of the muscles does not act as a distracting force on the edges of the fascial incision). The vertical midline incision can

be extended into the chest as a median sternotomy to improve exposure in the patient with traumatic injuries.

The Vertical Midline Incision (Fig. 44.2)

Technical Points

Cut cleanly through skin and subcutaneous tissue with a sharp knife, maintaining equal traction on both sides of the incision to ensure that the incision is straight. Make the incision in the upper midline or the lower midline, or extend it from xiphoid to pubis, depending on the expected findings. Curve

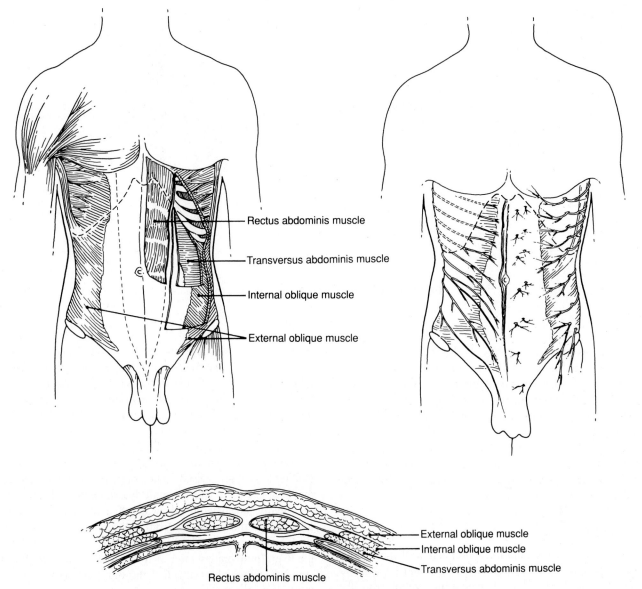

Rectus abdominis muscle

Transversus abdominis muscle

Internal oblique muscle

External oblique muscle

External oblique muscle
Internal oblique muscle
Transversus abdominis muscle

Rectus abdominis muscle

Figure 44.1 Anatomy of the anterior abdominal wall

the incision around to the left of the umbilicus to avoid dividing the ligamentum teres hepatis. As the incision deepens, place laparotomy pads on the subcutaneous fat and use strong traction and countertraction to assist in exposure. In massively obese patients, "pull" the fat apart by strong traction and countertraction. This seemingly brutal maneuver helps maintain orientation in the relatively avascular midline and leads directly to the linea alba. Clean the linea alba of fat for a few millimeters on each side of the midline to help define the exact midline and to facilitate closure. Confirm the midline by the visible decussation of fibers at the linea alba. Check the wound for hemostasis and use electrocautery to coagulate any bleeding points.

Incise the linea alba for the length of the incision and pick up the peritoneum. (Often, a transparent area can be identified in the upper midline through which intra-abdominal viscera can be seen.) It is helpful to lift up on the fascia as you incise it and the peritoneum. This maneuver creates negative pressure in the abdomen. As you enter the peritoneum, air will enter and any underlying bowel has a better chance of falling away from the knife. Conversely, pushing down on the fascia as you enter will increase pressure in the abdomen and cause the bowel to push out through any small incision, increasing the probability of injury. The preperitoneal fat becomes thicker below the umbilicus and, as the pubic bone is reached, the urinary bladder may be encountered. Therefore the abdomen should be entered in the upper midline, where the risk for injury to the bladder is eliminated, preperitoneal fat is least prominent, and the left lobe of the liver protects underlying hollow viscera from injury. Open the incision for its

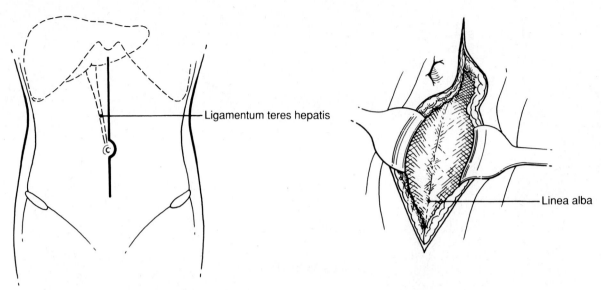

Figure 44.2 The vertical midline incision

entire length using electrocautery. If the incision extends to the lower midline, incise fascia first, bluntly pushing preperitoneal fat and bladder away from the fascia. After the fascia is opened, thin the preperitoneal fat by squeezing it between the thumb and the forefinger, feeling for the muscular wall of the bladder. If in doubt, feel for the balloon of the Foley catheter and pull it up to define the anterior extent of the bladder. Generally, the obliterated urachus will become visible as the fat is thinned out and a relatively free area lateral to the urachus can be identified.

Anatomic Points

Key dermatomes of the anterior abdominal wall include T5 and T6 (xiphoid), T9 and T10 (umbilicus), and L1 (pubis). Each dermatome receives supplemental innervation from the contiguous spinal nerves, both superiorly and inferiorly. Thus, an incision that results in a zone of denervated skin must section branches from at least two consecutive spinal nerves.

If a true midline incision is made, only minor nerves and arteries will be encountered. No named arteries or nerves occupy the midline because they enter the anterior abdominal wall laterally (in the case of spinal nerves and the intersegmental arteries) or are lateral to the midline (as is true of the superior and inferior epigastric arteries). Superficial veins are minimal, although one should expect a greater number as the umbilicus is approached. As usual, these vessels can be ligated or cauterized with impunity.

Deep to the linea alba and attached to the anterior body wall are remnants of two embryologically important structures. Superior to the umbilicus, the *ligamentum teres hepatis,* or round ligament of the liver, which is the obliterated left umbilical vein, passes in the free edge of the falciform ligament from the umbilicus to the fissure separating the left and right hepatic lobes. Because this fissure lies to the right of midline, the round

ligament deviates to the right. The falciform ligament is attached along its base to the midline, but it lies to the right. Thus, its left surface is in contact with the left lobe of the liver and its right side is in contact with the abdominal wall. Inferior to the umbilicus, the median umbilical ligament—the obliterated *urachus*—passes from the umbilicus to the vertex of the bladder. The urachus is a narrow canal, originating from the vesicourethral portion of the hindgut, which connects developing urinary bladder to allantois. Distally, the urachus is continuous, through the umbilical cord, with the entirely extraembryonic allantois.

Finally, one should be aware of abdominopelvic organs just deep to the linea alba from xiphoid to pubis. Most superiorly, and for a variable distance inferiorly, is the left lobe of the liver. Immediately inferior to the liver is the antrum of the stomach, to which is attached the thin gastrocolic ligament, through which the transverse colon is usually visible. From the inferior edge of the transverse colon (roughly midway between xiphoid and umbilicus, but quite variable in location), the greater omentum, which varies in both thickness and length, lies between the parietal peritoneum anteriorly and loops of small bowel, which should extend inferiorly to, or almost to, the pelvic brim. As the pelvic brim is approached, the extraperitoneal urinary bladder will be encountered. When the bladder is empty, its vertex typically is still superior to the pubis; thus, it may be encountered even if the urinary bladder is adequately drained.

Opening the Abdomen in the Case of Previous Abdominal Surgery (Fig. 44.3)

Technical and Anatomic Points

Adhesions are generally most prominent where there is foreign material (sutures, lint, talc) or at areas of injury or ischemia.

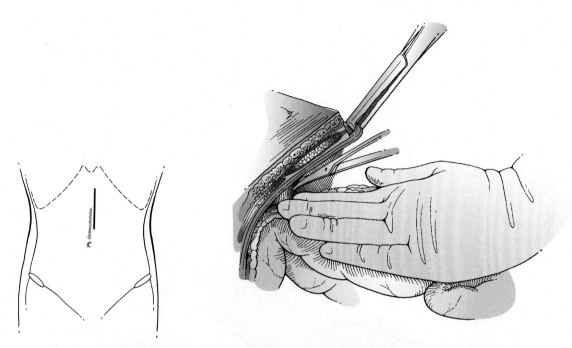

Figure 44.3 Opening the abdomen in the case of previous abdominal surgery

Generally, there will be adhesions from any old incision to the underlying viscera or omentum. If possible, enter the abdomen through a virgin area, above or below the old incision. If this is not possible, it is generally advisable to enter the upper pole of the incision where the underlying left lobe of the liver, rather than the colon or small bowel, is likely to be encountered first.

After you have made an opening into the peritoneal cavity, place Kocher clamps on the fascia and lift up. Use a laparotomy pad in your nondominant hand to pull down and provide countertraction. Lyse adhesions between loops of bowel or omentum and abdominal wall using Metzenbaum scissors or a knife. Do not cut fascia, dense fibrous adhesions, or old suture material with the Metzenbaum scissors; rather, reserve these scissors for cutting soft tissue to avoid dulling the blades. As you free up bowel and omentum from the underside of the incision, extend the peritoneal incision until more adhesions are encountered.

When you have opened the entire incision, place Kocher clamps on the fascia of one side and have your assistant pull up on the fascia. Apply downward countertraction with a laparotomy pad on bowel and omentum adherent to the underside of the abdominal wall. Sharply lyse adhesions; if necessary, take a small amount of peritoneum with a loop of bowel to avoid inadvertent injury. Generally, the adhesions will become less dense as you progress laterally away from the incision, and it may be possible to pass the fingers of the left hand behind adherent bowel to define the anatomy more clearly and to provide exposure. Adhesions are usually relatively avascular (in the absence of portal hypertension); bleeding from the serosal surface of the bowel can often be stopped with pressure from a laparotomy pad and bleeding from the abdominal wall can be controlled with electrocautery.

Alternatives to the Vertical Midline Incision (Fig. 44.4)

Technical Points

Alternative incisions are discussed in detail with the operations for which they are most commonly used. The following is simply a list of commonly used incisions, along with the advantages and disadvantages of each. All share the potential advantage of creating an incision directly over the pathology to be dealt with and the potential disadvantage of accordingly limiting exposure of other areas.

Kocher Incision

The Kocher incision is an oblique right upper quadrant incision made about 4 cm below and parallel to the costal margin. It provides excellent exposure for surgery of the liver and biliary tract (see Chapter 72), and it can be extended partially or completely across the midline, as a chevron, and used for surgery of the pancreas (Fig. 44.4A).

Disadvantages of this incision include pain (because muscles are cut) and the potential for inducing muscular weakness of the abdominal wall if several segmental nerves are cut in a long Kocher incision.

A left-sided Kocher-type incision provides excellent exposure for elective splenectomy of the small or only moderately enlarged spleen (see Chapter 70).

McBurney and Rocky-Davis Incisions

These two closely related incisions are the standard incisions used for appendectomy (see Chapter 94). Extended, they afford adequate exposure for pelvic surgery and right colon resection, should this be required. These incisions heal very well, with

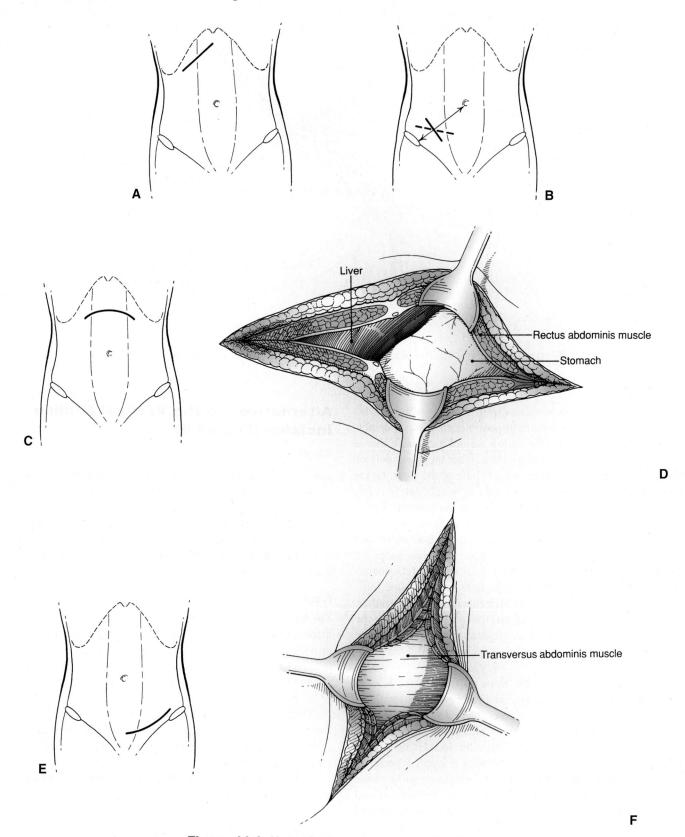

Figure 44.4 Alternatives to the vertical midline incision

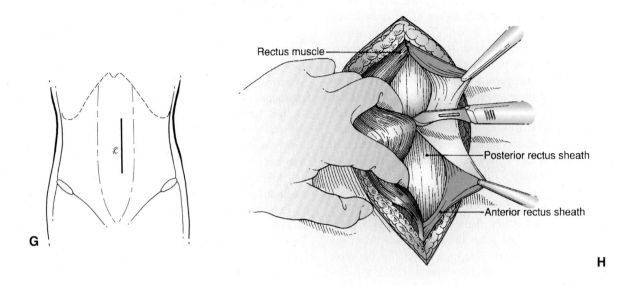

Figure 44.4 *Continued*

minimal chance of hernia formation because each muscular or aponeurotic layer of the abdominal wall is split in the direction of its fibers; hence, muscle contraction tends to close further, rather than to pull apart, the incision. The only disadvantage is the limited exposure, particularly of the upper abdomen. Use these incisions only when the pathology is known to be localized to the right lower quadrant (Fig. 44.4B).

Transverse Incisions

Transverse incisions afford excellent exposure for right colon resections (see Chapter 99). They are of limited use in other abdominal procedures in the adult but are commonly employed in infants. A transverse incision generally heals well because the pull of the abdominal wall muscles tends to close the incision (Fig. 44.4C,D). A potential disadvantage is the difficulty in siting ostomies, if required.

Lateral or Oblique Left Lower Quadrant Incisions

These incisions provide excellent exposure for left colon resections and may be preferred in obese patients or in instances in which surgery is performed with the patient in the lateral position (see Chapter 101). Exposure of the right upper quadrant is particularly poor; hence, these incisions are used only under very special circumstances (Fig. 44.4E,F).

Paramedian Incisions

Paramedian incisions are vertical incisions made parallel to the midline a few centimeters to the right or the left of the linea alba (Fig. 44.4G,H). The anterior rectus sheath is incised, and the rectus muscle is then retracted laterally to expose the posterior rectus sheath. The posterior sheath is then incised to enter the midline.

One of the advantages of a paramedian incision is that it is a vertical incision that is closed in two layers (rather than

one, as is the case with a midline incision), affording perhaps some extra strength. Also, there may be a slight advantage, in terms of exposure of structures to the left or right of the midline, gained by moving the incision from the midline to the paramedian position. The left paramedian incision may be used for left colon resections, for splenectomy, and for some gastric surgery. A high right paramedian incision may be used for biliary tract surgery in the patient with a narrow costal angle. Lower abdominal paramedian incisions heal poorly because the posterior rectus sheath is weak and, thus, are used relatively infrequently. A low right paramedian incision is used by some when the etiology of right lower quadrant pain is uncertain. The potential advantage of this approach is that the incision can be extended to gain exposure of the upper abdomen. Generally, this incision is not favored for appendectomy because it is associated with a high incidence of wound complications. In dubious cases, a vertical midline is preferred.

A major disadvantage of the paramedian incision is the increased time it takes to enter the abdomen. Closure is also slower than with other incisions because two layers must be sutured. Hence it is not an appropriate choice for emergency situations. Long paramedian incisions limit the options for access when a second abdominal operation is performed; if a midline incision is chosen for the subsequent operation, the strip of abdominal wall between the old paramedian and new midline incisions may have inadequate blood supply for proper healing.

Anatomic Points

Kocher Incision

The Kocher incision divides the rectus abdominis muscle at about a right angle to its fibers. Fibers of the lateral abdominal wall muscles are also cut. The superior epigastric artery, which is typically located on or in the deep aspect of the muscle and more medially than laterally, is divided. This incision almost always will cut the eighth thoracic nerve, which continues inferomedially to a position just inferior to the ninth costal cartilage. This is of little consequence; however, owing to overlapping of the segmental innervation. If the larger ninth thoracic nerve is also severed, then part of the rectus is denervated, and muscle weakness can be expected. As these nerves are encountered, it must also be noted that they are one component of a neurovascular bundle, and it may be necessary to use electrocautery or ligatures to control bleeding.

McBurney and Rocky-Davis Incisions

Classically, these incisions are made over McBurney's point (junction of the middle and outer thirds of a line from the umbilicus to the anterosuperior iliac spine), which is the most probable location of the appendix. Because these are muscle-splitting rather than muscle-dividing incisions, it is necessary to remember the direction of muscle fibers at this location. The external oblique fibers run inferomedially, the internal oblique fibers run superomedially (almost at right angles to the external oblique fibers), and the transversus abdominis muscle fibers are approximately transverse; these usually can be split as a unit with the internal oblique muscle fibers because the direction of their fibers at this point is quite similar. Keep in mind that neurovascular bundles occupy the plane between the internal oblique and transversus abdominis muscles.

Transverse Incisions

Transverse incisions are usually somewhat oblique, so that the skin incision approximates the direction of Langer's lines, affording excellent cosmetic results. When muscle layers are encountered, they can be split in the direction of their fibers rather than divided, thus achieving the same goals as the McBurney incision. In addition, transverse incisions approximate the course of the neurovascular bundles, thus destroying fewer nerves and blood vessels.

Lateral or Oblique Left Lower Quadrant Incisions

These incisions also involve splitting the rectus sheath inferior to the arcuate line (of Douglas), where there is no posterior rectus sheath. The inferior epigastric vessels enter the rectus sheath from an inferolateral direction at this line and must be ligated and divided.

Paramedian Incisions

These vertical incisions are made in the same direction as the fibers of the rectus abdominis muscle. The tendinous inscriptions of the rectus muscle are attached to the anterior rectus sheath but not to the posterior sheath. Care should be taken to retract all of the rectus muscle laterally, especially if the desired exposure is extensive, to prevent denervation to a median strip of the rectus muscle. Retraction of this muscle medially is not an accepted procedure because neurovascular bundles enter laterally and can be inadvertently disrupted.

Exploration of the Abdomen: Elective Laparotomy (Fig. 44.5)

Technical and Anatomic Points

Laparotomy provides the unique opportunity to observe and systematically palpate all of the intra-abdominal viscera. A thorough, systematic exploration is the first step in laparotomy. Do not "zero in" on known pathology before carefully checking the entire abdomen for unexpected findings. Similarly, resist the urge to place fixed retractors until thorough exploration has been performed.

Begin in the left upper quadrant. Place a Richardson retractor on the left upper abdominal wall and have an assistant retract it. Pass your dominant hand up under the left hemidiaphragm and feel the spleen, assessing it for size, mobility, and the presence of nodules. Note that the spleen is generally anchored to the diaphragm superiorly, the retroperitoneum posteriorly, and the stomach and colon medially and inferiorly. The spleen is a pulpy, blood-filled organ with a capsule of little tensile strength. It is easily damaged by vigorous retraction or palpation.

Next, pass the dominant hand under the left lobe of the liver, anterior to the stomach, and run the hand up toward the esophageal hiatus. Strong pulsations in the abdominal aorta (which should be assessed for size) assist in orientation. The esophagus lies anterior and slightly to the left of the aorta. An indwelling nasogastric tube, placed for most laparotomies, should be readily palpable and helps in the identification of the esophagus. The esophageal hiatus through which the esophagus passes should accept, at most, one finger. It may be dilated if the patient has a hiatal hernia; if so, make note of its approximate size by determining how many fingers it will admit easily. Next, feel the esophagogastric junction and stomach for masses, passing your hand down to the pylorus. Note any thickening or scarring that may be indicative of ulcer disease.

Feel the left lobe of the liver between the fingers of your dominant hand, assessing it for consistency and the presence of nodules or masses. Do not neglect to feel the underside of the diaphragm, a common site of metastases in patients with ovarian carcinoma.

Progress in a counterclockwise fashion to the right lobe of the liver. Place the retractor on the right upper abdominal wall and pass your dominant hand under the right hemidiaphragm as far as it will go. Normally, this potential space is clear, but sometimes adhesions from previous peritonitis limit access to this region; alternatively, a subphrenic abscess, by producing adhesions anteriorly between the right lobe of the liver and the diaphragm, may prevent palpation. The gallbladder should be felt and the presence or absence of stones noted. Passing a finger into the epiploic foramen (of Winslow) allows limited palpation of the common bile duct and hepatic artery. The head of the pancreas should also be felt for masses. (For systematic exploration of the entire pancreas, follow the procedure described in Chapter 84.) Next, feel the right kidney, noting its size and degree of mobility.

Progress down into the right lower quadrant and feel the terminal ileum, appendix, and cecum. Palpate the right colon up to

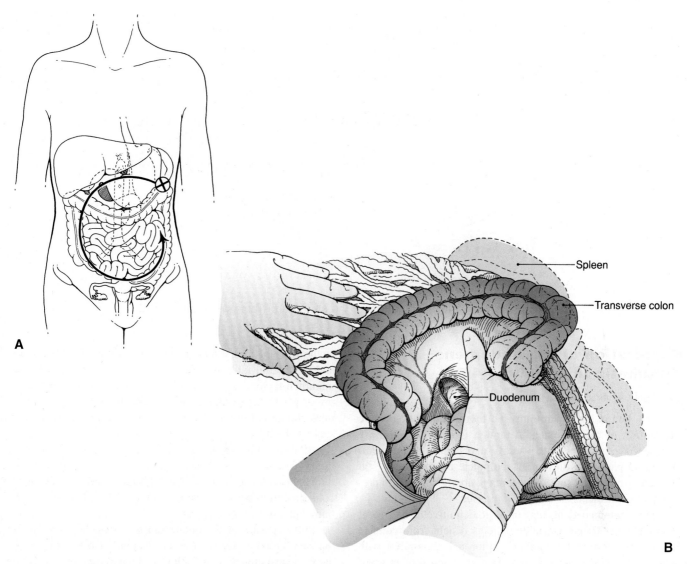

Figure 44.5 Exploration of the abdomen: Elective laparotomy. **A:** Schematic showing one method of systematic exploration of the entire abdomen. **B:** Evisceration of transverse colon and omentum to allow palpation of splenic flexure of colon, descending colon, and left retroperitoneum.

the hepatic flexure. Lift the greater omentum out of the abdomen. Feel the omentum, assessing it for metastatic deposits or cysts. Note that the transverse colon runs on the undersurface of the greater omentum and hence must be approached from this surface. Assess the hepatic flexure both by feeling up the ascending colon and by coming across from the midtransverse colon along the underside of the omentum. Lesions in the hepatic and splenic flexures are easy to miss because the flexures pass higher and more laterally (becoming almost retroperitoneal) than one might expect. Follow the transverse colon over to the left side of the abdomen and assess the splenic flexure, then palpate the descending and sigmoid colon. Feel the left kidney for size and mobility.

Follow the sigmoid colon into the pelvis and palpate the upper rectum. Assess the bladder and confirm the position of the balloon of the Foley catheter. In the female patient, assess the uterus, ovaries, and fallopian tubes. Feel for nodular metastatic deposits on the pelvic peritoneum.

Next, identify the duodenum at the ligament of Treitz. Then "run" the small bowel, with the aid of your first assistant, in the following manner: Grasp a 10- to 15-cm length of small intestine in two hands and inspect it first on one side and then on the other. Then pass this section of bowel to your assistant, who then holds the loop as you grasp the next section. In this manner, your assistant helps you keep track of your progress, thereby avoiding missing segments or losing your point of reference as you pass distally. Check the entire small intestine to the ileocecal valve. Replace the omentum and small and large intestines into the abdomen in an orderly fashion.

Finally, feel the abdominal aorta and left and right common, internal, and external iliac arteries, assessing each for strength of pulsations, atherosclerotic plaque, and aneurysmal dilatation. Retroperitoneal lymphadenopathy (enlargement of para-aortic or iliac nodes) should be noted, if present.

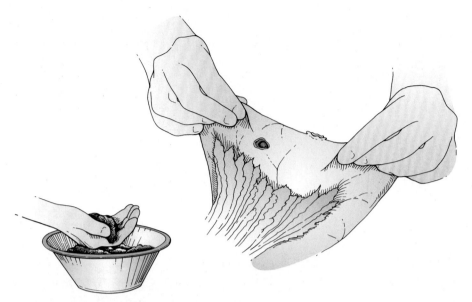

Figure 44.6 Exploration of the abdomen: Traumatic injury

Exploration of the Abdomen: Traumatic Injury (Fig. 44.6)

Technical and Anatomic Points

The first step in any laparotomy is a thorough and systematic exploration of the abdomen. Although it may be necessary to proceed expeditiously to identify and control active hemorrhage in patients with injuries, complete exploration is still mandatory before closure. A systematic approach helps to prevent the disastrous error of missed injuries.

Stable trauma patients may undergo definitive management of any injuries found. Unstable patients benefit from damage control laparotomy. This combines a thorough exploration with maneuvers designed to provide temporary control of injuries. Because it can be accomplished rapidly, it allows the surgeon to minimize time in the operating room and perform a planned return for more definitive management a day or two later when the patient is warm, resuscitated, and in optimum condition. Sometimes several sequential operations are required. This is discussed at the end of this section and in the references at the end.

First, note the character and distribution of blood or peritoneal fluid. Remove large quantities of blood, peritoneal fluid, or debris by suction or by scooping clots and semisolid material out into a basin. Identify and rapidly control any active bleeding or holes in hollow viscera to decrease contamination. Culture the peritoneal fluid if contamination by enteric contents has occurred. Then, irrigate the abdomen copiously and explore in a systematic fashion (Fig. 44.5), keeping in mind the additional considerations listed below.

Laparotomy in cases of trauma is performed with knowledge of the mechanism of injury. The probable course of the missile is known or suspected in cases of penetrating trauma. Be aware; however, that this is of limited predictive value. The relative positions of victim and assailant, the phase of respiration at the time of injury (and hence, the height of diaphragms), and the overall mobility of the intra-abdominal viscera are all unknown factors. Search for clues, such as blood or bile staining or gas in the retroperitoneum, and investigate not only the intra-abdominal organs but also the retroperitoneal structures, such as the duodenum.

Mobilize viscera as needed to expose possible sites of injury. The anterior surface of the stomach is immediately visible; expose the posterior surface by widely opening the gastrocolic omentum between clamps and ties. This also exposes the body and tail of the pancreas.

Full exposure of the duodenum is obtained by mobilizing the right colon as for right hemicolectomy. Do this by cutting along the avascular line of Toldt just lateral to the colon. This line is the result of fusion of the embryologic visceral peritoneum of the antimesenteric and right surface of the colon with the parietal peritoneum. By recreating the embryonic condition, few, if any, significant vessels will be encountered. Sweep the colon and small bowel mesentery to the midline and superiorly (toward the patient's left shoulder) to expose the entire duodenum. If colonic injury is a possibility, mobilize the involved segment of colon as for colon resection, so that all sides can be checked.

Approach retroperitoneal hematomas with respect. Contained hematomas secondary to pelvic fractures should be left alone. Obtain vascular control of the renal artery and vein before opening perinephric hematomas. Localized hematomas may be the only clue to retroperitoneal duodenal, pancreatic, or colonic injuries.

Always search for both entry and exit sites of the penetrating instrument in injuries to viscera. Be highly suspicious whenever you find an odd number of holes because you may have inadvertently missed one.

Damage control laparotomy uses packing to control liver injuries, resects damaged bowel but does not reanastomose segments, and may use a skin stapler to close small holes in the gut. At the conclusion, the abdomen is packed open to facilitate repeat access (see Fig. 44.8 below). A plan is made for return to surgery, usually 24 hours or so later.

Closure of Laparotomy (Fig. 44.7)

Technical and Anatomic Points

Check carefully for hemostasis and make sure that no foreign bodies (e.g., laparotomy pads, clamps) have been left behind. Pull the greater omentum down and interpose it between the viscera and the incision if possible.

Place Kocher clamps on the fascia. Often the incision can be closed with a running suture. An alternative that may be preferred for selected cases is the Smead-Jones closure shown here. This closure places bites in a staggered fashion and incorporates a sort of "internal retention" suture that may help resist fascial dehiscence. This closure can also be placed in a running fashion.

The ideal suture material would hold an incision together until it is fully healed, and then completely dissolve. Currently, monofilament absorbable materials such as PDS best fulfill these criteria. Choose a sufficiently heavy gauge—usually no. 1 or no. 0—to provide adequate strength.

To perform a classic Smead-Jones closure, imagine each suture as an asymmetric figure-of-eight which incorporates both "far bites" (which act as buried retention sutures) and "near bites" (which provide accurate fascial apposition). Blunt-tipped needles pierce the fascia effectively and minimize chance of injury during closure. Alternatively, use a "fish" (a flexible plastic visceral retractor) or one end of a malleable retractor to displace the viscera rather than using your hands.

As your assistant retracts skin and subcutaneous fat to expose as much fascia as possible, take your first far bite from out to in; this bite should pass at least 2 cm back from the cut edge of the fascia. Then cross over and place a second far bite, from in to out, on the opposite side. Progress about 1 cm down the incision and place a near bite from out to in (about 1 cm back from the edge). Complete the stitch by passing another near bite from in to out on the opposite side.

As noted, there are many other ways to close the abdomen, and a paucity of actual data as to which technique is best. A running suture suffices for many closures, provided the bites are taken at appropriate distance from the fascial edge and placed at appropriate intervals. Many surgeons favor a double-looped synthetic monofilament absorbable suture for this purpose.

A limited number of absorbable sutures may be placed in the subcutaneous tissues to obliterate dead space. Only do this to prevent a large cavity. The presence of foreign material (e.g., sutures) significantly reduces the inoculum of bacteria needed to cause infection.

Temporary Abdominal Wall Closure (Fig. 44.8)

Damage control principles are widely applied in trauma and increasingly considered in other emergency situations where repeated access may be required or where primary closure results in unacceptable rise in intra-abdominal pressure.

A variety of systems have been devised. The vacuum closure system described here allows maximum decompression, controls secretions (facilitating nursing and tracking output), is quick, allows repeated imaging studies, and can be changed at the bedside in SICU. This section describes how to construct a device from readily-available components. Commercial prepackaged vacuum dressing systems are also available and widely used.

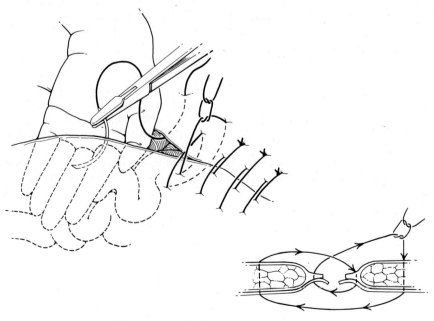

Figure 44.7 Closure of laparotomy

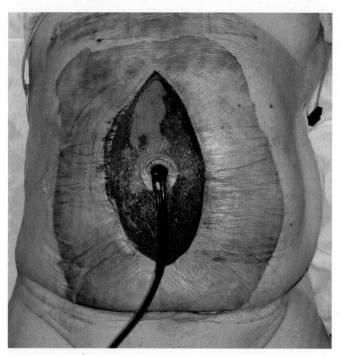

Figure 44.8 Temporary abdominal wall closure with commercial vacuum sponge device. Photograph courtesy of Evgeny V. Arshava, MD.

First, take care to arrange the viscera so that any anastomoses are protected with omentum and placed away from the midline. If injuries have been packed, take careful note of the location and number of packs. Next, bring omentum (if possible) over the viscera.

Cut holes in a large plastic drape (sometimes called a "10-10" drape) and place this over the omentum and under the abdominal wall. Place a green surgical towel over this. Place two large diameter closed suctions catheters, one on each side, in the natural gutters that form between the fascial edge and the towel. Cover the entire thing with an adhesive surgical drape, taking care to avoid wrinkles so that the entire thing is watertight. This watertight closure helps assure that secretions are efficiently collected by the suction catheters, making it easier to keep the patient dry and comfortable, and allowing accurate measurement of wound drainage output.

If definitive closure can then be achieved within a couple of days, primary closure as described above is often possible. When closure has been delayed, fascial edges generally retract and a more complex closure (such as separation of parts, or temporary closure with mesh) may be needed. See Chapter 47 for discussion of these techniques.

REFERENCES

1. A-Malik R, Scott NA. Double near and far Prolene suture closure: A technique for abdominal wall closure after laparostomy. *Br J Surg.* 2001;88:146–147.
2. Ballinger WF. Unexpected findings at laparotomy. *Probl Gen Surg.* 1984;1:1. (The entire issue is devoted to the unforeseen and how to deal with it.)
3. Bjorck M, D'Amours SK, Hamilton AE. Closure of the open abdomen. *Am Surg.* 2011;77(suppl 1):S58–S61.
4. Cattell RB, Braasch JW. The surgeon at work: Technique for the exposure of the third and fourth portions of the duodenum. *Surg Gynecol Obstet.* 1960;111:378–379. (Discusses wide exposure of the right retroperitoneum and entire duodenum.)
5. Cohn SM, Giannotti G, Ong AW, et al. Prospective randomized trial of two wound management strategies for dirty abdominal wounds. *Ann Surg.* 2001;233:409–413. (Reaffirms value of delayed primary closure for dirty wounds.)
6. Cothren CC, Moore EE, Johnson JL, et al. One hundred percent fascial approximation with sequential abdominal closure of the open abdomen. *Am J Surg.* 2006;192:238–242.
7. Fantus RJ, Mellett MM, Kirby JP. Use of controlled fascial tension and an adhesion preventing barrier to achieve delayed primary fascial closure in patients managed with an open abdomen. *Am J Surg.* 2006;192:243–247.
8. Franchi M, Ghezzi F, Benedetti-Panici PL, et al. A multicentre collaborative study on the use of cold scalpel and electrocautery for midline abdominal incision. *Am J Surg.* 2001;181:128–132. (Reports that the incidence of complications is similar.)
9. Miller PR, Meredith JW, Johnson JC, et al. Prospective evaluation of vacuum-assisted fascial closure after open abdomen: Planned ventral hernia rate is substantially reduced. *Ann Surg.* 2004;239:608–614.
10. Miller PR, Thompson JT, Faler BJ, et al. Late fascial closure in lieu of ventral hernia: The next step in open abdomen management. *J Trauma.* 2002;53:843–849.
11. Parantainen A, Verbeek JH, Lavoie MC, et al. Blunt versus sharp suture needles for preventing percutaneous exposure incidents in surgical staff. *Cochrane Database Syst Rev.* 2011;9:CD009170. (Confirms decreased injuries with blunt needles.)
12. Roberts DJ, Zygun DA, Grendar J, et al. Negative-pressure wound therapy for critically ill adults with open abdominal wounds: A systematic review. *J Trauma Acute Care Surg.* 2012;73:629–639.
13. Seiler CM, Bruckner T, Diener MK, et al. Interrupted or continuous slowly absorbable sutures for closure of primary elective midline abdominal incisions: A multicenter randomized trial (INSECT: ISRCTN24023541). *Ann Surg.* 2009;249:576–582.
14. Shapiro MB, Jenkins DH, Schwab CW, et al. Damage control: Collective review. *J Trauma.* 2000;49:969–978.
15. Soteriou MC, Williams LF Jr. Unexpected findings in gastrointestinal tract surgery. *Surg Clin North Am.* 1991;71:1283–1306.

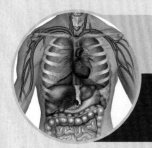

45

Open Drainage of Abdominal Abscesses

Most intra-abdominal abscesses are now managed by image-guided percutaneous drainage and antibiotics. Open drainage is used when percutaneous drainage fails or is not available, or when abscesses are encountered during open surgery. Access for open drainage may be obtained transperitoneally or extraperitoneally.

Extraperitoneal drainage is primarily used to drain an isolated abscess, such as an isolated subphrenic abscess. The major advantage is that the peritoneal cavity is not violated; this is, in fact, also the drawback of this approach. The abdomen cannot be explored and any underlying cause of the abscess cannot be addressed. Most abscesses that would have been amenable to extraperitoneal drainage are now managed percutaneously.

Transperitoneal drainage is used when there are multiple abscesses or an underlying problem (such as a perforation or anastomotic leak) must be addressed surgically.

This chapter demonstrates the recesses of the peritoneal cavity, a concept introduced in Chapter 42, and describes transperitoneal and extraperitoneal approaches to several common types of abscess. References at the end discuss management of less common kinds of abscesses, and Chapter 87 discusses drainage of infected pancreatic sequestrums.

SCORE™, the Surgical Council on Resident Education, classified open drainage of abdominal abscess as an "ESSENTIAL UNCOMMON" operation.

STEPS IN PROCEDURE

Intraperitoneal drainage of subphrenic abscess
Explore the abdomen
Place retractors to expose the right upper quadrant
Explore the line of adhesion between free edge of liver and diaphragm
Gently mobilize the liver down from the diaphragm
Take care to avoid entering the capsule of the liver
Have suction ready to deal with pus
Enter and explore the subphrenic space
Culture purulence
Break down loculations
Irrigate and place drains

Extraperitoneal Drainage—Anterior Approach
Incision 2 cm below and parallel to costal margin

Enter extraperitoneal space
Gently mobilize peritoneum downwards
Aspirate through peritoneum to identify abscess
Enter abscess and proceed as above

Extraperitoneal Drainage—Posterior Approach
Lateral position
Incision over twelfth rib
Elevate periosteum from rib and resect it
Push pleural reflection cephalad
Develop the extraperitoneal space
Aspirate to identify the abscess, and proceed as above

HALLMARK ANATOMIC COMPLICATIONS

Injury to liver
Missed second abscess
Injury to intercostal nerves

Inadvertent entry into pleural space (posterior approach)

LIST OF STRUCTURES

Liver
Diaphragm
Peritoneum

Twelfth rib
Eleventh and twelfth intercostal nerves

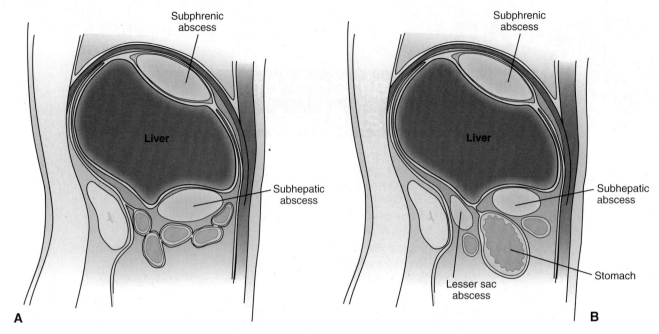

Figure 45.1 A: Potential spaces for abscess formation in the upper abdomen on the right include the very large right subphrenic and right subhepatic spaces. **B:** Potential spaces on the left include a left subphrenic, left subhepatic space (anterior to the stomach), and lesser sac (posterior to the stomach).

In the upper abdomen, there is a space between the underside of the diaphragm and the diaphragmatic surface of the liver, termed the right and left subphrenic spaces. Suction during inspiration draws fluid from anywhere in the abdomen into this space, where it is normally cleared by diaphragmatic lymphatics. This suction effect explains how abscesses can form in these spaces after infectious processes in the lower abdomen. The right side has the large right subphrenic space (Fig. 45.1A) and a subhepatic space. On the left, there is a smaller left subphrenic space and a subhepatic space. There is also a space in the lesser sac (Fig. 45.1B). In the mid abdomen, abscesses may form along the lateral gutters or between loops of bowel (termed interloop abscesses). In the pelvis, abscesses form in the deep recesses between the rectum and bladder (in the male) and the rectum and uterus (in the female).

Intraperitoneal Drainage of Right Subphrenic Abscess (Fig. 45.2)

Technical and Anatomic Points

The normally free edge of the right lobe of the liver adheres to the undersurface of the diaphragm to form the anterior boundary of the space containing purulent material. After thoroughly exploring the abdomen and excluding other pathology, gently explore the line of adhesion and begin to peel back the edge of the liver. It is best to avoid the region of the gallbladder, to avoid injuring it. Generally it is best to begin lateral to the gallbladder.

Have an assistant ready with suction as purulent material may gush out at any point. As you peel back the liver, ensure that you do not get into the capsule of the liver. Persistent careful dissection will eventually produce an opening into the subphrenic abscess cavity. Aspirate and culture the pus. Pass a finger of your nondominant hand into the hole and sweep it laterally and medially to complete mobilization of the liver and create a sufficiently wide opening. It is not necessary to completely mobilize the liver; but it is important to be certain that all loculations are opened up and the cavity thoroughly irrigated out. Place closed suction drains in the cavity.

Extraperitoneal Drainage of Right (or Left) Subphrenic Abscess—Anterior Approach (Fig. 45.3)

Technical and Anatomic Points

Make an incision 2 cm below and parallel to the costal margin, beginning just medial to the tip of the eleventh rib and extending medially for about 10 to 15 cm and deepen this through the muscular and fascial layers to the preperitoneal space. Gently develop the preperitoneal space by pushing the peritoneum down away from the diaphragm until the peritoneum and underlying liver are pushed down. The region of the abscess will generally be firmer and more indurated. Once adequate exposure has been achieved, confirm the location of the pus by aspirating through the peritoneum with a large gauge needle, then fenestrate the peritoneum to gain access to the cavity.

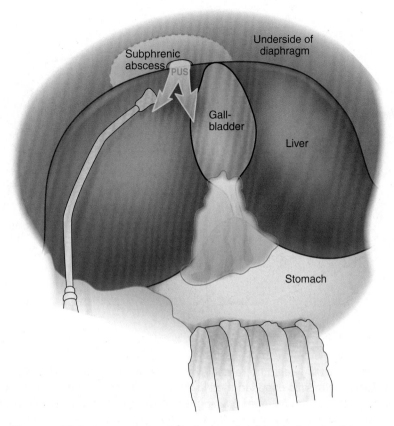

Figure 45.2 Intraperitoneal drainage of right subphrenic abscess

Explore the cavity for loculations, irrigate, and place drains. Partially or fully close the incision.

Extraperitoneal Drainage of Right (or Left) Subphrenic Abscess—Posterior Approach (Fig. 45.4)

This approach allows true dependent drainage and hence is desirable when closed suction drainage fails and larger drains must be placed. Access through this route can also be used to drain perinephric abscesses and some intrahepatic abscesses. It is a difficult approach to the right subphrenic space because, as shown in Figure 45.1, that space is actually quite anterior; but it may be the easier way to approach the left subphrenic space.

Technical and Anatomic Points

Place the patient in the lateral position with the affected side up. Make an incision over the twelfth rib and dissect down to the rib (Fig. 45.4A). Elevate the periosteum medially and laterally. Divide and resect a long segment of the rib. The pleural reflection will be encountered in the cephalad aspect of your field (Fig. 45.4B). Gently push it upward out of harm's way. Develop the plane between the retroperitoneal structures and the muscular abdominal wall.

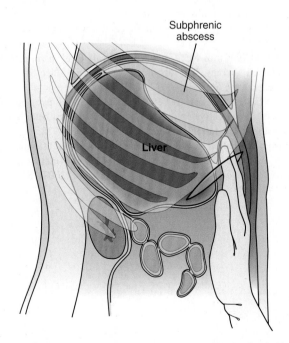

Figure 45.3 Extraperitoneal drainage of right (or left) subphrenic abscess—anterior approach

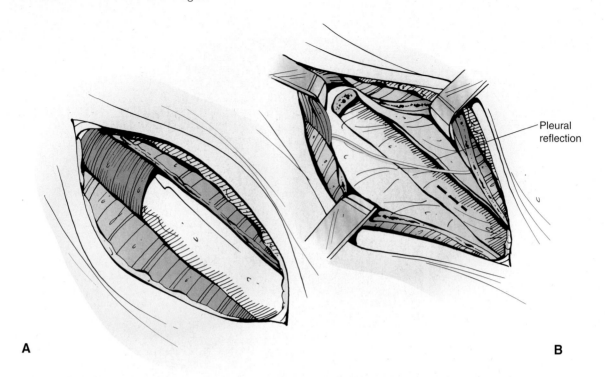

Pleural
reflection

A

B

Figure 45.4 Resection of twelfth rib to achieve posterior extraperitoneal drainage of abscesses. **A:** The incision has exposed the twelfth rib. **B:** Entry into the extraperitoneal space is made through the bed of the rib, after pushing the pleura gently cephalad. It may be necessary to divide an intercostal nerve, shown crossing over the field (from Alexander JW. Chapter 107. Drainage of hepatic, subphrenic, and subhepatic abscesses. In: *Fischer's Mastery of Surgery*. Philadelphia, PA: Wolters Kluwer Lippincott Williams & Wilkins; 2011).

Similarly, move cephalad to drain a subphrenic abscess. Identify the abscess by aspiration. Enter and drain the cavity as previously described. Generally the incision is left open.

REFERENCES

1. Alexander JW. Chapter 107. Drainage of hepatic, subphrenic, and subhepatic abscesses. In: *Fischer's Mastery of Surgery*. Philadelphia, PA: Wolters Kluwer Lippincott Williams & Wilkins; 2011:1182.
2. Bosscha K, Roukema AJ, van Vroonhoven TJ, et al. Twelfth rib resection: A direct posterior surgical approach for subphrenic abscesses. *Eur J Surg.* 2000;166:119–122.
3. Boyd DP. The subphrenic spaces and the emperor's new robes. *N Engl J Med.* 1966;275:911–917. (Classic description of the left and right subphrenic spaces.)
4. Scott-Conner CEH (ed), Chapter 108. Operations for infected abdominal wound dehiscence, necrotizing fasciitis, and intra-abdominal abscesses. In: Scott-Conner (ed), *Chassin's Operative Strategy in General Surgery.* 4th ed. Springer Verlag; (inpress)
5. Spain DA, Martin RC, Carrillo EH, et al. Twelfth rib resection. Preferred therapy for subphrenic abscess in selected surgical patients. *Arch Surg.* 1997;132:1203–1206.
6. Yu SC, Ho SS, Lau WY, et al. Treatment of pyogenic liver abscess: Prospective randomized comparison of catheter drainage and needle aspiration. *Hepatology.* 2004;39:932–938.
7. Zerem E, Hadzic A. Sonographically guided percutaneous catheter drainage versus needle aspiration in the management of pyogenic liver abscess. *AJR Am J Roentgenol.* 2007;189:W138–W142.

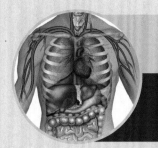

46

Laparoscopy: Principles of Access and Exposure

Laparoscopic surgery requires intense attention to the details of the equipment used. Become familiar with the equipment used in your operating room. Ensure that it is in working order and that the supplies that you will need for the procedure are at hand or readily available. An equipment troubleshooting chart, such as that produced by Society of American Gastrointestinal Endoscopic Surgeons (SAGES) (referenced at the end), can be invaluable when problems arise.

SCORE™, the Surgical Council on Resident Education, classified diagnostic laparoscopy as an "ESSENTIAL COMMON" procedure.

STEPS IN PROCEDURE

Position patient and monitor
Surgeon should stand opposite site of pathology (operative field)
Primary monitor is placed directly across from surgeon
Choose entry site
Closed entry
Make a small incision at entry site
Lift fascia
Pop Veress needle into peritoneal space (usually two pops are felt)
Aspirate and confirm absence of blood or succus

Saline should flow freely
Drop of saline in hub of needle should be sucked into peritoneum
Insufflate to desired pressure
Open entry with Hasson cannula
Make minilaparotomy incision and enter peritoneum
Place sutures on each side of peritoneal/fascia incision
Insert trocar and laparoscope
Inspect abdomen

HALLMARK ANATOMIC COMPLICATIONS

Injury to bowel during initial entry
Injury to retroperitoneal vessels during entry

Poor choice of trocar sites, room setup, causing difficulty with subsequent procedure

LIST OF STRUCTURES

Linea alba
Rectus abdominis muscle
Umbilicus

Median umbilical fold (urachus)
Falciform ligament
Inferior epigastric artery and vein

Patient positioning and layout of equipment can facilitate a laparoscopic procedure or immensely complicate it. Locate the primary monitor directly opposite the surgeon in a straight line of sight. Figure 46.1A shows the typical setup for surgery in the right upper quadrant (laparoscopic cholecystectomy, plication of perforated ulcer, liver biopsy or similar procedures). A secondary monitor may be located across from the first assistant, who will generally stand on the opposite side of the table. Arrange the insufflator, light source, cautery and other energy sources, suction irrigator, and so on, and the associated cords in such a fashion that you are free to move from one side of the table to the other if necessary.

For lower abdominal procedures, such as laparoscopic appendectomy (Chapter 95), it is best to tuck the arms at the side. This allows the surgeon and first assistant to move as far cephalad as needed without being cramped by the arm boards (Fig. 46.1B). Gynecologic laparoscopists will generally place the patient in stirrups to allow manipulations from below, for example, elevating the cervix to enhance visualization of the pelvic organs (see Figure 104.2A in Chapter 104).

Advanced laparoscopic procedures performed around the esophageal hiatus, such as laparoscopic fundoplication (Chapter 53) or esophagomyotomy (Chapter 55) are also best performed with the patient's legs spread to enable the surgeon to stand between the legs (Fig. 46.1C). This provides the straightest possible line of sight to the operative field and enables two assistants to stand comfortably, one on each side. Further information is given in the chapters for specific procedures.

ORIENTATION

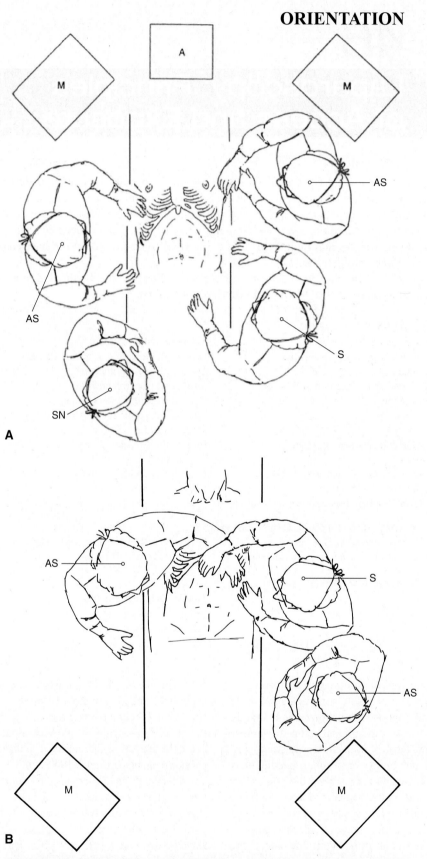

Figure 46.1 A: Setup for laparoscopic surgery in the right upper quadrant. **B:** Setup for laparoscopic surgery in the right lower quadrant. Note how "tucking" both arms allows surgeon and assistant to move cephalad without hindrance. **C:** Setup for surgery in region of esophageal hiatus.

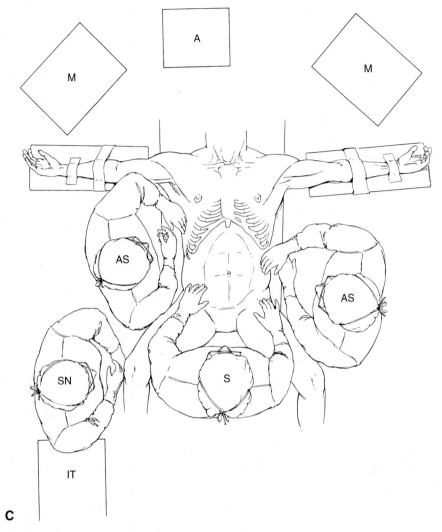

Figure 46.1 *Continued*

References at the end give additional information about equipment setup and troubleshooting.

Access to the Abdomen—Closed, with Veress Needle (Fig. 46.2)

Technical Points

The umbilicus is the usual site of initial entry. An infraumbilical "smile" or supraumbilical "frown" incision made in a natural skin crease is virtually invisible when healed (Fig. 46.2A). If conversion to open laparotomy is a strong possibility, a vertically oriented circumumbilical incision gives equally good access and is easily incorporated into a vertical midline incision.

Visualize the probable site of the pathology within the abdomen and consider the location of the umbilicus relative to this site. The level of the umbilicus varies considerably from individual to individual—do not hesitate to make the entry site slightly above or below the umbilicus, if necessary. If the umbilicus is low on the abdomen and the target site is in the upper abdomen, an incision above the umbilicus may be necessary. Conversely, an incision below the umbilicus may provide the best visualization for laparoscopic cholecystectomy in a small patient. If all other things are equal, it is a bit easier to enter the abdomen through a smile incision because this avoids the falciform ligament. Make the incision a millimeter or two longer than the diameter of the trocar you plan to use. Deepen the incision through skin and subcutaneous tissue until the fascia at the base of the umbilicus is encountered. If the patient is obese, place a Kocher clamp on the underside of the umbilicus and pull up. Because skin is adherent to fascia at the umbilicus, this will elevate the fascia. Place Kocher clamps side by side on the fascia. Hold one in your nondominant hand and have your first assistant hold the other.

Test the Veress needle and confirm that the tip retracts easily (Fig. 46.2B). Introduce the Veress needle with steady controlled pressure, attentive to the popping sensations as it passes through the fascia and then the peritoneum (Fig. 46.2C). When the Veress needle is properly positioned, the tip should move freely from side to side as the hub is gently moved back and forth.

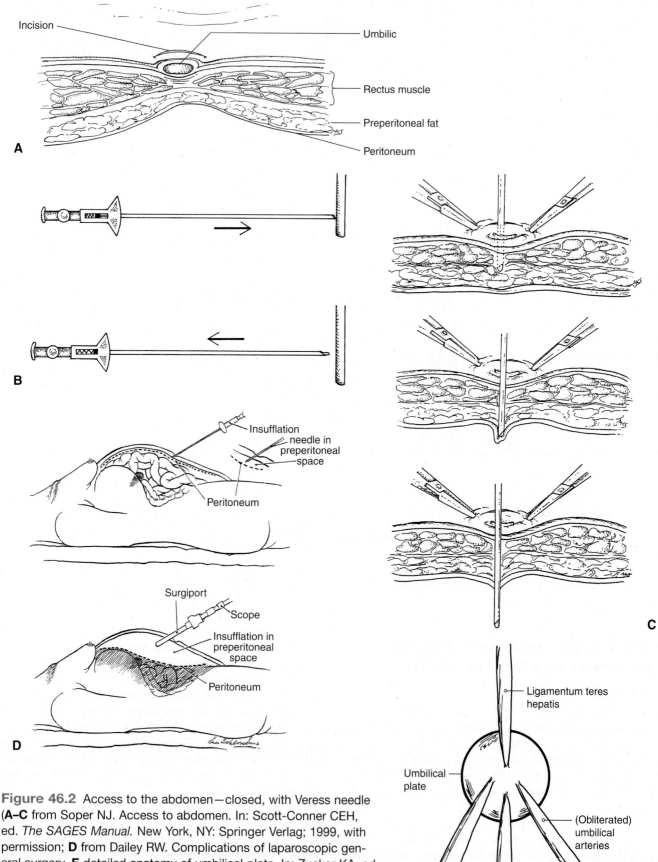

Figure 46.2 Access to the abdomen—closed, with Veress needle (**A–C** from Soper NJ. Access to abdomen. In: Scott-Conner CEH, ed. *The SAGES Manual.* New York, NY: Springer Verlag; 1999, with permission; **D** from Dailey RW. Complications of laparoscopic general surgery. **E** detailed anatomy of umbilical plate. In: Zucker KA, ed. *Surgical Laparoscopy.* 1st ed. St. Louis: Quality Medical Publishing; 1991:311–346, with permission).

Attach a syringe filled with saline. Aspirate, observing for gas, blood, or succus entericus. If the needle is properly positioned, a vacuum will be created. Inject saline; there should be no resistance to injection. Leave a meniscus of saline within the hub of the needle when you remove the syringe. Elevate both Kocher clamps while observing the meniscus. The saline should be drawn into the abdomen by the negative pressure thus created, confirming proper intraperitoneal positioning of the needle. Insufflate the abdomen. It is extremely important to take the time to ascertain proper placement to avoid visceral injury. On the other hand, if the Veress needle is not deep enough, the preperitoneal space can absorb an amazing amount of CO_2, making subsequent entry into the abdomen more difficult (Fig. 46.2D).

Anatomic Points

The umbilicus is an easy entry site because skin, fascia, and peritoneum lie in close apposition with minimal intervening fat, even in obese patients. Converging on the umbilicus are four structures, all remnants of fetal development (Fig. 46.2E).

Cephalad, the ligamentum teres hepatis, with its obliterated umbilical vein enters, potentially complicating supraumbilical access in two ways. First, the fat-laden ligamentum teres and falciform ligaments must be traversed. Difficulty increases as one moves slightly cephalad from the umbilicus. Second, dilated venous collaterals form in patients with portal hypertension, in whom the umbilical vein remains patent or recanalizes, acting as an outflow conduit by anastomosing with the systemic circulation (veins in the anterior abdominal wall). Profuse bleeding may accompany attempted supraumbilical (or even infraumbilical) access in these patients.

Inferiorly, the median umbilica fold (urachus) and paired obliterated umbilical arteries converge but represent less of a mechanical problem.

If a vitelline duct remnant persists, it will be encountered in this region as well.

The proximity of the anterior abdominal wall to the underlying great vessels is accentuated by the manner in which the sacral promontory juts anteriorly (see Figure 42.1). Directing the Veress needle toward the pelvis helps minimize the danger of vascular injury.

Open Entry with Hasson Cannula (Fig. 46.3)

Technical and Anatomic Points

A Hasson cannula allows open entry by minilaparotomy. Make a circumumbilical incision, as described previously. The skin incision should be several centimeters long, to allow easy exposure of the fascia. Make the fascial incision about 2 cm long. Attain careful hemostasis and place retractors (Fig. 46.3A). Elevate and incise the peritoneum (Fig. 46.3B). Confirm peritoneal entry by direct vision or by inserting your index finger. Place two figure-of-eight anchoring sutures, one on each side of the incision. These will be used to anchor the cannula during laparoscopy and will be tied when the cannula is removed, providing fascial closure.

Insert the cannula and push the tapered obturator into the fascia so that it is snugly engaged. Anchor the stay sutures by winding them into the retaining grooves on the obturator (Fig. 46.3C). This helps to minimize leakage of CO_2.

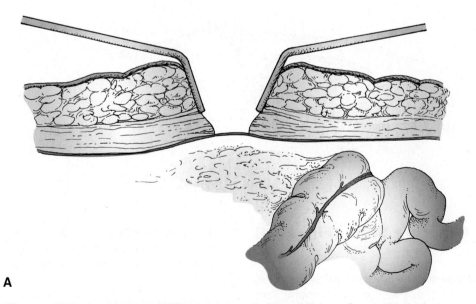

A

Figure 46.3 Open entry with Hasson cannula (**A** and **B** from Soper NJ. Access to abdomen. In: Scott-Conner CEH, ed. *The SAGES Manual.* New York, NY: Springer Verlag; 1999, with permission; **C** from Wind GG. *Special Operative Considerations.* Baltimore: Williams & Wilkins; 1997, with permission). (*continued*)

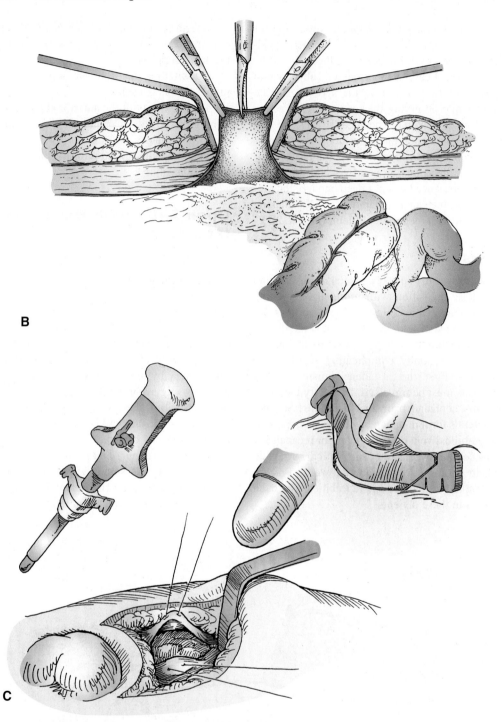

B

C

Figure 46.3 *Continued*

Alternative Puncture Sites (Fig. 46.4)

Technical Points

The left and right upper quadrants, where the costal margin elevates the anterior abdominal wall, may be used for alternative Veress needle puncture sites in cases in which the midline is inaccessible (Fig. 44.4 A and B). Choose a site close to the costal margin and remote from old scars, ideally in the midclavicular line. Make a transverse incision long enough to accommodate the planned trocar. Deepen the incision to fascia. Elevate the abdominal wall below the incision by grasping the full thickness of the abdominal wall with your nondominant hand. Insert the Veress needle as previously described and confirm intraperitoneal placement.

Anatomic Points

This method depends on the lower costal arch to provide counterpressure and resistance against which the Veress needle can be driven. Most often, the left upper quadrant site is employed because only stomach (decompressed with a nasogastric tube)

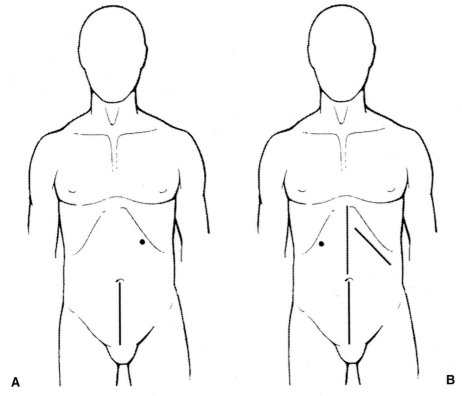

Figure 46.4 Alternative puncture sites. **A:** Left subcostal puncture site for lower abdominal incision. **B:** Right subcostal puncture site for midline or left subcostal incisions.

should lie beneath the site. In the right upper quadrant, liver, gallbladder, or colon may be encountered. This entry site is commonly employed in morbidly obese patients because the pannus is generally thinner in the upper abdomen, or when surgery is being done in the lateral decubitus position.

Exploration of the Abdomen and Placement of Secondary Trocars (Fig. 46.5)

Technical Points

Insert the laparoscope and inspect the abdomen in a systematic fashion. Place secondary trocars as needed to palpate and manipulate loops of bowel. The optimum location of secondary trocars depends on the specific pathology anticipated or the procedure to be performed. Become familiar with the use of angled (30- and 45-degree) as well as straight (0-degree) laparoscopes. The angled scopes allow the surgeon to look at structures from several viewpoints (Fig. 46.5A). If the view you are obtaining with the straight scope is inadequate, try an angled scope. Alternatively, move the laparoscope to another location for a different point of view.

Conceptualize your working space within the abdomen as a triangle. The laparoscope forms the apex of the triangle and corresponds to your eyes. Working ports to left and right of the laparoscope, and generally closer to the surgical target than the port for the laparoscope, are at your left and right hands. If the

ports are placed too close together, it will be difficult to manipulate instruments (Fig. 46.5B). Each laparoscopic chapter in this text describes the usual port locations. Sometimes, these locations must be modified according to individual anatomy.

Adjust the table and monitors so that a monitor is in the direct line of sight of both the surgeon and first assistant (Fig. 46.5C). Make sure the operating table is at a comfortable height; this will generally mean dropping it to a lower height than normal because of the length of the instruments.

In the upper abdomen, ports can be placed essentially anywhere without significant risk for bleeding. Below the umbilicus, ports should either be placed in the midline or lateral to the rectus sheath in order to avoid the inferior epigastric vessels. Although injury to a patent urachus is a theoretical possibility in the lower midline, it does not appear to be a problem in practice. Injury to the bladder is best avoided by preoperative decompression by an indwelling catheter.

For exploration of the upper abdomen, place the table in steep reverse Trendelenburg position to allow gravity to retract the viscera caudad. Examine the diaphragm (a common site of metastatic deposits), liver, gallbladder, stomach, and spleen.

Turn the patient into a right-side-up position to examine the right colon, cecum, and appendix. The transverse colon can only be seen if the greater omentum is elevated.

The entire small bowel can be systematically run between two atraumatic graspers or Babcock clamps.

Turn the patient to a left-side-up position to examine the descending colon. Steep Trendelenburg positioning is crucial

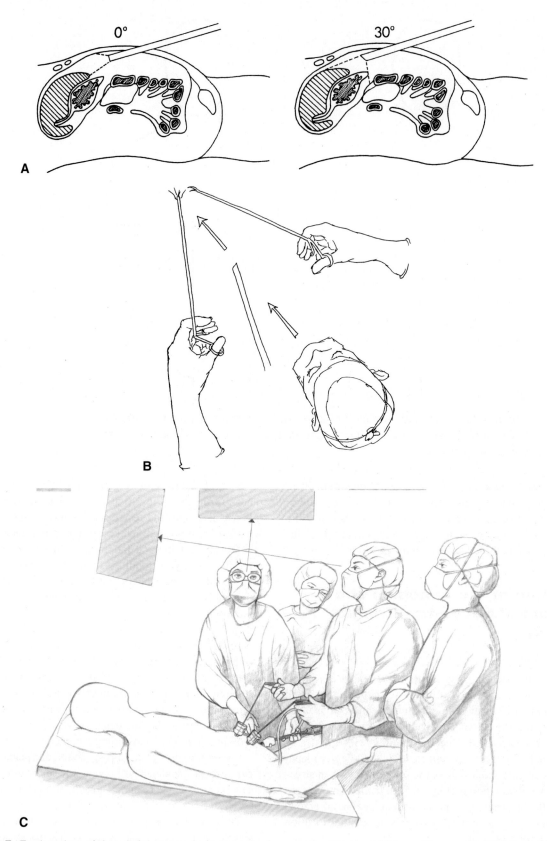

Figure 46.5 Exploration of the abdomen and placement of secondary trocars (**A** from Romanelli JR, Litwin DEM. Hand-assisted laparoscopic surgery. *Probl Gen Surg.* 2001;18:45–51, with permission; **B** from Wind GG. *Special Operative Considerations.* Baltimore: Williams & Wilkins; 1997, with permission; **C** from Scott-Conner CEH. Choice of laparoscope: Straight versus angled? In: *Chassin's Operative Strategy in General Surgery.* 3rd ed. New York, NY: Springer; 2002, with permission; **D** from Scott-Conner CEH, Cuschieri A, Carter FJ. Anterior abdominal wall. In: *Minimal Access Surgical Anatomy.* Philadelphia, PA: Lippincott Williams & Wilkins; 2000:1–5, with permission).

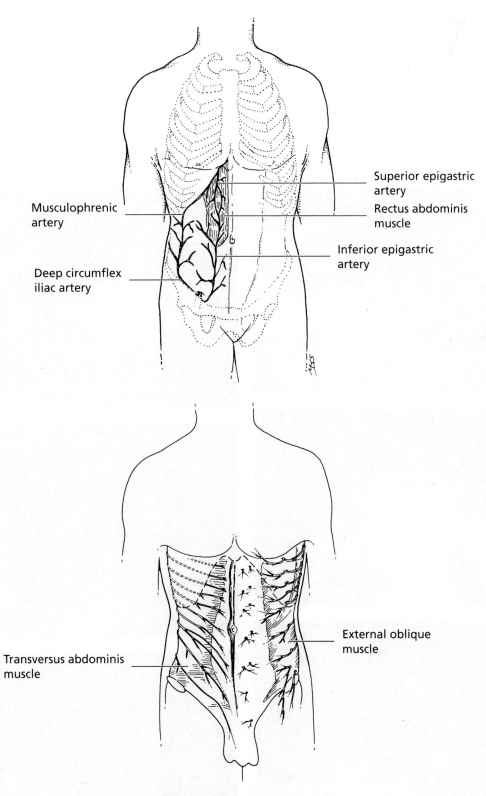

Figure 46.5 *Continued*

for adequate visualization of pelvic structures. The detailed normal laparoscopic anatomy of each region is shown in the specific chapters that follow.

Anatomic Points

The superior and inferior epigastric vessels run in the rectus sheath, posterior to the rectus abdominis muscles. Generally, only the inferior epigastric vessels are problematic.

Laterally, the musculophrenic arteries are noted (Fig. 46.5D), but these are rarely encountered during laparoscopic surgery.

Laparoscopic Landmarks (Fig. 46.6)

Technical and Anatomic Points

Develop a systematic approach similar to the approach you would use to explore the abdomen during open surgery (Fig. 44.5).

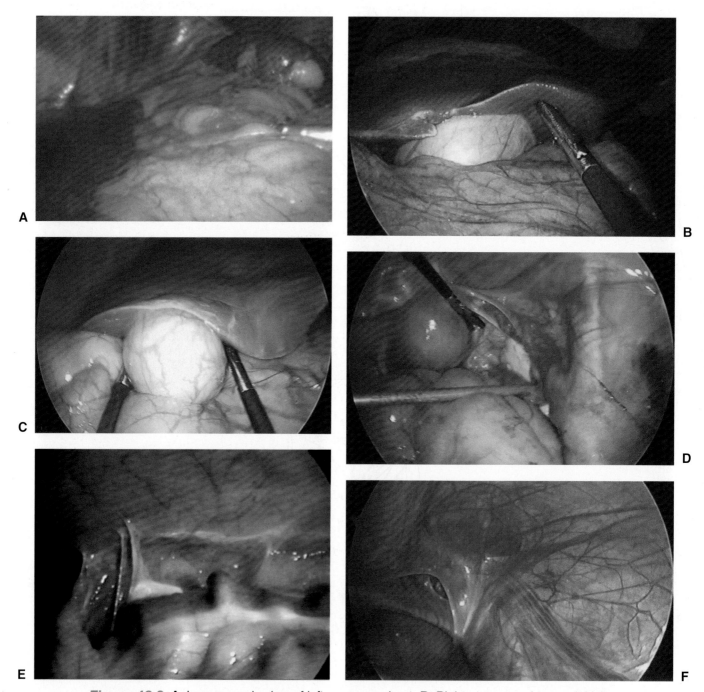

Figure 46.6 A: Laparoscopic view of left upper quadrant. **B:** Right upper quadrant as initially seen. **C:** Right upper quadrant with liver elevated. **D:** Female pelvis. **E:** Left colon. **F:** Incidental finding of indirect Inguinal hernia. Photos courtesy of Hui Sen Chong, MD, University of Iowa.

Insufflation will have produced a space between the viscera and the anterior abdominal wall. The first step in any laparoscopic procedure should be a routine check for evidence of injury during trocar placement. Thus, sweep the laparoscope around and look for blood or succus, particularly directly under the entry site. Then begin with a careful inspection of the left upper quadrant (Fig. 46.6A) where stomach, spleen, and diaphragm are visible. This area is best viewed with the patient in a slight head-up tilt (to allow gravity to pull the viscera down and out of the way). If not already done, have the anesthesiologist pass a temporary orogastric tube to decompress the stomach.

In the right upper quadrant (Fig. 46.6B), the initial view shows the upper aspect of the liver and gallbladder. The subhepatic space including first part of the duodenum are visualized only when the liver is elevated with a liver retractor or by lifting up on the ligamentum teres (Fig. 46.6C).

Follow the right colon down to the right lower quadrant. This view is improved by switching the operating table to a head-down tilt with the right side up. The female pelvis (Fig. 46.6D) is seen best by either gently lifting each adnexa or by manipulating the cervix from below.

Complete your inspection by following the left colon up (Fig. 46.6E) to the left upper quadrant. Run the small bowel between graspers.

Asymptomatic groin hernias (Fig. 46.6F) are common findings. Make note of these and inform the patient, but do not attempt to close these unless they are related to the problem at hand.

REFERENCES

1. Ahmad G, O'Flynn H, Duffy JM, et al. Laparoscopic entry techniques. *Cochrane Database Syst Rev.* 2012;2:CD006583.
2. Blichert-Toft M, Koch F, Neilson OV. Anatomic variants of the urachus related to clinical appearance and surgical treatment of urachal lesions. *Surg Gynecol Obstet.* 1973;137:51–54.
3. Easter DW. Diagnostic laparoscopy for acute and chronic abdominal pain. In: Zucker KA, ed. *Surgical Laparoscopy.* 2nd ed. Philadelphia, PA: Lippincott Williams & Wilkins; 2001: 97–102.
4. Jiang X, Anderson C, Schnatz PF. The safety of direct trocar versus Veress needle for laparoscopic entry: A meta-analysis of randomized clinical trials. *J Laparoendosc Adv Surg Tech A.* 2012;22:362–370.
5. MacVay CB, Anson BJ. Composition of the rectus sheath. *Anat Rec.* 1940;77:213–217.
6. Milloy FJ, Anson BJ, McFee DK. The rectus abdominis muscle and the epigastric arteries. *Surg Gynecol Obstet.* 1960;110: 293–302.
7. O'Malley E, Boyle E, O'Callaghan A, et al. Role of laparoscopy in penetrating abdominal trauma: A systematic review. *World J Surg.* 2013;37:113–122.
8. Orda R, Nathan H. Surgical anatomy of the umbilical structures. *Int Surg.* 1973;58:454–464.
9. Oshinsky GS, Smith AD. Laparoscopic needles and trocars: An overview of designs and complications. *J Laparoendosc Surg.* 1992;2: 117–125.
10. Riza ED, Deshmukh AS. An improved method of securing abdominal wall bleeders during laparoscopy. *J Laparoendosc Surg.* 1995; 5:37–40.
11. Romanelli JR, Litwin DE. Hand-assisted laparoscopic surgery: Problems in general surgery. *Probl Gen Surg.* 2001;18:45–51.
12. SAGES Guidelines for the optimum placement and adjustment of the operating room table and the video monitor during laparoscopic surgery. Available online at: www.sages.org.
13. SAGES Laparoscopy Troubleshooting Guide. Available online at: www.sages.org.
14. Schafer M, Lauper M, Krahenbuhl L. A nation's experience of bleeding complications during laparoscopy. *Am J Surg.* 2000;180: 73–77. (Describes major vascular injuries.)
15. Scott-Conner CEH, Cuschieri A, Carter FJ. Anterior abdominal wall. *Minimal Access Surgical Anatomy.* Philadelphia, PA: Lippincott Williams & Wilkins; 2000:1–5.

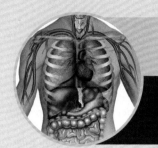

47

Open Repair of Ventral Hernias

Evgeny V. Arshava

Ventral hernias are classified as either spontaneous (epigastric, umbilical, Spigelian, lumbar) or postoperative. Most ventral hernias are postoperative (incisional) and occur at the site of previous laparotomy incisions. Many asymptomatic and minimally symptomatic hernias, especially with large defects in high risk patients, may be safely observed. Most symptomatic hernias are usually repaired electively. Others present with an acute incarceration and may need to be operated on urgently. Always optimize medical comorbidities, encourage smoking cessation and, if necessary, weight loss before the elective operation.

Multiple repairs have been described and none are perfect. Choice of repair depends on the size of the defect, tissue quality, comorbidities of the patient, previous surgical history and circumstances of the operation. Small defects may be closed by reopening the incision, clearing and reapproximating the fascial edges as one would close the laparotomy incision. Frequently, multiple defects may be present; thus, it is important to explore the entire incision. If the fascial defect is large and closure cannot be accomplished without excessive tension, synthetic or biologic implants may need to be used for a durable repair. A variety of such implants are available, each with its own advantages and disadvantages. It is important to be familiar with characteristics of these different products, since one mesh does not serve all purposes.

Tailor the implant to the specific patient and circumstances of the operation. For example, synthetic materials are contraindicated in the contaminated field (active infection, bowel resection, or history of infection) at the site. To cite another example, mesh without nonadhesive layer should not be used in direct apposition to the bowel.

The technique of separation of components lengthens the musculoaponeurotic flaps, allowing them to reach the midline, and may be used in combination with or as an alternative to placement of an implant.

This chapter highlights the anatomy of the abdominal wall and describes contemporary open approaches to the management of ventral hernias. The wide variety of techniques available attests to difficulties with recurrence even after the most meticulous repair. Literature sources discussing further details on various techniques, outcomes and materials are referenced at the end.

Laparoscopic ventral hernia repair is an increasingly popular alternative to an open herniorrhaphy with improved outcomes in selected patients (see Chapter 49). The laparoscopic approach should not be used for hernia defects larger than 10 cm.

SCORE™, the Surgical Council on Resident Education, classified open repair of ventral hernia as an "ESSENTIAL COMMON" procedure. SCORE™ classified component separation abdominal wall reconstruction and repair of miscellaneous hernias as "ESSENTIAL UNCOMMON" procedures.

STEPS IN PROCEDURE

Make incision over the hernia (usually through old scar) with extension beyond it

Try to stay in preperitoneal plane to avoid damage to adherent bowel

Raise skin flaps in all directions for adequate exploration and identification of all defects

Reduce the hernia and free the fascial edges from adhesions. Preserve the hernia sac if possible

Choose method of repair—avoid the use of prosthetic material if reasonable

Primary Repair

Close the facial defect in the direction of the
least tension

Repair by Separation of Components

Widely develop skin flaps or alternatively
perform short lateral counter incisions

Create relaxing incisions through the EOA

Close fascia in the midline

Place closed suction drains under skin flaps

**Repair with the Prosthetic or
Biologic Implant**

Secure the mesh to fascia

Close fascia over implant if possible

Umbilical Hernia Repair

Make incision in umbilical crease or excise the
stretched skin as needed

Identify and reduce hernia contents. Preserve
sac if possible

Close fascia in the direction of least tension

Use prosthetic for a large defect

Tack underside of umbilicus to fascia to
recreate normal appearance

HALLMARK ANATOMIC COMPLICATIONS

Surgical site infection

Injury to bowel during dissection

Recurrence due to excessive tension during
closure or to unidentified secondary defects

The anatomy of the abdominal wall is complex. The abdominal wall layers are shown in Figure 47.1.

The terminology used in the literature for description of subcutaneous tissue is not consistent and may be confusing. The superficial fascia (Scarpa's) is a distinct fibrous layer identifiable during dissection and imaging. This membranous layer stretches across entire abdomen and continues on to the back toward the spinous processes. It is less distinct along the midline and around umbilicus. In most individuals, the superficial adipose layer (frequently referred to as Camper's fascia) is thicker, consists of large fat lobes with high structural stability and elastic proper-

ties, and is encased in between the perpendicular oriented fibrous septa. The deep adipose layer has smaller fat lobes that deform much easier and may not be well developed in slender individuals. Obliquely oriented deep fibrous septa make this layer more amenable to surgical separation during dissection and are prone to traumatic separation (degloving) from the underlying muscle.

Paired rectus abdominis muscles, "masters of the abdomen," form the spine of the abdominal musculature. They stretch from the xiphoid process and fifth, sixth, and seventh ribs to the symphysis crest. They are joined in the midline by the linea alba. The linea alba is a continuous aponeurotic bridge, stretched from the xiphoid process to the symphysis pubis that joins musculoaponeurotic structure of both sides. It is recognized by the intersection of crossing fibers ("decussation") from each side. Overall, the linea alba is wider above the umbilicus, making initial laparotomy access on virgin abdomen easiest in this location. Insignificant pyramidalis muscles are found next to the lower part of the recti muscles, attach to the pubic crest and insert to the linea alba as well.

The external oblique muscle is the most superficial of the three flat lateral muscles. Superiorly, the muscular part attaches to the lower eight ribs intertwining with the bellies of the serratus anterior and latissimus dorsi muscles. Inferiorly, muscle fibers descend onto the iliac crest. While its muscular part occupies the lateral region of the abdomen, its aponeurosis extends medially, joining the fibers from the opposite side in the midline at the linea alba. Superiorly, aponeurosis extends over the costal margin, fusing with the origin of lower fibers of the pectoralis major muscle. Inferiorly, aponeurosis extends from pubic tubercle to the anterior superior iliac spine forming the inguinal ligament.

The internal oblique muscle is thinner and smaller than the external one. Its muscle fibers arise and run in a fan-like manner from the lower three ribs, thoracolumbar fascia, iliac crest and the lateral half of the inguinal ligament. Its aponeurosis is narrow. In the inguinal canal, it gives origin to the cremaster muscle. Medially, it continues into a narrow aponeurosis along the lateral border of rectus muscle.

Figure 47.1 Computed tomography of the abdomen at the level of the L5 vertebral body. SF, superficial fascia; SAL, superficial adipose layer; DAL, deep adipose layer; EOM, eternal oblique muscle; IOM, internal oblique muscle; TAM, transversus abdominis muscle; RAM, rectus abdominis muscle; X, linea semilunaris (sites of the division of external oblique aponeurosis during the components separation).

The transversus abdominis muscle is the most internal of the flat muscles. Its muscle fibers arise from the cartilages of the lower six ribs, lumbodorsal fascia, iliac crest and lateral third of the inguinal ligament. Medially it forms aponeurosis, almost as wide as an external oblique one. Above the internal ring, the dense lower edge of the transversus aponeurosis is supplemented by the mostly fleshy lower edge of the internal oblique muscle to form the falx inguinalis and the "roof" of the inguinal canal.

Together all three flat abdominal muscles form the sheath of the rectus muscles. The tendinous line along the lateral edge of rectus muscle stretches from the cartilage of the ninth rib to the pubic tubercle and is called linea semilunaris. In the upper abdomen, the aponeuroses of the internal oblique muscle split at the linea semilunaris into anterior and posterior layers and fuse around each rectus muscle with other flat muscles forming a dense sheath joined together by the linea alba. In the lower abdomen, all three aponeuroses pass completely anterior to the rectus muscle. This transition occurs along the concave arcuate (semicircular) line (Fig. 47.10A). The top of this arch is usually located 3 to 5 cm below the umbilicus. The absence of the posterior rectus sheath below the arcuate line makes the structure of the lower abdomen relatively deficient. The point of intersection of arcuate and semilunaris lines is the classic location of Spigelian hernias (discussed briefly in the end).

The abdominal wall is innervated by the lower five intercostal nerves (T7 to T11), subcostal (T12), iliohypogastric (T12 / L1) and ilioinguinal (L1) nerves. The intercostal nerves travel within the chest between the innermost intercostal and internal intercostal muscles. Within the abdominal wall, this plane naturally continues between the internal oblique and transversus abdominis muscles (Fig. 47.2A). The subcostal, ilioinguinal and iliohypogastric nerves, before piercing the the transversus abdominis muscle, travel within the abdomen on top of the quadratus lumborum muscle. Along the anterior axillary line, intercostal nerves give off the lateral cutaneous branches that penetrate the musculature and branches within the subcutaneous plane. Intercostal and other nerves, as they travel between internal oblique and transversus abdominis muscles, innervate flat muscles. Medially, the nerves penetrate posterior rectus sheath, innervate rectus muscle and then exit through the anterior sheath under the skin as sensory anterior cutaneous branches.

The rectus abdominis muscles are supplied by the superior and inferior epigastric vessels that travel within the rectus sheath and anastomose in the periumbilical area. Below the arcuate line, the inferior epigastric vessels lie directly on the posterior surface of rectus muscle and may be subject to injury during open or laparoscopic procedures.

The flat muscles of the abdomen are supplied by the rich network of lower intercostal, subcostal, musculophrenic, lumbar and deep circumflex iliac arterial and venous branches. This network is located between internal oblique and transversus abdominis muscles, giving off perforating vessels to surrounding tissues. This network also anastomoses with epigastric vessels through perforators in the rectus sheath. Such abundant

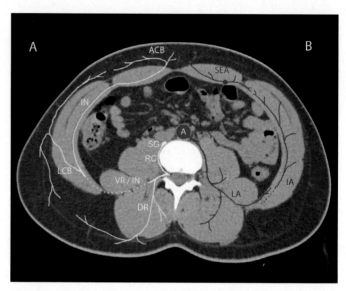

Figure 47.2 Anatomy of the abdominal wall at the level of L3 vertebral body. **A:** Innervation of the abdominal wall. DR, dorsal ramus; VR/IN, ventral ramus (intercostal nerve) of the spinal nerve; RC/SG, rami communicantes/sympathetic ganglion; LCB, lateral cutaneous branch; ACB, anterior cutaneous branch. **B:** Blood supply of the abdominal wall. A, aorta; SEA, superior epigastric artery; IA, intercostal artery; LA, lumbar artery. Dotted lines schematically represent the descending course of the intercostal nerves and arteries from the thorax onto the abdomen.

blood supply makes bleeding complications much more likely than ischemic (Fig. 47.2B).

It is thus clear that oblique and lateral transverse incisions through flat muscles divide nerves and may not only produce sensory disturbances, but also denervate muscles and may result in bothersome bulges. This is the anatomic reason that the division of the external oblique aponeurosis during components separation, with preservation of the internal oblique muscles, does not disturb underlying nerves and blood supply of the abdominal wall.

Ventral Hernia Repair

Selected small hernias may be repaired under local and spinal anesthesia. Large defects require general anesthesia with muscle relaxation and appropriate lines and tubes. Meticulous skin preparation and draping are essential. Consideration using transparent incise drapes, especially if there is a possibility of using the synthetic mesh. Appropriate intravenous antibiotics should be completed within 1 hour prior to the incision. Mechanical bowel preparation may be considered for some cases to decrease abdominal distention. Preoperative computed tomography of the abdomen may be very helpful for preoperative planning in complex cases to evaluate the location of the fascial defects, integrity of the linea semilunaris, rectus and oblique muscles in order to choose the appropriate method of repair.

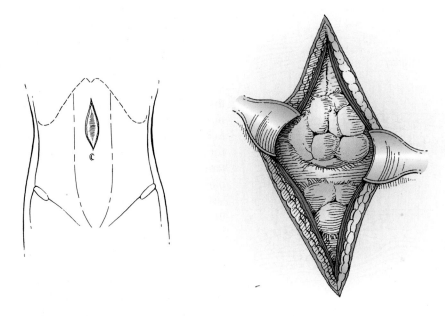

Figure 47.3 Exposure of fascia and identification of adjacent defects

Exposure of Fascia and Definition of the Defect (Fig. 47.3)

Most commonly the skin incision is performed over the existing scar. Elliptic excision of the wide scar frequently facilitates healing of the wound and improves the postoperative appearance. In cases of palpable Spigelian and epigastric hernia, it may be acceptable to orient the incision transversely in the direction of the relaxed skin tension lines. In selected cases, abdominal panniculectomy may be performed simultaneously during the same operation.

Deepen the incision cautiously until the hernia sac is encountered. Often, the sac lies quite close to the skin surface and may be adherent to the old scar. Usually the plane around the hernia is avascular and easy to dissect. Herniation of the preperitoneal fat in the absence of true sac looks somewhat like a lipoma and is easily "shelled out" of the surrounding tissues as well. Dissect circumferentially around the sac and then down to the fascia to visualize the hernia neck. Clean the intact fascia around the edge of the defect, raising flaps of subcutaneous tissue and skin as far as needed. In most cases, the entire length of the old incision should be explored in order not to miss frequently coexisting multiple defects. Lateral defects, which may occur at points where previous retention sutures may have cut through the fascia, must be ruled out as well.

If possible, dissect the sac away from the fascia. Preserve or repair the sac and reduce it with the hernia. This allows totally extraperitoneal repair, if mesh is to be used. Frequently this is not possible and the hernia sac needs to be excised. Debride the hernia sac and scar tissue until healthy fascia is exposed circumferentially around entire defect. Both for primary and mesh repair, it is critical to clean the underside of the fascia carefully so that the bowel is not caught in a stitch during the repair.

Generally, multiple adjacent defects should be joined into a single one by dividing the intervening bridges.

Primary Closure of the Hernia Defect

If the defect is of a small (less than 3 cm) or long, but narrow, and there is no tension, it can be closed with nonabsorbable sutures in the direction of the least tension. Use of the running or interrupted closure depends on the surgeon's preference. Either way suture length/wound length ratio should be at least 4:1. Be careful to avoid tension. If tension is required to appose the fascial edges, the repair will most likely fail. Remember that it is difficult to assess the tension of the repair under the conditions of muscle relaxation associated with general or spinal anesthesia. Therefore, if there is any tension or question about quality of the tissues, consider performing components separation or mesh repair.

Mesh Repair of Ventral Hernia (Figs. 47.4–47.6)

Use of mesh is associated with the improved success of repair of large ventral and recurrent incision hernia compared to primary closure technique. The most important prognostic factor for success may be the width of mesh overlap with the hernia defect. The circumferential, at least 5-cm overlap, is required for best outcomes.

The reduction of hernia and mobilization of the fascial edges are identical to primary repair.

Mesh can be used in several positions (Fig. 47.4). Neither overlay (Fig. 47.4A) nor inlay (Fig. 47.4B) positions are reliable and best avoided due to high failure rate. The underlay

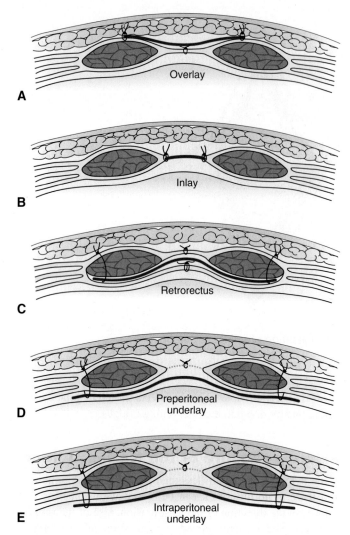

Figure 47.4 Mesh positions: **A:** Overlay (onlay). **B:** Inlay. **C:** Retrorectus. **D:** Preperitoneal (extraperitoneal) underlay. **E:** Intraperitoneal underlay.

position is associated with the lower recurrence rates and is currently the recommended approach. The so called "sandwich" (combination of the overlay and underlay meshes) repairs are rarely used at the present time.

The underlay position may be further classified on the basis of its relationship to the peritoneum and fascia as intra- and extra-peritoneal and retrorectus positions. Erosion of the mesh into bowel and development of enteric fistulae may occur even years after the index operation. Thus, to decrease the risks of this devastating complication, do not place synthetic mesh, lacking a nonadherent layer or coating, in the intraperitoneal position against the viscera.

Retrorectus Mesh Repair

The classic retrorectus repair (Fig. 47.4C) is a very durable method with a low recurrence rate and avoids the contact of viscera with nonprotected meshes such as straight polypropylene and polyester. The edges of the rectus sheaths are incised with

electrocautery on both sides of the defect for the full length of the defect. Dissect the plane to the lateral edge of the muscle between the posterior rectus sheath and muscle above the arcuate line and between the muscle and the peritoneum below it.

Sometimes, the integrity of the rectus muscle has been significantly compromised by previous operations and the width of the retrorectus plane is not sufficient for an optimal 4- to 5-cm mesh underlay. In such cases, the plane of the dissection needs to be continued outside of the rectus sheath. Two options exist for such cases. For the extraperitoneal position, incise the posterior rectus sheath medial to linea semilunaris and continue the plane of dissection between the peritoneum and the transversus abdominis muscle. For the intermuscular approach, incise the lateral edge of the rectus sheath and continue dissection in the plane between the transversus abdominis and internal oblique muscles. Note that the perforating vessels and nerve branches are encountered at the lateral edge and intermuscular extension of the retrorectus approach may permanently denervate the rectus muscles. To assure the adequate underlay both above and below the defect, continue dissection, if needed, behind the xiphoid and pubis. It is best to completely dissect the plane for mesh deployment before closing the posterior sheath to be able to repair defects in the peritoneum from inside of the abdomen and avoid injury to the underlying bowel.

Once the necessary space is developed circumferentially, pull the omentum over the bowel and close the peritoneum and the posterior rectus sheath as a separate layer of a running suture. Then fashion a sheet of mesh to the appropriate size to assure wide underlay circumferentially of at least 5 cm avoiding folding and wrinkling. Well fit flat mesh will be kept in place between the musculoaponeurotic layers by pressure and only a few fascial suture are needed along the mesh periphery. Suture the mesh under modest tension. The stretch across the midline will prevent mesh from folding inward once the fascial closure over it. Suturing the mesh to the posterior rectus sheath is an option, but carries the risk of injury to the underling bowel. A safer option is to place a series of U-stitches using large curved or Reverdin needle through the mesh and the rectus muscle and the anterior sheath. Consider placement of retrorectus drains in selected cases with the extensive dissection. Then close the anterior rectus over the prosthetic.

The modification of this method may be used for the laterally located incisional hernias. In such cases, make a transverse incision over the hernia. Define the hernia defect and develop the plane intermuscular between the transversus abdominis and internal oblique or between oblique muscles, depending on the hernia anatomy (Fig. 47.5). If needed, extend the plane medially incising the lateral edge of the rectus sheath and developing the retrorectus plane within its sheath.

Extraperitoneal Mesh Repair

In cases where the hernia sac can be preserved to cover intraabdominal organs and retrorectus method is not possible or practical, mesh may be placed extraperitoneally (Fig. 47.4D). In this case, develop the plane outside of the peritoneum

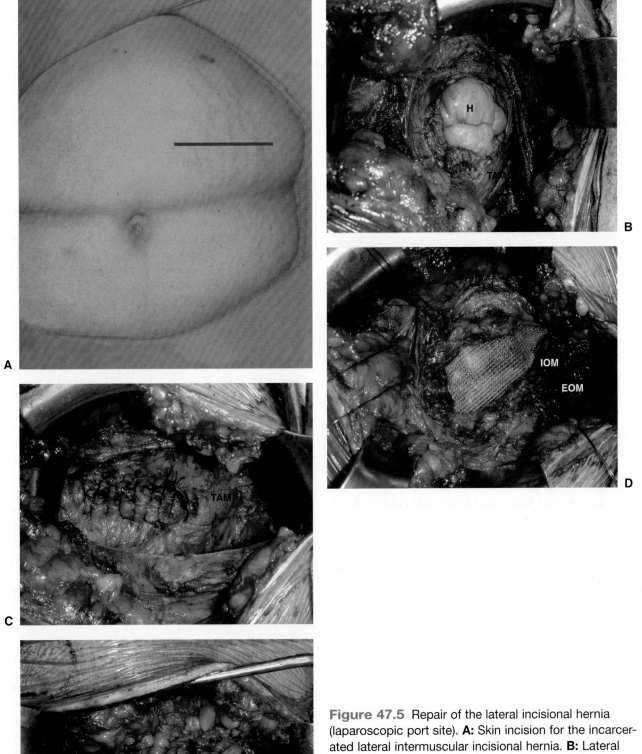

Figure 47.5 Repair of the lateral incisional hernia (laparoscopic port site). **A:** Skin incision for the incarcerated lateral intermuscular incisional hernia. **B:** Lateral abdominal wall defect dissected, hernia sac excised and colon reduced (TAM, transversus abdominis muscle; IOM, internal oblique muscle; H, herniating colon). **C:** Closure of the peritoneum and transversus abdominis muscle. **D:** Placement of the mesh in the previous hernia space over the transversus abdominis muscle. Securing U-stitches placed through the overlying oblique muscles. **E:** Closure of the oblique muscles over the mesh.

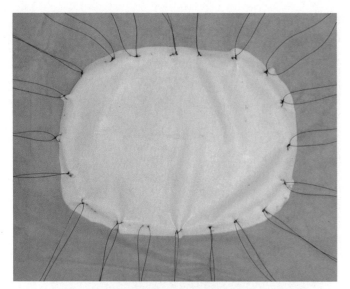

Figure 47.6 Placement of sutures on the periphery of the biologic mesh prior to the intraperitoneal implantation.

circumferentially around the defect to assure adequate overlap under the fascia. Secure the mesh circumferentially to the overlying musculoaponeurotic layer with transfixing sutures and close fascia over it.

Intraperitoneal Mesh Repair

With the improvement of the quality of the meshes with nonadhesive internal surfaces, the less cumbersome intraperitoneal underlay method has become more popular (Fig. 47.4E). Mesh can be secured under the fascia using either running or interrupted suture. Running suture in a vertical mattress fashion completely closes the space between the mesh and the fascia and eliminates the risk of interparietal herniation in early postoperative period. With the running technique; however, it may be difficult to adequately unfold the mesh and provide adequate overlap. Therefore, mesh is usually secured using multiple transfascial U-stitches. In contrast to retrorectus position, the mesh placed intraperitoneally will not be held in place by pressure and friction between fascial layers. For intraperitoneal attachment of the mesh, place a larger number of sutures along its periphery to prevent migration. In addition, do not space them wider than 1.5 to 2 cm apart, to avoid bowel herniation under the overlap of the mesh and peritoneum.

Fixation of the Mesh in Retrorectus, Retroperitoneal, and Intraperitoneal Positions (Figs. 47.6 and 47.7)

Flat position of the mesh with adequate overlap and its durable fixation to the abdominal wall is mandatory to prevent mesh migration and assure its incorporation into tissues. Since in most cases fascia will be closed over the mesh, it is important to stretch the mesh across the midline under a modest tension. This will prevent mesh from folding inside and will distribute the intra-abdominal pressure more evenly across the entire abdominal wall after fascial closure.

During the mesh placement it is best first to place stitches in 9-, 12-, 3-, and 6-o'clock positions or even all stitches. This unfolds the mesh well from very beginning and helps to better determine the number and location of additional sutures needed. Before tying these sutures, they are held on hemostats and the needed additional transfascial stitches are placed under direct vision in between them. Use a needle with a large curvature or a Reverdin needle.

For all three repairs, the useful technique is to place all the stitches along the edge of the mesh prior to its implantation (Fig. 47.6). Several types of laparoscopic port-site closure instruments can be used during the subsequent step to pull needless ties through the fascia. After the tails of the individual suture are passed through the fascia, they are held with hemostat until all are ready to be sequentially tied. Before tying these final transfascial sutures, it is mandatory to ensure visually and by palpation that no viscera are caught between the mesh and the fascia and confirm that the gaps between the stitches are not too wide or loose.

To assure that the mesh is stretched across the defect and there is at least a 5-cm overlap requires that the transfascial sutures exit remote from the fascial edge. It is not an issue, if earlier during the case wide skin flaps were produced to mobilize and reduce the hernia, and adequately expose good fascial edges. These large wound surfaces; however, increase the morbidity of the operation and require placement of closed suction drains.

If skin remains attached to fascia close to the defect, it may be best not to mobilize the skin flaps of the fascia. In such cases, place multiple small stab incisions with no. 11 blade 6 to 8 cm circumferentially around the fascial defects. Pass the tails of the sutures individually through the full thickness of the abdominal wall and tie the knots below the skin level. Make sure that this brings mesh into snug apposition against the abdominal wall with no gaps for the bowel to herniate (Fig. 47.7). This is the method used during the laparoscopic approach to incisional hernia repair.

It is best to close the fascia over the mesh after implantation. Even in the absence of hernia defect, there may be some bulging in the area of the implant, associated with either suboptimal sizing of the synthetic mesh or stretching of the biologic implant. Closure of the fascia may provide a better contour of the abdominal wall long term. In addition, this adds an additional strength to closure and creates another tissue plane between prosthetics and external environment in dreaded case of postoperative wound infection.

Mesh Patch Repair (Fig. 47.8)

Placing, unfolding, and securing the mesh evenly beneath the fascia frequently requires the extension of the hernia defect. Currently, several mesh devices of different sizes exist in shape

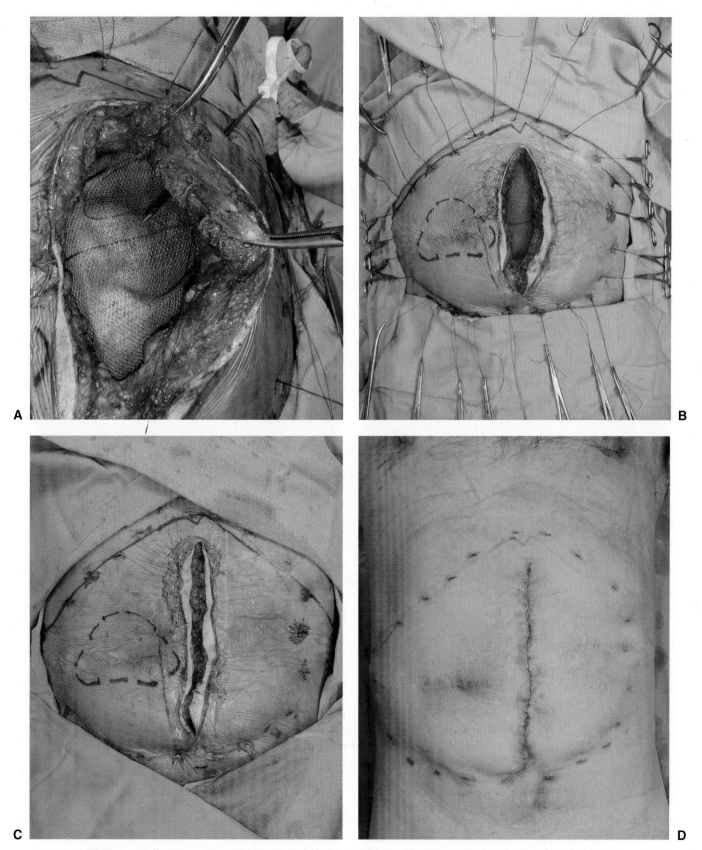

Figure 47.7 Placement of a large coated synthetic mesh in the intraperitoneal underlay position in a patient with multiple midline and lateral abdominal wall hernias. **A:** Passing sutures on periphery of the mesh through the full thickness of the abdominal wall. **B:** All sutures placed and mesh pulled against abdominal wall before tying. **C** and **D:** Fascia and all skin incisions are meticulously closed over the mesh.

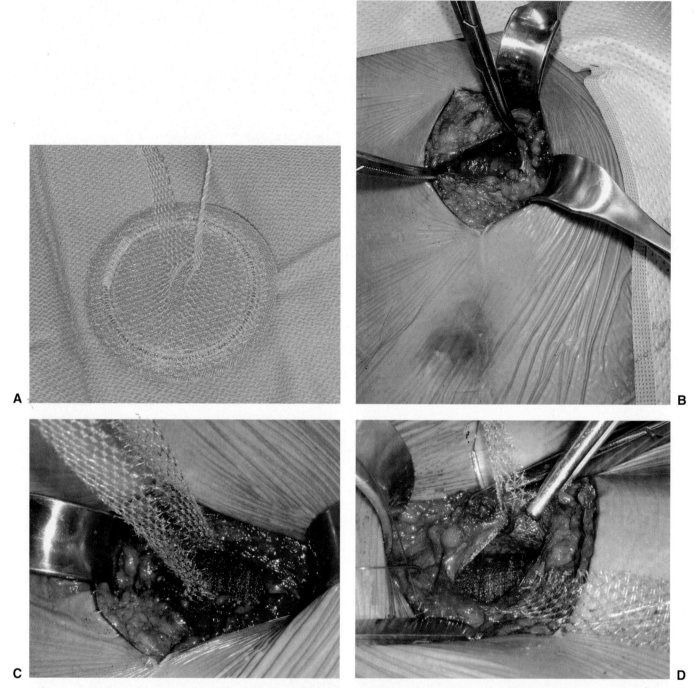

Figure 47.8 Incisional hernia repair with a hernia device. **A:** Example of a hernia patch device. **B:** The edges of the fascial defect are dissected and preperitoneal space developed. **C:** Mesh deployed in preperitoneal space. **D:** Outer layer of the mesh is incorporated into running fascial closure.

of the "mushroom" or "umbrella" for smaller hernia defects to minimize the dissection (Fig. 47.8). These devices may have a self-expanding "memory" disk or rings, partially absorbable structure or nonadherent coating on the side of the disk facing the viscera. Thus, they can be placed both in extra- and intra-peritoneal positions. The unprotected synthetic materials

face the undersurface of the fascia for better incorporation into tissues.

Dissect the hernia defect and preserve the sac if possible. Develop the preperitoneal space using blunt dissection with the finger or sponge wide enough to accommodate the disk of the device. For intraperitoneal position assure absence of adhesion

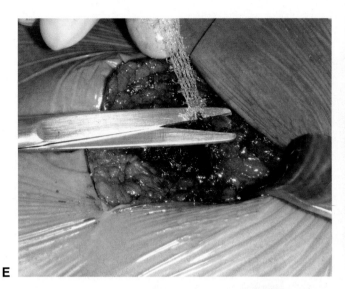
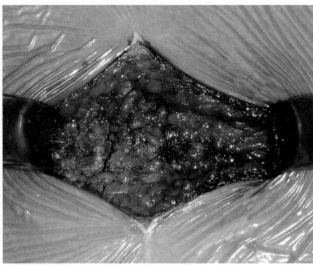

Figure 47.8 *Continued.* **E:** Outer tails are cut. **F:** Fascia is closed.

to the fascial edge. Select the mesh of appropriate diameter to assure sufficient overlap with the defect. Fold the disk and introduce it below the fascia, holding the outer tails outside of the wound as a handle. Assure flat expansion of the disk without folding. Close the fascia in vertical or transverse fashion with running or interrupted suture over the mesh, incorporating the remnants of the tails. Cut the outer tails above the stitches flush with the level of the fascia. Leaving parts of mesh in the subcutaneous plane may lead to its infection in cases of even minor superficial wound problems. Close the wound as for the primary repair.

Such devices may also be used with success for repair of umbilical, epigastric, and Spigelian hernias.

Components Separation Technique (Figs. 47.9–47.11)

The technique of separation of components is based on the multilayered anatomy of the abdominal wall lateral to the rectus abdominis muscles. Division of the external oblique muscle and its aponeurosis along the linea semilunaris lengthens the musculoaponeurotic flap on this side, allowing it to reach midline with less tension. Integrity of the abdominal wall is maintained by other components of the abdominal wall; specifically, the intact internal oblique and transversus abdominis muscles. Main vascular network and nerve pathways remain undisturbed under the internal oblique muscle.

The fascia defect is dissected and the hernia contents are reduced as described previously. Hernia sac is either preserved or resected. Excise the scar tissue to the edge of healthy fascia.

Using electrocautery and traction develop the subcutaneous flaps in the plane where the subcutaneous fat is loosely adherent to the fascia (Fig. 47.9A). These flaps should extend out past the lateral edge of the rectus muscle. Few encountered perforating vessels may be divided as needed. External oblique

aponeurosis is incised with electrocautery or scissors 1 to 2 cm lateral and parallel to the edge of the rectus muscle (Fig. 47.10). Care should be taken not to go inadvertently medial to the fusion of the aponeurosis of flat muscle, as this may result in full thickness fascial defect. Avascular plane is entered between the oblique muscles and relaxing incision is extended with electrocautery inferiorly and superiorly. This results in prompt and easy mobilization of the aponeurosis laterally (Fig. 47.9B). Do not cut the internal oblique muscle. This may weaken the abdominal wall and predispose to delayed development of hernia in this location.

Since superiorly the external oblique aponeurosis stretches over the costal margin, to achieve optimal mobility depending on the size of the hernia defect, its release may need to be extended over the lower ribs.

Once the release is completed, mobility of the fascial edges is reassessed. Remember that any tension that is evident with muscle relaxation under general anesthesia will be accentuated when the patient is awake and assumes upright position. If the closure is still tight, additional relaxing incisions can be on the posterior rectus sheath (Fig. 47.9C). This additional maneuver; however, may further compromise already weakened fascia and is rarely indicated.

Location of an old or existing ostomy site should also be taken into consideration, especially if it does not pass through the rectus muscle and is located on the linea semilunaris or lateral to it. In such case, it is best to perform asymmetric or even incomplete release of the external oblique on this side.

Most commonly, separations of the components are performed bilaterally. Complete release of the external oblique aponeurosis on both sides may allow closure of the fascial defects of over 15 cm in width. Once the desired relaxation has been achieved, fascia is closed in the midline using running or interrupted suture (Fig. 47.9D). Closed suction drains are placed above the fascia on each side prior to skin closure and removed when output is minimal.

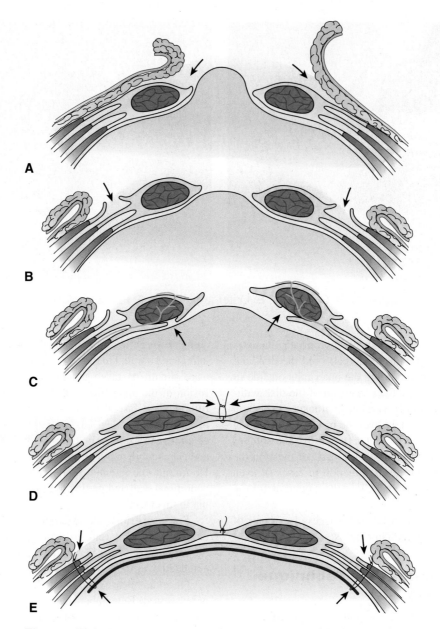

Figure 47.9 Components separation technique. **A:** Dissection of the hernia defect and development of skin flaps past the linea semilunaris. **B:** Incision of the external oblique aponeurosis. **C:** Posterior rectus sheath is incised if needed. **D:** Closure of the fascia in the midline. **E:** Mesh reinforcement may additionally be performed in the underlay position with transfixing sutures places lateral to the division of the external oblique aponeurosis.

Alternatively, full release of the external oblique aponeurosis may be performed through 2 to 3 cm transverse counter incisions on each side placed lateral to the linea semilunaris on each side of the mid abdomen (Fig. 47.11). If the lateral border of the rectus muscle is not palpable, site for placement of the incisions can be determined on preoperative computed tomography. Deep narrow retractors are used for cephalad and caudad skin retraction and allow to perform the division of the aponeurosis from the costal margin to the level of the arcu-

ate line under direct vision in most patients. These tracts ideally should not communicate with the midline incision, in case one of the wounds develops infection postoperatively. Lateral counter incisions are closed separately and drains are generally unnecessary. This is an easier and a less expensive approach than recently described endoscopic-assisted components separation with balloon dissection.

Separation of the components is an excellent technique to close retracted fascial edges walls in cases of delayed abdominal

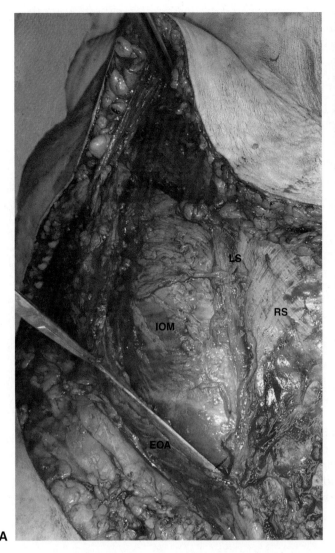

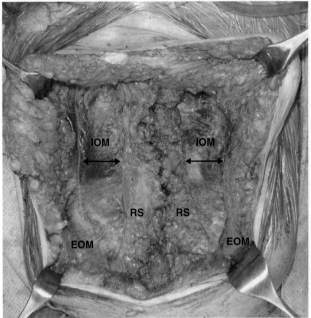

Figure 47.10 A: Components separation on the right. EOA, external oblique aponeurosis; IOM, internal oblique muscle; RS, rectus sheath; LS, linea semilunaris. **B:** Bilateral components separation and closure of the midline fascial defect. Arrows point to the edges of the divided aponeurosis of the external oblique muscle.

closure or cases with large defects where the use of synthetic material is contraindicated. It should be noted; however, that the repair of large incision hernias with this technique alone may be associated with recurrence in up to third of the patients.

Frequently this technique is used in combination with implantation of synthetic or biologic implant. In such cases, the implant may be placed in the underlay fashion to reinforce the entire abdominal wall. Secure the underlay mesh with the transfascial sutures exiting through all the three flat muscles lateral to the line of release of the external oblique aponeurosis (Fig. 47.9E). Transfixing sutures, either full thickness of transfascial, should be placed lateral to the line of division of the external oblique aponeurosis.

Anatomic Points

The rectus muscle is wider in the upper abdomen and while performing extension inferiorly, relaxing incision needs to follow its curved contour. Although, internal oblique and transversus abdominal muscles extend to the inguinal ligament and the iliac crest, posterior rectus sheath is absent below the

arcuate line. This makes the integrity of the lower abdominal wall relatively deficient. To avoid iatrogenic hernias at the site of the release, the division of the external oblique aponeurosis should not extend caudate to the arcuate line (Fig. 47.11).

Closure of the Incision

With any of the above methods used, but especially if the synthetic mesh repair has been performed, meticulous closure of the incision is of great importance. Inadequate apposition of the skin edges, their ischemia or breakthrough of underlying seroma, may lead to wound breakdown and subsequent contamination of prosthetic and its loss. Avoid placement of drains over mesh and close fascia if at all possible, even as attenuated flaps over it.

Excise the redundant skin flaps liberally. This improves the abdominal contour, decreases the dead space and most importantly assures that the residual skin edges have an optimal blood supply. It is wise to close the deep layer of subcutaneous tissue or superficial fascia as a separate layer to obliterate the dead space. Meticulous skin closure should complete the operation.

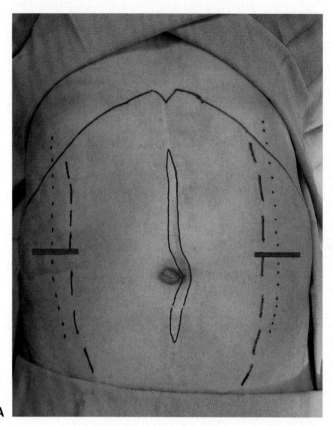
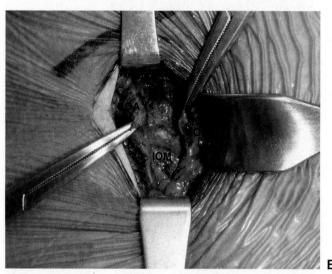

Figure 47.11 Minimally invasive separation of components. **A:** Thin red line—skin incision to excise an old scar and manage the midline incisional hernia. Black dashed line—contours of the lateral edges of the rectus abdominis muscles. Broad red lines—lateral skin incisions for bilateral EOA release without flap dissection. Black dotted lines—possible bilateral EOA release. Blue line—projection of the arcuate line. **B:** EOA release. Retraction the skin flaps cephalad and caudal is performed as needed for exposure.

Umbilical Hernia Repair (Figs. 47.12–47.14)

Incision

Small umbilical hernias, especially in slender patients, can be repaired through a small curvilinear incision placed just outside the umbilicus. This nicely hides the scar. Large umbilical hernias with stretched bulging skin or hernias in obese patients may require elliptic excision of the entire umbilicus (Figs. 47.12A and 47.14A).

Identification and Dissection of the Hernia Defect

The incision is deepened through the subcutaneous tissues until the hernia sac is identified. In cases of paraumbilical hernias there may be herniation of preperitoneal fat only, without the hernia sac. The umbilical skin is dissected free from the hernia and fascia. Continue the dissection around the hernia down to the fascia, exposing the entire fascial defect (Fig. 47.12B).

Adhesions to the fascia are divided circumferentially preserving the sac if possible. Occasionally, the sac or herniating peritoneal fat may need to be excised (Fig. 47.14B). In cases with the incarcerated bowel, the fascial defect may need to be enlarged dividing fascia on one or both sides of the hernia to reduce the hernia and to convert a round defect into a transverse slit that can be closed more easily.

Primary Closure of the Fascial Defect

Clean the fascial edges as described for ventral hernia repair above.

Classically, large umbilical hernias were repaired with interrupted nonabsorbable vertical mattress sutures in a transverse "vest-over-pants" fashion (Fig. 47.13).

First, bites are taken outside-in through the upper flap 1 to 1.5 cm from the edge. The bite is then taken outside-in through the lower flap again 1 to 1.5 cm from the edge. The suture is then returned inside-out through the top flap about 1 cm from the original entrance. Once all sutures are placed, they are then tied pulling the upper flap down over the lower flap. A second

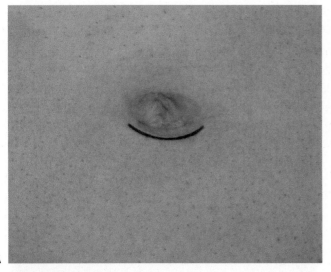

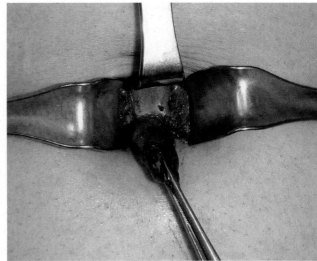

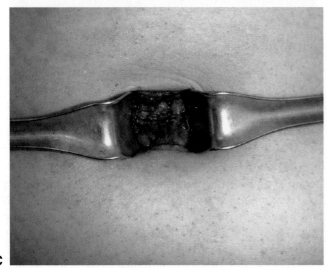

Figure 47.12 Repair of a small umbilical hernia.
A: Curvilinear incision (may be either infra or supraumbilical).
B: Hernia sac circumferentially dissected and fascial defect
defined. **C:** Hernia sac reduced and fascial defect closed
with interrupted sutures in transverse fashion.

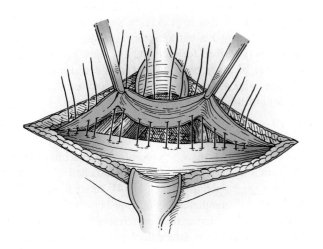

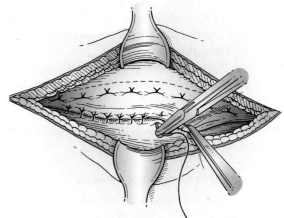

Figure 47.13 Mayo repair of the umbilical hernia

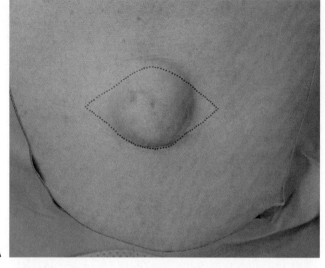

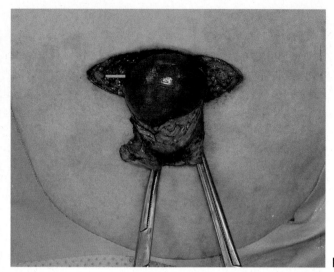

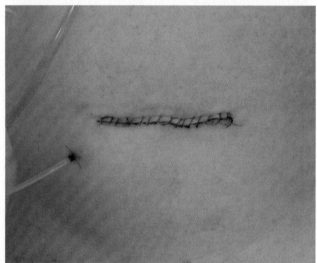

Figure 47.14 Repair of acutely incarcerated umbilical hernia in patient with cirrhosis. **A:** Elliptical incision placed to excised redundant skin and hernia sac. **B:** Incarcerated bowel assessed for viability and fascia incised transversely or vertically as needed to facilitate bowel reduction (marked with the line). **C:** Fascia and skin closed in layers after placement of the intraperitoneal drain.

row of interrupted sutures is placed to tack down the free edge of the upper flap. Care should be taken not to injure underlying bowel.

The underside of the umbilicus is tacked down to the fascia to recreate its shape. Close subcutaneous tissue and skin and place a compressing dressing inside umbilicus to obliterate the dead space and maintain an inverted contour.

The traditional "vest-over-pants" repair is less frequently utilized now given its high failure rate in large hernias. For umbilical hernias with the defect of less than 3 cm, closure of the defect with simple interrupted or running suture in the direction of lesser tension is less cumbersome and is associated with reasonable results.

Mesh Repair of the Umbilical Hernia

Primary repair of umbilical hernias with larger defects or poor tissue quality is associated with a high recurrence rates. When case is appropriate, mesh repair may be used to lower the risk of failure.

When the mesh repair is chosen, the general principles are similar to the incisional hernia repair. The best outcomes are achieved with underlay position of the prosthetic and closure of the fascia over it. For large defects, the mesh may be secured in the intraperitoneal of extraperitoneal position using transfixing sutures as described for incisional hernias. Periumbilical incisions may be more prone to maceration and breakdown. It is best not to leave prosthetic in the subcutaneous plane to avoid risk of infection in case of incision breakdown.

Patients with Cirrhosis

Patients with cirrhosis who present with an acute incarceration of an umbilical hernia or ascitic leak are challenging cases and require urgent operation (Fig. 47.14). In such patients, excise the umbilicus completely using transverse elliptic incision to facilitate healing. Incise the fascia transversely in the corner of the defect if unable to reduce the bowel. Synthetic mesh should not be used for the repair in the setting of enterotomy or bowel resection.

All the efforts should be made to decrease the risk of ascitic leak. Prior to closure, place the peritoneal drain through a separate stab incision laterally and keep it for 7 to 10 days postoperatively. Consider closing peritoneum as a separate layer with running absorbable suture. Assure meticulous hemostasis of the venous collaterals. Close the fascia in "vest-over-pants" fashion or with a running suture. Close well the subcutaneous tissue and use running suture for skin closure. Aggressive medical management of portal hypertension is of paramount importance.

Due to high mortality and morbidity of emergent operation, consider elective repair of umbilical hernias for selected medically optimized patients with cirrhosis.

Anatomic and Embryologic Points

The umbilicus is a midline fusion of the rectus abdominis aponeuroses around the cord components. Around the sixth week of gestation, the midgut migrates outside of abdominal cavity into the umbilical cord. As the midgut undergoes rotation, it returns into abdomen during tenth to twelfth weeks of gestation. After separation of the cord, umbilical ring contracts and during the subsequent healing forms a dense umbilical plate. The lower part of the plate is usually stronger, being supported by obliterated arteries and urachus as opposed to only round ligament superiorly. There is also a variable degree of reinforcement of the umbilical ring by the thickened part of transversalis fascia called umbilical fascia from behind. The umbilicus is the one place in the anterior abdominal wall where the skin is adherent to fascia without subcutaneous fat layer.

Two special kinds of congenital abdominal wall defects are encountered only in the neonates. Omphalocele results from the failure of intestinal loops to return into the abdomen during the gestational development. The bowel loops herniated into the umbilical cord are protected by amnion and peritoneum. Unless this sac is ruptured, the repair is an elective operation. By contrast, gastroschisis is herniation of bowel loops through a muscular defect of the anterior abdominal wall, usually to the right of the umbilicus, void of any protective covering. This herniation needs to be addressed and the threatened bowel protected emergently.

Congenital umbilical hernias develop if umbilical ring fails to close appropriately. They are always located within the umbilicus and have a peritoneal sac covered directly by the skin. By the age of two, most of them close spontaneously as the healing progresses.

The acquired umbilical and paraumbilical hernias are thought to develop in the weak area of the umbilical plate after repeated stress or chronically increased intra-abdominal pressure with advancing age, obesity, multiple pregnancies, or ascites. They are usually present in weaker upper area of umbilical plate and are only partially covered directly by the umbilical skin. Diastasis recti is a frequently coexisting condition. Apart from this, there is little practical difference between congenital and acquired umbilical hernias in adults.

Periumbilical subcutaneous tissue is more vascular than other regions of the anterior abdominal wall. Although this periumbilical plexus is primarily venous, small arterial branches are also present and can be cauterized, if needed. In the setting of portal venous hypertension, periumbilical veins act as important portosystemic collaterals. In patients with cirrhosis, multiple engorged veins may be encountered and result in significant bleeding.

Note on Repair of Other Types of Hernias

Epigastric Hernia Repair

Epigastric hernias occur through the linea alba anywhere between the xiphoid process and the umbilicus. Typically, epigastric hernias contain only preperitoneal fat, have no true hernia sac and may not be visualized during laparoscopy. Uncommon hernias with the large defects and peritoneal sacs most commonly contain only omentum.

Exposure of the hernia may be either through vertical or transverse incision. The defects commonly have a form of a transverse ellipse. Once the fascial edges are cleared, the incarcerated fat may need to be excised or reduced. Small defects are closed in a transverse fashion with several interrupted stitches. Epigastric hernias may coexist with the diastasis recti and the fascia quality may be poor. In such situations or with large defects, mesh repair may be performed as described for umbilical hernias.

Spigelian Hernia Repair

Spigelian hernias occur at the widest and the weakest area of linea semilunaris where it intersects with the arcuate line. During the early stages of development, these are the interparietal hernias and may not be palpable until after the break through the aponeuroses of all the three flat muscles.

Oblique incisions along the relaxed skin tension lines over the defect provide good exposure and an improved appearance of the scar. During the early stages of hernia evolution, external oblique aponeurosis, frequently attenuated, may need to be opened. Hernia sac is dissected free and the fascial defect is defined. Management of the hernia sac follows general principles described for other ventral hernias. If primary repair is performed, nonabsorbable material is used to suture the flat muscles laterally to the rectus sheath medially. Previously described mesh techniques may be used for the cases at high risk for hernia recurrence. In obese patients, the hernia may not be palpable and laparoscopic approach may provide a better visualization of the defect.

Parastomal Hernia

Parastomal hernia can be repaired in several ways, but with either approach there is over 50% risk of recurrence. These are best avoided in the first place.

For the local fascial repair method, make an incision transversely next to ostomy. Dissect down to the fascia and reduce the hernia and sac, not disturbing adhesions of the ostomy to the fascia itself. Using several interrupted sutures narrow the fascia ring with care not to make it so tight to compromise perfusion and patency of the bowel. This is a simplest, but also a very unreliable method. Close the skin around the ostomy. Placement of a small closed suction drain or leaving the corner of the incision for healing by secondary intention may be considered if the large skin flaps were developed.

Midline laparotomy incision is required for the ostomy relocation method. Make a midline laparotomy incision, enter abdomen and perform necessary adhesiolysis. Perform circumferential incision around ostomy itself, complete its mobilization in the avascular plane and reduce hernia and ostomy itself into the abdomen. Stomas site is closed as per surgeon's preference and a new tunnel of appropriate size is created through the rectus sheath in a different location.

Mesh repair is performed through midline incision with careful draping the ostomy away and not disturbing it. Perform adhesiolysis and reduce the hernia from inside of the abdomen. The fascial defect may be then tightened from the inside of the abdomen. Place the single sheath of an appropriate synthetic or biologic mesh intraperitoneally over an ostomy tunnel providing good overlap in all directions. The bowel should be emerging from under one side of the mesh. Do not cut any openings in the mesh. This would simply serve as a new area of weakness and may increase the risk of mesh erosion and fistula development. Secure the mesh circumferentially to the fascia. During laparoscopic repair mesh is placed in the same fashion.

REFERENCES

1. Arroyo A, García P, Pérez F, et al. Randomized clinical trial comparing suture and mesh repair of umbilical hernia in adults. *Br J Surg.* 2001;88(10):1321–1323.
2. Berry MF, Paisley S, Low DW, et al. Repair of large complex recurrent incisional hernias with retromuscular mesh and panniculectomy. *Am J Surg.* 2007;194:199–204.
3. Chan G, Chan CK. A review of incisional hernia repairs: Preoperative weight loss and selective use of the mesh repair. *Hernia* 2005;9(1):37–41.
4. den Hartog D, Dur AH, Tuinebreijer WE, et al. Open surgical procedures for incisional hernias. *Cochrane Database Syst Rev.* 2008; 16(3):CD006438. (Extensive review on outcomes of incisional hernias repair by technique used, position and types of the mesh from several large studies.)
5. Dietz UA, Hamelmann W, Winkler MS, et al. An alternative classification of incisional hernias enlisting morphology, body type, and risk factors in the assessment of prognosis and tailoring of surgical technique. *J Plast Reconstr Aesthet Surg.* 2007;60:383–388.
6. Halvorson EG. On the origins of components separation. *Plast Reconstr Surg.* 2009;124(5):1545–1549.
7. Harth KC, Rosen MJ. Endoscopic versus open component separation in complex abdominal wall reconstruction. *Am J Surg.* 2010; 199(3):342–346; discussion 346–347.
8. Mayo WJ. An operation for the radical cure of umbilical hernia. *Ann Surg.* 1901;34(2):276–280. (Original description of the technique.)
9. Paul A, Korenkov M, Peters S, et al. Unacceptable results of the Mayo procedure for repair of abdominal incisional hernias. *Eur J Surg.* 1998;164(5):361–367.
10. Ramirez OM, Ruas E, Dellon AL. "Components separation" method for closure of abdominal-wall defects: An anatomic and clinical study. *Plast Reconstr Surg.* 1990;86:519–526.
11. Sauerland S, Walgenbach M, Habermalz B, et al. Laparoscopic versus open surgical techniques for ventral or incisional hernia repair. *Cochrane Database Syst Rev.* 2011;16(3):CD007781.
12. Shah BC, Tiwari MM, Goede MR, et al. Not all biologics are equal! *Hernia.* 2011;15(2):165–171. Epub 2010 Dec 28.
13. Skandalakis PN, Zoras O, Skandalakis JE, et al. Spigelian hernia: Surgical anatomy, embryology, and technique of repair. *Am Surg.* 2006;72(1):42–48. Review.
14. Shell DH 4th, de la Torre J, Andrades P, et al. Open repair of ventral incisional hernias. *Surg Clin North Am.* 2008;88(1):61–83, viii.
15. Stumpf M, Conze J, Prescher A, et al. The lateral incisional hernia: Anatomical considerations for a standardized retromuscular sublay repair. *Hernia.* 2009;13(3):293–297. Epub 2009 Feb 12.
16. Sugarbaker PH. Peritoneal approach to prosthetic mesh repair of paraostomy hernias. *Ann Surg.* 1985;201(3):344–346.
17. Varshney S, Manek P, Johnson CD. Six-fold suture: Wound length ratio for abdominal closure. *Ann R Coll Surg Engl.* 1999; 81(5):333–336.
18. Williams RF, Martin DF, Mulrooney MT, et al. Intraperitoneal modification of the Rives-Stoppa repair for large incisional hernias. *Hernia.* 2008;12(2):141–145.
19. Xourafas D, Lipsitz SR, Negro P, et al. Impact of mesh use on morbidity following ventral hernia repair with a simultaneous bowel resection. *Arch Surg.* 2010;145(8):739–744.

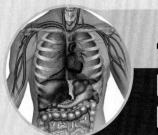

48

Pediatric Umbilical Hernia Repair

Raphael C. Sun and Graeme J. Pitcher

Umbilical hernias are the most common hernias seen in children. They occur as a result of a large or weak umbilical ring that persists after birth. For unknown reasons, these hernias are more common in African American children. The majority of pediatric umbilical hernias will, if given time, close spontaneously and require no surgical intervention. Thus the general rule is to wait until the child is of school-going age before repair. If the hernia defect is large enough to accommodate two fingers or more, it is unlikely to close, and repair can be done earlier when the child is 2 to 3 years old. The risk of incarceration and strangulation is extremely low, so it is reasonable to be conservative.

SCORE™, the Surgical Council on Resident Education, classified umbilical hernia repair in children as an "ESSENTIAL COMMON" procedure.

STEPS IN PROCEDURE

Make incision in the umbilical crease, guided by the location of fascial defect
    Usually inferior crease
    Superior crease in some situations (high fascial defect)
Dissect through the dermis to the subcutaneous tissue
Develop the plane between the hernia sac and the rectus sheath, clearly defining the edges of the musculofascial defect
Divide sac just anterior to the fascial edge
Dissect the sac off the skin if this can be easily accomplished

Control all bleeding points
Assure that the fascia is free from the sac and/or bowel contents
Close the fascia transversely or longitudinally in an interrupted fashion
    Many surgeons prefer a purse-string closure for smaller hernias.
Tack the base of the umbilical skin to the fascial closure to invert the umbilicus
Close the skin

HALLMARK ANATOMIC COMPLICATIONS

Injury to bowel
Failure to identify fascial edge correctly resulting in weak repair using the sac tissue

Fenestrating the skin during dissection of hernia sac from skin

Skin Incision and Initial Dissection (Fig. 48.1)

Technical Points

First, palpate the fascial defect to determine whether an incision above or below the umbilicus will give the best exposure. Accordingly, plan an infra- or supraumbilical curvilinear incision in the typical skin crease (Fig. 48.1).

Continue the incision through the subcutaneous tissue with a combination of electrocautery and blunt dissection. Identify the dissection plane between the subcutaneous tissue and the hernia sac. Take this dissection down to the level of the fascia. Next, identify the hernia sac and dissect circumferentially (Fig. 48.2). In some cases, dissecting with a hemostat between the fascia cranially and the sac allows the sac to be opened and the anatomy better defined. Adequate muscle relaxation or sufficient depth of anesthesia facilitates this step by preventing extrusion of loops of bowel into the wound. Carefully dissect the hernia sac off the skin in order to avoid fenestrating the skin.

Excise the sac down to the level of fascia (Fig. 48.3). Gain control of the fascial plane by placing a hemostat on each side.

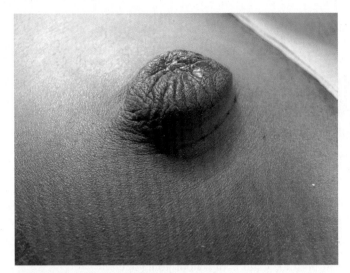

Figure 48.1 Infraumbilical skin crease incision

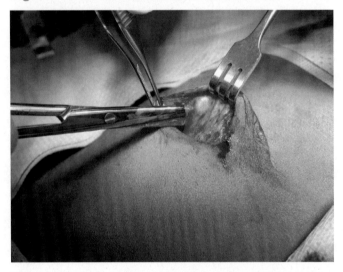

Figure 48.2 Dissection with scissors around circumference of intact hernia sac.

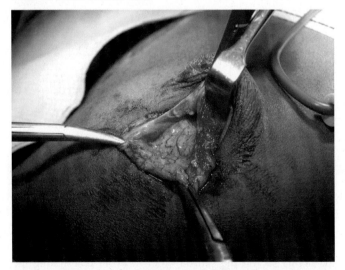

Figure 48.3 Excision of hernia sac at the base showing good quality healthy fascial edges triangulated preparatory to placement of purse-string suture.

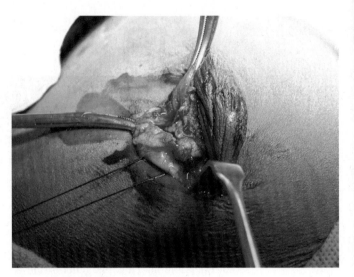

Figure 48.4 Tying the purse-string suture

Anatomic Points

Pediatric umbilical hernias are congenital and occur due to a persistent umbilical ring that has not spontaneously closed after birth. The hernia sac is the peritoneum and adheres to the dermis of the umbilical skin. Often times you will find a large "proboscis"-like protrusion of skin but this does not correlate with the size of the fascial defect.

If the correct plane is dissected, few bleeding vessels will be encountered and these can generally be cauterized. The only significant vessels encountered tend to be on the undersurface of the peritoneal margin of the defect. Care should be taken to either cauterize or include them in the repair for hemostasis.

The embryologic remnant structures of the falciform ligament (umbilical vein) and medial umbilical ligaments (umbilical arteries) are usually not seen at the time of hernia repair unless a large defect necessitates greater exposure.

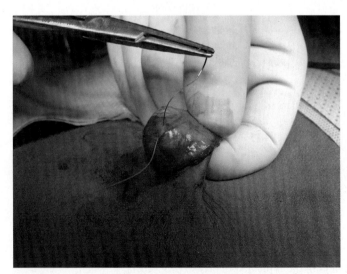

Figure 48.5 Placement of tacking absorbable suture to undersurface of the sac—this will be snugged down to the previous fascial closure to obliterate any dead space.

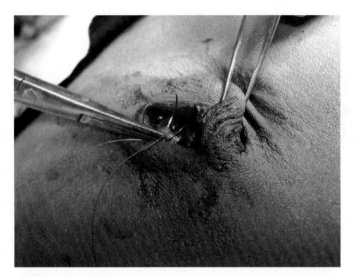

Figure 48.6 Closure of the subcutaneous layer

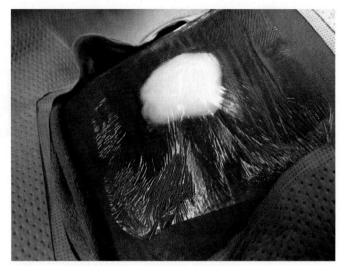

Figure 48.8 Occlusive pressure dressing with sponge pad over site of repair.

Repair of Fascial Defect and Closure

Technical and Anatomic Points

An absorbable suture-like PDS (polydioxanone) is ideal but vicryl (polyglactin) is an acceptable alternative. For small hernias a single continuous PDS suture placed through the fascial edge in a purse-string fashion and tied securely is sufficient (Fig. 48.4). For larger defects (greater than 2 cm diameter) close the defect with a series of interrupted sutures placed either horizontally or vertically (Fig. 48.5). Do not tie the sutures until all of them are placed. Holding tension on the previous sutures will allow for easier placement of any additional sutures. Most umbilical hernias are small enough to be closed primarily and mesh or prosthetic material is usually not required.

Reconstruct the umbilicus by suturing down the undersurface of the redundant skin to the fascia (Fig. 48.6). It is rarely necessary to excise skin. A better cosmetic result is usually obtained by preserving (rather than excising) the redundant skin (Fig. 48.7). A pressure dressing prevents a hematoma or seroma in extreme cases (Fig. 48.8). Close the skin with a subcuticular suture.

REFERENCE

1. Zendejas B, Kuchena A, Onkendi EO, et al. Fifty-three-year experience with pediatric umbilical hernia repairs. *J Pediatr Surg.* 2011; 46:2151–2156.

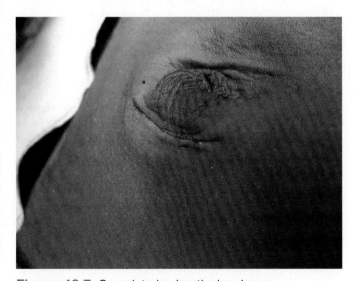

Figure 48.7 Completed subcuticular closure

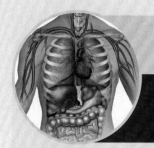

49

Laparoscopic Repair of Ventral Hernias

The theory behind laparoscopic ventral hernia repair is that because the problem is a defect in the fascia, an approach from inside the abdomen makes perfect sense. The role of this technique is still being defined. At present, it appears particularly appropriate for patients with relatively small defects who have not had previous mesh repair (hence no dense adhesions). It is considered relatively contraindicated in obese patients and is generally not considered appropriate for strangulated hernias.

SCORE™, the Surgical Council on Resident Education, classified laparoscopic repair of ventral hernia as an "ESSENTIAL COMMON" procedure.

STEPS IN PROCEDURE

Obtain laparoscopic access to the abdomen

Lyse any adhesions to anterior abdominal wall

Identify all fascial defects

Mark these on the anterior abdominal wall using a spinal needle to increase accuracy

Cut a dual mesh patch of sufficient size to provide overlap and cover all defects

Mark the patch so that you can identify the side to be placed next to the fascia and roll it up

Place horizontal mattress suture in each corner of the mesh

Pass mesh and sutures into abdomen

Unfurl the mesh and lay it flat upon the viscera

Take the suture corresponding to one of the far corners and pass it through the abdominal wall and tie it

Repeat this procedure with the other three sutures

Secure the spaces between the sutures using tacks

Close any trocar site greater than 5 mm diameter

HALLMARK ANATOMIC COMPLICATIONS

Visceral injury during entry or adhesiolysis

Missed defects or recurrence

Chronic pain due to sutures and tacks in peritoneum

LIST OF STRUCTURES

Linea alba

Rectus abdominis muscle

Inferior epigastric vessels

Initial Entry and Lysis of Adhesions (Fig. 49.1)

Technical and Anatomic Points

Choose an entry site remote from the defect and any old incision. This may require open entry with a Hasson cannula (see Chapter 46, Figure 46.3). Blind entry with a Veress needle in the left upper quadrant is an alternative in properly selected patients. This depends on the costal margin to provide resistance as the Veress needle is inserted and can only be used in patients in whom this area is free of old scars or probable adhesions from previous surgery in the region (e.g., splenectomy).

To perform blind left upper quadrant entry, select a point at the left costal border (Fig. 49.1A) well away from the hernia sac. Elevate the abdominal wall below the proposed insertion site with a towel clip and rely on counterpressure from the costal margin to elevate the cephalad portion. Make an incision and insert the Veress needle, checking for peritoneal entry in the usual fashion. Insert a laparoscope and explore the abdomen. An angled laparoscope facilitates inspection of the anterior abdominal wall.

The hernia may contain omentum or bowel that is adherent to the sac. Place secondary ports and gently attempt to reduce the contents into the abdomen (Fig. 49.1B). Divide omental adhesions with cautery or ultrasonic scalpel. Often, the abdominal expansion caused by the pneumoperitoneum will have reduced the hernia. Inspect the undersurface of the anterior abdominal wall and identify all defects; frequently, multiple defects are present.

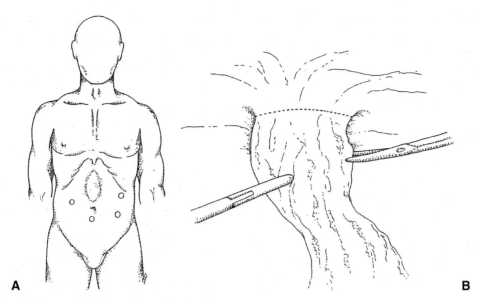

A   **B**

Figure 49.1 Initial entry and lysis of adhesions (**A** and **B** from Larson GM. Laparoscopic repair of ventral hernia. In: Scott-Conner CEH, ed. *The SAGES Manual.* New York, NY: Springer Verlag; 1999:379–385, with permission).

Preparing and Securing the Patch (Fig. 49.2)

Technical and Anatomic Points

Take a small-gauge spinal needle and pass it through the abdominal wall at the approximate edge of the hernia defect to confirm that the skin location corresponds to the actual edge of the fascial defect. Mark this point on the skin with a skin marking pen. Repeat the procedure at several points around the circumference, producing a map on the skin surface of the underlying fascial defect. Repeat this procedure for any additional defects (Fig. 49.2A).

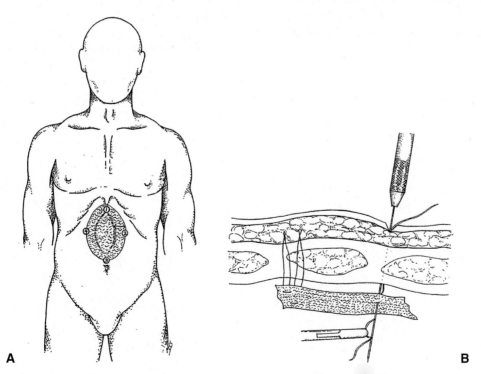

A   **B**

Figure 49.2 Preparing and securing the patch (**A** and **B** from Larson GM. Laparoscopic repair of ventral hernia. In: Scott-Conner CEH, ed. *The SAGES Manual.* New York, NY: Springer Verlag; 1999:379–385, with permission).

Cut a dual mesh patch large enough to cover all defects with an overlap of 2 cm on each side. Unless the shape is circular, mark the four corners as 1, 2, 3, and 4 with a skin marker. Mark the side that should face the peritoneal surface (and hence be visible to the laparoscope) as well. Mark the corresponding corners on the skin with the same numbers. Confirm that the mesh will be properly oriented, with the peritoneal surface facing the omentum and bowel and with the appropriate corners matched.

Place a horizontal mattress suture through each of the four corners of the mesh. Mark the locations on the skin where these sutures should exit when the mesh is properly situated. Then roll the mesh up into a narrow cylinder and introduce it through a trocar. Unroll the mesh and orient it so that the numbers correspond and the proper side of the mesh faces the bowel. There will be a tendency for the mesh to obscure visualization, much like a sail. Work with the two corners closest to the laparoscope first.

Select the first corner. Make a skin incision about 1 cm in length over the site previously identified. Pass a needle passer through the incision and the fascia at one side of the incision. Maneuver one end of the suture into the needle passer and bring it out through the abdominal wall. Do the same thing with the second end, taking care to allow about 1 cm of fascia between the two entry sites (Fig. 49.2B). Tie the knot; it should bury itself in the subcutaneous fascia. Observe through the laparoscope as you snug the knot down; the patch should rise to the abdominal wall and lie comfortably against it. Complete the knot, securing the first corner of the patch.

Repeat the process with the remaining three corners. The patch should now be secured against the abdominal wall, completely covering the defect. The peritoneal side of the mesh should face the intra-abdominal viscera.

Use a hernia tacking device to place tacks or staples between the four sutures so that there are no gaps through which bowel could herniate.

Withdraw the laparoscope. Close the trocar sites and skin incisions.

REFERENCES

1. Brill JB, Turner PL. Long-term outcomes with transfascial sutures versus tacks in laparoscopic ventral hernia repair: A review. *Am Surg.* 2011;77:458–465.
2. Deeken CR, Faucher KM, Matthews BD. A review of the composition, characteristics, and effectiveness of barrier mesh prostheses utilized for laparoscopic ventral hernia repair. *Surg Endosc.* 2012;26:566–575.
3. Fortelny RH, Petter-Puchner AH, Glaser KS, et al. Use of fibrin sealant (Tisseel/Tissucol) in hernia repair: A systematic review. *Surg Endosc.* 2012;26:1803–1812.
4. Gurusamy KS, Allen VB, Samraj K. Wound drains after incisional hernia repair. *Cochrane Database Syst Rev.* 2012;2:CD005570.
5. Larson GM. Laparoscopic repair of ventral hernia. In: Scott-Conner CEH, ed. *The SAGES Manual.* New York, NY: Springer Verlag; 1999:379–385.
6. LeBlanc KA. Laparoscopic incisional hernia repair: Are transfascial sutures necessary? A review of the literature. *Surg Endosc.* 2007;21:508–513. (Because transfascial sutures can cause chronic pain, alternatives have been sought. This article details alternatives and problems.)
7. Sauerland S, Walgenbach M, Habermalz B, et al. Laparoscopic versus open surgical techniques for ventral or incisional hernia repair. *Cochrane Database Syst Rev.* 2011;16:CD007781.
8. Selzer DJ. Taking LVHR beyond the learning curve. *Contemp Surg.* 2005;61:224–233.
9. Tong WM, Hope W, Overby DW, et al. Comparison of outcome after mesh-only repair, laparoscopic component separation, and open component separation. *Ann Plast Surg.* 2011;66:551–556.

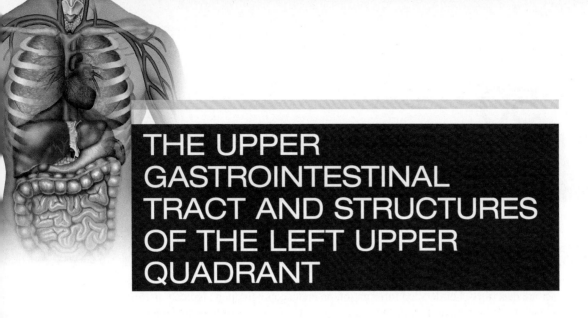

THE UPPER GASTROINTESTINAL TRACT AND STRUCTURES OF THE LEFT UPPER QUADRANT

It is evident that if the abdomen is divided into quadrants, the left upper quadrant includes more than the upper gastrointestinal tract and spleen (such as the pancreas) and that the pylorus and duodenum pass out of this quadrant. Nevertheless, it is convenient to group these structures together. Perhaps because these are the structures palpated when this region of the abdomen is manually explored (see Chapter 44), along with the left lobe of the liver, these structures are commonly considered together by surgeons.

The region of the lower esophagus, including the esophageal hiatus, stomach, duodenum, vagus nerves, and spleen, is described in this section. First, the procedure of upper gastrointestinal endoscopy (Chapter 50) is described to present the general topography of the esophagus, stomach, and duodenum as well as a view from inside. Hiatal hernia repair (Chapters 51–54) introduces the anatomy in the region of the esophageal hiatus, the opening in the diaphragm through which the esophagus enters the abdomen. Chapter 55 describes laparoscopic esophagomyotomy, continuing the description of the distal esophagus. The discussion of this region is concluded in the chapter on vagotomies (Chapter 65e).

The section on gastric surgery begins with the simplest procedure, feeding gastrostomy (Chapters 57 and 58e). Surgical, laparoscopic, and endoscopic techniques are described, and a related procedure, feeding jejunostomy, is included for convenience. Chapters on plication of perforated ulcers introduce the anatomy of the pylorus and the first portion of the duodenum as well as the subhepatic and subphrenic spaces from the traditional and laparoscopic approaches (Chapters 59 and 60). Gastric resections (Chapters 61 and 62), two operations performed for trauma, pyloric exclusion, and duodenal diverticulization (Chapter 66), and gastric procedures for obesity (Chapters 68 and 69), complete the discussion of anatomy and surgery of the stomach and duodenum (transduodenal sphincteroplasty and choledochoduodenostomy are included in the next part).

Finally, Chapters 70 and 71, open and laparoscopic splenectomy and splenorrhaphy (repair of injury), conclude the discussion of this region.

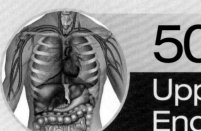

50

Upper Gastrointestinal Endoscopy

Upper gastrointestinal endoscopy, also known as esophagogastroduodenoscopy, is performed for diagnostic and therapeutic purposes. In this chapter, the endoscopic anatomy and the technical maneuvers necessary for safe visualization of the upper gastrointestinal tract are described. For detailed information on endoscopic findings, indications, and technique of biopsy, as well as therapeutic endoscopy of the upper gastrointestinal tract, the reader is referred to several excellent texts listed in the references.

SCORE™, the Surgical Council on Resident Education, classified esophagogastroduodenoscopy as an "ESSENTIAL COMMON" procedure.

STEPS IN PROCEDURE

Produce adequate topical anesthesia of the oropharynx

Intravenous sedation is generally used

Position patient with left side down

Gently introduce scope into mouth, with slight curve to facilitate passage into esophagus (controls unlocked)

The esophagus may be seen as a slit at the "base" of the "triangle" formed by the vocal cords

Pass the scope through the sphincter as the patient swallows

The esophageal lumen should then be visible—pass the scope under direct vision to the distal esophageal sphincter

Gentle pressure passes the scope into the stomach

Inflate the stomach with air and check all areas, including retroflexion to visualize the cardia

Hug the lesser curvature and pass through the pylorus to visualize the duodenum

Intraoperative small bowel endoscopy:
  Surgeon creates a balloon of air around the tip of the scope
  Pass the scope by gently reefing the bowel over the scope
  Mark any pathology with a fine silk suture on the outside of the bowel

HALLMARK ANATOMIC COMPLICATIONS

Perforation

Missed lesions resulting from incomplete examination

LIST OF STRUCTURES

Pharynx

Nasopharynx

Oropharynx

Laryngopharynx

Esophagus

Stomach

Cardia

Body

Fundus

Pylorus

Duodenum

Small intestine

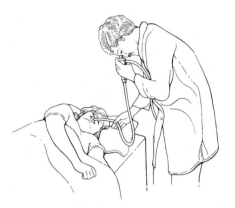
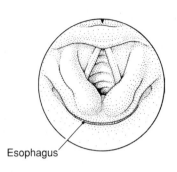

Esophagus

Figure 50.1 Position of the patient and initial passage of the endoscope

Position of the Patient and Initial Passage of the Endoscope (Fig. 50.1)

Technical Points

Thorough topical anesthesia of the pharynx is essential. This is best produced with the patient sitting facing the examiner and holding a basin.

The patient should then be placed in the left lateral decubitus position. Intravenous sedation is a useful adjunct and may be used at this point. In addition to the suction channel of the endoscope, a Yankauer suction apparatus should be available at the patient's head to avoid aspiration if the patient vomits.

Place a bite block over the endoscope. Check to make certain that the controls of the endoscope are not locked. Pass the endoscope into the posterior pharynx. Use the index and middle fingers of your nondominant hand to guide the endoscope and keep it in the midline. Ask the patient to swallow. Gently advance the endoscope as you feel the sphincter open as swallowing is initiated. Because this maneuver is done essentially blindly, it must be done gently. If the endoscope deviates from the midline, it will probably enter the left or right piriform sinus, a blind diverticulum. Forced attempts at passage may then result in perforation. Occasionally, the endoscope will enter the larynx; this generally results in coughing.

Anatomic Points

The pharynx, which is the vertical, tubular passage extending from the base of the skull to the beginning of the esophagus, is in open communication with the nasal, oral, and laryngeal cavities. It is customarily considered to have three components: The nasopharynx (superior to the soft palate), the oropharynx (the area extending from the soft palate superiorly to the hyoid bone inferiorly), and the laryngopharynx (the region extending from the hyoid bone to the lower border of the cricoid cartilage).

The nasopharynx communicates with the auditory tubes (whose ostia open into its lateral wall) and with the nasal cavities (through the choanae). The pharyngeal tonsils (adenoids) are located on the posterior wall of the nasopharynx. The cavity

of this portion of the pharynx is always patent and is the widest part of the pharynx.

The oropharynx, sometimes called the *posterior pharynx,* widely communicates anteriorly with the mouth, where the cavity faces the pharyngeal aspect of the tongue. The palatine tonsils are on the lateral wall between the anterior palatoglossal arch and the posterior palatopharyngeal arch. These lymphoid tissue masses, in conjunction with the pharyngeal tonsil in the nasopharynx and with the lymphoid tissue on the pharyngeal part of the tongue (lingual tonsil), form Waldeyer's ring. The oropharyngeal isthmus can be closed by approximation of the palatoglossal arches, accompanied by retraction of the tongue. This lingual movement also occludes the lumen of the oropharynx above the bolus during swallowing.

The laryngopharynx communicates anteriorly with the opening of the larynx. Lateral to the laryngeal aditus (inlet), on either side is an elongated fossa, the piriform recess. Inferiorly, the laryngopharynx is continuous with the esophagus. This junction is the narrowest part of the pharynx.

At the pharyngoesophageal junction, the pharyngeal musculature consists of the inferior pharyngeal constrictor, the thickest of the three pharyngeal constrictors. This muscle can be logically subdivided into a superior thyropharyngeus, whose fibers arise from the thyroid cartilage and are directed superomedially to insert on a posterior median raphe, and an inferior cricopharyngeus, whose fibers originate from the cricoid cartilage and pass horizontally to insert on the median raphe. During swallowing, contraction of the thyropharyngeus propels the bolus, whereas the cricopharyngeus acts as a sphincter. Failure of the cricopharyngeus to relax during swallowing can result in herniation of the mucosa between the two parts of the inferior constrictor (Zenker's diverticulum; see Chapter 12e), or a predisposition to perforation of the esophagus with the endoscope.

The Esophagus (Fig. 50.2)

Technical Points

After the endoscope is within the esophagus, visualize the lumen and advance the endoscope to the cardioesophageal

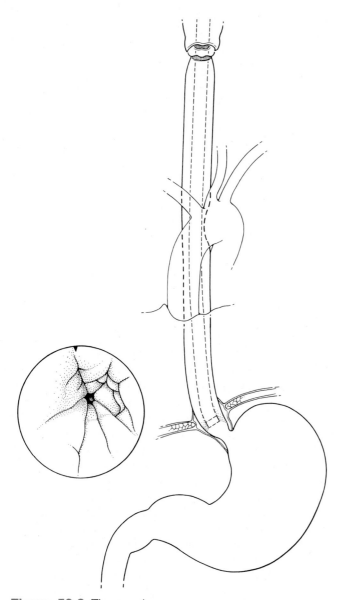

Figure 50.2 The esophagus

thorax just anterior to the vertebral bodies. It passes through the diaphragm at about the level of the tenth thoracic vertebra, and ends by opening into the cardia of the stomach at about the level of the eleventh thoracic vertebra. It lies in the median plane at its origin, but deviates slightly to the left until the root of the neck. At the root of the neck, it gradually deviates to the right so that, by the level of the fifth thoracic vertebra, it is once again midline. At the seventh thoracic vertebra, it again deviates to the left, and ultimately turns anteriorly to pass through the esophageal hiatus of the diaphragm. The thoracic esophagus also has anterior and posterior curves that follow the curvature of the vertebral column. The intra-abdominal esophagus turns sharply to the left to become continuous with the stomach.

The anatomic relationships of the esophagus are important. In the neck, the esophagus is posterior to the trachea and anterior to the cervical vertebra and the prevertebral muscles. Lateral to the cervical esophagus and trachea on both sides are the recurrent laryngeal nerve (in or near the tracheoesophageal groove), the common carotid artery, and the thyroid lobes. In the lower neck, the thoracic duct ascends to the left of the trachea. In the mediastinum, from superior to inferior, the esophagus has the following relationships.

Anterior: Trachea, left mainstem bronchus, right pulmonary artery, left atrium within the pericardial sac, and diaphragm

Posterior: Vertebral column and prevertebral muscles, right intercostal arteries of aortic origin, thoracic duct, azygos vein and the termination of the hemiazygos and accessory hemiazygos veins, and, as it approaches the diaphragm, the aorta

Right lateral: Right parietal pleura and intervening arch of the azygos vein and the right vagus nerve, which will principally form the posterior esophageal plexus

Left lateral: Left subclavian artery and thoracic duct, left recurrent laryngeal nerve, terminal portion of the aortic arch, left parietal pleura, left vagus nerve (which will principally form the anterior esophageal plexus), and the descending aorta

In the abdomen, the esophagus is anterior to the left crus of the diaphragm and the left inferior phrenic artery.

Four narrow areas of the esophagus are described. These are the cricoesophageal junction (15 cm from the incisors); the point at which the aortic arch crosses the esophagus (22 cm from the incisors); the point at which the esophagus is crossed by the left mainstem bronchus (27 cm from the incisors); and the point at which the esophagus traverses the diaphragm (40 cm from the incisors).

Although the distal esophageal sphincter cannot be identified anatomically, it can be demonstrated as a manometric high-pressure zone about 2 cm proximal to the gastroesophageal junction. Just distal to this physiologic sphincter, the gastroesophageal junction (ora serrata or Z line) can be recognized. The abrupt transition from esophageal squamous epithelium to gastric columnar epithelium is visualized endoscopically as a color change from gray-pink (esophageal mucosa) to yellow-orange (gastric mucosa).

junction under direct vision. This is a fairly straight shot and should require minimal motion of the controls. Periodic light puffs of air keep the lumen open and assist in the passage of the instrument. Recognize the cardioesophageal junction by the change in color at the squamocolumnar junction (the Z line). Generally, the cardioesophageal junction lies about 40 cm from the incisor teeth. The lower esophageal sphincter, a physiologic high-pressure zone without any consistent anatomic landmark, will generally be closed. Gentle pressure with the endoscope will allow the endoscope to pass into the stomach unless the distal esophagus is narrowed by a stricture or tumor.

Anatomic Points

The esophagus, which begins at the lower border of the cricoid cartilage, is about 25 cm long. It descends through the neck and

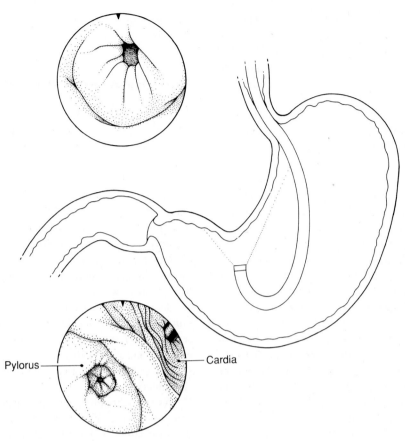

Figure 50.3 The stomach

The Stomach (Fig. 50.3)

Technical Points

First inflate the stomach by insufflating air, noting the mobility of the gastric walls as the stomach distends. Identify the gastric notch (incisura angularis) on the lesser curvature. Advance the scope to the notch. At this point, the scope may be passed distally toward the pylorus or retroflexed to visualize the cardioesophageal junction from below. It is helpful to think of a double-barreled configuration at this point. As you look at the incisure, one "barrel" is the view toward the pylorus and the second barrel is the retroflexed view up toward the cardia. Distention of the stomach with air pushes the greater curvature out and away from the incisure. The relatively fixed lesser curvature of the stomach looks like a septum, creating the double-barreled appearance. Slight changes in angulation of the tip of the endoscope will allow you either to proceed to the pylorus or to retroflex.

First retroflex the scope by entering the barrel leading back to the cardia. Push both control wheels away from you and pull back on the scope as you sharply angulate the tip. Look for the black tube of the endoscope as it emerges from the cardia. Twist and angulate the tip of the scope to visualize fully the cardia and fundus. Then return to the region of the incisure by advancing the scope and straightening the tip.

Identify the antrum by the relative paucity of folds. Advance the scope, hugging the lesser curvature, toward the pylorus and inspect the pylorus. Unless the pylorus is distorted by ulcer or tumor, it will open and close in a rhythmic fashion and will appear to be roughly circular. Advance the endoscope to visualize the pylorus face on. As the pylorus opens, gently push the scope through the pylorus. At this point, visualization of the lumen is generally lost as the scope enters the confines of the duodenal bulb. Note the numbers on the scope at the patient's incisor teeth. If a length of more than 60 cm of scope has been introduced, pull back on the scope gently to straighten the redundancy in the stomach.

Anatomic Points

The stomach is highly variable in its morphology and changes size and shape when full or empty. However, certain anatomic features can always, or almost always, be described. The greater curvature is directed to the left and inferiorly, whereas the lesser curvature is directed to the right and superiorly.

The esophagus opens into the stomach at the cardiac orifice. The immediate postesophageal part of the stomach is dilated in comparison to the esophagus and is referred to as the *cardiac antrum*. The left margin of the esophagus, at its junction with the stomach, makes an acute angle with the beginning of the greater curvature; this junction is the cardiac incisure. The fundus is that portion of the stomach that is superior to the cardiac incisure or cardiac notch. Along the lesser curvature, nearer to its distal end than to its proximal end, there is usually a distinct notch, the angular incisure. A line drawn from the angular incisure perpendicular to the axis of the stomach demarcates the proximal body from the distal, slightly dilated, pyloric antrum. The pyloric antrum is limited on the right by a slight groove, the sulcus terminalis. Immediately distal to the sulcus terminalis, the short segment of terminal stomach is termed the *pyloric canal*. The pyloric canal terminates at the pyloric sphincter, the restricted lumen of which is termed the *pyloric channel*. The pyloric channel is the terminal part of the stomach lumen and is continuous with the lumen of the duodenum.

Internally, the mucosa and submucosa of the stomach are characterized by thick folds and rugae. Along the lesser curvature and in the pyloric canal, the rugae are oriented longitudinally. It is the part of the lumen of the stomach that is referred to as the *gastric canal*. Elsewhere, the rugae assume a honeycomb pattern.

On endoscopic examination, the gastric notch can be identified as a crescentic fold projecting into the lumen from the lesser curvature. In passing the endoscope distally, the antrum is entered, identified on the basis that, here, as more distally, the relatively few rugae are aligned parallel to the longitudinal axis, rather than having a honeycomb appearance. The pylorus can be distinguished because the walls of the stomach converge at this point, severely restricting the diameter of the lumen, and a rhythmic opening and closing of the pyloric channel is noted. When the endoscope is retroflexed, the endoscope can be seen passing through the gastroesophageal sphincter, also characterized by a sudden reduction in luminal diameter as well as by the so-called cardiac rosette, which is a cluster of mucosal folds radiating from the gastroesophageal junction.

The Duodenum (Fig. 50.4)

Technical Points

Withdraw the endoscope slightly to advance the tip by straightening the scope in the stomach. After the scope is straight, advance it gently while insufflating air; the circumferential folds of the duodenum should be visible. If the scope pops out of the pylorus and back into the stomach, traverse the pylorus again. Clear bile is generally visible in the duodenum. The normal ampulla of Vater, frequently covered by a fold of mucosa, is rarely seen with the end-viewing endoscope. Pass the scope down the duodenum as far as possible, keeping in mind that most pathologic processes are found in the first and second portions of the duodenum.

As the scope is withdrawn, carefully inspect the duodenal bulb. This arrowhead-shaped chamber lacks the circular folds seen in the remainder of the duodenum. Because this region is small and poorly distensible, it may be necessary to make several passes through the pylorus to visualize this region adequately.

As you withdraw the scope, inspect the stomach and esophagus again. Use the suction channel of the endoscope to decompress the stomach when visualization is complete.

Anatomic Points

The duodenum, which is the widest, shortest, and most fixed portion of the small intestine, is usually 20 to 25 cm long. Beginning at the pylorus, it passes posteriorly, superiorly, and to the right

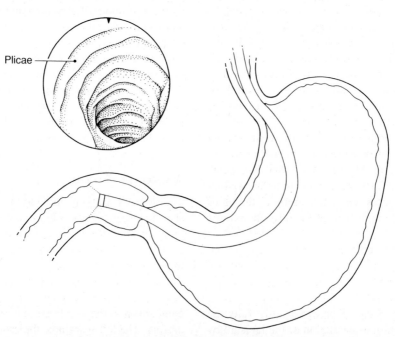

Plicae

Figure 50.4 The duodenum

(the first or superior part) for about 5 cm. This portion is comparatively mobile and is the duodenal bulb of radiologists. In contrast to the stomach, where the mucosa is yellow-orange, the mucosa of the duodenum is yellow-gray. Proximally, mucosal folds are lacking, but as the second part is approached, the beginnings of the characteristic plicae circulares of the small intestine appear.

The duodenum then makes an abrupt curve inferiorly, forming the superior duodenal flexure, and passes to the right of the vertebral bodies and head of the pancreas for a distance of 8 to 10 cm. This part, the second or descending portion, receives the united common bile and pancreatic duct (ampulla of Vater or hepatopancreatic ampulla), which has an oblique intramural path on the medial aspect of the duodenum. The ampulla of Vater opens on the summit of the major duodenal papilla, about 10 cm from the pylorus and often protected by a mucosal hood. Distal to the papilla, a single or bifid longitudinal mucosal fold can frequently be seen. Elsewhere, typical plicae circulares should be noted. About 2 cm proximal to the major duodenal papilla, a minor duodenal papilla may frequently be noted; at its apex, the accessory pancreatic duct (duct of Santorini) empties into the duodenum.

The third or horizontal portion of the duodenum starts at the inferior duodenal angle (flexure), another sharp bend to the left and across the vertebral bodies. The third portion is about 10 cm long, containing plicae circulares and nothing else of endoscopic or anatomic significance.

The ascending or fourth part of the duodenum is short (about 2.5 cm in length). Just before its termination, it makes an abrupt turn anteriorly to end at the duodenojejunal flexure. The duodenojejunal flexure is held in position by the suspensory muscle or ligament of the duodenum, commonly termed the *ligament of Treitz.*

The Postgastrectomy Stomach (Fig. 50.5)

Technical and Anatomic Points

Gastric surgery alters the appearance of the stomach. Pyloroplasty and partial gastrectomy using the Billroth I reconstruction both result in a patulous or nonexistent pylorus. (The Billroth I and II reconstructions are described in Chapter 53; pyloroplasty is described in Chapter 56.) Endoscopy in such situations proceeds normally, with the scope traversing a surgically altered "pylorus" to enter the duodenum. Pay special attention to the appearance of the anastomosis (if it can be identified). Generally, only the first portion of the duodenum will have been altered surgically.

A Billroth II reconstruction can generally be recognized by a septum with two identifiable outlets (afferent and efferent limbs). Although it is often difficult to ascertain which limb is which, the afferent limb generally contains copious bile, whereas the efferent limb does not. Cannulate and inspect both limbs.

A simple gastrojejunostomy (with antrum and pylorus left in situ) has a similar endoscopic appearance, but frequently, the antrum and pylorus can also be identified.

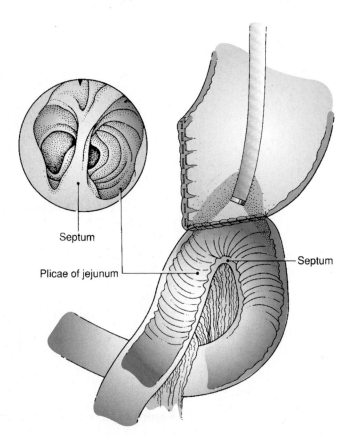

Figure 50.5 The postgastrectomy stomach

Intraoperative Upper Gastrointestinal Endoscopy (Fig. 50.6)

Technical Points

Operative upper gastrointestinal endoscopy is performed when urgent laparotomy for upper gastrointestinal bleeding of unknown origin is necessary. It is particularly helpful for identifying bleeding sites within the small intestine.

Safe passage of the endoscope in an unconscious, intubated patient requires skill and a firm but gentle touch. The anesthesiologist must hold and guard the endotracheal tube against accidental dislodgment. Pass your nondominant hand deep into the posterior pharynx above the endotracheal tube and displace the endotracheal tube, mandible, and tongue anteriorly. Pass the scope into the posterior pharynx and guide it in the midline between the fingers of the nondominant hand. An indwelling esophageal stethoscope or nasogastric tube can sometimes be "followed" into the esophagus, but this is not always easy.

Traverse the upper esophageal sphincter by applying gentle pressure and pass the scope as previously described (Figs. 50.2–50.5). Remember that endoscopic relationships will be altered by the supine position of the patient. If the abdomen is open, the inflated stomach will rise up into the wound, further distorting the angle between the stomach and the duodenum; moreover, the pylorus will appear to lie much more posterior than usual.

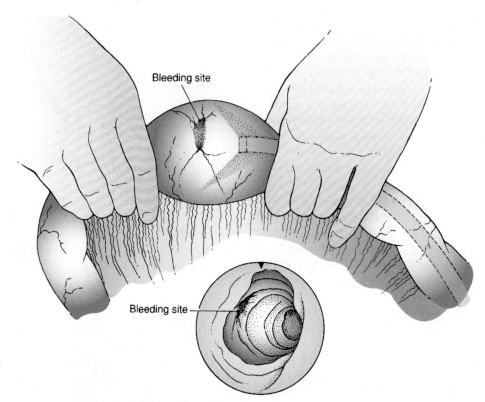

Figure 50.6 Intraoperative upper gastrointestinal endoscopy

An assistant within the sterile field of the abdomen should gently compress the proximal jejunum to limit passage of air into the small bowel. If the small bowel is allowed to become distended with air, closure of the abdomen will be difficult. If no source of bleeding is found proximal to the ligament of Treitz, endoscopy of the small intestine is often helpful. Often, the assistant can facilitate passage of the scope around the duodenum and into the proximal small intestine. A long scope, such as a colonoscope, can be passed by mouth and threaded through the small intestine to the ileocecal valve. The assistant should use both hands to "reef" the intestine over the scope as it is advanced. It is unnecessary and undesirable to distend the entire small intestine with air. Have your assistant maintain a sausage-shaped segment of air-filled intestine at the tip of the scope by occluding the bowel proximally and distally using gentle digital pressure. Look through the scope for fresh bleeding as the assistant inspects the transilluminated serosal surface of the intestine for prominent vessels or other abnormalities. Have your assistant mark any suspicious areas with silk sutures.

Anatomic Points

The predominant feature of the entire small bowel will be the plicae circulares. In addition, the diameter of the small bowel will be noted, both endoscopically and directly, to decrease progressively from the beginning of the jejunum to the ileocecal valve.

REFERENCES

1. Freeman RK, Ascioti AJ, Mahidhara RJ. Palliative therapy for patients with unresectable esophageal carcinoma. *Surg Clin North Am.* 2012;92:1337–1351.
2. Holster IL, Kuipers EJ. Management of acute nonvariceal upper gastrointestinal bleeding: Current policies and future perspectives. *World J Gastroenterol.* 2012;18:1202–1207.
3. Jairath V, Barkun AN. Improving outcomes from acute upper gastrointestinal bleeding. *Gut.* 2012;61:1246–1249.
4. Laine L, Jensen DM. Management of patients with ulcer bleeding. *Am J Gastroenterol.* 2012;107:345–360.
5. Mellinger JD, Ponsky JL. Endoscopic evaluation of the postoperative stomach. *Gastrointest Endosc Clin N Am.* 1996;6:621–639. (Gives specific pointers relevant to postsurgical anatomy.)
6. Pearl RK, ed. *Gastrointestinal Endoscopy for Surgeons.* Boston: Little, Brown; 1984:21.
7. Richardson JF, Lee JG, Smith BR, et al. Laparoscopic transgastric endoscopy after Roux-en-Y gastric bypass: Case series and review of the literature. *Am Surg.* 2012;78:1182–1186. (Describes a way to access the bypassed stomach and duodenum).
8. Stanley AJ. Update on risk scoring systems for patients with upper gastrointestinal haemorrhage. *World J Gastroenterol.* 2012;18:2739–2744.

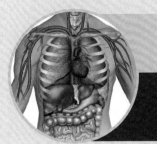

51

Hiatal Hernia Repair

The purpose of hiatal hernia repair is to generate a functional lower esophageal sphincter mechanism that will effectively prevent reflux of gastric contents into the esophagus but will allow swallowing, belching, and vomiting.

Most hiatal hernia repairs are now performed laparoscopically (see Chapter 53). Open repair is still necessary when the laparoscopic approach fails or is not feasible. The transabdominal Nissen procedure is presented in this chapter. For this repair, a 360-degree wrap of gastric fundus is placed around the distal esophagus, producing a functional valve. As intragastric pressure increases, the pressure in the wrap increases as well, closing off the distal esophagus. The open management of paraesophageal hernias is described in Chapter 52, and other surgical techniques for hiatal hernia repair are detailed in the references.

SCORE™, the Surgical Council on Resident Education, classified open antireflux procedure as an "ESSENTIAL UNCOMMON" operation.

STEPS IN PROCEDURE

Expose esophageal hiatus (this may require mobilizing the left lobe of the liver)
Incise the peritoneum over the esophagus
Gently isolate the esophagus from surrounding tissues and pass Penrose drain behind it
Divide short gastric vessels to fully mobilize fundus of stomach
Pass dilator transesophageally (or place dilator in operative field—see below)

Pass stomach behind esophagus
Place Hegar dilator next to esophagus (if dilator not passed previously)
Suture stomach to itself over esophagus and dilator
Anchor with one or two sutures that include esophageal wall

HALLMARK ANATOMIC COMPLICATIONS

Injury to esophagus
Injury to vagus nerves
Injury to spleen

Bleeding from short gastric vessels
Entry into either or both pleural cavities

LIST OF STRUCTURES

Xiphoid process
Costal margin

Diaphragm
Median arcuate ligament
Esophageal hiatus
Mediastinum
Pericardium
Phrenic nerve
Left and right pleural cavities
Thoracic duct
Inferior vena cava

Aorta
Left inferior phrenic artery (and vein)

Celiac trunk
Left gastric artery
Splenic artery
Short gastric arteries
Left gastroepiploic artery
Superior epigastric artery

Liver
Left lobe
Left triangular ligament
Esophagus

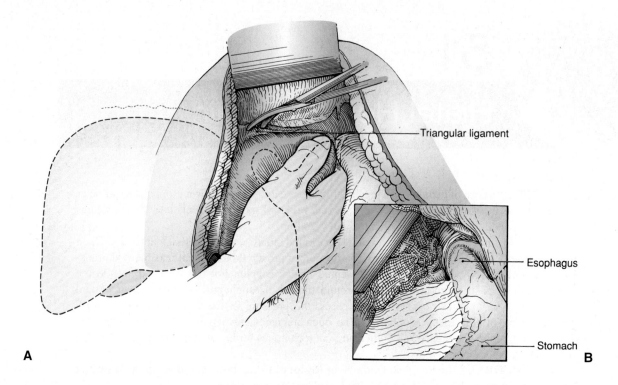

Figure 51.1 Exposure of the cardioesophageal junction. **A:** Mobilize the left lobe of the liver to expose the hiatus. **B:** With the liver retracted, incise the lesser omentum along the esophagogastric junction.

Exposure of the Cardioesophageal Junction (Fig. 51.1)

Technical Points

The right-handed surgeon should stand on the right side of the patient. Make an upper midline laparotomy incision. Extend the incision up and to the left of the xiphoid process for a little additional exposure. Clamp and ligate the small vessels that are frequently encountered in the angle between the xiphoid and the costal margin. Do not divide the xiphoid: This adds little to the exposure and may stimulate heterotopic bone formation within the incision. Explore the abdomen and confirm the position of a nasogastric tube at the cardioesophageal junction. Place a fixed retractor (such as the Omni system) to provide strong cephalad retraction of the left costal margin, placing additional blades to hold the incision open in the midportion. If this type of retractor is not available, a satisfactory alternative is an "upper-hand" type of retractor in the left upper margin of the incision and a Balfour retractor in the middle of the incision. Reverse Trendelenburg position assists as gravity pulls the upper abdominal viscera caudad into the field.

In most cases, adequate exposure can be obtained by placing a liver blade under the left lobe and retracting it upward. If this exposure is not sufficient, mobilize the left lobe of the liver by incising the triangular ligament. Pass your left hand around the inferior edge of the left lobe of the liver, grasp it, and pull down. The triangular ligament will be seen as a thin, tough, membranous structure passing along the posterosuperior aspect of the liver. Divide the small vessel at the free edge

between hemoclips. Use electrocautery to divide the triangular ligament. As you progress to the right, an anterior and posterior leaf of the triangular ligament will become apparent, with loose areolar tissue between. At this point, continue the dissection cautiously with Metzenbaum scissors until the left lobe of the liver can be folded down to expose the cardioesophageal junction. Place a moist laparotomy pad and Harrington retractor over the left lobe of the liver to hold it out of the way.

The inferior aspect of the diaphragm and the cardioesophageal junction should now be clearly visible. Confirm the location of the esophagus by palpating the nasogastric tube, which is anterior and a little to the left of the aorta at the esophageal hiatus. Incise the peritoneum overlying the cardioesophageal junction to expose the esophagus. Take care to avoid injury to the vagal nerve trunks.

Anatomic Points

Anteriorly, the diaphragm arises from the inner surface of the xiphoid process by two fleshy slips (sternal origin). Its costal origin is from the inner surfaces of the costal cartilages and adjacent bone of ribs 7 to 12. The costal cartilage of the seventh rib is the last to attach directly to the sternum at the xiphisternal articulation. The superior epigastric artery, a terminal branch of the internal thoracic (mammary) artery, enters the sheath of the rectus in the interval (termed the *foramen of Morgagni* or *space of Larrey*) between the sternal and costal origins of the diaphragm. This "defect" permits a retrosternal or parasternal hernia to occur. A paraxiphoid incision, then, will almost assuredly sever the superior epigastric artery or its branches. The artery anastomoses with the inferior epigastric artery in the substance of the rectus abdominis muscle and its division are of no consequence if bleeding is controlled.

Divide the free edge of the left triangular ligament between clamps. This ligament often contains vascular structures and may have both bile canaliculi (80%) and liver stroma (60%) present. Medially, the posterior layer of the left triangular ligament is continuous with the mesoesophagus, a more or less vertically disposed peritoneal reflection. Thus careful division of the left triangular ligament should lead one to the esophagus.

Divide the peritoneum at the cardioesophageal junction, taking care to avoid the anterior and posterior vagal trunks. Typically (88% of the time), there are a single anterior vagal trunk and a single posterior vagal trunk at the esophageal hiatus. Both trunks lie to the right of the esophageal midline, with the anterior vagal trunk lying on the esophagus and the posterior vagal trunk lying either immediately posterior to the esophagus or up to 2 cm to the right of the esophagus; thus, great care must be taken to avoid trauma to the vagi, especially the posterior vagal trunk.

Mobilization of the Esophagus (Fig. 51.2)

Technical Points

Mobilize the distal esophagus by blunt dissection in the mediastinum. Do not clear much of the lesser curvature of the stomach because tissue here will help to prevent the wrap from slipping. Encircle the mobilized esophagus and vagal trunks with a long Penrose drain to assist in subsequent dissection.

Anatomic Points

Dissection into the mediastinum requires some knowledge of the anatomy of the region of the esophageal hiatus, both on the abdominal and on the thoracic side of the diaphragm. The left inferior phrenic artery and vein lie on the left crus of the diaphragm and pass behind the esophagus. Occasionally, the left phrenic vein passes anterior to the esophageal hiatus, terminating in the inferior vena cava. The median arcuate ligament separates the aortic hiatus from the esophageal hiatus. The celiac trunk arises from the aorta in the region of the arcuate ligament. The inferior vena cava lies on the right crus of the diaphragm. The thoracic duct lies in areolar and adipose tissue just to the right of the aorta.

Superior to the esophageal hiatus, the right and left pleurae are approximated between the esophagus and the aorta, forming a mesoesophagus. This is a rather broad ligament, with an abundance of areolar tissue between the left and right pleurae. If perforation occurs, it is usually the right pleural cavity that is compromised because this is in contact with the lower esophagus, whereas the left is somewhat more removed. Only rarely are both pleural cavities perforated. The pericardial sac is immediately anterior to the esophagus at the level of the esophageal hiatus, and the left phrenic nerve is just to the left of the pericardium. Blunt dissection should not harm either of

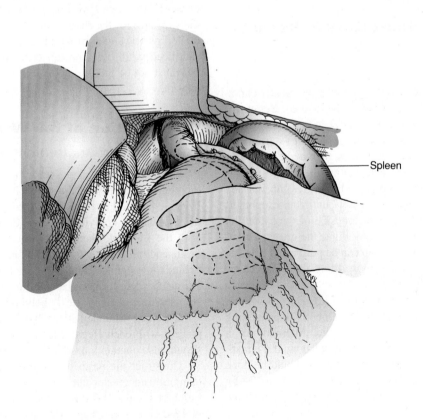

Figure 51.2 Mobilization of the esophagus

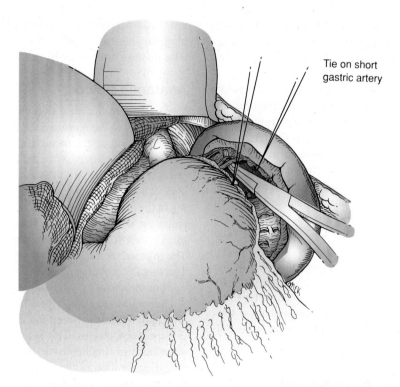

Figure 51.3 Division of the short gastric vessels

Tie on short gastric artery

these structures; however, later, if the anterior margin of the hiatus is to be approximated, care must be taken not to include them in the suture.

Division of the Short Gastric Vessels (Fig. 51.3)

Technical Points

Three or four short gastric vessels that tether the greater curvature of the stomach to the spleen must be divided. Begin this dissection at the lowest short gastric vessel and progress toward the esophagus. Identify the point on the greater curvature where the right gastroepiploic artery terminates, then make a window into the lesser sac by dividing and ligating the pair of vessels above. Through this window, continue to progress up, serially clamping, dividing, and ligating vessels until the esophagus is reached. Take care not to tear the capsule of the spleen by excessive traction on the stomach. Mobilize the greater curvature fully to ensure that a good wrap can be performed. Elevate the stomach and esophagus to expose filmy gastropancreatic folds. Divide these sharply.

The wrap is generally performed over a calibrated bougie. There are two ways to accomplish this. One involves passing a 40-French esophageal dilator from above. Alternatively, a Hegar dilator may be placed next to the esophagus. If a Hurst–Maloney dilator is to be passed from above, it should be done at this time and its position within the esophagus confirmed by direct palpation. Generally, it will be necessary to remove the nasogastric tube.

Anatomic Points

The short gastric arteries are branches of the splenic artery or one of its terminal divisions. These arteries run through the gastrosplenic (lienogastric) ligament to supply the fundus; in the substance of the fundus, they anastomose with branches of the left gastric and gastroepiploic arteries. These arteries can be sacrificed within the substance of the gastrosplenic ligament, but must not be pulled for fear of avulsing the delicate splenic capsule.

Construction of the Wrap (Fig. 51.4)

Technical and Anatomic Points

Pass a Babcock clamp posterior to the esophagus and grasp the greater curvature of the stomach, well down into the mobilized segment. Feed the mobilized greater curvature behind the esophagus, applying only gentle traction on the stomach with the Babcock clamp. Pull down and out on the Penrose drain, encircling the esophagus to facilitate passage of the wrap behind the esophagus and above the cardioesophageal junction. Do not hesitate to mobilize additional greater curvature if the stomach does not pass easily behind the esophagus.

If a Hurst–Maloney dilator has not been passed from above, place a 40-French Hegar dilator next to the esophagus (which should also contain a nasogastric tube).

Construct the wrap by suturing stomach on the left side to mobilized greater curvature on the right with four or five Lembert sutures of 0-0 or 2-0 silk. The lower two sutures may include bites of esophagus, but should not enter the esophageal

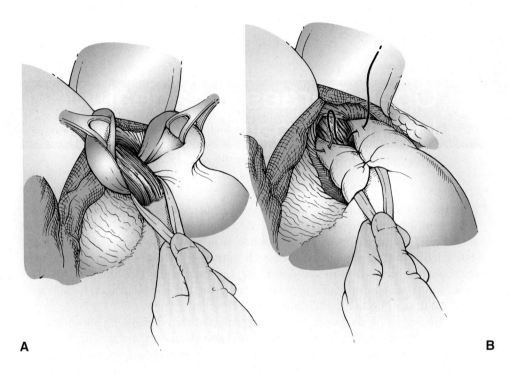

A   B

Figure 51.4 Construction of the wrap. **A:** With the esophagus retracted inferiorly, pull the fundus behind the esophagus to create a floppy wrap. **B:** The top suture incorporates a bite of esophageal muscle, to anchor the wrap.

lumen. Tie the sutures, confirming that the wrap is patulous and not under tension. Remove the Hegar or Hurst–Maloney dilator. Reinsert the nasogastric tube, if it was removed earlier. Check hemostasis and close the abdomen.

REFERENCES

1. Deschamps C, Trastek VF, Allen MS, et al. Long-term results after reoperation for failed antireflux procedures. *J Thorac Cardiovasc Surg.* 1997;113:545–550.
2. Draaisma WA, Rijnhart-de Jong HG, Broeders IA, et al. Five-year subjective and objective results of laparoscopic and conventional Nissen fundoplication: A randomized trial. *Ann Surg.* 2006; 144:34–41.
3. Gray SW, Rowe JS Jr, Skandalakis JE. Surgical anatomy of the gastroesophageal junction. *Am Surg.* 1979;45:575–587.
4. Horgan S, Pohl D, Bogetti D, et al. Failed antireflux surgery: What have we learned from reoperations? *Arch Surg.* 1999;134:809–815.
5. Houghton SG, Deschamps C, Cassivi SD, et al. The influence of transabdominal gastroplasty: Early outcomes of hiatal hernia repair. *J Gastrointest Surg.* 2007;11:101–106.
6. Luostarinen ME, Isolauri JO. Randomized trial to study the effect of fundic mobilization on long-term results of Nissen fundoplication. *Br J Surg.* 1999;86:614–618.
7. McLean TR, Haller CC, Lowry S. The need for flexibility in the operative management of type III paraesophageal hernias. *Am J Surg.* 2006;192:e32–e36.
8. Ohnmacht GA, Deschamps C, Cassivi SD, et al. Failed antireflux surgery: Results after reoperation. *Ann Thorac Surg.* 2006;81: 2050–2053.
9. Peillon C, Manouvrier JL, Labreche J, et al. Should the vagus nerves be isolated from the fundoplication wrap? A prospective study. *Arch Surg.* 1994;129:814–818.
10. Peters MJ, Mukhtar A, Yunus RM, et al. Meta-analysis of randomized clinical trials comparing open and laparoscopic antireflux surgery. *Am J Gastroenterol.* 2009;104:1548–1561.
11. Polk HC Jr. Fundoplication for reflux esophagitis: Misadventures with the operation of choice. *Ann Surg.* 1976;183:645–652. (Provides excellent review of technical pitfalls.)
12. Richardson JD, Larson GM, Polk HC Jr. Intrathoracic fundoplication for shortened esophagus: Treacherous solution to a challenging problem. *Am J Surg.* 1982;143:29–35.
13. Rieger NA, Jamieson GG, Britten-Jones R, et al. Reoperation after failed antireflux surgery. *Br J Surg.* 1994;81:1159–1161.
14. Salminen PT, Hiekkanen HI, Rantala AP, et al. Comparison of long-term outcome of laparoscopic and conventional Nissen fundoplication: A prospective randomized study with an 11-year follow-up. *Ann Surg.* 2007;246:201–206.
15. Wald H, Polk HC Jr. Anatomical variations in hiatal and upper gastric areas and their relationship to difficulties experienced in operations for reflux esophagitis. *Ann Surg.* 1983;197:389–392.

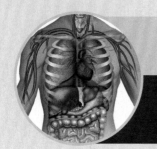

52

Open Paraesophageal Hernia Repair

Kevin A. Bridge and Hui Sen Chong

The vast majority of patients with paraesophageal hernias are asymptomatic. However, for those who are symptomatic despite medical treatment, surgical repair should be undertaken. The goal of operative intervention is to reduce the herniated contents and create a functional lower esophageal sphincter to prevent further reflux. In this era, most paraesophageal hernias repairs are performed laparoscopically (see Chapter 54). This chapter will present the operative steps for a transabdominal paraesophageal hernia repair with a 360-degree Nissen fundoplication.

Paraesophageal hernias occur due to enlargement of the esophageal hiatus in the diaphragm with herniation of intra-abdominal viscera into the thoracic cavity. The three common types of hiatal hernias is shown in Figure 52.1. Note that the pure paraesophageal hernia (type II), in which the gastroesophageal junction retains its normal anchorage posteriorly, is quite rare, accounting for only about 3% to 5% of hiatal hernias. There is also a type IV hernia, in which the defect is so large that essentially all of the stomach herniates up into the chest, sometimes with other viscera. All of these but type II involve displacement of the gastroesophageal junction with associated reflux. This is the rationale for adding an antireflux procedure to the hiatal repair.

SCORE™, the Surgical Council on Resident Education, has classified open repair of paraesophageal hernia as an "ESSENTIAL UNCOMMON" procedure.

STEPS IN PROCEDURE

Retract left lobe of liver exposing hiatus
Incise gastrohepatic and phrenoesophageal ligaments (please align them uniformly)
Dissection of hernia sac
Divide gastrosplenic ligament and ligate short gastric vessels
Mobilize distal esophagus
Close hiatal defect
Consider need for biologic mesh reinforcement
Pass fundus of the stomach behind esophagus
Insert bougie
Complete fundoplication
Consider need for anchoring wrap and gastric fixation

HALLMARK ANATOMIC COMPLICATIONS

Injury to:
    Esophagus
    Vagus nerves
    Stomach
    Colon
    Spleen
Bleeding from short gastric vessels
Excessively tight wrap
Herniation through hiatal defect

LIST OF STRUCTURES

Xiphoid process
Costal margin
Diaphragm
Esophagus
Esophageal hiatus
Liver
Left lobe of liver
Caudate lobe of liver
Left triangular ligament
Gastrohepatic ligament
Mediastinum
Stomach
Angle of His
Pericardium
Phrenic nerve
Vagus nerve
Left and right pleural cavities
Inferior vena cava
Aorta
Left and right gastroepiploic arteries
Short gastric arteries/veins
Splenic artery
Left inferior phrenic artery and vein
Left gastric artery

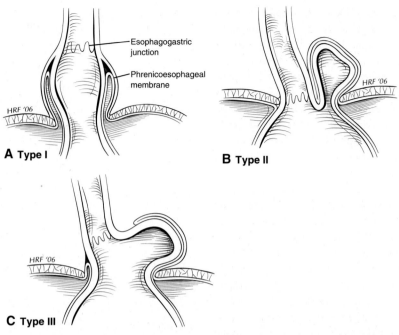

Figure 52.1 Types of hiatal hernia. **A:** Type I is a sliding hiatal hernia. **B:** Type II is a pure paraesophageal hernia. **C:** Type III is a combined sliding and paraesophageal hernia. Type IV (not shown) is a large hernia with most or all of the stomach and associated viscera in the chest. Figure reproduced from Melvin WS, Kyle A. Chapter 62, Open repair of paraesophageal hernia. In: *Fischer's Mastery of Surgery.* Philadelphia, PA: Wolters Kluwer Lippincott Williams & Wilkins; 2013:760.

Exposure of the Esophageal Hiatus

Technical Points

Position the patient supine with slight reverse Trendelenburg to allow gravity to provide retraction on the abdominal viscera. The primary surgeon should stand to the right of the patient. Make an upper midline laparotomy incision, extending it cephalad to the left of the xiphoid process, if necessary. Explore the abdomen, have an orogastric tube passed, and confirm placement within the stomach. Place a fixed retractor to provide cephalad retraction of the costal margins.

Identify the left lobe of the liver and retract it to expose the hiatus. If this maneuver does not provide adequate visualization of the hiatus, the left lobe may be further mobilized by incising the left triangular ligament (see Figure 51.1). The gastrohepatic ligament is identified. Seek and identify any anomalous hepatic vasculature and preserved it before incising the gastrohepatic ligament. After incising the gastrohepatic ligament, identify the esophagus by palpating the orogastric tube. Incise the peritoneum overlying the right crus to dissect the right crus away from the esophagus. This will allow entrance into the mediastinum for dissection of the hernia sac and reduction of the herniated viscera. General mobilization of the esophagus proceeds as outlined in Chapter 51, Figure 51.2 either at this point or after reduction of the sac (below).

Anatomic Points

The diaphragm is a dome-shaped muscle separating the thoracic and abdominal cavities. During respiration, the central portion of the diaphragm moves while the peripheral attachments of the diaphragm remain fixed. The diaphragm has three origins: The second and third lumbar vertebrae, the costal cartilage of ribs 7 to 12, and the inner part of the xiphoid process. The fibers of the diaphragm converge to form a trifoliate central aponeurosis named the central tendon. The inferior vena cava (IVC) passes through the central tendon to enter the heart.

The superior and inferior surfaces of the diaphragm are supplied by different vasculature. The superior surface of the diaphragm is supplied by the superior phrenic arteries and branches of the internal thoracic arteries (pericardiacophrenic and musculophrenic arteries). The inferior surface of the diaphragm is supplied by the inferior phrenic arteries which are branches of the abdominal aorta. The venous drainage of the superior surface is via the pericardiacophrenic and musculophrenic veins which ultimately drain back into the IVC. The inferior phrenic veins provide drainage of the inferior surface of the diaphragm via the IVC and the left suprarenal vein. The diaphragm is innervated by the phrenic nerve, which originates from the ventral rami of cervical nerves three, four, and five.

In about 65% of patients, the anomalous left hepatic artery that travels in the gastrohepatic ligament is a replaced left hepatic artery. They are easily identified in the gastrohepatic ligament if the surgeon is aware of this aberrant anatomy. When encountered, one should incise the gastrohepatic ligament above the aberrant artery, and extend the dissection toward the hiatus. Most of the time, the anomalous left hepatic artery is easily retracted out of the field, thus, allowing the surgeon to preserve the vascular supply to the left lobe of the liver. If the artery has to be ligated to allow for improved exposure of the hiatus, it can be temporarily clamped. This will allow the surgeon to evaluate for any ischemic changes in the left liver lobe before proceeding with its transection.

Most of the time, there is a single anterior and a single posterior vagal trunk at the esophageal hiatus. The left vagal trunk is usually found anterior to the esophagus, and could be partially embedded in the esophagus' muscular wall. The right vagal trunk lies posterior to the esophagus and has a more variable location. It usually lies within a 2 cm vicinity of the distal esophagus. In most patients, it is a band-like structure that travels separately from the distal portion of the esophagus. However, it could also be lying adjacent to the posterior portion of the esophagus. This anatomic variability, along with the mediastinal adhesions in the paraesophageal hernia cases, makes the right vagus nerve more susceptible to iatrogenic injury.

Dissection of Hernia Sac and Isolation of the Esophagus (Fig. 52.2)

Technical Points

Attempt to reduce the hernia by gentle traction on the stomach. Gentle manual downward traction on the stomach, as shown, facilitates this. It may be difficult to completely reduce the hernia especially with type III hernias. Dissect the right and left crura of the diaphragm away from the hernia sac. Incision of the peritoneum over the right crus allows entry into the right mediastinum. Free the hernia sac from the mediastinum with a combination of electrocautery and blunt dissection to completely reduce the herniated viscera. An incarcerated stomach can be friable; handle it with care to minimize iatrogenic injury.

Once the herniated viscera are reduced, mobilize the distal esophagus. Place a Penrose drain around the gastroesophageal junction to provide atraumatic retraction. This will aid in further circumferential mobilization of the distal esophagus to allow for adequate intra-abdominal esophageal length. The esophagus must be mobilized to the level of the aortic arch to allow the presence of adequate intra-abdominal esophageal length without tension.

To avoid inadvertent injury to the esophagus during mediastinal dissection, adhere to the following: (1) avoid direct grasping of the esophagus with a surgical instrument; (2) dissect away from the esophagus to minimize the risk of devascularizing it; (3) proper dissection in the anatomic plane, especially when attempting to create the retroesophageal window; (4) proper gentle passage of nasogastric tube or bougie. If you suspect a tear, test for air bubbles under saline. Repair the tear in a layered fashion and buttress it with the subsequent Nissen fundoplication.

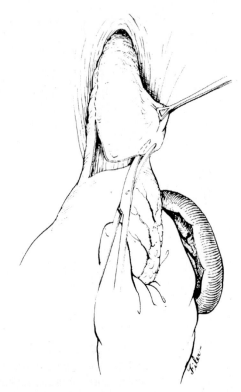

Figure 52.2 Gentle traction on the stomach is maintained while the sac is gradually reduced and dissected free of the mediastinum. Figure reproduced from Melvin WS, Kyle A. Chapter 62, Open repair of paraesophageal hernia. In: *Fischer's Mastery of Surgery*. Philadelphia, PA: Wolters Kluwer Lippincott Williams & Wilkins; 2013:760.

Anatomic Points

The esophageal hiatus is an oval-shaped aperture in which the esophagus and anterior and posterior vagal trunk passes through. In the majority of cases, it is formed from the muscle of the right crus at the level of T10 vertebra. Occasionally, the superficial bundle of the left crus contributes to the formation of the right border of the esophageal hiatus. The esophageal hiatus is superior to and to the left of the aortic hiatus. It is important to understand the location of the aorta during mobilization of the esophagus to prevent iatrogenic injury.

The esophageal wall is composed of striated muscle in the upper third, smooth muscle in the lower third, and a mixture of the two in the middle. Unlike the bowel, the esophagus has no serosa.

Mobilizing Greater Curvature of the Stomach (See Chapter 51, Figure 51.3)

Technical Points

Part of the greater curvature of the stomach is attached to the spleen by the gastrosplenic ligament. The short gastric vessels are located within the gastrosplenic ligament. The short gastric vessels must be ligated and transected to mobilize the greater curvature of the stomach in order to create a tension free Nissen fundoplication. The point where the right gastroepiploic artery terminates along the greater curvature of the stomach should be identified. A window into the lesser sac can be created by incising the gastrosplenic ligament at this level. Moving in a cephalad direction, the short gastric vessels within the gastrosplenic ligament can then be ligated until the angle of His is reached.

Anatomic Points

The greater omentum is a fold of peritoneum attached to the greater curvature of the stomach. It is anatomically divided into the gastrosplenic and gastrocolic ligaments. The stomach is perfused via multiple collateral blood vessels including the right and left gastric arteries, the right and left gastroepiploic arteries, and the short gastric arteries. The short gastric arteries and veins are branches of the splenic artery and vein. They course through the gastrosplenic and gastrocolic ligaments (divisions of the omentum) to anastomose with branches of the left gastric and left gastroepiploic arteries. The spleen is an end organ perfused mainly by the splenic artery which is a branch of the celiac trunk. There are multiple collateral vessels from the gastric, omental, and pancreatic arteries which perfuse the periphery of the spleen. Rare complications of splenic ischemia have been reported after ligation of the short gastric vessels during Nissen fundoplication.

Hiatal Repair, Fundoplication, and Gastropexy (Fig. 52.3)

Technical and Anatomic Points

After fully mobilizing the fundus of the stomach, identify the borders of the right and left crura. Remove the orogastric tube and Penrose drain and carefully pass a 56- to 58-French bougie into the stomach.

Select either primary or mesh repair based upon the surgeon's preference and the size of the defect. *Primary repair* is performed by carefully approximating the left and right crura with multiple simple interrupted nonabsorbable sutures. Carefully approximate the left and right crura behind the esophagus with multiple simple interrupted permanent sutures as shown in Figure 52.3A.

If the hiatal defect is large, consider *primary repair followed by mesh reinforcement*. Select a piece of biologic mesh and cut it to form a U-shaped patch around the esophagus for posterior reinforcement over the repaired hiatal defect (Fig. 52.3B). Alternatively, simply place a patch of mesh over the crural repair as shown in Figure 52.3C (this option is more commonly selected if a nonbiologic mesh is employed, to avoid mesh erosion into the esophagus).

Once the hiatus is reapproximated, perform a Nissen fundoplication by passing the mobilized fundus of the stomach behind the esophagus in a left to right direction (see Chapter 51, Figures 51.3 and 51.4). A shoeshine maneuver is performed to

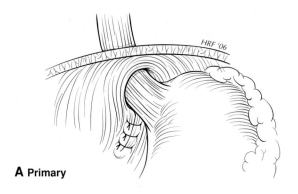

A Primary

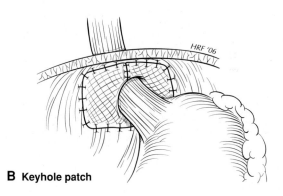

B Keyhole patch

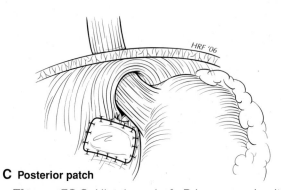

C Posterior patch

Figure 52.3 Hiatal repair. **A:** Primary repair with interrupted sutures. **B:** U-shaped reinforcement with mesh. **C:** Patch over hiatal repair only. Figure reproduced from Melvin WS, Kyle A. Chapter 62, Open repair of paraesophageal hernia. In: *Fischer's Mastery of Surgery.* Philadelphia, PA: Wolters Kluwer Lippincott Williams & Wilkins; 2013:760.

ensure the wrap is not twisted. The wrap is then constructed over the gastroesophageal junction and distal esophagus with approximately three 2-0 silk Lembert sutures. The Lembert sutures should incorporate superficial bites of the esophagus to anchor the wrap. Full thickness bites of the esophagus should be avoided since this can lead to an increased risk of a leak.

If the stomach is floppy, the surgeon may elect to perform an anterior gastropexy to reduce the risk of reherniation. The gastropexy may either be fixated using primary sutures to the anterior abdominal wall or by a gastrostomy tube. One study demonstrated a series of 28 patients who underwent repair with anterior gastropexy without any recurrences at 2-year follow-up.

Remove the bougie, attain hemostasis, and close the abdomen in the usual fashion. A nasogastric tube is not required. Some surgeons perform an esophagram ("swallow") on the first postoperative day as a baseline and to exclude leaks.

REFERENCES

1. Evans S. *Surgical Pitfalls: Prevention and Management.* 1st ed. Philadelphia, PA: Saunders Elsevier; 2009:175–189.
2. Ferri LE, Feldman LS, Stanbridge D, et al. Should laparoscopic paraesophageal hernia repair be abandoned in favor of the open approach? *Surg Endosc.* 2005;19:4–8.
3. Lee YK, James E, Bochkarev V, et al. Long-term outcome of cruroplasty reinforcement with human acellular dermal matrix in large paraesophageal hiatal hernia. *J Gastrointest Surg.* 2008;12:811–815.
4. Melvin WS, Kyle A. Chapter 62, Open repair of paraesophageal hernia. In: *Fischer's Mastery of Surgery.* Philadelphia, PA: Wolters Kluwer Lippincott Williams & Wilkins; 2013:760.
5. Moore KL, Dalley AF. *Clinically Oriented Anatomy.* Philadelphia, PA: Lippincott Williams & Wilkins; 1999:289–295.
6. Ponsky J, Rosen M, Fanning A, et al. Anterior gastropexy may reduce the recurrence rate after laparoscopic paraesophageal hernia repair. *Surg Endosc.* 2003;17:1036–1041.
7. Schauer PR, Meyers WC, et al. Mechanisms of gastric and esophageal perforations during laparoscopic Nissen fundoplication. *Ann Surg.* 1996;223:43–52.
8. Scott-Conner CE, Dawson DL. *Operative Anatomy.* 3rd ed. Philadelphia, PA: Lippincott Williams & Wilkins; 2009:319–323.
9. Wilkinson NW, Edwards K, Adams ED. Splenic infarction following laparoscopic Nissen fundoplications: Management strategies. *JSLS.* 2003;7(4):359–365.

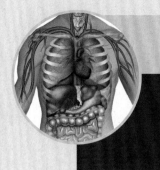

53

Laparoscopic Nissen Fundoplication and Hiatal Hernia Repair

Isaac Samuel

Patients with gastroesophageal reflux disease (GERD) who have failed medical therapy have developed complications of GERD (Barrett's esophagus, peptic stricture) or have persistent pulmonary symptoms are candidates for antireflux surgery. Some patients may opt for surgery in spite of the success of medication for reasons such as inconvenience or expense of medication or quality of life. Preoperative evaluation must include esophagogastroduodenoscopy to evaluate esophagitis, metaplasia, dysplasia, hiatal hernia, esophageal shortening and stricture, and for biopsies as needed. Esophageal manometry is not essential but may help to demonstrate a defective lower esophageal sphincter and to assess esophageal motility. A 24-hour pH study to confirm exposure of the lower esophageal sphincter to acid pH is essential only if esophagogastroduodenoscopy does not show esophagitis and if manometry is normal, but some surgeons perform this preoperative investigation routinely. A barium swallow is useful when a large hiatal hernia is associated with a shortened esophagus. A gastric emptying study helps evaluate patients undergoing revisions where vagal nerve injury may be suspected.

The laparoscopic Nissen fundoplication, described here, is a minimal access technique very similar to the open Nissen fundoplication (see Chapter 51), an operation that has proved highly successful and durable. Partial fundoplication is reported to have significantly lower incidence of dysphagia, bloating, flatulence, and reoperation rate compared after 5 years with total fundoplication, while achieving equivalent control of GERD, but long-term data are still awaited. Techniques of partial fundoplication are described in Chapter 55 (laparoscopic esophagomyotomy). The minimally invasive management of paraesophageal hernias is covered in Chapter 54. In morbidly obese patients (BMI > 35 kg/m^2) with GERD the Roux-en-Y gastric bypass is the procedure of choice as fundoplication has a high failure rate.

SCORE™, the Surgical Council on Resident Education, classified laparoscopic antireflux procedure as an "ESSENTIAL COMMON" procedure.

STEPS IN PROCEDURE

Obtain laparoscopic access—five ports are generally used

Retract liver up toward diaphragm

Assistant grasps esophageal fat pad and retracts it inferiorly to expose esophageal hiatus

Incise phrenoesophageal ligament and transparent portion of lesser omentum

Clean both left and right crura of overlying peritoneum, visualizing the vagus nerves and retracting esophagus gently

Pass instrument behind the esophagus, follow this with short segment of Penrose drain

Close defect in esophageal hiatus with interrupted sutures

Divide short gastric vessels

Pass bougie into stomach

Pass gastric fundus behind esophagus

Suture stomach to itself (include esophagus in two of these sutures)

Close trocar defects if indicated

HALLMARK ANATOMIC COMPLICATIONS

Injury to esophagus

Injury to vagus

Injury to stomach

Pneumothorax

Injury to spleen

Excessively tight wrap

Herniation through hiatal defect

Injury to inferior vena cava or aorta

> **LIST OF STRUCTURES**
>
> **Diaphragm**
> Crura, right and left
> Esophageal hiatus
> Phrenoesophageal ligament
> Gastrosplenic ligament
> Gastrophrenic ligament
>
> **Stomach**
> Fundus
> Mediastinum
>
> Left inferior phrenic artery (and vein)
> Short gastric arteries
> Esophagus
> Vagus nerves
>
> **Liver**
> Left lobe
> Segments II and III
> Caudate lobe (segment I)
> Left triangular ligament

Hiatal Dissection and Crural Closure (Fig. 53.1)

Technical and Anatomic Points

Five ports are used (Fig. 53.1A). The size of these ports depends on the instruments used. Five ports are usually needed, one for the camera, one for the liver retractor, one for the assistant, and two for the primary surgeon; if 5-mm instruments are available (e.g., 5-mm liver retractor, camera), correspondingly smaller trocars may be used.

Place the midline port for the laparoscope well above the umbilicus. This is crucial for adequate visualization of the hiatus. Use a 45-degree angled laparoscope for hiatal dissection. Place a right subcostal port along the anterior axillary line for a liver retractor (or epigastric incision for a Nathanson retractor), and a left subcostal port along the anterior axillary line for the assistant surgeon. The final two ports are inserted on either side of the camera port along the midclavicular line 3 inches below the costal margin. These allow the operating surgeon to work using both hands with good triangulation with the camera and operative field. Alternatively, the camera port may be placed to the left of the midline with both surgeon's ports in the right upper quadrant. Incline the patient into 35 to 45 degrees of reverse Trendelenburg position. Stand to the right side of the patient with the assistant to the left. Some surgeons prefer to stand in between the patient's legs with the patient in a modified lithotomy position.

Using a liver retractor, gently retract the left lobe of the liver up against the diaphragm. It is not necessary to divide the left triangular ligament. The stomach and undersurface of the diaphragm should come into view below the liver. A fat pad generally marks the gastroesophageal junction and obscures visualization of the esophagus.

The assistant surgeon grasps the esophageal fat pad and retracts it inferiorly to expose the phrenoesophageal membrane. When the hiatal defect is large, an opening into the chest will be seen. Divide the phrenoesophageal membrane to display the apex of the hiatus. Continue the dissection toward the right crus of the diaphragm, reducing any associated hiatus hernia (Fig. 53.1B). Focus attention on dissecting and defining the right crus of the diaphragm.

Divide the transparent part of the lesser omentum over the caudate lobe of the liver. Take care to avoid injury to the hepatic

branch of the anterior vagus nerve. Because some patients may have an aberrant left hepatic artery arising from the left gastric artery, exercise caution during this part of the dissection. With the stomach retracted inferiorly and to the left by the assistant surgeon, dissect the peritoneum off the abdominal surface and hiatal border of the right crus.

Gently dissect the loose connective tissue in the posterior mediastinum to visualize the distal esophagus. Next, gently displace the distal esophagus anteriorly and the right crus laterally to identify the right vagal nerve trunk. Use the shaft of an instrument to displace the esophagus gently forward; do not grasp it directly. Occult injury to the esophagus with peritonitis or mediastinitis is a potentially lethal complication. Similarly dissect and define the left crus of the diaphragm by working behind the esophagus from the right side, displacing the esophagus toward the anterior abdominal wall.

Retract the esophagus to the right to approach the left crus of the diaphragm from the left side. Retract the gastric fundus inferiorly and complete the circumferential dissection of the distal esophagus by dividing the peritoneum along the left crus of the diaphragm, the angle of His, and the gastric fundus. Retract the stomach carefully, by grasping the fundus very gently with atraumatic forceps; gastric perforations have occurred after vigorous retraction. Avoid injury to the phrenic vessels near the hiatus.

Pass a short segment of Penrose drain into the abdomen and use it to encircle the distal esophagus (Fig. 53.1C). Apply traction on this drain in such a way as to retract the esophagus anteriorly and to the left. Complete the hiatal dissection by cleaning away any loose connective tissue and defining the hiatal borders (Fig. 53.1D). To avoid pleural injury and resulting pneumothorax, do not transgress unnecessarily high into the posterior mediastinum.

Approximate the crura behind the esophagus with three to four interrupted nonabsorbable sutures, working from below upward (Fig. 53.1E). This step is generally omitted during open Nissen fundoplication if not associated with a significant hiatal hernia. It is required during the laparoscopic procedure because extensive crural dissection and lack of adhesion formation combine to permit postoperative herniation through the hiatus.

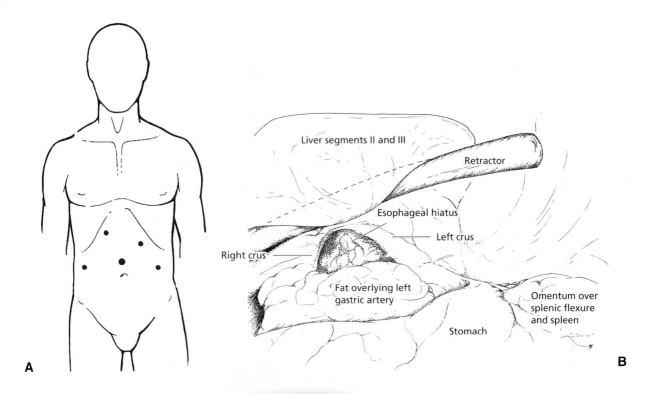

A

B

Liver segments II and III

Retractor

Esophageal hiatus

Left crus

Right crus

Fat overlying left gastric artery

Omentum over splenic flexure and spleen

Stomach

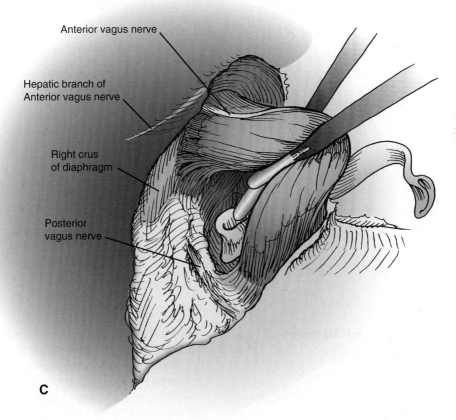

Anterior vagus nerve

Hepatic branch of Anterior vagus nerve

Right crus of diaphragm

Posterior vagus nerve

C

Figure 53.1 Hiatal dissection and crural closure (**B** and **D** from Scott-Conner C, Cuschieri A, Carter FJ. Diaphragm, hiatus, and esophagus. In: *Minimal Access Surgical Anatomy.* Philadelphia, PA: Lippincott Williams & Wilkins; 2000, with permission; **C** and **E** from Wind GG. The stomach. In: *Applied Laparoscopic Anatomy: Abdomen and Pelvis.* Baltimore, MD: Williams & Wilkins; 1997, with permission). (*continued*)

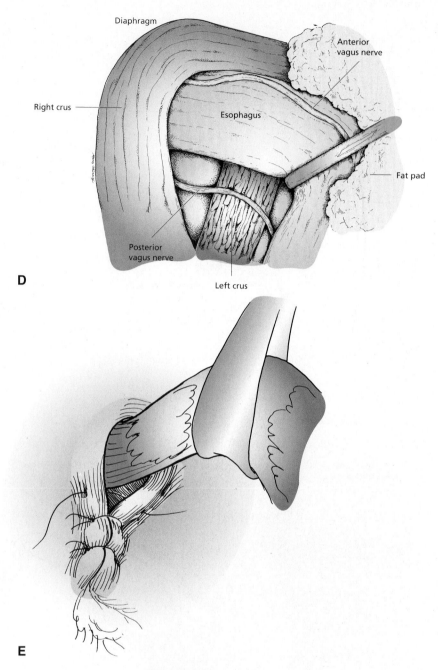

Diaphragm

Right crus

Esophagus

Anterior
vagus nerve

Fat pad

Posterior
vagus nerve

D

Left crus

E

Figure 53.1 *Continued*

Fundic Mobilization and Nissen Fundoplication (Fig. 53.2)

Technical and Anatomic Points

It is essential to mobilize the gastric fundus completely in order to produce a tension-free Nissen fundoplication. This entails meticulous division of the short gastric vessels (Fig. 53.2A), the gastrosplenic ligament, and the gastrophrenic ligament.

Retract the gastric fundus inferiorly and to the right. Begin dividing the short gastric vessels in the upper third of the greater curvature of the stomach and progress superiorly (Fig. 53.2B). The ultrasonic dissecting shears are ideal for this

purpose. Confirm that sufficient fundus has been mobilized by pulling it anteriorly across to the patient's right side.

Pass a Babcock forceps behind the esophagus and grasp the mobile portion of the fundus (Fig. 53.2C). Bring the posterior wall of the fundus behind the esophagus and around to the right side. Suture this to the anterior wall of the fundus in such a manner as to wrap the distal esophagus and gastroesophageal junction (Fig. 53.2D). Use nonabsorbable interrupted sutures. Include a bite of the esophagus with one stitch at the level of the gastroesophageal junction, and a second stitch placed 0.5 to 1 cm above it. Take care to avoid the left vagus nerve. Complete the wrap with an additional stitch

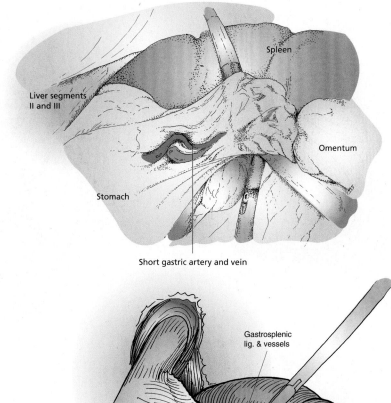

A

Short gastric artery and vein

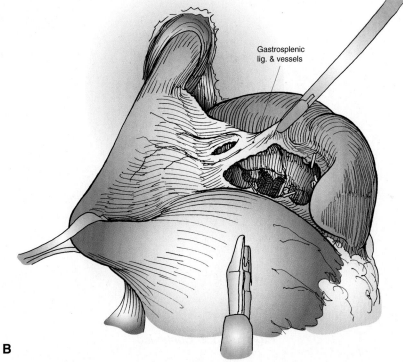

B

Figure 53.2 Fundic mobilization and Nissen fundoplication (**A** from Scott-Conner C, Cuschieri A, Carter FJ. Stomach and duodenum. In: *Minimal Access Surgical Anatomy.* Philadelphia, PA: Lippincott Williams & Wilkins; 2000, with permission; **B–D** from Wind GG. The stomach. In: *Applied Laparoscopic Anatomy: Abdomen and Pelvis.* Baltimore, MD: Williams & Wilkins; 1997, with permission; **E** from Scott-Conner C, Cuschieri A, Carter FJ. Diaphragm, hiatus, and esophagus. In: *Minimal Access Surgical Anatomy.* Philadelphia, PA: Lippincott Williams & Wilkins; 2000, with permission). (*continued*)

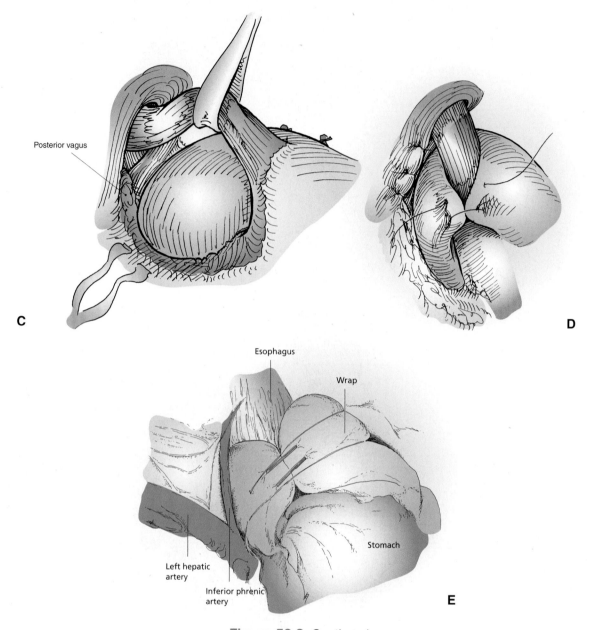

Figure 53.2 *Continued*

above, and one below, these sutures (Fig. 53.2E). Do not include the esophagus in these latter two sutures. The completed wrap should include both vagus trunks. Some surgeons leave the right (posterior) vagal trunk outside the wrap, but this tends to restrict the size of the posterior window. Use a 56-French bougie (+/−4F) to size the wrap, and do not create a wrap longer than 2 cm. If the wrap is too tight or too long, dysphagia may result. Avoid tension on the wrap by completely mobilizing the fundus. Ensure that the wrap is not twisted and that the posterior lip of the wrap has not been rendered ischemic by a narrow posterior window.

Remove the bougie and place a nasogastric tube. Suture the trocar sites closed if indicated.

REFERENCES

1. Allaix ME, Herbella FA, Patti MG. Laparoscopic total fundoplication for gastroesophageal reflux disease. How I do it. *J Gastrointest Surg.* 2012 Nov 6 (epub ahead of print).
2. Lubezky N, Sagie B, Keidar A, et al. Prosthetic mesh repair of large and recurrent diaphragmatic hernias. *Surg Endosc.* 2007;21: 737–741.
3. McKernan JB, Champion JK. Minimally invasive antireflux surgery. *Am J Surg.* 1998;175:271–276.
4. Mickevicius A, Endzinas Z, Kiudelis M, et al. Influence of wrap length on the effectiveness of Nissen and Toupet fundoplications: 5-year results of prospective, randomized study. *Surg Endosc.* 2013;27:986–991.

5. Peters JH, DeMeester TR, Crookes P, et al. The treatment of gastroesophageal reflux disease with laparoscopic Nissen fundoplication: Prospective evaluation of 100 patients with "typical" symptoms. *Ann Surg.* 1998;228:40–50. (Provides detailed description of patient selection, preoperative evaluation, surgical technique, and assessment of postoperative physiologic alterations.)

6. Peters JH, Heimbucher J, Kauer WK, et al. Clinical and physiologic comparison of laparoscopic and open Nissen fundoplication. *J Am Coll Surg.* 1995;180:385–393.

7. Ringley CD, Bochkarev V, Ahmed SI, et al. Laparoscopic hiatal hernia repair with human acellular dermal matrix patch: Our initial experience. *Am J Surg.* 2006;192:767–772.

8. Scott-Conner C, Cuschieri A, Carter FJ. Diaphragm, hiatus, and esophagus. In: *Minimal Access Surgical Anatomy.* Philadelphia, PA: Lippincott Williams & Wilkins; 2000. (Provides extensive illustration and description of regional laparoscopic anatomy.)

9. Trus TL, Peters JH. Gastroesophageal reflux disease. In: Zinner MJ, Ashley SW, eds. *Maingot's Abdominal Operations.* 11th ed. New York, NY: The McGraw-Hill Companies, Inc.; 2007: 231–270.

10. Varin O, Velstra B, De Sutter S, et al. Total vs partial fundoplication in the treatment of gastroesophageal reflux disease: A meta-analysis. *Arch Surg.* 2009;144:273–278. (This paper and several other useful publications are referenced on the Society of American Gastrointestinal and Endoscopic Surgeons' website under the "Publications" tab in "Guidelines for surgical treatment of GERD.")

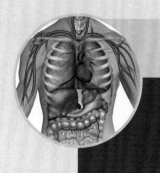

54

Laparoscopic Paraesophageal Hernia Repair

Hui Sen Chong and Samy Mokhtar Maklad

Paraesophageal hiatus hernias allow the stomach or other viscera to ascend through the hiatus into the mediastinum (see Chapter 52, Fig. 52.1). Laparoscopic repair is increasingly the preferred method, as it has less morbidity when compared to the open abdominal and thoracic approaches. The minimally invasive technique for repair described in this chapter follows the same principles as the open repair described in Chapter 52. The key principle of a successful paraesophageal hernia repair is as follows: Complete reduction of herniated viscera, adequate mobilization of the esophagus to allow 3 cm of distal esophagus to lie without tension in the abdominal cavity, tension-free crural repair, and an antireflux procedure. In this chapter we will only discuss the technical aspect of the laparoscopic paraesophageal repair; please consult Chapter 52 for the relevant anatomic points.

SCORE™, the Surgical Council on Resident Education, classified laparoscopic repair of paraesophageal hernia as an "ESSENTIAL UNCOMMON" procedure.

STEPS IN PROCEDURE

Obtain five-port laparoscopic access
Retract left lobe of liver exposing hiatus
Incise gastrohepatic and phrenoesophageal ligaments
Excise hernia sac and mediastinal adhesions
Reduce herniated viscera from chest
Expose and define right and left crura
Divide the short gastric vessels
Mobilize distal esophagus and create retroesophageal window
Assess esophageal length and need for modified Collis gastroplasty
Approximate esophageal hiatus with interrupted permanent sutures
Consider the need for biological mesh reinforcement
Perform Nissen fundoplication with bougie in place
Perform intraoperative esophagogastroduodenoscopy (EGD) if needed

HALLMARK ANATOMIC COMPLICATIONS

Injury to:
    Accessory or replaced left hepatic artery
    Left gastric artery
    Stomach
    Esophagus
    Vagus nerve
    Spleen
    Heart, lung, or aorta
Inadequate mobilization of esophagus
Inadequate closure of hiatus
Excessively tight wrap
Herniation through hiatal defect

LIST OF STRUCTURES

Diaphragm
    Left and right crura
    Esophageal hiatus
Gastrohepatic ligament
Accessory or replaced left hepatic artery
Gastrosplenic ligament
Short gastric arteries and veins
Fundus of the stomach
Pleura
Aorta
Esophagus
Left and right vagus nerves
Left lobe of liver (segments II and III)
Caudate lobe of liver (segment I)

Patient Positioning and Laparoscopic Port Placement (Figs. 54.1 and 54.2)

Technical Points

Position the patient in the modified lithotomy or split leg position with both arms extended. Perioperative antibiotics and SQ heparin should be administered. After padding all pressure points and securing the patient, a total of five laparoscopic ports using a combination of 5-mm and 10-mm trocars are positioned as follows. One supraumbilical 5-mm port to accommodate a 5-mm 30-degree laparoscope. Place this port about halfway between the xiphoid and the umbilicus, just slightly off to the left of the midline to avoid the falciform ligament. Place a 5-mm port at the right anterior axillary line, about 3 to 4 inches below the costal margin to accommodate a self-forming liver retractor.

Inspect the abdomen in the usual fashion. Place a liver retractor to elevate the left lobe of the liver to expose the hiatus and secure it to a stationary holding device (Fig. 54.2). In most patients, the liver retractor should provide adequate hiatal exposure and the left triangular ligament can be left in place. Next, position a 5-mm right and a 10-mm left subcostal port along the midclavicular lines. These are used as the main dissecting ports and should be placed as cephalad as possible to allow for dissection in the mediastinum. Place the 5-mm right subcostal port just to the left of the falciform ligament and below the lower

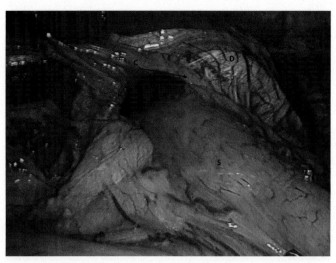

Figure 54.2 Exposure of the hiatus. With the left lobe of the liver (LL) elevated, one can identify the diaphragm (D), the caudate lobe (CL), the left and right crura (C), the left triangular ligament (LTL) as well as a large hiatal defect (HD). The portion of the herniated stomach (S) that is reducible is reduced back into the abdominal cavity.

edge of the elevated left liver lobe. Lastly, place a 5-mm port in the left anterior axillary line for the assistant.

If an additional port is needed for retraction, a second 5-mm port may be placed in the left lower quadrant region, just slightly lower than the camera port. The surgeon stands in between the legs to allow for ergonomic dissection, while the assistant stands on the left side of the table as shown in Chapter 46, Figure 46.1C.

Hiatal Dissection and Reduction of Gastric Fundus (Fig. 54.3)

Technical Points

Using atraumatic graspers passed through the main dissecting ports, gently reduce the easily reducible portion of the herniated stomach back into the abdominal cavity. The assistant provides lateral retraction to the herniated stomach while the surgeon divides the gastrohepatic ligament using the Harmonic scalpel (Fig. 54.3). The gastrohepatic ligament is the avascular tissue that joins the lesser curvature of the stomach to the liver. In 10% to 15% of the population, a replaced or accessory left hepatic artery arising from the left gastric artery may be present within the gastrohepatic ligament. It is easily identified as the vessel that travels horizontally within the gastrohepatic ligament. Oftentimes, the gastrohepatic ligament can be divided with the Harmonic scalpel, cephalad to the aberrant left hepatic artery. This maneuver will allow the artery to fall away from the surgical field while maintaining exposure of the hiatus. Take care also to avoid injury to the left gastric artery, which lies just posterior to the gastrohepatic ligament.

Next, further expose the right crus and define it from the right side by incising the right phrenoesophageal ligament (see Chapter 53, Figure 53.1). The phrenoesophageal ligament is the

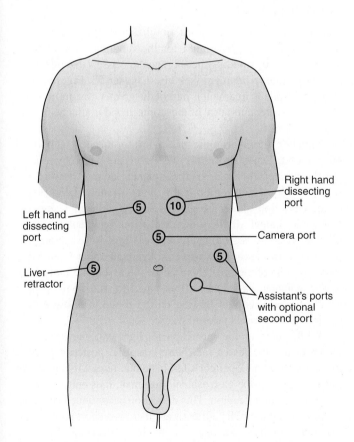

Left hand dissecting port

Liver retractor

Right hand dissecting port

Camera port

Assistant's ports with optional second port

Figure 54.1 Position of ports relative to anatomic landmarks.

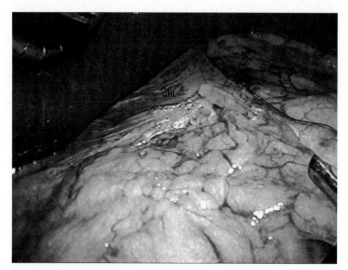

Figure 54.3 Exposure of the gastrohepatic ligament. The left lobe of the liver is elevated with a self-forming retractor exposing the gastrohepatic ligament (GHL), the GE junction, and lesser curvature of the stomach (S) as outlined by the black line; liver (L).

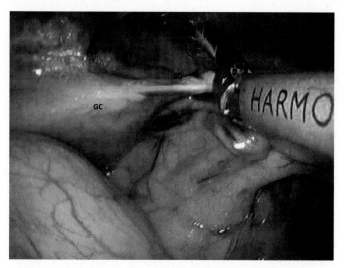

Figure 54.4 Division of the short gastric (SG) vessels from the greater curvature (GC) using the Harmonic scalpel.

avascular tissue that attaches the esophagus to the diaphragm at the gastroesophageal (GE) junction. Begin this dissection by incising the superficial layer of the right phrenoesophageal ligament, as plunging the harmonic scalpel into this area might lead to iatrogenic thermal or puncture injury to the adjacent esophagus. Bluntly dissect the esophagus away from the right crus as the phrenoesophageal ligament is divided. This allows access into the mediastinum for further dissection of the hernia sac and reduction of viscera. The mediastinal dissection is accomplished using a combination of blunt dissection with an Endo Peanut and sharp dissection with the Harmonic scalpel.

Dissection should then be carried toward the anterior mediastinum, advancing over the anterior surface of the herniated stomach, and directed toward the left crus.

During mediastinal dissection, the assistant's grasper should place continuous gentle but firm caudal retraction on the herniated stomach while the hernia sac is dissected away from the mediastinum. The direction of retraction should be caudal and opposite to the site of operation; that is, when mediastinal dissection is carried out on the right side, the herniated stomach should be retracted caudally and toward the left lower quadrant.

While dissecting in the mediastinum, the surgeon should pay close attention to the tissue planes. It is crucial to identify the esophagus to avoid inadvertent injury of it. Laterally, the parietal pleura is often attached to the hernia sac. To avoid violation of the pleural space which leads to CO_2 pneumothorax, the surgeon should perform blunt dissection by pushing the pleura away from the operative field. Lastly, some patients will have thick band-like adhesions within the mediastinum. These adhesions should be taken down in layers to avoid inadvertent transection of the vagus nerve.

At this stage, the majority of the hiatal dissection is complete and most of the herniated stomach is reduced back into the abdomen with the exception of the posterior wall of the stomach and its attachment to the posterior mediastinum.

Mobilization of the Gastric Fundus (Fig. 54.4)

Technical Points

Attention is now turned toward mobilization of the gastric fundus and cardia in preparation for the fundoplication. This is accomplished by dividing the short gastric vessels that lie within the gastrosplenic ligament (see also Chapter 53, Figure 53.2). The gastrosplenic ligament is part of the greater omentum found along the greater curvature of the stomach and is attached to the splenic hilum.

Transfer the Harmonic scalpel into the left subcostal 10-mm port. Exposure for this dissection is obtained by retracting the greater curvature of the stomach laterally toward the right lower quadrant region while the assistant surgeon places counter traction along the gastrosplenic ligament. Using the Harmonic scalpel, divide the gastrosplenic ligament along the greater curvature beginning at the level of the lowest short gastric vessel. Incise the gastrosplenic ligament about 1 cm away from the edge of the greater curvature to prevent thermal injury to the stomach wall. During this time, the Harmonic scalpel should be held without tension on the tissue to allow proper sealing of the vessels prior to transection.

While incising the gastrosplenic ligament, one will gain entrance into the lesser sac. Now grasp the posterior wall of the stomach by the operator's left hand and retract it laterally to further splay out the gastrosplenic ligament, thus enhancing the visualization in the region. This dissection is continued cephalad toward the angle of His. Oftentimes, there is a short gastric vessel in the vicinity of the angle of His. In some patients, the gastrosplenic ligament has been stretched over time, allowing easy visualization and ligation of this vessel. However, in others, the space between the angle of His and the splenic hilum is limited. Bleeding from this region may be difficult to control as a result of poor visualization. If bleeding occurs, promptly regrasp the vessel with the Harmonic scalpel toward the spleen for further thermal application. Any delay will result in blood obscuring the surgical field, diminishing the chances of locating the bleeder. Surgical clips, sponges, and hemostatic agents should always be at the ready during this step of the operation. Once the short gastric vessels are taken down, part of the superior pole of the spleen may appear ischemic. This is not a matter for concern.

Lastly, the fundus is retracted toward the right lower quadrant region and the remainder of the left phrenoesophageal ligament is incised, mobilizing the stomach from the left crus. Take care not to dissect into the left crus or compromise the peritoneum covering the left crus.

Retroesophageal Dissection and Crural Repair (Fig. 54.5)

Technical Points

At this point, the fundus and distal esophagus have been mobilized with the exception of the retroesophageal attachments. To create the retroesophageal window, the assistant's grasper is placed behind the esophagus and the assistant bluntly retracts the GE junction cephalad and laterally to expose the right crus. Next, perform blunt dissection under direct visualization to reach the left crus from the right side. Take care to keep the dissection anterior to the plane of the left crus. If this dissection is carried out too cephalad, the left chest cavity or the posterior wall of the esophagus may be entered inadvertently. In addition, care should be taken to avoid injuring the right vagal trunk that is located posterior to the esophagus. Next, pass a Penrose

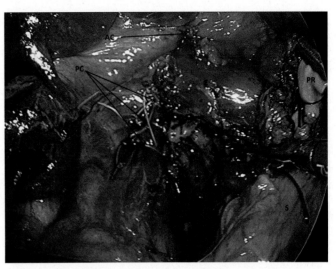

Figure 54.6 Accomplish the crural repair by placing interrupted permanent sutures to approximate the left and right crura, starting posteriorly, working toward the esophagus (E). Here three permanent sutures approximate the crural posterior (PC) and one anterior (AC) to the esophagus; stomach (S).

drain behind the esophagus under direct visualization via the retroesophageal window, encircling the GE junction (see also Chapter 53, Figure 53.2C). Use an Endoloop or clip applier to tie both ends of the Penrose drain together. The assistant may now grasp the Penrose drain to further retract the GE junction anteriorly and caudally. This provides the exposure needed to complete the remaining posterior mediastinal dissection and mobilization of the distal esophagus. Once completely dissected, the V-shaped decussation of the left and right crural fibers will be defined posteriorly, from where the crural repair will begin.

Once there is adequate intra-abdominal esophageal length (at least 3 cm), the crural repair is accomplished by placing interrupted permanent sutures to approximate the left and right crura (Fig. 54.6). It should be noted that the aorta is in close proximity to the V-shaped decussation of the crura. Place all stitches under direct visualization, especially the first posterior stitch. If the hiatal defect is large, one or two crural stitches may also be placed anteriorly to approximate the left and right crura. Pass a 56- to 58-French bougie into the stomach to allow the distal esophagus to distend. Evaluate the crural repair at this time to ensure adequate approximation of the crus. The repair should be snug enough to allow only the tip of a blunt grasper to slip in between the crural repair and the esophagus. If the repair is overly tight, this can lead to prolonged postoperative dysphagia.

Mesh Reinforcement of Crural Repair

Technical Points

Recent evidence points toward lower recurrence rate when mesh is used for paraesophageal hernia repair. The author recommends using biological mesh to perform posterior reinforcement

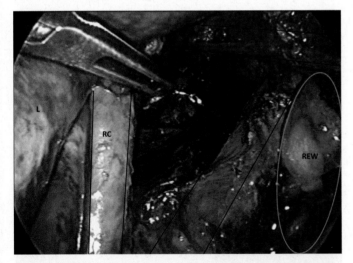

Figure 54.5 The esophagus (E) is retracted anteriorly to allow exposure of the posterior mediastinum (M) and retroesophageal window (REW). Once the distal esophagus is completely dissected and defined, the right crus (RC) and the left crus (LC) will reveal the V-shaped decussation of crural fibers posteriorly; liver (L).

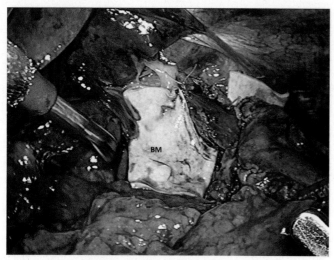

Figure 54.7 Mesh reinforcement with U-shaped piece of biologic mesh (BM); stomach (S); esophagus (E).

of the crural repair. The mesh should not encircle the hiatus circumferentially to avoid postoperative dysphagia.

A piece of mesh approximately 6 × 8 cm in size is brought into the field. A U-shaped hole is cut out to encompass the esophagus and placed as shown in Chapter 52, Figure 52.3B. The mesh is introduced into the abdomen through the 10-mm port. It is then laid over the posterior crus and secured in place using three permanent stitches, two on either side of the mesh and one at the posterior midsection of the mesh (Fig. 54.7). These stitches should incorporate the underlying crura and care should be taken to avoid tearing the underlying diaphragm when tying down these stitches. The mesh can be further adhered in place by spraying Tisseel between the mesh and the diaphragm.

Assessment of Esophageal Length and Need for Modified Collis Gastroplasty

Technical Points

One of the greatest pitfalls of this surgery is insufficient esophageal mobilization with inadequate intra-abdominal esophageal length. This is seen in the setting of chronic esophagitis which results in scarring and a foreshortened esophagus. After complete circumferential distal esophageal mobilization, the intra-abdominal esophagus should measure at least 3 cm in length before proceeding with the Nissen fundoplication. If this cannot be accomplished despite maximal distal esophageal mobilization, then a modified Collis gastroplasty is recommended to lengthen the esophagus.

First, the assistant's left subcostal port should be upsized to a 12-mm port. A bougie is passed into the stomach and is held against the lesser curvature. With lateral traction of the fundus, multiple firings of blue load 3.5-mm Endo GIA staplers are used to remove a wedge of the gastric fundus to create a distal neoesophagus (Fig. 54.8). Prior to each firing, the bougie

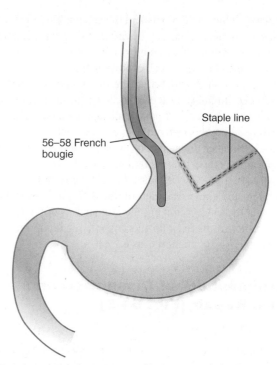

Figure 54.8 Modified Collis gastroplasty lengthens the esophagus with a tube of stomach.

should be slid in and out to ensure that it is not caught within the jaws of the stapler.

Nissen Fundoplication (Figs. 54.9 and 54.10)

Technical and Anatomic Points

Once adequate intra-abdominal esophageal length is obtained, remove the Penrose drain. The retroesophageal window is

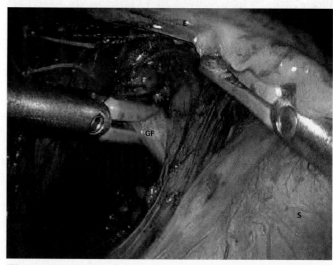

Figure 54.9 Retroesophageal window exposed from the right side, where the gastric fundus (GF) is grasped and brought behind the esophagus (E). Also shown is the crural repair (CR) and stomach (S).

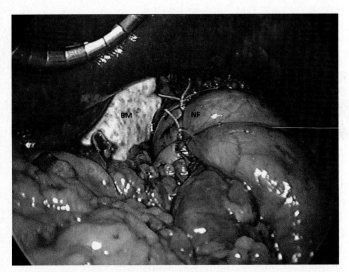

Figure 54.10 Completed Nissen fundoplication. The left lobe of the liver (L) is elevated, showing the completed Nissen fundoplication (NF), and the biologic mesh (BM); esophagus (E).

exposed from the right side, where the fundus is grasped behind the esophagus (Fig. 54.9). A shoeshine maneuver should be performed to ensure that the 360-degree wrap is not twisted. A floppy 2-cm wrap is then created over the bougie at the level of the GE junction using three nonabsorbable stitches to approximate the two ends of the fundus (Fig. 54.10).

A partial thickness bite of the esophagus should be included in the superior most stitch to prevent the wrap from migrating. If mesh repair of the crura is not performed, the authors recommend suturing the sides of the fundus to its respective crura, or performing gastropexy to possibly decrease the risk of reherniation of stomach into the mediastinum.

Intraoperative Esophagogastroduodenoscopy

Technical Points

At this point, the surgeon may elect to perform intraoperative EGD. First, evaluate the esophageal lumen for blood which may indicate iatrogenic esophageal injury. Next, the Z line which marks the GE junction should be noted and the fundoplication confirmed to be at this level. The scope is retroflexed and should show an appropriately tight wrap. Lastly, a leak test may be performed to rule out any occult full thickness injury to the stomach or esophagus.

Once the stomach is completely suctioned out, the endoscope is removed. Hemostasis is ensured and the liver retractor is withdrawn under direct visualization. All ports are removed under direct visualization and the pneumoperitoneum is evacuated. All port sites are closed.

REFERENCES

1. Andujar JJ, Papasavas PK, Birdas T, et al. Laparoscopic repair of large paraesophageal hernia is associated with a low incidence of recurrence and reoperation. *Surg Endosc.* 2004;18(3):444–447.
2. Awais O, Luketich JD. Management of giant paraesophageal hernia. *Minerva Chir.* 2009;64(2):159–168.
3. Evans RTS. *Surgical Pitfall: Prevention and Management.* Philadelphia, PA: Saunders Elsevier Health Sciences; 2009.
4. Fischer J. *Mastery of Surgery.* Philadelphia, PA: Lippincott Williams & Wilkins; 2007.
5. Kaiser L, Kron I, Spray T. *Mastery of Cardiothoracic Surgery.* Philadelphia, PA: Lippincott Williams & Wilkins; 2007.
6. Nason KS, Luketich JD, Witteman BP, et al. The laparoscopic approach to paraesophageal hernia repair. *J Gastrointest Surg.* 2012;16(2):417–426.
7. Oelschlager BK, Pellegrine CA, Hunter JG, et al. Biologic prosthesis to prevent recurrence after laparoscopic paraesophageal hernia repair: Long-term follow-up from a multicenter, prospective, randomized trial. *J Am Coll Surg.* 2011;213(4):461–468.

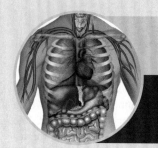

55

Laparoscopic Esophagomyotomy

Laparoscopic esophagomyotomy uses the magnification and precise dissection of minimally invasive surgery to divide the hypertrophied distal esophagus associated with esophageal achalasia. This operation has largely supplanted the older transthoracic Heller myotomy, which required a left thoracotomy. The laparoscopic procedure is often referred to as a "Heller" myotomy even though it is performed through the abdomen. References at the end of this chapter give details of the transthoracic myotomy (now generally performed thoracoscopically), which is still useful when a long-segment myotomy must be performed. Because achalasia is generally limited to the distal esophagus, the exposure attained at laparoscopy is usually ample.

Addition of a partial fundoplication is optional. The technique described here brings the fundus of the stomach anteriorly, where it may serve as a buttress for the myotomy. It is particularly useful if inadvertent entry into the esophagus has been made and repaired.

SCORE™, the Surgical Council on Resident Education, classified laparoscopic Heller myotomy as a "COMPLEX" procedure.

STEPS IN PROCEDURE

Obtain laparoscopic access—five ports are generally used

Retract liver up toward diaphragm

Excise esophageal fat pad and clean peritoneum from anterior surface of esophagus

Begin myotomy at convenient place in thickened distal esophagus

Extend distally 1.5 to 2 cm on stomach, proximally to thin muscle of esophagus

Confirm adequacy of myotomy by passing esophagogastroduodenoscope

Consider adding partial fundoplication—Dor or Toupet

Dor—roll stomach up over myotomy and suture to edges

Toupet—Mobilize Posterior to Esophagus and Bring Fundus Behind

Suture stomach to edges of myotomy

LIST OF STRUCTURES

Diaphragm
Crura, right and left
Esophageal hiatus
Median arcuate ligament
Esophagus
Stomach

Belsey's Fat Pad
Artery of Belsey
Phrenoesophageal ligament

Liver
Segment I—caudate lobe
Left lobe
Segments II and III

Coronary ligaments
Left triangular ligament

Ligamentum Teres Hepatis
Falciform ligament
Subphrenic space
Greater omentum
Lesser omentum
Colon
Pericardium
Phrenic nerves
Inferior phrenic artery and vein
Left gastric artery
Left and right vagus nerves

HALLMARK ANATOMIC COMPLICATIONS

Injury to esophagus
Injury to vagus nerves

Injury to stomach

Exposure of Distal Esophagus and Proximal Stomach (Fig. 55.1)

Technical Points

Set up the room as described for laparoscopic fundoplication (see Chapter 53). The trocar sites and initial exposure are identical. Avoid extensive dissection posterior to the esophagus; rather develop just enough of a window behind the esophagus to allow a Penrose drain to be passed behind for traction (Fig. 55.1A,B). The remainder of the dissection is performed on the anterior and lateral aspects of the esophagus with downward traction on the Penrose drain.

Visually confirm the thickened, narrowed segment of esophagus and mobilize the esophagus into the abdomen until dilated proximal esophagus is seen.

Excise Belsey's fat pad with electrocautery or ultrasonic shears (Fig. 55.1C,D). This allows unimpeded access to the gastroesophageal junction.

Anatomic Points

This dissection is largely confined to the anterior and lateral esophagus, in contrast to laparoscopic Nissen fundoplication, in which a more extensive dissection includes creation of an ample window behind the esophagus. As for Nissen fundoplication, dissection proceeds by outlining the crura of the diaphragm. These crura combine to form a muscular tunnel 2- to 3-cm long through which the esophagus and vagus nerves pass into the abdomen. There is considerable variability in the manner in which the fibrous and muscular parts of the esophageal hiatus form a sling around the esophagus; in actuality, dissection of the anterior and lateral parts of the hiatus is rarely affected by these variants. The median arcuate ligament crosses over the aorta just cephalad to the origin of the celiac axis and is not generally seen.

The left inferior phrenic artery runs along the left crus of the diaphragm and may give rise to an aberrant branch passing across the distal esophagus. The right inferior phrenic artery passes behind the inferior vena cava and is generally not encountered.

The phrenoesophageal ligament, which is more of a membrane than a ligament, covers the anterior surface of the esophageal hiatus and distal esophagus. It consists of a condensation of endoabdominal fascia and must be divided to expose the esophagus. Exposing the muscular fibers of the hiatus at its margins will automatically involve division of this structure, allowing exposure of the esophagus.

Belsey's (subhiatal) fat pad covers the gastroesophageal junction and contains Belsey's artery, a minor transversely oriented collateral channel between the left gastric and left inferior phrenic arteries.

Performance of Myotomy (Fig. 55.2)

Technical Points

Begin the myotomy at a convenient point in the middle of the thickened, narrow segment of distal esophagus, taking care to avoid the vagus nerve. Using hook cautery to progress distally and laparoscopic scissors to progress proximally, create a line of incision on the anterior surface of the esophagus in a direction parallel to the longitudinal fibers. Placement of a bougie in the esophagus may facilitate subsequent dissection by elevating and splaying out the layers of the esophagus and ensuring complete division. Use an atraumatic grasper to grasp the longitudinal fibers gently on each side of the myotomy and pull out and down (Fig. 55.2A).

Divide the thickened circular muscle in a similar fashion until the mucosal tube is seen (Fig. 55.2B). This is easily identified by its pale color and the absence of muscle fibers. Continue the myotomy, proximal and distal, until an ample myotomy has been created (Fig. 55.2C). This will generally require a dissection 1.5 to 2 cm down on the stomach and extension proximal until the muscle layers thin out (Fig. 55.2D). If the myotomy extends too far down on the stomach, gastroesophageal reflux is more likely. There does not appear to be any adverse consequence if the myotomy extends too far proximally. If the myotomy is incomplete, relief of symptoms is likely to be inadequate. Confirm adequacy of the myotomy by passing an esophagogastroduodenoscope down and directly inspecting the distal esophagus. Absence of blood confirms the absence of gross injury, and the gastroesophageal junction should appear patulous. Pass the scope with great caution to avoid perforation. Do not shine the laparoscope at the distal esophagus during this maneuver because light from the laparoscope, transmitted through the thin esophageal mucosa, will complicate viewing from above.

Next, confirm absence of injury by insufflating air into the distal esophagus while observing under saline in the abdomen. Methylene blue may be of assistance in identifying small injuries. Repair any injury and perform a partial fundoplication (see later section) to provide additional security. Do not hesitate to convert the procedure to an open operation if this appears to be the best way to manage an injury.

Irrigate the abdomen, ensure hemostasis, and close the trocar sites in the usual manner.

Anatomic Points

The esophagus is not covered by peritoneum. The outer layer consists of longitudinal muscle and rarely exceeds 1 mm in thickness at the distal esophagus. The distal esophageal sphincter is a physiologic rather than an anatomic structure and normally there is no distinct thickening to the distal esophagus. The circular muscle layer in the normal esophagus is generally about 1 mm. This layer is considerably thickened in achalasia. Beneath the circular muscle lies a submucosal layer containing a well-developed plexus of veins. The epithelial tube (squamous mucosa) is white and easily identified by three characteristics:

1. The white color, which contrasts with the pink-red of the muscle layers
2. The tendency to "pout out" after the constricting circular muscle fibers are released
3. The overlying submucosal plexus of small veins

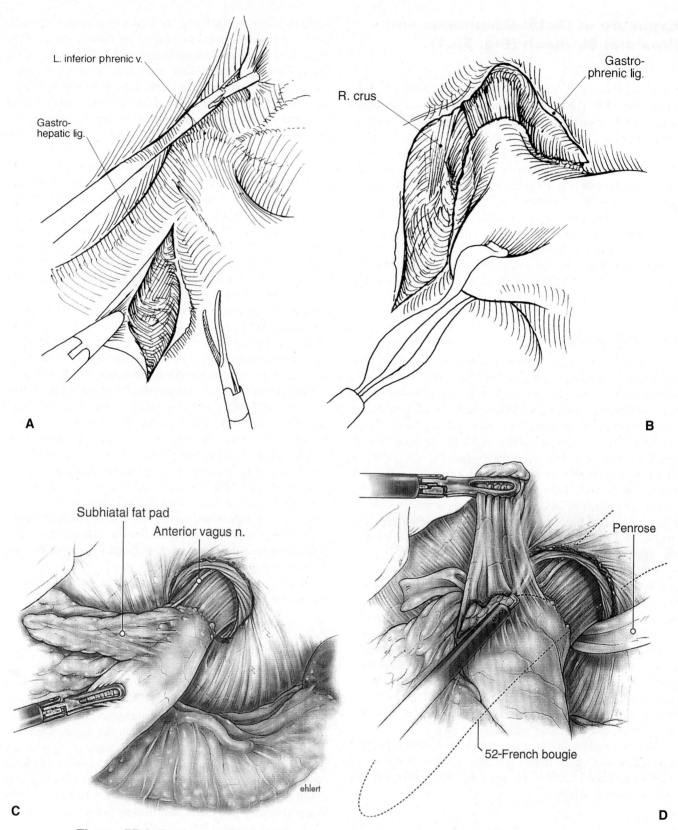

Figure 55.1 Exposure of distal esophagus and proximal stomach (**A** and **B** from Wind GG. The stomach. In: *The Applied Laparoscopic Anatomy: Abdomen and Pelvis.* Baltimore, MD: Williams & Wilkins; 1997, with permission; **C** and **D** from Pellegrini CA, Eubanks TR. Minimally invasive treatment of achalasia and other esophageal dysmotility. In: Baker RJ, Fischer JE, eds. *Mastery of Surgery.* 4th ed. Philadelphia, PA: Lippincott Williams & Wilkins; 2001:803–812, with permission).

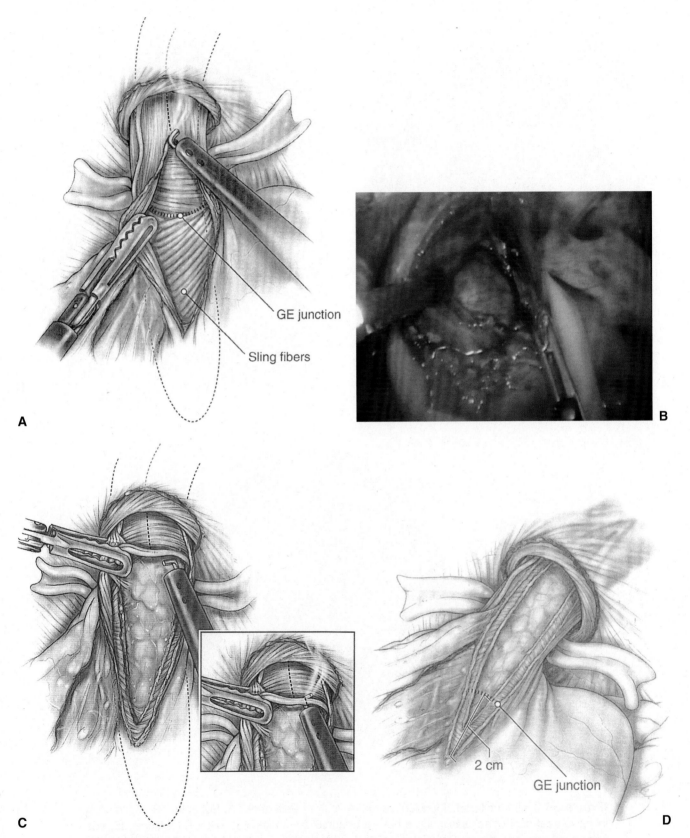

Figure 55.2 Performance of myotomy (**A,C** and **D** from Pellegrini CA, Eubanks TR. Minimally invasive treatment of achalasia and other esophageal dysmotility. In: Baker RJ, Fischer JE, eds. *Mastery of Surgery.* 4th ed. Philadelphia, PA: Lippincott Williams & Wilkins; 2001:803–812, with permission).

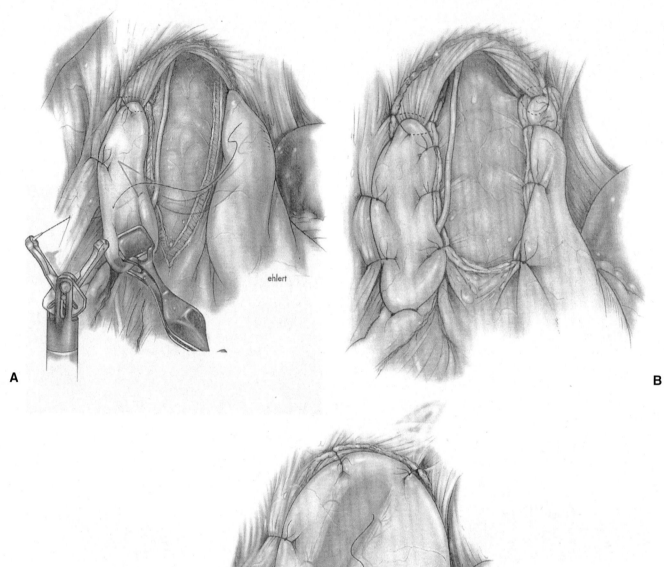

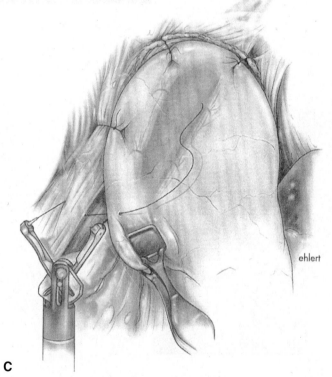

Figure 55.3 Optional partial fundoplication (**A–C** from Pellegrini CA, Eubanks TR. Minimally invasive treatment of achalasia and other esophageal dysmotility. In: Baker RJ, Fischer JE, eds. *Mastery of Surgery.* 4th ed. Philadelphia, PA: Lippincott Williams & Wilkins; 2001:803–812, with permission).

The vagus nerves coalesce into an anterior trunk and a posterior trunk in the vicinity of the esophageal hiatus in most individuals. The anterior vagus nerve may be visible on the surface of the esophagus as a white band with a small vessel running on it; if seen, it is easily avoided. The posterior vagus is generally not seen and is not at risk.

Optional Partial Fundoplication (Fig. 55.3)

Technical and Anatomic Points

Proponents of this procedure believe that the partial fundoplication helps keep the muscle layers apart during healing, lessening the chances of recurrence. It also may provide some protection against gastroesophageal reflux. In addition, this form of fundoplication is useful as a buttress when an injury has been repaired. Minimal mobilization of the stomach is required and it may be necessary to divide some short gastric vessels.

Ensure that the esophagus is circumferentially mobilized and that an adequate posterior window has been created. Divide short gastric vessels if necessary to generate sufficient mobility of the fundus (see Chapter 53). Pull the fundus of the stomach behind the esophagus and suture the fundus to the edges of the myotomy, rather than to each other (Fig. 55.3A). This provides a partial wrap and helps hold the edges of the myotomy apart. Take care during suture not to lacerate the delicate epithelial layer (Fig. 55.3B).

Next, roll the floppy region of the anterior fundus over the myotomy and suture it to the right side of the wrap with several interrupted sutures (Fig. 55.3C). Do not place sutures in the epithelial tube—it is fragile and prone to laceration. Rather, suture the stomach to the muscular walls of the esophagus.

REFERENCES

1. Anselmino M, Perdikis G, Hinder RA, et al. Heller myotomy is superior to dilatation for the treatment of early achalasia. *Arch Surg.* 1997;132:233–240.
2. Beck WC, Sharp KW. Achalasia. *Surg Clin North Am.* 2011;91:1031–1037. (Excellent review.)
3. Boeckxstaens GE, Annese V, des Varannes SB, et al. Pneumatic dilation versus laparoscopic Heller's myotomy for idiopathic achalasia. *N Engl J Med.* 2011;364:1807–1816.
4. Kashiwagi H, Omura N. Surgical treatment for achalasia: When should it be performed, and for which patients? *Gen Thorac Cardiovasc Surg.* 2011;59:389–398.
5. Nussbaum ME. Chapter 73. Minimally invasive treatment of achalasia and other dysmotility. In: Fischer J, et al. eds. *Fischer's Mastery of Surgery.* 6th ed. Philadelphia, PA: Wolters Kluwer Lippincott Williams & Wilkins; 2007:875–885. (Excellent review.)
6. Oddsdottir M. Laparoscopic cardiomyotomy (Heller myotomy). In: Scott-Conner CEH, ed. *The SAGES Manual: Fundamentals of Laparoscopy, Thoracoscopy, and GI Endoscopy.* 2nd ed. New York, NY: Springer-Verlag; 2006:238–246.
7. Wiener DC, Wee JO. Chapter 8. Minimally invasive esophageal procedures. In: Ashley SW (editorial board chair) *ACS Surgery: Principles & Practice.* BC Decker; 2012. Available at: http://www.acssurgery.com
8. Pechlivanides G, Chrysos E, Athanasakis E, et al. Laparoscopic Heller cardiomyotomy and Dor fundoplication for esophageal achalasia: Possible factors predicting outcome. *Arch Surg.* 2001;136:1240–1243.
9. Rosati R, Fumagalli U, Bonavina L, et al. Laparoscopic approach to esophageal achalasia. *Am J Surg.* 1995;169:424–427. (Describes the use of dilated balloon to facilitate myotomy, with a clear illustration of Dor fundoplication.)
10. Vogt D, Curet M, Pitcher D, et al. Successful treatment of esophageal achalasia with laparoscopic Heller myotomy and Toupet fundoplication. *Am J Surg.* 1997;174:709–714. (Discusses the use of Toupet fundoplication.)

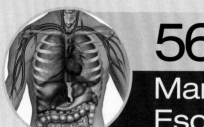

56

Management of Esophageal Perforation

A wide spectrum of strategies exists for management of esophageal perforation. Location (cervical, thoracic, or abdominal), nature of injury (iatrogenic, emetogenic), nature of esophageal tissue (normal or diseased), and length of time since perforation (immediate versus delayed) all influence choice of management. This chapter introduces some basic concepts of repair. It is included with material about surgery around the esophageal hiatus because any surgeon who operates in this region should be able to manage iatrogenic injuries that may occur during dissection. Wide drainage without repair or esophageal resection with immediate or delayed reconstruction are also options (see Chapters 30 to 32).

SCORE™, the Surgical council on Resident Education, classified procedures for esophageal perforation—repair/resection—as "ESSENTIAL UNCOMMON" operations.

STEPS IN PROCEDURE

Identify site of perforation
Extend opening in muscularis, if necessary, to expose entire extent of mucosal laceration
Perform layered repair

Reinforce the repair with adjacent well-vascularized tissue
Stomach, if lower esophagus
Pleural flap, if thoracic esophagus
Drain

HALLMARK ANATOMIC COMPLICATIONS

Failure to completely repair the laceration
Inadequate visualization of full extent of mucosal laceration

Mucosal laceration may be considerably longer than muscular laceration
Failure to adequately reinforce the repair

LIST OF STRUCTURES

Esophagus
Stomach
Fundus

Short gastric vessels
Parietal pleura
Intercostal muscles

Management of Distal Esophageal Perforation (Fig. 56.1)

Distal esophageal perforation may occur during dissection around the esophageal hiatus such as surgery for esophageal hiatus hernia. In these circumstances, the injury is fresh and the tissue is of good quality. Immediate recognition and repair with reinforcement of the suture line is appropriate. This is described here.

Mobilize the esophagus completely so that the perforation can be visualized. First ensure that you can see the full length of the mucosal laceration. The initial view of the injury may underestimate the length of the laceration (Fig. 56.1A). Do not hesitate to extend the laceration in the muscular layers until the

full extent of the mucosal laceration can be seen (Fig. 56.1B). Perform a hand-sutured two-layer anastomosis.

Buttress the repair with the fundus of the stomach by performing a Nissen, Dor, or Toupet fundoplication (see Chapters 51 and 53). Alternatively, a flap of diaphragm can be developed and sutured over the laceration. This latter method is rarely used.

Perforations in this region may also occur after vomiting (emetogenic perforation or Boerhaave syndrome). These cases require different management, as there is often massive contamination of the mediastinum and a delay in surgery. Generally wide drainage with diversion is appropriate.

Iatrogenic perforation during stricture dilatation or biopsy may also occur. If the esophagus is diseased, resection may be the best course.

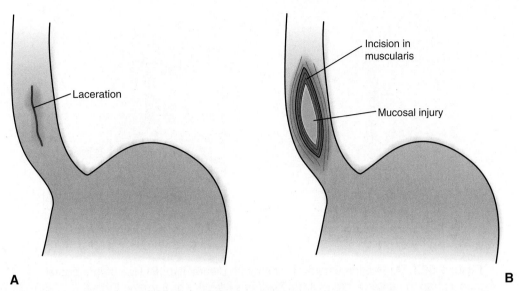

Figure 56.1 **A:** Obvious extent of injury in muscular layer is shorter than actual mucosal laceration. **B:** Full extent of injury is only revealed when muscular laceration is extended cephalad and caudad.

Repair of Midesophageal (Thoracic) Perforation (Fig. 56.2)

The thoracic esophagus is best approached through the right chest. Most repairs are performed by open rather than thoracoscopic surgery. Mobilize the esophagus as described for esophageal resection (Chapter 32e). Elevate the injured segment with Penrose drains (Fig. 56.2A). Fully visualize the per-

foration and extend the muscular incision cephalad and caudad as previously mentioned (Fig. 56.2B). Repair the perforation in two layers (Fig. 56.2C).

If the tissues are friable, diversion and drainage may be a better approach. Some perforations not amenable to repair may be managed by placement of a T-tube into the perforation and wide drainage. This converts the injury into a controlled fistula.

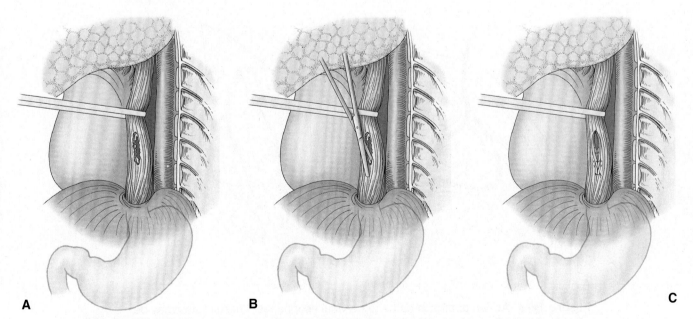

Figure 56.2 **A:** Exposure of perforation. **B:** Extension of muscular laceration to expose the full extent of the mucosal injury. **C:** Repair in two layers (from *Fischer's Mastery of Surgery*. 6th ed. Philadelphia, PA: Lippincott Williams & Wilkins, 2012).

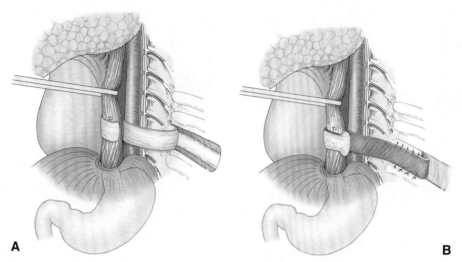

A

B

Figure 56.3 **A:** Reinforcement of repair with pleural flap. **B:** Use of intercostal muscle flap to reinforce repair (from *Fischer's Mastery of Surgery*. 6th ed. Philadelphia, PA: Lippincott Williams & Wilkins, 2012).

Reinforcement of Thoracic Repair (Fig. 56.3)

Then buttress the repair with adjacent well-vascularized tissue. Either develop a flap of pleura and suture it around the repair as shown in Figure 56.3A or similarly develop a flap of intercostal muscle as shown in Figure 56.3B. In either case, gently wrap the repair and tack the reinforcing patch in place with multiple sutures.

Drain the repair with a large diameter chest tube.

Approach to Cervical Esophageal Perforations (Fig. 56.4)

Injuries to the cervical esophagus may occur as a result of external trauma (see Chapter 13) or instrumental perforation. Drainage is the most common strategy. Two possible paths for drainage are shown in Figure 56.4A. The cervical esophagus exposed for repair or drainage is shown in Figure 56.4B. It may be exposed through either side of the neck.

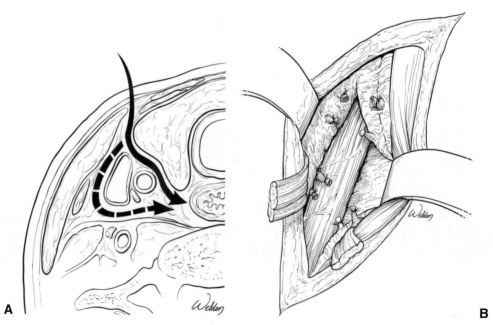

A

B

Figure 56.4 **A:** Two approach paths to cervical esophagus. These routes may be used for surgical exposure or for drain placement. **B:** Esophagus exposed in neck (from Wu J, Mattox K, Wall MJ Jr. Esophageal perforations: New perspectives and treatment paradigms. *J Trauma*. 2007;63(5):1173–1184, with permission).

REFERENCES

1. Bufkin BL, Miller JI Jr, Mansour KA. Esophageal perforation: Emphasis on management. *Ann Thorac Surg.* 1996;61:1447–1451.
2. Gupta NM, Kaman L. Personal management of 57 consecutive patients with esophageal perforation. *Am J Surg.* 2004;187:58–63.
3. Panieri E, Millar AJ, Rode H, et al. Iatrogenic esophageal perforation in children: Patterns of injury, presentation, management, and outcome. *J Pediatr Surg.* 1996;31:890–895.
4. Salminen P, Gullichsen R, Laine S. Use of self-expandable metal stents for the treatment of esophageal perforations and anastomotic leaks. *Surg Endosc.* 2009;23:1526–1530.
5. Vogel SB, Rout WR, Martin TD, et al. Esophageal perforation in adults: Aggressive, conservative treatment lowers morbidity and mortality. *Ann Surg.* 2005;241:1016–1021.
6. Wu JT, Mattox KL, Wall MJ Jr. Esophageal perforations: New perspectives and treatment paradigms. *J Trauma.* 2007;63:1173–1184.
7. Younes Z, Johnson DA. The spectrum of spontaneous and iatrogenic esophageal injury: Perforations, Mallory-Weiss tears, and hematomas. *J Clin Gastroenterol.* 1999;29:306–317.

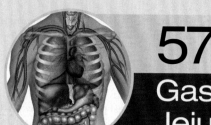

57

Gastrostomy and Jejunostomy

Gastrostomy may be performed for feeding or for decompression. The simplest open technique for creation of a gastrostomy is the Stamm procedure. Percutaneous endoscopic gastrostomy (PEG), an alternative to open gastrostomy, is also described in this chapter. Laparoscopic gastrostomy is described in Chapter 58e (which also describes the Janeway gastrostomy, a method of creating a permanent, mucosa-lined tube). Other techniques are included in the references.

After the tract has matured, a low-profile "button"-type device may be substituted for the catheter. These low-profile devices are often easier for patients and families to deal with. The exchange is made in the office or clinic and does not require anesthesia.

Jejunostomy is sometimes preferred over gastrostomy in patients in whom free gastroesophageal reflux, mental obtundation, or abnormal upper gastrointestinal motility makes aspiration of gastric feedings likely. It has been difficult to prove conclusively any advantage for this procedure over gastrostomy.

SCORE™, the Surgical Council on Resident Education, classified open and percutaneous gastrostomy, and open jejunostomy, as "ESSENTIAL COMMON" procedures.

LIST OF STRUCTURES

Stomach
Fundus
Antrum
Pylorus
Lesser curvature
Greater curvature
Duodenum
Suspensory ligament of duodenum
   (ligament of Treitz)

Jejunum
Ileum
Cecum

Liver
Left lobe
Greater omentum
Transverse colon
Gastrocolic ligament

Gastrostomy

The Incision (Fig. 57.1)

Technical and Anatomic Points

The patient is positioned supine, and an upper midline, short upper left paramedian, or left transverse incision is used. The choice of incision depends on the patient's body habitus. If an old midline scar is present, a left transverse incision provides good access through a space that is often free of adhesions.

STEPS IN PROCEDURE—GASTROSTOMY

Short upper abdominal incision
Identify and deliver stomach into wound
Two concentric purse-string sutures (2-0) silk
   on anterior stomach wall, leave tails long
Choose exit site on anterior abdominal wall
Create small skin incision and deliver catheter
   into peritoneal cavity
Incise stomach in center of purse-string
   sutures and insert catheter
Tie sutures, inkwelling stomach around catheter

**Tack Stomach to Anterior Abdominal
   Wall at Four Sites Around Catheter
   Entry Site**
Use previously placed purse-string sutures for
   two of these tacking stitches
Stomach should completely hide catheter from
   view when completed
Bring omentum into region
Close incision and anchor the catheter

HALLMARK ANATOMIC COMPLICATIONS—GASTROSTOMY

Injury to colon or even insertion of gastrostomy tube into colon	Site too close to pylorus with obstruction of pylorus if Foley catheter is used as tube

General anesthesia is preferred; however, in the cachectic, weakened patient, local anesthesia may be safer. If the procedure is to be performed using local anesthesia, use a midline incision because it requires minimal muscle manipulation. Infiltrate the skin and subcutaneous tissues with local anesthesia. As dissection progresses, inject additional local anesthesia just under the fascia to numb the peritoneum.

Choice of Site on Stomach Wall and Placement of Sutures (Fig. 57.2)

Technical Points

Identify the stomach with certainty by observing its thick muscular wall, absence of haustral folds and taeniae, and the vessels entering the greater and lesser curvatures. Grasp the stomach with a Babcock clamp and pull it into the wound. Choose a site well proximal to the pylorus on a mobile, accessible part of the anterior wall.

Place two concentric purse-string sutures of 2-0 silk, leaving the needles on. Begin and end one purse-string suture at the cephalad end of the incision and the other suture at the caudad end.

Anatomic Points

Remember the disposition of major organs in the upper abdomen, their attachments, and how to distinguish one from the other. On a surface projection, the stomach is located in the left hypochondriac and epigastric regions, with the pylorus just to the right of the vertebral column. The lesser curvature and the adjacent part of the stomach lie deep to the left lobe of the liver. The body of the stomach lies just deep to the parietal peritoneum of the anterior body wall. The free edge of the left lobe of the liver typically lies about halfway between the umbilicus and the xiphoid in the midline and then angles upward and to the left to pass behind the eighth costal cartilage. The greater omentum is attached to the greater curvature of the stomach. It is normally draped over the transverse colon and the numerous loops of small intestine.

The transverse colon is attached to the greater curvature of the stomach by the gastrocolic ligament (developmentally, the anterior "root" of the great omentum) and to the posterior body wall by the transverse mesocolon. It can lie anywhere in the upper abdomen, depending on the degree of redundancy of this organ and the lengths of its peritoneal attachments. Although it is classically described to be immediately inferior to the stomach and superior to the small intestine, it may be interposed between the stomach and the body wall, or conversely, it may sag inferiorly into the pelvis. To visualize small bowel, the greater omentum and often the transverse colon and transverse mesocolon must be reflected cranially.

Through the porthole of this small laparotomy incision, large bowel can be differentiated from other viscera by the presence of haustra, taenia coli, and fatty epiploic appendages.

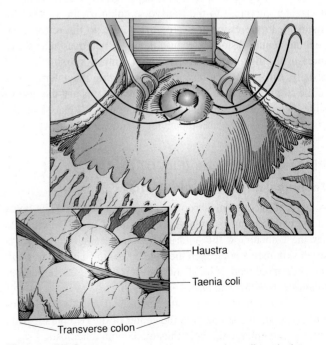

Figure 57.2 Choice or site on stomach wall and placement of sutures

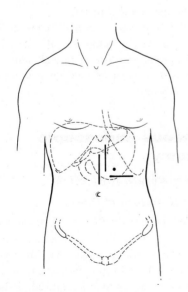

Figure 57.1 The incision

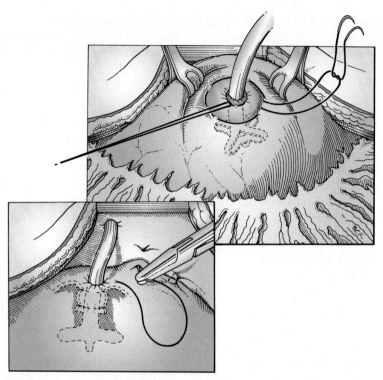

Figure 57.3 Placement of tube

Small bowel can be differentiated from stomach by its narrow diameter and from large bowel by the lack of the characteristics of large bowel just mentioned.

Unlike the colon, stomach lacks haustra and taeniae. Although the stomach is highly distensible and somewhat mobile, it should be remembered that it is attached along its lesser curvature to the liver by the hepatogastric ligament, along its greater curvature to the transverse colon by the gastrocolic ligament, to the esophagus proximally, and to the retroperitoneal duodenum distally. Because there are neurovascular structures in the ligaments and visceral continuity proximally and distally, care should be taken when delivering the anterior wall of the stomach into the wound to ensure that it is just the distensible anterior wall, and that undue traction is not placed on the viscus wall or on the accompanying neurovascular structures.

Placement of Tube (Fig. 57.3)

Technical and Anatomic Points

A large Malecot or mushroom catheter can be used. The holes in the catheter can be enlarged if desired. Choose an exit site for the catheter on the anterior abdominal wall and make a small skin incision. Deepen the hole by poking a clamp through the abdominal wall. If local anesthesia is being used, remember to anesthetize this site also.

Pass the catheter through the abdominal wall. With electrocautery, open the stomach in the center of the two purse-string sutures and enlarge the hole thus made with a hemostat.

Stretch and straighten the bulbous end of the catheter over a Kelly clamp and push it into the hole. Confirm proper placement within the gastric lumen by irrigating and aspirating saline freely.

Tie the inner purse string as an assistant dunks the hole in. Then tie the outer purse string. Do not cut the needles off; these two sutures will be used to anchor the gastrostomy site to the undersurface of the anterior abdominal wall. Properly placed and tied, these two sutures should "inkwell" the stomach over the tube.

Place retractors to visualize the site where the catheter enters the peritoneal cavity. Place a 2-0 silk suture to approximate the far side of the stomach to the underside of the anterior abdominal wall beyond the catheter.

Then use the "top" and "bottom" purse-string sutures to tack the stomach above and below. Finally, place a suture anterior to the catheter entrance site and tie all sutures. Omentum, if available, can be packed around the gastrostomy and the incision can then be closed.

Percutaneous Endoscopic Gastrostomy

The Pull Technique (Fig. 57.4)

Technical and Anatomic Points

PEG capitalizes on the fact that the distended stomach lies immediately under the anterior abdominal wall, displacing the colon inferiorly, where it can be directly cannulated. Topical anesthesia of the oropharynx and local anesthesia of the gastrostomy site are all that is required. Sedation may be helpful.

STEPS IN PROCEDURE—PERCUTANEOUS ENDOSCOPIC GASTROSTOMY

Pass esophagogastroduodenoscopy into stomach and insufflate

Turn off operating room lights and look for transilluminated spot on anterior abdominal wall

Confirm this by pressing with a finger; endoscopist should see stomach wall indent

Anesthetize this area with local anesthesia

Introduce needle supplied with PEG kit into stomach, confirm by visualization (endoscope) and rush of air

Endoscopist positions polypectomy snare around needle but does not tighten snare

Enlarge skin hole and fascial opening around needle using no. 11 blade

Pass monofilament suture (supplied with kit) into needle and allow endoscopist to snare it

Endoscopist pulls suture out through mouth, removing scope at the same time

PEG tube is looped onto suture by endoscopist and pulled back into stomach by surgeon

Endoscopist can follow PEG tube by looping it with snare before allowing it to be positioned

Endoscopist confirms good position and desufflates stomach

Secure tube in position

HALLMARK ANATOMIC COMPLICATIONS—PERCUTANEOUS ENDOSCOPIC GASTROSTOMY

Injury to colon

Early dislodgement of tube, resulting in peritonitis

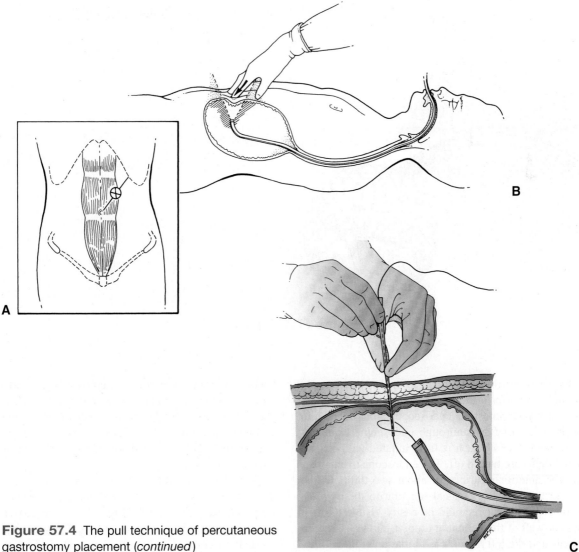

Figure 57.4 The pull technique of percutaneous gastrostomy placement (*continued*)

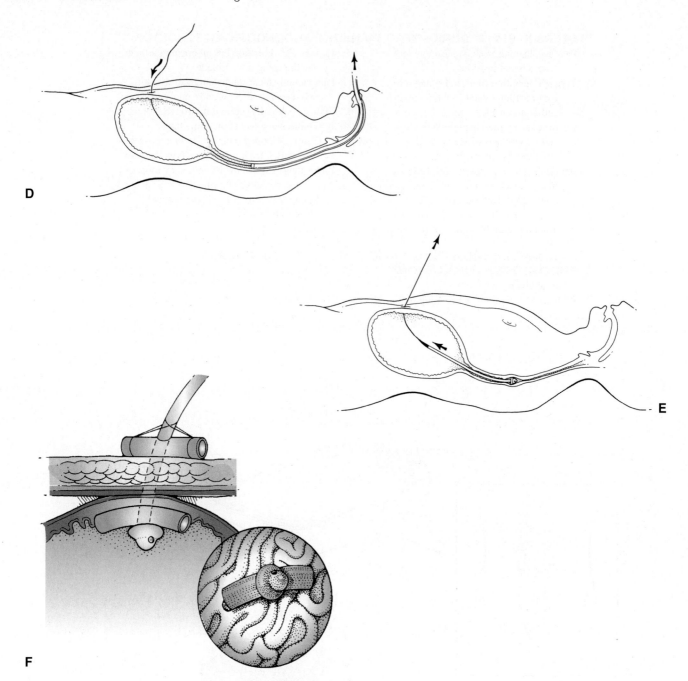

Figure 57.4 *Continued*

An assistant is positioned at the head of the table outside the sterile field to perform the upper gastrointestinal endoscopy. The upper gastrointestinal endoscope is introduced into the stomach and a brief but thorough endoscopic examination is performed. The stomach is fully inflated with air and the overhead lights are turned off. The endoscopist visualizes a point on the anterior gastric wall about two-thirds of the distance from the cardioesophageal junction to the pylorus. The light of the endoscope should be easily visible through the abdominal wall of the patient at a point midway between the umbilicus and the left lateral costal margin (Fig. 57.4A).

Touch the point of maximum light intensity, indenting the skin and anterior abdominal wall repeatedly (Fig. 57.4B). The endoscopist should see the wall of the stomach move in direct correspondence. This ensures that the gastric wall is up against the anterior abdominal wall without interposed viscera.

Turn the overhead lights back on and infiltrate the point that has just been identified with local anesthesia. Then introduce the needle supplied with the PEG kit into the stomach with a firm, straight, slightly screwing motion. Entry into the stomach is usually accompanied by a faint rush of air from the needle.

The endoscopist then visualizes and confirms the position of the needle in the stomach.

Use a no. 11 blade to enlarge the skin hole and the fascial opening adjacent to the needle. Pass a stout monofilament suture, supplied with the PEG kit, down through the needle into the stomach. The endoscopist must then grasp the end of the suture with biopsy forceps or snare it with a polypectomy snare (Fig. 57.4C) and pull endoscope and suture out through the patient's mouth (Fig. 57.4D). The PEG tube is then tied securely to the suture by the endoscopist. Pull the suture slowly and firmly back through the abdominal wall until the PEG tube emerges and is snug against the stomach (Fig. 57.4E).

The endoscopist should pass the scope and visualize the PEG tube to confirm that the mushroom of the PEG tube is up against the anterior gastric wall, snug, but not so tight as to produce pressure necrosis of the stomach (Fig. 57.4F). The PEG tube should be well secured in place because premature dislodgment (before a tract has formed) causes leakage of gastric juice and feedings into the peritoneal cavity and is often fatal.

Feeding Jejunostomy

The standard technique for creation of a Witzel jejunostomy is described here, followed by a derivation of the technique known as needle catheter jejunostomy.

Incision and Identification of the Jejunostomy Site (Fig. 57.5)

Technical Points

A feeding jejunostomy is frequently performed as an adjunct to complicated upper gastrointestinal surgery. When done as an isolated procedure, a midline or a left paramedian incision may be used. The incision must be long enough to identify proximal jejunum with certainty by palpation of the suspensory ligament of the duodenum (ligament of Treitz). General anesthesia is usually required, although in exceptional circumstances, the procedure can be performed using local anesthesia.

STEPS IN PROCEDURE—JEJUNOSTOMY

Upper abdominal incision

Identify proximal jejunum by palpating suspensory ligament of duodenum (ligament of Treitz)

Find a loop that will reach comfortably to the anterior abdominal wall

Place a purse-string suture

Identify exit site on anterior abdominal wall; create opening and pass catheter

Incise center of purse string and pass catheter distally into small bowel

Tie purse-string suture around catheter

Place Lembert sutures over the catheter entry site and along the course of catheter in such a way as to create a tunnel through which the catheter passes; take care to avoid narrowing the bowel too much

Tack small intestine to anterior abdominal wall in such a way that it cannot twist and the catheter is completely hidden

Bring omentum into area

Close incision and secure catheter

HALLMARK ANATOMIC COMPLICATIONS—JEJUNOSTOMY

Cannulation of ileum rather than jejunum

Torsion around fixation site resulting in small bowel obstruction

Bowel obstruction due to Witzel tunnel (tube too large, sutures taken too wide)

Find the small bowel in the left upper quadrant by displacing the colon and the omentum cephalad. Follow the small bowel up to the suspensory ligament of duodenum (ligament of Treitz) and identify a mobile segment of proximal jejunum, generally 40 to 60 cm from the suspensory ligament of duodenum (ligament of Treitz).

Choose a site on the anterior abdominal wall that can easily and comfortably be reached by the jejunum without kinking, and pass a red rubber catheter or Broviac-type catheter through the skin surface. Elevate the jejunal loop with a pair of Babcock clamps and place a single purse-string suture of 3-0 silk on the antimesenteric border at the point selected. Open the jejunum and introduce the catheter, taking care to pass it distally, in the direction of normal peristalsis. Confirm intraluminal passage rather than dissection in the submucosal plane by free injection

and aspiration of air into the lumen of the jejunum. Tie the purse-string suture, leaving the needle in place.

Anatomic Points

Not only do physiologic functions of the small bowel differ in different locations along its length, but the anatomy changes as well. The diameter of the small bowel is largest at the suspensory ligament of duodenum (ligament of Treitz) and gradually tapers distally, so that it is narrowest at the ileocecal junction. The mesenteric attachment of the small bowel runs along a diagonal line from the suspensory ligament of duodenum (ligament of Treitz) (in the left upper quadrant) to the ileocecal junction (in the right lower quadrant). The feeding tube needs to be placed as far proximal as possible. This will ensure the maximum length of bowel downstream for absorption of

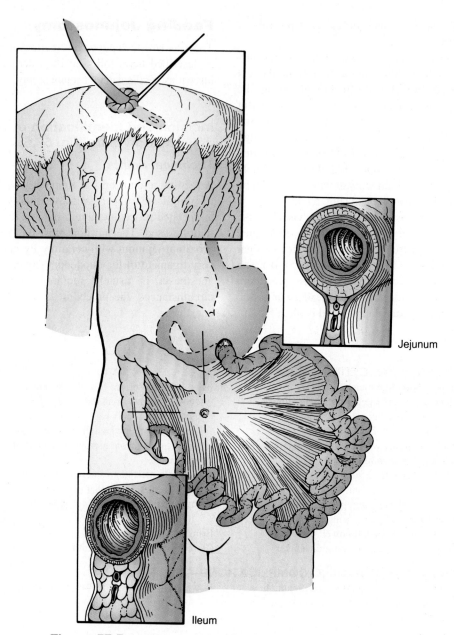

Figure 57.5 Incision and identification of the jejunostomy site

nutrients. Fortuitously, it also allows placement of the tube at the point in the bowel that is of greatest caliber.

Creating a Witzel Tunnel and Anchoring the Jejunostomy (Fig. 57.6)

Technical and Anatomic Points

Construct a Witzel tunnel by placing multiple interrupted Lembert sutures in such a way as to pull the sides of the small bowel over and across the catheter, burying it from view. Tie these, leaving the needles on. Place several sutures past the entrance point of the catheter into the bowel. Take care that these sutures, tied over the catheter, do not unduly restrict the lumen of the jejunum.

Suture the jejunostomy to the underside of the abdominal wall by tacking the Witzel sutures sequentially. Place the sutures in the anterior abdominal wall in such a way that the bowel lies naturally and is not kinked. Anchor the bowel for 1.5 to 2 cm to minimize the risk for volvulus around a point.

Needle Catheter Jejunostomy (Fig. 57.7)

Technical and Anatomic Points

This rapidly performed technique is a useful adjunct to complicated upper gastrointestinal surgery when temporary nutritional support is required. Because the catheter is small (#5 French), only elemental diets can be used. It is not a useful technique when prolonged nutritional support is likely to be needed.

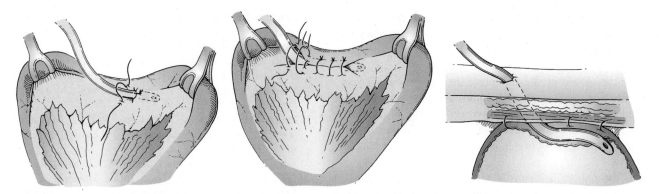

Figure 57.6 Creating a Witzel tunnel and anchoring the jejunostomy

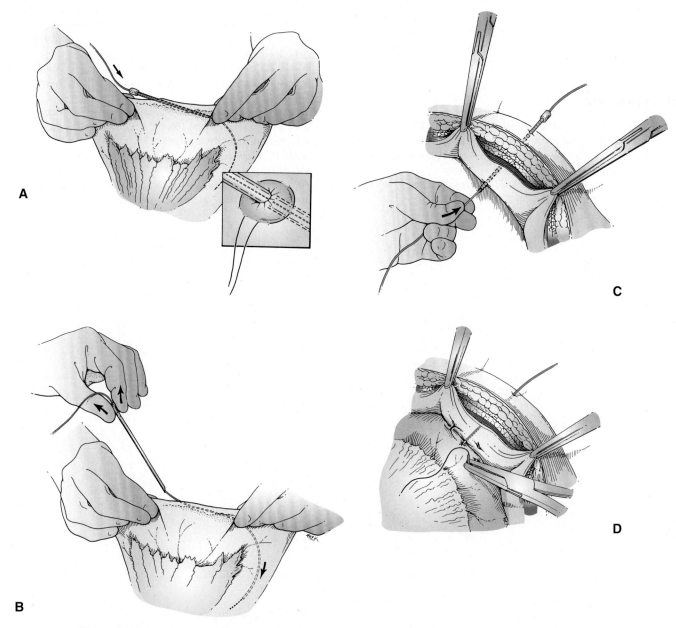

Figure 57.7 Needle catheter jejunostomy. **A:** Guidewire passed into jejunum. Note purse-string suture around entry site into jejunum. **B:** Guidewire passed distally. **C:** Catheter passed through abdominal wall. **D:** Jejunum tacked to parietal peritoneum along a line to prevent torsion around site.

Identify a loop of jejunum and place a purse-string suture (Fig. 57.5). Use the needle supplied with the catheter to pass the catheter through the abdominal wall, "floppy" guidewire first.

Take the second needle and pierce the seromuscular layers of the intestine in the center of the purse-string suture, passing the needle with its bevel down to decrease the risk for penetrating the lumen. Tunnel the needle for 2 to 3 cm in the submucosal plane, then pop it through into the lumen, first turning its bevel up.

Pass the catheter and guidewire through the needle into the lumen. Use the guidewire to facilitate passage of the tube into the small intestine and thread it 20 or 30 cm downstream.

Remove the guidewire and confirm intraluminal placement by injecting air. Suture the jejunum to the underside of the abdominal wall in several places to avoid volvulus. Secure the catheter to the skin using the device supplied by the manufacturer.

REFERENCES

1. Bergstrom LR, Larson DE, Zinsmeister AR, et al. Utilization and outcomes of surgical gastrostomies and jejunostomies in an era of percutaneous endoscopic gastrostomy: A population-based study. *Mayo Clin Proc.* 1995;70:829–836.
2. Castagnetti M, Patel S. A simple adjunct for safer change of PEG. *Pediatr Surg Int.* 2006;22:274–276.
3. Cosentini EP, Sautner T, Gnant M, et al. Outcomes of surgical, percutaneous endoscopic, and percutaneous radiologic gastrostomies. *Arch Surg.* 1998;133:1076–1083.
4. Fujita K, Ozaki M, Obata D, et al. Simple and safe replacement technique for a buried percutaneous endoscopic gastrostomy tube using a laparoscopic surgery device. *Surg Laparosc Endosc Percutan Tech.* 2012;22:546–547.
5. Heberer M, Bodoky A, Iwatschenko P, et al. Indications for needle catheter jejunostomy in elective abdominal surgery. *Am J Surg.* 1987;153:545–552.
6. Joehl RJ. Gastrostomy. In: Ritchie WP Jr, ed. *Shackelford's Surgery of the Alimentary Tract.* 3rd ed. Philadelphia, PA: WB Saunders; 1991:121. (Provides good description of Janeway gastrostomy and other techniques for creating permanent, mucosa-lined tubes.)
7. Morrison JJ, McVinnie DW, Suiter PA, et al. Percutaneous jejunostomy: Repeat access at the healed site of prior surgical jejunostomy with US and fluoroscopic guidance. *J Vasc Interv Radiol.* 2012;23:1646–1650.
8. Ponsky JL, Gauderer MW. Percutaneous endoscopic gastrostomy: Indications, limitations, techniques, and results. *World J Surg.* 1989; 13:165–170.
9. Steichen FM, Ravitch MM. *Stapling in Surgery.* Chicago: Year Book Medical Publishers; 1984:95. (Shows Janeway gastrostomy construction with GIA stapler.)
10. Yarze JC. One-step button PEG. *Gastrointest Endosc.* 2007;65: 556–557.
11. Zickler RW, Barbagiovanni JT, Swan KG. A simplified open gastrostomy under local anesthesia. *Am Surg.* 2001;67:806–808.

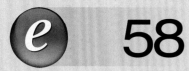

58 Laparoscopic Gastrostomy and Jejunostomy

This chapter can be accessed online at www.lww.com/eChapter58.

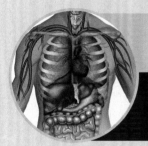

59

Plication of Perforated Duodenal Ulcer

Small anterior perforations of duodenal ulcers are treated by Graham patch plication, which may sometimes be performed laparoscopically (see Chapter 52). Larger perforations may require excision and closure by pyloroplasty or gastric resection for control.

In this chapter, the anatomy of the subhepatic space and its contents is introduced. The subphrenic spaces, frequent sites of associated abscess formation, are also demonstrated.

SCORE™, the Surgical Council on Resident Education, did not classify plication of perforated ulcer.

STEPS IN PROCEDURE

Upper midline or right paramedian incision
Explore and cleanse entire abdomen, especially subphrenic spaces and pelvis
Elevate liver and expose duodenum, suction away contamination
Visualize perforation; consider Graham patch only if perforation is small and anterior

Identify and, if necessary, mobilize tongue of omentum that reaches comfortably to perforation
Suture omentum over perforation using interrupted 2-0 silks
Irrigate abdomen and close

HALLMARK ANATOMIC COMPLICATIONS

Failure of seal (hole too large)

LIST OF STRUCTURES

Liver
Coronary ligament
Triangular ligaments
Falciform ligament
Ligamentum teres
Left and right subphrenic spaces

Subhepatic space
Lesser sac
Duodenum
Greater omentum
Gastroepiploic vessels

Identification of Perforation Site (Fig. 59.1)

Technical Points

Enter the abdomen through an upper midline or right paramedian incision (Fig. 59.1A) and thoroughly explore the abdomen. Often the site of perforation will have been sealed off by the overhanging liver and the omentum. Leave this seal undisturbed as you explore the left subphrenic space (over the stomach and spleen), the right subphrenic space (over the dome of the liver), and the rest of the abdomen. Culture the peritoneal fluid and remove as much contamination as possible by irrigation and suction. Then gently elevate the liver to expose the duodenum.

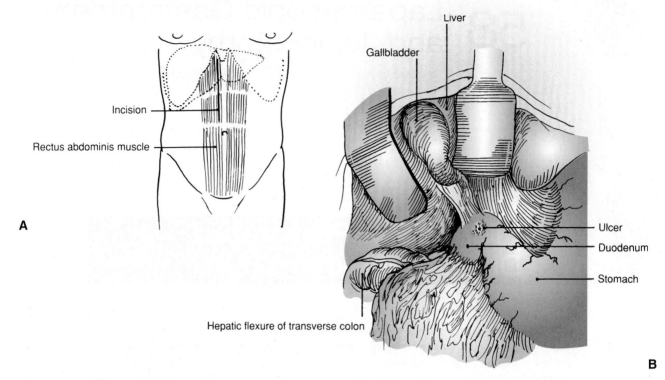

Figure 59.1 Identification of perforation site. **A:** Incision. **B:** Typical site of perforation.

Place a Harrington retractor on the liver, lift it up, and expose the subhepatic space by applying gentle downward traction on the stomach and the duodenum (Fig. 59.1B). Frequently, the left lobe of the liver will have "sealed" the perforation, which is typically located at the pylorus or first portion of the duodenum. This seal must be gently broken to expose the perforation. A flow of clear bile into the field usually results.

If the perforation is located on the gastric wall or is large, plication is not appropriate and resection (see Chapter 61) or closure as a pyloroplasty (see Chapter 65e) may be more appropriate.

Anatomic Points

Topographically, the liver divides the upper abdominal region from the diaphragm superiorly to the transverse colon and mesocolon inferiorly into the smaller subphrenic space and subhepatic spaces. Each of these smaller spaces can be further subdivided, by peritoneal folds and reflections, into three spaces, each of which has clinical importance because abscesses can form in any of them. Immediately superior to the liver and anterior to the anterior layer of the coronary and triangular ligaments, the falciform ligament, with its contained ligamentum teres, divides that space into a *left superior space* and a *right subphrenic space*. The *right subphrenic space* is limited by the anterior layer of the coronary ligament, the diaphragmatic surface of the liver, and the body wall.

The inferior aspect of the liver is divided by the ligamentum teres of the liver and the ligamentum venosum and associated mesenteric folds into a right and a left side. To the right of these structures is a large *right subhepatic space,* bounded

by the liver, transverse mesocolon and colon, and ligamentum teres. On the left side, a similar space lies between the liver and the anterior surface of the stomach and lesser omentum. The lesser sac (*lesser omental bursa*) is bounded superiorly by liver, anteriorly by stomach and lesser omentum, and posteriorly by parietal peritoneum over the parietes and structures in the retroperitoneal space. It is in this latter space that perigastric abscesses are most likely to form following perforation of a peptic ulcer. If the perforation is through the anterior stomach or duodenum, abscess formation can occur in either or both of the other two subphrenic spaces.

Placement of Sutures (Fig. 59.2)

Technical Points

Typically, bile will flow continuously into the field from the perforation. Have an assistant; maintain a clear field by suctioning the area. Select an appropriate piece of omentum from the free edge, mobilizing it, if necessary, to reach the site of perforation.

Place three or four interrupted 2-0 silk simple or Lembert sutures across the perforation (Fig. 59.2A, B). Pass the tongue of the omentum under the silk sutures and tie the sutures over the omentum (Fig. 59.2C). Do not try to approximate the edges of the hole with the sutures because the tissue adjacent to the site of perforation is generally inflamed and edematous and the sutures may cut through. If desired, test the plication by filling the upper abdomen with sterile saline and having the anesthesiologist insufflate the nasogastric tube with air. No air bubbles should be seen.

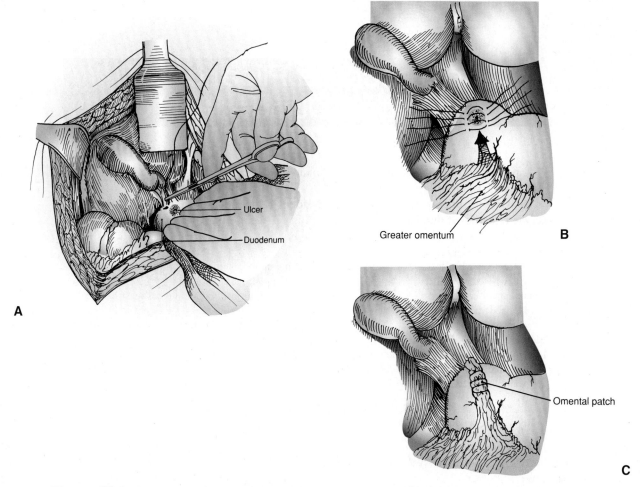

Figure 59.2 Placement of sutures. **A:** Initial suture placed in duodenum on one side of perforation. **B:** All sutures placed but not tied. **C:** Sutures tied over omentum.

If a highly selective vagotomy is to be performed, it may be done now. Recheck the patch after completing the highly selective vagotomy to ensure that the patch has not become dislodged during the course of the dissection.

Irrigate the abdomen again before closure and confirm that there is no leakage of bile from the patch. Place a closed suction drain in the subhepatic space if a true abscess was found in association with the perforation.

Anatomic Points

The blood supply of the greater omentum is based on several, rather long, descending branches from the gastroepiploic arcade. Mobilization of a pedicle flap of omentum can be accomplished with little danger as long as continuity with the gastroepiploic arcade is maintained.

References

1. Bonin EA, Moran E, Gostout CJ, et al. Natural orifice transluminal endoscopic surgery for patients with perforated peptic ulcer. *Surg Endosc.* 2012;26:1534–1538. (Completely new approach to the problem.)

2. Donovan AJ, Berne TV, Donovan JA. Perforated duodenal ulcer: An alternative therapeutic plan. *Arch Surg.* 1998;133:1166–1171. (Discusses role of therapy for *Helicobacter* species and other intensive medical therapy versus vagotomy.)

3. Graham RR. The treatment of perforated duodenal ulcers. *Surg Gynecol Obstet.* 1937;64:235–238. (Presents original description of the technique that bears the author's name.)

4. Ng EK, Lam YH, Sung JJ, et al. Eradication of *Helicobacter pylori* prevents recurrence of ulcer after simple closure of duodenal ulcer perforation: Randomized controlled trial. *Ann Surg.* 2000; 231:153–158.

5. Sharma R, Organ CH Jr, Hirvela ER, et al. Clinical observation of the temporal association between crack cocaine and duodenal ulcer perforation. *Am J Surg.* 1997;174:629–632.

6. Stabile BE. Redefining the role of surgery for perforated duodenal ulcer in the *Helicobacter pylori* era. *Ann Surg.* 2000;231:159–160.

7. Svanes C, Lie RT, Svanes K, et al. Adverse effects of delayed treatment for perforated peptic ulcer. *Ann Surg.* 1994;220:168–175.

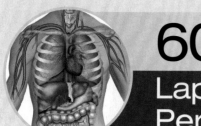

60

Laparoscopic Plication of Perforated Duodenal Ulcer

Laparoscopic plication is an easy way to manage a simple small anterior perforation of a duodenal ulcer.

SCORE™, the Surgical Council on Resident Education, did not classify laparoscopic plication of duodenal ulcer.

STEPS IN PROCEDURE

Set up room as with laparoscopic cholecystectomy

Obtain laparoscopic access

Explore abdomen and suction/irrigate any contamination

Elevate left lobe of liver

Identify perforation and determine suitability for simple plication (small hole on anterior wall of duodenum, edges well-defined)

Bring up mobile tongue of omentum

Suture over perforation

Test with air insufflation into nasogastric tube under saline

Consider placing closed suction drain in subhepatic space

Close any trocar sites larger than 5 mm

HALLMARK ANATOMIC COMPLICATIONS

Injury to viscera during laparoscopic entry

Inadequate closure of perforation

LIST OF STRUCTURES

Liver
    Falciform ligament
    Ligamentum teres
    Segment II
    Segment III
    Segment IV
Gallbladder

Left and right subphrenic spaces
Subhepatic space
Lesser sac
Duodenum
Prepyloric vein (of Mayo)
Greater omentum

Initial Exposure of the Right Upper Quadrant and Subhepatic Space (Fig. 60.1)

Technical Points

Set up the room as you would for laparoscopic cholecystectomy (see Figure 64.1A). Enter the abdomen through an infra-umbilical puncture site and explore. Aspirate and irrigate all four quadrants of the abdomen. Frequently, the perforation is sealed by overlying liver. Leave this seal intact until you are finished irrigating and inspecting the rest of the abdomen. Be alert to the possibility of another etiology for the problem (e.g., appendicitis, diverticulitis). If the appearance is consistent with a perforated duodenal ulcer, place secondary trocars as shown (Fig. 60.1A).

Gently elevate the liver to expose the perforation. An easy way to obtain initial exposure is to pass a grasper (closed) under the liver from the right lateral port and carefully lift up on liver and falciform ligament. Elevating the falciform ligament will lift the liver. Inspect the subhepatic space. Place a liver retractor to obtain a stable working field.

Anatomic Points

The initial laparoscopic view of the left upper quadrant demonstrates the liver, falciform ligament, omentum, colon, and gallbladder (Fig. 60.1B). As the liver is elevated, stomach and duodenum come into view (Fig. 60.1C). The prepyloric vein of Mayo provides a convenient visual dividing point between the stomach and the duodenum. Branches of the supraduodenal

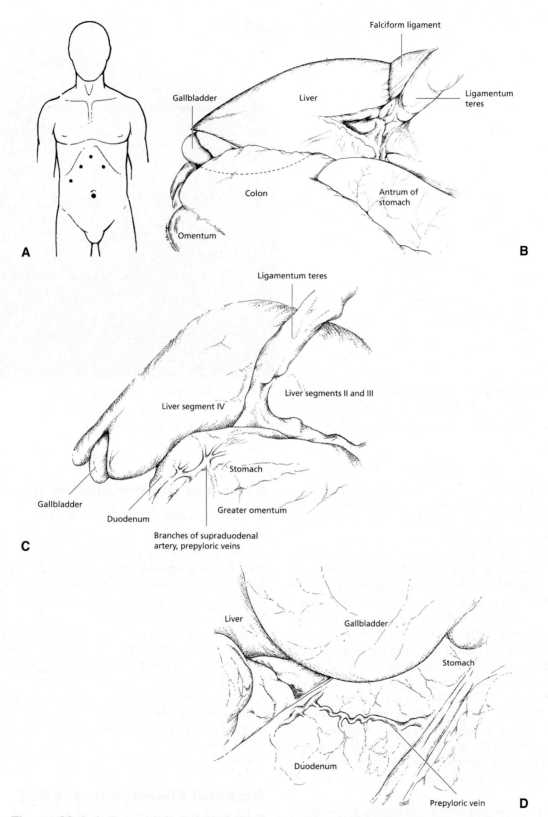

Figure 60.1 **A:** Trocar sites. **B:** Initial laparoscopic view. **C:** Elevation of liver to expose subhepatic space. **D:** Prepyloric vein (of Mayo) separates duodenum and stomach. (**B** from Scott-Conner CEH, Cushieri A, Carter FJ. Right upper quadrant: Liver, gallbladder, and extra-hepatic biliary tract. In: *Minimal Access Surgical Anatomy.* Philadelphia, PA: Lippincott Williams & Wilkins; 2000:101–137, with permission; **C** from Scott-Conner CEH, Cushieri A, Carter FJ. Stomach and duodenum. In: *Minimal Access Surgical Anatomy.* Philadelphia, PA: Lippincott Williams & Wilkins; 2000:79–100, with permission).

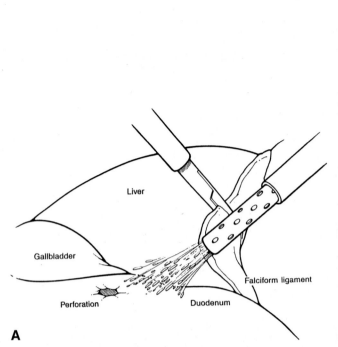

A

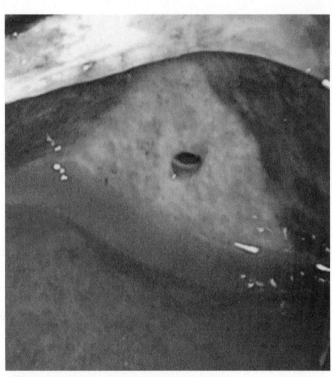

B

Figure 60.2 Exposing the perforation (**A** from Thompson AR, Hall TJ, Anglin BA, et al. Laparoscopic plication of perforated ulcer: Results of a selective approach. *South Med J.* 1995;88:185–189, with permission. **B:** Photo courtesy of Hui Sen Chong, MD).

artery are sometimes found in this region. As the laparoscope is brought closer, the manner in which gallbladder and segment IV of the liver overly the first and second portions of the duodenum becomes apparent (Fig. 60.1D).

The duodenum is conventionally divided into four parts. The first part of the duodenum extends from the pylorus to the point where the gallbladder overlies the duodenum. This is the portion that is easily accessible laparoscopically. Most simple anterior perforated duodenal ulcers are found in the first portion of the duodenum and are easily visualized when the liver is elevated. The second part of the duodenum extends from the gallbladder to approximately the right side of L3 or L4. It contains the ampulla of Vater. The third part of the duodenum runs from right to left, obliquely across to the left side of the aorta. The fourth part of the duodenum then ascends to the suspensory ligament of duodenum (ligament of Treitz). To expose the duodenum fully, it is necessary to mobilize the right colon, as described in Chapter 81. A perforated duodenal ulcer that requires extensive mobilization is best managed by open surgery.

Gastric ulcers that perforate are frequently on the lesser curvature. Identify this situation by the location relative to the prepyloric vein. These are best managed by open surgery.

The relations of the various spaces of the upper abdomen, including the subhepatic space and lesser sac, are described in Chapter 46. Laparoscopic exposure of the lesser sac is described in Chapter 64.

Exposing the Perforation (Fig. 60.2)

Technical and Anatomic Points

Gently elevate the liver with a retractor or with traction on the falciform ligament and use a laparoscopic irrigator to remove fibrinous debris and expose the perforation (Fig. 60.2A). Carefully visualize the perforation and confirm that it is small and localized to the anterior surface of the duodenum (Fig. 60.2B). Ascertain that the entire circumference of the perforation is visualized by washing or picking away any fibrin debris from the edge. Be aware that, occasionally, large perforations extend over the superior aspect of the duodenum into the retroperitoneum. In this situation, it is difficult to obtain secure closure. It is essential that the entire perforation be well visualized. Switch to a 30-degree angled laparoscope if necessary to view the anterior surface of the duodenum.

Omental Plication (Fig. 60.3)

Technical and Anatomic Points

Choose a mobile portion of omentum that reaches easily to the site of perforation. Generally, the omentum close to the ulcer will be inflamed and thickened; it is better to use omentum from the edge, distant from the perforation, because the texture is more pliable.

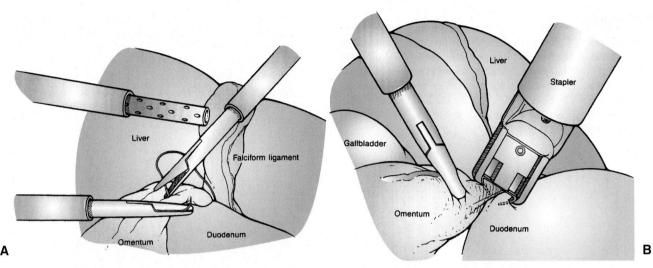

Figure 60.3 Omental plication (**A** and **B** from Thompson AR, Hall TJ, Anglin BA, et al. Laparoscopic plication of perforated ulcer: Results of a selective approach. *South Med J.* 1995;88:185–189).

Suture Fixation of Patch

Suture the patch in place with three or four interrupted sutures of 2-0 or 3-0 silk, beginning with the apex (farthest from the scope) and progressing toward the scope (Fig. 60.3A). Place all the sutures first, then lay the omentum in place and tie the sutures. Secure the omentum with additional sutures if desired (Fig. 60.3B).

Staple Fixation of Patch

A hernia stapler (not a helical tacker) can be used to secure the patch either as an adjunct to sutures or instead of sutures (Fig. 60.3).

Completed Plication (Fig. 60.4)

Technical and Anatomic Points

The completed plication should completely cover the perforation (Fig. 60.4). Confirm adequacy of the patch by having the anesthesiologist instill air into the nasogastric tube while you watch for bubbles under saline. Reinforce the patch if necessary.

Irrigate and aspirate until returns are clear. Place a closed suction drain in the subhepatic space and leave the nasogastric tube in place. Maintain nasogastric suction for 24 hours to allow the patch to seal.

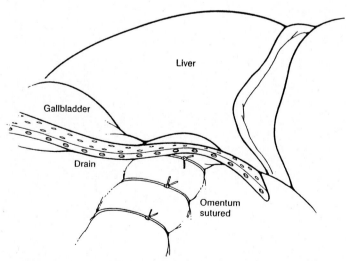

Figure 60.4 Completed plication (from Gadacz TR. Laparoscopic plication of perforated ulcer. In: Scott-Conner CEH, ed. *The SAGES Manual: Fundamentals of Laparoscopy and GI Endoscopy.* New York, NY: Springer-Verlag; 1999: 233–235, with permission).

REFERENCES

1. Androulakis J, Colborn GL, Skandalakis PN, et al. Embryologic and anatomic basis of duodenal surgery. *Surg Clin North Am.* 2000;80:171–199. (Provides excellent review of relevant anatomy.)
2. Gadacz TR. Laparoscopic plication of perforated ulcer. In: Scott-Conner CEH, ed. *The SAGES Manual: Fundamentals of Laparoscopy and GI Endoscopy.* New York, NY: Springer-Verlag; 1999:233–235.
3. Thompson AR, Hall TJ, Anglin BA, et al. Laparoscopic plication of perforated ulcer: Results of a selective approach. *South Med J.* 1995;88:185–189.
4. Scott-Conner CEH, Cushieri A, Carter FJ. Stomach and duodenum. In: *Minimal Access Surgical Anatomy.* Philadelphia, PA: Lippincott Williams & Wilkins; 2000:79–100. (Provides laparoscopic photographs and drawings illustrating regional anatomy.)

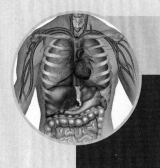

61

Gastric Resection – Subtotal Gastrectomy for Benign Disease

Gastric resection, or gastrectomy, is now performed mainly for treatment of gastric carcinoma. Benign ulcer disease, formerly a major indication, is still sometimes treated by gastrectomy, often in emergency circumstances or neglected cases. Many modifications of the operation exist, differing in the extent of resection and the method of reconstruction of gastrointestinal continuity. This chapter describes basic techniques of gastric resection and reconstruction, primarily as performed for benign disease. The chapter which follows (Chapter 62) describes gastric resection for carcinoma.

SCORE™, the Surgical Council on Resident Education, classified partial gastrectomy as an "ESSENTIAL UNCOMMON" procedure.

STEPS IN PROCEDURE

Subtotal Gastrectomy for Benign Disease

Upper midline incision and thorough abdominal exploration

Identify prepyloric veins of Mayo and evaluate extent of scarring from ulcer disease

Serially clamp, tie, and divide branches of the right gastroepiploic vessels, taking greater omentum from greater curvature

Elevate stomach and divide gastropancreatic folds

Similarly clear an area on the lesser curvature by dividing branches of left gastric artery and vein

Divide stomach with two straight clamps and 4.8-mm linear stapler

Dissect down past pylorus and divide duodenum

For Billroth I Reconstruction

Suture end of duodenum to opening in stomach (two-layer anastomosis)

For Billroth II Reconstruction

Close duodenal stump with staples or sutures

Identify loop of proximal jejunum (20 to 30 cm past ligament of Treitz) and pass antecolic or through hole in transverse mesocolon (retrocolic)

Anastomosis side of loop of jejunum to end of gastric remnant

Close abdomen in the usual fashion without drains

HALLMARK ANATOMIC COMPLICATIONS

Injury to common bile duct

Gastric remnant necrosis if splenectomy combined with high ligation of left gastric artery

Retained antrum (dissection not carried down past pylorus and BII performed)

LIST OF STRUCTURES

Esophagus

Stomach
Lesser curvature
Greater curvature
Antrum
Cardioesophageal junction
Pylorus

Duodenum
Ampulla of Vater
Ligament of Treitz
Spleen

Colon
Epiploic appendices

Right Gastric Vein
Prepyloric veins of Mayo
Transverse mesocolon
Greater omentum

Lesser Omentum
Hepatoduodenal ligament

Middle Colic Artery
Marginal artery of Drummond

Pancreas Accessory pancreatic duct Common bile duct	Left gastroepiploic artery Left gastric vein (coronary vein) Portal vein
Celiac Artery Common hepatic artery Proper hepatic artery Gastroduodenal artery Right gastroepiploic artery Left gastric artery	**Liver** Left lobe of liver Triangular ligament of liver Splenorenal (lienorenal) ligament Gastrosplenic ligament

The extent of resection is determined by the pathology. An antrectomy (resection of the antrum of the stomach) is performed for peptic ulcer disease, usually with a concomitant truncal vagotomy. A subtotal gastrectomy involves resection of additional stomach and is generally quantitated according to the approximate amount removed as shown in Figure 61.1A (e.g., a 60% gastrectomy). For radical subtotal gastrectomy, which is performed for carcinoma, resection of the omentum and regional lymph nodes is added (see Chapter 62). Regional lymph nodes lie along the greater and lesser curvatures and along named blood vessels. Total gastrectomy, also generally performed for carcinoma, entails removal of the entire stomach and surrounding node-bearing tissue. The spleen may also be removed during operations for gastric cancer to resect regional lymph nodes in the splenic hilum.

The simplest method of reconstruction after partial gastrectomy is by direct anastomosis of the gastric remnant to the duodenum (Billroth I reconstruction) as shown in Figure 61.1B. This creates what morphologically resembles a small stomach and is applicable when the gastric remnant and the duodenum can be brought together without tension. It is not used in operations for gastric carcinoma because the extent of resection generally precludes it and because recurrent disease can obstruct the new outlet.

The Billroth II reconstruction (Fig. 61.1C) eliminates problems with tension after an extensive resection, as well as the potential for recurrent disease, by closing the duodenal stump and draining the gastric remnant by a gastrojejunal anastomosis. The two limbs of a Billroth II are termed the *afferent limb,* which drains the duodenal stump, and the *efferent limb,* through which food exits the stomach into the small intestine. Bile and pancreatic juice from the afferent limb continually pass the stoma and sometimes cause gastritis; the Roux-en-Y reconstruction is designed to surmount this.

In this chapter, partial or subtotal gastrectomy for benign disease is presented first with discussion of the Billroth I and Billroth II methods of reconstruction. Radical subtotal gastrectomy and total gastrectomy are discussed in the chapter which follows (Chapter 62). Less common procedures (rarely performed at present), such as proximal gastric resection, are discussed in the references at the end of the chapter.

Subtotal Gastrectomy

Mobilization of the Greater Curvature (Fig. 61.2)

Technical Points

Enter the abdomen through an upper midline incision and explore it. Note the location of the pylorus by its landmark prepyloric veins of Mayo and determine the extent to which scarring and old or active ulcer disease have altered the anatomy, particularly in the region of the pylorus and duodenum. Verify the position of the nasogastric tube. If a vagotomy is to be performed, do this first (see Figure 65e.1 in Chapter 65e). Then commence mobilizing the stomach by serially dividing and ligating multiple branches of the right gastroepiploic artery and vein running to the greater curvature of the stomach. An opening into the free space of the lesser sac should become apparent. This free space is easier to enter to the left than to the right because multiple filmy layers of omentum can be difficult to separate from the antrum and transverse mesocolon.

Be aware of the close proximity of the transverse mesocolon (and middle colic artery) to gastrocolic omentum, and verify that you are in the correct plane by identifying the transverse mesocolon and pulling it inferiorly. Carry the dissection proximally on the greater curvature to the chosen point of transection of the stomach. The transition point between the left and right gastroepiploic arcades forms an easily recognizable landmark on the greater curvature, corresponding to about a 60% gastric resection.

Continue the dissection distally as far as it will go easily. As the pylorus is reached, chronic inflammation from ulcer disease may render the dissection more difficult. If so, it is best to delay this phase of the dissection until after the stomach is divided proximally. The added mobility will greatly facilitate dissection in the region of the pylorus and duodenum.

Place a Babcock clamp on the distal greater curvature and lift up. Divide multiple avascular adhesions between pancreas and posterior gastric wall with Metzenbaum scissors or electrocautery. A posterior gastric ulcer that is densely adherent to the pancreas is best managed by "buttonholing" the ulcer crater on the pancreas, rather than by attempting excision (which may result in injury to the pancreas).

ORIENTATION

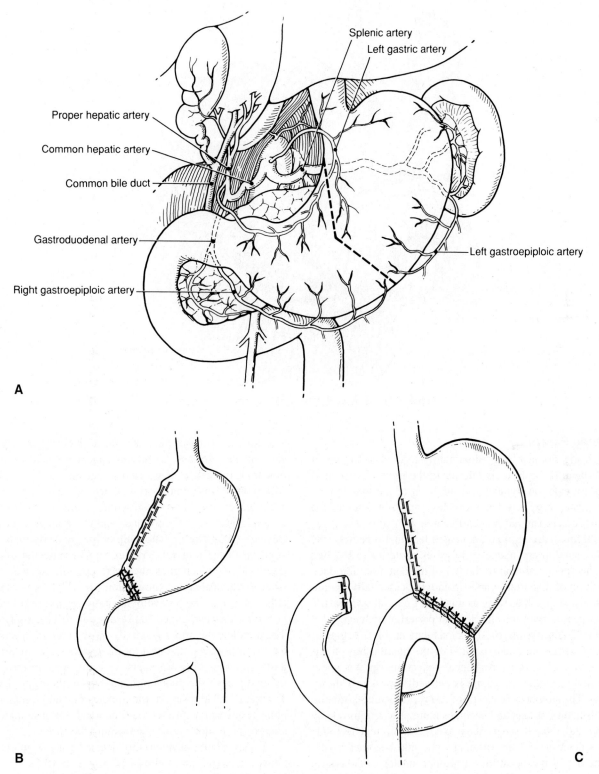

Splenic artery

Left gastric artery

Proper hepatic artery

Common hepatic artery

Common bile duct

Gastroduodenal artery

Right gastroepiploic artery

Left gastroepiploic artery

A

B

C

Figure 61.1 A: Regional anatomy and extent of resection for typical partial gastrectomy.
B: Billroth I reconstruction. **C:** Billroth II reconstruction.

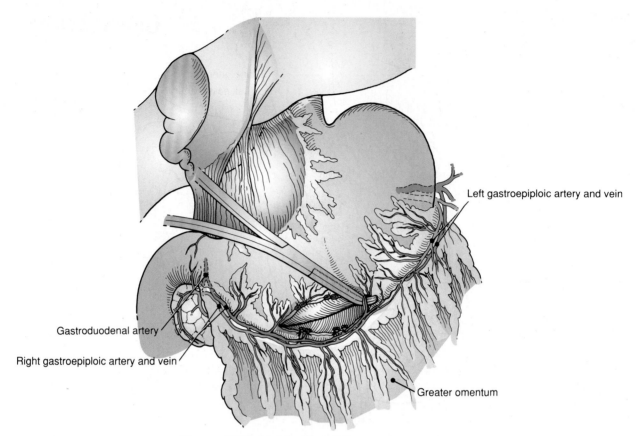

Figure 61.2 Mobilization of the greater curvature

Left gastroepiploic artery and vein

Gastroduodenal artery

Right gastroepiploic artery and vein

Greater omentum

Anatomic Points

Although the stomach is predominantly located in the upper left abdomen, the pylorus is inferior to the right seventh sternocostal articulation, typically at the level of the first lumbar vertebra. The prepyloric veins of Mayo are tributaries of the right gastric vein and aid in identification.

The right gastroepiploic artery is a terminal branch of the gastroduodenal artery that usually arises posterior to the first part of the duodenum and to the left of the common bile duct. The position of this artery varies from lying essentially in contact with the stomach to lying as much as 1 cm inferior; gastric branches pass to both the anterior and posterior stomach.

A brief description of the development of the greater omentum enables an understanding of the relationship of this structure and of various peritoneal reflections in the upper abdomen. The greater omentum is derived from dorsal mesogastrium. The stomach rotates from its original sagittal orientation to its adult position and becomes more or less transversely disposed and rotated on its long axis. The original left side becomes anterior and the original right side becomes posterior. The dorsal mesogastrium disproportionately increases in length and drapes anterior to the transverse colon. The portion of the dorsal mesogastrium that is in contact with the posterior parietal peritoneum fuses to it, and the apposed serosal layers degenerate. Dorsal mesogastrium in contact with transverse mesocolon and transverse colon then fuses to these serosal surfaces, and again, apposed serosal surfaces degenerate. Both the

anterior and posterior inner serosas of the bursal recess contact each other, fuse, and as before, degenerate. Thus the greater omentum typically has no cavity, but instead has a bloodless fusion plane between the original anterior and posterior leaves. This leaves the short gastrocolic ligament connecting the greater curvature of the stomach and the transverse mesocolon. Because of the close relationship of the greater curvature of the stomach to the transverse colon, and because the gastrocolic ligament (in which runs the gastroepiploic arcade) and one layer of the transverse mesocolon (in which runs the middle colic artery) are both developmentally related to dorsal mesogastrium, one can expect these arteries to be closely related. The middle colic artery generally passes into the mesocolon at the lower border of the neck of the pancreas, whereas the right gastroepiploic artery arises just superior to the lower border of the first part of the duodenum, slightly to the right of midline. The spatial relationship of the middle colic and right gastroepiploic arteries may, in fact, be functional, because there can be a large anastomotic artery connecting the two.

Texts and atlases invariably depict a gastroepiploic arcade. However, a true anastomosis is absent in 10% of the cases. Typically, when no anastomosis occurs, there is no definitive left gastroepiploic artery; instead, there are several small branches that unite with similar-sized branches of the right gastroepiploic. In the other 90% of cases, the transition between the left and right gastroepiploic supply is discerned by the change in angle of origin of the gastric branches.

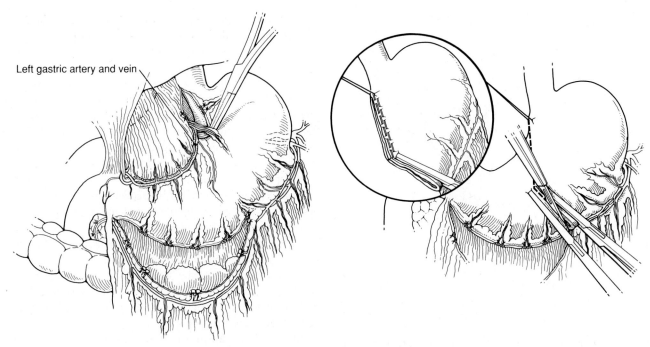

Figure 61.3 Mobilization of the lesser curvature

Mobilization of the Lesser Curvature (Fig. 61.3)

Technical Points

Identify the descending branch of the left gastric artery in the lesser omentum. Pass a right angle clamp under it and double ligate and divide it. Clean the lesser curvature as high up as desired. Place a 2-0 silk Lembert suture at the upper end of the cleared lesser curvature for traction. Verify the position of the nasogastric tube, high in the gastric pouch and well above the line of proposed transection. Place two Kocher clamps across the greater curvature at the selected point of division and cut between the clamps with a knife. This will form the new outlet of the gastric remnant and should be sized accordingly (about 3 cm, or about the size of the duodenum, for a Billroth I reconstruction, and about 4 to 5 cm for a Billroth II procedure).

Construct a Hofmeister shelf by passing a linear stapling device (with 4.8-mm staples) into the opened crotch of the divided stomach, angling it as high up on the lesser curvature as possible. Use traction on the lesser curvature suture to define the upper extent of resection of the lesser curvature. Fire the stapler and divide the lesser curvature between the stapling device and a Kocher clamp. Check the staple line for bleeding points. Place a moist laparotomy pad over the proximal gastric remnant and allow it to retract into the left upper quadrant, out of the way.

Anatomic Points

The most important vascular structure in the lesser omentum is the left gastric artery. This, the smallest branch of the celiac artery, initially has a retroperitoneal course that runs superiorly and to the left. It then runs anteriorly to approach the gastro-esophageal junction. Here, it gives rise to esophageal branches,

turns inferiorly to follow the lesser curvature of the stomach, and terminates by anastomosing with the much smaller right gastric artery. Frequently (25% of the time), it gives rise to the left hepatic artery or to accessory left hepatic arteries, which course through the superior part of the lesser omentum. Even more commonly (42%), it divides into anterior and posterior branches.

The right gastric artery is usually a branch of the common or proper hepatic artery, although it frequently arises from the left hepatic or gastroduodenal artery. As with the left gastric artery, it frequently divides into anterior or posterior branches.

Gastric veins parallel the arteries and empty into the portal vein or its components at different levels, rather than as a single vessel. There are no functional valves in these veins, and because the left gastric vein (coronary vein) has free anastomoses with the caval system through the esophageal veins, it assumes great importance in portal hypertension.

Anterior and posterior vagal nerve components are also found within the lesser omentum. One or more hepatic branches from the anterior vagal trunk pass through the superior part of this ligament, from the level of the esophagus to the porta hepatis. Gastric branches from the anterior vagus either radiate from an origin at the cardioesophageal junction (in which case they are not found in the lesser omentum) or pass from the nerve of Latarjet (which accompanies the left gastric artery) to the stomach with the vessels. A posterior nerve of Latarjet also parallels the lesser curvature of the stomach, although its length as a discrete nerve is not as long as the anterior nerve. A major celiac branch (including more than half of the total nerve fibers) accompanies the left gastric artery to the celiac plexus. Gastric branches reach the stomach in a manner similar to the anterior gastric branches.

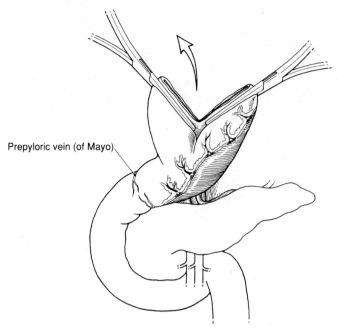

Prepyloric vein (of Mayo)

Figure 61.4 Dissection of the distal antrum and duodenal stump

The extreme right part of the lesser omentum connects the duodenum and liver; hence, it is termed the *hepatoduodenal ligament*. This part of the lesser omentum forms the anterior wall of the epiploic foramen and contains the common bile duct, hepatic artery, and portal vein. The portal vein is posterior, the hepatic artery is anterior and somewhat to the left of the vein, and the common bile duct is anterior and somewhat to the right in the free edge of the ligament.

Dissection of the Distal Antrum and Duodenal Stump (Fig. 61.4)

Technical Points

Dissect circumferentially around the distal antrum and down the duodenum until soft, pliable tissue is encountered. Recognize the pylorus by direct palpation of the doughnut-shaped pyloric sphincter or by the overlying prepyloric veins of Mayo. If severe scarring from ulcer disease or previous surgery has distorted the anatomy, confirm that the duodenum has been reached by examining a frozen section of the resection margin. Brunner's glands are characteristic of the duodenum and are readily seen on histologic examination.

The gastroduodenal artery will be encountered if the dissection progresses more than about 1 cm down the duodenum. Dissection beyond this point should be done with extreme care lest the accessory pancreatic duct or common bile duct be damaged. Remove the stomach by transecting the duodenum.

Anatomic Points

Mobilization of the stomach, including the antrum, presents no further problems if none have been encountered with mobilization of the greater and lesser curvatures. This is not true with respect to the duodenum, which becomes a retroperitoneal organ

shortly distal to the pyloric sphincter. Difficult anatomic relationships that can lead to complications also begin at this point. If the dissection proceeds from left to right and inferior tension is placed on the distal portion of the stomach, control of the right gastric vein superior to the pylorus will control bleeding from the prepyloric veins of Mayo. Further mobilization inferiorly and to the right should expose, posterior to the first part of the duodenum, the common hepatic artery and two of its branches, the proper hepatic and gastroduodenal arteries. Remember that the common bile duct should be located to the right of the common hepatic artery and anterior to the portal vein, both in the gastroduodenal ligament and immediately posterior to the duodenum, and that it is in the retroduodenal region that the common bile duct either becomes surrounded by pancreatic tissue or lies in the fascial plane between the pancreas and the duodenum. It, too, should be treated with utmost care.

If the second part of the duodenum is approached in this circumferential dissection, the surgeon should remember the significant features of pancreatic development. The superior part of the pancreatic head plus the neck and body of the pancreas develop from the dorsal pancreatic bud, initially a diverticulum of the original dorsal aspect of the duodenum. The elongated diverticulum forms the duct of Santorini. The ventral pancreatic bud begins as a diverticulum of the developing common bile duct. As a result of foregut rotation and differential growth, the ventral pancreatic bud migrates to a position immediately caudal to the dorsal pancreatic bud, where it develops into the uncinate process and lower part of the head of the pancreas. Its attachment (duct of Wirsung) to the common bile duct is retained. Later, the duct systems fuse, and the definitive pancreatic duct is derived distally (neck, body, and tail) from the duct of Santorini and proximally (head and uncinate process) from the duct of Wirsung. In the adult, this main pancreatic duct opens into the duodenum, typically through the chamber (ampulla of Vater) that is common to the terminal common bile duct, at the major duodenal papilla, which is located somewhat posteriorly on the concave side of the duodenal lumen at about the level of the second lumbar vertebra. The proximal end of the duct of Santorini usually persists as the accessory pancreatic duct (in 70% of cases), opening into the duodenum somewhat more anteriorly than the major pancreatic duct and typically about 2 cm superior to the major duodenal papilla. In about 10% of cases, the accessory duct is the only grossly visible duct draining the pancreas.

This region is the site of many variations in the configuration and anatomic relationships of the biliary apparatus; blood supply to the liver, duodenum, and pancreas; and tributaries of the portal vein. A general rule that will help to prevent complications secondary to variant anatomy is to define carefully and identify accurately all tubular structures in this region before ligation and division.

Billroth I Reconstruction (Fig. 61.5)

Technical Points

Mobilize the duodenum by performing a Kocher maneuver (see Figure 72.5 in Chapter 72). Place a posterior row of interrupted

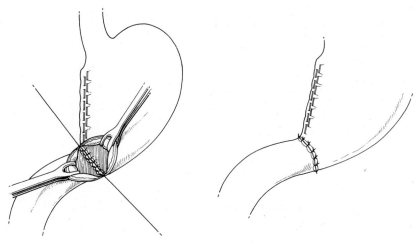

Figure 61.5 Billroth I reconstruction

silk Lembert sutures to anastomose the duodenum to the gastric remnant. At the superior angle, where the Hofmeister shelf intersects the suture line, place a three-corner stitch, as shown in Figure 61.7C. Visualize the three bites of this stitch as defining the sides of a triangle drawn around the "angle of sorrows." Place the inner suture line as a running lock-stitch of 3-0 absorbable suture, beginning at the midline of the back wall, and continue this anteriorly as a running Connell suture to achieve careful mucosal apposition. Then place an anterior row of interrupted Lembert sutures of 3-0 silk to complete the anastomosis.

Anatomic Points

The Kocher maneuver returns the duodenum and pancreas to their embryologic midline position. The duodenum originally is a midline segment of gut suspended by a dorsal mesoduodenum in which the dorsal bud of the pancreas (destined to become the upper part of the head plus the neck and body of the pancreas) develops. As a result of rotation of the upper gastrointestinal organs, the original right side of the duodenum and pancreas come to lie in contact with the dorsal parietal peritoneum. The apposing serosal surfaces then fuse and degenerate, leaving an avascular plane posterior to the now retroperitoneal duodenum and pancreas. In addition, on the original antimesenteric (convex) side of the duodenum, the parietal peritoneum and serosa of the original left side of the duodenum fuse.

Positional changes of the midgut loop (secondary to rotation, physiologic herniation and reduction, and fixation of those segments destined to become retroperitoneal) occur after fixation of the foregut-derived duodenum. Consequently, the root of the transverse mesocolon is frequently attached to the anterior surface of the second part of the duodenum and anterior surface of the pancreas. The hepatic flexure of the colon should be pulled inferiorly and medially to expose the superior part of the C loop of duodenum. At this point, one should identify the middle colic vessels because they frequently course immediately anterior to the second part of the duodenum. With these vessels identified, incision of the peritoneum along the lateral

edge of the duodenum, followed by blunt finger dissection in the avascular fusion plane posterior to the duodenum and head of pancreas, should result in adequate mobilization of these structures with little or no blood loss.

Billroth II Reconstruction: Closure of the Duodenal Stump (Fig. 61.6)

Technical and Anatomic Points

If Billroth II reconstruction is planned, first close the duodenal stump in two layers in the following manner. Start a Connell suture at the inferior end of the duodenal stump and run it superiorly. At the top, either terminate the suture line by tying the suture to itself or turn the suture line back and invert again by running back to the point of origin as a running horizontal mattress suture. Then place an outer layer of interrupted 3-0 silk Lembert sutures. Alternatively, an easy duodenal stump can be closed with a linear stapling device loaded with 3.5-mm staples.

The difficult duodenal stump, scarred by duodenal ulcer disease, can be closed by one of a variety of methods. Generally, pliable anterior duodenal wall is rolled down and over, with subsequent suturing to the pancreatic capsule if necessary. A tube duodenostomy can be placed through a separate stab wound and secured with an absorbable purse-string suture as an extra precaution. This creates a controlled fistula.

Pack omentum over the duodenal stump before closure. Place a closed-suction drain in the vicinity of the tube duodenostomy, if one was placed. Otherwise, do not drain the stump.

Billroth II Reconstruction—Sutured Gastrojejunostomy (Fig. 61.7)

Technical Points

The gastrojejunostomy may be performed in an antecolic or retrocolic fashion. Here, the basic antecolic gastrojejunostomy is described, with comments on the alternative retrocolic version.

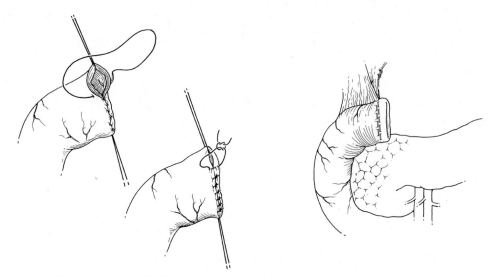

Figure 61.6 Billroth II reconstruction: Closure of the duodenal stump

Identify the proximal jejunum at the ligament of Treitz. Trace it down 20 to 30 cm and locate a loop of proximal jejunum that will reach to the gastric remnant without tension. The loop should be as close to the ligament of Treitz as possible. The jejunal loop will be routed to the left of the main bulk of the greater omentum, which will pass to the right and be used to pack off the duodenal stump and surround the gastrojejunostomy.

Suture the jejunal loop to the gastric remnant with a standard two-layer technique. Take special care to clamp and ligate multiple small arterial branches in the gastric submucosa that can cause gastrointestinal bleeding in the postoperative period. Place a three-corner suture at the "angle of sorrows." The afferent limb should exit to the left, whereas the efferent limb should exit to the right. Allow the gastrojejunostomy to rise into the left upper quadrant, where it should lie comfortably without tension or kinking.

Anatomic Points

Technically, the antecolic anastomosis is the simpler of the two procedures. The gastrojejunal anastomosis is placed anterior to the colon, so that additional dissection is unnecessary. If a retrocolic anastomosis is to be performed, the transverse mesocolon must be incised. This should be done to the left of the middle colic artery and vein and to the right of the superior branch of the inferior mesenteric artery, taking care not to insult the marginal artery close to the mesenteric border of the colon. This area is essentially avascular.

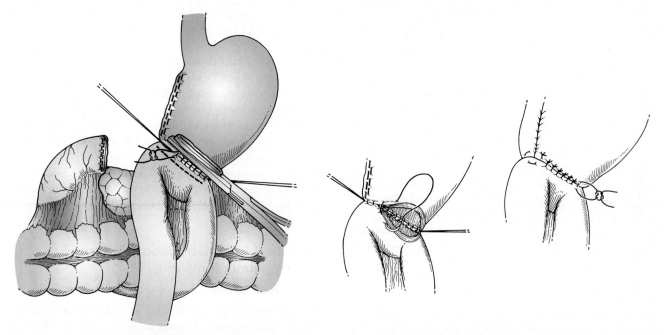

Figure 61.7 Billroth II reconstruction—sutured gastrojejunostomy

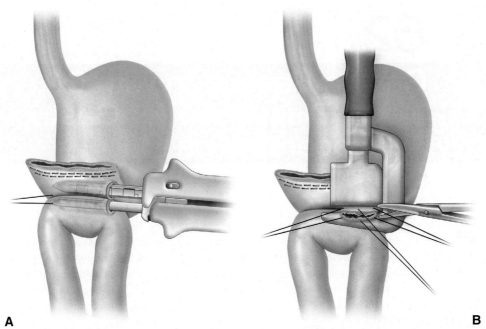

A　　　　　　　　　　　　　　　　　　　　　　**B**

Figure 61.8 Billroth II reconstruction—stapled gastrojejunostomy. **A:** Insertion of limbs of stapler into the stomach and jejunum. **B:** Closure of stab wounds (from Chapter 17: Subtotal gastrectomy and D2 resection. In: Nussbaum MS, ed. *Master Techniques in Gastric Surgery.* Philadelphia, PA: Wolters Kluwer Lippincott Williams & Wilkins; 2013).

Stapled Gastrojejunostomy (Billroth II) (Fig. 61.8)

Many surgeons preferred a stapled reconstruction. In this case, mobilize the proximal stomach as previously described. Fire a long linear stapler obliquely across the proximal stomach, angling it in such a fashion as to include the antral tongue of lesser curvature without creating a separate Hoffmeister shelf. Make stab wounds in the proximal stomach and jejunum (Fig. 61.8A) and insert a GIA-type stapler. Fire the stapler. Check the inverted staple line for hemostasis and carefully secure any arterial bleeders with figure-of-eight sutures of PDS.

Then close the stab wounds with suture or stapler (Fig. 61.8B) in the usual fashion.

REFERENCES

1. Besson A. The Roux-Y loop in modern digestive tract surgery. *Am J Surg.* 1985;149:656. (Describes the history and multiple applications of this technique.)
2. Burch JM, Cox CL, Feliciano DV, et al. Management of the difficult duodenal stump. *Am J Surg.* 1991;162:522–526. (Compares various techniques.)
3. Dempsey D. Chapter 24. Bile (alkaline Reflux) Gastritis. In: Nussbaum MS, Fischer JE, eds. *Master Techniques in Gastric Surgery.* Philadelphia, PA: Wolters Kluwer Lippincott Williams & Wilkins; 2013:253.
4. Eagon JC, Miedema BW, Kelly KA. Postgastrectomy syndromes. *Surg Clin North Am.* 1992;72:445. (Provides good review of problems that occur after gastric resection and their management.)
5. Gingrich GW. The use of the T-tube in difficult duodenal stump closures. *Am Surg.* 1959;25:639. (Provides good description of tube duodenostomy.)
6. Harrower HW. Closure of the duodenal stump after gastrectomy for posterior ulcer. *Am J Surg.* 1966;111:488.
7. Hermann RE. T-tube catheter drainage of the duodenal stump. *Am J Surg.* 1973;125:364.
8. Powers JC, Fitzgerald JF, McAlvanah MJ. The anatomic basis for the surgical detachment of the greater omentum from the transverse colon. *Surg Gynecol Obstet.* 1976;143:105.
9. Steichen FM, Ravitch MM. Operations on the stomach. In: Steichen FM, ed. *Stapling in Surgery.* Chicago: Year Book Medical Publishers; 1984:173. (Describes a variety of procedures by pioneers in surgical stapling.)

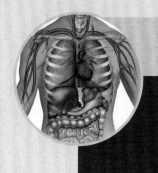

62

Gastric Resection with D2 Nodal Dissection for Gastric Adenocarcinoma

Hisakazu Hoshi

As the incidence of gastric cancer declines, gastrectomy for gastric carcinoma is becoming one of the rarely performed operations for general surgeons. The extent of nodal dissection associated with the operation is a topic of debate but current national guidelines recommend resection of regional lymph nodes. This chapter reviews anatomy and technique of both distal and total gastrectomies with D2 nodal dissection. Additional material on technique of gastrectomy and BI and BII reconstructions is given in Chapter 61.

SCORE™, the Surgical Council on Resident Education, classified partial and total gastrectomies as "ESSENTIAL UNCOMMON" procedures.

STEPS IN PROCEDURE

Gastrectomy with D2 Nodal Dissection (Common Portion)

Upper midline incision and through abdominal exploration

Assess resectability, undetected metastatic disease

Retract greater omentum cephalad and detach from transverse colon, preserving mesentery to colon

Dissect infrapyloric nodal station and ligate right gastroepiploic vessels

Ligate right gastric artery and dissect suprapyloric nodal station

Divide duodenum with stapler

Divide lesser omentum to the GE junction

Dissect nodes along the hepatic artery

Elevate stomach and divide left gastric artery at its origin

Dissect celiac and proximal splenic nodal stations

Distal Gastrectomy

Dissect right paracardiac nodes and lesser curvature nodes toward resection line

Ligate left gastroepiploic vessels and dissect greater curvature nodes toward resection line

Divided stomach with 3 to 5 cm margin

Total Gastrectomy

Ligate left gastroepiploic vessels and divide gastrosplenic ligament by ligating all short gastric arteries

Isolate distal esophagus and divide

For Roux-en-Y Reconstruction

Divide upper jejunum 20 to 30 cm past ligament of Treitz

Pass jejunum to stomach or esophagus (if total gastrectomy)

Antecolic, or through hole in transverse mesocolon (retrocolic)

End-to-side esophagojejunostomy with circular staple or end-to-end gastrojejunostomy (stapled or sutured)

Jejunojejunostomy (stapled or sutured)

Side-to-side jejunojejunostomy 40 to 45 cm from anastomosis

HALLMARK ANATOMIC COMPLICATIONS

Injury to
   common bile duct
   celiac artery branches
   portal or splenic vein
   spleen
   pancreas

Gastric remnant necrosis from splenic artery injury

LIST OF STRUCTURES

Esophagus
Right diaphragmatic crus
Stomach

Lesser curvature
Greater curvature
Antrum

Esophagogastric junction	Pancreas
Pylorus	Common bile duct
Duodenum	Celiac artery
Ligament of Treitz	Common hepatic artery
Spleen	Proper hepatic artery
Transverse colon	Splenic artery
Transverse mesocolon	Posterior gastric artery
Greater omentum	Left gastric artery
Lesser omentum	Left gastric vein (coronary vein)
Lesser sac	Left gastroepiploic artery
Hepatoduodenal ligament	Portal vein
Middle colic vessels	Splenic vein
Right accessory colic vein	Liver
Right gastroepiploic vein	Left lateral lobe of liver
Gastro colic trunk	Caudate lobe
Right gastroepiploic artery	Gastrosplenic ligament
Right gastric artery	Short gastric arteries

Definition of the Nodal Stations and the D1 and D2 Nodal Dissections

The nodal stations around the stomach are anatomically defined and numerically classified by the Japanese Classification of Gastric Carcinoma published by Japanese Gastric Cancer Association (JGCA) (Fig. 62.1, Table 62.1). Perigastric nodal stations are numbered 1 to 6 and regional nodal stations are 7 to 12. Nodal stations numbered higher than 12 are generally considered "distant" nodal stations and are not dissected for the standard D2 nodal dissection except nodal station 14v.

The level of the nodal dissection, known as D number, is defined by the guidelines from JGCA. While the classic D1 nodal dissection is defined by complete dissection of the first-tier nodal stations (which are determined by the location of the primary lesion and is most compatible with current concept of the "D1 nodes, perigastric nodes [stations 1 to 6]" in western literature), current (2010) definition of D1 nodal dissection in Japan includes left gastric artery node station (station 7) in addition to the perigastric nodal stations due to the observed high rate of metastasis in this nodal station by the early gastric cancer.

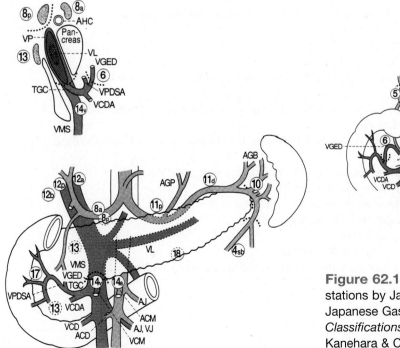

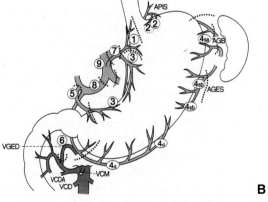

Figure 62.1 **A** and **B:** Location and border of lymph node stations by Japanese Gastric Cancer Association (from Japanese Gastric Cancer Association. Figure 7. In: *Japanese Classifications of Gastric Carcinoma.* 14th ed. Tokyo, Japan: Kanehara & Co. Ltd., with permission).

Table 62.1 Anatomical Definitions of Lymph Node Stations

No.	Definition
1	Right paracardial LNs, including those along the first branch of the ascending limb of the left gastric artery
2	Left paracardial LNs including those along the esophagocardiac branch of the left subphrenic artery
3a	Lesser curvature LNs along the branches of the left gastric artery
3b	Lesser curvature LNs along the second branch and distal part of the right gastric artery
4sa	Left greater curvature LNs along the short gastric arteries (perigastric area)
4sb	Left greater curvature LNs along the left gastroepiploic artery (perigastric area)
4d	Right greater curvature LNs along the second branch and distal part of the right gastroepiploic artery
5	Suprapyloric LNs along the first branch and proximal part of the right gastric artery
6	Infrapyloric LNs along the first branch and proximal part of the right gastroepiploic artery down to the confluence of the right gastroepiploic vein and the anterior superior pancreatoduodenal vein
7	LNs along the trunk of the left gastric artery between its root and the origin of its ascending branch
8a	Anterosuperior LNs along the common hepatic artery
8p	Posterior LNs along the common hepatic artery
9	Celiac artery LNs
10	Splenic hilar LNs including those adjacent to the splenic artery distal to the pancreatic tail, and those on the roots of the short gastric arteries and those along the left gastroepiploic artery proximal to its first gastric branch
11p	Proximal splenic artery LNs from its origin to halfway between its origin and the pancreatic tail end
11d	Distal splenic artery LNs from halfway between its origin and the pancreatic tail end to the end of the pancreatic tail
12a	Hepatoduodenal ligament LNs along the proper hepatic artery, in the caudal half between the confluence of the right and left hepatic ducts and the upper border of the pancreas
12b	Hepatoduodenal ligament LNs along the bile duct, in the caudal half between the confluence of the right and left hepatic ducts and the upper border of the pancreas
12p	Hepatoduodenal ligament LNs along the portal vein in the caudal half between the confluence of the right and left hepatic ducts and the upper border of the pancreas
13	LNs on the posterior surface of the pancreatic head cranial to the duodenal papilla
14v	LNs along the superior mesenteric vein
15	LNs along the middle colic vessels
16a1	Para-aortic LNs in the diaphragmatic aortic hiatus
16a2	Para-aortic LNs between the upper margin of the origin of the celiac artery and the lower border of the left renal vein
16b1	Para-aortic LNs between the lower border of the left renal vein and the upper border of the origin of the inferior mesenteric artery
16b2	Para-aortic LNs between the upper border of the origin of the inferior mesenteric artery and the aortic bifurcation
17	LNs on the anterior surface of the pancreatic head beneath the pancreatic sheath
18	LNs along the inferior border of the pancreatic body
19	Infradiaphragmatic LNs predominantly along the subphrenic artery
20	Paraesophageal LNs in the diaphragmatic esophageal hiatus
110	Paraesophageal LNs in the lower thorax
111	Supradiaphragmatic LNs separate from the esophagus
112	Posterior mediastinal LNs separate from the esophagus and the esophageal hiatus

Adapted from: Japanese Gastric Cancer Association. Table 5. In: *Japanese Classifications of Gastric Carcinoma.* 14th ed. Tokyo, Japan: Kanehara & Co. Ltd., with permission.

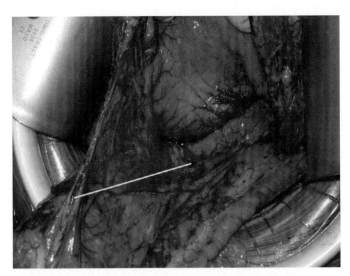

Figure 62.2 Right side border of lesser sac. The yellow line indicates peritoneal incision to further separate the greater omentum and the transverse colon mesentery (from Hoshi H. Standard D2 and modified nodal dissection for gastric adenocarcinoma. *Surg Oncol Clin N Am.* 2012; 21(1):57–70).

The Technique of the D2 Nodal Dissection (Common Portion for Both a Distal and a Total Gastrectomy) (Figs. 62.2 and 62.3)

Greater Curvature and Infrapyloric Node Dissection

Technical Points

Typically, a D2 nodal dissection starts from the greater curvature of the stomach. An omentectomy is an integral part of the D2 nodal dissection. Enter the lesser sac by detaching the greater omentum from the transverse colon. Once it is widely separated, note that the greater omentum is fused with the anterior surface of the transverse colon mesentery on the right side (Fig. 62.2). This portion is considered "right side border" of the lesser sac. Gain access to the station 6 (infrapyloric) nodes by dividing this "right side border" to further separate the omentum from the transverse colon mesentery by separating peritoneum along the yellow line shown in Figure 62.2.

This complete separation allows the middle colic vessels and a right accessory colic vein to be seen (Fig. 62.3). Trace the middle colic vessels to the anterior surface of the superior mesenteric vein (SMV). The soft tissue covering the anterior surface of the SMV below the lower edge of the pancreas is classified as station 14v. If the tumor is located in the antrum of the stomach, then this station may be included in the resection (see later discussion).

Nodal station 6 is located proximal to the junction of the right accessory colic vein and the right gastroepiploic vein (see Anatomical Points). For complete dissection of station 6, ligate the right gastroepiploic at this junction point. Then dissect all the soft tissues covering the anterior surface of the pancreas head off toward the pylorus.

About 5 mm to 1 cm cephalad to the right gastroepiploic vein, note that a right gastroepiploic artery can be seen emerging from the pancreatic head parenchyma (Fig. 62.4). Ligate this and clear all the soft tissues from the pancreas toward the inferior wall of the duodenum. This concludes infrapyloric portion of the dissection.

Anatomic Points

Lesser sac (bursa omentalis) is a blind pouch formed by the posterior gastric wall anteriorly, the anterior surface of the pancreas posteriorly, the left side of transverse colon mesentery inferiorly, and the caudate lobe of the liver superiorly. It communicates

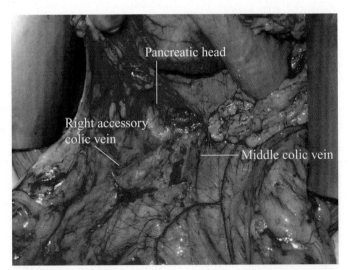

Figure 62.3 Middle colic vein and right accessory colic vein (from Hoshi H. Standard D2 and modified nodal dissection for gastric adenocarcinoma. *Surg Oncol Clin N Am.* 2012;21(1):57–70).

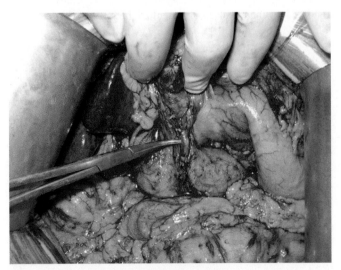

Figure 62.4 Right gastroepiploic artery (from Hoshi H. Standard D2 and modified nodal dissection for gastric adenocarcinoma. *Surg Oncol Clin N Am.* 2012;21(1):57–70).

with peritoneal cavity through the foramen of Winslow behind the hepatoduodenal ligament. The lesser sac can be accessed by dividing the greater omentum from the left side of the transverse colon in avascular plane. The right limit of the lesser sac is formed by the fusion of greater omentum and anterior surface of the transverse colon mesentery. Once this "right side border" is separated by incising peritoneum, then transverse colon and its mesentery can be completely separated from greater omentum, antrum, and even pancreatic head.

In this portion of the transverse colon mesentery, middle colic vessels and right accessory colic vein can be identified (Fig. 62.3). The right accessory colic vein is located in the right side of the transverse colon mesentery and this joins with the right gastroepiploic vein, and the venous drainage from pancreatic head then forms a gastrocolic trunk. This relatively large vein then drains directly into the SMV (Fig. 62.5). Some articles call this right accessory vein an "accessory middle colic vein"; however, in this chapter the naming by the JGCA, "right accessory colic vein" is used.

Right gastroepiploic artery is the end branch of gastroduodenal artery and is located at the inferior edge of the junction of pancreatic head and duodenum. This artery should be ligated at the level of pancreatic head, and soft tissue around the artery should be separated from inferior duodenal wall and dissected toward pylorus (infrapyloric nodal dissection).

Suprapyloric Nodal Dissection and Division of Duodenum (Fig. 62.5)

Technical Points

At the lesser curvature of the stomach, incise the lesser omentum along the attachment about 1 cm away from the liver. The incision extends all the way up to the esophageal hiatus. An accessory (or replaced) left hepatic artery should be recognized in the area if this is present. It can be preserved by dissecting all the surrounding soft tissues if the gastric cancer is relatively early and has low chance of involvement of the left gastric nodes.

On the left side of the hepatoduodenal ligament, dissect the soft tissue covering the proper hepatic artery toward the common hepatic artery (station 12a). As the dissection progresses toward the common hepatic artery, the origin of the right gastric artery can be seen. Ligate this at its origin and separate the suprapyloric portion of the soft tissue along this artery (station 5) from hepatoduodenal ligament and head of the pancreas toward superior duodenal wall.

Now the duodenum is ready to be divided by mobilizing it from the neck of the pancreas. Management of the duodenal stump is discussed in detail in Chapter 61 and illustrated in Figure 61.6.

Anatomic Points

The lesser omentum extends from the lesser curvature of the stomach to the hepatoduodenal ligament and the liver in between the left lateral lobe and the caudate lobe. The remnant of ductus venosus (Arantius' duct) which used to connect the left portal vein and the IVC is the portion where the lesser omentum attaches to the liver. In this thin membranous structure, hepatic branch of the vagus nerve and occasionally left accessory or replaced artery originating from the left gastric artery are running. Once this is divided then the upper portion of the lesser sac can be accessed and caudate lobe of the liver, right diaphragmatic crus, common hepatic artery and celiac axis, and body of the pancreas are exposed.

Right gastric artery typically branches off of proper hepatic artery, however, if proper hepatic artery divides into right and left hepatic arteries low in hepatoduodenal ligament then it can arise from the left hepatic artery and this can be mistaken as a right gastric artery in this situation.

Completion of Nodal Dissection for Subtotal or Total Gastrectomy (Figs. 62.6–62.9)

Technical Points

A retroperitoneal dissection can be performed without transecting the duodenum but the exposure is better after the transection. The retroperitoneal dissection starts as a continuation of the previous proper hepatic artery node dissection. Divide the

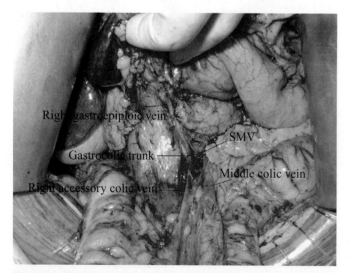

Figure 62.5 Anatomy of the gastrocolic trunk

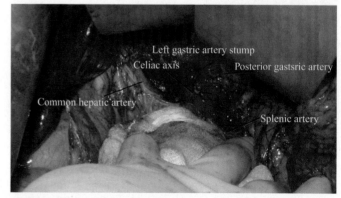

Figure 62.6 Celiac, hepatic artery, and splenic artery dissection (Stations 8a, 9, 11p)

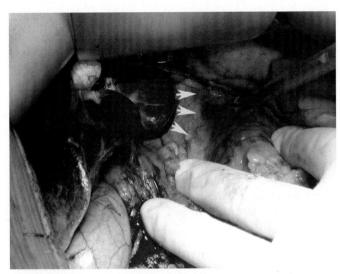

Figure 62.7 Upper border of retroperitoneal dissection. Yellow arrows point out the retroperitoneal incision line along the right diaphragmatic crus (from Hoshi H. Standard D2 and modified nodal dissection for gastric adenocarcinoma. *Surg Oncol Clin N Am.* 2012;21(1):57–70).

peritoneum along the superior border of the pancreas toward left and dissect away the soft tissue covering the common hepatic artery (station 8a). The superior border of the dissection is the right crus of the diaphragm.

Once the origin of the left gastric artery is identified, dissect the soft tissue surrounding the artery distally and ligate this vessel at the origin. Dissection then proceeds along the splenic artery. Nodal tissue proximal to the origin of the posterior gastric artery (station 11p) should be dissected for all gastric cancers except early gastric cancers (Fig. 62.6). For a total gastrectomy, remove the nodal tissue distal to the posterior gastric

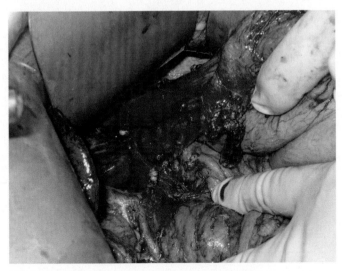

Figure 62.8 Retroperitoneal appearance after completion of the dissection (from Hoshi H. Standard D2 and modified nodal dissection for gastric adenocarcinoma. *Surg Oncol Clin N Am.* 2012;21(1):57–70).

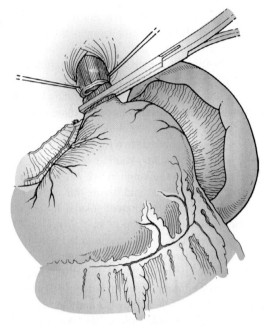

Figure 62.9 Complete a total gastrectomy by dividing the esophagus. Stay sutures on the esophagus help avoid retraction.

artery (station 11d). This portion of the dissection is easier after the fundus has been mobilized for total gastrectomy by ligating short gastric arteries.

In the retroperitoneum, identify the border of the right diaphragmatic crus and divide the peritoneum covering the crus (Fig. 62.7, yellow arrows). This will provide access to the space between the anterior surface of the aorta and the nodal tissue along the lesser curvature of the stomach. Dissection of this plane in right to left direction mobilizes node stations 1 (right cardiac), 3 (lesser curvature), 7 (left gastric artery), and 9 (celiac) toward the stomach. In the end, the left side of esophageal hiatus will be completely exposed and the dissection plane should connect to the previous left gastric artery and the splenic artery dissection plane (Fig. 62.8).

At the greater curvature side, continue to separate the greater omentum from the transverse colon to the splenic flexure. Use caution not to pull the greater omentum to expose this area to avoid splenic capsular tears until lower pole of the spleen is completely separated from the specimen. At the lower pole of the spleen and the tail of the pancreas, the origin of the left gastroepiploic artery and vein can be identified. Ligate these to completely clear the left greater curvature nodal tissue (station 4sb).

For the *distal subtotal gastrectomy,* both lesser curvature and greater curvature of the stomach need to be cleared with nodal tissue for transection. Along the greater curvature, all the terminal branches from the left gastroepiploic artery should be ligated on the wall of the stomach starting from the first branch of the left gastroepiploic artery to planned transection point. Preserved short gastric arteries can prevent gastric remnant necrosis.

On the lesser curvature, the previously dissected nodal packet needs to be separated from the stomach wall. This can be accomplished by ligating left gastric artery terminal branches on the gastric wall from the esophagogastric junction to the transection point or vice versa.

Once this portion of the dissection is completed, then the stomach should be ready to be divided to remove all the nodal tissue en bloc with the main specimen. For the clean and complete dissection of the nodes in the correct plane, en bloc resection of the celiac nodes is recommended except left gastric artery preservation is required for a replaced left hepatic artery.

For the *total gastrectomy*, routine splenectomy for nodal clearance is currently not recommended. After ligating the left gastroepiploic vessels, ligate and divide the short gastric vessels close to the splenic attachment. Nodal tissue located in gastrosplenic ligament is classified as station 4sa. Once the short gastric vessels are ligated and divided, the gastric fundus can be mobilized completely from the retroperitoneum and spleen. Finally, nodal tissues along the distal splenic artery (station 11d) and the hilum of spleen (station 10) are dissected. To avoid injury to the splenic vessels and the tail of the pancreas, the dissection should follow the previous dissection plane identified at the celiac axis. The esophagus is encircled and both anterior and posterior vagus nerves are divided. All nodal tissues can now be removed en bloc with the stomach by dividing the esophagus (Fig. 62.9).

Anatomic Points

While dissecting hepatic artery nodes, there is a distinctive plane between the nodal tissue and the pancreas parenchyma, and this should be recognized and the dissection should be maintained in this plane to avoid injury to the pancreas. There are multiple small vessels present between these nodes and the upper border of the pancreas and these should be recognized and coagulated before transection. The dissection plane can also be maintained just outside the perivascular nerve plexus unless gross metastatic nodes present along the artery.

The left gastric vein is typically present around the common hepatic artery but may be located in front of the common hepatic artery. The left gastric vein drains into either splenic vein or portal vein, and it makes arcade along the lesser curvature with the right gastric vein running along the right gastric artery, thus this arcade of vein is often referred to as the coronary vein. Injury to this vein will create a bleeding situation that is difficult to control. Careful dissection and vessel control prior to division is recommended.

The left gastric artery is one of the three branches of celiac axis and is the major blood supply to the stomach. About 10% to 15% of the cases have accessory or replaced left hepatic artery arising from the left gastric artery and this should be recognized before transection. By ligating this artery in distal gastrectomy, remnant stomach becomes dependent on blood supply from splenic artery/short gastric arteries. About 40% to 97% of patients have a posterior gastric artery supplying posterior portion of the gastric fundus that arises from the middle portion of the splenic artery. Nodal tissue proximal (celiac artery side) to this artery along the splenic artery is classified as 11p (proximal) and distal (splenic hilum side) as 11d (Fig. 62.6).

The left gastroepiploic artery is a branch of splenic artery and sometimes originates from the most caudal branch of splenic artery tributary in the splenic hilum. It emerges from the lower edge of the pancreatic tail near the lower pole of the spleen.

The left gastric artery has ascending and descending branches which supply GE junction and lesser curvature of the stomach correspondingly. Right paracardial nodal station locates around this ascending branch. For distal gastrectomy, it is important to completely dissect this nodal station by ligating terminal branches on the wall of the esophagus and stomach. The left gastric artery has anterior and posterior branches which terminate corresponding surfaces of the stomach, thus both branches need to be ligated.

Roux-en-Y Reconstruction After Gastrectomy (Figs. 62.10 and 62.11)

Technical and Anatomic Points

The simplest reconstruction is to create a Roux-en-Y loop of jejunum. Even for reconstruction for distal gastrectomy, Roux-en-Y caries lower incidence of anastomotic leak and bile gastritis. If Billroth II reconstruction is desired, perform this as described in Chapter 61.

To create a Roux-en-Y anastomosis, first identify the proximal jejunum and trace it to the ligament of Treitz. Measure down 20 to 30 cm distal to the ligament of Treitz and isolate a

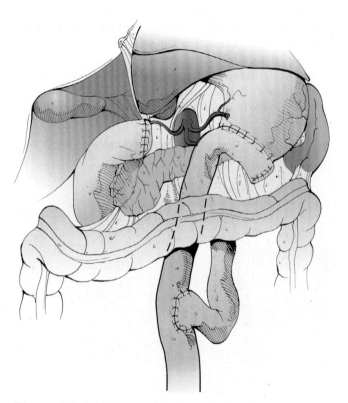

Figure 62.10 Roux-en-Y reconstruction after distal subtotal gastrectomy (from Merado MA. Chapter 83. Distal gastrectomy. In: *Fischer's Mastery of Surgery.* Philadelphia, PA: Lippincott Williams & Wilkins; 2012, with permission).

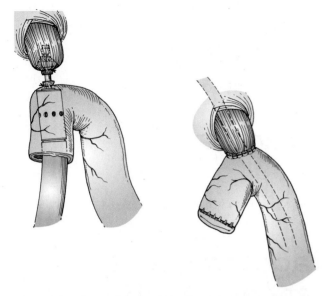

Figure 62.11 Reconstruction after total gastrectomy

loop of jejunum. Hold the loop up and inspect its mesentery, looking for the pattern of the jejunal arcades. Plan to divide the jejunum at the midpoint of the arch of an arcade so that there is a good blood supply to both ends. Make a window through the mesentery and divide the mesentery for a total distance of about 10 cm, or until the root of the mesentery is reached. Divide the jejunum with a linear stapling device.

The Roux limb (distal limb) should pass comfortably up to the esophagus or to the remnant stomach. The shortest path is retrocolic, through a small window in the transverse mesocolon. However, this may predispose the patient to obstruction if tumor recurs in the gastric bed. If possible, route the Roux limb in an antecolic path especially for distal gastectomy.

The end-to-end sutured gastrojejunostomy then can be created with single-layer Gambee sutures or double-layer standard technique (Fig. 62.10).

The esophagojejunal anastomosis may be sutured using a standard single-layer suture technique. Generally, it is preferable to sew the end of the stomach to the side of the jejunum along the antimesenteric border, several centimeters from the end of the loop. Complete the back wall, then have the anesthesiologist advance the nasogastric tube through the anastomosis and suture the front layer over the nasogastric tube.

Alternatively, a stapled anastomosis (end-esophagus to side-jejunum) may be fashioned using a circular stapling device

(Fig. 62.11). Have the anesthesiologist advance the nasogastric tube slowly as you guide it through the anastomosis and down 10 to 15 cm into the jejunum.

Close the end of the loop with a linear stapling device using 3.5-mm staples.

Place two closed-suction drains, one on each side, in close proximity to the esophagojejunal anastomosis.

Finally, complete the Roux-en-Y reconstruction by suturing or stapling the proximal blind Roux loop (draining pancreatic and biliary secretions) 40 to 45 cm below the esophago(gastro) jejunostomy. Close the mesenteric defect.

Part of the technical description is adapted from Surgical Oncology Clinics of North America, 2012 Jan;21(1): 57–70, Hoshi, Standard D2 and Modified Nodal Dissection for Gastric Adenocarcinoma

REFERENCES

1. Hoshi H. Standard D2 and modified nodal dissection for gastric adenocarcinoma. *Surg Oncol Clin N Am.* 2012;21(1):57–70.
2. Japanese Gastric Cancer Association. Japanese classification of gastric carcinoma: 3rd English edition. *Gastric Cancer.* 2011;14:101–112.
3. Japanese Gastric Cancer Association. Japanese gastric cancer treatment guidelines 2010 (ver. 3). *Gastric Cancer.* 2011;14:113–123.
4. Kawasaki K, Kanaji S, Kobayashi I, et al. Multidetector computed tomography for preoperative identification of left gastric vein location in patients with gastric cancer. *Gastric Cancer.* 2010;13:25–29.
5. Loukas M, Wartmann CT, Louis RG Jr, et al. The clinical anatomy of the posterior gastric artery revisited. *Surg Radiol Anat.* 2007;29:361–366.
6. Natsume T, Shuto K, Yanagawa N, et al. The classification of anatomic variations in the perigasric vessels by dual-phase CT to reduce intraoperative bleeding during laparoscopic gastrectomy. *Surg Endosc.* 2011;25(5):1420–1424.
7. Okabayashi T, Kobayashi M, Nishimori I, et al. Autopsy study of anatomical features of the posterior gastric artery for surgical contribution. *World J Gastroenterol.* 2006;12(33):5357–5359.
8. Sasako M. D2 nodal dissection. *Oper Tech Gen Surg.* 2003;5:36–49.
9. Songun I, Putter H, Kranenbarg EM, et al. Surgical treatment of gastric cancer: 15-year follow-up results of the randomized nationwide Dutch D1D2 trial. *Lancet Oncol.* 2010;11(5):439–449.
10. Yamaguchi S, Kuroyanagi H, Milson JW, et al. Venous anatomy of the right colon: Precise structure of the major vein and gastrocolic trunk in 58 cadavers. *Dis Colon Rectum.* 2001;45:1337–1340.

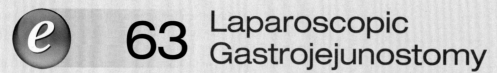

63 Laparoscopic Gastrojejunostomy

This chapter can be accessed online at www.lww.com/eChapter63.

64 Laparoscopic Gastric Resection

This chapter can be accessed online at www.lww.com/eChapter64.

65 Truncal Vagotomy and Pyloroplasty and Highly Selective Vagotomy

This chapter can be accessed online at www.lww.com/eChapter65.

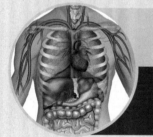

66

Pyloric Exclusion and Duodenal Diverticulization

Injuries of the duodenum can be difficult to manage. In this chapter, exposure of the duodenum from the pylorus to the suspensory ligament of duodenum (ligament of Treitz) and two useful maneuvers for managing complex injuries to the duodenum are covered.

Duodenal injuries are rarely isolated, due to the central location of the duodenum (Fig. 66.1). Careful assessment of the adjacent pancreas, bile duct, colon, and neighboring vascular structures is an essential component of management.

Sometimes primary repair is all that is needed, particularly for clean isolated cuts limited to less than 50% of the circumference of the duodenum. The procedures described here are used when more severe injuries require management. A standard grading system has been developed and this facilitates classification of duodenal injuries (see references at the end).

Duodenal diverticulization is the first procedure described. It is essential for a distal gastric resection with BII reconstruction. It is rarely used, having generally been replaced by the less invasive pyloric exclusion operation. The goal of both procedures is to allow the enteric contents to bypass the duodenal repair. When properly performed, pyloric exclusion provides this bypass with less dissection in a fully reversible fashion.

SCORE™, the Surgical Council on Resident Education, classified management of duodenal trauma as an "ESSENTIAL UNCOMMON" procedure.

LIST OF STRUCTURES

Stomach
Pylorus

Duodenum
First portion (duodenal ampulla or bulb)
Second portion
Third portion
Fourth portion

Pancreas
Head of pancreas
Suspensory ligament of duodenum (ligament
　of Treitz)

Gallbladder
Bile duct

Colon
Ascending (right) colon
Hepatic flexure
Cecum
Transverse colon

Embryologic Terms
Foregut
Midgut
Hindgut

Exposure of the Duodenum (Fig. 66.2)

Technical Points

First, mobilize the hepatic flexure of the colon by incising the lateral peritoneal attachments at the hepatic flexure. Make a small window in the peritoneum with Metzenbaum scissors, then pass the fingers of the nondominant hand behind the colon, sweeping the peritoneum up and thinning it out. Divide it with electrocautery. Often, there are filmy adhesions extending to the gallbladder; divide these by sharp dissection.

If you anticipate the need to expose the entire duodenum, pass your nondominant hand down behind the ascending (right) colon and divide the lateral peritoneal reflection all the way down past the cecum. Lift the ascending (right) colon with its mesentery, sharply dividing any filmy adhesions between the colon and the retroperitoneum. The third portion of the duodenum will be visible as the colon is swept medially. Elevate the ascending (right) colon and the mesentery of the small intestine

ORIENTATION

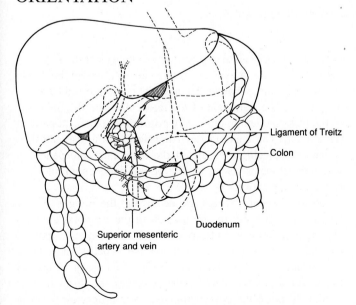

Figure 66.1 Anatomic relations of the duodenum

(carefully preserving the superior mesenteric vessels) and swing them toward the left shoulder of the patient. The anterior surface of the duodenum from the pylorus to the suspensory ligament of duodenum (ligament of Treitz) should now be visible.

Mobilize the duodenum and head of the pancreas using a wide Kocher maneuver to gain access to the lateral and posterior surfaces of the duodenum in these regions. The fourth portion of the duodenum may be similarly mobilized by incising the antimesenteric border.

Anatomic Points

This procedure is made necessary, as well as technically possible, by the embryologic rotation of the gut. A knowledge of this developmental process enables a rational approach to the procedure.

The gut can be divided into foregut, midgut, and hindgut. For the purposes of the general surgeon operating on the abdomen, these divisions can be defined as follows: The foregut is that portion of the gut supplied by the celiac artery, the midgut is that portion supplied by the superior mesenteric artery, and the hindgut is that portion supplied by the inferior mesenteric artery. Foregut derivatives in the abdomen include the distal esophagus, the stomach, and the duodenum to just distal to the major duodenal papilla. The liver and biliary apparatus arise as the hepatic diverticulum from the terminal foregut, whereas the pancreas arises from a diverticulum of the hepatic diverticulum and from a separate dorsal pancreatic bud. Midgut derivatives include the rest of the duodenum, all of the small intestine, the appendix, the cecum, the ascending colon, and the proximal two-thirds of the transverse colon. Hindgut derivatives include the distal one-third of the transverse colon, the descending colon, the sigmoid colon, the rectum, and the anal canal to the anal valves.

The development of the abdominal gastrointestinal tract can be understood as a consequence of two phenomena. One of these is differential growth of the gut components in comparison to each other and to the developing peritoneal cavity. The other is the fusion and later degeneration, of apposed serosal surfaces. What follows is a conceptual description of some of

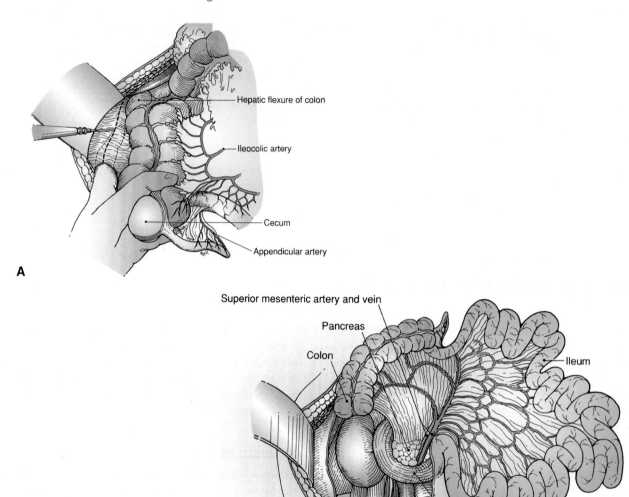

A

- Hepatic flexure of colon
- Ileocolic artery
- Cecum
- Appendicular artery

B

- Superior mesenteric artery and vein
- Pancreas
- Colon
- Ileum
- Jejunum
- Duodenum

Figure 66.2 Exposure of the duodenum

the surgically relevant facets of the development of the infra-diaphragmatic gastrointestinal system.

Initially, the gut is a midline intraperitoneal tube suspended from the dorsal body wall along its entire length by the dorsal mesentery. A ventral mesentery attaches the foregut to the anterior body wall from the umbilicus to the diaphragm, carrying the left umbilical vein from the umbilicus to its ultimate union with the caval system. As the fusiform dilatation destined to become stomach begins to develop by rapid elongation, the duodenum assumes the form of a C-shaped loop, with its convexity directed ventrally. Soon after these structures begin to be recognizable, the stomach changes its position by rotating 90 degrees to the right about its longitudinal axis. The end result of this rotation is that the right side of the stomach becomes the definitive posterior side and the left side becomes the definitive anterior side. Moreover, the original dorsal border becomes the greater curvature and the ventral border becomes the lesser

curvature. As a result of the positional changes of the stomach, the C-loop of the duodenum rotates about a longitudinal axis so that the convex border becomes its definitive right border. This causes the right side of the duodenum and the right leaf of the mesoduodenum to be in apposition to the dorsal parietal peritoneum. The apposed serosal surfaces soon fuse and then degenerate, placing the bulk of the duodenum and pancreas, which develops primarily within the mesoduodenum, in a retroperitoneal position.

While foregut changes are occurring, the midgut rapidly lengthens, especially in comparison to the vertebral column. The midgut forms a ventrally directed loop that is suspended by the dorsal mesentery containing the superior mesenteric artery and vein. The proximal limb of the loop is cranial to the superior mesenteric artery, whereas the distal loop is caudal. Because the developing liver and urogenital systems occupy most of the abdominal space, the midgut loop rotates

90 degrees counterclockwise around the superior mesenteric artery axis (as viewed anteriorly) and herniates into the umbilical cord. While herniated, the gut diverticulum destined to become vermiform appendix and cecum becomes recognizable, and the proximal limb, which elongates more than the distal limb, is thrown into numerous coils. At the same time, the abdominal cavity expands, resulting in a peritoneal cavity with sufficient room for the "herniated" midgut. The "herniation" is then reduced in an orderly fashion, and rotation (ultimately through a total of 270 degrees) of the midgut loop continues.

When the midgut returns to the abdominal cavity, the pattern of return progresses in a craniocaudal sequence, with the most cranial portions passing to the left upper quadrant and the rest of the midgut following obliquely toward the right lower quadrant. As the midgut returns into the peritoneal cavity, it forces the intraperitoneal hindgut (descending and sigmoid colon) to the left. As a consequence of this pattern of return, the left side of the descending colon and the left leaf of its mesentery come to lie in contact with the parietal peritoneum, and the inevitable fusion and degeneration of apposed serosal surfaces occur. The end result of this is that the descending colon and its blood supply, contained in the mesentery, become retroperitoneal to a greater or lesser degree. The sigmoid colon retains its mesentery because midgut loops have entered the left upper quadrant (not the left lower quadrant), and consequently, the apposition of serosal surfaces necessary to allow fusion and degeneration is not achieved.

The last part of the midgut loop to return is the ascending and transverse colon. The ascending colon and its mesentery, similar to the descending colon, are fixed to the parietal peritoneum, and subsequent fusion and degeneration of apposed serosal surfaces again occur. Because the transverse colon is the last to return, it must pass anterior to the midgut loops that entered earlier; hence, it retains its mesentery. Later, a leaf of greater omentum, derived from dorsal mesogastrium, fuses with the cranial leaf of the original transverse mesocolon, so that the definitive transverse mesocolon develops from the original transverse mesocolon plus the original dorsal mesogastrium.

The procedure for exposure of the duodenum just described simply recreates the earlier developmental stage when the gut was an intraperitoneal structure. Fusion and degeneration of apposed serosal surfaces result in relatively avascular planes that allow massive mobilization with minimal blood loss.

Inspection of the dorsal side of the duodenum and head of the pancreas allows visualization of the terminal bile duct, as this duct passes posterior to the duodenum and, in its "intrapancreatic" course, is more posterior than anterior with respect to pancreatic tissue. The same is true of the pancreatic duct; although embedded in pancreatic tissue, it is more posterior than anterior. In addition, the beginning of the portal vein, formed by the confluence of the superior mesenteric vein and splenic vein, should be visible.

The third portion of the duodenum lies in the angle between the root of the superior mesenteric artery (and its accompanying vein) and the aorta. The leftward mobilization of duodenum and pancreas is thus limited by the superior mesenteric artery.

Duodenal Diverticulization as a Means of "Defunctionalizing" the Duodenum and Converting a Leak into an End-Duodenal Fistula (Fig. 66.3)

Technical and Anatomic Points

First, debride and repair the injury. Because enteric contents will bypass the duodenum, a considerable amount of narrowing can be tolerated, if necessary, to achieve a secure repair. A standard two-layered suture technique is preferred. Confirm the integrity of the biliary and pancreatic ducts and cannulate them, performing contrast studies if necessary.

HALLMARK ANATOMIC COMPLICATIONS—DUODENAL DIVERTICULIZATION
Leakage from duodenal closure

STEPS IN PROCEDURE—DUODENAL DIVERTICULIZATION

Explore abdomen and expose duodenum by mobilizing ascending (right) colon
Repair the duodenal injury
Mobilize the distal stomach and pylorus
Perform distal gastrectomy with Billroth II reconstruction

Divide Pylorus with Linear Stapler
Create gastrojejunostomy (stapled or sutured)
Place omentum over duodenal repair
Consider closed suction drains
Close abdomen in usual fashion

Next, "defunctionalize" or diverticulize the duodenum by performing a limited gastric resection using the Billroth II reconstruction. Perform a truncal vagotomy. Place omentum over the duodenal suture line and duodenal stump closure. If closure of the duodenal stump has been difficult, a tube duodenostomy is a prudent additional step. Place drains in the region of the duodenal suture line.

Note that duodenal diverticulization is, in essence, gastric resection with vagotomy. This is a lengthy operation that results in permanent anatomic changes. Pyloric exclusion (Fig. 66.4) accomplishes the same objective but is a much shorter procedure and results in only temporary diversion. In many patients, pyloric exclusion is the preferred alternative.

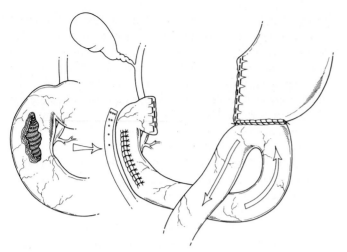

Figure 66.3 Duodenal diverticulization as a means of "defunctionalizing" the duodenum and converting a leak into an end-duodenal fistula

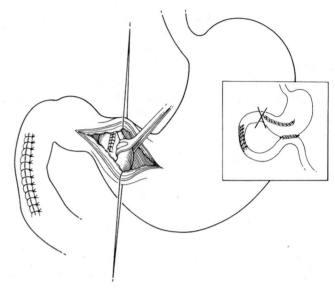

Figure 66.4 Pyloric exclusion

Pyloric Exclusion (Fig. 66.4)

Technical and Anatomic Points

Repair the duodenal injury as described in Fig. 66.3. There are two ways to close the pylorus: Suture from within the stomach or stapled closure.

To close from within the pylorus, first create a low anterior gastrotomy. Pass Babcock clamps into the stomach and grasp the pylorus, everting it through the gastrotomy. Close the pylorus firmly with a running suture of 2-0 synthetic absorbable suture. Take large bites through the pyloric ring. This has the potential advantage of speed and ease of correction if pylorus does not reopen on schedule. The suture can be cut and removed endoscopically. It also avoids additional dissection in the region of the duodenal repair.

STEPS IN PROCEDURE—PYLORIC EXCLUSION

Thoroughly explore abdomen and identify injuries
Mobilize ascending (right) colon to expose duodenum
Close injury
Create anterior gastrotomy

Close Pylorus (Choose Method):
Mobilize pylorus and fire a noncutting linear stapler across

Grasp pylorus through gastrotomy and close with purse-string suture (2-0 synthetic absorbable suture)
Create gastrojejunostomy, incorporating gastrotomy in anastomosis
Cover duodenal repair with omentum and consider placing closed suction drains
Close abdomen in the usual fashion

HALLMARK ANATOMIC COMPLICATIONS—PYLORIC EXCLUSION

Leakage from duodenal closure
Duodenal obstruction

Failure of pylorus to reopen; alternatively pylorus may reopen before repair is healed

---

Alternatively, mobilize the pylorus and fire a noncutting linear stapler across it. Create an anterior gastrotomy.

Construct an anterior gastrojejunostomy by bringing up a loop of jejunum and suturing it at the site of the gastrotomy.

Place omentum over the duodenal suture line and place drains in close proximity to it. The pylorus will generally remain closed for only a few weeks. Even if a nonabsorbable suture is used, the pylorus will reopen spontaneously in most cases. If it does not, the suture can be cut endoscopically after the duodenal suture line has healed satisfactorily.

Severe combined duodenal and pancreatic injuries, particularly when accompanied by profuse bleeding, may require pancreaticoduodenectomy.

REFERENCES

1. Androulakis J, Colborn GL, Skandalakis PN, et al. Embryologic and anatomic basis of duodenal surgery. *Surg Clin North Am.* 2000;80:171–199. (Provides excellent review of anatomy and embryology.)

2. Asensio JA, Demetriades D, Berne JD, et al. A unified approach to the surgical exposure of pancreatic and duodenal injuries. *Am J Surg.* 1997;174:54–60. (Presents comprehensive review of management options.)

3. Cattell RB, Braasch JW. A technique for the exposure of the third and fourth portions of the duodenum. *Surg Gynecol Obstet.* 1960;111:379. (Describes wide exposure of entire duodenum.)

4. Clendenon JN, Meyers RL, Nance ML, et al. Management of duodenal injuries in children. *J Pediatr Surg.* 2004; 39:964.

5. Martin TD, Feleciano DV, Mattox KL, et al. Severe duodenal injuries: Treatment with pyloric exclusion and gastrojejunostomy. *Arch Surg.* 1983;118:631.

6. Moore EE, Cogbill TH, Malangoni MA, et al. Organ injury scaling, II: Pancreas, duodenum, small bowel, colon and rectum. *J Trauma.* 1990;30:1427.

7. Moore EE, Moore FA. American Association for the Surgery of Trauma Organ Injury Scaling: 50th Anniversary Review. *J Trauma.* 2010;69:1600.

8. Walley BD, Goco I. Duodenal patch grafting. *Am J Surg.* 1980; 140:706.

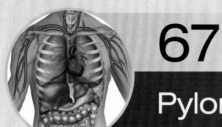

67

Pyloromyotomy

Infants with hypertrophic pyloric stenosis typically develop symptoms in the first month or two of life. The history of progressive nonbilious vomiting, occurring right after feeding, is classic. Palpation of a rounded "olive" in the epigastrium is diagnostic, and this may be confirmed by ultrasound examination. The treatment is myotomy. Both open and laparoscopic techniques are available. This chapter explores both.

Hypochloremic hypokalemic metabolic acidosis is a characteristic. Always correct the associated dehydration and electrolyte abnormalities before performing either of these procedures.

SCORE™, the Surgical Council on Resident Education, classified pyloromyotomy as an "ESSENTIAL UNCOMMON" procedure.

STEPS IN PROCEDURE

Open Pyloromyotomy (Ramstedt Procedure)

Umbilical or right upper quadrant transverse incision

Deliver hypertrophied pylorus into incision

Longitudinal incision along anterior wall of thickened portion

Spread and divide all circular muscle fibers using pyloromyotomy spreader

Confirm that submucosa pouts out and that it is intact

Close incision

Laparoscopic Pyloromyotomy

Trocars at umbilicus, left and right upper quadrants

Pass atraumatic grasper through right upper quadrant trocar; sweep liver cephalad and grasp duodenum just below pylorus

Make incision on anterior surface of thickened portion of pylorus using laparoscopic pylorotome

Use laparoscopic spreader to split hypertrophied fibers

Confirm adequate myotomy and absence of perforation

HALLMARK ANATOMIC COMPLICATIONS

Inadequate myotomy

Perforation (usually at the duodenal end of the myotomy)

LIST OF STRUCTURES

Stomach

Duodenum

Pylorus

Liver

Open Pyloromyotomy (Ramstedt Procedure) (Fig. 67.1)

Technical and Anatomic Points

Make a small incision in the umbilical fold or a short transverse right upper quadrant incision. Reach in, palpate, and deliver the thickened pylorus. Make a longitudinal incision over the anterior surface of the thickened portion. Deepen this incision through the hypertrophied circular fibers. A special spreader assists in opening the myotomy to display the herniated submucosa. Carry the myotomy from the stomach down onto the duodenum, taking care not to injure the mucosa. Perforation is most likely to occur at the duodenal end, because the duodenum is thinner than the stomach. The myotomy must completely divide all fibers of the hypertrophied pylorus.

Check the myotomy for completeness, and ensure that the submucosa is uninjured. Close the small incision.

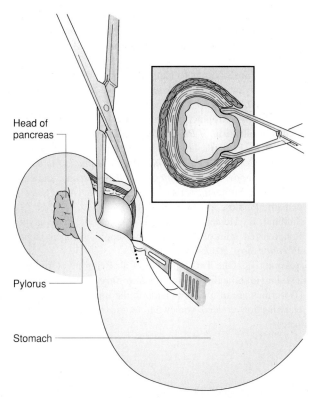

Figure 67.1 Open pyloromyotomy (Ramstedt procedure) (from Sato TT, Oldham KT. Pediatric abdomen. In: Mulholland MW, Lillemoe KD, Dohert GM, et al., eds. *Greenfield's Surgery: Scientific Principles and Practice.* Philadelphia, PA: Lippincott Williams & Wilkins; 2006, with permission).

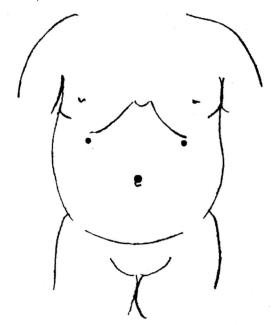

Figure 67.2 Laparoscopic pyloromyotomy: Patient position and trocar placement (from Scott-Conner CEH (ed.). *The SAGES Manual: Fundamentals of Laparoscopy, Thoracoscopy and GI Endoscopy.* 2nd ed. New York, NY: Springer Verlag; 2006).

Laparoscopic Pyloromyotomy: Patient Position and Trocar Placement (Fig. 67.2)

Technical and Anatomic Points

Position the patient supine with a small roll under the spine to elevate the pylorus. Three trocars are used. The laparoscope is placed through a supraumbilical incision and two working ports are placed just to the left and right of the umbilicus.

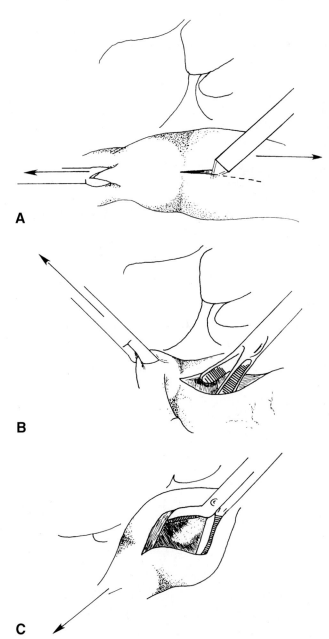

Figure 67.3 Laparoscopic pyloromyotomy: Performing the myotomy. **A:** Initial incision on stomach. **B:** Longitudinal muscle divided to expose circular muscle. **C:** Division of circular muscle (from Scott-Conner CEH (ed.). *The SAGES Manual: Fundamentals of Laparoscopy, Thoracoscopy, and GI Endoscopy.* 2nd ed. New York, NY: Springer Verlag; 2006).

Laparoscopic Pyloromyotomy: Performing the Myotomy (Fig. 67.3)

Technical and Anatomic Points

Pass a small atraumatic grasper through the right-hand port, elevate the liver with the shaft of the grasper, and gently grasp the first portion of the duodenum. Pass a laparoscopic myotome through the left-hand port and create a longitudinal incision on the anterior surface of the duodenum, extending it across the pylorus (Fig. 67.3A). It is safest to begin this incision on the distal part of the thickened portion and extend it proximally. Use a laparoscopic pyloromyotomy spreader to spread and split the hypertrophied fibers. This spreader has serrations on the outside edges which help anchor the instrument in the myotomy, increasing the mechanical effectiveness (Fig. 67.3B). Continue this proximally and distally until submucosa pouts out freely (Fig. 67.3C). Do not continue this down onto the normal duodenum, because perforation may result. Check for small perforations under saline, if necessary.

REFERENCES

1. Alberti D, Cheli M, Locatelli G. A new technical variant for extra-mucosal pyloromyotomy: The Tan-Bianchi operation moves to the right. *J Pediatr Surg.* 2004;39:53–56.

2. Aldridge RD, MacKinlay GA, Aldridge RB. Choice of incision: The experience and evolution of surgical management of infantile hypertrophic pyloric stenosis. *J Laparoendosc Adv Surg Tech A.* 2007;17:131–136.

3. Dozier K, Kim S. Vascular clamp stabilization of pylorus during laparoscopic pyloromyotomy. *Pediatr Surg Int.* 2007;23:1237–1239.

4. Leclair MD, Plattner V, Mirallie E, et al. Laparoscopic pyloromyotomy for hypertrophic pyloric stenosis: A prospective, randomized controlled trial. *J Pediatr Surg.* 2007;42:692–698.

5. Meehan JJ. Pediatric laparoscopy: Specific surgical procedures. In: Scott-Conner CEH, ed. *The SAGES Manual: Fundamentals of Laparoscopy, Thoracoscopy, and GI Endoscopy.* 2nd ed. New York, NY: Springer Verlag; 2006:500–502. (Also gives other pediatric laparoscopic procedures.)

6. Siddiqui S, Heidel RE, Angel CA, et al. Pyloromyotomy: Randomized control trial of laparoscopic vs open technique. *J Pediatr Surg.* 2012;47:93–98.

7. Yokomori K, Oue T, Odajima T, et al. Pyloromyotomy through a sliding umbilical window. *J Pediatr Surg.* 2006;41:2066–2068. (Describes use of a skin incision in the umbilical fold, with fascial incision created somewhat to the right, improving open access.)

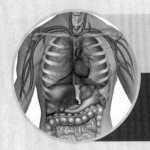

68

Laparoscopic Adjustable Gastric Banding

The adjustable gastric band is designed to divide the stomach into a small upper pouch of approximately 15 mL that can empty only gradually into the rest of the stomach. This bariatric surgical procedure is used in selected patients. It has the advantage of reversibility and causes minimal metabolic derangements. Early problems with band erosion, inadequate weight loss, and slippage are gradually being eliminated as the technique evolves.

This chapter presents the basic steps for implantation. Currently, two such devices are in use around the world, and the procedure has some nuances depending upon which device is being used. It is essential to be completely familiar with the device being used, and to follow recommended steps specific for that particular device.

With any bariatric surgery procedure, the surgery is just a small part of the overall care of the patient. Careful patient selection, preoperative preparation, and postoperative care are ideally delivered by a dedicated and experienced bariatric team. References at the end describe these parts of care in greater detail.

SCORE™, the Surgical Council on Resident Education, classified laparoscopic operations for morbid obesity as "COMPLEX" procedures.

STEPS IN PROCEDURE

Position patient with legs spread, reverse Trendelenburg

Access abdomen with Veress needle, left upper quadrant at midclavicular line

Additional trocars along left and right costal margins

Elevate left lobe of liver to expose lesser omentum and hiatus

Grasp stomach and pull it inferiorly and caudally

Identify and grasp Belsey's fat pad

Incise peritoneum over left crus

Pull stomach to left and caudally

Open lesser omentum at cephalad aspect, where diaphragm and gastrophrenic ligament converge

Dissect plane behind gastroesophageal junction, exiting through opening in the left crural peritoneum

Introduce band passer into laparoscopic field and pass it through tunnel

Select appropriate size band, and similarly pass through tunnel

Have anesthesiologist inflate calibrating balloon with 25 mL of air and withdraw it, pulling stomach up against hiatus

Adjust band

Pass attached tubing through fascia

Secure hemostasis and desufflate abdomen

Place port in subcutaneous location

Secure all trocar sites

HALLMARK ANATOMIC COMPLICATIONS

Injury to esophagus or stomach

Band slippage

Band erosion into stomach

Gastric pouch dilatation

LIST OF STRUCTURES

Stomach

Esophagus

Diaphragm

Left crus

Right crus

Lesser omentum

Pars flaccida

Patient Position and Initial Dissection (Fig. 68.1)

Technical and Anatomic Points

Position the patient with legs spread. Place the operating table in reverse Trendelenburg position. Stand between the patient's legs so that you are directly facing the operating field (Fig. 68.1A). Note how the operating room setup shown allows the surgeon (S) unobstructed access to the field. The monitors (M) should face surgeon and assistant (A) while the camera operator (CO) stands to the patient's right side. An instrument table (IT) completes the setup.

Obtain access to the abdomen with a Veress needle inserted in the left upper quadrant at the midclavicular line. This location

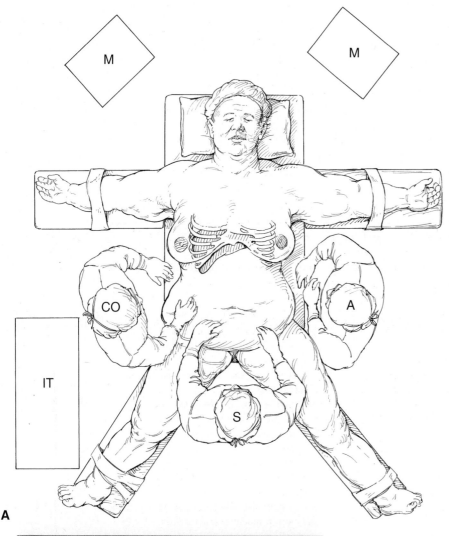

A

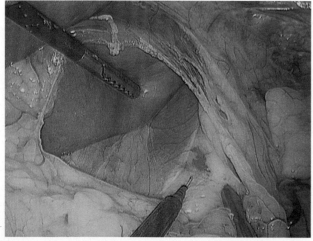

B

Figure 68.1 A: Patient position and initial dissection (from Soper NJ, Swanstrom LL, Eubanks WS (eds.). *Mastery of Endoscopic and Laparoscopic Surgery.* 2nd ed. Philadelphia, PA: Lippincott Williams & Wilkins; 2005, with permission). **B:** Dissection in pars flaccida of the lesser omentum (from Fischer JE, Jones DB, Pomposelli FB, et al. *Fischer's Mastery of Surgery.* 6th ed. Philadelphia, PA: Wolters Kluwer Lippincott Williams & Wilkins, with permission).

generally avoids the thickest part of the pannus as well as the liver (which is often fatty and significantly enlarged in these patients). The lower costal margin helps to provide support as the needle enters the peritoneum, minimizing the chance of visceral injury.

Place a camera port in the midline near the hiatus. Place four or five additional ports as needed along the left and right costal margins. Elevate the left lobe of the liver and identify the fatty lesser omentum and the esophageal hiatus.

Grasp the stomach and pull it gently, inferiorly and caudally. Identify and grasp the fatty pad of tissue overlying the gastroesophageal junction (Belsey's fat pad). Incise the peritoneum overlying the right crus.

Next, find the most cephalad portion of the fatty lesser omentum. The area for dissection is demarcated by the diaphragm, the gastrophrenic ligament, and the esophagus. Detach the pars flaccida of the lesser omentum to expose the right crus (Fig. 68.1B). Dissect gently along this plane behind the gastroesophageal junction to identify the left crus. Keep this dissection high enough to avoid entering the lesser sac. The goal is to atraumatically create a tunnel behind the stomach without producing an opening large enough to allow the band to slip or the stomach to herniate.

Gently develop the tunnel behind the stomach and the confluence of the crura to allow the band to be passed. Take care not to injure the esophagus. A variety of articulating dissectors are available for this purpose.

Band Placement and Adjustment (Fig. 68.2)

Technical and Anatomic Points

The band device consists of a collar that fits around the stomach, connected by a tubing to a subcutaneous port that is used to access the device (Fig. 68.2A). Through this port, the collar around the esophagus can be adjusted by injecting or withdrawing fluid.

Introduce the band passer into the laparoscopic field by passing it through one of the larger ports. Place the blunt tip of the passer into the opening in the pars flaccida and gently pass it through the retrogastric tunnel until it emerges from the opening overlying the right crus. Select the appropriate size band, based upon the position of the placer, and introduce it into one of the 15-mm ports. Pass it behind the stomach.

Have the anesthesiologist introduce the tube with the calibrating balloon down into the stomach. The balloon should be inflated with 25 mL of air and the tube is withdrawn to pull the stomach up against the hiatus. This is used to judge final placement site for the band. It may be necessary to excise the fat pad to adequately expose the anterior gastric wall.

Deflate the balloon and adjust the band. Close the band when satisfied with position and size (Fig. 68.2B). Tighten the band, taking care that it is not too tight. The buckle is generally placed on the right anterior side of the stomach (Fig. 68.2C) Most surgeons anchor the band with sutures to the gastric wall, essentially pulling the wall of the stomach below the band up over and suturing it to the small pouch to cover and secure the band (Fig. 68.2D).

Pass the tubing out through the 15-mm port. Check hemostasis and withdraw all trocars, allowing the abdomen to desufflate. Develop a subcutaneous pocket for the fill port and mate it to the tubing. Secure the port to the fascia. The completed assemblage is shown in Figure 68.2E.

Close wounds in the usual fashion.

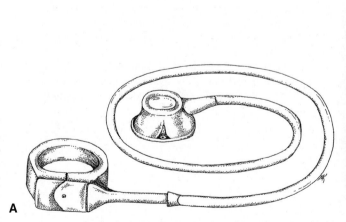

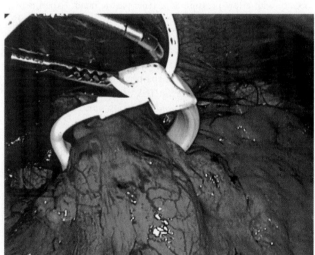

Figure 68.2 **A:** Band placement and adjustment (from Scott-Conner CEH (ed.). *The SAGES Manual: Fundamentals of Laparoscopy, Thoracoscopy, and GI Endoscopy.* 2nd ed. New York, NY: Springer Verlag, 2006). **B:** Band passed around stomach (from Nussbaum M. *Master Techniques in Surgery: Gastric Surgery.* Philadelphia, PA: Lippincott Williams & Wilkins; 2013, with permission). *(continued)*

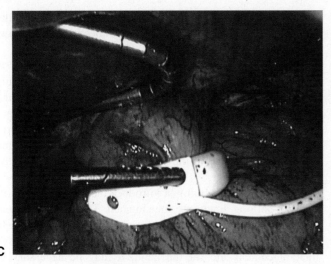

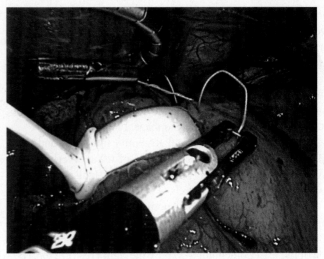

C   D

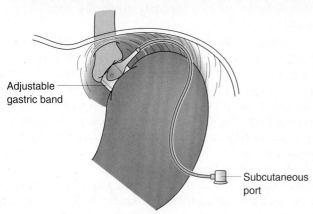

Adjustable gastric band

Subcutaneous port

E

Figure 68.2 *Continued.* **C:** Band tightened in place (from Nussbaum M. *Master Techniques in Surgery: Gastric Surgery.* Philadelphia, PA: Lippincott Williams & Wilkins; 2013, with permission). **D:** Sutures placed to cover and anchor the band (from Nussbaum M. *Master Techniques in Surgery: Gastric Surgery.* Philadelphia, PA: Lippincott Williams & Wilkins; 2013, with permission). **E:** Completed assemblage (from Mulholland MW, Lillemoe KD, Doherty GM, et al. *Greenfields' Surgery: Scientific Principles & Practice.* 4th ed. Philadelphia, PA: Lippincott Williams & Wilkins, 2006).

REFERENCES

1. Ceelen W, Walder J, Cardon A, et al. Surgical treatment of severe obesity with a low-pressure adjustable gastric band. Experimental data and clinical results in 625 patients. *Ann Surg.* 2003;237:10–16.
2. DeMaria EJ, Sugerman JH, Meador JG, et al. High failure rate after laparoscopic adjustable silicone gastric banding for treatment of morbid obesity. *Ann Surg.* 2001;233:809–818.
3. Kellogg TA, Ikramuddin S. Laparoscopic gastric banding. In: Scott-Conner CEH, ed. *The SAGES Manual: Fundamentals of Laparoscopy, Thoracoscopy, and GI Endoscopy.* New York, NY: Springer Verlag; 2006:293–302.
4. Mizrahi S, Avinoah E. Technical tips for laparoscopic gastric banding: 6 years' experience in 2800 procedures by a single surgical team. *Am J Surg.* 2007;193:160–165.
5. Nguyen NT, Smith BH. Laparoscopic adjustable gastric banding. In: Nussbaum MS, ed. *Master Techniques in Gastric Surgery.* Philadelphia, PA: Lippincott Williams & Wilkins; 2013:327.
6. O'Brien PE. The laparoscopic gastric band technique of placement. In: Fischer JE, Bland KI, eds. *Mastery of Surgery.* 6th ed. Philadelphia, PA: Lippincott Williams & Wilkins; 2013:1104.
7. Ren CJ, Fielding GA. Laparoscopic adjustable gastric banding: Surgical technique. *J Laparoendosc Adv Surg Tech A.* 2003; 13(4):257–263.
8. Suter M, Calmes JM, Paroz A, et al. A 10-year experience with laparoscopic gastric banding for morbid obesity: High long-term complication and failure rates. *Obesity Surg.* 2006;16: 829–835.
9. Zinzindohoue F, Chevallier J-M, Douard R, et al. Laparoscopic gastric banding: A minimally invasive surgical treatment for morbid obesity. Prospective study of 500 consecutive patients. *Ann Surg.* 2003;237:1–9.

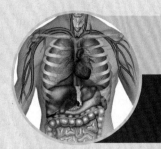

69

Laparoscopic Roux-en-Y Gastric Bypass

Christine J. Waller and Jessica K. Smith

Laparoscopic Roux-en-Y gastric bypass is one of the most technically demanding laparoscopic procedures and is the preferred method for treating morbid obesity when non-surgical therapy has failed. As with all bariatric procedures, the surgery is only part of a comprehensive team effort that requires careful patient selection, preoperative preparation, and postoperative care for optimal results.

SCORE™, the Surgical Council on Resident Education, classified laparoscopic operation for morbid obesity as "COMPLEX" procedures.

STEPS IN PROCEDURE

Place patient in supine position.
Obtain laparoscopic access in the following way:
    Grasp the umbilicus with two towel clamps and elevate the abdominal wall anteriorly. Introduce a Veress needle in Palmer's point, and establish pneumoperitoneum to 15 mm Hg.
Place trocars as demonstrated in Figure 69.1.
Identify the omentum; retract it cephalad and tuck it under the liver.
Grasp the transverse colon by an epiploic appendage and retract it cephalad to expose the ligament of Treitz.
Divide the jejunum 30 cm distal to the ligament of Treitz with an endoscopic linear cutting stapler.
Mark the distal bowel with suture to avoid confusion.
Trace the jejunum for an additional 75 cm distal to the point of transaction and approximate antimesenteric border of

proximal bowel to antimesenteric border of this region.
Anastomose with endoscopic cutting linear stapler, place additional antiobstruction suture, and close mesenteric defect.
Place patient in steep reverse Trendelenburg position.
Divide the omentum to allow passage of the antecolic Roux limb.
Divide the gastrohepatic ligament and enter the lesser sac.
Fashion a 30-cc gastric pouch with an endoscopic linear cutting stapler.
Anastomose the Roux limb to the gastric pouch with a double-layer stapled and hand-sewn anastomosis.
Place closed suction drain behind gastrojejunostomy, bringing it out through a lateral trocar site.

HALLMARK ANATOMIC COMPLICATIONS

Injury to bowel or viscera during laparoscopic access
Injury to esophagus
Injury to stomach

Injury to spleen
Confusion as to proximal or distal loop of jejunum

LIST OF STRUCTURES

Stomach
Fundus
Incisura
Cardial notch (angle of His)
Greater curvature
Lesser curvature

Esophagogastric Junction

Esophagus

Greater Omentum

Lesser (Gastrohepatic) Omentum

Jejunum

Suspensory Ligament of Duodenum (Ligament of Treitz)

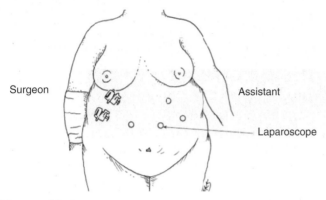

Figure 69.1 Patient position and trocar positioning

Patient Position and Trocar Position (Fig. 69.1)

Technical and Anatomic Points

A Foley catheter is inserted into the bladder. A nasogastric tube is placed. Position the patient supine on the table with the right arm tucked to the side. Position the left arm on an arm board. Apply a footboard to the end of the table to facilitate placement of the patient in reverse Trendelenburg position to aid exposure in the upper abdomen.

The surgeon stands on the patient's right, the assistant and scope holder on the patient's left. Elevate the umbilical plate with two penetrating towel clamps and insert a Veress needle into the abdomen approximately 15 cm below the xiphoid and 2 to 3 cm to the left of the midline. Do not use the umbilicus as a landmark because it is displaced inferiorly in many morbidly

obese patients. Insufflate the abdomen with a high-flow insufflator to an intra-abdominal pressure of 15 mm Hg.

The first 12-mm trocar, the camera port, is inserted 15 to 20 cm below the xiphoid process just to the left of midline using a Visiport technique. This trocar will be used for the 10-mm, 45-degree scope throughout the procedure. Insert a 12-mm port at the same level in the right epigastrium; this will serve as one of the surgeon's operating ports. Take care not to place this port too inferior because this may compromise the ability of the instruments to reach the operating area. Next insert a 5-mm trocar in the left upper quadrant. The next trocar is a 5-mm trocar inserted in the right upper quadrant laterally to allow liver retraction. Next place the liver retractor. Retract the liver superiorly and fix the retractor to the table with a retractor holder to provide stable exposure. Insert another 5-mm trocar into the right upper quadrant as the second operating port. Take care to place this port below the liver retractor and free of the round ligament. Inserting a long needle through the abdominal wall in the proposed trocar site may help prevent misplacement of this trocar. Finally, place the fourth 5-mm trocar in the left upper quadrant as a second port for the assistant.

Identification of the Ligament of Treitz and Division of Jejunum (Fig. 69.2)

Technical Points

Retract omentum and transverse colon superiorly into the upper abdomen where it is held by the assistant.

Identify the suspensory ligament of duodenum (ligament of Treitz) (see Figure 63.1D). Next, trace the jejunum 30 cm

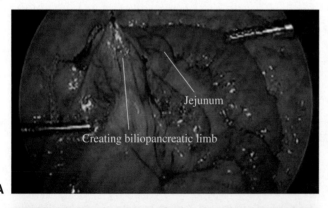

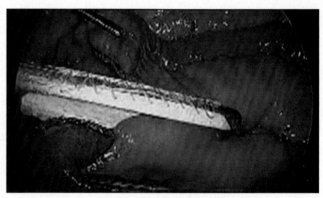

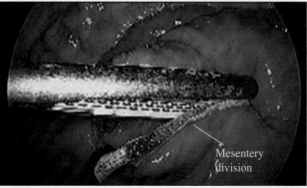

Figure 69.2 A: Creating biliopancreatic limb. **B:** Division of small bowel mesentery. **C:** Completed small bowel mesentery division.

(Fig. 69.2A) distal to the suspensory ligament of duodenum (ligament of Treitz) and divide it with a linear cutting stapler. Use a second firing of the linear stapler to divide small bowel mesentery further if necessary (Fig. 69.2B,C). Mark the distal bowel with a stitch to avoid confusion with the proximal end of the bowel.

Fashioning the Enteroenterostomy (Fig. 69.3)

Technical Points

Measure the jejunum 75 cm distal to the point of transection. Approximate this point on its antimesenteric border to the antimesenteric border of the proximal bowel with a single stitch (Fig. 69.3A, B). The assistant holds up on this stitch and enterotomies are made with the harmonic scalpel. Insert a linear cutting stapler and fire it to fashion the side-to-side stapled anastomosis (Fig. 69.3C–E).

Approximate the two edges of the staple line with another stitch (Fig. 69.3F,G). With the assistant holding up on this stitch, close the enterotomies (Fig. 69.3H) with a second firing of the stapler, taking care not to compromise the lumen of the in-continuity bowel (Fig. 69.3I). Place sutures at the distal end of the enteroenterostomy (Fig. 69.3J) staple line to prevent kinking by taking tension off the anastomosis and between the proximal jejunum and the incontinuity jejunum (the so-called "antiobstruction" stitch). Close the mesenteric defect with a running suture (Fig. 69.3K).

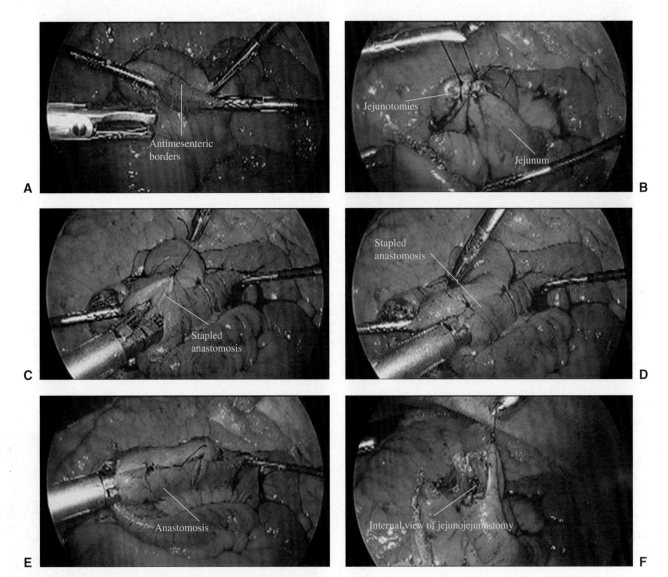

Figure 69.3　A: Approximation of jejunal antimesenteric borders. **B:** Jejunostomies created in preparation for jejunojejunal anastomosis. **C:** Linear cutting stapler insertion for jejunojejunostomy. **D:** Jejunal side-to-side anastomosis. **E:** Completed jejunojejunostomy side-to-side anastomosis. **F:** Internal view of stapled jejunojejunostomy prior to closure. (*continued*)

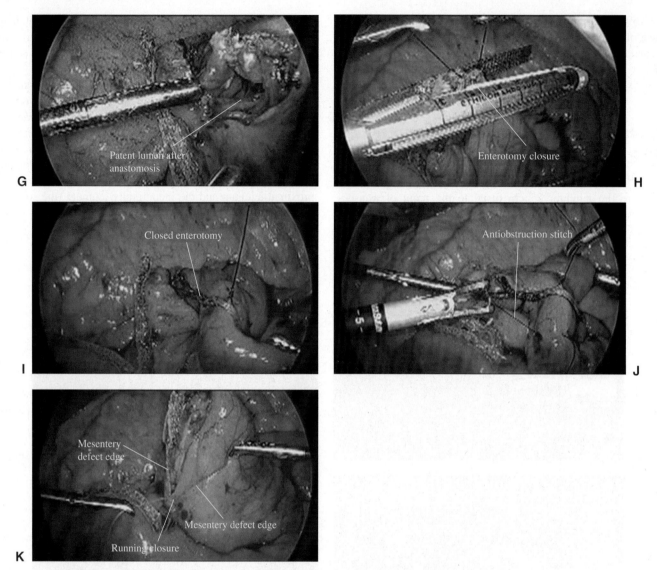

Figure 69.3 *Continued.* **G:** Ensuring jejunojejunostomy patency. **H:** Stapled closure of jejunojejunostomy with linear cutting stapler. **I:** Completed closure of jejunal anastomosis. **J:** Placement of antiobstruction stitch. **K:** Closure of mesentery defect with running suture.

Division of Gastrocolic Ligament (Fig. 69.4)

Grasp the greater omentum and divide with harmonic scalpel until the clear space in the gastrocolic ligament is reached. Next create a 4-cm transverse defect in the clear space of the gastrocolic ligament to allow passage of the antecolic Roux limb.

Dissection of the Lesser Curve (Fig. 69.5)

Technical Points

Place table in steep reverse Trendelenburg position and allow the colon and omentum to fall into the lower abdomen. The incisura is identified by the crow's foot on the lesser curvature. The

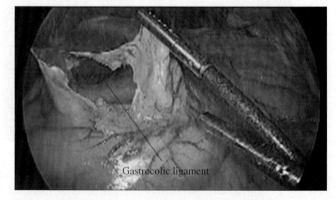

Figure 69.4 Division of gastrocolic ligament

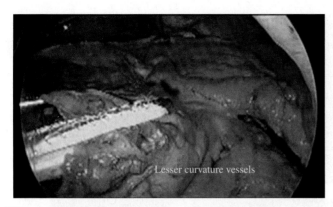

Figure 69.5 Division of lesser curvature vessels

lesser short gastric vessels are counted from the gastroesophageal junction. The first gastric pouch staple line will be between the third and fourth lesser curvature vessels. Grasp the gastrohepatic omentum to give medial traction with the left hand while using the ultrasonic shears in the right. Work through the fatty lesser omentum until, eventually, the lesser sac is entered.

Anatomic Points

Recall that the blood supply to the proximal stomach is derived from the left gastric artery, which is the smallest branch of the celiac artery (see Figure 53.1). Potential collateral circulation coming from the short gastric vessels will be divided in the course of developing the pouch. Care must be taken to keep the left gastric artery and vein superior to the opening into the lesser sac.

Dividing the Stomach (Fig. 69.6)

Technical Points

Have the nasogastric tube and any other devices that may have been inserted into the stomach withdrawn. Use an endoscopic linear cutting stapler to transect the stomach. Orient the first stapler load transversely, then direct subsequent loads toward the cardial notch (angle of His) until division of the stomach is

complete (Fig. 69.6A,B). Obtain hemostasis with electrocautery or suture ligatures as needed.

The Gastrojejunostomy (Fig. 69.7)

Technical and Anatomic Points

Grasp the marked end of the Roux limb and use it to draw the attached jejunum into the appropriate position in the upper abdomen. Take care that the jejunum is not twisted on its mesentery. The Roux limb may be traced back to the jejunojejunostomy to ensure proper orientation.

Attach the jejunum to the distal gastric staple line with a single stitch. Attach the jejunum to the posterior aspect of the gastric pouch using a running suture that begins at the distal corner of the second staple line and ends at the lesser curvature. This will be the posterior layer of the gastrojejunostomy (Fig. 69.7A,B).

Next choose a suitable site for the gastrotomy and jejunotomy and make these with the harmonic scalpel or L-hook cautery (Fig. 69.7C,D). Insert a 45-mm linear stapler into the two openings. Fire the stapler, creating a 3-cm side-to-side anastomosis (Fig. 69.7E,F).

An Ewald tube is passed by the anesthetist until it is visible through the gastrojejunostomy. This will later be used for the air insufflation test.

Close the enterotomy with a running full-thickness stitch (Fig. 69.7G). Cover the gastric staple line from lesser to greater curve with a second running layer of Lembert sutures (Fig. 69.7H). This completes the anastomosis (Fig. 69.7I). Clamp the bowel distal to the anastomosis with a bowel clamp and use the irrigator to fill the left upper quadrant with fluid.

The anesthetist administers oxygen via Ewald tube at 1 to 1.5 L/min while the assistant carefully looks for any bubbling that might indicate a leak. If none is found, aspirate the insufflated air and remove the bowel clamp and Ewald tube.

Insert a Jackson-Pratt drain and place it behind the gastrojejunostomy (Fig. 69.7J,K). Bring this drain out through the right upper quadrant trocar site. The drain will remain in place for 5 days to detect and potentially manage any possible anastomotic leak. Inspect all port sites for hemostasis prior to trocar removal. Close the skin in the usual fashion.

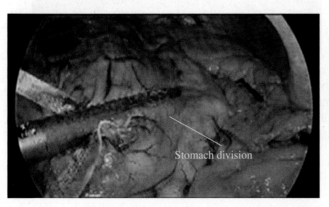

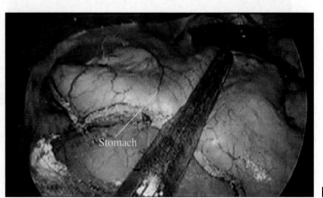

Figure 69.6 A: Division of stomach. **B:** Completing division of gastric pouch.

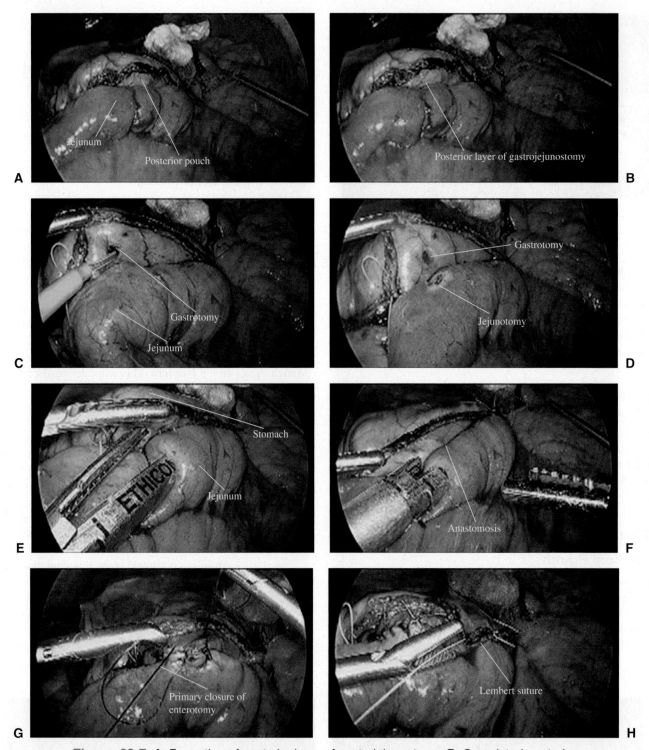

Figure 69.7 **A:** Formation of posterior layer of gastrojejunostomy. **B:** Completed posterior layer of gastrojejunostomy. **C:** Gastrotomy with L-hook cautery. **D:** Gastrotomy and jejunotomy with cautery. **E:** Forty-five–millimeter stapler into gastrotomy and jejunotomy. **F:** Stapled portion of gastrojejunostomy. **G:** Primary closure of first anterior layer of gastrojejunal anastomosis. **H:** Running Lembert suture placed at second anterior layer of gastrojejunal anastomosis.

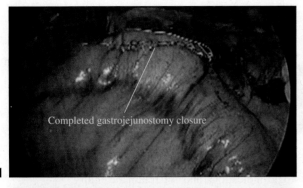

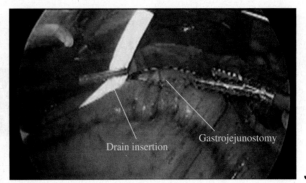

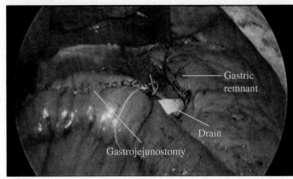

Figure 69.7 *Continued.* **I:** Completed gastrojejunostomy closure. **J:** Insertion of drain tunneling under gastrojejunostomy. **K:** Drain end and gastric remnant.

Acknowledgment

Thanks to Paul Jose, MD and Mohammad Jamal, MD, University of Iowa Hospital, Iowa City, IA for providing the video from which the figures were extracted.

REFERENCES

1. Abdel-Galil E, AA Sabry. Laparoscopic Roux-en-Y gastric bypass—evaluation of three different techniques. *Obes Surg.* 2002;12(5):639–642.

2. Maher JW, et al. Four hundred fifty consecutive laparoscopic Roux-en-Y gastric bypasses with no mortality and declining leak rates and lengths of stay in a bariatric training program. *J Am Coll Surg.* 2008;206(5):940–944.

3. Maher JW, et al. Drain amylase levels are an adjunct in detection of gastrojejunostomy leaks after Roux-en-Y gastric bypass. *J Am Coll Surg.* 2009;208(5):881–884.

4. Schauer PR, Ikramuddin S. Laparoscopic surgery for morbid obesity. *Surg Clin North Am.* 2001;81:1145–1179.

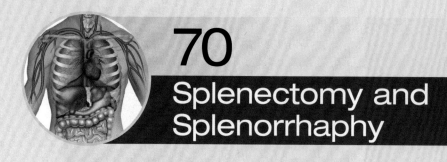

70

Splenectomy and Splenorrhaphy

Total splenectomy is performed for hematologic indications and for traumatic injury. Special techniques for repairing the injured spleen are discussed in Figures 70.8 and 70.9. A staging laparotomy procedure for Hodgkin disease is discussed in Figure 70.10. Laparoscopic splenectomy, an increasingly attractive alternative for elective splenectomy, is described in Chapter 71.

SCORE™, the Surgical Council on Resident Education, classified open splenectomy as an "ESSENTIAL COMMON" procedure and splenorrhaphy as an "ESSENTIAL UNCOMMON" procedure.

STEPS IN PROCEDURE—SPLENECTOMY

Left subcostal, upper left paramedian, or upper midline incision

Early Ligation of Splenic Artery (Optional)

Divide gastrocolic omentum and enter lesser sac

Identify splenic artery and ligate

Incise peritoneum lateral to spleen and gently develop the plane deep to spleen and tail of pancreas

Divide attachments to splenic flexure of colon and short gastric vessels

Identify tail of pancreas and protect it from harm

Ligate and divide splenic artery and vein and remove spleen

Check hemostasis; seek accessory spleens

Close abdomen without drainage

HALLMARK ANATOMIC COMPLICATIONS—SPLENECTOMY

Injury to tail of pancreas

Injury to stomach

Injury to colon

Missed accessory spleen

LIST OF STRUCTURES

Spleen

Splenic artery

Splenic vein

Stomach

Short gastric vessels

Left gastroepiploic artery

Transverse mesocolon

Celiac nodes

Hepatoduodenal nodes

Para-aortic nodes

Iliac nodes

Mesenteric nodes

Pancreas

Gastrosplenic ligament

Gastrocolic ligament

Splenorenal ligament

Lesser sac (omental bursa)

Splenic Exploration and Assessment of Mobility (Fig. 70.1)

Technical Points

Position the patient supine on the operating table. If the spleen is small, place a folded sheet under the left costal margin to elevate the operative field. A left subcostal incision (Fig. 70.1A) provides the best exposure for a small- or normal-sized spleen. However, this incision divides muscles and may result in

wound hematoma in patients with profound thrombocytopenia. As the spleen enlarges, it descends from the left upper quadrant, displacing the hilar vascular structures medially. Thus, in a patient with an enlarged spleen, use a midline or left paramedian incision for splenic exposure (Fig. 70.1B).

Explore the abdomen. Pass your nondominant hand up over the spleen and assess its mobility and size, as well as the nature and location of the attachments to the diaphragm and retroperitoneum.

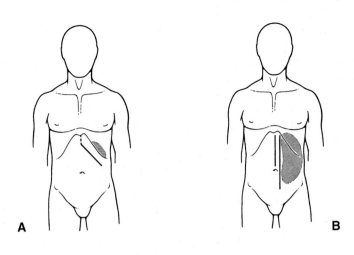

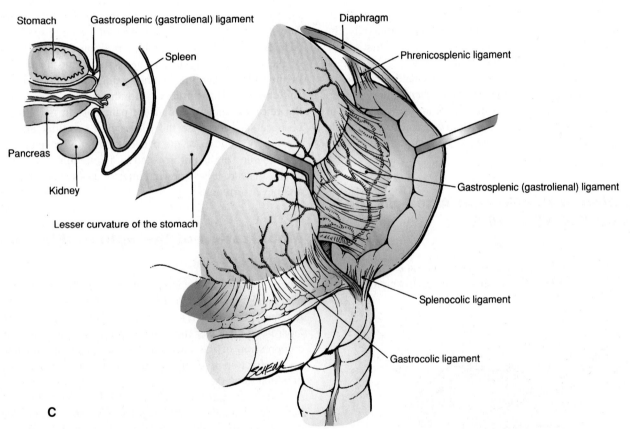

Figure 70.1 Splenic exploration and assessment of mobility. **A:** Left subcostal incision used for small spleen. **B:** Midline or left paramedian incision for large spleen. **C:** Regional anatomy and initial assessment of mobility.

At this point, decide whether or not to proceed with preliminary ligation of the splenic artery in the lesser sac. This maneuver decreases splenic blood flow and should be considered in the patient with a large spleen, particularly when difficulty in mobilization is anticipated.

Anatomic Points

The spleen develops embryologically in the dorsal mesogastrium. As the stomach rotates, the greater omentum develops as an elongation and subsequent redundancy of the dorsal mesogastrium. The pancreas (also initially within the dorsal mesogastrium) becomes retroduodenal. The spleen comes to lie in the left hypochondriac region, interposed between the diaphragm and the left kidney posteriorly and the fundus of the stomach anteriorly. Unlike the pancreas, it does not become retroperitoneal, but instead retains its intraperitoneal status, at the left extremity of the lesser sacromental bursa.

Short bilaminar peritoneal folds attach the spleen to the fundus of the stomach (gastrosplenic or gastrolienal ligament) and to the left kidney and diaphragm (splenorenal or phrenico-splenic ligament) (Fig. 70.1C). The gastrosplenic ligament is really the left extremity of the gastrocolic ligament; thus, there is also a splenocolic ligament. The splenorenal ligament is the left extremity of the transverse mesocolon. The attachments of spleen to colon are avascular.

The sides of these ligaments (gastrosplenic and splenorenal) that contribute to the walls of the lesser sac are continuous at the hilum, whereas the sides that are part of the boundary of the general peritoneal cavity are separated by the visceral peritoneal investment of the spleen. In other words, the spleen is invested with the general peritoneal layer of the embryologic dorsal mesogastrium. Both gastrosplenic and splenorenal ligaments are vascular. The splenorenal ligament supports the splenic artery and vein (and their splenic ramifications), whereas the gastrosplenic ligament supports those branches of the splenic artery (and the accompanying veins)—namely, the left gastroepiploic artery and short gastric arteries—that supply the greater curvature and fundus of the stomach.

The left gastroepiploic artery may originate from one of the splenic branches, rather than from the splenic artery proper. The short gastric arteries, of which there are typically four to six, can arise from the left gastroepiploic artery, the splenic artery proper, the splenic branches of the splenic artery, or any combination thereof.

Ligation of the Splenic Artery in the Lesser Sac (Fig. 70.2)

Technical Points

Enter the lesser sac by dividing the gastrocolic omentum. Serially clamp and ligate multiple branches of the gastroepiploic artery

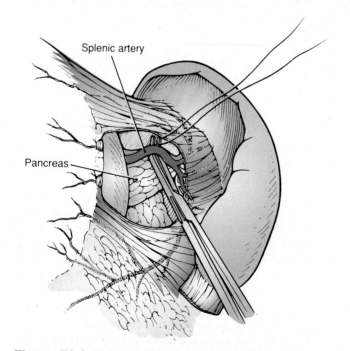

Figure 70.2 Ligation of the splenic artery in the lesser sac

Splenic artery

Pancreas

and vein until you have created a window in the gastrocolic omentum that is of sufficient size to admit retractors. Elevate the stomach, dividing the filmy avascular gastropancreatic folds as necessary to expose the pancreas. Identify the splenic artery where it loops along the upper border of the pancreas and pass a right-angle clamp under it. Ligate the splenic artery with a heavy silk tie.

Anatomic Points

Make the gastrocolic window either between the stomach and gastroepiploic arcade or between the gastroepiploic arcade and colon. Nothing will be devascularized in either case owing to the free and abundant anastomoses in this area. After entering the lesser sac (omental bursa), observe the pancreas through the parietal peritoneum of the posterior wall of the lesser sac. The characteristic corkscrew course of the large splenic artery (which is about 5 mm in diameter) along the superior border of the pancreas is related to age. The tortuosity is maximal in the elderly, minimal in the young, and absent in infants and children. This tortuosity lifts the splenic artery up out of the retroperitoneum behind the pancreas. In a child, it may be necessary to incise the peritoneum carefully and elevate the superior border of the pancreas to find the splenic artery. The splenic vein is not invested in a common sheath with the artery. Instead, it is somewhat inferior, always retropancreatic, and never tortuous.

Mobilization of the Spleen (Fig. 70.3)

Technical Points

Place retractors on the left costal margin. Pass your nondominant hand up over the spleen and hook the posterior edge, pulling the spleen down strongly and rolling it medially. Use a laparotomy pad over the spleen to improve traction. By strong compression of the spleen and steady traction, coupled with good retraction up on the costal margin, one can create a space in which to work.

Incise the peritoneum lateral to the spleen (Fig. 70.3A). Pass your nondominant hand under the medial leaf of the peritoneum and develop the plane deep to the spleen, the splenic vessels, and the tail of the pancreas. Mobilize the splenic flexure of the colon with the lower pole of the spleen. Mobilization of the spleen into the operative field will then be limited by the short gastric vessels and splenocolic ligaments (Fig. 70.3B).

Check the retroperitoneum and bed of the spleen for bleeding. Pack two laparotomy pads into the bed of the spleen.

Anatomic Points

Mobilization of the spleen should not exceed the limits imposed by the gastrosplenic ligament, as it is possible to avulse the short gastric blood vessels running in this ligament. The maneuver described partially recreates the embryonic

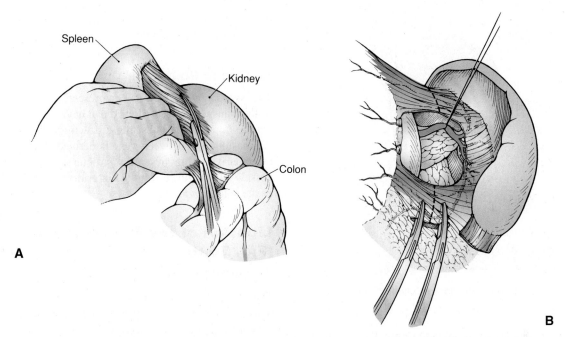

Figure 70.3 Mobilization of the spleen. **A:** Division of splenorenal ligament. **B:** Division of gastrosplenic ligament and exposure of splenic artery.

midline position of the spleen in the dorsal mesogastrium. Incision of the peritoneum lateral to the spleen allows access to the relatively avascular fusion plane formed by fusion and subsequent degeneration of the original left leaf of dorsal mesogastrium with posterior parietal peritoneum. As the spleen, splenic vessels, and pancreas all begin their development in the dorsal mesogastrium, this fusion plane is posterior to these structures. The splenic flexure of the colon is mobilized with the spleen because of the variable presence of small vessels in this ligament. Placing traction on the short splenocolic ligament can tear the delicate splenic capsule. Although the spleen is to be removed, capsular damage at this point can result in a bloody operative field.

Division of the Short Gastric Vessels (Fig. 70.4)

Technical Points

Typically, three to four short gastric arteries (with accompanying veins) connect the spleen to the greater curvature of the stomach high up near the cardioesophageal junction. The highest of these is generally the shortest, and the gastric wall closely approximates the upper pole of the spleen. With the spleen mobilized into the operative field, pass a right-angle clamp behind the highest short gastric vessels and doubly ligate and divide them. Be careful not to include the wall of the stomach in the tie. Then, sequentially ligate and divide the remaining short gastric vessels. Inspect the ties on the greater curvature of the stomach. If the gastric wall has been injured or included in a tie, the area should be imbricated with a 3-0 silk Lembert suture.

Anatomic Points

As discussed earlier (Fig. 70.1C), the origin of the short gastric arteries is variable. As can be expected, the number of short gastric vessels is also variable. There may be as few as 2 or as many as 10. Often, these can be divided into a superior group and an inferior group. The superior group is shorter than the inferior one, and downward traction of the spleen, without concomitant movement of the gastric fundus, can result in troublesome bleeding at the time of operation. It is best to ligate and

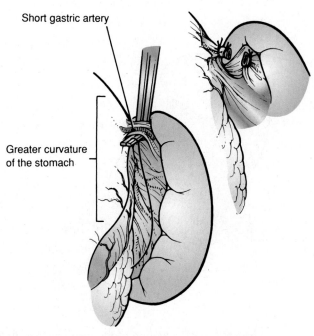

Figure 70.4 Division of the short gastric vessels

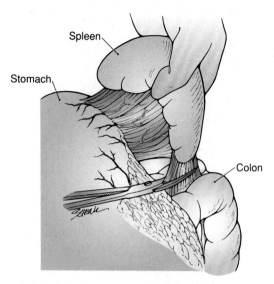

Figure 70.5 Division of the gastrocolic ligament

divide the most superior short gastric vessels first, working in an inferior direction. Because of the variability in the origin of the arteries, it is easier to ligate and divide them as close to the stomach as possible, rather than trying to ligate and divide them at their origin.

Division of the Gastrocolic Ligament (Fig. 70.5)

Technical Points

The gastrocolic ligament commonly contains small, unnamed vessels that may cause troublesome bleeding. Thus, even if no vessels are visible in the fatty tissue connecting the lower pole

of the spleen with the splenic flexure of the colon, divide this tissue with clamps and ties.

Anatomic Points

The gastrocolic ligament, when present, is the left continuation of the transverse mesocolon. It can have small vessels supplying the fat and other mesenteric structures, but there should be no anastomoses between vessels derived from the spleen and those derived from mesenteric structures. In all probability, the vessels will originate from the inferior proper splenic divisions of the splenic artery.

Ligation of the Hilar Vessels (Fig. 70.6)

Technical Points

The hilar vessels are best approached from the posterior aspect, with the spleen well mobilized into the field. The tail of the pancreas extends for a variable extent into the region of the splenic hilum and may be difficult to differentiate from fatty and nodal tissue in the hilum. Individually ligate the terminal branches of the splenic artery and splenic vein close to the spleen. Suture-ligate the large branches.

Some surgeons prefer to ligate the splenic vein close to its juncture with the superior mesenteric vein, especially in cases of massive splenomegaly. This has the theoretical advantage of preventing thrombus within the stump of the splenic vein from propagating into the portal or superior mesenteric vein. To perform a more proximal ligation of the splenic vein, trace the vein along the back of the mobilized tail of the pancreas and pass a right-angle clamp behind the vein at the desired point. Ligate the vein with a heavy silk tie.

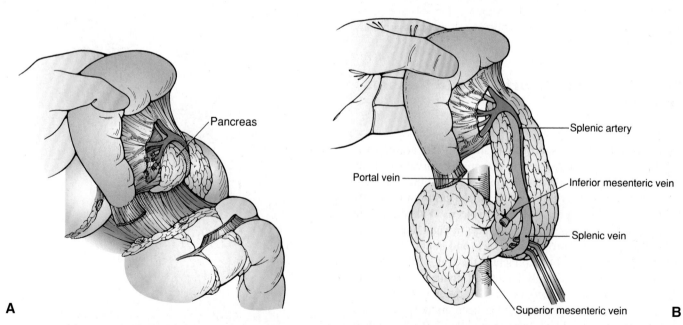

Figure 70.6 Ligation of the hilar vessels. **A:** Exposure of hilar vessels (note proximity of tail of pancreas). **B:** High ligation of splenic vein in cases of splenomegaly.

Anatomic Points

Ligate the hilar vessels as close as possible to the spleen because the tail of the pancreas is frequently supplied by a recurrent branch from one of the segmental divisions of the splenic artery, usually an inferior segmental division. Although this recurrent artery, a caudal pancreatic artery, is frequently illustrated as anastomosing with pancreatic arteries that are more medial, the fact that necrosis of the tail of the pancreas is a recognized complication of splenectomy suggests that the anastomosis is either variable or potential.

With respect to ligation of the splenic vein, it is advisable, on the basis of anatomic arrangements, to locate the termination of the inferior mesenteric vein and ligate distal to this. As expected, this termination is variable. It can terminate by draining into the superior mesenteric vein, confluence of the superior mesenteric and splenic veins, or into the splenic vein. Regardless of where this termination occurs, it is always retropancreatic.

Searching for Accessory Spleens and Subsequent Closure (Fig. 70.7)

Technical Points

Because many patients who undergo elective splenectomy have coagulation defects, hemostasis must be especially meticulous. The time spent double-checking for bleeding can also be used to conduct a search for accessory spleens which, if not found and removed, may cause a recurrence of the symptoms for which elective splenectomy was initially recommended.

Check the sites of ligation of the hilar vessels and the region of the tail of the pancreas for bleeding. Remove the laparotomy pads that were placed in the bed of the spleen. Suture-ligate any persistent bleeding points in the retroperitoneum. If bleeding from the cut edges of the peritoneal reflection is a problem, oversew these edges with a running lockstitch.

Search for accessory splenic tissue in the hilum of the spleen, in the gastrocolic omentum, around the tail of the pancreas, in the mesentery of the bowel, and in the pelvis. Most accessory spleens are found close to the spleen.

Anatomic Points

Accessory splenic tissue has been reported to be present in the abdominal cavity of 10% to 35% of individuals. Rarely, it has been reported found in the liver, scrotum, and pancreas. If an accessory spleen is present, there is typically only one; however, multiple accessory spleens have been reported. As stated earlier, most accessory spleens are located in the region of the spleen proper (Fig. 70.7A). The retroperitoneal region around the tail of the pancreas should be examined with great care, as this is an area in which accessory splenic tissue is often overlooked. The splenic tissue is usually less than 3 cm in diameter. It is usually dark purple, a similar color to the spleen itself (Fig. 70.7B), but sometimes small nodules of accessory splenic tissue resemble lymph nodes. In addition, a careful examination of the left ovary and uterine tube in the female, and the scrotum in males, is warranted because the spleen develops in close contact with the genital ridge.

Splenorrhaphy (Fig. 70.8)

Technical and Anatomic Points

Repair of the damaged spleen is often possible and should be attempted in patients who can tolerate the somewhat longer operative time required and the greater blood loss associated with it as compared with total splenectomy.

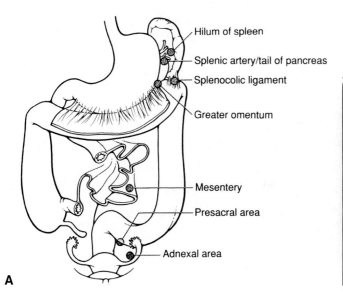

Hilum of spleen

Splenic artery/tail of pancreas

Splenocolic ligament

Greater omentum

Mesentery

Presacral area

Adnexal area

A

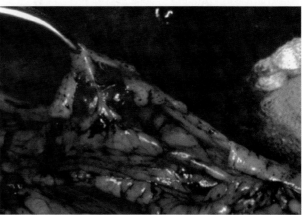

B

Figure 70.7 Searching for accessory spleens and subsequent closure. **A:** Common locations for accessory spleens. **B:** Accessory spleen in greater omentum showing typical location, size, and color (acute myelogenous leukemia).

First, mobilize the spleen up into the operative field. Use the same procedure that is used for elective splenectomy. Ligate the short gastric vessels, if necessary, to mobilize the spleen fully. Use extreme care not to damage the spleen further. Obtain temporary control of any bleeding by applying direct pressure to the bleeding site using a laparotomy pad. It may be necessary to occlude the splenic vessels in the hilum with an atraumatic vascular clamp.

Capsular avulsion injuries occur when traction on the colon or stomach stretches the splenic capsule. These are common iatrogenic injuries. In such cases, apply direct pressure to the injury for 5 minutes. Then apply a piece of microfibrillar collagen sponge and again apply direct pressure. Do not use electrocautery; episodes of rebleeding are common. The argon beam coagulator is an ideal thermal hemostatic device for this situation.

Large capsular avulsion injuries or simple capsular lacerations (Fig. 70.8A) may require suturing. Choose a monofilament suture, such as 4-0 chromic catgut, and a fine taper point needle. This particular suture is good because it is very soft when wet and hence is less likely than other monofilaments to saw through the capsule. Place a series of horizontal mattress

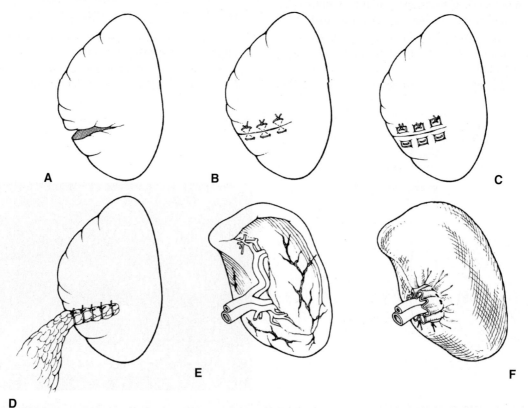

Figure 70.8 Splenorrhaphy. **A:** Simple splenic laceration amenable to suture. **B:** Closure with mattress sutures. **C:** Use of pledgeted sutures. **D:** Omentum used to buttress repair. **E:** Shattered spleen with intact hilar vessels suitable for wrap. **F:** Completed mesh wrap of shattered spleen.

sutures in such a way as to close the defect (Fig. 70.8B). As the capsule of the spleen is thin and flimsy, place sutures with precision and pull each suture through gently to avoid damaging the capsule. These sutures may be tied over pledgets, if desired, to decrease the chance of the suture's cutting through the capsule of the spleen (Fig. 70.8C). Tie the sutures gently. Use omentum to buttress the repair, if necessary (Fig. 70.8D).

If there is considerable damage to the spleen but the hilar vessels are intact, it may be possible to salvage the spleen by wrapping it in absorbable mesh (Fig. 70.8E, F). Debride the injured parenchyma and cut a piece of mesh large enough to enclose the spleen completely. Place a purse-string suture around the edge to create a bag. Tighten the purse-string around the hilum. Take care not to compromise venous return from the spleen. Make the wrap a little loose initially, then place a running suture on the outer aspect to tighten it. As the wrap works by compression, it must be snug and work to pull lacerated edges together in order to be effective. Check the completed wrap for hemostasis.

Partial Splenectomy (Fig. 70.9)

Technical Points

Extensive damage to one pole of the spleen, or damage to one of the hilar vessels, can be managed by partial splenectomy (Fig. 70.9A). Ligate the splenic artery branch or branches supplying the injured segment. The bleeding should stop or slow

significantly. The spleen should turn dark and develop a line of demarcation. Cut through the spleen along this line of demarcation (Fig. 70.9B). Suture-ligate occasional bleeding points. If necessary, close the transected edge with a series of horizontal mattress sutures to ensure hemostasis (Fig. 70.9C, D).

Anatomic Points

As the portal venous system lacks functional valves, it is necessary to ligate splenic segmental tributaries of the splenic vein, as well. These segmental tributaries drain segments supplied by corresponding arteries and are not intersegmental, as is the case in some other segmental organs.

Staging Laparotomy for Hodgkin Disease (Fig. 70.10)

Technical Points

A staging laparotomy for Hodgkin disease consists of splenectomy, liver biopsy, and biopsy of multiple intra-abdominal node groups; in addition, it may include biopsy of the iliac crest bone and oophoropexy (in the female). The procedure has largely been abandoned for noninvasive staging with scans. It is included in this chapter because it illustrates the regional anatomy.

Use a long midline incision, as all four quadrants of the abdomen must be explored.

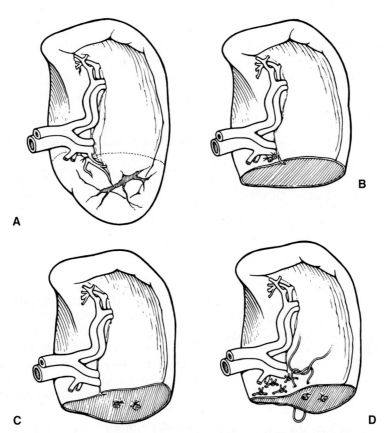

Figure 70.9 Partial splenectomy. **A:** Complex laceration limited to inferior pole of spleen. **B:** Amputation of lower pole. **C:** Suture ligation of vessels and any open renal calyces. **D:** Mattress closure of remaining portion of kidney.

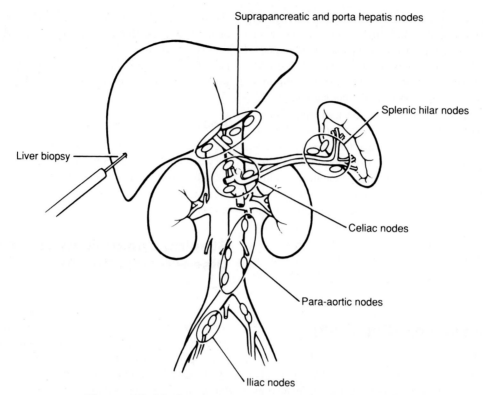

Figure 70.10 Staging laparotomy for Hodgkin disease

STEPS IN PROCEDURE—STAGING LAPAROTOMY FOR HODGKIN DISEASE

Midline laparotomy
Splenectomy (see Section 70.1)
Liver biopsy

Biopsy of Nodes
Celiac (upper para-aortic)
Hepatoduodenal
Para-aortic
Iliac

Mesenteric
Iliac crest bone marrow biopsy

Consider Oophoropexy in Young Females
Incise lateral peritoneal attachments of adnexae
Gently mobilize and tack ovaries to posterior surface of uterus
Mark lateral border of each ovary with metal clip

HALLMARK ANATOMIC COMPLICATIONS—STAGING LAPAROTOMY FOR HODGKIN DISEASE
Same as splenectomy (Section 70.1)

Liver Biopsy

Perform a liver biopsy first to minimize changes in liver histology caused by operative trauma. Obtain a biopsy specimen from any suspicious nodules. Take a wedge biopsy specimen from one lobe and a deep core biopsy specimen (using a liver biopsy needle) from the other lobe.

Splenectomy

Next, proceed with splenectomy. Include the splenic hilar lymph nodes with the specimen. Send the spleen in the fresh state to the pathologist. If the spleen shows obvious involve-ment by Hodgkin disease, the tedious search for and biopsy of intra-abdominal node groups can be curtailed. Mark the hilum of the spleen with a hemoclip.

Next, systematically expose and palpate the para-aortic, celiac, hepatoduodenal, mesenteric, and iliac lymph nodes. Obtain biopsy specimens from representative nodes from each group, as well as from any suspicious masses.

Celiac Nodes

Expose the celiac (or upper para-aortic) nodes by opening a window through the lesser omentum along the lesser curvature of the stomach. This can usually be done through an avascular region, which can easily be identified in thin patients. Palpate the region of the celiac axis and excise or obtain biopsy specimens from any enlarged nodes, or take a representative sample. Be careful not to damage the celiac artery or its branches.

Hepatoduodenal Nodes

Palpate the region of the hepatoduodenal ligament. Divide the filmy adhesions between the gallbladder and omentum or colon, if necessary, to expose the region. Nodes are commonly found in the region of the cystic duct and porta hepatis.

Para-aortic Nodes

Expose the abdominal aorta by lifting the omentum and transverse colon. Reflect the small bowel to the right, eviscerating the intestines, if necessary, to improve exposure. Palpate the abdominal aorta for the presence of enlarged nodes. Incise the peritoneum from just below the ligament of Treitz to the region just above the inferior mesenteric artery. If nodes are palpable behind the fourth portion of the duodenum at the ligament of Treitz, mobilize the fourth portion of the duodenum by incising the peritoneum lateral to the duodenum, then reflect the duodenum upward to expose the nodes.

If no nodes are palpable, explore the region to the left and deep in the groove adjacent to the abdominal aorta, excising fatty tissue from this area. Avoid the nearby sympathetic trunk.

Iliac Nodes

Incise the peritoneum overlying the iliac vessels. Identify the ureter as it crosses the common iliac artery at the bifurcation of the iliac vessels. Iliac nodes lie lateral and deep to the iliac vessels, just past the bifurcation of the iliac artery.

Mesenteric Nodes

Nodes are commonly palpable in the mesentery of the terminal ileum and elsewhere along the mesentery of the small intestine. Incise the peritoneum overlying the largest of these nodes and carefully shell out a node or two for biopsy. In addition, remove any enlarged or suspicious node, regardless of its location.

Biopsy of the Iliac Crest Bone

Expose the anterior iliac crest. Use a periosteal elevator to strip the periosteum. Use a small electric saw to remove a segment of the iliac crest that includes bone marrow.

Oophoropexy

Mobilize the tubes and ovaries gently by incising their lateral peritoneal attachments. Tack the ovaries to the posterior surface of the uterus with nonabsorbable suture. The ovaries and tubes should lie comfortably in the pouch of Douglas. Mark the lateral border of each ovary with a metal clip.

Anatomic Points

Celiac Nodes

The celiac nodes are the last in a chain of preaortic nodes that drain the gastrointestinal system. The para-aortic nodes in approximately the same location are terminal nodes in a chain that drain the lower extremities, parietes, and paired retroperitoneal and genitourinary organs.

Hepatoduodenal Nodes

The hepatoduodenal nodes are in the hepatoduodenal ligament, near the free right edge of the lesser omentum in close proximity to the hepatic artery. These nodes drain those structures supplied by the hepatic artery, and send efferents to the celiac nodes.

Para-aortic Nodes

Nodes in the para-aortic region (as described earlier in the section on technical points) are part of the chain draining the lower extremities, parietes, and genitourinary organs. They are close to the abdominal sympathetic chain, and care should be taken not to confuse them with these ganglia. Gentle palpation and attention to their size and their more "peritoneal" than "parietal" location should allow one to distinguish them.

Iliac Nodes

Nodes along the common and external iliac artery drain the extremities, parietes, and skin of the lower trunk. Nodes along the internal iliac artery are responsible for drainage of pelvic viscera.

Mesenteric Nodes

The mesenteric nodes drain the portion of bowel supplied by the intestinal artery (e.g., specific jejunal or ileal) with which they are associated.

Oophoropexy

The neurovascular supply to the ovaries and distal part of the uterine tubes runs through the suspensory ligament, that portion of the broad ligament extending from the pelvic wall to the uterine tube and ovary. Consequently, when these ligaments are incised, care must be taken to permit medial mobilization of the ovaries and uterine tubes.

REFERENCES

1. Cahill CJ, Wastell C. Splenic conservation. *Surg Annu.* 1990;22: 379. (Describes multiple techniques for splenic salvage.)
2. Cannon WB, Kaplan HS, Dorfman RF, et al. Staging laparotomy with splenectomy in Hodgkin's disease. *Surg Annu.* 1975;7:103.
3. Cioffiro W, Schein CJ, Gliedman ML. Splenic injury during abdominal surgery. *Arch Surg.* 1976;111:167. (Discusses mechanisms of iatrogenic splenic injury based on attachments of the spleen and mechanical forces exerted during surgery.)

4. Dawson DL, Molina ME, Scott-Conner CE. Venous segmentation of the human spleen. A corrosion case study. *Am Surg.* 1986;52:253. (Venous segmentation is similar to arterial segmentation.)

5. Dixon JA, Miller F, McCloskey D, et al. Anatomy and techniques in segmental splenectomy. *Surg Gynecol Obstet.* 1980;150:516.

6. Gospodarowicz MK. Hodgkin's lymphoma – patient's assessment and staging. *Cancer J.* 2009;15:138.

7. Lee J, Moriarty KP, Tashjian DB. Less is more: Management of pediatric splenic injury. *Arch Surg.* 2012;147:437.

8. Michels NA. The variational anatomy of the spleen and the splenic artery. *Am J Anat.* 1942;70:21.

9. Millikan JS, Moore EE, Moore GE, et al. Alternatives to splenectomy in adults after trauma. Repair, partial resection, and reimplantation of splenic tissue. *Am J Surg.* 1982;144:711.

10. Mitchell RI, Peters MV. Lymph node biopsy during laparotomy for the staging of Hodgkin's disease. *Ann Surg.* 1973;178:698.

11. Morgenstern L. Technique of partial splenectomy. *Probl Gen Surg.* 1990;7:103.

12. Oyo-Ita A, Ugare UG, Ikpeme IA. Surgical versus non-surgical management of abdominal injury. *Cochrane Database Syst Rev.* 2012;11:CD007383.

13. Pemberton LB, Skandalakis LJ. Indications for and technique of total splenectomy. *Probl Gen Surg.* 1990;7:85.

14. Uranus S, Kronberger L, Kraft-Kine J. Partial splenic resection using the TA-stapler. *Am J Surg.* 1994;168:49. (Describes useful technique for small soft spleens.)

15. Waizer A, Baniel J, Zin Y, et al. Clinical implications of anatomic variations of the splenic artery. *Surg Gynecol Obstet.* 1989; 168:57.

16. Zonies D, Estridge B. Combat management of splenic injury: Trends during a decade of conflict. *J Trauma Acute Care Surg.* 2012; 73(2 suppl 1):S71.

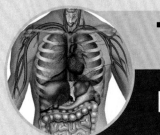

71

Laparoscopic Splenectomy

Laparoscopic splenectomy is easiest for small spleens (e.g., the normal-sized spleen associated with idiopathic thrombocytopenic purpura [ITP]). Techniques have been developed for moderate- to large-sized spleens, but in general, the larger the spleen the more difficult the surgery. The first laparoscopic splenectomies were performed with the patient supine, in a manner similar to that used during open splenectomy. The technique described here, in which the patient is placed in the lateral position and the peritoneal attachments of the spleen are used to suspend it in place is sometimes termed the *"hanging spleen"* technique. References at the end give details of other techniques and modifications for large spleens, as well as techniques for partial splenectomy and excision of splenic cysts.

SCORE™, the Surgical Council on Resident Education, classified laparoscopic splenectomy as an "ESSENTIAL COMMON" procedure.

STEPS IN PROCEDURE

Place patient in lateral decubitus position, left side up
Obtain laparoscopic access and explore abdomen
Rotate colon medially and inferiorly out of field
Divide gastrocolic ligament and short gastric vessels
Rotate stomach medially out of field
Isolate and divide hilar vessels
Incise lateral peritoneal attachments and remove spleen
Check for accessory spleens
Close any trocar sites (or small incision for spleen removal) greater than 5 mm

HALLMARK ANATOMIC COMPLICATIONS

Injury to bowel or viscera
Injury to tail of pancreas
Injury to stomach
Injury to colon
Missed accessory spleens

LIST OF STRUCTURES

Spleen
Splenic artery
Superior polar artery
Inferior polar artery

Colon
Descending colon
Splenic flexure

Greater omentum
Splenocolic ligament
Phrenicocolic ligament
Splenophrenic ligament
Lesser sac

Stomach
Short gastric vessels

Initial Exposure (Fig. 71.1)

Technical Points

Place the patient in the full lateral decubitus position, with the left side up. The general trocar pattern is shown in Figure 71.1A. A 30- or 45-degree laparoscope gives optimum visualization. Place the laparoscope through an umbilical port. Operating trocars need to be large enough (generally 12 mm) to accommodate the endoscopic linear cutting stapler, if that is

planned. Reverse Trendelenburg positioning allows gravity to assist in retraction.

Use the ultrasonic scalpel to mobilize and detach the splenic flexure of the colon from the spleen by first dividing the peritoneal reflection of the descending colon. Start inferiorly at a convenient point and progress cephalad (Fig. 71.1B). Fully divide the phrenicocolic ligament, and then the splenocolic ligament (Fig. 71.1C). Leave the splenophrenic ligament intact, to allow the spleen to "hang" from this ligament during subsequent dissection.

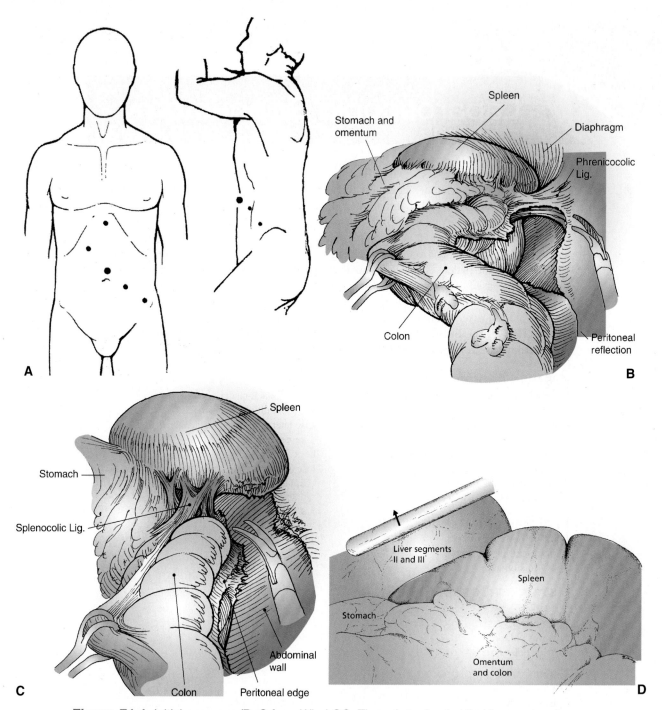

Figure 71.1 Initial exposure (**B, C** from Wind GG. The spleen. In: *Applied Laparoscopic Anatomy: Abdomen and Pelvis.* Baltimore, MD: Williams & Wilkins; 1997:187–216, with permission; **D** from Scott-Conner CEH, Cuschieri A, Carter FJ. Spleen and pancreas. In: *Minimal Access Surgical Anatomy.* Philadelphia, PA: Lippincott Williams & Wilkins; 2000:139–163, with permission).

Rotate the colon medially and inferiorly out of the field. Then sequentially divide the anterior peritoneal folds and short gastric vessels (see Figure 47.2A,B in Chapter 47). This creates an opening into the lesser sac through which the splenic hilum should be visible. Mobilize and rotate the stomach medially out of the field.

Anatomic Points

The peritoneal attachments and topographic relations of the spleen were discussed in Chapter 61. The shape of the spleen gives the laparoscopic surgeon a clue as to the pattern of vessels in the hilum. The rounded shape shown in Figure 71.1A–C correlates with late branching (within 1 or 2 cm of the hilum) of the splenic artery and vein. This implies a single, well-defined vascular pedicle that is easy to identify and control. This magistral splenic artery pattern occurs in only approximately 30% of individuals.

In the remainder, the splenic artery and vein divide into branches at a distance from the hilum and multiple vessels must be identified and controlled, often in close proximity to the tail of the pancreas. The sharply notched border of the spleen shown in Figure 71.1D correlates with early branching of the splenic vessels. A superior polar splenic artery is found in 13%, an inferior polar artery in 31%, and both are identified in 16% of normal individuals.

Division of Hilar Vessels (Fig. 71.2)

Technical and Anatomic Points

Ideally, identify the splenic artery near the hilum of the spleen but before it branches. Look for the tip of the pancreas and find a site on the splenic artery that is beyond the tip of the pancreas. Seek the splenic vein deep to splenic artery and pancreas, and generally a little inferior to the splenic artery (Fig. 71.2A). Multiple vessels associated with a notched splenic border are best individually ligated or clipped (Fig. 71.2A,B).

If the hilar vessels form a neat packet near the splenic hilum, use an endoscopic linear stapler to secure them (Fig. 71.2C).

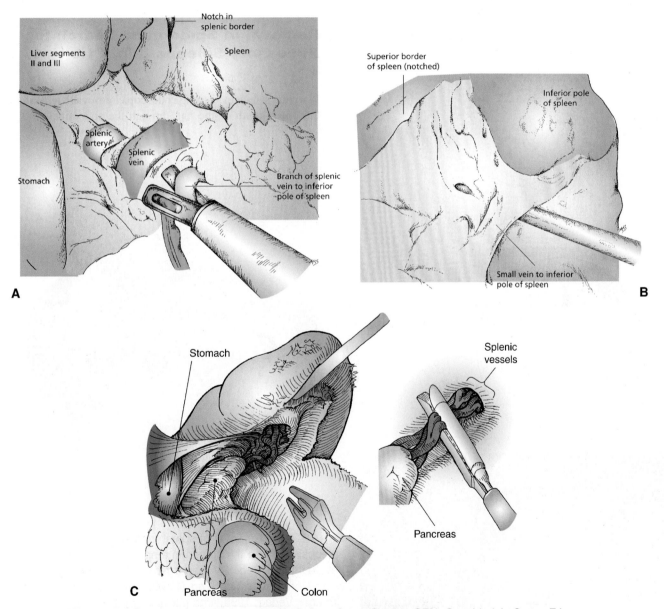

Figure 71.2 Division of hilar vessels (**A, B** from Scott-Conner CEH, Cuschieri A, Carter FJ. Spleen and pancreas. In: *Minimal Access Surgical Anatomy.* Philadelphia, PA: Lippincott Williams & Wilkins; 2000:139–163, with permission; **C, D** from Wind GG. The spleen. In: *Applied Laparoscopic Anatomy: Abdomen and Pelvis.* Baltimore, MD: Williams & Wilkins; 1997:187–216, with permission). *(continued)*

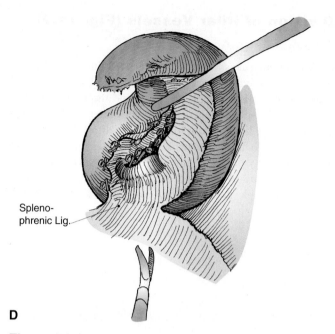

Spleno-phrenic Lig.

D

Figure 71.2 *Continued*

It may be necessary to place a fan retractor and gently elevate the spleen to secure adequate visualization of the hilum. Manipulate the spleen with extreme gentleness to avoid bleeding; even a small amount of bleeding can obscure visualization.

Develop the plane above and below the hilar vessels. The vessels may be taken in a single firing of the stapler if located close to each other. Avoid superimposing one vessel on the other because postoperative arteriovenous fistula may complicate mass ligation or stapling. Gently insert the endoscopic cutting linear stapler (vascular cartridge) and manipulate splenic artery and vein within the jaws. Fire and remove the stapler.

Divide the remaining peritoneal attachments with an ultrasonic scalpel (Fig. 71.2D).

Removal of Spleen and Search for Accessory Spleens (Fig. 71.3)

Technical Points

Place the spleen in a strong endoscopic retrieval bag. Withdraw the open mouth of the bag through the abdominal wall. Use

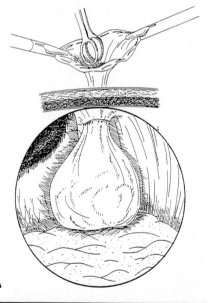

A

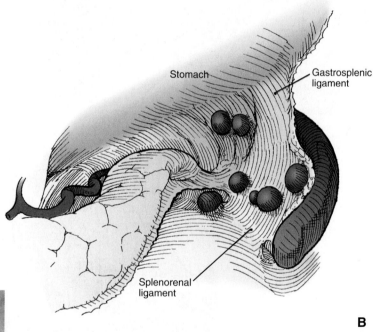

Stomach

Gastrosplenic ligament

Splenorenal ligament

B

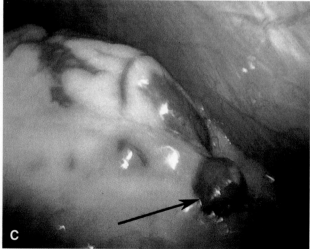

C

Figure 71.3 Removal of spleen and search for accessory spleens. **A:** Place the spleen in a specimen bag and morcellate it (from Rege RV. Laparoscopic splenectomy. In: Scott-Conner CEH, ed. *The SAGES Manual.* New York, NY: Springer-Verlag; 1999, with permission). **B:** Common locations of accessory spleens in vicinity of splenic hilum (from Wind GG. The spleen. In: *Applied Laparoscopic Anatomy: Abdomen and Pelvis.* Baltimore, MD: Williams & Wilkins; 1997:187–216, with permission). **C:** Laparoscopic appearance of accessory spleen (from *Fischer's Mastery of Surgery.* Philadelphia, PA: Lippincott Williams & Wilkins; 2013, with permission).

a ring forceps, your fingers, a suction irrigator, or specially designed morcellator to fragment and suck out the spleen (Fig. 71.3A). Remove the bag.

Search again for accessory spleens in the usual locations before desufflating the abdomen and closing the trocar sites.

Anatomic Points

There has been a suggestion that accessory spleens are more difficult to find during laparoscopic splenectomy. The most common location is in the splenic hilum, as previously discussed (see Chapter 61). Throughout the dissection, remain alert to the possibility of accessory spleens, particularly when the splenic hilum is first exposed, as shown in Figure 71.3B,C.

REFERENCES

1. Hery G, Becmeur F, Mefat L, et al. Laparoscopic partial splenectomy: Indications and results of a multicenter retrospective study. *Surg Endosc.* 2008;22:45–49.
2. MacFadyen BV, Litwin D, Park A, et al. Laparoscopic splenectomy. II. Technical considerations. *Contemp Surg.* 2000;56: 398–407.
3. Musallam KM, Khalife M, Sfeir PNM, et al. Postoperative outcomes after laparoscopic compared with open splenectomy. *Ann Surg.* 2012 (epub ahead of print).
4. Rescorla FJ, Breitfeld PP, West KW, et al. A case controlled comparison of open and laparoscopic splenectomy in children. *Surgery.* 1998;124:670–676.
5. Romano F, Gelmini R, Caprotti R, et al. Laparoscopic splenectomy: Ligasure versus EndoGIA: A comparative study. *J Laparoendosc Adv Surg Tech A.* 2007;17:763–768.
6. Schwaltzberg SD. Chapter 176. Laparoscopic splenectomy. In: Fischer, ed *Fischer's Mastery of Surgery.* Philadelphia, PA: Wolters Kluwer Lippincott Williams & Wilkins; 2012:1859.
7. Silvestri F, Russo D, Fanin R, et al. Laparoscopic splenectomy in the management of hematological diseases. *Haematologica.* 1995; 80:47–49.
8. Tatarov A, Muggia-Sullam M. A simple technique for deploying a laparoscopic bag during splenectomy: Two-point anchoring to the abdominal wall. *J Laparoendosc Adv Surg Tech A.* 2007;17: 329–330.
9. Vargun R, Gollu G, Fitoz S, et al. En-bloc stapling of the splenic hilum in laparoscopic splenectomy. *Minim Invasive Ther Allied Technol.* 2007;16:360–362.
10. Vecchio R, Marchese S, Intagliata E, et al. Long-term results after splenectomy in adult idiopathic thrombocytopenic purpura: Comparison between open and laparoscopic procedures. *J Laparoendosc Adv Surg Tech A* 2012 (epub ahead of print).
11. Wind GG. The spleen. In: *Applied Laparoscopic Anatomy: Abdomen and Pelvis.* Baltimore, MD: Williams & Wilkins; 1997:187–216. (Provides an excellent description of embryology and anatomy from the laparoscopist's viewpoint.)

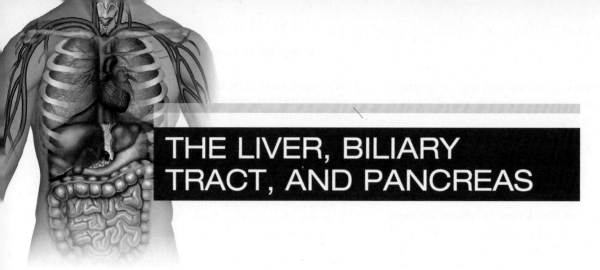

THE LIVER, BILIARY TRACT, AND PANCREAS

This section is organized into two parts: The extrahepatic biliary tract (and liver) and the pancreas. Within each part, simple procedures are described first, followed by a discussion of more complex procedures. The extrahepatic biliary tract is introduced in Chapters 72 and 73, which are devoted to cholecystectomy, bile duct exploration, and liver biopsy. Both open and laparoscopic cholecystectomies are described. Operations to bypass an obstructed bile duct by direct anastomosis to the gut, either by anastomosis to the duodenum (choledochoduodenostomy) or to a defunctionalized loop of jejunum (choledochojejunostomy) are then detailed (Chapters 75 to 77). A related procedure—transduodenal sphincteroplasty (Chapters 78

and 79e)—illustrates the anatomy of the ampulla of Vater. More complex procedures that demonstrate the anatomy of the portal venous system (Chapter 80) and liver (Chapters 81 and 82) are then presented.

Pancreatic resections are described in Chapters 84 and 85e, continuing the discussion of portal venous anatomy, celiac artery anatomy, the spleen, and the anatomy of the duodenum begun in earlier sections. Finally, chapters on operations for drainage of pancreatic pseudocysts and pancreatic necrosectomy (Chapters 86 and 87) conclude this section. More complex hepatobiliary and pancreatic procedures are detailed in the references at the end of each chapter.

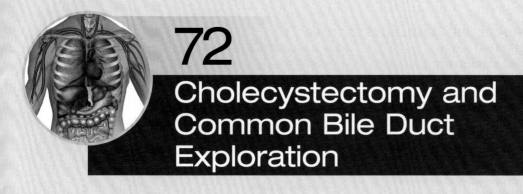

72

Cholecystectomy and Common Bile Duct Exploration

The safest way to perform an open cholecystectomy is from the top down, rather than retrograde (bottom up), as is done during laparoscopic cholecystectomy. This is particularly important because open cholecystectomy is generally reserved for the most difficult situations, where there is a lot of inflammation, or for failure of the laparoscopic approach. Top-down dissection reserves division of the cystic duct until the gallbladder is fully mobilized, minimizing the chance of injury to the bile duct.

The traditional top-down approach to open cholecystectomy as described here uses early ligation and division of the cystic artery to minimize bleeding. A tie is then placed around the cystic duct to minimize the chance of stone passage into the bile duct, but the duct is not divided until late in the dissection. These steps are not always safe or feasible in cases of severe inflammation. In that case, do not hesitate to simply dissect from top down, ligating the artery and duct as encountered. This chapter also details an important bail-out option, subtotal cholecystectomy, which is useful in the most difficult cases.

SCORE™, the Surgical Council on Resident Education, classified open and laparoscopic cholecystectomies with or without cholangiography as "ESSENTIAL COMMON" procedures, and open common duct exploration and choledochoscopy as "ESSENTIAL UNCOMMON" procedures.

HALLMARK ANATOMIC COMPLICATIONS—CHOLECYSTECTOMY
Bile duct injury
Bleeding from cystic artery or hepatic artery
Retain bile duct stone

LIST OF STRUCTURES
Liver

Gallbladder
Infundibulum (Hartmann's pouch)
Cystic duct
Common hepatic duct
Bile duct

Ligamentum teres hepatis
Right and left hepatic arteries
Cystic artery
Cholecystoduodenal ligament
Cystohepatic (Calot's) triangle

Incision and Exposure of the Gallbladder (Fig. 72.1)

Technical Points

In most patients, a right-sided subcostal (Kocher) incision provides the best exposure. If the subcostal angle is very acute, a right paramedian incision may be chosen instead, especially in a slender patient.

Make the incision two fingerbreadths below the right costal margin and parallel to it. Divide the anterior rectus sheath sharply. Pass a long Kelly hemostat under the rectus abdominis muscle and divide it with electrocautery. Occasional small arteries may require suture ligation. Pick up and incise the posterior rectus sheath and preperitoneal fat to enter the abdomen. Medially, the ligamentum teres hepatis may need to be divided, particularly if exposure is difficult and surgery on the bile duct is anticipated.

STEPS IN PROCEDURE—CHOLECYSTECTOMY

Right subcostal (Kocher) incision

Divide ligamentum teres hepatic

Kelly clamp on fundus of gallbladder (decompress first, if tense)

Divide adhesions to omentum, pack omentum and colon down

If dissection is difficult because of inflammation, do not attempt to find cystic artery and duct at this point

Incise peritoneum over gallbladder several millimeters from liver and dissect in submucosal plane of gallbladder, working from the top down

Divide peritoneum over Calot's triangle and posterior peritoneum

Identify and Divide Cystic Artery

Identify and Divide Cystic Duct

If cholangiogram is needed, do not completely divide cystic duct

Make small nick in anterior surface of cystic duct

Insert catheter and secure in cystic duct

Remove gallbladder

If Adhesions are Severe, Consider Subtotal Cholecystectomy

Leave as much of back wall of gallbladder as necessary

Remove anterior part of gallbladder as far down as possible

Secure cystic duct from inside gallbladder with purse-string suture

Destroy remaining mucosa of gallbladder with electrocautery

Place omentum and closed suction drain into subhepatic space

Close incision in usual fashion

Explore the abdomen. Pass a hand over the right lobe of the liver and pull down, allowing air to enter the subphrenic space and providing increased exposure of the subhepatic region. Filmy adhesions between the gallbladder and the gastrocolic omentum or transverse colon may need to be cut.

If the gallbladder is tense and acutely inflamed, preliminary decompression with a trocar will decrease the chance of uncontrolled spillage of infected bile during dissection. Place a purse-string suture of 3-0 silk on the top of the gallbladder in an easily accessible location. Support the gallbladder with the left hand and insert a trocar through the center of the purse string. Aspirate bile and calculous material from the gallbladder. Withdraw the trocar, taking care not to spill bile, and tie the purse string suture to close the hole. Obtain a culture of the bile.

If the gallbladder is not tense, place a Kelly clamp on the fundus of the gallbladder and pull down and out. Use the clamp to gain traction and expose the cystohepatic (Calot's) triangle. Place packs to depress the colon and to hold the stomach and duodenum medially out of the field.

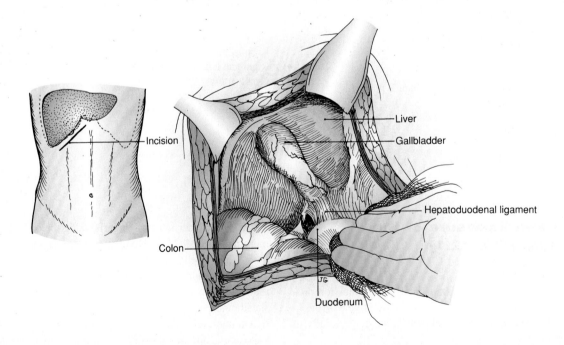

Figure 72.1 Incision and exposure of the gallbladder

Anatomic Points

A short Kocher incision does not cause any functional deficit of the rectus abdominis muscle. However, a very long Kocher incision may result in weakness of the rectus, especially if several segmental nerves are divided. The superior epigastric artery and vein lie posterior to the rectus abdominis muscle, about halfway (at this level) between the linea alba and the costal margin. These vessels are generally small and are either divided with electrocautery or ligated and divided.

The falciform ligament (and its contained ligamentum teres hepatis, in the free edge of the falciform ligament) runs from the umbilicus to the fissure separating the right and left lobes. This lies to the right of the midline, so the falciform ligament is oriented with its left surface in contact with liver and its right in contact with the anterior parietal peritoneum. If the falciform and round ligaments must be divided, this should be done between clamps. The reasons for this are twofold. First, the round ligament, which is the obliterated left umbilical vein, may retain a patent lumen. Second, paralleling the round ligament are a variable number of paraumbilical veins, which provide a potential collateral circuit between the portal vein and the caval system via the superficial veins of the abdomen.

The right and left hepatic ducts leave their corresponding liver lobes and unite close to the porta hepatis to form the common hepatic duct, typically the most anterior tubular structure in this region. The cystic duct, which drains the gallbladder, joins the common hepatic duct at a variable distance from the porta hepatis and at a variable angle. This union forms the bile duct.

The gallbladder is a diverticulum of the extrahepatic biliary tree. From the cystic duct, the gallbladder is divided into a narrow neck (in which spirally arranged folds of mucosa form the so-called valve of Heister), a tapering body, and an expanded fundus that extends beyond the inferior border of the liver. Frequently, an asymmetric bulging of the right side of the neck may occur. This bulge, known as the infundibulum of the gallbladder (or Hartmann's pouch), may be bound down toward the first part of the duodenum by a cholecystoduodenal ligament, the right edge of the lesser omentum. This ligament must be divided and the infundibulum (Hartmann's pouch) mobilized to clearly identify the cystic duct.

Identification of the Cystic Artery and Cystic Duct (Fig. 72.2)

Technical Points

Divide any filmy adhesions that remain between the gallbladder and the colon or omentum. Place a second Kelly clamp farther down on the gallbladder; be careful to clamp the gallbladder and not the cystic or bile duct. Incise the peritoneum overlying the cystohepatic (Calot's) triangle and dissect bluntly with a Kitner dissector. Push fatty and areolar tissues away from the gallbladder to expose the bile duct, cystic duct, and cystic artery.

Sometimes the gallbladder is so inflamed that it is adherent to the duodenum or bile duct. If this appears to be the case, abandon the attempt to identify and ligate the cystic artery and

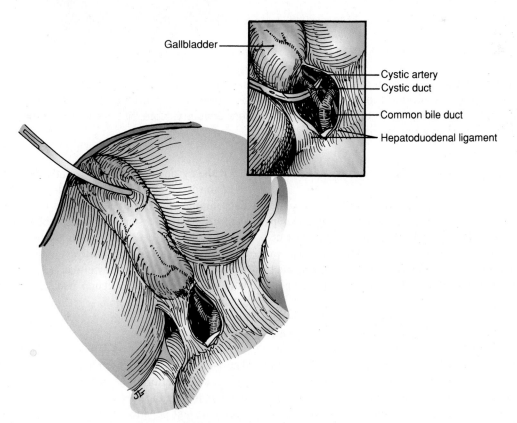

Gallbladder

Cystic artery
Cystic duct
Common bile duct
Hepatoduodenal ligament

Figure 72.2 Identification of the cystic artery and cystic duct

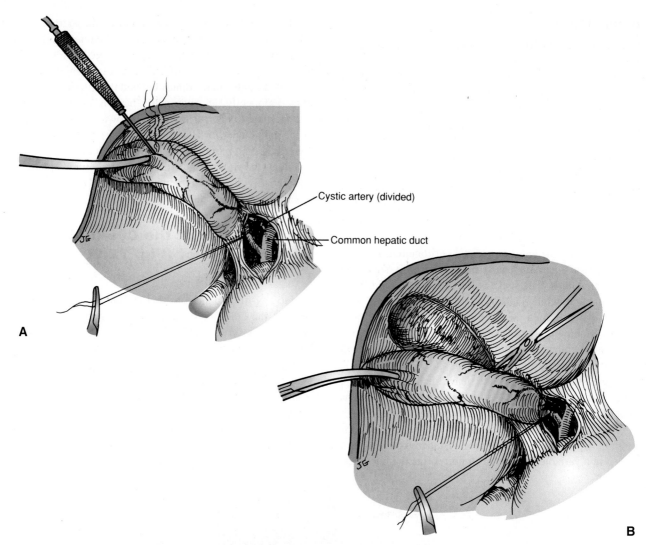

Figure 72.3 Removal of the gallbladder. **A:** Cystic artery has been ligated and divided, and a tie placed around the cystic duct. Dissection begins at the fundus of the gallbladder. **B:** Gallbladder being taken off the liver bed with electrocautery. Note that cystic duct remains intact until gallbladder is completely freed.

cystic duct and simply proceed directly to top-down removal of the gallbladder (Fig. 72.3).

Identify the cystic duct passing from the gallbladder to the bile duct. Clean the duct gently and pass a right-angle clamp behind it. Double-loop the duct with a 2-0 silk suture to provide temporary but atraumatic occlusion of the duct. This helps to prevent small stones from being forced down into the bile duct during the dissection and facilitates the performance of a cholangiogram of the cystic duct.

Next, identify the cystic artery, which typically passes superior to the cystic duct and runs along the anterior surface of the gallbladder. Clean the cystic artery and divide it, securing the ends with 3-0 silk ligatures. Anomalies are common in this area; an unusually large cystic artery should raise the suspicion that the vessel may, in fact, be an anomalous right hepatic artery. Dissect along the course of the vessel to see whether it terminates on the gallbladder or loops back up into the liver.

If the cystic artery is inadvertently divided, do not attempt to clamp it. Blind clamping in a bloody field may cause bile duct injuries. Simply pass the index finger of your nondominant hand into the space behind the bile duct and duodenum and compress the pedicle including the bile duct, hepatic artery, and portal vein (Pringle maneuver) with your fingers, slowing the bleeding so that the vessel can be identified and clamped with surety. A vascular clamp may also be used to provide secure temporary occlusion.

Anatomic Points

The boundaries of the cystohepatic (Calot's) triangle are the cystic duct inferiorly, the common hepatic duct medially, and the right lobe of the liver superiorly. It contains the right hepatic duct and right hepatic artery (usually posterior to the duct) in the superior part of the triangle, and the cystic artery more inferiorly. Anomalous vessels and bile ducts are common. The right hepatic artery can lie anterior to the right hepatic duct, or it may be up to 1 cm distant from the duct. Because its course briefly parallels the cystic artery, it can be mistaken for the latter vessel. The cystic artery, typically a branch of the right hepatic artery, can arise from any artery in the vicinity (e.g., the left hepatic, common hepatic, gastroduodenal, superior mesenteric). However, regardless of its origin, it usually passes through the cystohepatic (Calot's) triangle.

Skeletonization of the cystic duct from the neck of the gallbladder to the bile duct is necessary, because it allows the surgeon to verify its identity. Variations in the biliary apparatus are also common. There can be accessory hepatic ducts (usually from the right), which can be mistaken for the cystic duct; bifurcated cystic ducts; multiple cystic ducts; and even absence of a cystic duct.

Removal of the Gallbladder (Fig. 72.3)

Technical Points

With the cystic artery and cystic duct controlled, dissection now progresses from the fundus of the gallbladder down. Incise the peritoneum overlying the gallbladder until the blue submucosal plane, which is superficial to a network of small vessels, is identified. Dissection in this plane will allow removal of the gallbladder without injury to the liver and with a minimum of blood loss. Carry the peritoneal incisions laterally as far as exposure will allow. After the correct plane has been identified, use electrocautery to incise the peritoneum over a right-angle clamp.

Hold the Kelly clamp and the gallbladder with your nondominant hand, moving the gallbladder from side to side as required to expose the attachments between the gallbladder and the liver. Cut these attachments sharply, remaining as much as possible in the submucosal plane.

As the dissection progresses, connect the peritoneal incision over the gallbladder with that made previously over the cystohepatic (Calot's) triangle. Hold the gallbladder in your nondominant hand and work on the edge of the gallbladder.

Lift the gallbladder and incise the posterior peritoneum. Push fatty and areolar tissue overlying the gallbladder downward with a Kitner dissector. Although most of the dissection in the critical region close to the bile duct is done from the front, mobility gained by clearing peritoneum posteriorly will greatly facilitate the remaining phase of dissection. Ideally, the bile duct should be visualized and the common duct/cystic duct juncture clearly identified.

Occasionally, severe inflammation or the presence of hepatic cirrhosis renders dissection of the back wall of the gallbladder from the liver difficult, hazardous, or almost impossible. In this case, leave the back wall of the gallbladder in place where it attaches to the liver (subtotal cholecystectomy). Remove the gallbladder by cutting through the full thickness of the wall as shown for the peritoneal incision. As you extend the dissection downward, attempt to reenter the wall of the

gallbladder and dissect within the wall for the terminal 1 to 2 cm. This maneuver facilitates identification and ligation of the cystic duct. If inflammation is so severe that dissection within the wall of the gallbladder cannot be attempted, then remove the gallbladder and suture-ligate the cystic duct orifice from within. Thoroughly obliterate the mucosa of the gallbladder remnant with electrocautery and pack the area with omentum. Drain the subhepatic space with a closed suction drain.

Anatomic Points

Do not remove the gallbladder until you have clearly identified all ancillary structures, components of the biliary apparatus, and associated vasculature. As you dissect the gallbladder from the liver bed, stay as close as possible to the gallbladder rather than to the liver surface. This avoids injury to subvesicular bile ducts (which are blind ducts, present in as many as 35% of gallbladder fossae, that do not communicate with the gallbladder but that can be a source of bile leakage) or to the intrahepatic anterior segmental branch of the right hepatic artery, which is very close to the subvesicular surface of the liver. Occasionally, there can be small accessory cystohepatic ducts in the gallbladder fossa or in the vicinity that must be controlled to prevent bile leakage. Moreover, the right, left, or both hepatic ducts can empty directly into the gallbladder.

Operative Cholangiogram (Fig. 72.4)

Technical and Anatomic Points

At this point, the gallbladder should be attached only by the cystic duct, which has a 2-0 silk double-looped around it. Place a hemostatic clip on the gallbladder to prevent spillage of bile when the cystic duct is opened. Choose a catheter appropriate to the size of the cystic duct. Soft Silastic pediatric feeding tubes are safe, atraumatic, and available in several sizes. An 8-French feeding tube is a good catheter to use when the cystic duct is large. A 5-French feeding tube can generally be placed in even the smallest cystic duct. Commercially available kits with stiffer catheters are convenient, but one must be very careful not to injure the bile duct when a stiff catheter is used.

Flush the catheter and connecting tubes with sterile saline and remove any bubbles. While maintaining slight traction on the cystic duct, make a small incision in the upper surface with a no. 11 blade. A small drop of bile should appear at the site of incision, confirming entry into the biliary tree. Pass the catheter gently into the cystic duct and tie the silk suture around it. Confirm that bile can be aspirated and that saline can be injected easily, without extravasation.

Exchange the syringe of saline for one containing dilute water-soluble contrast medium. Generally, the contrast material should be diluted 1:1 or 1:2 so that small stones will not be hidden in a dense column of contrast medium. Check to make

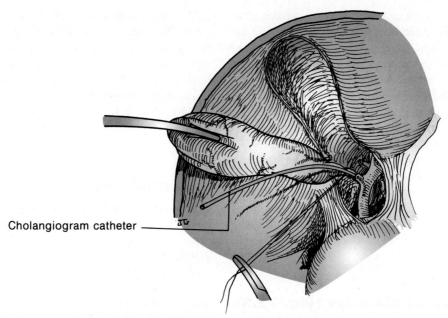

Cholangiogram catheter

Figure 72.4 Operative cholangiogram

sure that no air bubbles have been introduced. Remove all packs and retractors, taking care not to dislodge the catheter. Obtain two exposures, one after a small amount of contrast medium has been instilled and the second after a larger amount. For a small common duct, 8 to 12 mL of contrast material are appropriate. If the common duct appears to be large, use correspondingly larger amounts. The common duct and intrahepatic biliary tree should be able to be well visualized, with good definition of the distal common duct. If too much contrast material is used initially, spillage of contrast into the duodenum may obscure visualization of the terminal common duct. On the second film, contrast material should be seen to flow into the duodenum.

After checking the cholangiograms, remove the gallbladder in the following fashion. Cut the suture holding the cholangiogram catheter in the cystic duct. Then pull the catheter out while an assistant clamps the cystic duct close to its juncture with the bile duct. Suture-ligate the cystic duct with 3-0 silk. Check the field for hemostasis.

Bile Duct Exploration (Kocher Maneuver) (Fig. 72.5)

Technical and Anatomic Points

A recent, good-quality cholangiogram is critical; preferably, this should be obtained on the operating table, either as part of the preliminary cholecystectomy or by direct puncture of the common duct with a small-caliber butterfly needle. The cholangiogram guides the subsequent exploration by showing the regional anatomy and the approximate number and location of stones. Even if a recent preoperative cholangiogram is available, consideration should be given to obtaining a preliminary operative radiograph, as the number and location of the stones may have changed.

Ascertain that the incision is long enough to allow adequate exposure of the bile duct. Because the gallbladder mobilizes upward in the course of the dissection, cholecystectomy can be done through a relatively short incision under favorable circumstances. Safe and thorough exploration of the bile duct requires generous exposure.

STEPS IN PROCEDURE—BILE DUCT EXPLORATION

Remove Gallbladder (If Not Already Performed)

If no recent cholangiogram, perform intraoperative cholangiogram to determine anatomy, number and location of stones

Mobilize hepatic flexure of colon downward to fully expose duodenum

Mobilize duodenum medially to expose inferior vena cava (Kocher maneuver)

Palpate hepatoduodenal ligament for stones, palpate head of pancreas for masses

Clean Anterior Surface of Bile Duct and Choose Site for Choledochotomy

If choledochoduodenostomy is planned, choose site low on bile duct

Place two stay sutures and open bile duct, observe character of bile (stones, pus, debris)

Explore distal duct first

Place nondominant hand behind duodenum and pull slightly downward to straighten duct, facilitating passage of instruments

Retrieve stones with scoops, stone forceps, or biliary Fogarty catheters

Pass no. 3 Bakes dilator through into duodenum

Explore proximal duct, taking care not to wedge
 stones high in intrahepatic biliary tree
Visualize proximal and distal duct with
 choledochoscope

**Close Bile Duct Around T-Tube and
 Perform Completion Cholangiogram**
No stones should remain and bile should flow
 freely into duodenum

Place closed suction drain near
 choledochotomy and place omentum into
 subhepatic space
Close incision in usual fashion, place T-tube
 to drainage

HALLMARK ANATOMIC COMPLICATIONS—BILE DUCT EXPLORATION
Retained bile duct stones
Injury to duodenum

Injury to hepatic artery

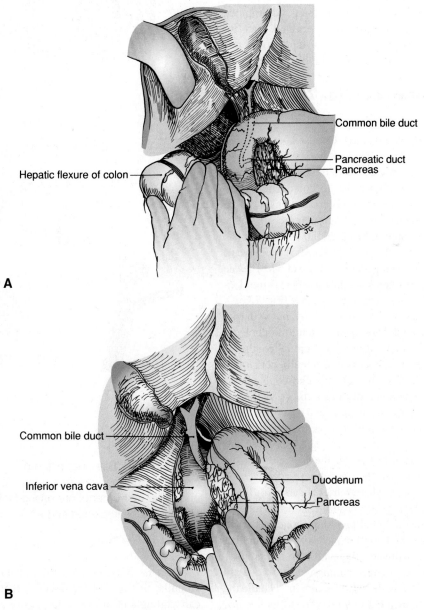

Figure 72.5 Bile duct exploration (Kocher maneuver). **A:** Initial exposure
and regional anatomy. **B:** Duodenum has been fully mobilized by performing
a Kocher maneuver.

Divide the ligamentum teres hepatis by doubly clamping and ligating the obliterated umbilical vessel in the free edge. Use electrocautery to divide the rest of this ligament.

Mobilize the hepatic flexure of the colon to expose the duodenum. Incise the peritoneum lateral to the duodenum. After creating an initial window large enough to admit a finger, pass the index finger of your nondominant hand into the retroperitoneum and elevate the remaining peritoneum, dividing it with electrocautery when it is thin enough to see through. Place traction on the duodenum with a laparotomy pad and incise the filmy, avascular adhesions between the duodenum and the retroperitoneum using Metzenbaum scissors. As the dissection progresses, elevate the duodenum and head of the pancreas and rotate them medially. Continue mobilization until you can pass your nondominant hand comfortably behind the head of the pancreas and can feel the terminal bile duct and ampulla. Palpate the hepatoduodenal ligament and terminal duct for stones and the pancreas for masses. Place a laparotomy pad behind the duodenum to elevate it into the field.

Bile Duct Exploration (Fig. 72.6)

Technical Points

Clean the upper surface of the bile duct. Choose a site for choledochotomy. If a choledochoduodenostomy (see Figures 75.1 and 75.2 in Chapter 75) is planned, make the choledochotomy low, just above the duodenum. Otherwise, a choledochotomy at about the level of the cystic duct stump is convenient.

Place two traction sutures of 4-0 silk through the superficial layers of the bile duct, avoiding entering the lumen, if possible. Bile is a detergent and will pass through small holes; hence, even a needle hole can be the site of postoperative leakage of bile. Elevate the common duct with these sutures and make a 2- to 3-mm longitudinal slit in the common duct with a no. 11 blade (Fig. 72.6A). Entry into the common duct must be made cleanly, but with care taken to avoid penetrating the back wall. Extend the choledochotomy with Pott's scissors until it is about 1 cm in length.

Exploration of the common duct is traditionally performed as a blind procedure. Because the choledochoscope allows direct visualization and manipulation under direct vision, its use has superseded many of the maneuvers described here. Nevertheless, these approaches are still useful and will be described briefly.

Often, a stone or two can be palpated in the duct and felt to be mobile. In this situation, one must be careful not to displace the stone into the intrahepatic tree, where retrieval can be difficult. Instead, it may be possible to gently push the stone up into the choledochotomy using gentle digital pressure. Stones retrieved from the duct should be saved and counted and their number and size compared to the estimates obtained from the preliminary cholangiogram. Stones in the common duct frequently acquire layers of muddy, easily dislodged sediment. Handle the stones gently to avoid fragmenting them. If the stones become fragmented, it is more difficult to ascertain whether all stones have been removed, and any debris left behind in the common duct may act as a nidus for further stone formation.

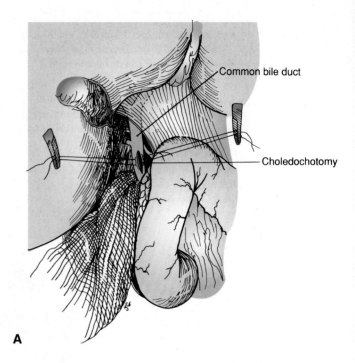

A

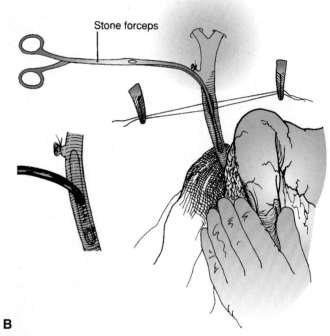

B

Figure 72.6 Bile duct exploration. **A:** Incision is made in common duct between two stay sutures. **B:** Stone forceps and other instruments are passed into the duct to retrieve stones; T-tube is placed in duct at conclusion of exploration.

Because most stones settle in the distal duct just above the ampulla, this part of the duct is generally explored first. Take care throughout not to dislodge stones from the lower part of the duct, where they are relatively easy to retrieve, into the intrahepatic biliary tree, where they may become impacted. Minimize the chance of this happening by temporarily occluding the proximal duct with a peanut sponge. Remove the sponge from the clamp and transfix it with a 2-0 silk suture. Tag the tails of the suture with a clamp, tails and remain outside of the duct and are used to retrieve the peanut sponge when the distal duct is clear.

When passing instruments into the distal bile duct, place your nondominant hand behind the duodenum and head of pancreas and pull down to straighten the terminal duct and palpate the ampulla. The nondominant hand will help you judge the direction and course of the terminal common duct and you will probably be able to feel instruments as they are being passed into the region above the ampulla. When you explore the upper duct, bend the malleable handle of the instruments to allow both the left and right intrahepatic ducts to be entered. Allow the instrument to find its own path into the duct; you will have a sensation that the instrument is following a tract when it is passing into the intrahepatic tree.

Scoops of various sizes on malleable handles are passed proximal and distal to lift up and retrieve stones. Pass the scoop along the back wall of the duct and concentrate on the sensation of stone against steel that indicates the presence of a stone. Try to pass the scoop under the stone and lift up, pulling the scoop and stone back into the choledochotomy. An assistant should hold a medicine glass of saline ready for you to wash the stone after each passage. Typically, mucus and debris will also be obtained; stones should be visible at the bottom of the glass.

A large stone in a large duct may be retrieved using a stone forceps (Fig. 72.6B). Such forceps are available with several degrees of curvature. To grasp a stone in the lower duct, choose a stone forceps that is relatively straight. Pass the forceps with the jaws open as wide as the common duct will allow; then, gently close the forceps periodically as the instrument is advanced. If successful, you will feel the forceps grip the stone. Pull stone and forceps back and out the choledochotomy.

Biliary Fogarty catheters may be passed proximal and distal with the balloon deflated; then they may be inflated and pulled back to drag out stones and debris. Particularly in the intrahepatic biliary tree, it is important not to inflate the balloon too much as it is easy to rupture small intrahepatic radicles. Adjacent branches of the portal vein may be injured, resulting in troublesome bleeding. Inflate the balloon with just enough saline to feel a slight resistance when the catheter is withdrawn. Vary the amount of saline in the balloon in response to the feel of the catheter as the Fogarty catheter is pulled back. Additional saline may be introduced as the catheter enters the larger bile duct. If the Fogarty catheter is passed through the ampulla, the balloon will catch on the ampulla as the catheter is withdrawn. It is then necessary to deflate the balloon, pull the catheter back through the ampulla, and reinflate the balloon.

Bakes dilators, which are calibrated dilators on malleable handles, are passed through the ampulla. Start with a small Bakes dilator (a no. 3 is usually the smallest available). Be extremely careful to feel the ampulla as the Bakes dilator is passed and to pass the dilator atraumatically. It is possible, and undesirable, to create a false passage with the use of these dilators. When the Bakes dilator passes into the duodenum, you will feel it pop through the ampulla, at which point you should be able to see the steel tip shining through the lateral wall of the duodenum if you stretch the duodenal wall over the dilator. Passage of successively larger Bakes dilators stretches and will ultimately tear the ampulla. There is a general lack of agreement as to what extent the ampulla should be dilated. Record the size of the largest Bakes dilator that is successfully passed. If it is not possible to pass even the no. 3 Bakes dilator, there is probably a stone lodged at the ampulla.

Finally, a large red rubber catheter can be passed proximally and distally to flush the duct out with saline. Observe the effluent and continue flushing until no stones or debris are obtained.

Anatomic Points

Proximal to the site of entrance of the biliary duct, the extrahepatic biliary apparatus consists of right and left hepatic ducts; these unite to form the common hepatic duct. This union is between 0.25 and 2.5 cm from the liver surface. Within the liver parenchyma, the right and left hepatic ducts are formed by the union of appropriate segmental ducts. As would be expected, there are several possible variations in this pattern. Accessory hepatic ducts, usually with a diameter that is about half that of the main pancreatic ducts, may be present. These are really normal segmental ducts that join the biliary tract extrahepatically, rather than intrahepatically.

From its formation in the hepatoduodenal ligament, the bile duct passes posterior to the first part of the duodenum, then passes posterior to or through the head of the pancreas, unites with the terminal pancreatic duct, and finally pierces the wall of the second part of the duodenum to open on the summit of the major duodenal papilla. The pancreatic part of the bile duct lies at a variable distance from the duodenum and may be entirely retroduodenal; alternatively and more commonly, it may be covered posteriorly by a small tongue or bridge of pancreatic tissue. In most cases, there is a fusion cleft to the right of the duct that permits exposure of this terminal duct. Rarely, the duct lies anterior to the pancreas rather than posterior to it.

As the bile duct approaches the duodenum, it is posterior and somewhat superior to the pancreatic duct. These ducts typically join extramurally, then follow an oblique course through the wall of the duodenum.

As the bile duct enters the wall of the duodenum, it narrows significantly (from about 10 mm to about 5 mm), sometimes resulting in the formation of an intraluminal ridge or step. This ridge can present problems during intraluminal procedures, and is an anatomic reason for the settling of common duct stones just proximal to the ampulla of Vater. The intramural part of its course can be as narrow as 2 mm. Here, the wall of the bile duct and pancreatic duct fuse, forming the ampulla of Vater, and both the biliary system and the exocrine pancreatic system open by the single ostium at the apex of the major duodenal papilla. The length of the common channel within the ampulla of Vater is variable. Typically, a variable septum separates the intra-ampullary bile duct from the pancreatic duct; this septum may be complete so that both ducts open independently on the apex of the papilla. The major duodenal papilla is normally on the posteromedial wall of the second part of the duodenum, approximately 7 to 10 cm distal to the pylorus.

Operative Choledochoscopy and Closure of Choledochotomy (Fig. 72.7)

Technical and Anatomic Points

Both rigid and flexible fiberoptic scopes are available and may be used for choledochoscopy. The rigid scope provides excellent optics, but demands that the duodenum be fully kocherized so that the duct can be straightened and the scope passed. The fiberoptic scope is considerably easier to pass. Its use is described here.

Pass the scope distally first. Use the controls of the scope to introduce a slight bend on the tip and pass it from above down through the choledochotomy. Cross the traction sutures over the scope to "close" the duct over the instrument and allow it to fill with saline. Allow saline to run freely into the duct through the instrument. The duct should become distended with saline, allowing the lumen to become visible. The ampulla will be visible as a sphincter at the terminal duct (Figure 72.7A). The central lumen of the ampulla may be visualized. Generally, it is not possible to pass the scope into the ampulla and duodenum. If a stone is seen, pass the biliary Fogarty catheter next to the scope and, under direct vision, attempt to engage the stone. A stone basket can also be used under direct vision. As the scope is pulled back, the common duct should be inspected.

The choledochoscope should then be passed into the right and left hepatic ducts. Several branches of the intrahepatic biliary tree may be visible. Retrieve any stones seen. Pull back the scope and inspect the common duct. It is easy to overlook stones in the region of the common duct adjacent to the choledochotomy unless you are especially careful.

Choose a T-tube of appropriate size. If the duct is large and multiple stones have been obtained, use at least a no. 14-French T-tube. A large tube will facilitate subsequent manipulation if stones are left behind at operation. If the duct is small, a smaller tube is appropriate. Cut the crossbars of the T short, and either cut out the back wall or cut a V into the back wall so that the crossarms bend easily when the tube is pulled. Confirm patency of both limbs by injecting saline. Place the T-tube in the common duct and push it to the upper margin of the choledochotomy. After it is in the common duct, it should slide freely, indicating that the crossbar of the T is not kinked within the lumen of the duct. Push the T-tube to the upper limit of the choledochotomy so that closure can proceed from below, where visualization is easiest.

Start a running lock-stitch of 4-0 Vicryl at the inferior margin of the choledochotomy and proceed up to the T-tube. Take full-thickness bites of the duct, but be careful not to narrow the lumen (especially if the duct is small). At the T-tube, close the choledochotomy snugly around the tube, taking care not to catch the rubber tube within a suture. Run the suture back as

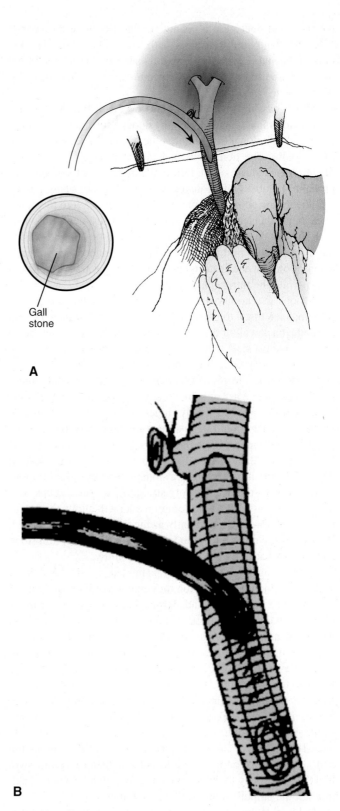

Gall stone

A

B

Figure 72.7 Operative choledochoscopy and closure of choledochotomy

a simple running stitch and tie it to itself (Fig. 72.7B). Inject saline to check for leaks.

Perform a completion cholangiogram by injecting dye into the T-tube to confirm that all stones have been removed and that the duct has not been narrowed. Place the omentum and a closed suction drain in the subhepatic space.

REFERENCES

1. Benson EA, Page RE. A practical reappraisal of the anatomy of the extrahepatic bile ducts and arteries. *Br J Surg.* 1976;63:853.
2. Bornman PC, Terblanche J. Subtotal cholecystectomy for the difficult gallbladder in portal hypertension and cholecystitis. *Surgery.* 1985;98:1–6.
3. Browne EZ. Variations in origin and course of the hepatic artery and its branches: Importance from surgical viewpoint. *Surgery.* 1940;8:424.
4. Gross RE. Congenital anomalies of the gallbladder: A review of 148 cases, with report of a double gallbladder. *Arch Surg.* 1936;32:131.
5. Johnston EV, Anson BJ. Variations in the formation and vascular relationships of the bile ducts. *Surg Gynecol Obstet.* 1952;94:669.
6. Linder HH, Green RB. Embryology and surgical anatomy of the extrahepatic biliary tree. *Surg Clin North Am.* 1963;44:1273.
7. Michels NA. The hepatic, cystic, and retroduodenal arteries and their relations to the biliary ducts with samples of the entire celiacal blood supply. *Ann Surg.* 1951;133:503.
8. Michels NA. Variational anatomy of the hepatic, cystic, and retroduodenal arteries: A statistical analysis of their origin, distribution, and relations to the biliary ducts in two hundred bodies. *Arch Surg.* 1953;66:20.
9. Moosman DA. Where and how to find the cystic artery during cholecystectomy. *Surg Gynecol Obstet.* 1975;133:769.
10. Sutton JP, Sachatella CR. The confluence stone: A hazardous complication of biliary tract disease. *Am J Surg.* 1967;113:719.

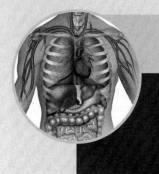

73

Laparoscopic Cholecystectomy and Common Bile Duct Exploration

Laparoscopic cholecystectomy introduced operative laparoscopy to most general surgeons, and is often the first laparoscopic procedure performed by surgical residents. Although the anatomy is identical to that described in Chapter 72, the significance of some biliary anomalies is greater for the laparoscopic procedure. Accordingly, this chapter stresses not only surgical technique but also ways in which specific anatomic pitfalls can be avoided. It should be read in conjunction with Chapter 72. The regional anatomy is shown in Figure 73.1A with the more limited laparoscopic view demonstrated in Figure 73.1B.

This chapter describes the classic four-trocar approach. Many uncomplicated laparoscopic cholecystectomies are now done through a single incision approach, and natural orifice surgery (NOTES) has been adapted to this procedure as well. References at the end give details of these more advanced approaches.

SCORE™, the Surgical Council on Resident Education, classified laparoscopic cholecystectomy with and without cholangiography as "ESSENTIAL COMMON" procedures, and laparoscopic common duct exploration as a "COMPLEX" procedure.

STEPS IN PROCEDURES—LAPAROSCOPIC CHOLECYSTECTOMY

Obtain laparoscopic access and inspect abdomen

Place grasper on fundus of gallbladder and pull up and over the liver

Lyse any adhesions to omentum

Place second grasper on gallbladder infundibulum (Hartmann's pouch)

Expose cystohepatic triangle

Incise peritoneum over distal gallbladder

Identify cystic duct and cystic artery

If cholangiogram is desired, insert catheter into cystic duct and secure it

Divide cystic duct and cystic artery

Dissect gallbladder from bed of liver, working in submucosal plane

Place gallbladder into retrieval bag and remove

Close trocar sites greater than 5 mm

HALLMARK ANATOMIC COMPLICATIONS—LAPAROSCOPIC CHOLECYSTECTOMY

Bile duct injury

Injury to duodenum

Injury to other surrounding viscera

Retained bile duct stone

LIST OF STRUCTURES

Bile Duct

Common hepatic duct

Right and left hepatic ducts

Cystic duct

Left and right subphrenic spaces

Subhepatic space

Lesser sac

Duodenum

Greater omentum

Hepatic artery

Cystic artery

ORIENTATION

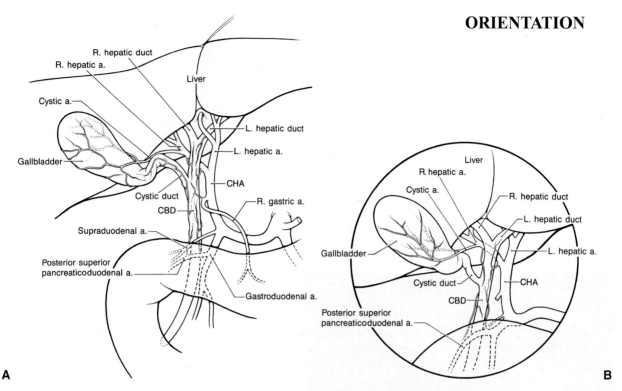

Figure 73.1 Regional anatomy. **A:** As seen during open surgery. **B:** The more limited laparoscopic view.

Initial Exposure (Fig. 73.2)

Technical Points

Introduce the laparoscope through an umbilical portal. Place a 10-mm port in the epigastric region and two 5-mm ports in the right midclavicular line and right anterior axillary line (Fig. 73.2A). Explore the abdomen. Cautiously lyse any adhesions of gallbladder to colon, omentum, or duodenum (Fig. 73.2B). Pass a grasping forceps through the anterior axillary line port and grasp the fundus of the gallbladder, pulling it up and over the liver. This will expose the subhepatic space (Fig. 73.2C). If the stomach and duodenum are distended, have suction placed on an orogastric or nasogastric tube. Reverse Trendelenburg positioning and tilting the operating table right side up will help increase the working space by allowing the viscera to move caudad and to the left.

Place a second grasping forceps through the midclavicular line port and grasp Hartmann's pouch. Pull out, away from the liver. This maneuver will open Calot's triangle and create a safe working space (Fig. 73.2D).

Take a moment to orient yourself. Frequently, there is an obvious color difference between the pale blue or green of the gallbladder (unless severely diseased) and the yellow fat of the Calot's triangle. This blue–yellow junction is a good place to begin dissection. A few filmy adhesions of omentum, transverse colon, or duodenum may need to be cautiously lysed to provide optimum visualization of the region. Calot's node, often enlarged in acute or resolving acute cholecystitis, nestles in Calot's triangle (Fig. 73.2E).

Another good landmark is the hepatic artery, which should be visible as a large pulsating vessel well to the left of the surgical field. This is a marker for the bile duct, which generally lies just to the right.

Anatomic Points

The cystic artery arises from the right hepatic artery in Calot's triangle and ascends on the left side of the gallbladder in approximately 80% of individuals. A fatty stripe or slight tenting of the peritoneum overlying the gallbladder may serve as a clue to its probable location. In a significant minority of individuals, the cystic artery arises directly from the hepatic artery. Other anomalies of the cystic artery of laparoscopic significance are described in Figure 73.3.

Calot's node is one of two fairly constant nodes in this region. The second node, termed the node of the anterior border of the epiploic foramen, lies along the upper part of the bile duct. Thus, simply noting the presence of a node in proximity to the bile duct does not guarantee a safe working distance from the bile duct.

Initial Dissection (Fig. 73.3)

Technical Points

Incise the peritoneum overlying the blue–yellow junction (Fig. 73.3A). The cystic duct should become evident as a tubular structure which runs into the gallbladder. It is generally

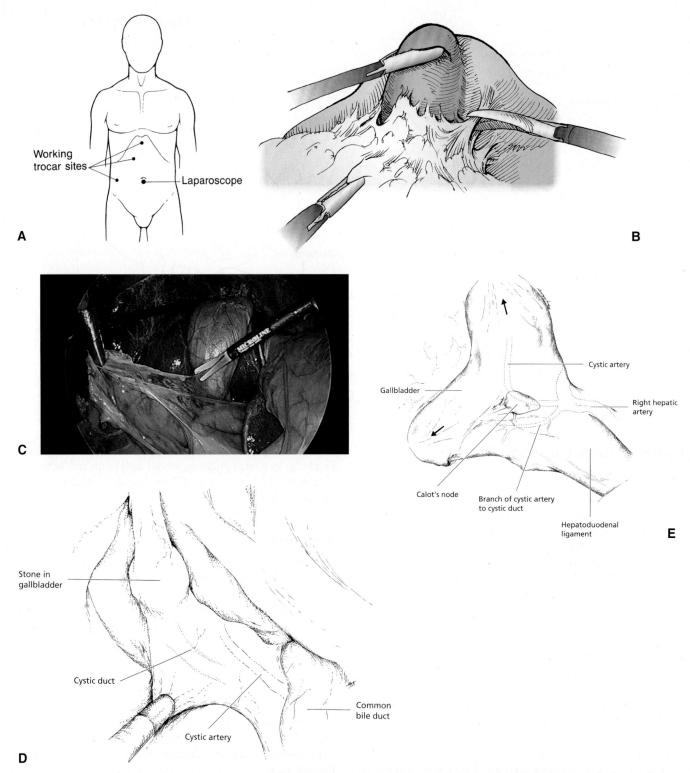

Figure 73.2 Initial exposure (**A** from Scott-Conner CEH, Brunson CD. Surgery and anesthesia. In: Embury SH, Hebbel RP, eds. *Sickle Cell Disease: Basic Principles and Clinical Practice.* New York, NY: Raven; 1994:809–827, with permission; **B** from: Wind GG. The biliary system. In: *Applied Laparoscopic Anatomy: Abdomen and Pelvis.* Baltimore, MD: Williams & Wilkins; 1997:13–83, with permission; **C:** Laparoscopic photograph kindly supplied by Evgeny V. Arshava, MD; **D** and **E** from: Scott-Conner CEH, Cushieri A, Carter F. Right upper quadrant: Liver, gallbladder, and extrahepatic biliary tract. In: *Minimal Access Surgical Anatomy.* Philadelphia, PA: Lippincott Williams & Wilkins; 2000:101–138, with permission).

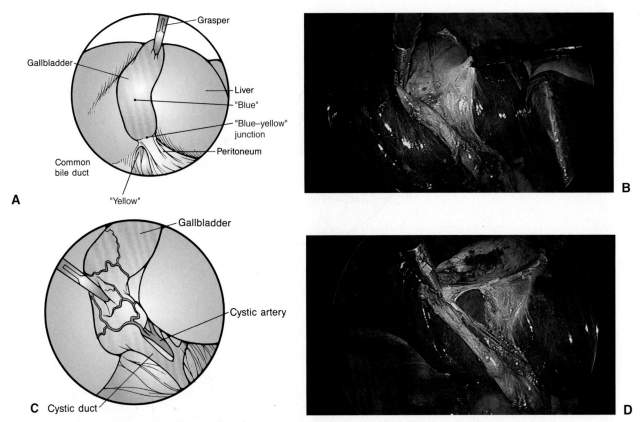

Figure 73.3 Initial dissection (**A, C** from Scott-Conner CEH, Brunson CD. Surgery and anesthesia. In: Embury SH, Hebbel RP, eds. *Sickle Cell Disease: Basic Principles and Clinical Practice.* New York, NY: Raven; 1994:809–827; **B, D:** Laparoscopic photographs kindly supplied by Evgeny V. Arshava, MD; **E, F** from Scott-Conner CEH, Hall TJ. Variant arterial anatomy in laparoscopic cholecystectomy. *Am J Surg.* 1992;163:590, with permission; **G** from: Cullen JJ, Scott-Conner CEH. Surgical anatomy of laparoscopic common duct exploration. In: Berci G, Cuschieri A, eds. *Bile Ducts and Bile Duct Stones.* Philadelphia, PA: WB Saunders; 1997:20–25, with permission). (*continued*)

the closest structure to the laparoscope, and hence the first structure which is encountered. Develop a window behind the gallbladder by incising the gallbladder peritoneum on the left and right sides and blunt dissecting behind cystic duct and gallbladder (Fig. 73.3B). The cystic artery should be visible to the left of the cystic duct (Fig. 73.3C). With good traction outward on Hartmann's pouch and an adequate peritoneal window, two tubular structures going to the gallbladder, the cystic duct and cystic artery, should be clearly seen (Fig. 73.3D).

Anatomic Points

The normal laparoscopic appearance is shown in Figure 73.3E. As previously mentioned, this textbook pattern is present in approximately 80% of individuals. In 6% to 16% of normal individuals, the right hepatic artery passes close to the gallbladder (Fig. 73.3F). In such cases, the artery may assume a tortuous or "caterpillar hump"; this redundancy, combined with small arterial twigs to the gallbladder rather than a single cystic artery, renders the right hepatic artery susceptible to injury. The artery may be mistaken for the cystic artery and ligated, or may be damaged when these small twigs are controlled. Suspect this abnormality when the "cystic artery" appears larger than normal. In up to 8% of normals, an accessory right hepatic artery may arise from the superior mesenteric artery or another vessel in the region pass in close proximity to Hartmann's pouch as it ascends to the liver. More commonly, the cystic artery arises from the gastroduodenal artery or superior mesenteric artery and ascends to the gallbladder. This "low-lying" cystic artery will be encountered closer to the laparoscope than the cystic duct and may be mistaken for it.

In 25% of individuals, the superficial and deep branches of the cystic artery have separate origins, and thus there appear to be paired or double cystic arteries. In this situation, one cystic artery may be identified in the normal position and the second may be a "low-lying" cystic artery encountered before the cystic duct (Fig. 73.3G). In the example shown, the cystic artery arises from the gastroduodenal artery. It may also originate from the superior mesenteric artery.

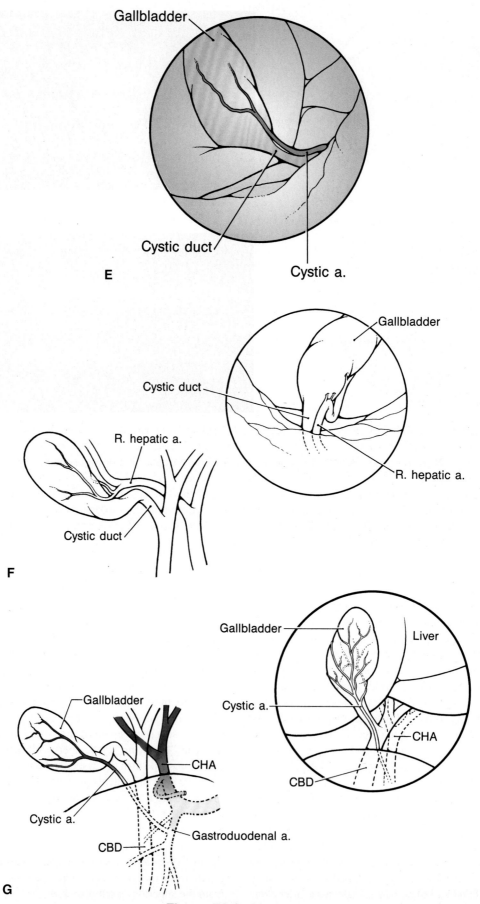

Figure 73.3 *Continued*

Division of Cystic Duct and Cystic Artery, Cholangiogram (Fig. 73.4)

Technical Points

Skeletonize the cystic duct by blunt dissection. Place a clip proximal on the cystic duct, high on the gallbladder. It is generally easiest to use the midclavicular port for the cholangiogram. Place a grasper in the subxiphoid port and grasp the gallbladder to release the midclavicular port. Pass scissors through the midclavicular port and incise the cystic duct. Bile should flow freely when an adequate ductotomy has been made. Gently use the shaft of the scissors to milk any stones from the distal cystic duct by pressing from below upward toward the ductotomy. Place a cholangiogram catheter through the midclavicular port and manipulate it into the cystic duct (Fig. 73.4A). Perform a cholangiogram in the usual fashion. It is fairly common to see small filling defects, presumed to be bubbles of carbon dioxide; for this reason fluorocholangiography (rather than taking films and waiting for them to be developed) and the capability to flush the duct with copious amounts of saline are advisable. Generally bubbles and small stones can easily be flushed through the ampulla and a clean cholangiogram obtained.

If the cholangiogram confirms both normal anatomy and the absence of stones in the bile duct, remove the cholangiogram catheter and clip the cystic duct with two clips proximally. Divide the cystic duct. The cystic artery will lie posterior and cephalad. Doubly clip and divide it.

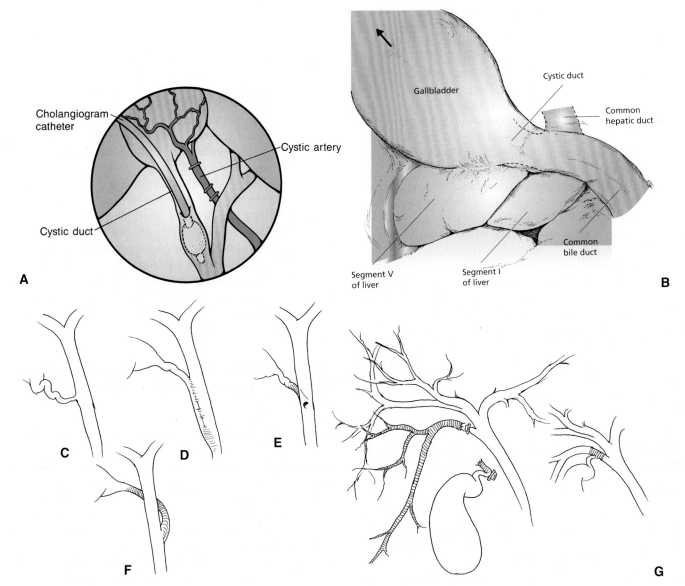

Figure 73.4 Division of cystic duct and cystic artery, cholangiogram (from Scott-Conner CEH, Brunson CD. Surgery and anesthesia. In: Embury SH, Hebbel RP, eds. *Sickle Cell Disease: Basic Principles and Clinical Practice.* New York, NY: Raven; 1994:809–827).

Anatomic Points

In the normal situation, there is an adequate length of cystic duct available for cannulation and ligation. The cystic duct may be abnormally short, either as a result of chronic inflammation or as an anomaly. In such cases, it is often abnormally thick as well (Fig. 73.4B). There are several anatomic pitfalls here. First, it is very easy to assume that the bile duct, which may appear as a visual continuation of the cystic duct and which may be similar in caliber, is the cystic duct. Traction on the gallbladder accentuates this tendency as shown. Second, it may be difficult or impossible to simply clip the cystic duct. Always confirm the anatomy by cholangiography in such situations and then secure the cystic duct by an alternative means—such as by stapler transection or by suturing the stump closed. The final anatomic pitfall may occur if this is encountered as a normal variant. The relatively large caliber and short cystic duct allows easy egress of stones into the bile duct; thus, an increased incidence of choledocholithiasis may be anticipated. This is another reason to perform cholangiography in these cases.

Most of the variants of the cystic duct that are stressed during open cholecystectomy are of little significance for the laparoscopic surgeon, provided the dissection is confined to the region of the gallbladder infundibulum. Although the normal situation in which a good length of cystic duct terminates obliquely but directly into the bile duct (Fig. 73.4C), occurs in only 60% to 75% of individuals, the other common variants (Fig. 73.4D–F) are generally associated with an adequate length of cystic duct near the gallbladder. Hence, in all of these cases, the cystic duct can be safely dissected and ligated or clipped if the laparoscopic surgeon works close to the gallbladder.

As laparoscopic surgeons have become more cognizant of the ways in which bile duct injury can occur, a lesser known variant has emerged as a major source of ductal injuries. When the cystic duct terminates onto the right hepatic duct rather than the bile duct, or when the right hepatic duct, the posterior or anterior segmental duct, or an accessory duct terminates onto the cystic duct, it is possible to clip or excise this part of the ductal system (Fig. 73.4G). Only careful dissection and liberal use of cholangiography can provide secure guidance in this region.

Dissection of Gallbladder from Liver; Removal of Gallbladder (Fig. 73.5)

Technical Points

Apply upward traction on the gallbladder and separate it from its bed by sharp and blunt dissection. The hook cautery is the instrument most commonly used (Fig. 73.5A). Be extremely careful in the initial phase of this dissection because of the proximity of the gallbladder to the right hepatic duct and right hepatic artery. As the dissection progresses, obtain better access to the dissection plane by flipping the gallbladder up and over the liver (Fig. 73.5B). Remove the gallbladder from the bottom up, obtaining hemostasis in the gallbladder bed with electrocautery as the dissection progresses (Fig. 73.5C). Before completely detaching the gallbladder, irrigate the subhepatic space and check hemostasis – remember that once you detach the gallbladder, you lose the ability to use it to retract the liver and provide easy exposure of the subhepatic region.

Move the laparoscope to the epigastric portal and pass grasping forceps through the umbilical portal. Pull the neck of the gallbladder up into the portal, engaging it firmly. Then pull both the portal and gallbladder out together. As the gallbladder neck appears in the incision, grasp it with Kelly clamps. Incise the gallbladder and decompress it with a suction, removing stones if necessary. It may be necessary to gently dilate the trocar site by introducing a ring forceps and opening it, taking care not to perforate the gallbladder (Fig. 73.5D). Do not hesitate to use a retrieval pouch if difficulties are anticipated due to inflammation or large stones. Secure all stab wounds with interrupted 2-0 Vicryl sutures in the fascia and subcuticular sutures on the skin.

Anatomic Points

Small bile ducts are occasionally encountered in the gallbladder fossa. Normally, vascular structures will be found in the peritoneal reflections, thus any small tubular structure should be assumed to be a bile duct. Many of these ducts are actually running parallel to the gallbladder fossa and can be left alone by careful dissection. These are simply small segmental ducts draining parts of the liver into the right hepatic ductal system. Other ductal structures drain directly into the gallbladder (Fig. 73.5E). Most of these can be clipped or ligated. If a large ductal structure is encountered, attempt cholangiography to confirm that the segment of liver drained by the duct has other, more central, drainage into the biliary tree. If these ducts are not recognized and are simply divided with cautery, significant leakage of bile may result.

Laparoscopic Bile Duct Exploration— Transcystic Exploration (Fig. 73.6)

Technical Points

There are two basic ways to explore the bile duct laparoscopically. The simplest, termed *transcystic bile duct exploration,* is done by passing catheters through the cystic duct into the bile duct. Success depends on the size of the stones and the angle formed between the cystic duct and the bile duct. This method works best with small stones and a cystic duct that enters the bile duct relatively high. Generally, it is only possible to explore the duct below the cystic duct entry point, because it is not feasible to steer the catheter up into the proximal ductal system. In the second method, a choledochotomy is created through which the duct is explored. Fluoroscopy and a flexible choledochoscope are essential for both.

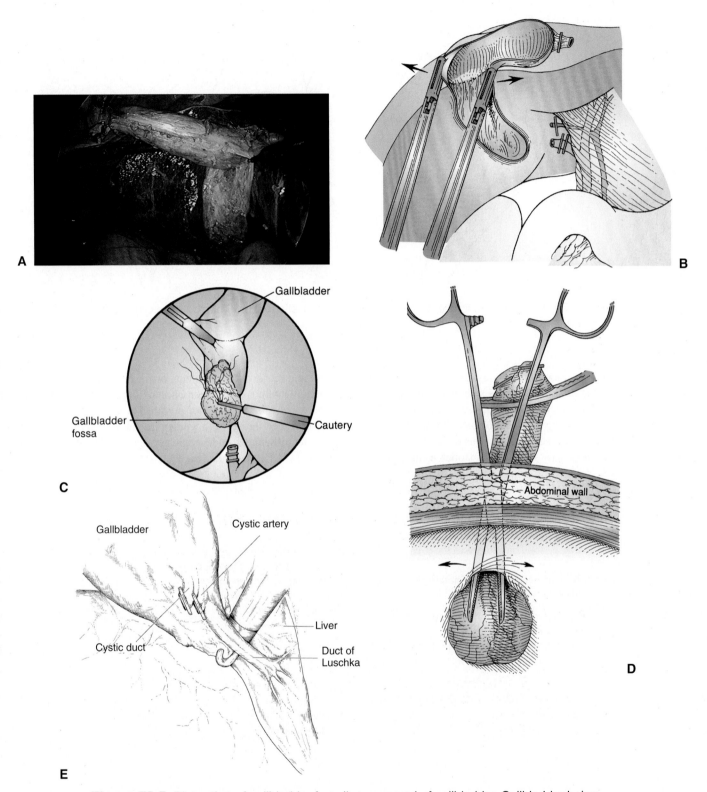

Figure 73.5 Dissection of gallbladder from liver; removal of gallbladder. Gallbladder being dissected from liver (laparoscopic photograph kindly supplied by Evgeny V. Arshava, MD). **B:** Completion of dissection from liver. **C:** Securing hemostasis in bed. **D:** Enlarging fascial hole to permit removal of gallbladder with stones. **E:** Duct of Luschka identified. Secure these ducts with ligatures or clips to avoid a bile leak.

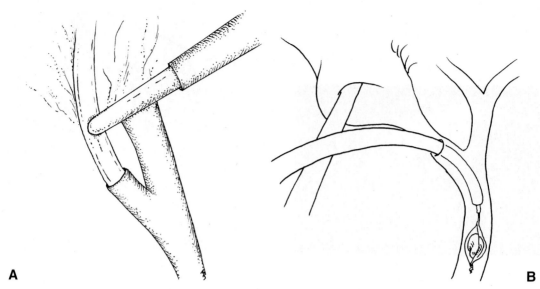

Figure 73.6 Laparoscopic bile duct exploration–transcystic exploration. **A:** Access to dilated cystic duct. **B:** Stone retrieval.

Pass a dilating balloon into the cystic duct and gently dilate it. Through the dilated duct, pass a choledochoscope and retrieve stones under direct vision ("picture in picture" video technology helps) using wire baskets or balloons (Fig. 73.6A, B). Alternatively, perform the manipulations under fluoroscopic control. It may be necessary to fragment stones using a litho-triptor and retrieve the fragments or flush them out through the ampulla. Obtain a completion cholangiogram and clip the duct at the conclusion. If it is not possible to completely clear the duct, consider threading a guidewire through the ampulla to facilitate subsequent endoscopic retrograde cholangiopancrea-tography (ERCP) cannulation.

STEPS IN PROCEDURE—LAPAROSCOPIC COMMON DUCT EXPLORATION–TRANSCYSTIC EXPLORATION

After performing cholecystectomy, cannulate cystic duct

Perform cholangiogram, if necessary

Dilate with dilating balloon

Pass Fiberoptic Choledochoscope, if Available

Retrieve stones with stone baskets under direct vision

If Fiberoptic Choledochoscope not Available, use Fluoroscopy

Retrieve stones with stone baskets

Completion cholangiogram

Secure cystic duct

Close all trocar sites over 5 mm

HALLMARK ANATOMIC COMPLICATIONS—LAPAROSCOPIC BILE DUCT EXPLORATION—TRANSCYSTIC

Damage to cystic duct–bile duct juncture during dilation

Retained bile duct stones, especially in proximal duct

Anatomic Points

The success of this depends upon ease of dilatation and cannulation of the cystic duct, and the extent of bile duct that can be explored depends upon how distal the cystic duct enters the bile duct. In a situation such as that shown in Figure 73.4D, where the cystic duct enters relatively low on the bile duct, only the most distal segment of bile duct is accessible for transcystic exploration.

Laparoscopic Choledochotomy (Fig. 73.7)

Technical Points

A 30-degree laparoscope works better than a straight (0-degree) scope for this operation, as it allows the surgeon to look "down" on the hepatoduodenal ligament.

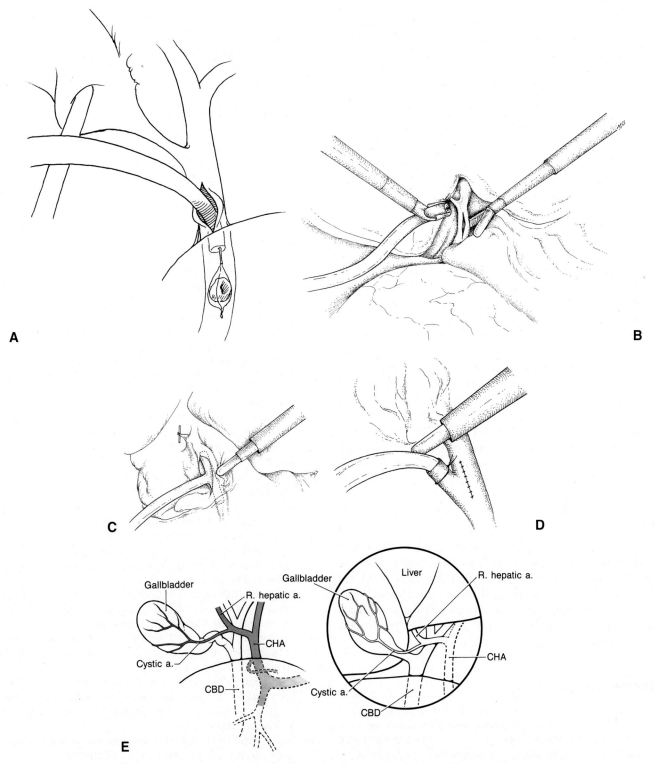

Figure 73.7 Laparoscopic choledochotomy. **A:** Use of basket to remove stone under visual guidance. **B:** Placement of T-tube into choledochotomy. **C:** T-tube in place prior to closure of choledochotomy. **D:** Alternatively, primary closure of choledochotomy with drain placed through cystic duct remnant may be performed. **E:** Regional anatomy.

Identify the bile duct immediately to the left of the hepatic artery. Clear the surface to expose 1 to 2 cm. Place two stay sutures and incise the anterior surface for approximately 0.5 to 1 cm (Fig. 73.7A). Pass balloon catheters and baskets proximal and distal to retrieve stones. A flexible choledochoscope can be used to inspect the duct. At the conclusion of the procedure, tailor a small T-tube to fit and place it in the choledochotomy. Secure it in place with two or three interrupted sutures of 3-0 or 4-0 Vicryl (Fig. 73.7B, C). Alternatively, some surgeons close the choledochotomy and drain the biliary tree with a catheter secured into the cystic duct stump (Fig. 73.7D). Obtain a completion cholangiogram. Place a closed suction drain in proximity to the choledochotomy and bring omentum up to lie within the subhepatic space.

Anatomic Points

When the right hepatic artery crosses anterior (rather than posterior) to the common hepatic duct (Fig. 73.7E), it may be injured during the cephalad aspect of choledochotomy. Avoid this pitfall by carefully observing the field for pulsations before making any incision, and by limiting the incision to the distal duct, after incising the peritoneum and clearly exposing the anterior surface of the duct.

REFERENCES

1. Davidoff AM, Pappas TN, Murray EA, et al. Mechanisms of major biliary injury during laparoscopic cholecystectomy. *Ann Surg.* 1992;215:196–202. (Reviews 12 cases of major duct injury and discusses causes and management of these complications.)
2. Dubois F, Icard P, Berthelot G, et al. Coelioscopic cholecystectomy: Preliminary report of 36 cases. *Ann Surg.* 1990;211:60–62.
3. Fine A. The cystic vein: The significance of a forgotten anatomic landmark. *JSLS.* 1997;1:263–266.
4. Franklin ME Jr. Laparoscopic choledochotomy for management of common bile duct stones and other common bile duct diseases. In: Arregui M, Fitzqibbons R, Katkhouda N, et al., eds. *Principles of Laparoscopic Surgery: Basic and Advanced Techniques.* New York, NY: Springer-Verlag; 197–204; 1995.
5. Gholipour C, Shalchi RA, Abassi M. Efficacy and safety of early laparoscopic common bile duct exploration as primary procedure in acute cholangitis caused by common bile duct stones. *J Laparoendosc Adv Surg Tech A.* 2007;17:634–638.
6. Huang SM, Wu CW, Chau GY, et al. An alternative approach of choledocholithotomy via laparoscopic choledochotomy. *Arch Surg.* 1996;131:407–411.
7. Kanamaru T, Sakata K, Nakamura Y, et al. Laparoscopic choledochotomy in management of choledocholithiasis. *Surg Laparosc Endosc Percutan Tech.* 2007;17:262–266.
8. Karaliotas C, Sgourakis G, Goumas C, et al. Laparoscopic common bile duct exploration after failed endoscopic stone extraction. *Surg Endosc.* 2008;22:1826–1831.
9. Kitano S, Iso Y, Moriyama M, et al. A rapid and simple technique for insertion of a T-tube into the minimally incised common bile duct at laparoscopic surgery. *Surg Endosc.* 1993;7:104–105.
10. Phillips EH, Toouli J, Pitt HA, et al. Treatment of common bile duct stones discovered during cholecystectomy. *J Gastrointest Surg.* 2008;12:624–628.
11. Rhodes M, Nathansom L, O'Rourke N, et al. Laparoscopic exploration of the common bile duct: Lessons learned from 129 consecutive cases. *Br J Surg.* 1995;82:666–668.
12. Robinson G, Hollinshead J, Falk G, et al. Technique and results of laparoscopic choledochotomy for the management of bile duct calculi. *Aust N Z J Surg.* 1995;65:347–349.
13. Scott-Conner CEH, Cushieri A, Carter F. Right upper quadrant: Liver, gallbladder, and extrahepatic biliary tract. In: *Minimal Access Surgical Anatomy.* Philadelphia, PA: Lippincott Williams & Wilkins; 2000:101–138.
14. Scott-Conner CEH, Hall TJ. Variant arterial anatomy in laparoscopic cholecystectomy. *Am J Surg.* 1992;163:590–592.
15. Topal B, Aerts R, Pennickx F. Laparoscopic common bile duct clearance with flexible choledochoscopy. *Surg Endosc.* 2007;21:2317–2321.
16. Wind GG. The biliary system. In: *Applied Laparoscopic Anatomy: Abdomen and Pelvis.* Baltimore, MD: Williams & Wilkins; 1997:13–83.

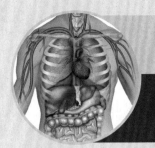

74

Extended Cholecystectomy for Gallbladder Carcinoma

Prashant Khullar and Hisakazu Hoshi

The operations for gallbladder carcinoma have a wide range of variety from simple cholecystectomy for T1a cancer to extended right hepatectomy with regional nodal dissection for locally advanced disease. The standard operation for gallbladder cancer is a radical cholecystectomy, which involves resection of the gallbladder fossa which overlies segments IVb and V of the liver along with regional lymphadenectomy. However, involvement of the infundibulum and the cystic duct with cancer may require more extensive resections to include the bile duct and major hepatic resections to achieve negative resection margins.

It is important to understand the pattern of the lymphatic drainage of gallbladder to perform a regional lymphadenectomy. The lymphatic channels from the gallbladder drain into the cystic and pericholedochal nodes first and subsequently can follow either of two pathways. Lymphatic channels can drain into the lower retroportal and retropancreatic nodes, and then to peri-SMA nodes (Fig. 74.1, yellow line) or to the proper hepatic artery nodes to common hepatic nodes and then to celiac axis nodes (Fig. 74.2, yellow line). However, the lymphatic dissemination of tumor cells is not always in an orderly fashion and skip metastases are common.

The operation should be modified depending on the clinical scenario in which gallbladder cancer presents. If the diagnosis is made on final pathologic examination after laparoscopic cholecystectomy and it is confined to the lamina propria (T1a), no additional operation may be necessary. For T1b or above, cystic duct stump excision, possible bile duct resection, regional lymphadenectomy, and liver resection are recommended for residual disease. On the other hand, extended resections including right hepatectomy, or right extended hepatectomy along with bile duct resection and reconstruction may be needed in case of locally advanced disease at initial presentation. Often times, intraoperative findings dictate the extent of the resection necessary to obtain R0 resection and the patient and surgeon should be prepared to take on this difficult task. Port site recurrences are regarded as stage IV disease and this category of patients may not derive any benefit from wide excision of port sites. The surgeon also has to keep in mind the variations in the origin of the hepatic artery, its branches and variations in bile duct anatomy.

SCORE™, the Surgical Council on Resident Education, classified operation for gallbladder cancer (when found incidentally) as an "ESSENTIAL UNCOMMON" procedure, and operation for gallbladder cancer (planned) as a "COMPLEX" procedure.

STEPS IN PROCEDURE

Bilateral subcostal incision or right subcostal incision with vertical extension up to the xiphoid process.

Abdominal exploration to look for locally advanced, unresectable disease or metastases.

Kocher maneuver to dissect posterior pancreaticoduodenal nodes and to sample aortocaval nodes.

Nodal dissection from celiac axis to the proper hepatic artery.

Identify aberrant arterial or bile duct anatomy.

Skeletonize porta hepatis to perform a portal lymphadenectomy. In case of prior hilar dissection or locally advanced disease, resection of the extrahepatic bile ducts may be required.

Assess for extent of hepatic resection depending on local extension of the disease.

Lower hilar plate by incising Glisson capsule at base of segment IVb.

Dissect inflow of segment IVb along the umbilical fissure.

Ensure low central venous pressure with anesthesiology assistance.

Pringle maneuver can be used intermittently to minimize blood loss.

Parenchymal division with appropriate device.

Identification and transection of middle hepatic vein with assistance of intraoperative ultrasound.

Identification and transection of segment V portal pedicle at the end of parenchymal transection.

HALLMARK ANATOMICAL COMPLICATIONS

Injury to portal vein, hepatic artery, or bile duct during portal dissection or hepatic parenchymal transection

Injury to middle hepatic vein during hepatic parenchymal transection

Parenchymal biliary leak

Postoperative bleeding or hematoma formation

Injury to duodenum or pancreas during portal lymphadenectomy

Aortic or caval injures during celiac or aortocaval lymph nodal dissection

LIST OF STRUCTURES

Gallbladder

Portal triad (portal vein, hepatic artery, common bile duct (CBD) and their branches)

Duodenum

Pancreas

Aorta

Inferior vena cava (IVC)

Left and right lobes of the liver

Ligamentum teres and umbilical fissure

Middle and right hepatic veins

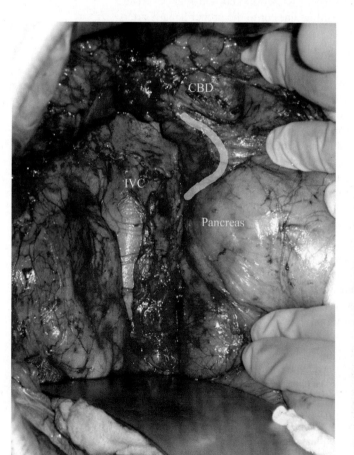

Figure 74.1 Operative photograph demonstrating lymphatic pathway from pericholedochal nodes to retropancreatic nodes (*yellow line*).

Extended (Radical) Cholecystectomy

Abdominal Exploration and Assessment of Resectability

Technical Points

Position the patient supine on the table. A roll can be placed under the right side of patient's torso to improve exposure. A right subcostal incision with an upward extension toward the xiphoid process provides adequate exposure to the relevant anatomy. Alternatively, a rooftop incision, or a vertical upper midline incision with a horizontal right lateral extension can

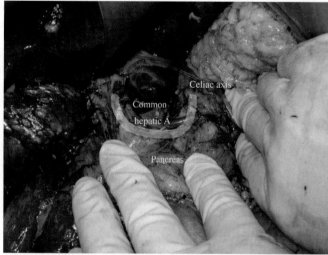

Figure 74.2 Operative photograph demonstrating lymphatic pathway from pericholedochal nodes along the hepatic artery to the celiac axis group of nodes (*yellow line*).

be made to provide a similar exposure. Perform a thorough abdominal exploration to rule out unresectable metastatic disease. Examine the liver by palpation. Use intraoperative ultrasound to identify vascular structures and lesions undetectable by preoperative radiologic imaging. Resectability of the tumor is also assessed by evaluating locoregional spread of the disease. Liver resection and a regional lymphadenectomy is the minimum operation required for any stage of gallbladder cancer beyond T1a. The extent of the tumor into the cystic duct will require resection of the bile duct and possibly an extended right hepatectomy for adequate margins.

Anatomic Points

It is imperative for the surgeon to have an extensive knowledge of hepatic segmental anatomy and aberrant vascular and ductal anatomy to safely perform operations for gallbladder cancer. The liver is divided by three scissurae, into four sectors, each of which receives a portal pedicle (Fig. 74.3). Each scissura is occupied by a hepatic vein. Each sector is further divided into segments. The middle hepatic vein which lies in the main portal scissura divides the liver into the right and left hemilivers. The right portal scissura is occupied by the right hepatic vein which divides the right hemiliver into the anterior and posterior sectors. The posterior sector comprises segment VI anteriorly and segment VII posteriorly. The anterior sector comprises segment VIII posteriorly and segment V anteriorly. The left hemiliver is divided by the left portal scissura into a posterior sector containing segment II and an anterior sector containing segment III laterally and segment IV medially. The division between segments III and IV is marked externally by the falciform ligament superiorly and the umbilical fissure inferiorly. The caudate lobe (segment I) lies over the IVC and is separated from the left lobe of the liver by the ligamentum venosum (Arantius ligament). The left lateral aspect of the caudate lobe is wedged between the left portal triad inferiorly and the confluence of the left and middle hepatic veins superiorly. The caudate lobe is unique since it drains directly into the IVC rather into the main hepatic veins. The inflow into the caudate lobe is through branches originating from the main, left, and right portal branches.

The gallbladder is located in the gallbladder fossa which occupies the undersurface of segments IV and V of the liver. The connective tissue between the gallbladder and the liver is an extension of the connective tissue which encompasses the hepatoduodenal ligament (hilar plate system) and is in close relation to the Glisson capsule which extends intrahepatically around the portal pedicles. The cystic duct arises from the neck of the gallbladder and joins the CBD. The cystic duct–common duct junction can be variable and determines the length and course of the cystic duct.

Several anatomical variations in bile duct anatomy are known. The bile ducts follow the arterial divisions intrahepatically, but have several variations extrahepatically. One of the common variations is triple confluence of the right anterior, right posterior, and the left hepatic duct. A second commonly encountered variation is ectopic drainage of a right posterior sectoral duct into the common hepatic duct, left hepatic duct, or the cystic duct, which therefore can be at risk for injury during portal dissection. Common variations in arterial anatomy are a replaced/accessory right hepatic artery which arises from the proximal superior mesenteric artery and travels posterior to the pancreatic head and portal vein. The accessory/replaced left hepatic artery arises from the left gastric artery and travels in the lesser omentum separately from the hepatoduodenal ligament.

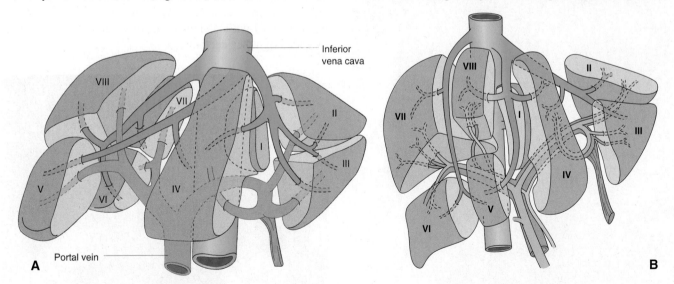

Figure 74.3 Surgical anatomy of the liver and its segments according to Couinaud's nomenclature. **A:** Branches of portal vein and hepatic veins interdigitate. **B:** Relationship between hepatic vein branches, liver segments, and branches of the portal vein, hepatic artery, and bile ducts (from Schulick RD. Hepatobiliary anatomy. In: Mulholland MW, Lillemoe KD, Dohert GM, et al., eds. *Greenfield's Surgery: Scientific Principles and Practice.* 5th ed. Philadelphia, PA: Lippincott Williams & Wilkins; 2011, with permission).

Regional Lymphadenectomy

Technical Points

Before commencing an extensive regional lymphadenectomy it is prudent to biopsy any enlarged aortocaval or celiac group of lymph nodes to rule out advanced regional disease. Involvement of the celiac or aortocaval lymph nodes indicates N2 disease, and further resection is generally not recommended. First, perform a Kocher maneuver to medially rotate the duodenum. Excise the lymphatic tissue toward the hepatoduodenal ligament and dissect the retropancreatic lymph nodes (Fig. 74.4). The retroportal nodes (located posterior aspect of hepatoduodenal ligament) are included in the resection. Continue the dissection of the common hepatic artery and the proper hepatic artery nodes from the celiac axis to the hilum of the liver (Fig. 74.2).

Connect these two dissection planes behind the portal vein and remove the specimen en bloc. Care should be taken to preserve sufficient connective tissue around the bile duct to ensure its vascularity. Bile duct resection may be necessary if there is tumor infiltration into the porta hepatis. The bile duct may also be involved in scar tissue post cholecystectomy, which makes the differentiation of scar tissue from malignant infiltration dif-ficult. In these situations, it is prudent to resect the duct to avoid potentially residual tumor in the porta hepatis.

Anatomical Points

The hepatoduodenal ligament contains the hepatic artery, the bile duct, and the portal vein, which except for some anatomical variations, occupy constant positions within the ligament. The portal vein lies posteriorly, while the proper hepatic artery lies left lateral and the CBD lies in the right lateral aspect of the hepatoduodenal ligament anterior to the portal vein. The CBD in its upper segment above the cystic duct junction is referred to as the common hepatic duct. The proper hepatic artery divides into the left and right hepatic arteries. The right hepatic artery usually crosses over to the right side posterior to the bile duct before entering the liver parenchyma. The cystic artery arises from the right hepatic artery and can cross the bile duct anteriorly or posteriorly. The left hepatic artery, along with the corresponding portal branch and left hepatic duct have a long extrahepatic course before entering the hepatic parenchyma at the umbilical fissure.

Hepatic Parenchymal Transection

Technical and Anatomic Points

Hepatic resection for gallbladder cancer can range from gallbladder bed wedge resection to right trisegmentectomy. Resection of segments IVb (caudal portion of segment IV) and V (Fig. 74.5) is anatomically appropriate and sound oncologic procedure for carcinoma involving the body and fundus of the gallbladder. It is important to determine the cystic duct margin by frozen section before commencing hepatic transection. The status of the cystic duct margin will determine the extent of hepatic and bile duct resection. Bile duct resection and Roux-en-Y hepaticojejunostomy may be required to achieve negative margins. Invasion of the right portal pedicle necessitates an extended right hepatectomy.

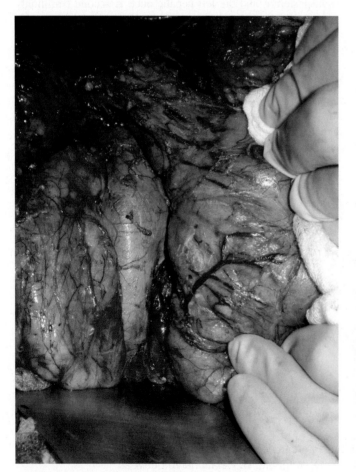

Figure 74.4 Operative photograph demonstrating the duodenum and the pancreatic head after complete lymph node dissection of the retropancreatic and retroportal group of lymph nodes.

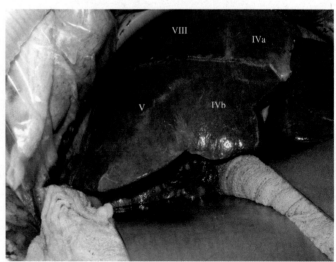

Figure 74.5 Operative photograph demonstrating planned extent of hepatic resection to include segments IVb and V.

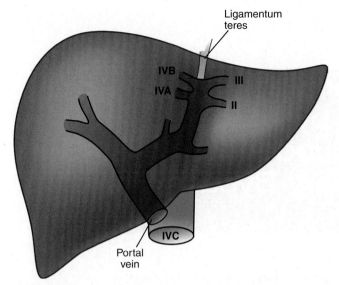

Figure 74.6 Illustration showing relationship of segments IVa and IVb portal pedicles with the falciform ligament.

Segment IVb resection commences with identification of the round ligament (ligamentum teres), which runs in the umbilical fissure till the termination of the left portal vein. Often, there is a bridge of liver tissue between segments IVb and III over the umbilical fissure that can easily be divided using electrocautery. The left portal pedicle can be identified entering the base of the umbilical fissure by lowering the hilar plate. This is done by lifting the quadrate lobe (segment IV) upward and incising the fusion line of the Glisson capsule with the connective tissue enveloping the left portal pedicle. Dissection of the round ligament on its right side leads to the segments IVb and IVa pedicles which arise from the left main trunk within the umbilical fissure. Segment IVb pedicle is usually located in the caudal position to the segment IVa pedicle (Fig. 74.6). Ultrasound can be used to confirm the distribution of each pedicle. The segment IVb pedicle is then dissected circumferentially, suture ligated and divided. It is not critical to isolate these pedicles within the umbilical fissure if the tumor does not reach up to the umbilical fissure. The pedicles can very well be isolated during parenchymal transection. Parenchymal transection starts along the attachment of falciform ligament until segment IVb pedicle is

encountered. Then the plane should be directed toward branching point of segments V and VIII of anterior sector pedicle which can be identified by ultrasound. The posterior limit of the resection is the transverse portion of left hepatic pedicle if bile duct resection is not necessary. Then, transection along the right hepatic vein up to the imaginary line extended from the left side of the transection line is performed (Fig. 74.5). Finally, the plane between segments V and VIII is developed and advanced toward the hilum of the liver. During this transection, branches of the right and middle hepatic veins (V5) will be encountered which can be ligated and divided while preserving main trunks of the right and middle hepatic veins. The pedicle of segment V is identified close to the base of the resection, is ligated and divided. Finally, the only connection is the extension of the hilar plate from the hilum to the gallbladder bed which is encircled at the base, ligated and divided.

Patients who have undergone a previous cholecystectomy can undergo a similar operation as described above. If the prior procedure was performed laparoscopically, excise all trocar sites. Pathologic findings on the gallbladder help to determine the most appropriate extent of operation, especially cystic duct margin. The location of the tumor (fundus vs. neck, serosal side vs. liver side) should be investigated on pathology specimen. Tumor stage above T1a mandates further curative surgery. Preoperative imaging is obtained to exclude distant metastases and unresectable local disease. Trocar site recurrence is a marker of stage IV disease and curative surgery is not feasible. Recurrent disease in the gallbladder fossa can be treated similar to primary gallbladder cancer. Resection of the bile duct depends on the extent of local disease and margin status of the cystic duct stump on frozen section. The presence of scar tissue in the hepatic hilum from prior operation, can make it difficult for the surgeon to differentiate between fibrosis and recurrent tumor. Bile duct resection and Roux-en-Y hepaticojejunostomy may be the only option in such situations.

REFERENCES

1. Blumgart LH. *Video Atlas. Liver, Biliary, & Pancreatic Surgery.* Philadelphia, PA: Elsevier Saunders; 2011.
2. Blumgart LH, Belghiti J, Jarnagin WR, et al., eds. *Surgery of the Liver, Biliary Tract, and Pancreas.* 4th ed. Philadelphia, PA: Elsevier Saunders; 2007.

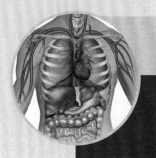

75

Choledochoenteric Anastomosis by Choledochoduodenostomy and Other Biliary Bypass Procedures

Choledochoduoenteric anastomosis is required when stones, stricture (including bile duct injury) and malignancy necessitate permanent drainage of the bile duct. This chapter includes choledochoduodenostomy, an operation that may be performed when multiple stones have been found in the common duct at exploration and when it appears unlikely that complete removal of all stones has been achieved. It is a simple side-to-side bypass procedure. In most cases, repeated clearance of the duct by endoscopic retrograde cholangiopancreatography (ERCP) has replaced this operation.

Choledochojejunostomy and cholecystojejunostomy are performed as part of reconstruction after bile duct injury (see Chapter 76), malignancy, or as palliative procedures performed for advanced malignant disease involving the periampullary region. In choledochojejunostomy, an anastomosis of the bile duct to a loop of jejunum is performed. Cholecystojejunostomy consists of anastomosis of the gallbladder to a jejunal loop. These have largely been superseded by endoscopic stent placement.

Hepaticojejunostomy and choledochojejunostomy are also performed for reconstruction after bile duct injuries. Finally, resection of tumors of the hepatic duct bifurcation (Klatskin tumors) necessitates high reconstruction. References at the end of the chapter detail these applications.

SCORE™, the Surgical Council on Resident Education, classified choledochoenteric anastomosis as an "ESSENTIAL UNCOMMON" procedure.

HALLMARK ANATOMIC COMPLICATIONS—CHOLEDOCHODUODENOSTOMY

Sump syndrome from debris in distal duct

LIST OF STRUCTURES

Bile duct

Gallbladder
Cystic duct
Pancreas
Duodenum

Jejunum
Transverse colon
Superior mesenteric artery
Jejunal branches
Middle colic artery

STEPS IN PROCEDURE—CHOLEDOCHODUODENOSTOMY

Clean anterior surface of distal bile duct
Place two stay sutures
Make longitudinal choledochotomy low on
    bile duct
Perform bile duct exploration
Create transverse incision on upper aspect of
    duodenum, centered on choledochotomy

Construct two-layered anastomosis between
    duodenum and bile duct
Place omentum around anastomosis
Consider placing closed suction drains
Close abdomen in usual fashion

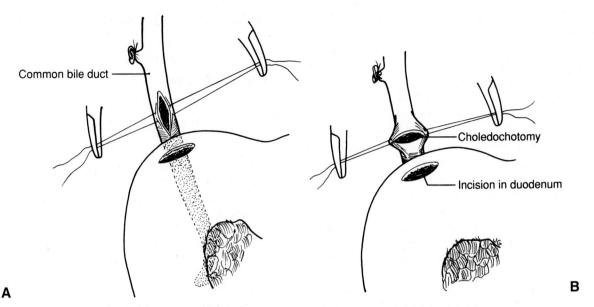

Figure 75.1 Choledochotomy and duodenotomy. **A.** Stay sutures placed. **B.** Tension placed upon stay sutures to prepare longitudinal incision for anastomosis to duodenotomy.

Choledochoduodenostomy

Choledochotomy and Duodenotomy (Fig. 75.1)

Technical Points

Expose and prepare the bile duct for exploration, as detailed in Chapter 72. Place two stay sutures and make a longitudinal incision in the lower third of the common duct. Make the incision approximately 2 cm in length and just above the appearance of the common duct over the superior aspect of the duodenum. Place the incision lower than you normally would for common duct exploration to facilitate construction of the choledochoduodenal anastomosis. Explore the common duct thoroughly.

Anatomic Points

The close proximity of the distal bile duct and duodenum make this anastomosis possible. Extra mobility of the duodenum may be obtained by performing a Kocher maneuver.

Anastomosis (Fig. 75.2)

Technical and Anatomic Points

Place stay sutures on the anterior duodenal wall just below the entry of the bile duct into the duodenum. Center a longitudinal duodenotomy above the choledochotomy on the anterior superior surface of the duodenum. Make this incision approximately the same length as the incision in the bile duct.

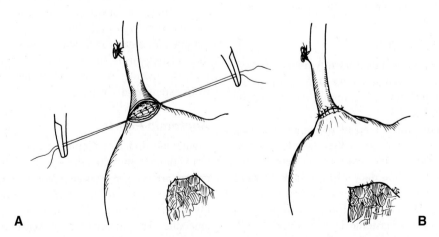

Figure 75.2 Choledochoduodenostomy—end-to-side anastomosis

The two incisions will be perpendicular to each other and will produce a diamond-shaped opening when sutured together. Place a posterior interrupted row of 4-0 silk Lembert sutures, beginning at the apex of the choledochotomy and continuing laterally in both directions. This will form the back wall of the anastomosis. Interrupted mucosal sutures of 4-0 Vicryl can be placed if desired. Next, suture the anterior row with interrupted sutures of 4-0 Vicryl on the inner layer and interrupted 4-0 silk on the outer layer. Alternatively, a single layer of interrupted 4-0 polydioxanone (PDS) sutures may be used.

Do not stent the anastomosis or place a T-tube or other drainage device in the common duct. A lumen should be palpable to the tip of the finger at the conclusion of the procedure. Place omentum around the choledochoduodenal anastomosis and then place two closed suction drains (generally, one on each side) in the vicinity of the anastomosis.

Choledochojejunostomy

Choledochotomy and Construction of a Roux-en-Y Anastomosis (Fig. 75.3)

Technical Points

When performed for malignant disease of the distal common duct or pancreas, the anastomosis should be made high enough to avoid tumor encroachment as the tumor enlarges. When benign biliary stricture is the indication for surgery, the anastomosis must be made to clean, healthy, unscarred duct. This may necessitate hepaticojejunostomy (see Chapter 76 and references at the end of the chapter).

These procedures are often performed in a previously operated, scarred field. Identify the common duct by needle aspiration of bile in the anticipated location (anterior to the portal vein and to the right of the hepatic artery) (Fig. 75.3A).

STEPS IN PROCEDURE—CHOLEDOCHOJEJUNOSTOMY

If Side-to-Side Anastomosis
Place stay sutures and make longitudinal choledochotomy

If End-to-Side Anastomosis
Gently dissect bile duct from surrounding structures
Place two stay sutures and divide bile duct, ligating or suturing distal duct

Create Roux-en-Y loop of jejunum
Anastomose blind end of jejunum to bile duct
Bring omentum to vicinity of anastomosis
Place closed suction drains
Close abdomen in the usual fashion

HALLMARK ANATOMIC COMPLICATIONS—CHOLEDOCHOJEJUNOSTOMY
Failure of bypass from growth of tumor

Identify the common duct and trace it proximally. Either a side-to-side duct-to-jejunum or an end-to-side anastomosis may be performed. Side-to-side anastomosis is usually reserved for patients in whom extensive tumor renders circumferential dissection of the duct hazardous.

Side-to-Side Anastomosis

Place stay sutures on the common duct and make a longitudinal choledochotomy approximately 2 cm in length. Explore the duct.

End-to-Side Anastomosis

Place stay sutures on the common duct. Gently dissect on both sides of the duct with a right angle clamp until it is possible to come behind it. Divide the duct, ligating or oversewing the distal segment (Fig. 75.3B).

Then construct a Roux-en-Y loop of the jejunum. Bring the blind end of the Roux loop up to the choledochotomy. Construct a two-layer, side-to-side anastomosis between the loop of jejunum and the common duct using a single layer of interrupted 4-0 PDS sutures. Construct the back wall of the anastomosis (Fig. 75.3C, D) and then roll the jejunum up and complete the front row of the anastomosis (Fig. 75.3E, F, G). Reinforce the anastomosis by inkwelling the jejunum up and

tacking it to tissues surrounding the proximal duct or the capsule of the liver with three or four sutures of 4-0 silk or Vicryl, taking care not to encroach on the lumen of the common duct.

Finish the Roux-en-Y by creating an anastomosis between the end of the proximal jejunum and the side of the distal segment (as described in Chapter 69).

As an alternative to the Roux-en-Y loop, the omega loop is simply a loop of jejunum (remaining in continuity) that is sewn in a side-to-side fashion to the common duct. An enteroenterostomy is constructed approximately 20 to 30 cm from the anastomosis to partially bypass the anastomosis. In some patients, an omega loop may be quicker or easier to construct than a Roux-en-Y, and it serves the same function. This procedure is generally reserved for patients with limited life spans from extensive disease.

Anatomic Points

Ligate and divide the jejunal branches of the superior mesenteric artery to mobilize the jejunum close to the superior mesenteric artery. The arterial arcades, which are relatively simple in the proximal bowel, provide a collateral route of blood supply for the Roux loop. This anastomosis is generally performed antecolic. This direct route is easier and less hazardous than a retrocolic route, because it avoids the transverse mesocolon

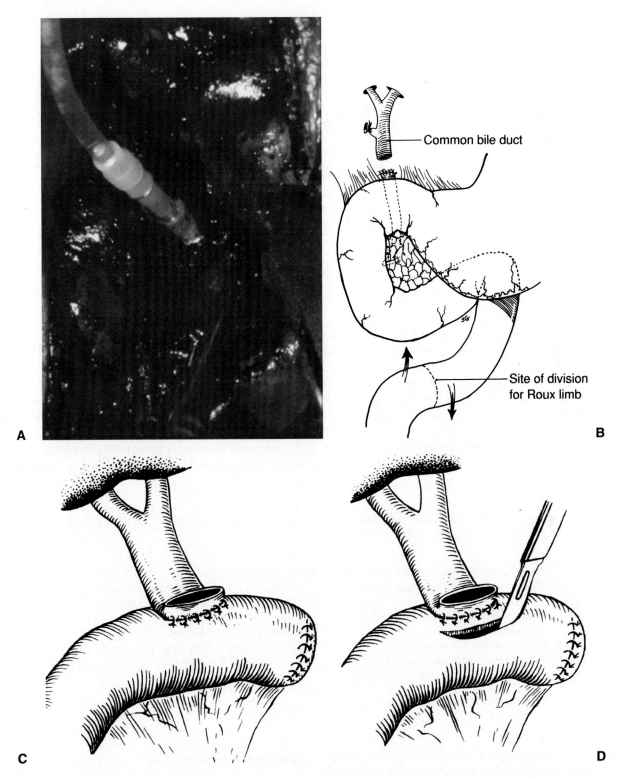

Figure 75.3 Choledochotomy and construction of a Roux-en-Y anastomosis. (Parts **C–F** are reproduced from Fischer JE. *Fischer's Mastery of Surgery.* 6th ed. Lippincott Williams & Wilkins; 2012. Parts **D–F** modified from Blumgart LH, ed. *Surgery of the Liver and Biliary Tract.* 2nd ed. London: Churchill Livingstone; 1994). (*continued*)

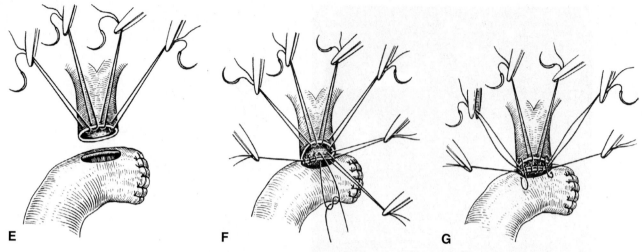

Figure 75.3 *Continued*

and its contained vasculature. Occasionally, a retrocolic approach may be necessary. In such cases, identify the middle colic vessels and take care not to damage them or the marginal arteries. The best place to pierce the transverse mesocolon is to the right of the middle colic artery, taking care to control all mesenteric vessels before dividing them. If you pass to the left of the middle colic artery, you will enter the lesser omental bursa, necessitating a circuitous route to bring the loop of jejunum up to the bile duct. This route is used only when a concomitant pancreatic bypass is performed.

Cholecystojejunostomy

Construction of the Anastomosis (Fig. 75.4)

Technical and Anatomic Points

Cholecystojejunostomy is performed for palliation of advanced carcinoma of the head of the pancreas. It should only be elected when the cystic duct is known to be patent or when a grossly enlarged (Courvoisier) gallbladder is found. If the cystic duct is not patent, this anastomotic procedure will not adequately decompress the obstructed biliary tree and should not be attempted.

HALLMARK ANATOMIC COMPLICATIONS—CHOLECYSTOJEJUNOSTOMY
Occlusion of cystic duct leading to bypass
    failure

STEPS IN PROCEDURE—CHOLECYSTOJEJUNOSTOMY

Explore abdomen and document extent of
    disease
Place purse-string suture and decompress
    gallbladder
Create Roux-en-Y loop of jejunum
Pass circular stapler into blind end of jejunum
    and spike it out through antimesenteric
    border of bowel
Place anvil on stapler and insert into gallbladder

Tie purse-string suture and check for gaps
Fire stapler and remove, check doughnuts
Close blind end of jejunum with linear stapler
Reinforce with a few sutures if desired
Consider closed suction drains
Evaluate need for concomitant
    gastrojejunostomy
Close abdomen in usual fashion

Place a purse-string suture of 4-0 silk on the apex of the distended gallbladder. Place this suture in the form of a small square measuring approximately 1 cm on each side. Introduce a gallbladder trocar through the purse-string, using the suture to control leakage. Decompress the distended gallbladder fully. Obtain a culture of the bile. Remove the trocar, taking care not to spill any bile as the trocar is removed. Place Babcock clamps on the gallbladder to maintain it in a high position within the operative field. Construct a Roux-en-Y loop of jejunum that will comfortably reach to the fundus of the gallbladder.

Sutured Anastomosis

Construct a two-layer anastomosis between the side of the Roux-en-Y loop of jejunum and the previously made opening in the gallbladder, using 4-0 silk for the outer layer and running 4-0 Vicryl for the inner layer. Interrupted single layer 3-0 PDS is an alternative preferred by some surgeons. Confirm that the anastomosis is patent and cover it with omentum at the conclusion of the surgical procedure. Place drains in proximity to any biliary enteric anastomosis.

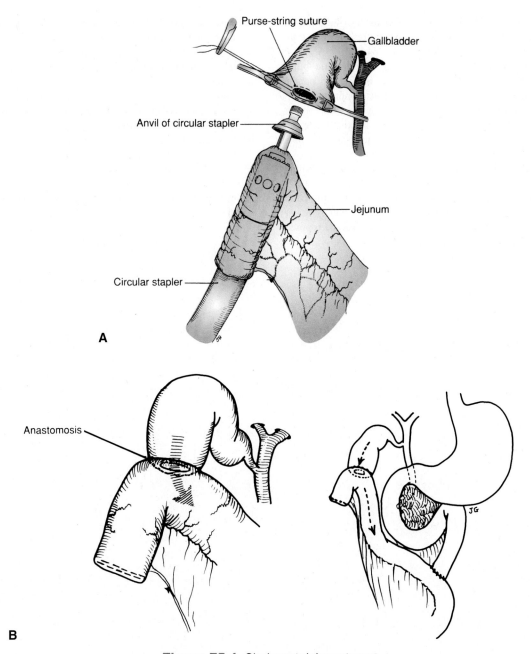

Figure 75.4 Cholecystojejunostomy

Stapled Anastomosis

Pass a small circular stapling device (EEA) stapler (the largest that will fit within the lumen of the Roux loop) through the open end of the jejunum and then spike it out through the antimesenteric border at the proposed site of anastomosis. Create a purse-string suture of 3-0 Prolene around the opening in the gallbladder made at the time of trocar decompression and introduce the anvil. Tie the purse string, connect the anvil to the EEA and fire the stapler. Confirm patency of the anastomosis by palpation and inspect the donuts. Reinforce the anastomosis with a few interrupted 4-0 silk sutures. Close the open end of jejunum with a TA-55 stapler and complete the Roux-en-Y as previously described.

Consider performing a gastroenterostomy if the tumor is encroaching on the duodenum or if preoperative gastric outlet obstruction is suspected.

References

1. Freund HR. Cholecystojejunostomy and choledocho/hepaticojejunostomy. In: *Fischer's Mastery of Surgery.* 6th ed. Philadelphia, PA: Wolters Kluwer Lippincott Williams & Wilkins; 2013: 1327.
2. Gerhards MF, van Gulik TM, Bosma A, et al. Long-term survival after resection of proximal bile duct carcinoma (Klatskin tumors). *World J Surg.* 1999;23:91–96.

3. Iwatsuki S, Todo S, Marsh JW, et al. Treatment of hilar cholangiocarcinoma (Klatskin tumors) with hepatic resection or transplantation. *J Am Coll Surg.* 1998;187:358–364.

4. Jarnagin WR, Burke E, Powers C, et al. Intrahepatic biliary enteric bypass provides effective palliation in selected patients with malignant obstruction at the hepatic duct confluence. *Am J Surg.* 1998;175:453–460.

5. Launois B, Terblanche J, Lakehal M, et al. Proximal bile duct cancer: High resectability rate and 5-year survival. *Ann Surg.* 1999;230:266–275.

6. Schein CJ, Gliedman ML. Choledochoduodenostomy as an adjunct to choledocholithotomy. *Surg Gynecol Obstet.* 1981;152:797.

7. Strasberg SM. Chapter 117. Reconstruction of the bile duct: Anatomic principles and surgical technique. In: *Fischer's Mastery of Surgery.* 6th ed. Philadelphia, PA: Wolters Kluwer Lippincott Williams & Wilkins; 2013:1288.

8. Taschieri AM, Elli M, Danelli PG, et al. Third-segment cholangio-jejunostomy in the treatment of unresectable Klatskin tumors. *Hepatogastroenterology.* 1995;42:597–600. (Describes alternative technique that is useful when tumor precludes access to ducts in the hilum.)

9. Tocchi A, Mazzoni G, Liotta G, et al. Management of benign biliary strictures: Biliary enteric anastomosis vs endoscopic stenting. *Arch Surg.* 2000;135:153–157.

10. van den Bosch RP, van der Schelling GP, Klinkenbijl JHG, et al. Guidelines for the application of surgery and endoprostheses in the palliation of obstructive jaundice in advanced cancer of the pancreas. *Ann Surg.* 1994;219:18–24. (Advocates use of surgical biliary bypass for patients with anticipated survival time longer than 6 months.)

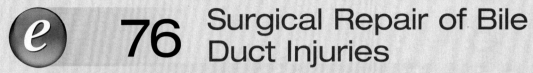

81

Liver Biopsy—Open and Laparoscopic

Liver biopsy is generally performed as part of another procedure in order to document pathology. Common indications include nodules suggestive of metastatic disease or the unexpected finding of hepatic cirrhosis. Wedge resection, which is also included in this chapter, may be used to remove a small benign lesion from the edge of the liver.

SCORE™, the Surgical Council on Resident Education, classified open and laparoscopic liver biopsy as "ESSENTIAL COMMON" procedures.

STEPS IN PROCEDURE

Liver Biopsy (Open or Laparoscopic)

Wedge biopsy
Identify area on free edge of liver
Place two sutures of 2-0 Chromic in such a fashion as to outline a triangle
Excise the tissue between the sutures
Attain hemostasis with electrocautery
Place apex suture if necessary

Needle biopsy
Choose entry site (on free edge if possible)
Insert needle and fire it

Take several biopsies through same entry site, angling the needle in different directions
Attain hemostasis with electrocautery
Place figure-of-eight suture across entry site if necessary

Forceps biopsy
Press forceps, with jaws open, against the lesion
Close the jaws and remove the biopsy
Attain hemostasis with electrocautery

LIST OF STRUCTURES

Liver
Left lobe
    Segments I, II, III, and IV

Right lobe
    Segments V, VI, VII, and VIII
Falciform ligament
Ligamentum teres

HALLMARK ANATOMIC COMPLICATIONS
Bleeding

Open Wedge and Needle Biopsy of the Liver (Fig. 81.1)

Technical and Anatomic Points

Carefully note the site of the biopsy, using a standard nomenclature for liver segments (see Chapter 82 for a thorough discussion of liver segments). At a minimum, document which lobe (right or left) and whether the abnormality is isolated, one of many similar nodules, or generalized. Clearly, if there is a focal abnormality, the biopsy should include part or all of that abnormality. For a generalized process, such as hepatic cirrhosis, liver biopsy is most easily performed at the free edge of the left or right lobe. If any obvious abnormalities are present, however, obtain the biopsy specimen from the affected area. If there are no visible or palpable masses, the free edge of the right lobe, away from any areas that may have been damaged in the course of dissection or by placement of retractors, should be selected. This area is selected because it is generally representative and easy to approach. It is relatively to get hemostasis with sutures if persistent bleeding is encountered.

Wedge Biopsy

The wedge biopsy technique provides a generous amount of tissue, but is limited in depth. To perform this procedure, place two sutures of 2-0 chromic in such a way as to outline a triangle. The sutures should overlap at the apex of the triangle for complete hemostasis.

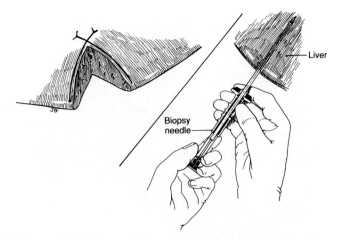

Figure 81.1 Open wedge and needle biopsy of the liver

If possible, place these as a figure-of-eight with a small bite near the free edge (to anchor the suture) and a wide deep at the apex. Tie the sutures and leave long ends. Cut a wedge of tissue from the inside of the triangle. Check the cut surface for hemostasis. Use electrocautery to control any small bleeding points. Persistent bleeding from the apex of the V-shaped defect may be controlled with a horizontal mattress suture placed above the apex. The long ends of the two lateral sutures may be tied together to close the defect. This should only be done after hemostasis has been achieved, as hidden bleeding may persist.

Needle Biopsy

Familiarize yourself with the mechanics of the biopsy needle that you plan to use. Spring-loaded needles are convenient and are easily operated with one hand. These needles vary in gauge (diameter of core taken) and "throw" (how far beyond the tip the needle projects to take the biopsy). The most basic kind of needle is not spring loaded and requires two hands to operate properly.

Stabilize the liver with your nondominant hand and stick the liver on the free edge, using a disposable, core-cutting needle. Pass the needle as deeply as desired and cut a core of tissue. Note that with either the spring-loaded or the manual needle, the core will be cut deeper than the tip of the needle.

Remove the needle, using your nondominant hand to compress the edge of the liver for hemostasis, and inspect the core. Cut several cores through the same entry point by inserting the needle at several different angles. Generally the bleeding will stop with pressure and with electrocautery. If bleeding persists from the puncture site, close the hole with a single 3-0 chromic suture placed across the hole in a figure-of-eight pattern.

Biopsy of Surface Nodule

A small nodule on the surface or just under the capsule of the liver can be excised with electrocautery or biopsied with a biopsy forceps (see section which follows). Cervical biopsy forceps work well for this purpose and are available in gynecologic kits in most operating room suites. These take a generous bite of tissue and are easily controlled. Central umbilication (depression) may be seen with larger nodules; if this is the case, take your biopsy from the edge as the center may be necrotic. Obtain hemostasis with electrocautery.

Laparoscopic Liver Biopsy—Wedge and Needle (Figs. 81.2 and 81.3)

Technical Points

Similarly, document the lobe from which the biopsy is taken (for focal abnormalities). Perform needle biopsy by passing a

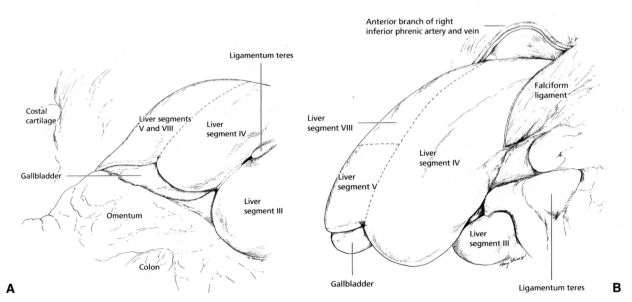

Figure 81.2 Laparoscopic view of segments of the liver. **A:** Segments III, IV, V, and VIII are easily seen. **B:** Segment VIII is seen to lie posterior to segment V. (*continued*)

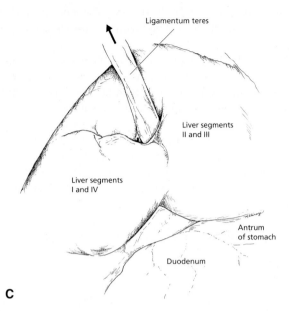

C

Figure 81.2 *Continued.* **C:** Elevation of the liver reveals segments I–IV.

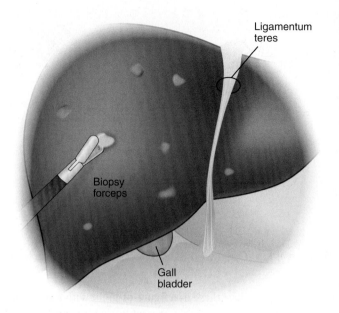

Figure 81.3 Use of biopsy forceps to obtain a sample of a liver nodule.

cutting biopsy needle directly through the abdominal wall and puncturing the liver under direct vision. Biopsy is performed as described above. Stabilize the free edge of the liver with a grasper and use the grasper to achieve temporary hemostasis while the core is unloaded before taking the next core. Wedge biopsy is best performed using the ultrasonic scalpel to divide a small portion of liver and secure hemostasis. It is rarely necessary to place sutures.

Anatomic Points

It is important to recognize laparoscopic landmarks in order to document the site of the biopsy. This can be a bit more difficult than it is during open surgery. The most obvious laparoscopic landmarks are the ligamentum teres with its associated falciform ligament, which divides segments II and III of the left lobe from the rest of the liver (Fig. 81.2A). A line drawn through the gallbladder fossa indicates the demarcation of segment IV of the left lobe from the right lobe. As the laparoscope is passed higher into the abdomen, segment VIII, which is more posterior, comes into view (Fig. 81.2B). There is no visual landmark to demarcate segment V from segment VIII. Laparoscopic ultrasound may be of some assistance. Elevation of the ligamentum teres exposes segment I (Fig. 81.2C), which may also be seen through the transparent part of the lesser omentum during dissection along the lesser curvature.

Biopsy of Liver Nodule (Fig. 81.3)

Technical and Anatomic Points

Diagnostic laparoscopy is often performed as part of staging for malignancy. Because this procedure is generally only performed when imaging studies are negative, any metastatic deposits found tend to be small and superficial.

Nodules of metastatic disease may be seen on the surface of the liver or on the peritoneal surface. A biopsy forceps provides a convenient way to obtain a sample in either case to document the presence of metastatic disease.

Obtain a laparoscopic biopsy forceps (generally available on a gynecologic laparoscopy tray if not readily at hand) or a cervical biopsy forceps. Pass the biopsy forceps through a trocar. Choose a nodule that is readily accessible, if possible. Take a generous bite of the nodule by digging the jaws of the biopsy forceps into the nodule and then closing the forceps. Remove the specimen. Attain hemostasis with electrocautery.

REFERENCES

1. Appel BL, Tolat P, Evans DB, et al. Current staging systems for pancreatic cancer. *Cancer J.* 2012;18:539.
2. Hoekstra LT, Bieze M, Busch OR, et al. Staging laparoscopy in patients with hepatocellular carcinoma: Is it useful? *Surg Endosc.* 2013;27(3):826–831.
3. Yamagata Y, Amikura K, Kawashima Y, et al. Staging laparoscopy in advanced gastric cancer: Usefulness and issues requiring improvement. *Hepatogastroenterology.* 2012. (Epub ahead of print.)

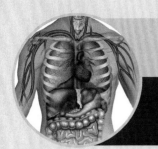

82

Major Hepatic Resection

Neal Wilkinson

Hepatic resections are performed for benign and malignant conditions. Hepatic adenoma, hemangioma, and focal nodular hyperplasia are all benign mass lesions that the surgeon may be asked to manage. With improved noninvasive imaging, to include computed tomography, ultrasound, and magnetic resonance imagery, resection for diagnostic purposes is seldom required. The treatment of cystic lesions: Simple, complex, neoplastic, and infectious needs to be individualized and may range from observation, simple marsupialization, to resection. Traumatic liver injury can lead to acute and delayed bleeding, infection, and bile leaks. Urgent surgical management is limited to obtaining control of ongoing bleeding. Damage control surgery is now recommended over anatomic resection at time of injury to avoid death from hypotension, hypothermia, and coagulopathy.

Major hepatic resections are most commonly performed for malignant tumors including primary hepatocellular carcinoma, primary biliary adenocarcinoma often referred to as intrahepatic cholangiocarcinoma, and a wide variety of metastatic lesions.

SCORE™, the Surgical Council on Resident Education, classified open segmentectomy/lobectomy of the liver as "COMPLEX" procedures.

STEPS IN PROCEDURE

Common Steps for All Resections
Right subcostal or bilateral subcostal (optional sternal split)
Divide falciform ligament cephalad to hepatic veins
Gently rotate left liver medially and down and incise triangular ligament
Roll liver medially to expose and divide right triangular ligament to hepatic veins
Elevate left lateral liver to expose caudate lobe and divide transparent part of lesser omentum
Completely surround porta hepatis through foramen of Winslow, place umbilical tape in case vascular control is later required (Pringle maneuver)

Wedge Resections
Confirm that lesion is amenable to wedge (as apposed to formal segmental) resection
Outline wide margins (1 to 2 cm) on lesion
Place through-and-through 2-0 chromic sutures just beyond planned margin and tie these gently
Sharply excise wedge of tissue
Obtain hemostasis

Left Lateral Bisegmentectomy (Segments II and III)
Elevate these segments up off of the caudate lobe to expose narrowest segment (transition point)

Divide small vascular pedicles to immediate left of falciform
Divide liver parenchyma from anterior to posterior along narrow transition point; secure left hepatic vein
Complete the transection and remove the specimen
Obtain hemostasis

Right Hepatectomy (Segments V to VIII)
Remove gallbladder and trace cystic duct to common hepatic duct (CHD)
Follow anterior surface of CHD to right hepatic duct, secure and divide
Identify and control right hepatic artery
Retract stumps of right hepatic duct and hepatic artery to the left to expose right portal vein
Carefully dissect, control, and divide the right portal vein
Reflect the entire liver medially to expose the vena cava; sequentially control and divide retrohepatic branches to cava
Divide parenchyma along line of demarcation, controlling any small vessels or bile ducts
Obtain hemostasis and bile stasis

Left Hepatectomy (Segments II through IV)
Remove gallbladder and trace cystic duct to CHD, then to left hepatic duct
Divide left hepatic duct

Expose, control, and divide left hepatic artery and left portal vein

Rotate liver downward to expose left and middle hepatic veins; control and divide these

Divide liver along line of demarcation, controlling any small vessels or bile ducts

Obtain hemostasis and bile stasis

Place omentum into operative field and close abdomen without drains

HALLMARK ANATOMIC COMPLICATIONS

Injury to artery, duct, or portal vein supplying remnant to be left behind

Massive bleeding from failure of vascular control

Hepatic insufficiency due to resection

Bile leak

LIST OF STRUCTURES

Left and right triangular ligaments
Diaphragm
Falciform ligament
Left, right, and middle hepatic veins

Portal Vein
Left and right portal veins
Common bile duct

Left and right hepatic ducts
Common and proper hepatic arteries
Left and right hepatic arteries
Glisson's capsule
Hepatic segmental anatomy

For malignant lesions, a safe and planned surgical intervention is required to ensure appropriate margins, adequate hepatic reserve, and low surgical morbidity and mortality. Key elements to a successful surgical plan must take into account both tumor extent and viability of the remnant liver. Indications and contraindications for surgery vary widely and are beyond the scope of this chapter. A balanced discussion between the patient and the surgeon should address the surgical risk involved, morbidity and mortality, and the anticipated results: Disease-free and overall survival.

The underlying liver parenchyma (cirrhosis, steatosis, or normal) dictates how the patient will tolerate the surgical insult. Careful history and physical examination may help predict the status of the liver parenchyma, but unanticipated cirrhosis and steatosis are still encountered. A history of hepatitis or drug and alcohol abuse should be documented. Cachexia, jaundice, ascites, and portal hypertension are all stigmata of cirrhosis. In the setting of metastatic colorectal cancer, the long-term effects of chemotherapy may alter hepatic reserve and regeneration potential. Safe surgical interventions are clearly possible, but steatosis and steatohepatitis increase the surgical risk. Despite a careful history and physical, unrecognized liver diseases and even subclinical cirrhosis can be encountered at the time of surgery. A needle biopsy of "normal" liver may be the best way to preoperatively evaluate for subclinical liver disease. The surgical plan and operative consent should be flexible enough to accommodate the unexpected.

The volume and quality of the liver must be sufficient to sustain the patient during and after surgery. A healthy arterial and portal inflow, venous outflow, and biliary drainage are required. Judicious use of cautery, sutures and intraoperative ischemia, and Pringle maneuver (see the following section) can minimize damage to the remaining liver parenchyma. Up to 66% of the liver can be safely resected if the remnant liver is healthy. With resections involving greater than 50%, transient jaundice and ascites may develop but typically resolve within 1 to 2 months. Efforts to predict postoperative liver failure still lack sensitivity and specificity. Clinical judgment and experience are required. In the diseased liver, the minimum volume of liver required to prevent liver failure is difficult to predict. In general, the cirrhotic liver with signs of end-stage liver failure such as portal hypertension or ascites will not tolerate an anatomic liver resection and strong consideration should be given to parenchyma-sparing surgery such as wedge resections or ablative procedures.

The appropriate radiographic studies (computed tomography or magnetic resonance imaging) must be obtained before initiation of chemotherapy and carefully studied. For metastatic colorectal cancer, treatment decisions should always be based on the pretreatment imaging. A careful assessment of the extent of disease needs to be done before embarking on major hepatic surgery. This should include evaluation of the extra- and intrahepatic disease burden as well as the quality of the liver parenchyma. Peritoneal disease, extensive nodal disease (of the primary cancer or within the hepatic nodal distribution), or numerous unanticipated hepatic lesions are all relative contraindications for hepatic resection. Preoperative chemotherapy, staged procedures, portal vein embolization, and ablative techniques can increase curative options and ensure margin-negative resections.

The Couinaud system numbers the anatomic segments of the liver (Fig. 82.1). A clear understanding of segmental liver anatomy is critical when planning a hepatic resection. This system is based on portal vein and biliary anatomy. It provides safe segmental anatomy on which to base surgical resection lines. Any surgical resection can be labeled numerically; for example, a right hepatectomy corresponds to resection of segments V to VIII and left hepatectomy segments II to IV. When

ORIENTATION

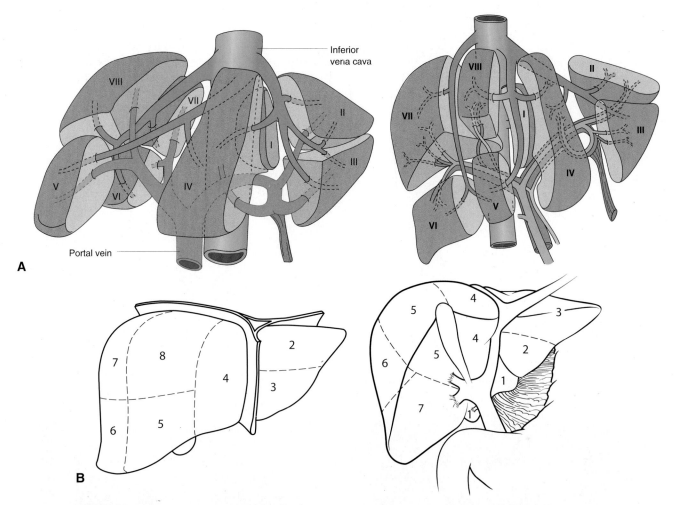

Figure 82.1 The segmental anatomy of the liver. **A:** The segmental anatomy is based upon portal units and is crossed by branches of the hepatic veins. **B:** Segmental anatomy relative to external landmarks (**A** from Schulick RD. Hepatobiliary anatomy. In: Mulholland MW, Lillemoe KD, Dohert GM, et al., eds. *Greenfield's Surgery: Scientific Principles and Practice.* Philadelphia, PA: Lippincott Williams & Wilkins; 2006, with permission).

segment I (caudate) is removed, this should be stipulated. Using the segmental (numerical) terminology can ensure that the radiologist, medical oncologist, and hepatic surgeon are communicating effectively.

This chapter provides the technical steps involved in performing a nonanatomic wedge resection, a left lateral bisegmentectomy (segments II and III), and left and right hepatectomies. These general techniques can be modified and combined as needed on the basis of tumor distribution, keeping in mind that the more extensive the resection, the higher the risk of transient or even possibly permanent liver failure (especially in the cirrhotic liver). Extended resection or trisegmentectomies will not be covered because these procedures are best performed by experienced hepatobiliary surgeons. These are covered in the references at the end of the chapter.

Incision and Initial Hepatic Mobilization (Fig. 82.2)

Technical Points

The liver fills the right upper quadrant of the abdomen and exposure is critical to safe surgery. A right subcostal with vertical midline extension or bilateral subcostal incision will provide wide exposure for most hepatic resections (Fig. 82.2A). A self-retaining retractor with rib elevation is helpful. Sternal split or right anterior thoracotomy is seldom required but must be kept within the surgical armamentarium for difficult situations (Fig. 82.2B). Small wedge resections or peripheral segmentectomies can be accomplished through upper midline incisions and laparoscopic mobilization and resections are now being accomplished safely.

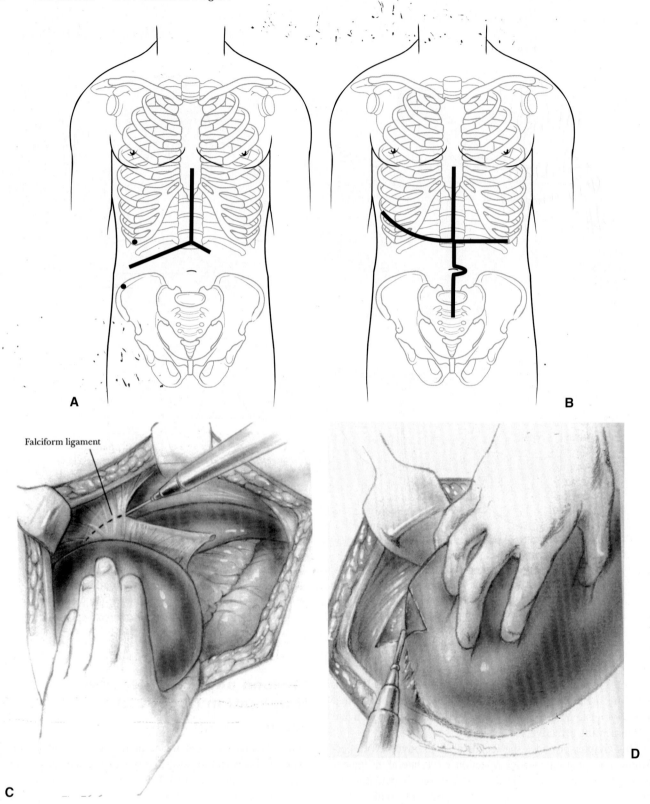

A

B

Falciform ligament

C

D

Figure 82.2 Incision and initial hepatic mobilization

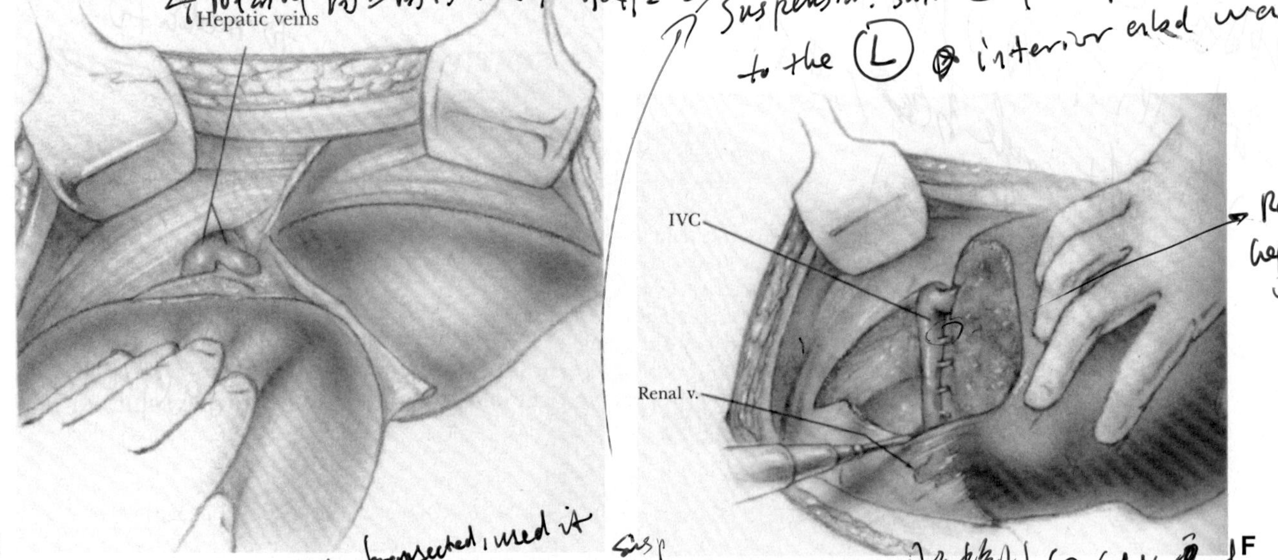

Handwritten (top): Right triangle ligament / roll liver ⇒ medrally ; then pull down to / roll liver upward. separate from liver

Handwritten: How to media rotate: ...

Handwritten: Suspension. suture falciform ligment / to the (L) @ interior ed wall.

Labels: Hepatic veins; IVC; Renal v.; E; F

Figure 82.2 Continued

Release the liver from supporting structures before embarking on major hepatic procedures. The falciform contains the obliterated umbilical vein and can be divided low and used for traction. Above the liver, the thin avascular ligament is divided with cautery (Fig. 82.2C). When the ligament nears the diaphragm it widens and will lead directly to the left and middle hepatic veins. The left triangular ligament can be divided laterally with cautery by gently pulling the lateral segments (II and III) downward and rotating medially. With thick or diseased livers, the lateral-most corner may be difficult to see, resulting in a lateral tear if too much traction is applied. If a lateral tear occurs, it is easily repaired after being completely released from the diaphragm. In these cases, begin medially by placing a finger or laparotomy sponge between the proximal stomach and push upward to expose the thin ligament between the diaphragm liver surfaces. Divide this medially and work laterally.

The right triangular ligament is divided by lifting and rolling the liver medially using a laparotomy pad to create gentle tension between the ligament and the diaphragm (Fig. 82.2D). Working close to the liver surface is safe because there are no major vascular structures until the right hepatic vein and retrohepatic veins are encountered entering the vena cava (Fig. 82.2E, F). At completion, the inferior vena cava can be visualized and small retrohepatic veins divided with care. For tumors invading the diaphragm, resection en bloc with the liver should be done and the diaphragm defect closed primarily. If bleeding from the diaphragm occurs, the vessels can retract into the muscular layers and should be controlled with suture ligature. After releasing the right and left triangular ligaments, the liver should be mobile within the abdomen. This is the best time to confirm the surgical plan and ensure the incision is adequate for the proposed procedure. Intraoperative ultrasound is a useful adjunct to identify lesions and ensure that planned segments to remain are disease free.

Anatomic Points

The liver is attached to the diaphragm relatively posteriorly by a series of peritoneal reflections, termed ligaments. As the peritoneal leaves of the falciform ligament reach the liver, they diverge to the left and right to form the coronary ligaments that surround the bare area of the liver. This region of the liver is described as bare because it is not covered by peritoneum. On the right, the coronary ligament consists of anterior (superior) and posterior (inferior) layers that are widely separated from each other. On the left, the anterior and posterior layers are quite close, separated from each other only by a modest amount of connective tissue. Within this connective tissue run some variable vessels, nerves, and, frequently, biliary radicles. The left triangular ligament forms the upper boundary of the superior recess of the omental bursa, whereas the superior layer of the right coronary ligament prevents the manual exploration of the diaphragmatic surface of the liver. Division of the coronary ligament and the right or left triangular ligament, or both, is necessary to mobilize the liver and expose the hepatic part of the inferior vena cava. The coronary and right triangular ligaments are simply peritoneal reflections and can be sharply divided with no special precautions. The long, narrow left triangular ligament always contains vessels or bile canaliculi, or both, and thus should be divided between the clamps. As the incision of these peritoneal reflections progresses medially, the hepatic veins will begin to appear.

Inflow Control (Pringle Maneuver) (Fig. 82.3)

Technical Points

Control of vascular inflow to the liver should be in the armamentarium of all general surgeons (Pringle maneuver). A medial to lateral mobilization of the porta hepatis is fast and safe. Begin

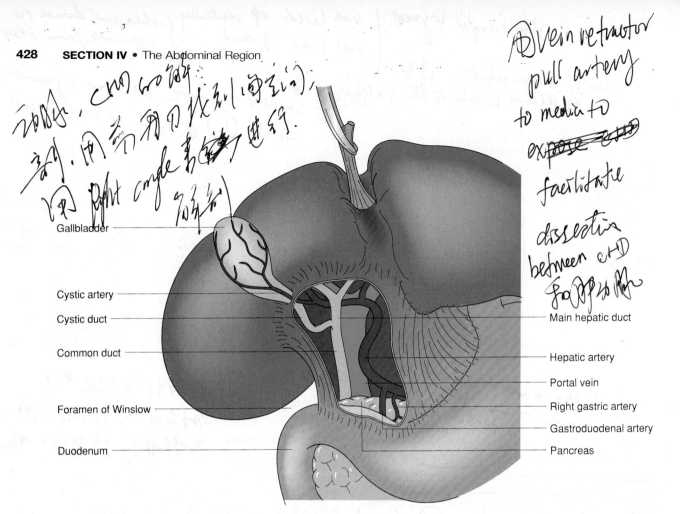

Gallbladder

Cystic artery

Cystic duct

Common duct

Foramen of Winslow

Duodenum

Main hepatic duct

Hepatic artery

Portal vein

Right gastric artery

Gastroduodenal artery

Pancreas

Figure 82.3 Inflow control (Pringle maneuver) (from Schulick RD. Hepatobiliary anatomy. In: Mulholland MW, Lillemoe KD, Dohert GM, et al., eds. *Greenfield's Surgery: Scientific Principles and Practice.* Philadelphia, PA: Lippincott Williams & Wilkins; 2006, with permission).

by lifting the left lateral liver (segments II and III) to expose the caudate lobe (segment I) and divide the lesser omentum (avascular tissue between the lesser curve of the stomach and liver). A finger placed directly on the caudate lobe can be swept to the right (above the inferior vena cava) to encircle the porta hepatis through the foramen of Winslow. Circumferential control of the hepatic artery and portal vein can be done without any dissection or mobilization. Palpation of the porta hepatis can define the right and left portal veins and hepatic arterial divisions. Arterial anomalous patterns are common. A left hepatic artery directly off the celiac axis or right hepatic arteries off the superior mesenteric artery are frequently encountered.

Anatomic Points

The relative relationships of the major structures within the hepatoduodenal ligament are maintained up into the hilum of the liver, forming a pattern that is followed throughout the liver. The portal vein is posterior in the hepatoduodenal ligament and at the porta hepatis. The CHD is anterior and to the right, whereas the hepatic artery is anterior and to the left.

Calot triangle is that triangle formed by the liver, CHD, and cystic duct. It usually contains the cystic artery and right hepatic artery and, when present, the accessory right hepatic

arteries and accessory hepatic ducts. Remember that, although the arteries usually are posterior to the biliary ducts, a common anomaly involves the hepatic artery crossing anterior to the CHD.

The CHD is formed by the confluence of the right and left ducts at the porta hepatis. This union may be intrahepatic or extrahepatic; therefore, parenchymal dissection may be necessary to allow ligation of the right duct. In about 28% of the cases, one of the two right segmental ducts crosses the interlobar plane to drain into the left hepatic duct.

Of the structures entering the porta hepatis, the arterial supply is probably the most variable. Typically, the common hepatic artery divides into left and right branches at the porta hepatis, before entering liver parenchyma. Thereafter, the right branch soon divides into anterior and posterior segmental branches. Seemingly, almost any conceivable variation from this pattern can—and does—occur. For example, the right hepatic artery frequently arises from the superior mesenteric artery (in 17% of cases), a middle hepatic artery (in reality, the artery supplying the left medial segment) may be visible extrahepatically and may arise from the right hepatic artery, and various accessory arteries can also be present.

The portal vein also usually divides into left and right branches extrahepatically. The right portal vein, as with the right hepatic artery, travels only a short distance within the substance of the liver before it divides into its segmental branches. Although there is less variation in the portal venous system than in either the arterial supply or the biliary apparatus, the intrahepatic course of the right portal vein tends to be more variable than that of the left, and caution should be exercised.

Wedge Resection (Fig. 82.4)

Technical and Anatomic Points

Wedge resections of the liver are safe and simple and can be done with minimal morbidity (Fig. 82.4A). Margins should wide (1 to 2 cm) if malignancy is suspected. An adequate incision and control of the surgical field (mobilized from the peritoneal and diaphragm attachments) is required for the region in question. There are regions of the liver that are poorly suited for wedge resection (Fig. 82.4B). Wedge resection of a hilar lesion may devascularize large regions of normal liver parenchyma if central vessels (veins or arteries) are inadvertently encountered. Central biliary injuries resulting in a leak or stricture can lead to serious postoperative sequela. A second danger zone for wedge resection is central and high

on the dome of the liver, where the hepatic veins enter the vena cava. Major bleeding and the risk of an air embolism make wedge resections of segments IV, VII, and VIII more dangerous than often anticipated. Segment II and III lesions are amenable to simple wedge resection if the dissection stays to the left of the falciform ligament. Inadvertent dissection or injury to the right of the falciform will place segment IV at risk.

After the lesion is identified and deemed adequate for limited resection, achieve circumferential hemostatic control. Placing blunt chromic sutures with overlapping bites around the lesion followed by sharp division of the parenchyma is safe and simple. Either use the needle with the curvature as provided, or bend it into a straighter configuration (for a deep yet straight bite). Tie these sutures to compress but not tear through the liver parenchyma. Resect the lesion sharply using knife or electrocautery set on "cutting." This is rapid and provides clean margins for histologic analysis. Direct pressure on the surrounding tissue will control any bleeding followed by direct suture ligation after the specimen is removed.

A Pringle maneuver, compression of the portal vein and hepatic artery, can be done but is seldom required. When there is a question of potential bleeding, pass an umbilical tape around the porta hepatis early in the procedure for easy and

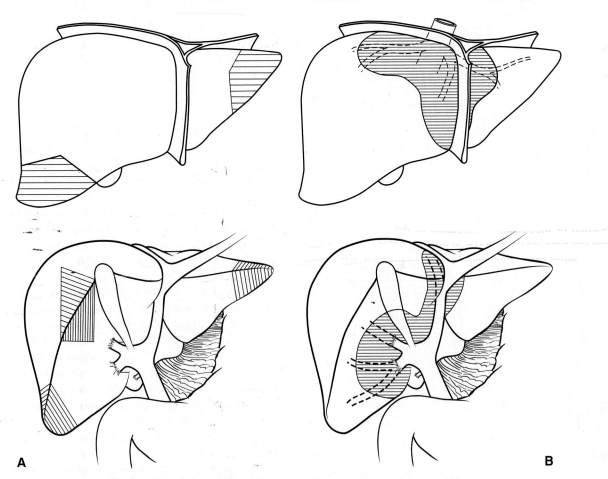

Figure 82.4 Suitable and unsuitable areas for wedge resection

fast control. The inexperienced surgeon should be cautioned against performing a wedge resection without an adequate incision and proper liver mobilization. A poorly thought-out wedge resection may result in inadequate margins, inadvertent tractions injuries, or injuring unrecognized deep vascular or biliary structures.

Left Lateral Bisegmentectomy (Fig. 82.5)

Technical Points

This resection removes segments II and III (those segments to the left of the falciform ligament). It will remove less than 40% of the normal liver and is well tolerated. A smaller upper midline incision and laparoscopic techniques are suitable for this procedure as long as adequate margins are maintained. The falciform and left triangular ligaments are released as described; laparoscopically this is easy to visualize. A bridge of liver may cover the falciform between segments III and IV; no major structures exist here and cautery can be used over a right-angle clamp.

The falciform ligament identifies the junction between segments II/III and IV. Elevate the left lateral liver off the caudate lobe to expose the narrowest transection plane. To the immedi-

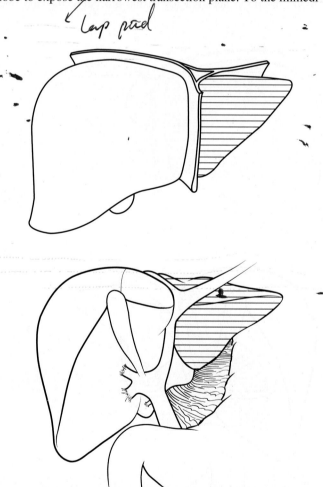

Figure 82.5 Left lateral bisegmentectomy

ate left of the falciform, small vascular pedicles can be identified and divided. Divide the liver parenchyma from anterior to posterior. As the posterior aspect is approached, divide the left hepatic vein to complete the transection. If the liver has a thin profile and the liver capsule is divided, the entire procedure can be done by sequential firing of cutting linear stapler. The division must stay to the left of the falciform to avoid injury to segment IV. If this cannot be done due to tumor location, a left hepatectomy (Fig. 82.8) is advised.

Anatomic Points

The segmental anatomy of the liver is based on ramifications of the portal triad structures. With few exceptions, the ramifications of these three structures (portal vein, hepatic artery, and biliary apparatus) accompany each other through the liver parenchyma. These triads interdigitate with the branches of the hepatic vein in much the way that the fingers of one hand, from above, might interdigitate with the fingers of the other hand from below.

On the basis of the first major division of portal triad structures, the liver can be divided into a right and left lobe of nearly equal size. The plane of division (line of Cantlie) runs from the inferior vena cava to the middle of the gallbladder fossa, parallel to the fissure of the round ligament.

Each of the two major lobes of the liver can be subdivided into segments. The left lobe is composed of medial and lateral segments, with the plane of division indicated by the falciform ligament and fissure of the round ligament. The right lobe is subdivided into anterior and posterior segments. Typically, no external features indicate the plane dividing the right lobe segments, although sometimes an intersegmental fissure is present.

Finally, each segment can be divided into superior and inferior subsegments. Because there are no external features that can be used to demarcate these superior and inferior subsegments, the surgical importance of subsegments is considered to be minimal.

Segments IV and I, the quadrate and caudate lobes, are apparent on visual inspection of the liver. However, these externally apparent lobes do not correspond to functional anatomic subunits. The quadrate lobe is a part of the medial segment of the left lobe. The caudate lobe receives its portal supply from both the right and left lobar branches. The interlobar plane passes through the middle of the caudate lobe. Thus this so-called lobe is not functionally distinct; rather, its right half is part of the right lobe, whereas its left half is part of the left lobe.

The caudate lobe has particular nuisance value during the performance of a side-to-side portacaval shunt (see Chapter 80e). Enlargement of this region secondary to cirrhosis may make it difficult to bring the portal vein down to the inferior vena cava during shunt construction. Sometimes, partial wedge excision of this lobe is necessary to allow the shunt to be constructed.

The venous drainage of the liver is through the hepatic veins. It does not follow these divisions. Three major branches of the hepatic veins define the corresponding major scissurae. Thus the right hepatic vein defines the right scissura between segments VI and VII to the right and V and VIII to the left of the right hepatic vein. The middle hepatic vein defines the main scissura between segments V and VIII to the right and segments I and IV to the left. This main scissura corresponds to the line of Cantlie dividing the true left and right lobes of the liver. Finally, the left hepatic vein defines the left scissura between segments I and IV to the right and segments II and III to the left.

For this particular resection, be careful to keep the dissection to the left of the umbilical fissure, rather than within the fissure. The umbilical part of the portal vein lies in the fissure and has branches on both the medial and lateral sides. Likewise, the arterial supply of the medial segment can be derived primarily from so-called retrograde branches arising from the left lateral segmental arteries. Thus resection and subsequent control of portal vein branches and arterial branches on the right side of the umbilical fissure can result in devascularization of the left medial segment.

Right Hepatectomy: Hilar Dissection (Fig. 82.6)

Technical and Anatomic Points

A right hepatectomy involves removing liver segments V to VIII and typically involves loss of greater than 50% of the liver volume (Fig. 82.6A). When segment IV is added, it becomes an extended resection and transient liver failure may result. The procedure will require an adequate incision, complete mobilization of the liver and hilar dissection.

Hilar Dissection

The hilar dissection for right hepatic resection can be done anatomically by identifying each structure individually (vein, artery, and bile duct) or regionally by taking the portal triad within the controlled Glissonian pedicle. Each technique is described and the pros and cons of the two techniques are listed in Table 82.1.

Anatomic Technique

Take the gallbladder down to facilitate identification of the cystic duct and CHD. Follow the anterior surface of the CHD until the right duct is clearly identified, taking care to avoid inadvertent injury or extensive mobilization (devasculariza-

tion). Circumferential control and ligation of the right hepatic duct must be accomplished without narrowing or compromising the left system. The right hepatic artery is identified and circumferentially controlled (Fig. 82.6B). Anomalous vasculature in this region is common and palpating the left hepatic arterial system before division will ensure that the left liver perfusion is preserved. After dividing the right bile duct and right hepatic artery, retract these to the left (Fig. 82.6C) and begin dissecting the portal vein. This dissection is safest when performed directly on the vein. Dissection on the vein traveling toward the hilum will expose the right and left branches. The right portal branch is dissected free by rolling the vein medially and laterally using Kittners until circumferential control is achieved under direct vision (Fig. 82.6B, inset). Do not pass a right-angle clamp blindly posterior to the vein; the resulting injury is both difficult to see and to repair. The posterior branch to segments V and VI and small caudate branches come off the right portal vein trunk and are prone to injury if excess traction or blind dissection is used. Divide the right portal vein at a point that ensures that the junction of the left and main portal veins is not narrowed. This can be done at the main trunk or at the anterior and posterior branches depending on exposure and margins. Division with a vascular load on a laparoscopic stapler is fast and simple. Division between vascular clamps and oversewing with running Prolene suture works equally well. Before dividing each structure it is prudent to visualize or palpate the protected contralateral vessel/duct to ensure that the remnant liver will remain healthy. At completion, the liver will demarcate clearly between the left and right liver. If a clear demarcation does not occur, suspect that the hilar dissection is incomplete or anomalous vascular inflow exists and must be identified.

Pedicle Technique

An alternative technique is to control the entire right portal system (vein, artery, and biliary system) through dissection along Glissonian pedicles. This is often referred to as "lowering the hilar plate" and can be done centrally or on either the right or left side. The gallbladder is removed early, but the CHD need not be dissected free. A small ligamentous band of tissue between the gallbladder fossa and the CHD needs to be divided. The dissection is begun centrally between the liver parenchyma and the connective tissue surrounding the pedicle. Identifying the avascular plane between the fibrous sheath (Glisson's capsule) and the liver parenchyma protects

Table 82.1 Comparison of Techniques of Hepatectomy

Technique	Pro	Con
Anatomic	Better visualization of artery, vein, and bile duct	Technically demanding and time consuming
	Better assessment of margins and enables reconstruction (biliary/portal) if needed	Increased dissection and risk of injury of contralateral hilar structures (remnant liver)
Pedicle	Simple and direct	
	Less dissection required	Not suitable for all tumor locations (hilar or central lesions) and tumor types (Klatskin)

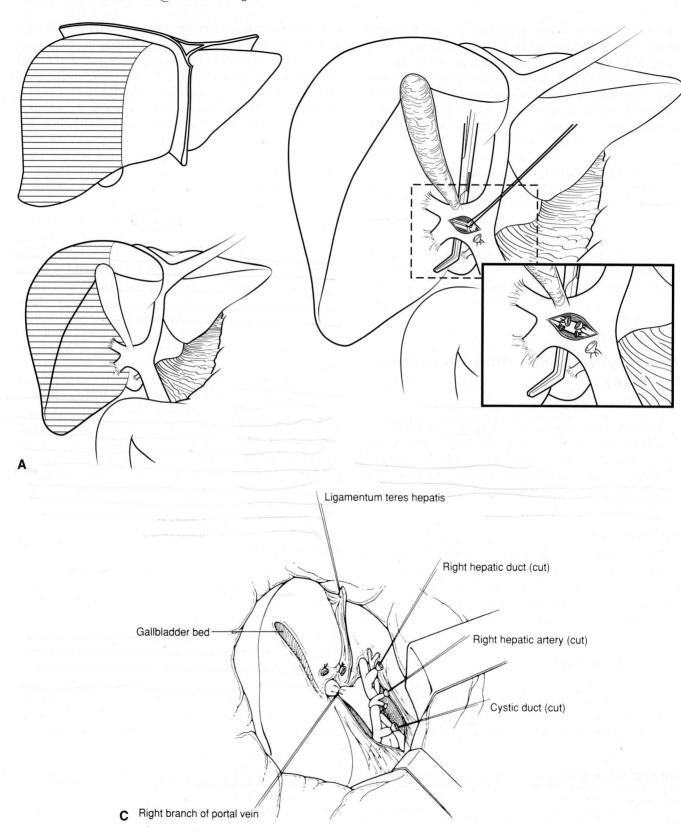

Ligamentum teres hepatis

Right hepatic duct (cut)

Gallbladder bed

Right hepatic artery (cut)

Cystic duct (cut)

Right branch of portal vein

Figure 82.6 Right hepatectomy: Hilar dissection

the major vascular structures from injury. By gently pulling the Glissonian fibrous sheath away from the liver parenchyma, circumferential control of the right pedicle can be obtained. At times, the subsegmental branches to segments VI and VII will branch from the right main pedicle low and at right angles to the dissection plane (Fig. 82.5B). The branch to segments V and VI may take off from the main right portal vein at right angles to the visible trunk. A small branch to the caudate lobe (segment I) is medial to dissection plane. The insert shows the anatomic technique with bile duct and artery divided in order to expose the right portal vein.

Both the anterior (segments V and VIII) and posterior (segments VI and VII) pedicles should be controlled. The right main pedicle (or the anterior and posterior pedicles) should be temporarily occluded to produce a clear demarcation line on the liver surface, which dictates the line of transection and also ensures that the contralateral side remains healthy prior to

division. The pedicle(s) can be suture ligated or divided using a laparoscopic vascular stapler.

Right Hepatectomy: Hepatic Vein Control and Parenchymal Dissection (Fig. 82.7)

Technical Points

The devascularized liver will demarcate clearly between segments IV and V. Before parenchymal dissection, control the right hepatic vein if technically feasible. With the liver rotated from right to left, the vena cava should be clearly seen and cleared of small vascular attachments. The assisting surgeon holds the liver upward while the operating surgeon identifies, controls, and divides the short retrohepatic branches (Fig. 82.7A). Clips are easy to dislodge from the vena cava

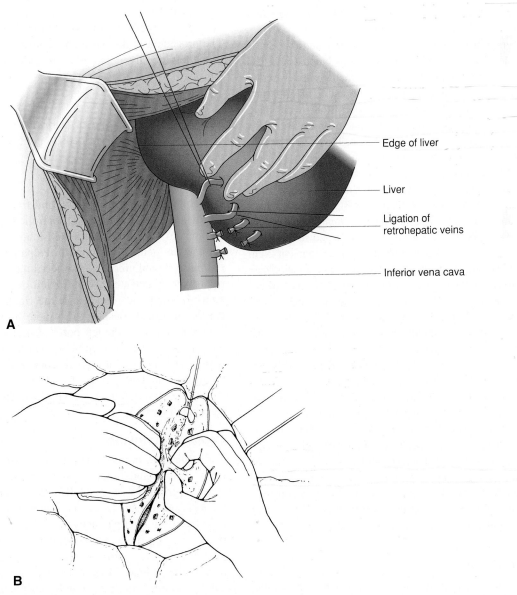

Figure 82.7 Right hepatectomy: Hepatic vein control and parenchymal dissection

when laparotomy sponges are placed posterior to the liver and for this reason should be used with appropriate caution. As the junction of the right hepatic vein and vena cava is approached from below, the retrohepatic ligament will need to be divided. It typically contains no vessels but will obscure visualization and control of the extrahepatic portion of the vein. A vascular stapler can then be used to divide the right hepatic vein. The hepatic vein can also be clamped and over sewn with running Prolene suture, but clamp slippage will result in major bleeding at a time when the right liver prevents clear visualization of the vena cava for repair. Control of the hepatic vein can be done at any time, but division should not be done until inflow to the liver is divided to prevent congestion. In certain circumstances, the extrahepatic vein cannot be safely visualized or divided. In these cases, parenchymal dissection is performed first and identification and control of the hepatic vein is done within the liver parenchyma. Circumferential control of the vena cava above and below the liver can be obtained in difficult cases and will limit unnecessary blood loss if parenchymal dissection proves difficult.

Parenchymal dissection after vascular inflow and outflow is controlled can proceed rapidly and relatively bloodlessly. The middle hepatic vein should be the only uncontrolled vascular structure encountered and should be protected if margins and tumor characteristics permit. Temporary occlusion of the main portal trial or Pringle maneuver can be done to limit blood loss during the parenchymal dissection. A clear, bloodless working field must be achieved to ensure proper line of division and safe adequate margins, and to protect the contralateral hilar structures. Short periods of hepatic inflow occlusion should not affect remnant liver function. Numerous techniques exist to divide the liver along the demarcation line. Classic finger or clamp fracture technique requires no special equipment and is safe and simple (Fig. 82.7B). Placement of straightened blunt chromic sutures at 2-cm intervals controls most parenchyma bleeders and division can proceed sharply. Sophisticated devices using ultrasound, water jet, and coagulation can be used to safely divide the parenchyma. Ablation devices and vascular staplers are now being used successfully. All techniques should achieve hemostasis on small vessels. Larger vascular pedicles should be identified and suture ligated. Biliary radicals should be identified and ligated to prevent postoperative bile leaks. Through a tagged long cystic duct left at the time of cholecystectomy, injection of saline or dye can assist with visualization of small leaking biliary ducts. Raw surfaces can be treated with argon beam coagulation if necessary. Other topical treatments for hemostasis are usually not needed. Ensuring that the remnant liver is placed in a suitable location is not a risk of torsion or tension on vascular or biliary pedicles completes the procedure. Drains are not recommended unless a complex biliary reconstruction or pancreatic procedure was also undertaken. Omentum may be packed over the raw surface and under the incision.

Anatomic Points

The liver drains through three major (right, left, and middle) veins and a variable number (12 to 15) of minor veins. The three major veins of the liver are intersegmental or interlobar. The right hepatic vein lies between the anterior and posterior segments of the right lobe, the middle hepatic vein lies in the true interlobar fissure, and the left hepatic vein is located in the superior aspect of the umbilical fissure. Thus the right hepatic vein must be ligated. Depending on the relationship of the resection plane to the middle hepatic vein, either tributaries or the middle vein itself will have to be ligated. Remember that in most cases (84%), the middle vein drains into the terminal part of the left hepatic vein, rather than into the inferior vena cava directly, because ligation of the common trunk could be disastrous.

Left Hepatectomy (Fig. 82.8)

Technical and Anatomic Points

A left hepatectomy involves removing liver segments II through IV (Fig. 82.8A). Typically, this involves loss of less than 50% of the liver volume and transient liver failure is rare. The procedure will require an adequate incision, mobilization of the left lobe liver, and hilar dissection.

Hilar Dissection

The hilar dissection for left hepatic resection can again be done anatomically or via pedicle control very similar to that described for the right hepatectomy.

Anatomic Technique

The gallbladder is taken down and the left hepatic duct and artery are circumferentially controlled (Fig. 82.8B, inset). Anomalous vasculature to the left lobe of the liver is common yet easy to identify and control. Palpating a strong right arterial pulse should precede left arterial ligation to ensure that the right liver is protected. With the left bile duct and left hepatic artery divided and retracted to the right, the left portal vein can be identified. Because of a more horizontal and extrahepatic path taken by the left portal vein, the dissection is easier and can be done farther from the right branch takeoff. Division with a vascular load on a laparoscopic stapler is fast and simple but division and oversewing with Prolene suture works equally well. At completion the liver will demarcate clearly separating segments IV and V.

Pedicle Technique

The pedicle technique controls the entire left portal system (vein, artery, and biliary system) as it travels horizontally below segment IV (Fig. 82.8B). By lowering the hilar plate, the Glissonian pedicle can be isolated as it travels horizontally free from liver parenchyma. Separating the fibrous sheath (Glisson's capsule) and liver parenchyma can be done by using a combination of sharp dissection and gentle downward traction on the pedicle. Circumferential control of the left pedicle can be obtained and temperately occluded to produce a clear demarcation line on the liver surface. The pedicle can be suture

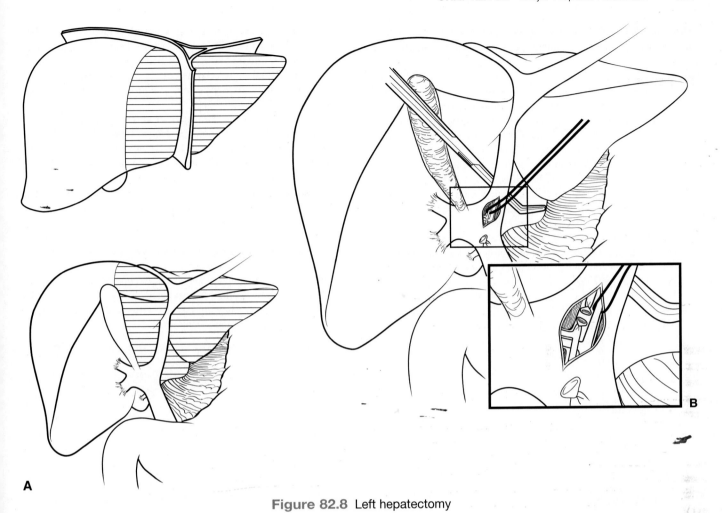

Figure 82.8 Left hepatectomy

ligated or divided using a laparoscopic vascular stapler or suture ligation.

Hepatic Vein Control and Parenchymal Dissection

The left and middle hepatic veins often arise from a common trunk and divide into separate branches within the liver parenchyma. This makes extrahepatic isolation of the left vein difficult and can place the middle branch at risk. At times it is safer to control the common trunk (left and middle), but not divide until after the liver parenchyma is split. When favorable anatomy allows, circumferential control of the left hepatic vein should be completed and again only divided after inflow control to prevent congestion. A vascular stapler can then be used to divide the hepatic vein. In certain circumstances, the extrahepatic vein cannot be safely visualized or divided. In these cases, parenchymal dissection is performed first and identification and control of the hepatic vein is done within the liver parenchyma. Circumferential control of the vena cava above and below the liver can be obtained in difficult cases to limit blood loss during parenchymal division. Parenchyma dissection once vascular inflow and outflow is controlled can proceed as described for right hepatectomy.

Closure

After the hepatic resection is completed, pathologic margin assessment is advised. The closest margin is marked and either gross or microscopic margins determined. Typically, frozen section analysis for a tissue diagnosis is not required because this will not have any immediate impact on the surgical procedure. Most hepatic resections are done with curative not diagnostic intent. If a margin is suboptimal and adequate parenchyma exists, then wider margins should be obtained. Every effort should be made to not violate a tumor or leave a positive margin.

Hemostasis is achieved and all transected surfaces inspected for bile. Liver remnant is inspected and inflow and outflow confirmed to be adequate. Layered closure of the facial and skin close completes the procedure. Drains are not recommended unless biliary reconstruction or pancreatic injury is suspected. Closely monitoring liver function in the postoperative period may predict hepatic insufficiency. Typically, liver function tests are monitored every 2 to 3 days until a downward or normalizing trend is documented. If hepatic dysfunction persists or acutely worsens, ultrasound evaluation of the intrahepatic bile ducts, portal vein, and hepatic artery and vein should be done. A subhepatic fluid collection may represent a biloma and can be percutaneously drained.

Most bile leaks will resolve spontaneously if the contralateral hepatic duct was protected and there is no distal obstruction.

REFERENCES

1. Blumgart LH. *Surgery of the Liver, Biliary Tract and Pancreas.* 4th ed. Philadelphia, PA: Saunders; 2006. (The basic reference used by all surgeons in this area. Contains a wealth of information including specialized and more difficult resections.)
2. The Brisbane 2000 Terminology of Liver Anatomy and Resections. Terminology Committee of the IHPBA. *HPB* 2000;2:333–339.
3. Chang YF, Huang TL, Chen CL, et al. Variations of the middle and inferior right hepatic vein: Application in hepatectomy. *J Clin Ultrasound.* 1997;25:175–182.
4. Cucchetti A, Cescon M, Ercolani G, et al. A comprehensive meta-regression analysis on outcome of anatomic resection versus non-anatomic resection for hepatocellular carcinoma. *Ann Surg Oncol.* 2012;19(12):3697–3705.
5. Delattre J-F, Avisse C, Flament J-B. Anatomic basis of hepatic surgery. *Surg Clin North Am.* 2000;80:345–362. (Presents excellent summary of surgical anatomy and embryology.)
6. Dirocchi R, Trastulli S, Boselli C, et al. Radiofrequency ablation in the treatment of liver metastases from colorectal cancer. *Cochrane Database Syst Rev.* 2012;6:CD006317.
7. Fong Y. Hepatic colorectal metastasis: Current surgical therapy, selection criteria for hepatectomy, and role for adjuvant therapy. *Adv Surg.* 2000;34:351–360.
8. Fong Y, Brennan MF, Brown K, et al. Drainage is unnecessary after elective liver resection. *Am J Surg.* 1996;171:158–162.
9. Kele PG, de Boer M, van der Jagt EJ, et al. Early hepatic regeneration index and completeness of regeneration at 6 months after partial hepatectomy. *Br J Surg.* 2012;99(8):1113–1119.
10. Starzl TE, Iwatsuki S, Shaw BW, et al. Left hepatic trisegmentectomy. *Surg Gynecol Obstet.* 1982;155:21. (Classic description of an uncommon resection.)
11. Starzl TE, Koep LJ, Weil R, et al. Right trisegmentectomy for hepatic neoplasms. *Surg Gynecol Obstet.* 1980;150:208. (Classic description of extensive resection.)
12. Takasaki K. *Glissonean Pedicle Transection Method of Hepatic Resection.* New York, NY: Springer Verlag; 2007. (Elegantly illustrated manual showing how the Glissonean pedicle method can be applied to various situations.)

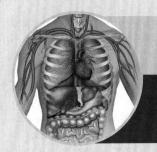

83

Drainage of Hepatic Abscess

James J. Mezhir

This chapter discusses open and laparoscopic approaches to the drainage of pyogenic hepatic abscess. Currently, most liver abscesses are drained percutaneously under ultrasound or computed tomography (CT) guidance. Several factors have been shown to correlate with failure of percutaneous drainage, including large size, the presence of multiple loculations, and communication with the biliary tree. Each patient is approached selectively and the treatment approach based on clinical status and imaging findings.

When percutaneous approaches are not available, the patient has failed percutaneous drainage, or if an abscess is not amenable to percutaneous drainage, operative drainage remains an essential treatment option for these patients. In some instances of refractory liver abscess or necrosis, liver resection may be necessary for definitive treatment. Knowledge of the principles of liver surgery essential for safe performance of major hepatic procedures is discussed elsewhere.

SCORE™, The Surgical Council on Resident Education, classified drainage of hepatic abscess as an "ESSENTIAL UNCOMMON" procedure.

STEPS IN PROCEDURE

Operative Drainage of Hepatic Abscess

Right subcostal incision

This incision can be extended to the midline (hockey-stick incision) or a bilateral subcostal incision may be utilized if necessary for safe exposure.

Localize the abscess by inspection, ultrasound, or with needle aspiration

Send cultures for bacteriology and antibiotic sensitivity

Unroof the abscess with electrocautery

Minimize contamination of the peritoneal cavity with suction and laparotomy pads

Disrupt loculations manually

Irrigate the abscess cavity

Evaluate for bile leak and hemostasis

Place drains to provide continued drainage of the abscess

A laparoscopic approach may also be utilized and the same principles are applied (safe access to the peritoneal cavity, identification of the abscess, unroofing and debridement, and wide drainage)

HALLMARK ANATOMIC COMPLICATIONS

Hemorrhage (from liver parenchyma or from major vascular injury)

Bile leak and/or biloma formation

Sepsis resulting from uncontrolled drainage

Liver necrosis

Diaphragm injury and resultant pneumothorax

Bile duct injury

Duodenal injury

Injury to colon or mesentery

LIST OF STRUCTURES

Liver (including knowledge of segmental anatomy and blood supply and venous drainage)

Portal veins and branches

Hepatic veins and branches

Diaphragm

Liver hilum including common bile duct, proper hepatic artery, and portal vein

Gallbladder

Duodenum

Right and transverse colon and mesentery

Operative Localization of Abscess (Fig. 83.1)

Technical and Anatomic Points

Carefully review all available imaging studies (Fig. 83.1A,B). Obtain access to the liver through a right subcostal incision. Extend this to include the upper midline or bilateral subcostal as needed for safe exposure. When entering the abdomen in the setting of a large abscess, the right upper quadrant may be severely inflamed depending on the etiology of the abscess. Take care to safely lower the right colon if it is stuck to the liver and gallbladder. This may also be necessary if the patient has had a prior cholecystectomy. Take care to not injure the duodenum or colon or mesentery. In the setting of severe inflammation, the colonic mesentery can be torn and this may result in significant hemorrhage from the superior mesenteric vein.

Identification and dissection of the porta hepatis is not necessary in most situations when drainage hepatic abscesses. However, if significant vascular injury were to occur, a Pringle maneuver may be necessary. This is performed by placing a finger behind the foramen of Winslow, opening the gastrohepatic ligament, and placing a vessel loop around the bile duct, portal vein, and hepatic artery to reduce inflow while obtaining control of any bleeding. If significant bleeding results from abscess drainage, it may be very difficult to obtain control in an inflamed cavity and therefore damage control with packing and temporary abdominal closure may be necessary.

Mobilize the liver if needed for exposure of the abscess. This should be done carefully and selectively since injury to the diaphragm would allow for contamination of the chest from the liver abscess. Carefully palpate the liver, seeking an area of firmness close to the capsule. If the abscess is not palpable, use intraoperative ultrasound or probe with a needle.

Perform needle aspiration with a long large-gauge needle such as a spinal needle (Fig. 83.1C). Send any purulent material for cultures and sensitivity. Take care to identify a site on the liver where aspiration does not yield a flash of blood.

Drainage of Abscess (Fig. 83.2)

Technical and Anatomic Points

Use electrocautery to enter the abscess, following the track of the aspirating needle (Fig. 83.2A). Unroof the abscess (Fig. 83.2B). Control contamination with laparotomy pads and suction. Disrupt any loculations manually using finger fracture and the suction device.

Irrigate the cavity and inspect it for hemostasis and for any evidence of bile leak (Fig. 83.2C). Control bile leaks with sutures or clips; however, major intrahepatic bile duct injury may require additional procedures for control.

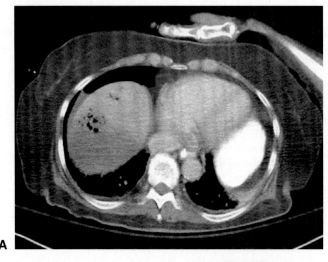

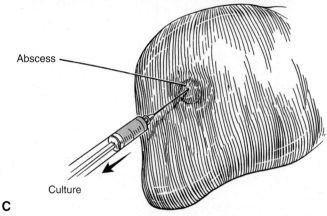

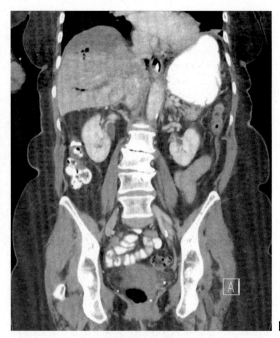

Figure 83.1 Pyogenic liver abscess in right lobe of liver. **A:** Large complex collection with gas bubbles in right lobe of liver, transverse CT section. **B:** Coronal reconstruction showing abscess. **C:** Aspiration to identify access site for drainage (**C** from RH Bell Jr, Rikkers LF, Mulholland MW. *Digestive Surgery: A Text and Atlas.* Philadelphia, PA: Lippincott Raven; 1996, with permission).

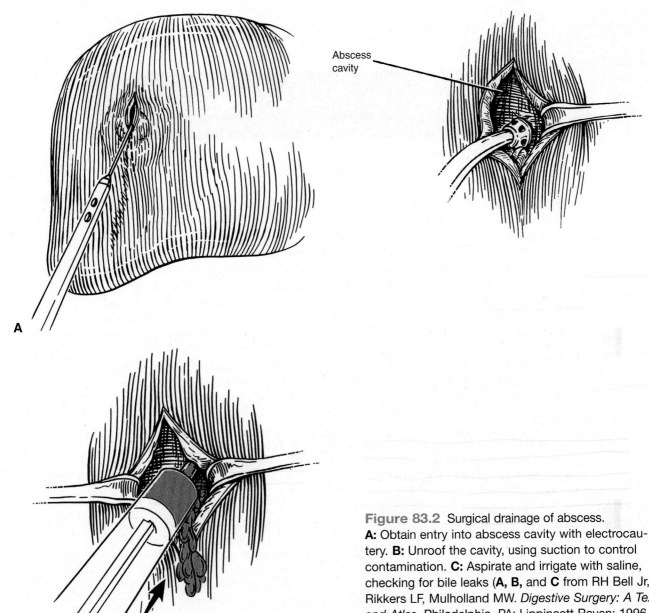

Abscess
cavity

A

B

C

Figure 83.2 Surgical drainage of abscess. **A:** Obtain entry into abscess cavity with electrocautery. **B:** Unroof the cavity, using suction to control contamination. **C:** Aspirate and irrigate with saline, checking for bile leaks (**A, B,** and **C** from RH Bell Jr, Rikkers LF, Mulholland MW. *Digestive Surgery: A Text and Atlas.* Philadelphia, PA: Lippincott Raven; 1996, with permission).

Place drains in the abscess cavity and bring these out away from the incision. Place these to gravity or closed suction drainage. Remove the drains once the patient has low output and no evidence for ongoing sepsis or bile leak.

The laparoscopic approach to drainage can also be applied selectively depending on abscess location and surgeon preference and comfort. The same principles are applied as in open drainage.

REFERENCES

1. Mezhir JJ, Fong Y, Jacks LM, et al. Current management of pyogenic liver abscess: Surgery is now second-line treatment. *J Am Coll Surg.* 2010;210(6):975–983.
2. Tan YM, Chung AY, Chow PK, et al. An appraisal of surgical and percutaneous drainage for pyogenic liver abscesses larger than 5 cm. *Ann Surg.* 2005;241(3):485–490.

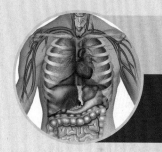

84

Pancreatic Resections

James J. Mezhir

This chapter discusses distal (left) pancreatectomy and pancreaticoduodenectomy (Whipple procedure). Because of the close anatomic proximity of the body and tail of pancreas to the splenic vessels, splenectomy is generally performed when the tail of the pancreas is resected for treatment of malignant disease. When this operation is performed for benign tumors, trauma, or highly select cancer cases, it is possible to preserve the blood supply of the spleen. The laparoscopic approach to distal pancreatectomy is described in Chapter 85e.

Resection of the head of the pancreas (pancreaticoduodenectomy) can be performed with or without pylorus preservation. References at the end of the chapter give additional details about total pancreatectomy and central pancreatectomy which are beyond the scope of this chapter.

For patients with pancreatic cancer, high quality contrast-enhanced imaging for staging is essential to prevent unnecessary laparotomy in these patients. Diagnostic laparoscopy is used selectively—in general those with any concern for M1 disease, body and tail lesions, and elevated Ca 19-9 (greater than 140 U/mL).

The regional anatomy is shown in Figure 84.1.

SCORE™, The Surgical Council on Resident Education, classified distal pancreatectomy as an "ESSENTIAL UNCOMMON" procedure, and other pancreatic resections as "COMPLEX" procedures.

HALLMARK ANATOMIC COMPLICATIONS

Tearing of the gonadal vein during Kocher maneuver

Inadvertent division of the hepatic artery

Injury to superior mesenteric vein (SMV) or branches during retraction (gastroepiploic or middle colic veins) or dissection (first jejunal branch, uncinate branch)

Accidental division of a replaced right hepatic artery coursing behind pancreas and/or common bile duct

Mesenteric bleeding during resection of first portion of jejunum

Inadvertent injury to the middle colic vessels or transverse mesocolon

Abdominal collection (sterile or infected)

Pancreatic leak/fistula/abscess

Bile leak, delayed gastric emptying (for pancreaticoduodenectomy)

Delayed hemorrhage (most commonly gastroduodenal artery [GDA] after a pancreatic leak)

LIST OF STRUCTURES

Pancreas
Head
Body
Tail
Uncinate process
Pancreatic duct

Spleen
Splenic artery
Splenic vein

Colon
Transverse mesocolon
Transverse colon
Middle colic artery and veins

Stomach
Greater curvature
Pylorus
Antrum

Duodenum
First, second, third, and fourth portions
Ligament of Treitz

Gallbladder
Cystic artery
Cystic duct
Bile duct
Porta hepatis
Right hepatic artery (and anatomic variants)

Portal vein
Superior mesenteric artery and vein
Inferior vena cava (IVC) and right gonadal vein
Left and right gastroepiploic arteries and veins

Inferior (transverse) pancreatic artery
Gastrocolic omentum (ligament)
Gastrosplenic ligament
Splenocolic ligament

ORIENTATION

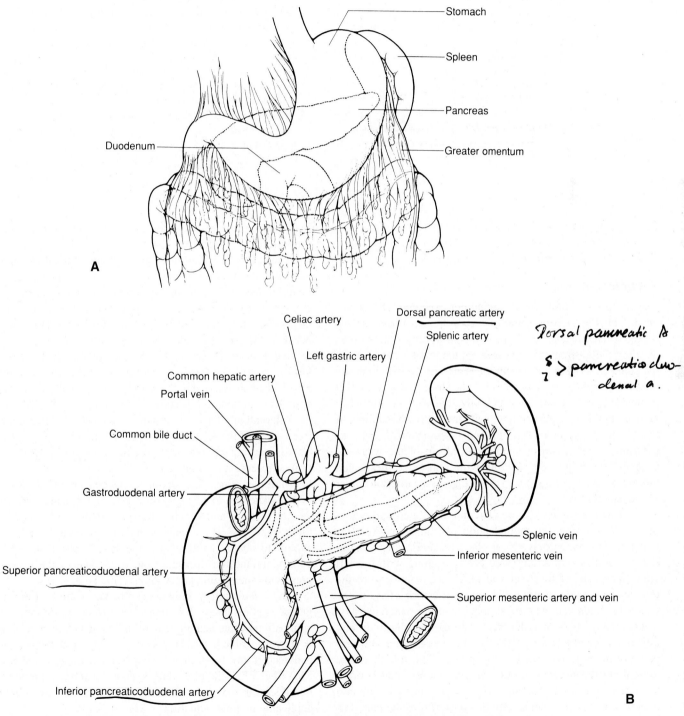

Figure 84.1 Regional anatomy. **A:** Pancreas is completely obscured by overlying viscera on initial exploration. **B:** Regional anatomy including vascular relationships.

Distal Pancreatectomy With or Without Splenectomy

STEPS IN PROCEDURE

Distal Pancreatectomy

Diagnostic laparoscopy (adenocarcinoma of body or tail)

Upper midline or extended left subcostal incision

Start with a small incision and palpate the liver and the remainder of the abdomen for M1 disease

Open the greater omentum and enter the lesser sac and lower right colon

Divide gastroepiploic vessels

Preserve short gastrics (for splenic preservation)

Mobilize back wall of stomach from pancreas and inferior border of pancreas from transverse mesocolon

Create a tunnel behind the pancreas over the SMV

Secure gastropancreatic arteries and divide pancreas

If splenectomy: Staple or suture ligate the splenic artery followed by the vein and move medial to lateral and perform splenectomy

If splenic preservation: Elevate distal remnant and gently dissect from splenic vessels

If splenic vessels need to be taken, the short gastric vessels must have been preserved (Warshaw procedure)

Check for a defect in the transverse mesocolon before closure

Consider using a drain if high risk features present (e.g., small duct, soft pancreas)

Exposure of the Body and Tail of the Pancreas and Resection of Distal Pancreas (Fig. 84.2)

Technical Points

Use an upper midline (most patients) or extended left subcostal or Chevron incision (morbidly obese patient). Explore for distant disease. Make a window in the gastrocolic omentum by dividing the gastroepiploic vessels on the greater curvature of the stomach. Divide these from the region of the distal antrum to the short gastric vessels. Preserve the short gastric vessels if planning splenic preservation and if the main splenic artery and vein are going to require resection (Warshaw modification). At this point, the greater omentum can be removed to enhance exposure or retraction or simply moved out of the way (see Chapter 80e, Figure 80.5). Protect the transverse mesocolon throughout the operation when dissecting on the inferior border of the pancreas.

Follow the gastroepiploic vein and middle colic down to the SMV to define the medial point of transection for formal left pancreatectomy. Now place retractors in to maintain the stomach in an elevated position along with the left lateral segment of the liver and take care to not injure the left gastric arcade. Retract the colon inferiorly. Divide the avascular folds between the stomach and the pancreas (gastropancreatic folds or Allen's veil) to expose the body and tail of the pancreas fully. The splenic vessels may be palpable in the region of the distal pancreas. The splenic artery runs along the superior surface of the pancreas and is often seen here and can be palpated. Be sure it is not the common hepatic artery. The splenic vein lies posterior to the pancreas and cannot be seen until the pancreas is mobilized. Incise the peritoneum along the inferior border of the pancreas with electrocautery and take care not to injure the inferior mesenteric vein (IMV).

Elevate the pancreas out of the retroperitoneum by blunt dissection in an avascular (normally) plane. The splenic artery and vein will be elevated along with the body and tail of the pancreas. Identify the point at which the pancreas is to be divided. Generally, this point will be over the SMV. Develop a plane between the pancreas and the splenic artery and splenic vein by careful blunt dissection. Use Silastic vessel loops on the two vessels to facilitate traction after the plane has been developed. Divide the pancreas using the technique of choice (stapler, sharp with duct ligation, radiofrequency ablation) (Fig. 84.2A).

Alternatively, in some situations, it may be simpler to mobilize the tail of the pancreas first and then divide it (Fig. 84.2B). This is particularly useful in trauma situations where a more limited resection is indicated.

Multiple, short, fine vessels connecting the body and tail of the pancreas to the splenic artery and splenic vein must then be isolated and serially clipped or ligated (Fig. 84.2C). If these small vessels are inadvertently avulsed, use fine Prolene sutures to obtain hemostasis in the splenic artery and splenic vein. Continue the dissection out to the tail of the pancreas, preserving the splenic artery and splenic vein.

The splenic artery and vein can be taken safely if the short gastric vessels were left intact (Warshaw procedure). The application of this technique to a limited distal pancreatectomy is shown in Figure 84.2D. As previously noted, formal distal pancreatectomy for tumor generally requires resection to the SMV, but when the procedure is done for trauma a more limited resection may be appropriate. The Warshaw procedure is applicable in either situation.

If splenic preservation is not planned, simply mobilize both the spleen and tail of the pancreas together. Divide the short

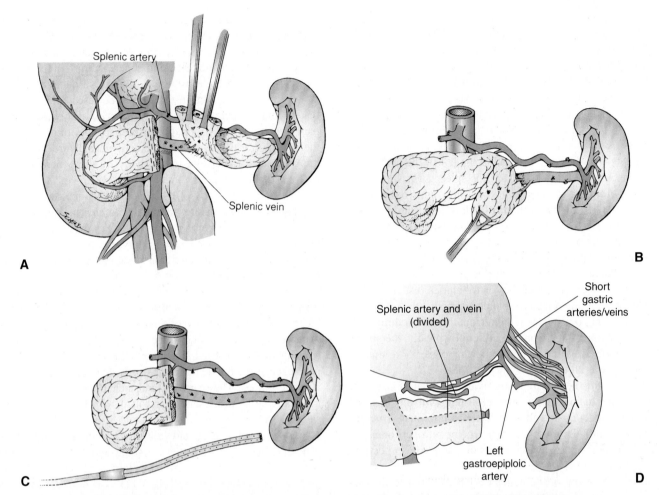

Figure 84.2 Resection of distal pancreas. **A:** Transection of pancreas, followed by mobilization of distal remnant. **B:** Mobilization, followed by transection. **C:** Completed resection. **D:** Warshaw modification (from Ferrone CR, Konstantinidis JT, Sahani DV, Wargo JA, et al. Twenty-three years of the Warshaw operation for distal pancreatectomy with preservation of the spleen. *Ann Surg.* 2011;253:1136, with permission).

gastric vessels. Secure the splenic artery and vein and transect the pancreas with stapler as previous noted.

Check the area for hemostasis and place omentum over the pancreatic stump if possible. Intraperitoneal drains may be placed to gravity selectively at the pancreatic stump.

Anatomic Points

The greater omentum is attached to the greater curvature of the stomach and the first part of the duodenum. On the left, it is continuous with the gastrosplenic ligament. The entire length of its posterior surface is adherent to the entire length of the transverse colon. That portion of the greater omentum connecting the stomach and transverse colon is the gastrocolic omentum (ligament). The gastroepiploic vessels, contained within the greater omentum, typically are close to the stomach, but may be 2 cm or more distant from the stomach.

On the left, the gastrosplenic and splenocolic ligaments are continuous with the greater omentum. Multiple, short, gastric

arteries (commonly, four to six) arise from the splenic artery or its branches and run through the gastrosplenic ligament to the greater curvature of the stomach at the fundus. The left gastroepiploic artery has a similar origin and similar course, except that it parallels the greater curvature, running from left to right, ultimately anastomosing with the right gastroepiploic artery. There are no vessels of consequence in the splenocolic ligament, although small communications may exist between the splenic vessels and branches of the middle or right colic vessels.

The lienorenal ligament attaches the spleen to the retroperitoneum. In this ligament are the major splenic vessels and the tail of the pancreas, which usually is either in contact with the splenic hilum or is no more than 1 cm distant from the hilum.

The gastropancreatic folds are formed by the left gastric artery as it passes from the celiac trunk to the upper part of the lesser curvature. Avascular, filmy connections can occur between the visceral peritoneum of the stomach and the parietal peritoneum covering the pancreas. These are common at the right extremity of the stomach, where the antrum is in close proximity to the head of the pancreas, and, on the left, where the posterior surface of the stomach is very close to the tail of the pancreas. These avascular folds tether the stomach to the posterior wall of the lesser sac, as the duodenum starts to become retroperitoneal, and to the gastrosplenic ligament and its contained vasculature.

The splenic artery runs along the superior border of the pancreas from its celiac trunk origin to the hilum of the spleen. The celiac trunk lies superior and to the left of the neck of the pancreas. As it progresses toward the spleen, it has a characteristically tortuous course (in the adult) owing to tethering by pancreatic branches, and it frequently dips downward posterior to the pancreas. By contrast, the splenic vein should not be visible until the pancreatic tail and splenic hilum are explored because this vein is posterior to the pancreas. As these vessels approach the splenic hilum, both artery and vein have a variable number of splenic branches or tributaries (usually two or three) that serve the different splenic segments; this branching most commonly occurs about 4 cm from the splenic hilum, but the distance may range from 1 to 12 cm. Typically, the splenic vein tributaries are inferior and somewhat posterior to the corresponding arterial branches.

Posterior to the pancreas, an avascular plane exists as a result of the fusion of the mesogastrium with the posterior parietal peritoneum and that those more proximal structures contained within the mesogastrium become retroperitoneal. As could be expected, the avascular fusion plane is also posterior to the splenic vessels.

The relationship of the major vessels posterior to the pancreas is also important. The portal vein, formed by the union of the superior mesenteric and splenic veins, lies to the right of the aorta and superior mesenteric artery (SMA). The splenic vein, which lies more or less in the transverse plane, joins the SMV by passing between the SMA and pancreas; thus, in this region, the splenic vein is the most anterior major vascular structure.

The pancreatic duct, in the area to be resected, is approximately midway between the superior and inferior borders of the pancreas. It is slightly more posterior than anterior but is nevertheless anterior to the major pancreatic vasculature. Normally, the diameter of the duct in the body of the pancreas varies between 2 and 4 mm.

Division of the body of the pancreas requires control of the intrapancreatic vasculature; to maintain a clear field, some control must be gained before sectioning. One major vessel is the inferior or transverse pancreatic artery; the origin of this artery is quite variable, but its inferodorsal course along the pancreas, either extraparenchymal or intraparenchymal, is fairly constant. The other main artery is a branch of the great pancreatic artery, a branch of the splenic artery that typically enters at the junction of the middle and distal thirds of this vessel; it then divides into one or more branches coursing to the tail and one or more branches coursing toward the head. The latter branches parallel the inferior pancreatic artery but lie more superiorly than the inferior pancreatic artery does. These arteries and their branches are the ones that must be hemostatically controlled with the figure-of-eight sutures.

As the splenic artery and vein travel along the length of the pancreas, several short, delicate radicles either supply or drain the pancreas. There are more pancreatic veins (15 to 31) than there are pancreatic arteries (4 to 11), and both appear to be distributed fairly evenly along the length of the vessels.

Pancreaticoduodenectomy

STEPS IN PROCEDURE

Pancreaticoduodenectomy (Whipple Procedure)

Use diagnostic laparoscopy selectively in high risk patients (high Ca 19-9, locally advanced disease)

Upper midline or Chevron incision (for morbidly obese patients). Start with a limited incision and palpate the liver and assess for M1 disease

Mobilize the hepatic flexure off of the liver, gallbladder, and duodenum and perform a Kocher maneuver

Identify and free up the SMV behind the pancreas

Now perform cholecystectomy and dissect out the porta hepatis structures—common duct laterally, hepatic artery medially, and portal vein posteriorly

Now that the tumor is deemed resectable, divide the bile duct

Suture ligate and clip the GDA

Divide the stomach

Identify ligament of Treitz and divide jejunum at a convenient point just beyond this structure

Decide on point of transection over the SMV and secure pancreatic arcades with figure-of-eight sutures

Divide pancreas and dissect uncinate process off of retroperitoneum, SMV, and SMA

Mark the retroperitoneal margin and send specimen for analysis

Once all margins are negative, begin reconstruction

Bring the jejunum through the transverse mesocolon to the right of the middle colic vessels

Create pancreaticojejunostomy, hepaticojejunostomy, and gastrojejunostomy

Close any mesenteric defects

Use intraperitoneal drain selectively

Determining Resectability and Freeing Up the Inferior Border of the Pancreas and SMV (Fig. 84.3)

Technical Points

This operation can be performed through an upper-midline incision in the vast majority of patients—bilateral subcostal incisions may provide better exposure in morbidly obese patients with truncated stature. Assess tumor resectability carefully before division of any major structures (in general the stomach, fourth portion of duodenum, and pancreas).

First, inspect the abdomen for metastatic disease. With modern imaging, still approximately 10% to 20% of patients with adenocarcinoma will be found to be unresectable due to M1 disease or vascular invasion. Determining resectability early in the operation will prevent unnecessary dissection or committing to resection too early to later find that the tumor is not resectable. If metastases are found in the liver, peritoneal surfaces/omentum, or distant nodes (e.g., aortacaval nodes), confirm these by frozen-section analysis. It is not necessary to routinely perform extended lymph node dissections for the treatment of pancreatic adenocarcinoma—distant nodes should be evaluated only if suspicious on high quality contrast enhanced CT imaging or MRI.

Once appropriately staged, mobilize the hepatic flexure downward to expose the duodenum and head of the pancreas. Perform a Kocher maneuver, incising the peritoneum lateral to the duodenum. Take care here not to inadvertently injure the right gonadal vein draining into the IVC—this will cause annoying bleeding. Reflect the duodenum and head of the pancreas medially so that the IVC is fully exposed. Palpate the head of the pancreas between your fingers. Note the size and consistency of the head of the pancreas and the size of the tumor mass. It has been demonstrated in multiple randomized controlled trials that doing an extended lymphadenectomy increases morbidity and mortality and does not confer a survival benefit to patients with pancreatic cancer.

Open the gastrocolic omentum by dividing it along the greater curvature of the stomach and remove the greater omentum off of the colon and pass it off of the field. Removing the greater omentum will greatly enhance exposure for the remainder of the operation. The senior surgeon should hold the colon in their hand and protect the transverse mesocolon during the dissection of the inferior border of the pancreas. The SMV is identified by following the middle colic and right gastroepiploic veins as they drain directly into the SMV in close proximity. The gastroepiploic vein can be divided after pancreatic transection—otherwise it often requires two divisions.

Identify the SMV passing deep to the body of the pancreas at the inferior border. By blunt dissection using a Kelly clamp, enter the adventitial plane of the vein and follow it upward under the pancreas. No collateral vein should enter the anterior surface of the SMV from the substance of the pancreas since this plane is normally avascular. Care should be taken to not injury the splenic vein. This maneuver is not done to determine resectability in most cases—this is typically evident on CT imaging. However, creating this tunnel will allow the vessels of the SMV and portal vein and the branches to be protected. It also allows for hemostatic division of the pancreas, which will occur while the SMV is completely protected.

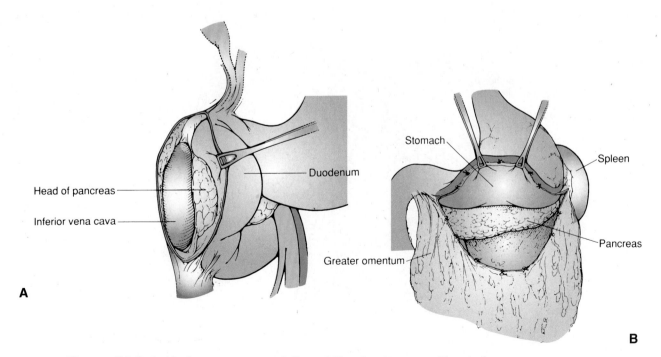

Head of pancreas

Inferior vena cava

Duodenum

A

Stomach

Spleen

Pancreas

Greater omentum

B

Figure 84.3 A: Kocher maneuver to fully mobilize duodenum and head of pancreas **B:** Assessment of resectability.

Anatomic Points

Mobilization of the right colon and performance of the Kocher maneuver should not result in significant bleeding. In both cases, incision and division of the peritoneum is made on the antimesenteric border in an avascular plane that allows blunt dissection and mobilization. As you reflect the duodenum and head of the pancreas, remember that the head of the pancreas and the third portion of the duodenum lie on the IVC, and use appropriate caution during their mobilization to avoid injury to the IVC and right gonadal vein.

The SMV unites with the splenic vein to form the portal vein, which then continues posterior to the duodenum to gain access to the gastroduodenal ligament. The plane between the anterior surface of the SMV or portal vein and the posterior surface of the neck of the pancreas is usually avascular. Small veins, which are smaller than the splenic or IMV but still large enough to cause hemostatic problems, often enter the lateral side of the superior mesenteric—portal vein axis. Thus caution is warranted. In addition, remember that variations in this region are legion; hence, almost any anatomic arrangement can and should be expected.

Dissection of the Porta Hepatis, Bile Duct Division, Hepatic Artery Exposure and Division of the Gastroduodenal Artery, and Stomach Division (Fig. 84.4)

Technical Points

Customary precautions in performing cholecystectomy are warranted—check for a replaced right hepatic artery before bile duct division. Remember that the cystic artery usually lies in the triangle of Calot, regardless of its origin (which is quite variable), and that the location of the union of cystic duct and common hepatic duct is also quite variable. For these reasons, the structures in this area should be dissected to allow adequate visualization before ligation or division. The cystic duct is suture ligated.

When dissecting out the common bile duct, take care to avoid inadvertent injury to the portal vein running posterior to the duct and the proper hepatic artery. Divide the bile duct above the substance of the pancreas—frozen section of the bile duct can be sent at this time to save time later. Stents should be removed and passed off the field—be careful with metal stents that may adhere to tumors distally and if forcefully removed may contaminate the field with tumor cells. The stent can be cut and the distal bile duct oversewed.

Division of the bile duct frees up the portal vein and allows completion of the mobilization of the pancreas off of the SMV. The hepatic artery is then dissected and carefully preserved until all structures are evident—common hepatic artery, GDA, and proper hepatic artery. Always check to be sure there is no GDA-dependent flow to the proper hepatic and suture ligate the GDA. It is important to leave a stump in the case of GDA bleeding or fistulization with the jejunal loop where coiling of the vessel would be required.

Classic pancreatectomy has been compared with pylorus-preserving pancreatectomy in many prospective randomized trials and have been shown to be equivalent with regard to complications and delayed gastric emptying. However, one study demonstrated that with resection of the pyloric ring and

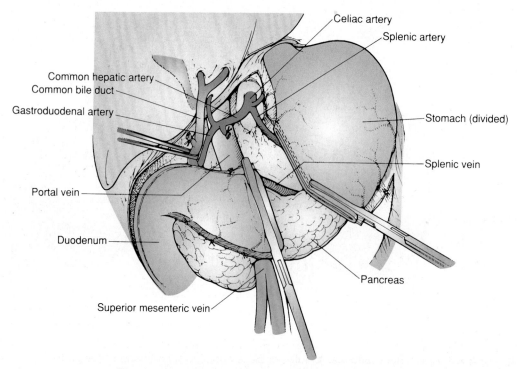

Figure 84.4 Division of the stomach and bile duct

stomach preservation, delayed gastric emptying was significantly reduced. For classic pancreaticoduodenectomy, choose a point of division in the greater curvature of the stomach and divide the stomach with a GIA green load stapler. Divide the vessels in the lesser curvature with the LigaSure device progressing down toward the pylorus. For pylorus preservation, staple just distal to the pylorus. For resection of the pyloric ring with preservation of the stomach, staple just proximal to the pyloric ring. Reconstruction is the same irrespective of the area of transection—an antecolic gastrojejunostomy.

Anatomic Points

The common hepatic artery runs superior to the pancreas and branches into the GDA and the proper hepatic artery. The common hepatic can run posterior to the pancreas and be confused with the GDA—it is critical to test for not only dependent flow to the proper hepatic from the GDA but also to delineate the arterial anatomy to avoid inadvertent injury or division of the proper hepatic artery. The hepatic artery node is found invariably where the common hepatic artery runs superior to the pancreas.

Division of the gastroepiploic arcade has already been accomplished, and because of the collateral circulation at this point, vascular control must be obtained on both sides of division. The same is true of division of the right gastric and left gastric vascular arcades, which lie in the lesser omentum. The arterial and venous arcades parallel the lesser curvature of the stomach and usually lie close to this border of the stomach. Bear in mind that frequently (20% to 35% of cases), this arterial arcade can consist of two parallel arteries because both right and left gastric arteries can divide. In addition, the left gastric artery can supply the left lateral segment of the liver; this variant may provide the major or sole blood supply to this segment. Other than the gastric arcade and portal triad structures in the hepatoduodenal ligament, the lesser omentum contains the vagally derived nerves of Latarjet (in close proximity to the arterial arcade) and the hepatic branch of the anterior vagal trunk. The nerves of Latarjet, which supply the stomach and pyloric region, also must be divided. The hepatic branch of the anterior vagal trunk; however, originates in the vicinity of the esophageal hiatus and traverses the lesser omentum very close to its hepatic attachment. It should not be at risk if the dissection is restricted to the lower, or gastric, part of the hepatogastric ligament.

Division of the Jejunum (Fig. 84.5)

Technical Points

Locate the ligament of Treitz at the base of the transverse mesocolon. Divide the jejunum at a convenient point just below the ligament of Treitz (typically, just lifting the jejunum up to reach the anterior abdominal wall will give enough length for retrocolic reconstruction) (Fig. 84.5A). Take care to avoid injury to the IMV. Mobilize the ligament of Treitz and as much of the duodenum as feasible from the left side of the abdomen. Pass the divided jejunum through, under the transverse mesocolon and mesenteric small bowel, so that it comes out on the same side as the rest of the duodenum. At this point, the duodenum will be swung to the right (Fig. 84.5B).

Anatomic Points

Mention has already been made of the fact that the ligament of Treitz also contains muscle, derived either from the crus of the diaphragm or from the jejunal wall. As a consequence, its mobilization can cause unwanted bleeding unless measures are taken (using clamps or electrocautery) to prevent this. The surface of the mesentery is taken with electrocautery to expose the underlying mesenteric vessels, which can then be divided with the LigaSure device or with suture ligation under direct vision.

Transection of the Body of the Pancreas and the Uncinate Process (Fig. 84.6)

Technical Points

Place figure-of-eight stay sutures in the upper and inferior border of the pancreas in the region of the superior and inferior pancreatic arcades (Fig. 84.6A). Divide the pancreas sharply or with electrocautery (Fig. 84.6B). Identify the pancreatic duct and take care not to cauterize it. Frozen section analysis of the pancreatic duct can be sent at this time from the specimen side. The uncinate process can now be separated from the retroperitoneal structures, SMV, and SMA. Multiple small tributaries in the region of the pancreatic head and uncinate process will need to be secured with fine ligatures or with the LigaSure device (Fig. 84.6C). Proceed with caution to avoid injuring the portal vein or SMV. The SMA is protected during this dissection by the senior surgeon.

The right hepatic artery occasionally arises from the SMA. In this case, it will be encountered in the surgical field. Therefore, identify the origin and termination of any anomalous vessel before division. If you encounter an aberrant right hepatic artery, preserve it especially in jaundiced patients.

Anatomic Points

The location of intrapancreatic arcades has already been discussed in this chapter, as has the location of the pancreatic duct. The multiple small portal tributaries in the pancreatic head and uncinate process drain into the lateral aspect of the SMV—portal vein axis. In addition, the right gastric vein may be encountered, again entering the lateral aspect of the portal vein. Frequently, one can identify the IMV, either entering the SMV or at the angle between the SMV and splenic vein.

The head and uncinate process of the pancreas fill the concavity formed by the C-loop of the pancreas. The head of the pancreas lies cranial and somewhat anterior to the root of the SMA and the termination of the SMV, whereas the uncinate process is inferior and more or less posterior to the superior mesenteric vessels. The blood supply to the head of the pancreas and duodenum is provided by the anastomosing superior pancreaticoduodenal artery (a terminal branch of the GDA, which arises either posterior to the duodenum or slightly more

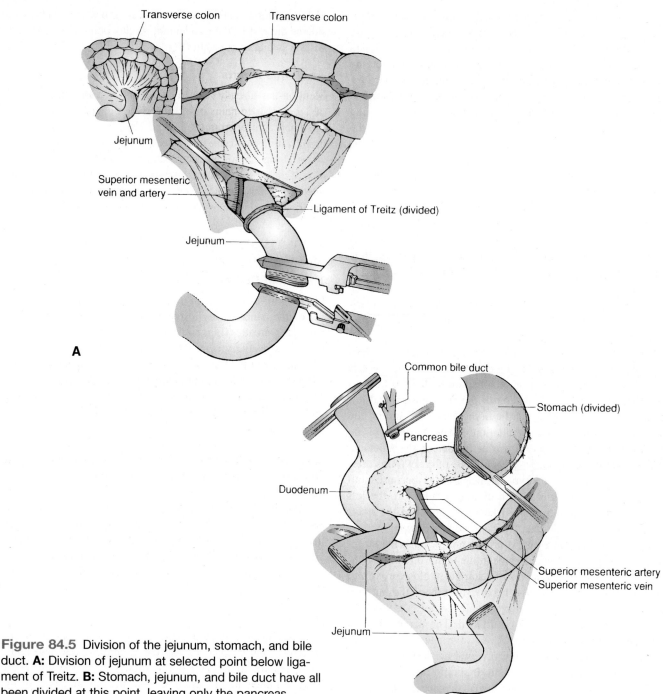

Figure 84.5 Division of the jejunum, stomach, and bile duct. **A:** Division of jejunum at selected point below ligament of Treitz. **B:** Stomach, jejunum, and bile duct have all been divided at this point, leaving only the pancreas.

inferior) and inferior pancreaticoduodenal artery (typically, the first branch of the SMA).

Reconstruction (Fig. 84.7)

Technical and Anatomic Points

Reconstruction is accomplished by a series of three anastomoses: Pancreaticojejunostomy, hepaticojejunostomy, and gastrojejunostomy. Generally, the tail of the pancreas is anastomosed onto the side of the jejunum (Fig. 84.7A). The second anastomosis in line is an end-to-side anastomosis of the bile duct to the jejunum. The third anastomosis consists of the gastrojejunostomy. There have been randomized controlled trials comparing both pancreaticogastrostomy and pancreatic invagination to the classic duct to mucosa pancreaticojejunostomy. Different techniques may be utilized to reduce fistula rates in selected patients at high risk for pancreatic leak.

The jejunum is brought through the transverse mesocolon to the right of the middle colic vein. Be careful not to tear

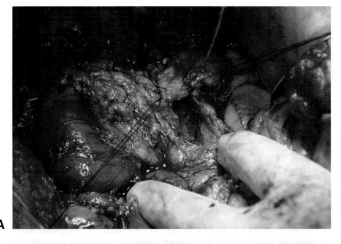

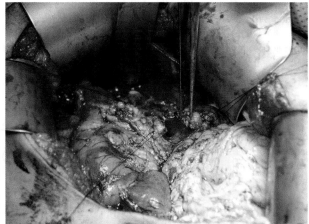

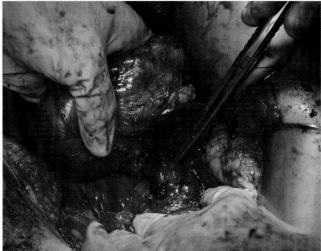

Figure 84.6 Division of the pancreas and mobilization of uncinate process. **A:** Pancreas prepared for division. **B:** Pancreas divided, revealing portal vein and superior mesenteric vein. **C:** Mobilization of uncinate process.

the middle colic vein during manipulation and retraction. The pancreaticojejunostomy is constructed with a duct to mucosa anastomosis. Using a technique described by Blumgart, transpancreatic interrupted 3-0 Vicryl sutures are placed and then through jejunum and back through pancreas and the needle is left in place. The jejunum is opened—take care not to make it too big—it often stretches. Using a pancreatic stent (internal or external) has been studied in several randomized trials with mixed results. The duct to mucosa anastomosis is fashioned with 4-0 or 5-0 PDS. Then the anterior layer is completed with the 3-0 Vicryl sutures—tie them on the pancreas side, go through the jejunum again and tie again.

Make an end-to-side hepaticojejunostomy distal to the pancreaticojejunostomy—be sure there is no tension—there is no specific distance required between these anastomoses (Fig. 84.7B). If the falciform ligament reaches, it can be utilized to cover the stump of the GDA to prevent fistulization or bleeding if there is a pancreatic leak. As the jejunum comes through the transverse mesocolon, fix it with interrupted Vicryl sutures to prevent herniation into the right upper quadrant. This is also a good time to check the transverse mesocolon for defects that

require closure. The ligament of Treitz does not require closure in all patients but should be checked for a large defect.

Construct the gastrojejunostomy 40 cm downstream from the biliary anastomosis in standard two-layer fashion (Fig. 84.7C). This can also be stapled. Position a drain to gravity if indicated in select patients and try to remove early if amylase levels are <5,000 U/mL. Double and triple check all anatomy before closure. Irrigate well if tumor was encountered during the resection either when dividing the pancreas, bile duct, or retroperitoneal margin or if the patient had a preoperative biliary stent. Reconstruction after pylorus-preserving pancreaticoduodenectomy is shown in Figure 84.8.

Central Pancreatectomy and Total Pancreatectomy

These procedures are beyond the scope of this chapter; however, they should be within the arsenal of all pancreatic surgeons. There are some references below that address these operations and their indications and technique.

Aspirate about 100 mL of cyst fluid and then inject 50 to 100 mL of water-soluble contrast material and obtain a radiograph. This will demonstrate the anatomy of the cyst and whether or not there are septations that must be treated. Depending on the adequacy of preoperative studies, this step may be omitted. Place stay sutures in the posterior gastric wall and prepare to make an incision into the back wall of the stomach.

Anatomic Points

The anatomic relationships of the pancreas, the location of the pancreatic pseudocyst, and the anatomic fusion of adjacent organs in response to inflammation allow internal drainage of pancreatic pseudocysts.

The head of the pancreas lies in the duodenal curve. Superiorly, it is overlapped anteriorly by the first part of the duodenum; elsewhere, its margin is indented by the duodenum. Its anterior anatomic relationships include the first part of the duodenum, the gastroduodenal artery (which makes a groove in the pancreas that delineates head from neck), the transverse mesocolon, and the jejunum. Posteriorly, the head of the pancreas lies on the right diaphragmatic crus, the inferior vena cava and terminal segments of the renal veins, and the aorta. The inferior part of the head is continuous with the uncinate process, which lies in the space between the superior mesenteric vessels and the aorta. The bile duct is either posterior to the head of the pancreas or embedded within the substance of this gland.

The neck of the pancreas begins on the right at the groove from the gastroduodenal artery and merges insensibly with the body. Anteriorly, it is related to the pylorus and omental bursa. Posteriorly, it is related to the superior mesenteric and splenic veins, which join to form the portal vein.

Anteriorly, the body of the pancreas is separated from the stomach by the omental bursa (lesser sac), and its peritoneal covering is continuous with the anterior leaf of the transverse mesocolon. Posteriorly, the body is in contact with the aorta, the beginning of the superior mesenteric artery, the left diaphragmatic crus, the left suprarenal gland, the left kidney and renal vessels, and the splenic vein. The inferior aspect of the body is in contact with the duodenojejunal flexure, coils of jejunum, and the left colic flexure. Where it is not in direct contact with these organs, the peritoneum covering it is directly continuous with the transverse mesocolon.

The tail of the pancreas is the narrow left termination of the pancreas. It extends to the splenic surface at the hilum. The tail lies in the lienorenal ligament and is in contact with the splenic flexure of the colon. Posteriorly, it is in contact with the left kidney.

In summary, remember that the pancreas is a retroperitoneal organ whose head is inferior to the root of the transverse mesocolon, but whose body and tail are predominantly superior to the transverse mesocolon. Thus the body and tail are posterior to the peritoneum of the lesser sac and to the stomach. Because of these anatomic relationships, inflammatory processes involving the body and tail of the pancreas can easily result in adhesions between the pancreas and the posterior wall of the stomach.

The major blood supply to the stomach is provided by the gastric artery arcade along the lesser curvature, the gastroepiploic arcade along the greater curvature, and the short gastric arteries to the fundus. Thus the anterior gastrotomy should be located about halfway between the greater and lesser curvatures to avoid dividing large vessels that could cause troublesome bleeding.

Construction of a Cyst Gastrostomy (Fig. 86.3)

Technical and Anatomic Points

Incise the back wall of the stomach and puncture through into the cysts with electrocautery or by poking through with a clamp. Decompress the cyst with suction. The retroperitoneal area should become completely flat so that no residual masses are palpable. If a residual mass is palpable, the possibility of a second pseudocyst should be considered. If a second pseudocyst is found, it, too, must be drained. Enlarge the opening in the back wall of the stomach until it is several centimeters across. Take a full-thickness piece of the back wall of the stomach and the anterior wall of the cyst for biopsy. Check the edges of the incision for hemostasis. Use electrocautery and suture ligatures to achieve hemostasis in the edge.

Place a running lockstitch of 2-0 Vicryl around the entire anastomosis to ensure adequate hemostasis. Note that this anastomosis is actually simply a fenestration. The inflammatory

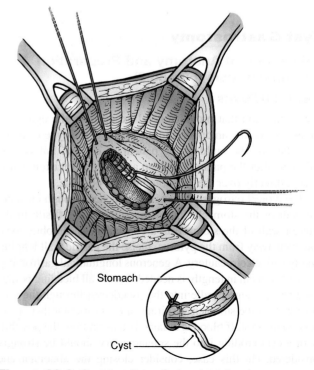

Stomach

Cyst

Figure 86.3 Construction of a cyst gastrostomy

process in the lesser sac creates a fusion between the anterior wall of the pseudocyst and the back wall of the stomach. The suture is placed purely for hemostasis. At the conclusion of the procedure, hemostasis must be absolute. The retroperitoneum should be collapsed, and no residual masses should be palpable. A nasogastric tube should lie comfortably within the stomach.

Close the gastrotomy in two layers by suture or by application of a linear stapling device. Place omentum over the gastrotomy.

Cyst Duodenostomy

Construction of Cyst Duodenostomy (Fig. 86.4)

Technical Points

Cyst duodenostomy is performed when a pseudocyst in the head of the pancreas is not in proximity to the back wall of the stomach. It is a procedure of second choice (after drainage to a Roux-en-Y loop of jejunum). It is more hazardous than cyst gastrostomy because of the potential for damage to the intraduodenal bile duct. Occasionally, it is the only way to drain a cyst.

STEPS IN PROCEDURE—CYST DUODENOSTOMY

Upper midline or chevron incision

Explore abdomen and confirm cyst adherent to duodenum but not stomach

Fully mobilize duodenum (Kocher maneuver)

Open bile duct and place no. 3 Bakes dilator or other cannula through ampulla

Two stay sutures on anterior surface of duodenum over ampulla

Generous longitudinal duodenotomy

Choose site for cyst duodenostomy away from ampulla (usually medial to ampulla)

Aspirate to confirm cyst and exclude blood in cyst

Create opening into cyst

Perform full-thickness biopsy of cyst wall

Running lockstitch to oversew cyst duodenostomy (avoid ampulla)

Close duodenostomy and cover with omentum

Close abdomen without drains

HALLMARK ANATOMIC COMPLICATIONS—CYST DUODENOSTOMY

Injury to bile duct

Premature closure with recurrence of cyst

Perform a Kocher maneuver, if possible, to elevate the duodenum and head of the pancreas into the surgical field. Open the bile duct and place a probe within it if there is any uncertainty about the relationship of the bile duct to the cyst. Incise the anterior wall of the duodenum over the cyst. Place stay sutures on the back wall of the duodenum. Make certain that you know where the bile duct lies within the surgical field.

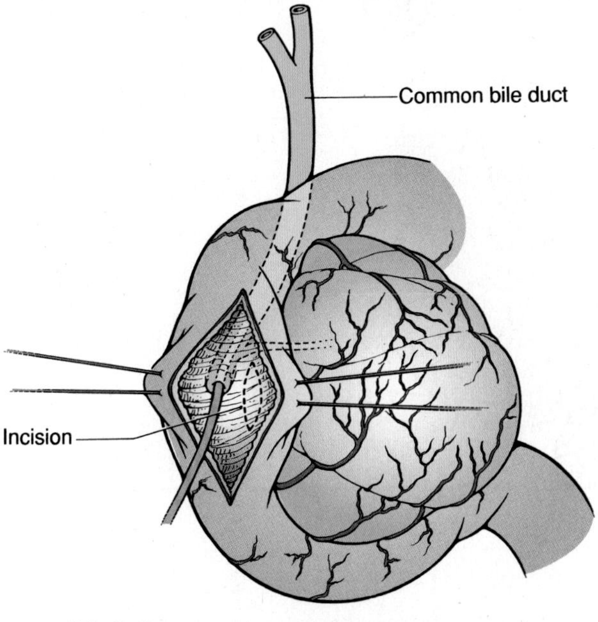

Make an opening into the pseudocyst through the back wall of the duodenum. Perform an anastomosis in a similar fashion to that outlined for cyst gastrostomy. Perform a cholangiogram at the conclusion of the procedure to verify that no injury to the bile duct has occurred.

Close the duodenostomy in two layers. Cover the duodenal suture line with omentum.

Anatomic Points

The infrapyloric segment of the bile duct is close to the duodenal edge of the pancreas. Here, it is either retropancreatic or, more commonly, bridged posteriorly by pancreatic tissue. When the duodenum and pancreas are mobilized by the Kocher maneuver, this duct can be seen to be more closely associated with the parietal surface of the pancreas than with the peritoneal surface.

Roux-en-Y Drainage of a Pseudocyst

Roux-en-Y Drainage of a Pseudocyst (Fig. 86.5)

Technical Points

Expose the pseudocyst, which is generally located in the inferior portion of the lesser sac. Elevate the transverse colon and examine an avascular portion of the transverse mesocolon. If the pseudocyst can be identified in this region, this is the most convenient area for anastomosis. Confirm the location of the pseudocyst by palpation and by aspiration with an 18-gauge needle.

Figure 86.4 Construction of cyst duodenostomy

Common bile duct

Incision

STEPS IN PROCEDURE—ROUX-EN-Y DRAINAGE OF PSEUDOCYST

Upper midline or chevron incision

Explore abdomen and confirm location of pseudocyst

   Ideal location is in inferior region of lesser sac, approachable through transverse mesocolon

Aspirate cyst to confirm location and exclude bloody contents

Identify mobile region of proximal jejunum and divide

Open pseudocyst, taking full-thickness biopsy of cyst wall

Anastomose jejunum to cyst wall

Complete construction of Roux-en-Y

Double check hemostasis

Place omentum around anastomosis

Consider closed-suction drains in proximity of anastomosis

Close abdomen in usual fashion

HALLMARK ANATOMIC COMPLICATIONS—ROUX-EN-Y DRAINAGE OF A PSEUDOCYST

Leakage from anastomosis

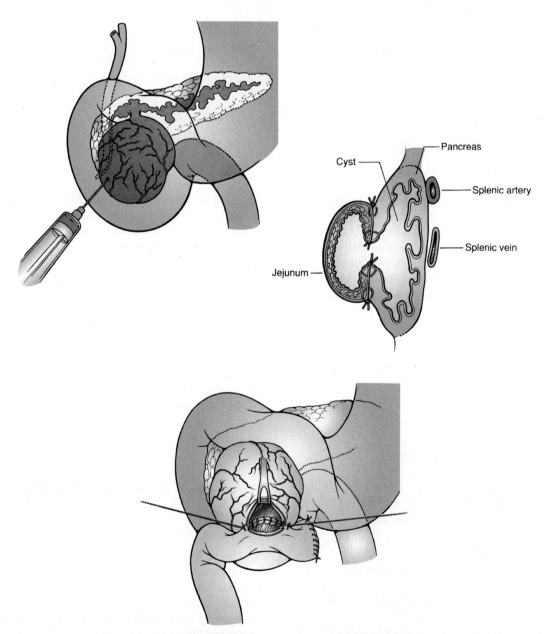

Figure 86.5 Roux-en-Y drainage of a pseudocyst

Construct a Roux-en-Y loop of jejunum. Place stay sutures into the pseudocyst in a dependent region. Make an opening into the pseudocyst and aspirate the cyst fluid. Obtain a full-thickness biopsy specimen of the wall of the pseudocyst. Construct a two-layer anastomosis between the pseudocyst and the blind end of the Roux loop. Use interrupted 3-0 silk for the outer layer and interrupted 3-0 Vicryl for the inner layer. In contrast to the cyst gastrostomy and cyst duodenostomy procedures previously described, this anastomosis is surgically created because previous fusion of the cyst to the Roux loop has not occurred. Therefore, the anastomosis must be constructed with the same meticulous care with which any intestinal anastomosis is performed. Do not stent the anastomosis.

Place omentum around the anastomosis. Closed-suction drains may be placed in the vicinity of the anastomosis, if desired, but are not necessary.

Anatomic Points

Because the pseudocyst is most often located in the inferior portion of the omental bursa, the most logical route to the cyst is through the posterior leaf of the transverse mesocolon. Exposure of the posterior leaf of transverse mesocolon is accomplished by elevating the transverse colon. If possible, place the Roux limb to the left of the middle colic artery, where the transverse mesocolon is essentially avascular.

REFERENCES

1. Aljarabah M, Ammori BJ. Laparoscopic and endoscopic approaches for drainage of pancreatic pseudocysts: A systematic review of published series. *Surg Endosc.* 2007;21:1936–1944.

2. Behrns KE, Ben-David K. Surgical therapy of pancreatic pseudocysts. *J Gastrointest Surg.* 2008;12:2231.

3. Bergman S, Melvin WS. Operative and nonoperative management of pancreatic pseudocysts. *Surg Clin North Am.* 2007;87:1447.

4. Cannon JW, Callery MP, Vollmer CM Jr. Diagnosis and management of pancreatic pseudocysts: What is the evidence? *J Am Coll Surg.* 2009;209:385.

5. Dissanike S, Frezza EE. Minimally invasive open cystgastrostomy for pancreatic pseudocysts. *Minerva Chir.* 2006;61:455–458.

6. Heniford BT, Iannitti Da, Paton BL, et al. Minilaparoscopic transgastric cystgastrostomy. *Am J Surg.* 2006;192:248–251.

7. Ito K, Perez A, Ito H, et al. Pancreatic pseudocysts: Is delayed surgical intervention associated with adverse outcomes? *J Gastrointest Surg.* 2007;11:1317–1321.

8. Johnson LB, Rattner DW, Warshaw AL. The effect of size of giant pancreatic pseudocysts on the outcome of internal drainage procedures. *Surg Gynecol Obstet.* 1991;173:171.

9. Kuroda A, Konishi T, Kimura W, et al. Cystopancreaticostomy and longitudinal pancreaticojejunostomy as a simpler technique of combined drainage operation for chronic pancreatitis with pancreatic pseudocyst causing persistent cholecystasis. *Surg Gynecol Obstet.* 1993;177:183.

10. Lohr-Happe A, Peiper M, Lankisch PG. Natural course of operated pseudocysts in chronic pancreatitis. *Gut.* 1994;35:1479.

11. Taghizadeh F, Bower RJ, Kiesewetter WB. Stapled cystogastrostomy: A method of treatment for pediatric pancreatic pseudocyst. *Ann Surg.* 1979;190:166.

12. Vitale GC, Lawhon JC, Larson GM, et al. Endoscopic drainage of the pancreatic pseudocyst. *Surgery.* 1999;126:616–623. (Presents alternative method of drainage.)

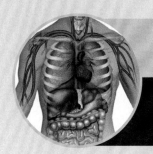

87

Pancreatic Necrosectomy (Open and Laparoscopic)

Severe (necrotizing) pancreatitis results in collections of necrotic tissue in the retroperitoneum. When these become infected, antibiotics and drainage are required. In the majority of cases, drainage can be accomplished percutaneously. When repeated percutaneous drainage fails, surgical debridement of the dead tissue and drainage is the next step.

Decision making is complex and is discussed in references at the end of the chapter.

This chapter presents open necrosectomy first, followed by laparoscopic necrosectomy. This is done to illustrate the nature of the problem. In practice, laparoscopic necrosectomy has been associated with a lower mortality rate than the equivalent open drainage and is the preferred method of management when possible. The laparoscopic procedure can be repeated multiple times, if necessary, to attain adequate control of the necrotizing infectious process.

Experienced gastrointestinal endoscopists have also employed another procedure—endoscopic transgastric drainage. This is referenced at the end.

SCORE™, the Surgical Council on Resident Education, classified open pancreatic debridement for necrosis as an "ESSENTIAL UNCOMMON" and laparoscopic/endoscopic debridement for necrosis as a "COMPLEX" procedure.

STEPS IN PROCEDURE

Open Drainage

Midline or chevron incision

Thorough exploration

Identify region where necrosis is "pointing" to the peritoneal cavity

    Avascular region of transverse colon mesentery

Enter the collection and obtain cultures

Follow all tongues of necrosis to obtain adequate drainage

    Lesser sac toward hilum of spleen

    Behind head of pancreas

Debride all easily removable tissue

Place drains or pack open

HALLMARK ANATOMIC COMPLICATIONS

Inadequate drainage

Fistula formation

Bleeding from splenic artery or other regional vessel

LIST OF STRUCTURES

Pancreas

Colon

    Transverse colon

    Middle colic artery and vein

Spleen

    Splenic artery

Stomach

    Gastroduodenal artery

Duodenum

Open Drainage of Pancreatic Necrosis (Fig. 87.1)

Technical and Anatomic Points

After induction of anesthesia, palpate the abdomen. Often an upper abdominal mass is palpable. Make an incision that will provide best access to this mass. In a very narrow-chested individual, an upper midline incision will work well. For the majority of patients, an extended left subcostal or bilateral subcostal incision will be the best approach.

Thoroughly explore the abdomen. Commonly there will be free fluid. Culture this. The peritoneal surfaces may be studded with nodules that resemble metastatic disease. These represent "fat necrosis" or "saponification" from pancreatic enzymes.

Generally, the necrotizing process is limited to the peripancreatic region, but in extreme cases it may extend down the right or left gutter behind the colon. Figure 87.1A shows the common extent of necrosis. Seek a place where the abscess appears to be "pointing", that is, where it is close to the peritoneal cavity.

Often this is at the root of the transverse colon. Lift the transverse colon and omentum to expose the root of the mesentery. Look for discoloration or a firm or (less likely) fluctuant area. Identify and avoid the middle colic artery and vein (use intraoperative Doppler ultrasound to find the artery, if

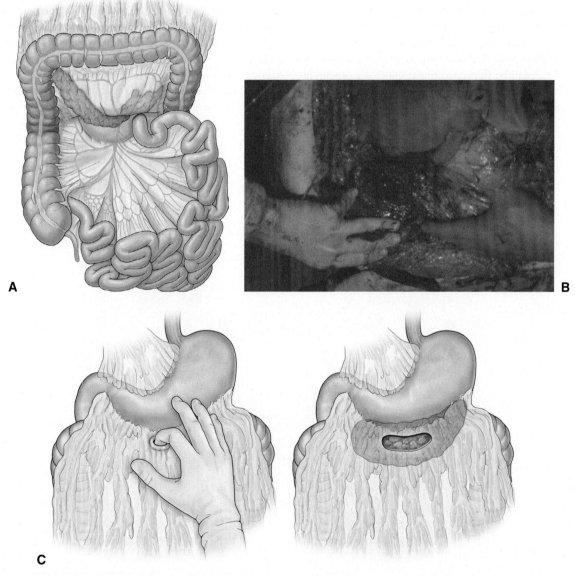

A

B

C

Figure 87.1 A: Extent of necrotizing process in the common situation. **B:** Debrided cavity at root of transverse colon mesentery. **C:** Alternative approach through the gastrocolic omentum (Figure **A** and **C** from Howard TJ. Chapter 130. Necrosectomy for acute necrotizing pancreatitis. In: Fischer JE, ed. *Fischer's Mastery of Surgery.* Philadelphia, PA: Wolters Kluwer Lippincott Williams & Wilkins, 2013, with permission).

necessary) and poke into the collection with a closed hemostat. Obtain cultures. The space is generally filled with semisolid necrotic tissue that needs to be wiped and pulled out. The tissue will have a texture between clay and fibrous seaweed. A sponge forceps is an excellent grasping tool for removing this tissue. Multiple vessels in the retroperitoneum (see Chapter 84, Figure 84.1), such as the splenic artery, may cross this space and thus debridement must be done firmly but carefully. It is rarely possible to remove all necrotic tissue (Fig. 87.1B). The goal is to open all of the fingers that extend into various recesses of the retroperitoneum.

Make sure that you identify any finger-like projection that follows the tail of the pancreas into the splenic hilum. Similarly, seek collections behind the head of the pancreas.

If the collection does not appear to "point" anywhere, then open the gastrocolic omentum into the lesser sac (Fig. 87.1C). Secure the branches of the gastroepiploic artery and vein with ties. Generally the transverse colon will have been pushed inferiorly, out of harm's way, but take care to keep the colon out of the way. There will be thickened tissue under the omentum and, once again, it is usually necessary to poke into the collection with a hemostat. Once you have gained entry into the collection, debride and explore all loculations as previously described.

Depending upon the extent of necrosis and the patient's physiologic condition, either place large-diameter suction drains or pack ("marsupialize") the cavity and leave the abdomen open (see Chapter 44). Packing can be changed at the bedside in intensive care. Marsupialization is associated with a high rate of fistula formation, but may be lifesaving in extreme cases.

Laparoscopic Drainage (Fig. 87.2)

Technical and Anatomic Points

Laparoscopic drainage commonly uses the laparoscope to provide visualization of a widened tract into the cavity, allowing debridement and irrigation and drain placement. It is more properly termed "minimally invasive video-assisted" drainage. It is most easily performed after a drain has produced access into the cavity. This drain demonstrates a safe window into the cavity that does not traverse viscera or vessels.

Position the patient with the entry site of the drain and the midline of the abdomen accessible. Generally this will involve

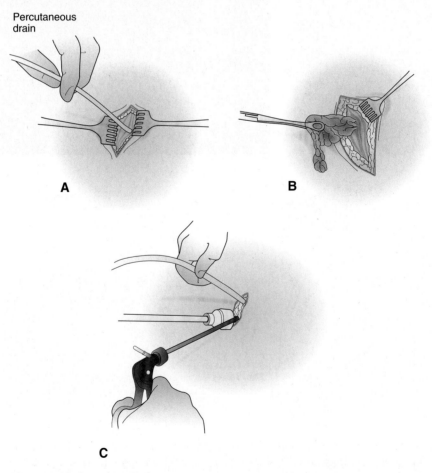

Figure 87.2 A: Small flank incision has been made around skin entry site of percutaneous drain. **B:** Drain tract has been enlarged and necrosis is being removed. **C:** Laparoscope is used to inspect and irrigate the resulting cavity.

placing the patient on a beanbag to elevate the entry site in a partial lateral position.

Make a small incision along the drain (Fig. 87.2A) and deepen this through muscle and fascia, always following the drain. Once sufficient depth has been attained, you will enter the necrotic cavity. Debride tissue with ring forceps and explore the cavity digitally as much as possible (Fig. 87.2B). Then use the laparoscope to guide further debridement, irrigation, and drain placement (Figure 78.2C).

REFERENCES

1. Castellanos G, Pinero A, Doig LA, et al. Management of infected pancreatic necrosis using retroperitoneal necrosectomy with flexible endoscope: 10 years of experience. *Surg Endosc.* 2012; 27:443–453 (epub ahead of print).
2. Freeman ML, Werner J, van Santvoort HC, et al. Interventions for necrotizing pancreatitis: Summary of a multidisciplinary consensus conference. *Pancreas.* 2012;41:1176. (Results of an international consensus conference.)
3. Horvath KD, Dao LS, Wherry KL, et al. A technique for laparoscopic-assisted percutaneous drainage of infected pancreatic necrosis and pancreatic abscess. *Surg Endosc.* 2001;15:1221.
4. Mouli VP, Sreenivas V, Garg PK. Efficacy of conservative treatment without necrosectomy, for infected pancreatic necrosis: A systematic review and meta-analysis. *Gastroenterology.* 2012 (epub ahead of print).
5. The Society for Surgery of the Alimentary Tract. SSAT Patient Care Guidelines. Treatment of Acute Pancreatitis. Available online at: http://www.ssat.com/cgi-bin/acupanc6.cgi (accessed December 2012).
6. Van Santvoort HC, Besselink MGH, Horvath KD, et al. Videoscopic assisted retroperitoneal debridement in infected necrotizing pancreatitis. *HPT (Oxford).* 2007;9:156.
7. Warshaw AL. Improving the treatment of necrotizing pancreatitis— a step up. *N Engl J Med.* 2010;362:1535.
8. Wong VW, Chan FK. Endoscopic pancreatic necrosectomy: Notes of excitement. *Gastroenterology.* 2012;143:1114.

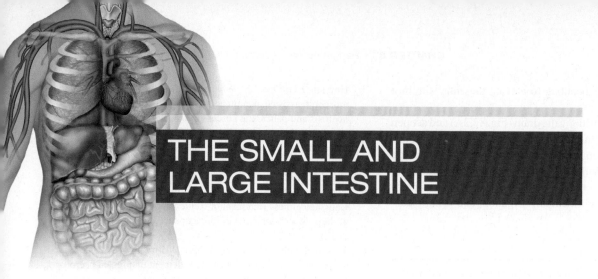

THE SMALL AND LARGE INTESTINE

In this section, common operations performed on the small and large intestine are described. First, operations for small bowel obstruction and superior mesenteric artery embolism are described. Small bowel resection and anastomosis are detailed in Chapter 90 in which the technique of double-layered, hand-sewn anastomosis is introduced; strictureplasty for Crohn disease is also described. Subsequent chapters deal with pediatric problems involving the small bowel, as well as with loop ileostomy and laparoscopic procedures. The general topography of the small intestine and the differences between the jejunum and the ileum have already been illustrated in previous chapters.

The appendix, a diverticulum of the gastrointestinal tract of uncertain significance, is described in Chapters 94 and 95 in which the common operations of traditional and laparoscopic appendectomy are presented. Because the operation for appendicitis sometimes discloses an unexpected Meckel diverticulum, the procedures for resection of this diverticulum are included in these chapters.

As in other sections, endoscopy is used to introduce the topography and general layout of the colon (Chapter 96). This introduction to the colon is further expanded in the discussions of colostomy and colostomy closure (Chapters 97 and 98e), often the first operations on the large intestine performed during surgical training. In Chapter 99, the blood supply and mesenteries of the colon are described. Finally, chapters on laparoscopic colostomy, open and laparoscopic colon resections, and right and left colon resections (Chapters 99 and 100) complete this part. Low anterior resection for carcinoma of the rectum is described in conjunction with abdominoperineal resection (Chapters 101 and 102e) in the next part, *The Pelvis*.

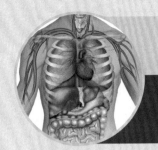

88

Operations for Small Bowel Obstruction

Adhesions are the most common cause of small bowel obstruction in the United States and other westernized countries. When adhesive small bowel obstruction fails to resolve with bowel rest and intravenous fluids, laparotomy or laparoscopy may be required. Surgery is generally required for the other causes (hernia, carcinoma, stricture). The first part of this chapter deals with open laparotomy for small bowel obstruction. The skills described here are also used whenever the abdomen must be opened after previous abdominal surgery. The chapter concludes with a discussion of laparoscopic lysis of adhesions.

SCORE™, the Surgical Council on Resident Education, classified open and laparoscopic adhesiolysis as "ESSENTIAL COMMON" procedures.

STEPS IN PROCEDURE

Open the abdomen through a site above or
    below the old incision if possible
      If necessary, open through upper part of
        old incision
Carefully lyse adhesions to underside of
    abdominal wall
Lyse adhesions between loops of
    bowel
Identify the obstructive mechanism
    and release it

Consider side-to-side bypass in difficult situations
    Choose a dilated proximal and collapsed
      distal segment
    Ensure there is no additional obstruction
      downstream
    Create sutured or stapled side-to-side
      anastomosis
Assess bowel for viability and injuries
Repair any injuries, resect nonviable bowel
Close incision in usual fashion

HALLMARK ANATOMIC COMPLICATIONS

Injury to bowel
Missed obstruction

LIST OF STRUCTURES

Small intestine
    Jejunum
    Ileum
Ligament of Treitz

Opening the Abdomen (Fig. 88.1)

If opening the abdomen after a previous midline incision, extend the incision into fresh territory cephalad or caudad if possible (Fig. 88.1A). Be sure that the incision will provide you with good access to the presumed point of obstruction on preoperative imaging studies. If the old incision extends from xiphoid to pubis, it is generally best to re-enter the abdomen through the upper aspect, where only the liver and stomach are likely to be encountered, rather than loops of small bowel.

If the previous incision was made elsewhere in the abdominal wall (e.g., a right lower quadrant incision for appendicitis), make a short midline incision near the likely site of obstruction.

Elevate the abdomen by lifting up strongly on the incision on your side (and have your assistant lift up opposite to you) and enter the peritoneal cavity with care, using scalpel (see Chapter 44). Be aware that adhesions tend to form to suture material, so there are often dense adhesions to the underside of the incision. In extreme cases, entering the abdomen just lateral to a dense adhesion (Fig. 88.1B) and allowing a small nubbin of fascia to remain adherent to a loop of bowel may prevent enterotomy. This nubbin can then be debrided during the enterolysis part of the operation.

Once a clear window has been formed, it may be possible to open the fascia with cautery in the usual fashion. Be aware

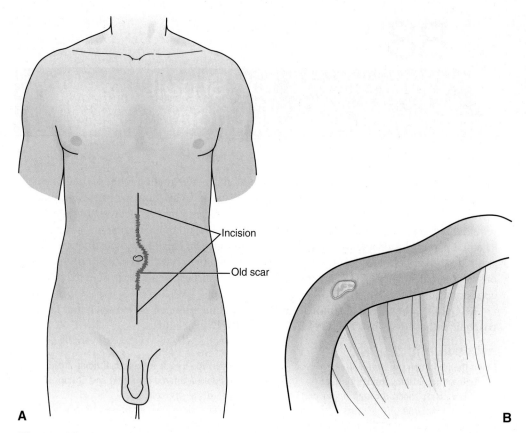

A   B

Figure 88.1 A: Enter the abdomen through a fresh area above or below the old incision. **B:** Leave a small nubbin of fascia adherent to the bowel to avoid injuring the bowel.

that a collapsed loop of bowel may be adherent to the inferior aspect of the incision where it is easily mistaken for peritoneum and injured during entry.

Enterolysis and Identification of Site of Obstruction (Fig. 88.2)

First, concentrate on lysing adhesions of bowel to abdominal wall. Have your assistant elevate the abdominal wall by pulling on Kocher or Allis clamps placed on the fascial edges and carefully take down the adherent loops of bowel with Metzenbaum scissors or scalpel, insinuating your hand behind each loop of bowel if possible. Gentle downward traction on the loop will then usually reveal the adhesion that needs to be divided (Fig. 88.2A). In most cases, the adhesions become less dense as the dissection progresses away from the incision. Once the block of small intestine has been freed from the abdominal wall, place fixed retractors.

It is prudent to keep the area you are working upon isolated with laparotomy pads, and to have a Yankauer suction close at hand. Inadvertant enterotomy during dissection may result in copious spillage of the liquid contents of the obstructed bowel.

Next, lyse adhesions between loops of bowel by similarly insinuating your finger behind the adhesion and displaying it for division with electrocautery or Metzenbaum scissors (Fig. 88.2B). At all times be alert for the point of obstruction.

If the preoperative imaging studies showed a clear transition between proximal dilated bowel and distal collapsed bowel, then a discrete point of obstruction (often a single adhesive band) will be found. Carefully inspect the bowel at the site of obstruction for viability; in extreme cases, pressure from the obstructing band will have caused localized necrosis (in a ring-like fashion) of the trapped bowel. Continue to lyse all adhesions from the ligament of Treitz to the ileocecal valve.

Wherever possible, keep the bowel within the abdomen and expose only the area that you are working upon. Bowel hanging out over the edge of the incision is apt to swell, making assessment of viability and subsequent closure difficult.

Inspect all the bowel for viability and injuries (see the following section). Injuries are best repaired after all bowel has been lysed, unless suture is necessary to prevent continued leakage of succus.

If the viability of the bowel is questionable, allow it to rest in a comfortable position within the peritoneal cavity. If the bowel is not viable, resect and perform an end-to-end anastomosis (see Chapter 90).

Repairing Injured Bowel (Fig. 88.3)

Partial and full-thickness injuries are unfortunately common and need assessment and repair. Repair is best performed after

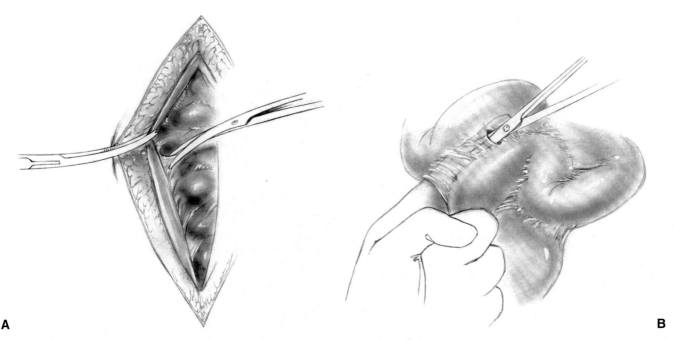

A   **B**

Figure 88.2 A: Lyse adhesions of bowel to underside of abdomen sharply. **B:** Then lyse adhesions between loops of bowel.

all adhesions have been lysed, and if a short segment of bowel is severely damaged, segmental resection may be the best approach.

Partial thickness injuries require repair if they extend into or through the submucosa. Assess this by holding the loop of bowel in your hands and gently squeezing to increase the intra-luminal pressure in the loop (Fig. 88.3A). If the bowel balloons out at the site of injury, repair it by reapproximating the outer layers with simple interrupted silk sutures (Fig. 88.3B). If the bowel does not balloon out, the injury may not be deep enough to require repair. It is better to err on the side of repair than to have to deal with a delayed perforation.

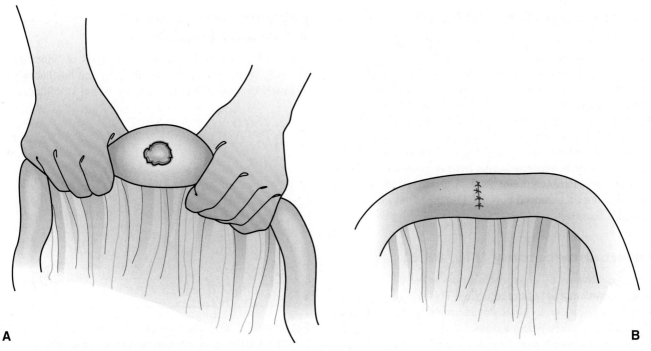

A   **B**

Figure 88.3 A: Test partial thickness injuries to assess need for repair. **B:** Repair with simple interrupted sutures.

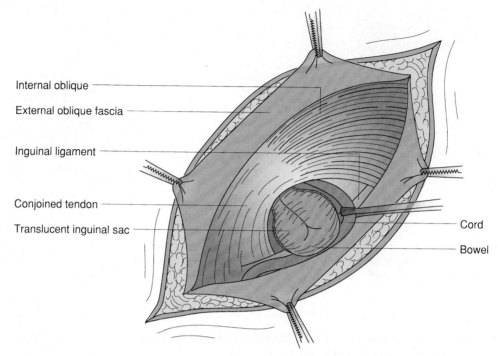

Figure 88.4 Trapped loop of bowel within groin hernia (from Mulholland MW, ed. *Greenfield's Surgery.* 5th ed. Philadelphia, PA: Lippincott Williams & Wilkins, 2011).

Full thickness injuries always require repair or resection. Small injuries may be debrided and closed with bowel sutures in the usual fashion. Larger injuries may be best treated by segmental resection.

Incarcerated Hernia (Fig. 88.4)

Generally, the diagnosis of an incarcerated hernia will have been made prior to surgery, either from physical examination or from imaging studies. Approach an incarcerated groin hernia through the groin. It may be necessary to enlarge the hernia ring to adequately assess the bowel and perform resection if necessary. See Chapter 115 for more tips on management.

Under rare circumstances, an undiagnosed hernia will be found at laparotomy to be the cause of obstruction. These may be internal hernias, incisional hernias, or hernias through unusual sites (such as obturator hernias). Gently dilate the hernia ring and reduce the trapped bowel. Close the hernia defect with a patch if necessary.

Enteroenterostomy (Fig. 88.5)

Sometimes bypass by enteroenterostomy is the wisest course, rather than attempt at lysis or resection. This is particularly true with obstruction due to nonresectable malignancy or in cases of radiation enteritis. Select a dilated loop just proximal to the obstruction and a collapsed loop distal to all obstruction. Make sure that these loops can be comfortable brought together and that there are no further obstructions distal to the chosen site.

One strategy to ensure this in difficult circumstances is to anastomose to transverse colon.

Place the two loops of bowel side by side and create a handsewn or stapled enteroenterostomy as shown.

Laparoscopic Lysis of Adhesions (Fig. 88.6)

The ideal candidate for laparoscopic lysis of adhesions has an easily identified point of obstruction and has had a period of bowel decompression (so that the bowel is collapsed). An

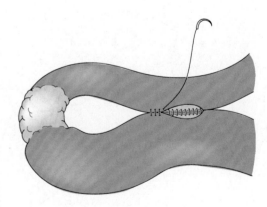

Figure 88.5 Bypass enteroenterostomy for complicated situations such as unresectable tumor or radiation damage (from Mulholland MW, ed. *Greenfield's Surgery.* 5th ed. Philadelphia, PA: Lippincott Williams & Wilkins, 2011).

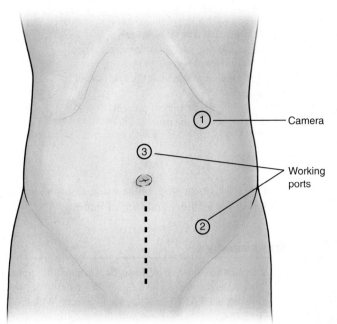

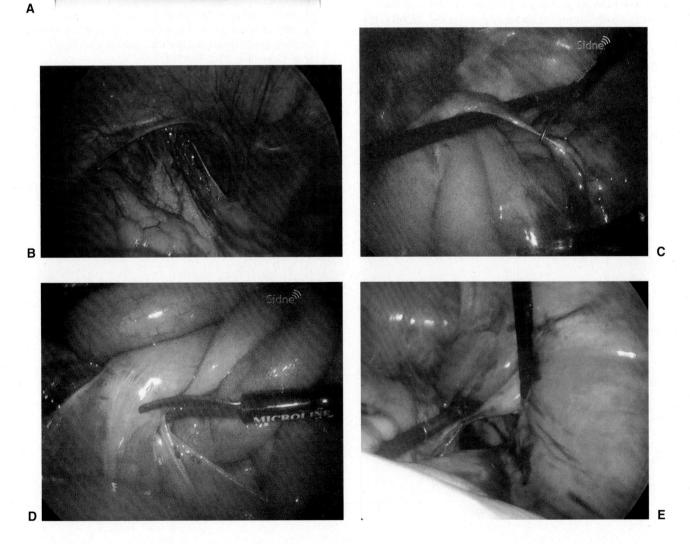

Figure 88.6 Laparoscopic lysis of adhesions. **A:** Place trocars away from old incision. **B:** Adhesions to underside of abdominal wall (incisional hernia). **C:** Dividing obstructing band. **D:** Dividing broad adhesion. **E:** Internal hernia (obstructed bowel has been reduced) (parts **A, C, D, E** from Fischer JF, ed. *Mastery of Surgery.* 6th ed. Philadelphia, PA: Lippincott Williams & Wilkins, 2012).

example of such a situation would be a patient with adhesive obstruction after gynecologic surgery.

Place trocars away from the incision (Fig. 88.6A), taking care not to create further damage as you enter the abdomen. Often, open entry with a Hasson cannula (see Chapter 46, Figure 46.2) is the safest approach. Explore the abdomen.

Adhesions to the underside of the abdominal wall are easily identified and lysed, as the pneumoperitoneum will increase the distance between bowel and peritoneum, allowing these to essentially "hang" from the abdominal wall (Fig. 88.6B). It is safest to divide these sharply, avoiding the use of hook cautery to avoid injury to the bowel.

After identifying and dividing the obstructing band (Fig. 88.6C) or adhesion (Fig. 88.6D), carefully run the bowel. Experienced laparoscopists can deal with more complex situations such as internal hernias (Fig. 88.6E). Remember that the hernia defect must be closed to prevent recurrence.

Close the trocar sites in the usual fashion after rechecking the bowel for viability and lack of injuries.

REFERENCES

1. Britt LD, Collins J, Pickelman JR. Chapter 142. Small and large bowel obstruction. In: *Fischer's Mastery of Surgery*. 6th ed. Philadelphia, PA: Wolters Kluwer Lippincott Williams & Wilkins; 2013:1542.
2. Maung AA, Johnson DC, Piper GL, et al. Evaluation and management of small-bowel obstruction: An Eastern Association for the Surgery of Trauma practice management guideline. *J Trauma Acute Care Surg*. 2012;73:S362.
3. Meissner K. Late radiogenic small bowel damage: Guidelines for the general surgeon. *Dig Surg*. 1999;16:169.
4. Simmons JD, Rogers EA, Porter JM, et al. The role of laparoscopy in small bowel obstruction after previous laparotomy for trauma: An initial report. *Am Surg*. 2011;77:185.

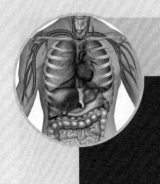

89

Mesenteric Revascularization with Superior Mesenteric Artery Embolectomy and Other Strategies

Rachael Nicholson and Jose E. Torres

Acute occlusion of the superior mesenteric artery (SMA) can be a result of embolic or thrombotic phenomena. No matter the offending cause, prompt evaluation and intervention is warranted because of the high morbidity and mortality associated with ischemic bowel. Etiology will often determine the approach to intervention. Options for restoration of blood flow fall within the wide spectrum of open, hybrid, and endovascular techniques, including open embolectomy, mesenteric bypass, retrograde stenting of the SMA, and endovascular revascularization.

SCORE™, the Surgical Council on Resident Education, classified superior mesenteric artery embolectomy as an "ESSENTIAL UNCOMMON" procedure.

STEPS IN PROCEDURE

SMA Embolectomy

Vertical midline abdominal incision

Retract omentum and transverse colon cephalad

Small bowel caudad and to right

Mobilize the ligament of Treitz

Palpate the middle colic artery and trace it to the root of the mesentery to locate the SMA

Incise the peritoneum longitudinally along the course of the SMA

Dissect the SMA, preserving branches, and loop with silastic bands

Assure systemic heparinization

Transverse arteriotomy with a 11-blade knife and extend it a few millimeters with Potts scissors

Pass an appropriately sized Fogarty catheter proximally, inflate the balloon and pull back to extract clot

Repeat distally

Flush the lumen with heparinized saline

Close the arteriotomy with interrupted 6-0 monofilament suture

If there is concern for narrowing the lumen, consider a vein patch for closure

Assess Doppler signals

Proximal and distal to the arteriotomy site

Site of arteriotomy

Intestinal branches

Evaluate the bowel for viability and consider a second look laparotomy depending on the appearance of the bowel

Pitfalls and Complications

Bowel perforation

Necrotic bowel

Ischemic stricture

Gastrointestinal bleed

Short gut syndrome

Abdominal compartment syndrome

Loss of abdominal domain

SMA dissection, thrombosis, spasm

Distal embolization

Percutaneous access complications of hemorrhage, pseudoaneurysm, dissection and thrombosis

LIST OF STRUCTURES

Superior mesenteric artery

Aorta

Middle colic artery

Transverse colon

Duodenum

Ligament of Treitz

Exposure of Superior Mesenteric Artery (Fig. 89.1)

Technical Points

Optimal exposure is provided by a vertical midline incision. Retract the transverse colon and omentum upward, and the small intestine, including mesentery, downward and to the right to expose the SMA. Mobilize the ligament of Treitz to provide wide exposure. Normally, the artery is easy to locate by its size and pulsation; however, when occluded it may be a bit difficult to find. Palpate the middle colic artery and trace it to the root of the mesentery to locate the SMA. Incise the peritoneum on the mesentery longitudinally along the course of the SMA (Fig. 89.1). Dissect the SMA, preserving its branches. Pass silastic vessel loops around the proximal artery, distal artery, and any branches in the field. The patient should already be systemically heparinized, but if not, administer heparin. Make a transverse arteriotomy with a 11-blade knife and extend it a few millimeters with Potts scissors. Typically, clot will be encountered in the artery (Fig. 89.2).

Pass an appropriately sized Fogarty catheter proximally (typically a 3-French catheter), inflate the balloon and pull back to extract clot (Fig. 89.3). Flush the vessel with heparinized saline and place a small Yassargil clamp proximal to the arteriotomy once blood return is established. In a similar manner, pass the Fogarty catheter distally to remove clot. Extreme care should be taken not to overinflate the balloon with this maneuver, as the mesenteric vessels are fragile and easily injured. Flush the vessel with heparinized saline and place a small Yassargil clamp distal to the arteriotomy once blood return is established. Close the arteriotomy with interrupted 6-0 monofilament suture. Flash the clamps and flush the lumen with heparinized saline prior to the suture line being tightened.

If the artery is stenotic or there is concern for narrowing the lumen, a longitudinal arteriotomy should be used rather than

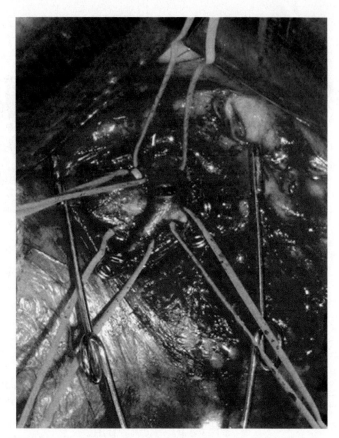

Figure 89.2 SMA exposed with transverse arteriotomy and embolus shown

a transverse one. A limited endarterectomy can be performed if there is a stenotic lesion by using a Freer elevator to remove the plaque. The distal endpoint of the endarterectomy site is inspected and any loose ends of intima are being trimmed and/or tacked using a 6-0 or 7-0 Prolene suture. The arteriotomy is closed by using a small piece of vein, usually harvested from the greater saphenous vein. The vein is opened longitudinally after being flushed with heparinized saline. Any valves are removed with fine Potts scissors. The vein is cut to length and sewn to the arteriotomy with 6-0 Prolene suture starting by tacking the vein patch in place at each apex and then running the suture line toward the middle of the patch on either side. Prior to the suture line being tied, the clamps are flashed and then reapplied. The lumen is flushed with heparinized saline and the suture line is then tightened.

Assess Doppler signals proximal and distal to the arteriotomy site as well as at the site itself. There should be Doppler signals within the intestinal branches and along the mesenteric and antimesenteric borders of the bowel. Evaluate the bowel for viability and consider a second look laparotomy depending on the appearance of the bowel.

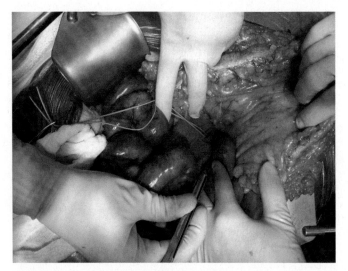

Figure 89.1 Exposure of SMA with transverse colon reflected cephalad, silastic loop around SMA, and proximal small bowel to the patient's left

Anatomic Points

The SMA supplies the distal duodenum, small intestine, large intestine to the splenic flexure, and the head and body of the

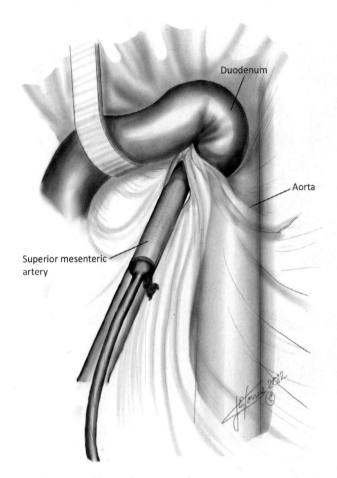

Superior mesenteric artery

Duodenum

Aorta

pancreas. It arises anteriorly from the aorta at the level of the first lumbar vertebral body at an acute angle, making it a particularly susceptible target for emboli relative to the celiac and inferior mesenteric arteries which originate off the aorta in more perpendicular conformations. Proximally, it lies posterior to the pancreas and then travels anterior to the fourth portion of the duodenum. Its first branch is the inferior pancreaticoduodenal artery, which has an anterior and posterior branch that anastomose with the anterior and posterior superior pancreaticoduodenal arteries, derived from the gastroduodenal artery, to form the pancreaticoduodenal arcades, providing a collateral pathway to the celiac artery distribution. There are then between 10 and 15 jejunal and ileal branches which come off the SMA as it travels toward the right lower quadrant. These branches create a series of arcades as they divide at right angles which then communicate with adjacent jejunal branches. Successive arcades then divide to supply the anterior and posterior surfaces of the intestine, oriented perpendicular to the long axis of the bowel.

Although its origin can vary, the middle colic artery usually comes off the SMA as its second major branch. It travels anteriorly and divides into right and left branches, the former connecting with the ascending branch of the right colic and the left branch anastomosing with the ascending branch of the left colic. The middle colic can be followed during embolectomy to locate the SMA, by lifting the transverse colon and tracing the middle colic artery to the root of the mesentery where it originates off the SMA.

Figure 89.3 Thromboembolectomy of SMA with a Fogarty catheter

STEPS IN PROCEDURE

Expose the supraceliac aorta by retracting the left lobe of the liver cephalad and opening the lesser sac. Then, divide the right crus of the diaphragm and the peritoneum overlying the aorta. Expose the supraceliac aorta along its anterior and lateral surfaces. Expose the infracolic SMA as described above

Create a retropancreatic tunnel from the aorta to the SMA by blunt-finger dissection behind the pancreas

Harvest the greater saphenous vein through a longitudinal incision on the medial aspect of the leg (see also Chapter 130 for information on harvesting saphenous vein for graft). Prosthetic graft material can be used if there is no bowel contamination. The saphenous vein may be used either in a reversed or a non-reversed fashion. If the vein is to be placed in a non-reversed fashion, lyse the valves with a valvulotome (see Chapter 133, Fig. 133.5).

Systemically heparinize the patient

Place a partial occlusion clamp, such as a Lemole–Strong on the supraceliac aorta

Make an aortotomy with either a 11-blade knife and Potts scissors or a 5- or 6-mm punch. Spatulate the proximal end of the vein graft and anastomose the graft to the aorta with a continuous 5-0 Prolene suture

Flush the graft

Inspect the proximal anastomosis for hemostasis

Pass the vein graft behind the pancreas with the vein distended, taking care to avoid twisting or kinking it

Make a longitudinal arteriotomy on the SMA

Cut the vein to proper length so that it reaches comfortably to the SMA without kinking or excess tension when all retraction is released

Spatulate the distal end and sew the vein to the SMA in an end-to-side manner using a running 6-0 monofilament suture

Release all vascular clamps and assure flow as noted below.

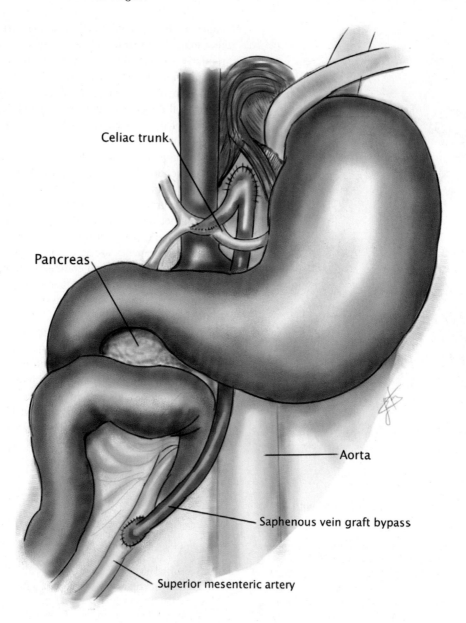

Celiac trunk

Pancreas

Aorta

Saphenous vein graft bypass

Superior mesenteric artery

Figure 89.4 Mesenteric bypass

Mesenteric Bypass (Fig. 89.4)

Technical Points

The abdomen is entered through a vertical midline incision. Expose the supraceliac aorta by retracting the left lobe of the liver cephalad and opening the lesser sac. Divide the right crus of the diaphragm with electrocautery. Open the peritoneum overlying the aorta longitudinally with sharp dissection. Dissect the supraceliac aorta along its anterior and lateral surfaces until enough room is available to place a clamp. Ideally, a side-biting, partial occlusion clamp, such as a Lemole–Strong, is used. However, if the aorta is severely diseased or there is not enough space for the partial occlusion clamp, enough dissection along the aorta will need to be done in order to place two separate clamps proximal and distal to the planned aortotomy.

Expose the infracolic SMA as described above. Choose a point on the SMA where the artery feels soft. This will generally be just distal to the origin of the middle colic artery. Create a retropancreatic tunnel from the aorta to the SMA by blunt-finger dissection behind the pancreas, anterior and to the left of the aorta and through the base of the small bowel mesentery.

Harvest the greater saphenous vein through a longitudinal incision on the medial aspect of the leg (see also Chapter 130 for information on harvesting saphenous vein for graft). Prosthetic graft material can be used if there is no bowel contamination. The saphenous vein may be used either in a reversed or a non-reversed fashion. If the vein is to be placed in a non-reversed fashion, lyse the valves with a valvulotome (see Chapter 133, Fig. 133.5).

Once the patient is systemically heparinized, clamp the supraceliac aorta. Make an aortotomy with either a 11-blade knife and Potts scissors or a 5- or 6-mm punch. Spatulate the proximal end of the vein graft and anastomose it to the aorta with a continuous 5-0 Prolene suture. Clamp the end of the vein graft with a Yassargil clamp and release the aortic clamp. Inspect the proximal anastomosis for hemostasis. Flash the Yassargil clamp to flush the graft and ensure good inflow. Replace the Yassargil clamp with a medium vascular clip at the end of the vein in order to pass the vein graft through the retropancreatic tunnel while distended, taking care to avoid twisting or kinking it.

Place Yassargil clamps proximal and distal to the planned arteriotomy on the SMA. Make a longitudinal arteriotomy with a 11-blade knife and Potts scissors. Cut the vein to the proper length so that it reaches comfortably to the SMA without kinking or excess tension when all retraction is released. Spatulate the distal end and sewn to the SMA in an end-to-side manner using a running 6-0 monofilament suture.

The clamps are released after flushing the vessels and flow is assessed as noted above.

Anatomic Points

In the setting of acute thrombosis of an underlying chronic stenosis, a mesenteric bypass should be considered. With acute on chronic mesenteric ischemia, often the amount of ischemic bowel involved is greater than that seen with an embolus. This is partly because the origin of the SMA is the most common location for atherosclerotic changes in the vessel, whereas an embolus commonly lodges slightly distal to the origin at the first branch point of the SMA. Furthermore, typically at least two of the three mesenteric vessels are involved with chronic mesenteric ischemia lowering the potential reserve through celiac and inferior mesenteric collaterals when there is an acute occlusion. Two-vessel revascularization is preferred, although in the acute setting certainly single-vessel revascularization is acceptable.

The inflow for the bypass can come from the supraceliac aorta, the adjacent infrarenal aorta or the iliac arteries. Often the supraceliac aorta is spared changes associated with severe atherosclerosis. Additionally, the supraceliac aorta provides a short and relatively straight, antegrade path for a bypass, especially when tunneled in a retropancreatic fashion. The tunnel is created with gentle, blunt-finger dissection from the supraceliac aorta behind the pancreas to the SMA. As with SMA embolectomy, the SMA arteriotomy is usually made just distal the middle colic takeoff as this area is relatively spared of chronic atherosclerotic disease. Autogenous conduit, specifically the greater saphenous vein, is preferred in the setting of necrotic bowel, although PTFE can be used if contamination is minimal. Often bypass of the celiac artery is needed as well in order to assure adequate revascularization, as shown in Figure 89.4.

STEPS IN PROCEDURE

Expose the SMA as described previously and perform thromboembolectomy

Place an umbilical tape or vessel loop around the proximal aspect of the vessel

Insert an 8- or 9-French sheath over a wire using Seldinger technique

Perform angiogram through the sheath

Cross occlusion/stenosis with a wire and catheter

Angioplasty and stent the stenotic lesion

Completion angiogram

Retrograde Open Stenting of the SMA

Technical Points (Fig. 89.5)

The hybrid technique of open retrograde stenting of the SMA is another method available for revascularization of the SMA. The infracolic SMA exposure is performed through a vertical midline incision in the same manner described previously for SMA embolectomy. The proximal infracolic SMA is controlled with an umbilical tape. Distally a silastic loop is placed. An arteriotomy is made in the SMA. Embolectomy is performed as described above. If an underlying chronic stenosis is found or known by preoperative imaging or if there is poor inflow after embolectomy, a sheath can be placed in a retrograde manner through the arteriotomy over a wire. The sheath is secured in place with the umbilical tape and a Rummel tourniquet. Contrast is injected to evaluate the proximal SMA. The stenosis is first attempted to be crossed with a combination of a 0.035-inch Glidewire and Glide catheter. If successful passage is obtained, a diagnostic catheter is placed over the wire and into the supraceliac aorta and used to perform a lateral and AP angiogram. The underlying stenosis is measured for length and the SMA is assessed for diameter. The diagnostic catheter is removed and the lesion is predilated with an appropriately sized angioplasty balloon. The balloon is removed over the wire and the lesion is stented with either a balloon expandable or self-expanding stent. The diagnostic catheter is replaced to perform a completion angiogram in lateral and AP views. If the lesion is successfully opened, the sheath is removed. The SMA just proximal to the arteriotomy is clamped with a Yassargil clamp and the arteriotomy is closed in the same manner described above.

Anatomic Points

Stenting of the SMA in a retrograde fashion via an open exposure of the vessel through a midline incision minimizes the distance from the sheath to the stenosis, thus in some ways removing many of the challenges that arise in the percutaneous, antegrade endovascular interventions from femoral or brachial access. Furthermore, cannulating the SMA from this location,

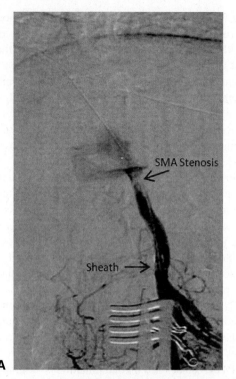
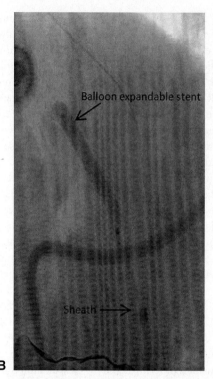
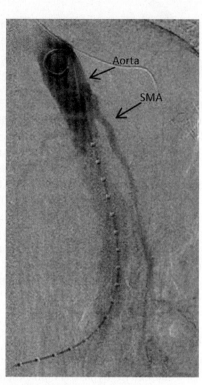

A   **B**   **C**

Figure 89.5 Retrograde stenting. **A:** Angiogram obtained through a sheath placed retrograde in the SMA following open thrombectomy demonstrating a chronic stenosis near the SMA origin. **B:** Deployment of balloon expandable stent across the stenosis. **C:** Completion angiogram demonstrating restoration of flow in the SMA.

provides a short, straight path for the passage of wires and catheters, eliminating the curves of the iliac arteries and the sharp turn of the SMA relative to the aorta when coming from the femoral artery and also the turn required when traveling through the left subclavian to the descending aorta during a left brachial approach. Passage of the wire from the true lumen of the SMA through the stenosis or occlusion and into the true lumen of the aorta can still be problematic from this approach. And at times, changing from a 0.035-inch system to a 0.018-inch or 0.014-inch system is sometimes necessary. However, the hybrid technique does minimize the possibility of a dissec-

tion in the distal SMA which can occur with interventions done from the standard percutaneous approach.

Endovascular Revascularization (Fig. 89.6)

Technical Points

Access the common femoral artery or the left brachial artery percutaneously with a 4- or 5-French micropuncture needle and exchange for a micropuncture sheath over a wire. Exchange the

STEPS IN PROCEDURE

Access the common femoral artery or the left brachial artery percutaneously

Place a long sheath or guide catheter into the visceral segment of the aorta

Perform an angiogram through a flush catheter in the visceral segment of the aorta in an anterior–posterior and a magnified lateral view

Select the origin of the SMA with a reverse curve catheter (if using a femoral approach), or an angled catheter (if using a brachial approach)

Embed the tip of a large end-hole catheter into the occlusion and perform suction thrombectomy

Consider other endovascular adjuncts such as catheter-directed thrombolytic or vasodilator therapy, pharmacomechanical or rheolytic thrombectomy, or angioplasty and stenting should suction thrombectomy yield inadequate revascularization

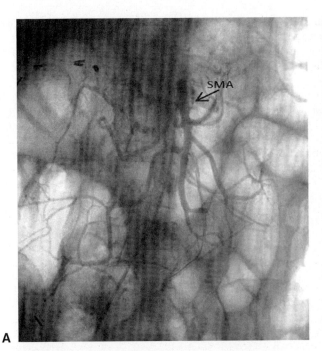
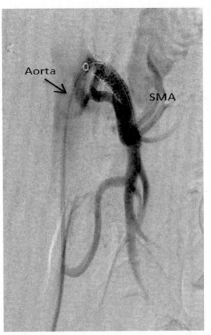

Figure 89.6 **A:** AP view angiogram of the SMA demonstrating distal branches. **B:** Lateral view angiogram of the SMA demonstrating a patent origin following successful thrombolysis and stenting of an acute thrombosis of a chronic stenosis.

sheath over a long 0.035-inch wire for a 6-French sheath long enough to reach the visceral segment of the aorta. Perform an angiogram through a flush catheter in the visceral segment of the aorta in an anterior–posterior and a magnified lateral view. Select the origin of the SMA with a reverse curve catheter (if using a femoral approach), or an angled catheter (if using a brachial approach). If there is acute clot, embed the tip of a large end-hole catheter into the occlusion, apply suction to the catheter with a 60-cc syringe and quickly withdraw the catheter into the sheath to perform the suction thrombectomy. Repeat this maneuver until there is no further return of clot. Perform an angiogram to assess the SMA. If there is residual clot or an underlying stenosis, consider other endovascular adjuncts such as catheter-directed thrombolytic or vasodilator therapy, pharmacomechanical or rheolytic thrombectomy, or angioplasty and stenting.

Anatomic Points

Endovascular interventions of the SMA can be challenging for a number of reasons. While the distal portion of the SMA is best imaged from an AP position, the more proximal portion is best seen through a lateral, or at least a steep anterior, oblique projection due to the vessel's origin coming off the anterior surface of the aorta (Fig. 89.6). Of course, with sharper angles, image quality is compromised due the poor x-ray penetration. Having the patient's arms raised above their head can improve the image quality in lateral projections, but is a demanding position for the patient to maintain for any length of time.

There is also a lot of movement in the area of the SMA, which adds further difficulty to obtaining adequate images.

The angulation of the vessel's origin increases the complexity of gaining secure, selective access to the vessel as well as maintaining a stable platform for intervention. This is particularly true for procedures done from the femoral approach, where attempts at antegrade movements of a catheter or wire tip in the SMA might result in unwanted, retrograde buckling of the catheter or wire into the aorta. Because of this, a severe angulation frequently requires a left brachial approach, most notably when there is an occlusion of the origin of the SMA flush with the aorta. While working from a brachial approach can improve the stability of an SMA intervention by reducing many potential paradoxical movements, it can be more cumbersome for the operator as most endovascular suites are designed to best accommodate the surgeon from a femoral approach with regards to the image intensifier, viewing screens and access to the equipment table.

REFERENCES

1. Acosta S, Ogren M, Sternby NH, et al. Clinical implications for the management of acute thromboembolic occlusion of the superior mesenteric artery: Autopsy findings in 213 patients. *Ann Surg.* 2005;241(3):516–522.
2. Kadir S, Lundell C, Saeed M. Celiac, superior, and inferior mesenteric arteries. In: *Atlas of Normal and Variant Angiographic Anatomy.* Philadelphia, PA: W.B. Saunders Company; 1991:297–364.
3. Kao GD, Whittington R, Coia L. Anatomy of the celiac axis and superior mesenteric artery and its significance in radiation therapy. *Int J Radiat Oncol Biol Phys.* 1993;25(1):131–134.

4. Lin PH, Bush RL, Lumsden AB. Treatment of acute visceral artery occlusive disease. In: Zelenock GB, Huber TS, Messina LM, Lumsden AB, Moneta GL, eds. *Mastery of Vascular and Endovascular Surgery.* Philadelphia, PA: Lippincott Williams & Wilkins; 2006:293–299.

5. Matsumoto AH, Tegtmeyer CJ, Angle JF. Endovascular interventions for chronic mesenteric ischemia. In: Baum S, Pentecost MJ, eds. *Abrams' Angiography Interventional Radiology. Vol III.* Boston, MA: Little, Brown and Company; 1997:326–338.

6. Pisimisis GT, Oderich GS. Technique of hybrid retrograde superior mesenteric artery stent placement for acute-on-chronic mesenteric ischemia. *Ann Vasc Surg.* 2011;25(1):132.e7–132.e11.

7. Resch TA, Acosta S, Sonesson B. Endovascular techniques in acute arterial mesenteric ischemia. *Semin Vasc Surg.* 2010;23:29–35.

8. Schneider PA. Chapters 9 & 10. *Endovascular Skills Guidewire and Catheter Skills for Endovascular Surgery.* 3rd ed. New York, NY: Informa Healthcare USA; 2009:134–136, 172–173.

9. Sharafuddin MJ, Nicholson RM, Kresowik TF, et al. Endovascular recanalization of total occlusions of the mesenteric and celiac arteries. *J Vasc Surg.* 2012;55(6):1674–1681.

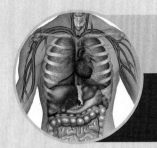

90

Small Bowel Resection and Anastomosis

Small bowel resection is performed when a segment of small intestine must be removed. The nature of the pathology dictates the extent of resection. Carcinoma of the small intestine is rare. Resection for carcinoma should encompass margins of at least 10 cm and a fan-shaped piece of mesentery containing regional nodes. Resection for benign disease is far more common. In the latter case, margins should be conservative, and as much bowel as possible should be preserved. This is particularly true when reoperations may be necessary (e.g., in patients with Crohn disease). Strictureplasty, a popular alternative to resection in patients with Crohn disease, is briefly presented at the end of this chapter.

When a significant length of small intestine must be removed, measure the length of the remaining bowel. Take a wet umbilical tape and measure the length along the antimesenteric border with the bowel under slight stretch. Record the measured length in the operative note.

SCORE™, the Surgical Council on Resident Education, classified open small bowel resection as an "ESSENTIAL COMMON" procedure.

STEPS IN PROCEDURE—SMALL BOWEL RESECTION

Midline laparotomy
Run small intestine from ligament of Treitz to
    ileocecal valve
Identify segment to resect and eviscerate it
    Return the rest of the bowel to the
        abdominal cavity
    Grasp the bowel and identify avascular
        window in mesentery adjacent to
        bowel at sites of proposed resection
    Extent of resection depends on pathology
    Wider resection with generous fan of
        mesentery is needed for malignancy

Create window under bowel
Divide bowel
Divide mesentery in V-shaped fashion
Check ends for viability (resect additional
    bowel, if necessary)
Create anastomosis (stapled or sutured)
Close mesenteric defect
Wrap omentum around anastomosis
Check hemostasis and close abdomen
    without drains

HALLMARK ANATOMIC COMPLICATIONS—SMALL BOWEL RESECTION
Anastomotic leak

LIST OF STRUCTURES
Jejunum
Ileum
Cecum

Ileocecal valve
Suspensory ligament of duodenum (ligament
    of Treitz)

Small Bowel Resection (Fig. 90.1)

Technical Points

Always "run" the entire small intestine before any resection. Grasp a section of small bowel and pass it from one hand to the other, "walking" your fingers proximally. You should be progressing in the general direction of the left upper quadrant. Identify the suspensory ligament of duodenum (ligament of Treitz). Progressing distally from the ligament of Treitz, elevate a section of small bowel about 10 cm in length. Flip each sec-

tion over so that both sides are examined. Then pass the section to your first assistant. Continue in this fashion to the ileocecal valve. If, by chance, the loop of bowel that you grasp in the beginning leads you to the ileocecal valve instead of the ligament of Treitz, it is perfectly acceptable to run the bowel from distal to proximal, finishing at the ligament of Treitz. Minimize the amount of time that the bowel is out of the abdomen. Interference with venous drainage, swelling, and hypothermia can result from prolonged evisceration. Return all bowel, with the exception of the segment to be resected, to the abdomen.

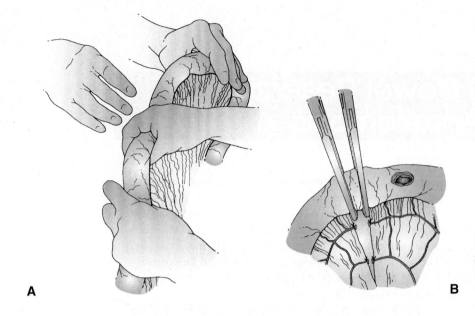

A

B

Figure 90.1 Small bowel resection. **A:** Running the bowel. **B:** Division of bowel on one side of injured area. Note that the mesentery is already divided.

Grasp the bowel between the thumb and the forefinger of your nondominant hand and use your thumb to feel the mesenteric border of the bowel at one of the planned resection margins. Take a fine-pointed mosquito hemostat and pass it under one of the small vessels that supply the bowel. Double clamp and ligate the vessel with fine silk. Do not try to break through on your first pass unless the mesentery is very flimsy. Divide the mesentery close to the bowel with precision to minimize the bulk of tissue included in ligatures next to the bowel. The mesenteric surface of the bowel will then be clean and ready for anastomosis.

Clamp the bowel with Allen clamps or similar straight clamps designed to hold bowel securely. Kocher clamps will work if nothing else is available. Divide the bowel between the clamps with a scalpel.

Repeat this process at the other end of the segment to be resected.

Lift the bowel up to display the mesentery and identify the line along which you plan to resect it. With the mesentery slightly stretched, place the opened blade of a pair of Metzenbaum scissors into the incision in the mesentery and lift up, elevating a flap of peritoneum with the tip of the blade. Push-cut the peritoneum by pushing with the crotch of the barely opened scissors, outlining a **V**-shaped segment of mesentery to be resected. This cut should not injure the underlying mesenteric vessels. Flip the bowel over and do the same thing on the other side of the mesentery. Use the thumb and forefinger of your nondominant hand to elevate the thin, fatty mesentery. A finger fracture technique is sometimes useful. Double clamp and divide all mesenteric vessels, and remove the resected segment.

Secure the mesenteric vessels with suture ligatures of 3-0 silk.

Anatomic Points

Running the bowel allows the surgeon to inspect the entire length of small bowel for disease or incidental developmental anomalies. The most common anomaly is Meckel diverticulum, which has been reported to be present (although is usually asymptomatic) as frequently as 4.5% of the time.

The ligament of Treitz, or the suspensory muscle of the duodenum, marks the beginning of the intraperitoneal jejunum. This ligament is present about 75% of the time. A band of smooth muscle running from the connective tissue around the celiac artery and right diaphragmatic crus blends with smooth muscle at the duodenojejunal flexure. It has little significance as a muscle, but functions as a ligament to maintain the duodenojejunal flexure. However, because it is muscular and thus vascular, division of this ligament, if necessary, must be done between clamps and with appropriate hemostatic control.

As you run the bowel, note the blood supply and venous drainage of the small bowel. Numerous jejunal and ileal branches arise from the left side of the superior mesenteric artery. A few centimeters from the intestinal border, these arteries branch, and contiguous branches of the superior mesenteric artery anastomose to form arcades. There tends to be one order of arcades for the proximal jejunum, several orders in the middle third of the small bowel, and then a decrease in the number of orders, so that the distal ileum may again be supplied by a single arcade. These anastomotic arches form the primary collateral blood supply for any given segment of small bowel. Multiple vasa recti of variable lengths arise from those arches closest to the bowel wall and directly supply the bowel. Each vasa recta typically (about 90% of the time) passes to one side of the bowel wall, rather than splitting to supply both sides; the side supplied alternates as one progresses along the bowel. The vasa recti are end arteries. An intramural plexus allows intestinal viability to be maintained for a small distance after division of these terminal vessels.

Intestinal veins follow a pattern similar to that of the arterial supply. Although there are no supporting statistics available, one gets the distinct impression that veins tend to lie on the upper side of the mesentery, whereas arteries tend to course on the lower side.

Although jejunum blends imperceptibly with ileum in the midportion of the small bowel, the following differences may help one to distinguish between jejunum and ileum.

1. Jejunum has a thicker wall and larger lumen than ileum; thus, the diameter of the small bowel decreases as one progresses distally.
2. In the jejunum, fat is restricted to the mesentery, but as one progresses distally, fat creeps up onto the wall of the ileum.
3. Jejunal arterial arcades tend to be less complex and vasa recti tend to be longer in the proximal jejunum; arcade complexity increases and vasa recta become shorter as one progresses distally. Arcade complexity reaches its maximum in the middle third of the small bowel, and then becomes simpler more distally. However, the vasa recti do not lengthen.

Anastomosis (Fig. 90.2)

Technical Points

Inspect both ends of the bowel and verify that the color is normal, indicating a good blood supply. Occasionally, division of the mesentery compromises the circulation to one or both of the ends. If the color becomes dusky or bluish adjacent to

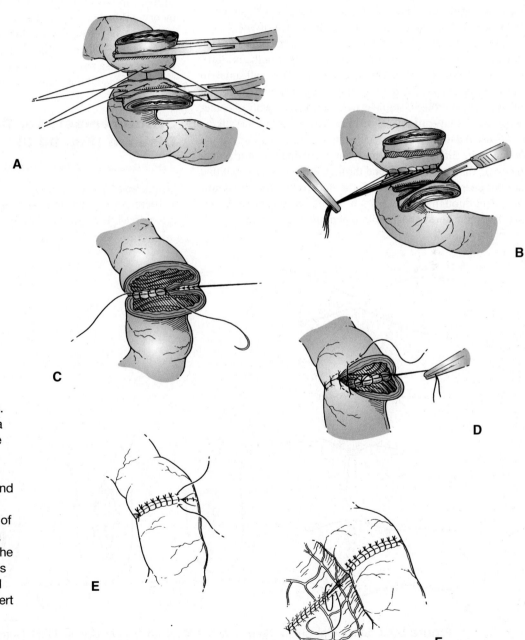

Figure 90.2 Anastomosis. **A:** Two corner sutures and a middle Lembert suture have been placed. **B:** The back row of interrupted Lembert sutures have been placed and tied and the bowel is being trimmed. **C:** The inner layer of the back wall is placed as a running locking suture. **D:** The inner layer of the front wall is placed as a running Connell suture. **E:** Interrupted Lembert sutures are placed to complete the front wall. **F:** The mesenteric defect is closed.

the clamps, suspect vascular compromise and resect additional bowel.

Check the mesenteric border. The bowel should be cleaned of mesenteric fat for a distance of 2 to 3 mm from the clamp. Extension of this is unnecessary and may result in ischemia.

Align the mesenteric borders and confirm that the bowel is not twisted by tracing the **V** of the mesentery. Some surgeons prefer to close the mesenteric defect first. This ensures that there are no twists and that vascular compromise does not occur in the process of mesenteric closure. Use wet laparotomy pads to isolate the two ends to be anastomosed.

Construct the anastomosis by placing a posterior row of interrupted Lembert sutures of 3-0 silk. Remove the clamps and excise the crushed ends of the bowel. It is advantageous to leave a small (0.5 mm) remnant of crush because it keeps all of the layers of the bowel wall together so that the mucosa does not "pout out."

Place the inner suture as a running lockstitch of 3-0 Vicryl, beginning at the middle of the back wall and progressing in each direction. Use two sutures and tie them together in the midline. Continue the suture line anteriorly as a running Connell suture to invert the outer row. Tie the two sutures together at the midpoint of the anterior row. Complete the anastomosis with an outer seromuscular layer of interrupted Lembert sutures of 3-0 silk.

Close the mesenteric defect by suturing the two sides of the **V** together. Either an interrupted or a continuous suture may be used. Take bites that extend through the peritoneum but that are not deep enough to "catch" the underlying vessels. Leave no defect through which a loop of small intestine could herniate. Wrap the anastomosis with omentum, if available.

Anatomic Points

The outer layer of the bowel wall is the serosa, which is visceral peritoneum. Just deep to this layer, one can see the vasculature to the bowel and, where appropriate, the fat encroaching on the ileal wall. The next layer is longitudinal smooth muscle, then circular smooth muscle; between them is Auerbach myenteric nerve plexus. These two layers comprise the tunica muscularis or muscularis externa. The next layer encountered is the submucosa, which is predominantly areolar connective tissue; it contains a plexus of blood vessels and Meissner submucosal nerve plexus. The innermost layer—the mucosa—can be divided into an outer muscularis mucosa, middle lamina propria, and inner epithelium.

Of the four layers, it is the submucosa that provides the strength in bowel repairs. Moreover, although a time-honored theory holds that proper healing of bowel wounds depends on apposition of serosal layers; this is, in fact, not the case. Rather, accurate and watertight apposition of one surface to another, whether serosa or mucosa, coupled with sufficient time allowed for healing, is all that is necessary.

Strictureplasty for Crohn Disease (Fig. 90.3)

Technical and Anatomic Points

Strictureplasty is an alternative to resection for management of a strictured segment. It is particularly useful for multiple strictured areas. It allows maximum preservation of bowel length

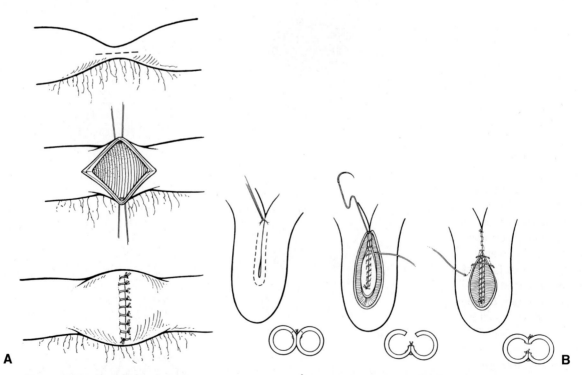

Figure 90.3 Strictureplasty for Crohn disease (**A, B** from Scott-Conner CEH. Current surgical management of inflammatory bowel disease. *South Med J.* 1994;87:1232–1241, with permission).

with restoration of a widely patent lumen. Use the Heineke-Mikulicz approach for short segments, the Finney approach for longer areas.

STEPS IN PROCEDURE—STRICTUREPLASTY

Midline laparotomy

Explore abdomen and identify all strictured regions

Decide whether resection is needed

If strictureplasty is planned:

Open strictured bowel in longitudinal fashion

Close transversely

Longer Strictures May Require Side-to-side (Finney-type) Strictureplasty

Open entire strictured area longitudinally

Loop bowel at midportion and approximate two limbs

Close as single long incision, anastomosing proximal and distal portions of loop

Confirm that all strictures have been addressed

Close abdomen in usual fashion without drains

HALLMARK ANATOMIC COMPLICATIONS—STRICTUREPLASTY

Missed stricture

Anastomotic leak

Heineke-Mikulicz Strictureplasty

Open the strictured portion of bowel in a longitudinal fashion (Fig. 90.3A). Place two stay sutures of 3-0 silk at opposite sides to hold the bowel open—these may be used as corner stitches if placed as Lembert sutures. Close the incision in a transverse fashion with a running suture of 3-0 Vicryl placed as a Connell suture, followed by a layer of interrupted 3-0 silk Lembert sutures.

Finney-type Strictureplasty

For longer strictured areas, again open the entire strictured area in a longitudinal fashion (Fig. 90.3B). Then loop the bowel at its midportion to approximate the proximal and distal edges of one side of the incision. Sew these together with interrupted 3-0 silk Lembert sutures. Begin an inner layer of running 3-0 Vicryl at the point where the bowel folds back on itself. Run this suture line as a locking stitch to the apex, and then use it to approximate the two open ends of bowel as a Connell suture. Complete this functional side-to-side anastomosis with an outer layer of 3-0 Lembert sutures.

REFERENCES

1. Asensio JA, Berne JD, Chahwan S, et al. Traumatic injury to the superior mesenteric artery. *Am J Surg*. 1999;178:235–239. (Discusses special considerations for management of rare injury.)

2. Barnes JP. The techniques for end-to-end intestinal anastomosis. *Surg Gynecol Obstet*. 1974;138:433–452.

3. Bulkley GB, Zuidema GD, Hamilton ST, et al. Intraoperative determination of small intestinal viability following ischemic injury: A prospective, controlled trial of two adjuvant methods (Doppler and fluorescein) compared with standard clinical judgment. *Ann Surg*. 1981;193:628–637.

4. Getzen LC. Intestinal suturing. I. The development of intestinal sutures. *Curr Probl Surg*. 1969;6:3–48.

5. Getzen LC. Intestinal suturing. II. Inverting and everting intestinal sutures. *Curr Probl Surg*. 1969;6:3–36.

6. Mulholland M. Atlas of small intestinal surgery. In: Bell RH Jr, Rikkers L, Mulholland M, eds. *Digestive Tract Surgery: A Text and Atlas*. Philadelphia, PA: JB Lippincott; 1996:1304–1305. (Discusses strictureplasty for Crohn disease.)

7. Poth EJ, Gold D. Technics of gastrointestinal suture. *Curr Probl Surg*. 1965;2:1–46.

8. Scott-Conner CEH. Current surgical management of inflammatory bowel disease. *South Med J*. 1994;87:1232–1241.

9. Townsend MC, Pelias ME. A technique for rapid closure of traumatic small intestine perforations without resection. *Am J Surg*. 1992;164:171–172. (Describes ingenious method of staple closure of perforations too large for primary closure.)

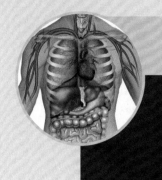

91

Pediatric Exploratory Laparotomy for Trauma, Malrotation, or Intussusception

Raphael C. Sun and Graeme J. Pitcher

While there are many different incisions for laparotomy in the adult population, the two most common approaches for exploratory laparotomy in a pediatric patient are the vertical midline and the transverse abdominal incision. In most situations, the pediatric surgeon prefers a transverse abdominal incision over the traditional vertical midline incision. However, it is important to consider the indication for surgery and take into account the area of concern when choosing an incision.

In general, a child younger than 5 years of age has a round or elliptical abdomen with the width being relatively longer than the length. The costal margin in children is proportionately higher from the iliac crest than the adult, making the abdominal cavity proportionately larger compared to the adult. Given these differences in body habitus and anatomy, it is understandable that the pediatric surgeon prefers the transverse abdominal incision.

Most of the time, a transverse abdominal incision provides adequate exposure for all four quadrants. However, in certain penetrating trauma situations, the traditional vertical incision is preferred. This incision can also be more easily extended into a sternotomy should that become necessary. It is important to understand the technical and anatomic points for each approach.

This chapter discusses the general conduct of exploratory laparotomy in infants and children, and then describes specific management of two common conditions: Malrotation and intussusception.

SCORE™, the Surgical Council on Resident Education, classified emergency operation for malrotation and emergency operation for intussusception as "ESSENTIAL UNCOMMON" procedures.

STEPS IN PROCEDURE

Make a vertical midline or transverse abdominal incision

Gain entry into the abdomen

Pack all four quadrants if there is severe bleeding

Inspect the entire abdomen by quadrants or organ systems

Perform the necessary procedure

Achieve hemostasis

Close fascia and skin or leave abdomen open if indicated

HALLMARK ANATOMIC COMPLICATIONS

Making a paramedian or off midline incision unintentionally

Injury to bowel or other organs upon entry

Missed injury or pathology

LIST OF STRUCTURES

External oblique muscle and aponeurosis

Internal oblique muscle and aponeurosis

Transversus abdominis muscle and transversalis fascia

Preperitoneal fat

Peritoneum

Linea alba

Remnant of the umbilical vein (falciform ligament)

The Vertical Midline Incision (Fig. 91.1)

The traditional vertical midline incision is most often used in trauma situations. The reason in choosing this incision is because it allows access to all four quadrants of the abdomen and provides better exposure to areas such as the aortic hiatus and the pelvis and can be performed quickly. There is usually minimal blood loss if the surgeon stays in the midline. The incision may be extended in either direction and can even be extended into the chest if a sternotomy is necessary.

The Transverse Abdominal Incision

There have been many clinical studies to observe the differences and outcomes between surgical incisions in the pediatric patient population. Studies have concluded that the transverse abdominal incision has decreased the occurrence of hernia defects, fascial or wound dehiscence compared to the vertical midline incision. The cosmetic appearance of the transverse incision is superior if placed accurately in the skin creases or Langer's lines. This incision allows all four quadrants to be exposed adequately and may easily be extended laterally if needed. Therefore, transverse abdominal incision is the preferred approach for exploratory laparotomy for nontraumatic indications in a child younger than 5 years of age.

Technical Points and Anatomic Points

Make the intended incision by using a knife to cut through the skin and dermis. The child's skin is much thinner and easier to cut compared to the adult. The subcutaneous layer and fat layer may be separated using electrocautery. If electrocautery is used, a low setting should be used in the "blend" mode. In general, the younger the patient is, the lower the electrocautery settings should be.

For a midline vertical incision, use the anatomic landmarks of the xiphoid and the pubic symphysis to guide the incision.

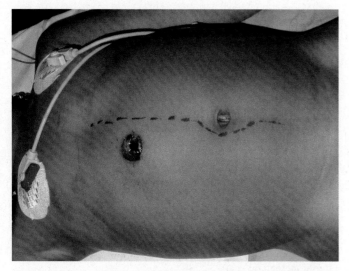

Figure 91.1 Midline incision preferred in small infant with penetrating abdominal trauma for ease of access to pelvis and aortic hiatus.

The incision should sweep gently around the umbilicus. If you anticipate the creation of an ostomy, the curvilinear incision should be placed on the opposite side of planned ostomy site. The linea alba is the reference landmark to confirm that the midline is reached and is seen more easily above the umbilicus than below. The midline incision may be superior or inferior to the umbilicus. When extending below the umbilicus in an infant, remember that the bladder occupies an intra-abdominal position and needs to be swept aside to avoid injury to it on entry.

Keep in mind that the umbilicus is lower in the abdomen compared to an adult, so a supraumbilical transverse incision will give excellent access to most structures in the upper and central abdomen. As you gain entry into the abdomen, the falciform ligament (remnant of the umbilical vein) is usually encountered, and will need to be ligated and divided to expose the liver, stomach, esophagus, and duodenum.

Close the fascia of a *midline incision* with absorbable sutures such as Vicryl or PDS. The fascia is normally closed in a standard running fashion from one end to the other. Make sure that each bite of fascia closure includes the anterior rectus sheath below the umbilicus and are adequately "deep" and closely spaced. The thin skin and subcutaneous tissues dictate that knots should be buried, even with absorbable material to prevent unsightly and uncomfortably prominent "bumps" during healing.

In situations where tension is encountered such as when closing the abdomen for abdominal wall defects, interrupted suturing techniques can be used. These sutures are usually simple or mattress sutures but some prefer the Smead-Jones technique. This technique is a double stitch on each side of the fascia in a far-near-near-far fashion as shown (for the adult case) in Chapter 44, Figure 44.6. Be careful not to injure bowel contents underneath the fascia. Retraction and exposure is important to allow the surgeon to visualize each bite of suture going through the fascia. This will help avoid injuries while closing the abdomen. A narrow malleable retractor placed on the bowel surface and projecting out of the abdomen (to ensure its removal) facilitates safe closure.

When closing a *transverse incision,* two options are available. Most surgeons prefer layered closure where the posterior rectus sheath, internal oblique and transversus abdominis muscles are approximated in the deep layer, and the external oblique muscles and the anterior rectus sheath are sutured in the second layer. A mass closure with a single running suture line encompassing all tissue layers is also acceptable and may in fact be preferable in very premature babies.

Skin closure is achieved by the use of absorbable sutures wherever possible in children to avoid the need for painful and fear-inducing suture removal postoperatively. Skin clips are generally avoided for this reason except for situations where hemostasis in skin edges is required. Running subcuticular sutures of Vicryl or Monocryl are commonly used. The choice of dressings is personal.

Drains or catheters need to be securely fixed to avoid premature removal by an often uncooperative child postoperatively. Ensure that all devices are covered by secure dressings before the patient emerges from anesthesia.

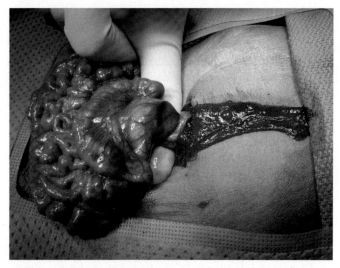

Figure 91.2 Operative findings in 2-day-old baby with classical midgut volulus showing the narrow mesenteric pedicle.

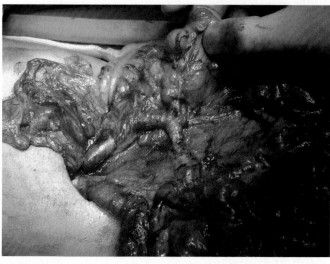

Figure 91.3 Configuration achieved after widening of the mesentery at the time of Ladd's procedure.

Management of Malrotation (Figs. 91.2–91.4)

The intestines undergo their first stages of development in an extracelomic position by lengthening around the superior mesenteric artery (SMA) pedicle at around the sixth to eighth week of gestation. Malrotation refers to a variety of anatomic abnormalities which are the result of failure of the intestinal tract to complete its normal rotation and fixation, following its return to the abdominal cavity between the eight and twelfth week of development. There are two distinct components:

■ Rotation and retroperitoneal fixation of the duodenum (270 degrees counterclockwise and posterior to the SMA) in the configuration of the normal "C loop" with the ligament of Treitz located to the left of the midline.

■ Rotation of the cecum (cranial to the SMA) into the normal retroperitoneal position in the right paracolic gutter. In malrotation, the cecum is displaced in a variety of positions from the subhepatic position, the epigastrium to the left lower quadrant.

The first or duodenal phase of development seems to be the most important from a clinical perspective as duodenal malrotation in tandem with an unfixed cecum results in the well-known and feared narrow-based mesentery which puts patients at risk for midgut volvulus. Any child who presents with bilious vomiting and is proven to have malrotation should be explored as a matter of urgency to prevent the loss of intestine due to volvulus.

It is thought that isolated abnormalities of the latter phase (typified by a high cecum with a mesentery) are fairly common and may not always place patients at risk for volvulus.

STEPS IN PROCEDURE

Transverse incision above the umbilicus
Gain entry into the abdomen
Inspect the peritoneal fluid
Eviscerate the abdomen contents
Identify the rotational anatomy by ascertaining the position of the ligament of Treitz and the degree of fixation of the cecum

Counterclockwise detorsion of the bowel if present
Divide the Ladd's bands
Broaden the base of the mesentery
Perform an appendectomy
Placement of small bowel in the right lateral gutter and colon along the left lateral gutter
Close the abdomen

HALLMARK ANATOMIC COMPLICATIONS

Injury to the mesenteric vessels during broadening of the base of the mesentery

Injury to a preduodenal portal vein

LIST OF STRUCTURES

Duodenum
Cecum
Appendix
Superior mesentery artery
Small bowel

Portal vein
Superior mesenteric vein
Inferior mesenteric vein
Ligament of Treitz

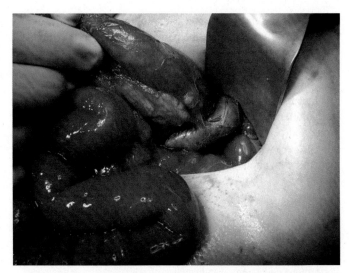

Figure 91.4 Preduodenal portal vein identified at the time of Ladd's procedure on a patient with symptomatic upper gastrointestinal (GI) obstruction, heterotaxia, and multiple cardiac anomalies.

Technical Points

A transverse incision is the standard approach for the traditional Ladd's procedure. A midline incision is another approach but this is not preferred. Any incision may be extended if necessary to gain adequate exposure. More importantly, the point is to gain adequate exposure to be able to identify the key structures listed above as well as derotate and inspect the small bowel in its entirety.

Once the abdomen is entered, inspect the peritoneal fluid. Sample and culture the peritoneal fluid. As in the case of any exploratory laparotomy, the character of the peritoneal fluid may suggest either ischemia or perforation.

Eviscerate the omentum, small bowel, and mesentery. Handle the small bowel with care, especially if it appears ischemic and is dilated from the obstruction. A *counterclockwise* detorsion of the bowel will relieve the volvulus and obstruction. A segment of bowel may have vascular compromise and detorsion will restore blood flow. Next, the breadth of the mesentery should be widened. The typically narrow mesenteric pedicle is shown in Figure 91.2. Widen the mesenteric base by releasing the cecum from any peritoneal attachments that may be anchoring it. The goal is to allow the mesentery of the SMA and its branches to be splayed out widely without any tension or torsion so that blood supply is not compromised. Broadening the mesentery helps prevent recurrence of midgut volvulus.

An important step of the operation is the straightening of the second and third parts of the duodenum. They are frequently found to be in a tortuous or "concertina" configuration as a result of congenital adhesions at this level. Full Kocherization of the duodenum facilitates dividing these, after which the duodenum should be placed directly into an unobstructed position in the right paracolic gutter. The completed procedure is shown in Figure 91.3. Perform an incidental appendectomy to avoid any diagnostic confusion in the future. The location of the cecum on the left side of the abdomen would otherwise make the diagnosis of acute appendicitis in a child with previous major abdominal surgery challenging.

Reinspect the intestines before closure. The duodenum and the small intestine should be positioned along the right abdomen and the colon positioned in the left abdomen along the gutters. Ensure that the bowel lies comfortably without any tension or torsion. It is not necessary to fix the bowel with any additional sutures.

If there is a limited segment of bowel that appears necrotic, a standard resection and anastomosis can be performed. In the event of a catastrophic loss of small bowel and resection of the entire midgut, immediate reanastomosis (of jejunum to colon) is not recommended. A stoma is the safer option and facilitates the management of the ensuing short bowel syndrome in the early stages. In some instances when intestinal viability is doubtful, the management of the patient with an open abdomen and scheduled re-exploration at 24 to 48 hours interval is a useful strategy. Bowel viability will be declared in this period and decompression facilitates intestinal recovery.

The fascia should be closed with a running suture. Close the subcutaneous fat and skin with running absorbable sutures in a subcuticular fashion.

Anatomic Points

It is important to understand the abnormal embryology and recognize the implications of the anatomic changes associated with malrotation. In practice, a spectrum of abnormalities is encountered, reflecting the degree of rotation of the duodenum and cecum respectively as well as the degree of narrowing of the mesenteric pedicle. The typical configuration, which we have described, is referred to as "classical malrotation" and when symptomatic, its management by Ladd's procedure is uncontroversial. Lesser degrees of abnormalities of duodenal rotation—"atypical malrotation"—are frequently encountered, especially in children with cardiac disease or other syndromes. The management of these children is more controversial. In these cases, the surgeon must be aware of the possibility of complete situs inversus or heterotaxia where there may be a bizarre configuration of the intra-abdominal organs such as a right-sided or retrohepatic stomach and polysplenia or asplenia depending on the type. Such patients can in addition have a preduodenal portal vein as shown in Figure 91.4. Awareness of this can prevent inadvertent injury.

Ladd's bands refer to the congenital bands crossing from cecum across the base of the mesentery to the liver. They may compress the underlying duodenum and although commonly implicated as the prime cause of obstruction, in reality the duodenum is usually obstructed by a combination of volvulus and anatomic distortion. A variation of Ladd's bands can be seen when the peritoneal bands attach higher up from the cecum in the ascending colon.

When volvulus occurs, it almost always occurs in a clockwise direction (usually two to three revolutions) of the bowel. Therefore, it is important to remember that detorsion involves a counterclockwise hand motion.

Intussusception (Figs. 91.5 and 91.6)

Intussusception occurs when one portion of the intestine invaginates into a usually distal portion as a result of peristaltic activity. It occurs most commonly in infants younger than 2 years of age.

Ileocolic is the most common form followed by ileoileal intussusception. After diagnosis, the patient should be resuscitated and if no contraindications exist, an attempt at air reduction should be performed. This is associated with a success rate between 60% and 80%. If the intussusception fails to reduce, surgery is generally the next step in management although in certain select cases a further attempt at reduction is appropriate. The potential for gangrene and perforation makes this a surgical emergency. Patients who present with acute peritonitis or signs of perforation should be explored without an attempt at reduction in the radiology suite.

STEPS IN PROCEDURE

Transverse incision in the right upper quadrant above the umbilicus
Gain entry into the abdomen
Deliver the cecum and terminal ileum out of the abdomen
Identify the lead point of the intussusception

Gently manipulate and reduce the intussusception
Resect bowel if necessary
Perform appendectomy if indicated
Close abdomen

HALLMARK ANATOMIC COMPLICATIONS

Injury to the bowel during aggressive reduction
Failure to resect an anatomic lead point

Failure to recognize a lead point perforation distal to the intraoperative location of the intussusception

LIST OF STRUCTURES

Cecum
Appendix

Ileum
Meckel diverticulum

Technical Points

Eighty percent to ninety percent of pediatric intussusceptions are ileocolic. A transverse muscle-cutting incision in the right upper quadrant, just above the umbilicus is the most common approach. However, this can be adjusted on the basis of the position of the intussusception. This may be determined using a combination of radiologic imaging and physical examination. Extend the incision if necessary to gain adequate exposure.

Once the abdomen is entered, the peritoneal fluid should be inspected. Cultures of the peritoneal fluid can be sampled and sent for cultures. Just like any exploratory laparotomy, the peritoneal fluid may suggest either ischemia or perforation.

Next, deliver the cecum and terminal ileum out of the abdomen. It is easier to reduce the intussusception outside of the abdomen as opposed to intra-abdominally. Manual reduction should be performed carefully and in an unhurried way. Note

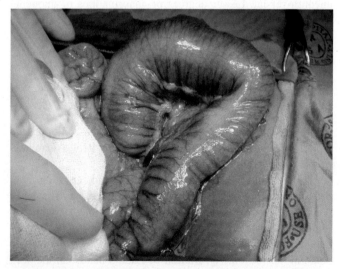

Figure 91.5 Intraoperative appearance of ileocolic intussusception showing right colon filled with intussusceptum.

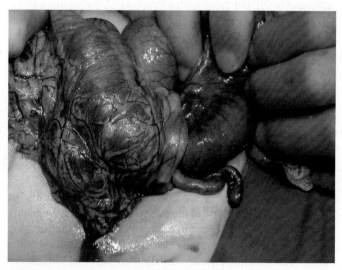

Figure 91.6 Patient in Figure 91.5 showing successful manual reduction in progress.

that in contrast to the adult situation (where there is generally a lead point such as a polyp or tumor that has caused the intussusception), resection is only performed in children if the bowel is necrotic. The apex of the intussusception is squeezed between the fingers and cup of the surgeon's hand at the distal end and gently massaged in a retrograde direction (Fig. 91.5). Using a piece of gauze may help gain traction during this procedure. Seventy percent of the force should be applied by pushing at the apex and 30% by pulling proximally at the intussusception. If reduction is not possible it may indicate that the bowel has strangulated. Under these circumstances resection is necessary. Do not attempt to reduce if the bowel appears edematous and vascular compromised.

During manual reduction, serosal or seromuscular tears may occur due to the edematous bowel. Serosal tears can generally be left alone; however, seromuscular flaps must be repaired with 5-0 or 6-0 sutures. Never use instruments to reduce bowel.

Once the intussusception is reduced, take some time to examine the bowel that has been reduced (Fig. 91.6). The segment of bowel is often edematous and dusky appearing. If there is a segment of bowel that appears necrotic or gangrenous or if a pathologic lead point lesion such as a Meckel diverticulum is identified, a standard resection and anastomosis should be performed.

An appendectomy should always be performed if the appendix is congested or contused. Performing an incidental appendectomy to eliminate any future diagnostic confusion in a patient with the right abdominal scar is optional.

It is not necessary to anchor the terminal ileum or the mesentery after successful reduction. Place the bowel back into the abdomen and assure no twisting or tension. Close the abdomen in standard fashion. The fascia is usually closed in two layers with a running suture. Close the subcutaneous fat and skin with running absorbable sutures in a subcuticular fashion.

Anatomic Points

Intussusception is most commonly ileocolic followed by ileoileal forms. Colocolic and jejunojejunal are other varieties that rarely occur. Intussusception can also be associated with feeding tubes in the duodenum and retrograde varieties occur sometimes under these circumstances. Infants can also be found to have asymptomatic small bowel intussusceptions on screening ultrasound done for other conditions. These are usually self-limiting and do not necessarily need treatment. Children with cystic fibrosis are frequently found to have silent small bowel intussusceptions at the time of laparotomy. Care should be taken to evaluate the extent of any intussusception. It can extend into the rectosigmoid region and may even be present extruding from the anus in severe cases.

When perforation occurs with intussusception, it usually occurs at the point where the apex of the intussusceptum causes necrosis on the downstream bowel wall. This point may be found in much more distal colon than the surgeon expects.

Idiopathic intussusceptions in infants are usually due to lymphoid hyperplasia within the lamina propria of the terminal ileum. After reduction, there may be a characteristic dimple site representing a Peyer's patch. It is not necessary to resect this lesion as it is considered a nonpathologic lead point. All other lead points including small bowel polyps in Peutz–Jeghers syndrome, Meckel diverticulum, submucosal hamartomas, lymphoma, or duplication cysts should be resected. These occur more often in patients outside the typical age range and surgeons should have a higher suspicion for these types of lead points with recurrent intussusception. Lastly, in some patients a very mobile cecum with a long mesentery, known as Waugh's syndrome, may predispose to intussusception and may be a cause for recurrent intussusception.

REFERENCES

1. Beasley S. Intussusception. *Pediatr Radiol.* 2004;34:302–304.
2. Brereton RJ, Taylor B, Hall CM. Intussusception and intestinal malrotation in infants: Waugh's syndrome. *Br J Surg.* 1986;73:55–57.
3. Burger JW, van't Riet M, Jeekel J. Abdominal incisions: Techniques and postoperative complications. *Scand J Surg.* 2002;91:315–321.
4. Daneman A, Navarro O. Intussusception. Part 2: An update on the evolution of management. *Pediatr Radiol.* 2004;34:97–108.
5. Gauderer MW. A rationale for routine use of transverse abdominal incisions in infants and children. *J Pediatr Surg.* 1981;16(4 suppl 1): 583–586.
6. Lampl B, Levin TL, Berdon WE, et al. Malrotation and midgut volvulus: A historical review and current controversies in diagnosis and management. *Pediatr Radiol.* 2009;39:359–366.
7. McVay MR, Kokoska ER, Jackson RJ, et al. Jack Barney Award. The changing spectrum of intestinal malrotation: Diagnosis and management. *Am J Surg.* 2007;194:712–719.
8. Millar AJ, Rode H, Cywes S. Malrotation and volvulus in infancy and childhood. *Semin Pediatr Surg.* 2003;12:229–236.
9. Ong NT, Beasley SW. The leadpoint in intussusception. *J Pediatr Surg.* 1990;25:640–643.
10. Patnaik VVG, Singla Rajan K, Bansal VK. Surgical incisions-their anatomical basis Part IV-abdomen. *J Anat Soc India.* 2001; 50(2):170–178.
11. Suri M, Langer JC. A comparison of circumumbilical and transverse abdominal incisions for neonatal abdominal surgery. *J Pediatr Surg.* 2011;46:1076–1080.
12. Waldhausen JH, Davies L. Pediatric postoperative abdominal wound dehiscence: Transverse versus vertical incisions. *J Am Coll Surg.* 2000;190:688–691.

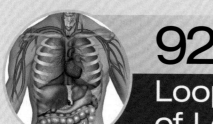

92

Loop Ileostomy and Closure of Loop Ileostomy

Jennifer Hrabe and John C. Byrn

Loop ileostomy is performed whenever fecal diversion is indicated. It is often done in conjunction with other abdominal or perineal procedures. Loop ileostomy affords a technically reliable form of complete fecal diversion that is well tolerated by the patient when constructed properly. Often criticized for the risk of dehydration and small bowel obstruction, its ease of closure, low rate of infection, and reduced risk of prolapse more than correct for these concerns. This form of proximal diversion is commonly indicated for high-risk anastomoses (such as with restorative proctectomy), hostile abdomen (e.g., obstruction, sepsis, or radiation enteritis), functional colonic constipation, and temporary management of colonic or perianal inflammatory bowel disease.

SCORE™, the Surgical Council on Resident Education, classified ileostomy and closure of ileostomy as "ESSENTIAL COMMON" procedures.

STEPS IN PROCEDURE

Loop Ileostomy
Mark location preoperatively

Lower Midline Laparotomy
Identify suitable loop of ileum

Create stoma aperture with a rectus-splitting technique
Exteriorize loop of ileum
Mature stoma

HALLMARK ANATOMIC COMPLICATIONS

Loop Ileostomy
Small bowel obstruction
Dehydration
Stomal necrosis or retraction

Closure of Loop Ileostomy
Small bowel obstruction
Anastomotic leak

LIST OF STRUCTURES
Rectus abdominis muscle
Rectus sheath

Terminal ileum and cecum

Loop Ileostomy

Preparation of Ileostomy Site and Ileal Loop (Fig. 92.1)

Technical Points

The patient's abdomen should be marked prior to surgery by either the surgeon or a trained stoma therapist. The location should avoid previous incisions, bony prominences, and skin creases. The ideal site is the right lower quadrant over the rectus muscle, but must be visible to the patient. If preoperative marking is not possible, consider placing the ostomy high on the right side of the abdomen where there will be fewer skin creases and the patient will be able to see and care for it appropriately. The stomal incision should be appropriately spaced from the midline incision; too close will make pouching

difficult, whereas a more lateral incision is likely to lie outside of the rectus muscle.

The patient should be positioned supine. If the abdomen is not already open, make a short vertical midline incision. Select the most distal ileal segment that reaches the desired site on the abdominal wall without tension. If necessary, mobilize the terminal ileum by incising any lateral peritoneal attachments. Avoid excess mobilization, however, as an overly mobile ileum may be at greater risk for volvulus. Using a hemostat, make a window in the mesentery adjacent to the portion of ileum that will be used for the stoma. Pass a Penrose drain through this defect and clamp the drain. The Penrose drain will provide atraumatic manipulation of the bowel through the abdominal wall. Mark the bowel with two seromuscular sutures to ensure maturation of the

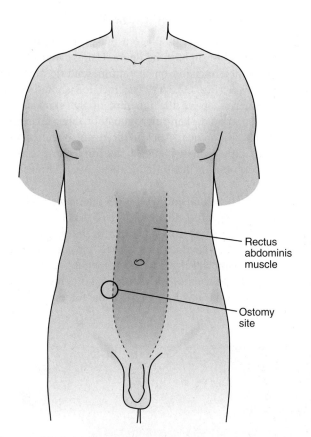

Figure 92.1 Ideal site for ileostomy

Rectus
abdominis
muscle

Ostomy
site

sheath, which is formed from the aponeuroses of the external and internal oblique and the transversus abdominis muscles. Ostomies located outside of the rectus sheath have been associated with higher rates of parastomal hernias.

Most of the ileum lies in the right lower quadrant. It is approximately 2 to 3 cm in diameter and several meters long. It is attached to the posterior abdominal wall by the mesentery. The terminal ileum is typically in the pelvis and then ascends to the medial portion of the cecum. A fold of peritoneum, the ileocecal fold, connects the antimesenteric terminal ileum to the cecum and vermiform appendix. The ileal blood supply is the superior mesenteric artery (SMA) which gives off arterial arcades that lead to the vasa recta. The terminal ileum is supplied by the ileal branch of the ileocolic artery. Venous drainage is via the superior mesenteric vein and mirrors the SMA.

Creating the abdominal defect of the stoma requires one to traverse all layers of the abdominal wall. Beneath the skin is the variably thick layer of Camper's fascia. Superior to the arcuate line, the rectus muscles are covered both anteriorly and posteriorly by the aponeuroses of the lateral abdominal wall muscles. The arcuate line position varies between individuals, but generally is one-third the distance from the umbilicus to the pubic symphysis. Inferior to the arcuate line, the rectus sheath covers only the anterior surface of the rectus abdominis muscles. Deep to the rectus sheath is the transversalis fascia and then the parietal peritoneum. It is this transversalis fascia that should be kept aligned with the overlying tissues to ensure alignment of

correct limb. Place a blue vicryl suture proximally and a brown chromic suture distally.

Before incising the stoma site skin, place one Kocher clamp on the midline incision fascia and one on the overlying dermis. These will keep the layers of the abdominal wall aligned during stoma creation. Hold the clamps in the palm of your nondominant hand and, with a laparotomy pad to protect intra-abdominal contents, elevate the abdominal wall with your fingers. Excise a 2-cm disc of skin at the marked ostomy site. Incise the subcutaneous tissue vertically and use right-angle retractors to reveal the underlying anterior rectus abdominis fascia. Make a 2-cm vertical incision in this fascia. Gently separate the rectus abdominis muscle fibers with a curved blunt instrument, then use right-angle retractors to retract the muscle and reveal the posterior rectus fascia. Incise the posterior fascia and underlying peritoneum. Check the opening diameter. It should be approximately two fingers' breadth.

To detect occult injuries to the inferior epigastric artery, pass a dry sponge through the stoma track. Clamp the ends of the sponge with a Peon and complete any remaining intra-abdominal portions of the procedure.

Anatomic Points

The rectus abdominis is significantly wider superiorly than inferiorly, transitioning from a broad, thin muscle to a narrow, thick one. Above the arcuate line, it is enclosed by the rectus

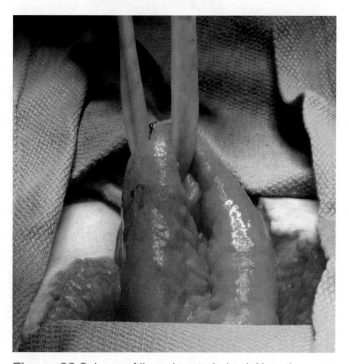

Figure 92.2 Loop of ileum is exteriorized. Note the Penrose drain used for gentle retraction, and the blue stitch (proximal) and brown chromic stitch (distal) to assure accurate orientation.

ostomy defects. The inferior epigastric artery runs superiorly in the transversalis fascia and enters the rectus sheath inferior to the arcuate line. It runs posterior to the rectus abdominis, and near the umbilicus, anastomoses with branches from the superior epigastric artery.

Exteriorization of the Ileum (Fig. 92.2)

Remove the previously placed sponge and check for bleeding. If none is apparent, pass a Peon clamp through the ostomy site and grasp the Penrose drain. Deliver the loop of ileum through the aperture, using limited tension on the Peon and Penrose to guide the bowel. The bowel should protrude approximately 3 to 5 cm above skin level. The brown suture should be at the inferior aspect, such that the proximal, or afferent, limb is cephalad. Before proceeding to maturing the ostomy, close the midline incision and apply a sterile towel or dressing to protect the wound from enteral spillage.

Maturation of Stoma (Fig. 92.3)

Remove the Penrose drain. Place a plastic bar through the mesenteric defect to support the ileum. Using electrocautery, make a transverse incision on the antimesenteric portion of the distal bowel (Fig. 92.3A). The incision should be just a few millimeters above the juncture of the skin and distal bowel and should span approximately three-quarters of the bowel circumference. Anchor the distal opening to the dermis with three equally spaced interrupted 3-0 chromic sutures, incorporating the full thickness of the bowel wall (Fig. 92.3B).

Anchor the proximal end with three interrupted 3-0 chromic sutures, taking a full-thickness bite of the bowel and then the dermis. Some surgeons take tripartite bites, passing the suture through the full-thickness bowel, seromuscular layer of the bowel at the level of the skin opening, and then the dermis. Clamp the ends of the sutures with hemostats without tying. Using the handle of an Adson forceps, evert the

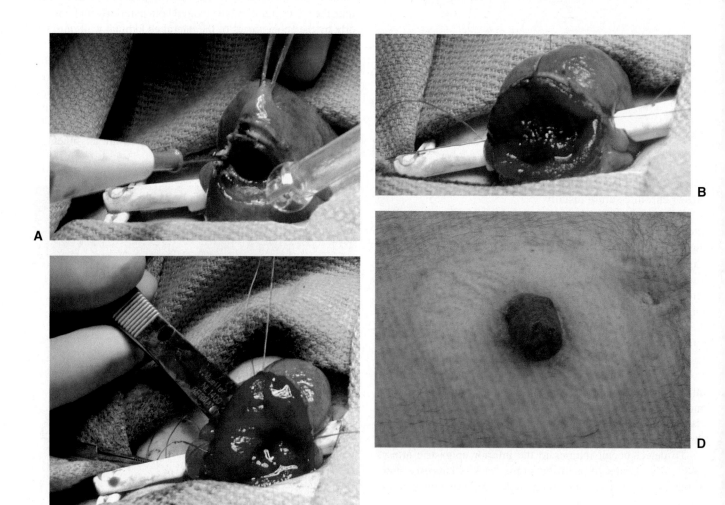

Figure 92.3 Maturation of stoma. **A:** Open the bowel low on the distal loop with electrocautery. **B:** Bowel completely opened with anchoring quadrant sutures in place. **C:** Eversion of the loop is assisted by the handle of a forceps. **D:** Example of well-formed loop ileostomy showing good protrusion of bowel.

afferent end (Fig. 92.3C), then tie down the sutures. Complete the maturation by placing interrupted sutures between each of the previously completed sutures, going from full-thickness open-edge bowel to dermis. The sutures should span the superior two-thirds of the stomal circumference.

Once this is complete, cover the stoma with a clear ostomy appliance.

The ideal loop ileostomy should, after maturation, protrude approximately 2 cm above skin level and have a centrally placed lumen (Fig. 92.3D).

STEPS IN PROCEDURE
Closure of Loop Ileostomy
Preoperatively determine integrity of
    downstream bowel or anastomosis
Circumstomal skin incision
Dissect bowel from subcutaneous tissue
    and fascia

Inspect bowel for injury
Re-establish continuity with hand-sewn or
    stapled anastomosis
Close fascia and purse-string dermis of
    wound

Ileostomy Closure

Ileostomy takedown is generally not performed before 8 to 12 weeks after construction to allow intestinal edema to resolve and adhesions to remodel. Prior to ileostomy closure, the downstream bowel should be assessed by radiographic water-soluble contrast enema or endoscopy, evaluating for patency and absence of anastomotic leak. Bowel preparation consists of limiting patients to clear liquids for 24 hours prior to surgery.

Dissection of the Stoma (Fig. 92.4)

Position the patient supine. The procedure is typically limited to the stoma site, though rarely a laparotomy is required. With a skin knife, make a circumstomal skin incision approximately 2 to 3 mm outside the mucocutaneous junction (Fig. 92.4A). With four hemostats on the skin edge, grasp and retract upward the stoma. Use handheld retractors to retract the wound from the bowel. Sharply dissect the bowel from the wound down to the anterior fascia. With appropriate tension, a white line should be evident between the bowel serosa and the subcutaneous tissue (Fig. 92.4B). Continue the dissection, separating the bowel from the fascia and rectus muscle. A finger may be inserted into the peritoneum to identify and gently sweep away any filmy adhesions. Mobilize an adequate length of bowel (Fig. 92.4C). If needed, the fascial opening can be enlarged with a vertical incision in the rectus fascia. Once the bowel is mobilized, and before re-establishing continuity, check the bowel for serosal tears and enterotomies. With a bulb syringe, irrigate each limb under pressure to examine for occult injuries.

Anatomic Points

When dissecting the bowel, stay on the serosal surface. The ileum, unlike the colon, has no fat appendages, so its antimesenteric border is smooth. Retracting upward will help with the dissection; however, judicious retraction is in order so as to avoid serosal injuries.

Re-establishing Continuity and Closure of Wound (Fig. 92.5)

Studies have demonstrated equivalence between stapled and hand-sewn anastomosis in terms of complication rate, return of bowel function, and length of hospital stay. However, a stapled side-to-side anastomosis may be preferred for its inherently larger diameter and for the speed with which it can be performed. See Chapter 90 for detailed information on various techniques of small bowel anastomosis.

For Hand-Sewn Anastomosis

Divide adhesions between the afferent and efferent limbs so that the loop lies in a straight line. Free the everted edges. Trim the open stomal edges to attain a healthy, clean bowel. Starting at one corner of the opening, place an interrupted full-thickness suture, taking minimal mucosa with each bite. Clamp the suture with a hemostat. Do the same at the other corner and again at the midpoint of the enterotomy. Complete the closure, working from each corner toward the midpoint. Once all sutures are in place, tie them sequentially and cut all but the outermost (corner) sutures. Examine the wound for defects; if a defect can accommodate the closed tip of an Adson pickup, place another stitch. Cut the remaining sutures once satisfied with the closure.

For Stapled Anastomosis

Trim the open stomal edges to attain a healthy, clean bowel; remove any attached skin as necessary. Approximate the antimesenteric borders of the ileum with a seromuscular stay suture placed approximately 6 cm from the apex. Grasp the open end and hold upright with Babcock clamps so as to minimize enteric spillage. Place one arm of the GIA stapler into each limb and join the stapler arms. The bowel must be oriented with the mesentery at the lateral-most aspect so that the staple line is through the antimesenteric surface. Fire the stapler and remove. With Allis clamps, grasp the

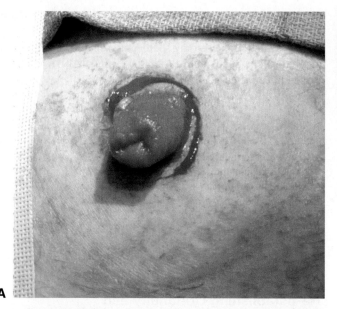

A

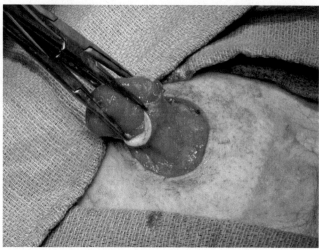

B

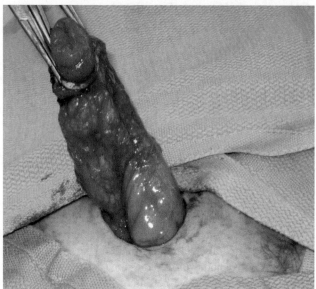

C

Figure 92.4 Closure of ileostomy. **A:** Incision around stoma. **B:** Initial dissection around bowel. **C:** Bowel fully mobilized.

corners of the staple line, then use several more Allis clamps to approximate the open edges. Place a linear or TA stapler directly beneath the row of Allis clamps and fire to complete the anastomosis.

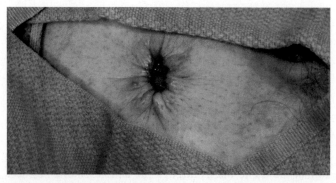

Figure 92.5 Purse-string suture closure of ostomy site

Wound Closure

Place the bowel back into the abdominal cavity. If this is difficult, consider enlarging the aperture with a vertical incision. Use absorbable suture to close the fascia in a single layer. The skin wound can be closed with staples or sutures. A running subcuticular purse string affords both an open wound to reduce wound infection and a smaller wound to speed closure.

REFERENCES

1. Beck DE, Roberts PL, Saclarides TJ, Senagore AJ, Stamos MJ, Wexner S (eds). *The ASCRS Textbook of Colon and Rectal Surgery.* 2nd ed. New York, NY: Springer Verlag; 2011.
2. Carlsen E, Bergan AB. Loop ileostomy: Technical aspects and complications. *Eur J Surg.* 1999;165(2):140–143; discussion 144.
3. Fazio VW, Church JM, Wu JS. *Atlas of Intestinal Stomas.* New York, NY: Springer; 2012.

4. Hasegawa H, Radley S, Morton DG, et al. Stapled versus sutured closure of loop ileostomy: A randomized controlled trial. *Ann Surg.* 2000;231(2):202–204.

5. Hultén L. Enterostomies–technical aspects. *Scand J Gastroenterol Suppl.* 1988;149:125–135.

6. Kaidar-Person O, Person B, Wexner SD. Complications of construction and closure of temporary loop ileostomy. *J Am Coll Surg.* 2005;201(5):759–773. Epub 2005 Sep 6.

7. Law WL, Chu KW, Choi HK. Randomized clinical trial comparing loop ileostomy and loop transverse colostomy for faecal diversion following total mesorectal excision. *Br J Surg.* 2002; 89(6):704–708.

8. Leung TT, MacLean AR, Buie WD, et al. Comparison of stapled versus handsewn loop ileostomy closure: A meta-analysis. *J Gastrointest Surg.* 2008;12(5):939–944.

9. Moore KL, Dalley AF. *Clinically Oriented Anatomy.* 4th ed. New York, NY: Lippincott Williams & Wilkins; 1999.

10. Phang PT, Hain JM, Perez-Ramirez JJ, et al. Techniques and complications of ileostomy takedown. *Am J Surg.* 1999;177(6):463–466.

11. Wexner SD, Taranow DA, Johansen OB, et al. Loop ileostomy is a safe option for fecal diversion. *Dis Colon Rectum.* 1993;36(4):349–354.

12. Wong KS, Remzi FH, Gorgun E, et al. Loop ileostomy closure after restorative proctocolectomy: Outcome in 1,504 patients. *Dis Colon Rectum.* 2005;48(2):243–250.

e 93 Laparoscopic Small Bowel Resection and Anastomosis

This chapter can be accessed online at www.lww.com/eChapter93.

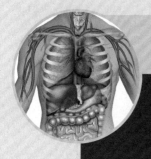

94

Appendectomy and Resection of Meckel Diverticulum

The anatomy of the lateral abdominal wall, including the rectus sheath and the right lower quadrant, is described in this chapter. The laparoscopic approach to the appendix and Meckel diverticulum is given in Chapter 95.

SCORE™, the Surgical Council on Resident Education, classified open appendectomy as an "ESSENTIAL COMMON" procedure.

STEPS IN PROCEDURE

Make small, obliquely oriented incision over McBurney point or over mass (if palpable)

Divide each layer by splitting or incising parallel to fibers

Deliver appendix into wound and confirm diagnosis

Serially clamp and tie appendiceal mesentery

Crush base of appendix with clamp and ligate with 0 chromic

Amputate appendix

Invert stump with purse string or Z stitch

Suction and irrigate field

Close incision in layers

If Appendix Appears Normal:

Remove appendix

Run small bowel for at least 1.2 m (4 feet)

Check pelvic organs (female), colon

Further exploration is determined by character of peritoneal fluid

HALLMARK ANATOMIC COMPLICATIONS

Missed pathology due to small incision when appendix normal

LIST OF STRUCTURES

Anterosuperior iliac spine
Umbilicus
McBurney point
Camper fascia
Scarpa fascia
External oblique muscle and aponeurosis
Rectus abdominis muscle
Rectus sheath
Semilunar line
Arcuate line (of Douglas)
Transversus abdominis muscle

Transversalis fascia
Iliohypogastric nerve
Subcostal nerves
Cecum
Appendix
Mesoappendix
Appendicular artery
Ileocolic artery
Ileocecal fold
Meckel diverticulum

Skin Incision (Fig. 94.1)

Technical Points

Always gently palpate the abdomen after the patient is intubated under anesthesia. You may be able to feel a mass that was inapparent while the patient was conscious and guarding. If a mass is palpable in the right lower quadrant after induction of anesthesia, make the incision over the mass.

More commonly, no mass is felt, and the skin incision is then centered by two fixed anatomic landmarks: The anterosuperior iliac spine and the umbilicus. Draw a line from the umbilicus to the anterosuperior iliac spine. McBurney point lies one-third of the distance from the anterosuperior iliac spine. The classic McBurney incision is made perpendicular to this line. The incision may be modified to follow the local lines of skin tension, as indicated, but it should pass through McBurney point. A Rockey-Davis incision is made over McBurney point, but is directed in a nearly transverse direction. This incision yields a good cosmetic result because it parallels Langer's lines. It also more nearly approximates the direction of the major cutaneous nerves of the region, and it is easy to extend this incision should unexpected pathology be encountered at laparotomy.

Anatomic Points

The anterosuperior iliac spine presents as a prominence in slender individuals, but may take the form of a depression in obese patients. It is a constant, palpable landmark. The lateral border of the rectus abdominis muscle may be visible as the semilunar line. This begins inferiorly at the pubic tubercle and curves laterally as it ascends. At the level of the umbilicus, the semilunar line is about 7 cm from the midline and lies about halfway between the midline and the side of the body.

Generally, in this region, one will be able to identify a distinct division of the superficial fascia into two layers: The more superficial layer of fatty areolar tissue, which is Camper fascia, and the deeper, membranous layer, which is Scarpa fascia.

Muscle-Splitting Incision (Fig. 94.2)

Technical Points

The external oblique muscle and its aponeurosis form the first layer of the abdominal wall (which is encountered as the incision is deepened). Open each layer of the abdominal wall by splitting, rather than cutting, the muscular and aponeurotic fibers. The resulting muscle-splitting incision is called a gridiron

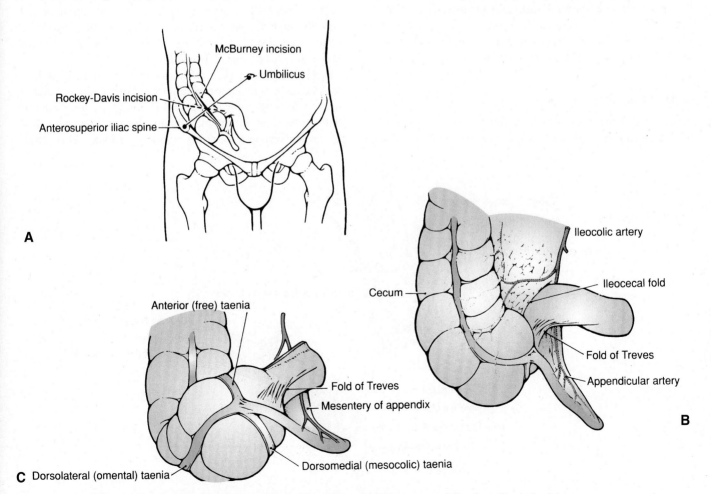

Figure 94.1 Skin incision. **A:** Typical location of McBurney and Rockey-Davis incisions. **B:** Regional anatomy. **C:** Relationship of appendix to taeniae of cecum.

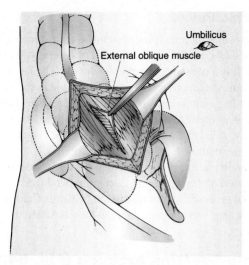

Figure 94.2 Muscle-splitting incision

incision. Because each layer is opened parallel to the muscle fibers and hence in the direction of maximum tension when the fibers contract, the resulting incision is very strong, and hernias are rare.

Medially, the external oblique aponeurosis contributes to the anterior rectus sheath. Usually, the rectus sheath forms the medial boundary of the fascial incision. If necessary, the rectus sheath may be incised. The rectus muscle can then be retracted medially to achieve additional exposure.

Anatomic Points

The fibers of the external oblique muscle run obliquely from above downward, and from lateral to medial (i.e., in the same direction as you would put your hands into your pockets). Fibers of the external oblique muscle terminate in its aponeurosis following a curved line from the semilunar line to approximately the anterosuperior iliac spine.

The major cutaneous nerves of the region are branches of the iliohypogastric and subcostal nerves.

Deepening the Incision (Fig. 94.3)

Technical Points

Split the fibers of the internal oblique and transversus abdominis muscles in turn by a combination of sharp and blunt dissection. Incise the fascia with a scalpel, cutting carefully, parallel to the fibers. Extend the cut by inserting partially closed Metzenbaum scissors and pushing, or by splitting bluntly with two fingers or a pair of hemostats. Medially, the sheath of the rectus abdominis muscle limits the extent of the split.

Anatomic Points

Note that the fibers of the internal oblique muscle are almost transverse at the level of this incision and that muscle extends much more medially than the muscular portion of the external oblique muscle. The aponeurosis of the internal oblique muscle contributes to the anterior rectus sheath along the entire length of this muscle and, by splitting, to the posterior rectus sheath above the arcuate line of Douglas.

Observe that fibers of the transversus abdominis muscle, in the operative field, almost parallel those of the internal oblique muscle. Muscle fibers proper terminate slightly more laterally than do those of the internal oblique muscle. The aponeurosis of the transversus abdominis muscle contributes fibers to the

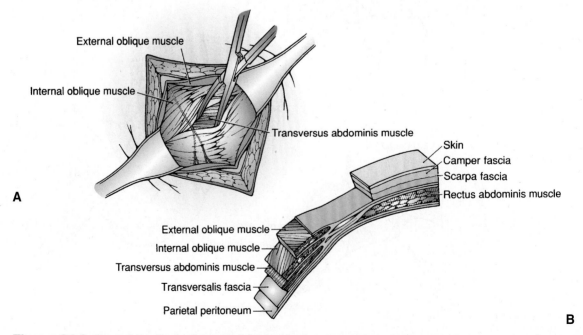

Figure 94.3 Deepening the incision. **A:** Incision is deepened by splitting muscles in the direction of their fibers. **B:** Cross-sectional anatomy of region.

anterior rectus sheath below the line of Douglas as well as to the posterior rectus sheath above.

The plane between the internal oblique and transversus abdominis muscles should be approached with caution because the main branches of the nerves that innervate the lower rectus abdominis muscle (T11, subcostal) and the skin of the lower abdominal wall (T11, subcostal, iliohypogastric) lie within this plane.

Entry into the Peritoneum and Delivery of the Appendix (Fig. 94.4)

Technical Points

Incise the peritoneum in any convenient direction. Generally, cutting in a vertical or oblique direction provides good exposure and avoids the possibility of inadvertent entry into the rectus sheath medially, injury to the inferior epigastric vessels medially, or injury to the cecum laterally. Obtain a culture of any turbid or purulent fluid that is encountered, and place retractors to obtain exposure.

In contrast with laparoscopic appendectomy, where dissection usually begins at the base of the appendix, open appendectomy starts with delivery of the appendix into the incision. It is not unusual to encounter difficulty finding the appendix in the depths of the small incision. Usually it is the tip of the appendix that is seen first, and the appendiceal mesentery must be divided to bring the base of the appendix up into the operative field (see next section).

If the appendix is not immediately visible, place the index finger of your nondominant hand into the incision and feel around for a firm tubular structure about the thickness of a pencil (sometimes much thicker!). Hook your finger around this and elevate it into the wound. It is likely to be the appendix. Double check that it is not the terminal ileum. Grasp the appendix with a Babcock clamp, taking great care not to cut

through tissues that are inflamed and edematous. Do not pull on the appendix; if it is close to perforation, it may come free in your hand, and the base will retract into the depths of the incision.

If you cannot find the appendix, locate the cecum which may be identified by its size, as well as the presence of taeniae, the terminal ileum, and the lateral peritoneal attachment (Fig. 94.4A). Cecum will commonly present into the wound, but occasionally, greater omentum, small intestine, or even sigmoid colon may be the first structure encountered. If small intestine presents into the incision and the cecum cannot be located easily, follow the small intestine distally to the terminal ileum, which leads to the cecum. Grasp the cecum firmly and pull it gently toward the patient's left shoulder with a rocking motion. If the cecum cannot be mobilized sufficiently by this maneuver, it may be necessary to incise the lateral peritoneal reflection and elevate the cecum from the retroperitoneum by blunt dissection (Fig. 94.4B).

Anatomic Points

Although typically transversalis fascia and peritoneum are fused at this point and thus can be cut as a unit, it is important to remember that these are two separate layers between which lie variable amounts of loose areolar connective tissue and fat. Note, too, that the peritoneum, which attaches the lateral side of the cecum and colon to the abdominal wall, is an embryonic fusion plane between parietal and visceral peritoneum. It is, therefore, an essentially bloodless plane and can be carefully cut with a minimum of bleeding.

The position of the appendix relative to the cecum and terminal ileum is extremely variable. The retrocecal and retroileal positions are most common (65%), but a pelvic position may also be found (31%).

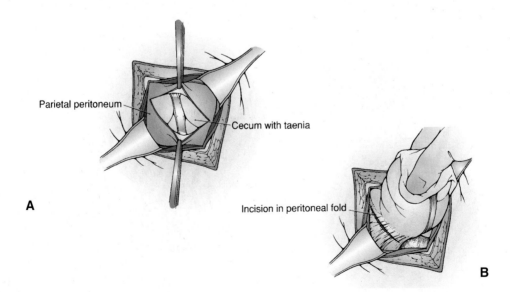

A

Parietal peritoneum

Cecum with taenia

Incision in peritoneal fold

B

Figure 94.4 Entry into the peritoneum. **A:** Initial exposure of cecum. **B:** Gentle traction on cecum to elevate and expose appendix.

Developmentally, the appendix represents the original apex of the cecum. As a result of asymmetric growth of the cecum, the origin of the appendix is usually on the posteromedial side of the cecum. The appendix is usually intraperitoneal, even when it is retrocecal. Although a retroperitoneal location for the appendix has been reported, this is generally the result of inflammation.

Regardless of location, the appendix can reliably be located by following the taeniae downward along the cecum to their junction with each other. The base of the appendix is always located at this point.

Mobilizing the Appendix (Fig. 94.5)

Technical Points

Clamp and ligate the mesentery of the appendix, starting at the part that is visible and progressing more proximally. As the mesentery is divided, the appendix will become more mobile, and the tip will come up into the wound. Sometimes, the appendix is sufficiently mobile that the appendicular artery can be secured with a single clamp, without preliminary division of the mesoappendix. Always ligate the appendicular artery separately from the appendiceal stump. If the artery is included in the stump ligature or inverted with the stump, troublesome postoperative bleeding may occur.

Anatomic Points

The mesoappendix transports the appendicular artery. This is a branch of the ileocolic artery, which arises from the superior mesenteric artery. The mesoappendix passes posterior to the terminal ileum and is of variable length. Commonly, it is so short that the appendix is significantly tethered behind the cecum and ileum and may be folded on itself. The appendicular artery frequently runs close to the base of the appendix and then passes away from the appendix to run in the free edge of the mesoappendix, sending out several small branches.

The mesoappendix forms the posterior wall of the inferior ileocecal fossa. A fold of fatty tissue (the inferior ileocecal fold or bloodless fold of Treves) commonly runs from the antimesenteric border of the terminal ileum to the cecum. This can be cut safely.

Appendectomy (Fig. 94.6)

Technical Points

The most common cause of acute appendicitis is obstruction of the appendiceal lumen by a fecalith. In such cases, the appendix distal to the fecalith becomes inflamed and edematous; however, the portion proximal to the fecalith remains relatively normal. Thus dissection of the appendix past the inflamed portion toward the cecum often yields a segment of appendix that may be ligated safely (Fig. 94.6A). Carefully dissect the appendix down to its origin from the cecum. Crush the appendix carefully with a clamp, and then clamp it just distal to the crushed portion. Ligate the appendix through the previously crushed portion, clamp above the ligature, and cut through the base of the appendix (Fig. 94.6B).

If desired, invert the appendiceal stump by use of a purse-string suture or Z stitch (Fig. 94.6C,D). The inverting suture should be placed wide enough to allow the cecum to cover the stump completely when the suture is tied; however, it should not impinge on the ileocecal valve or appendicular artery. Because there is maximal mobility laterally, the suture may be placed wider laterally, allowing the cecum to roll medially over the stump of the appendix.

Anatomic Points

The ileocecal valve represents a protrusion of the mucosa, submucosa, and circular muscle layers of the terminal ileum into

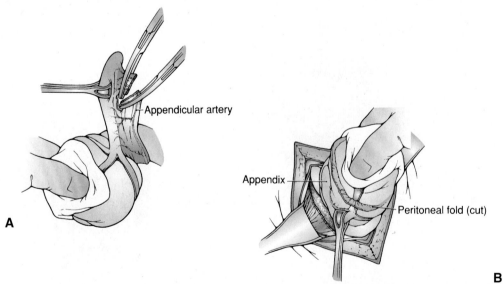

Figure 94.5 Mobilizing the appendix. **A:** Initial division of appendicular artery. **B:** Position of retrocecal appendix (note that peritoneum has been cut to expose appendix).

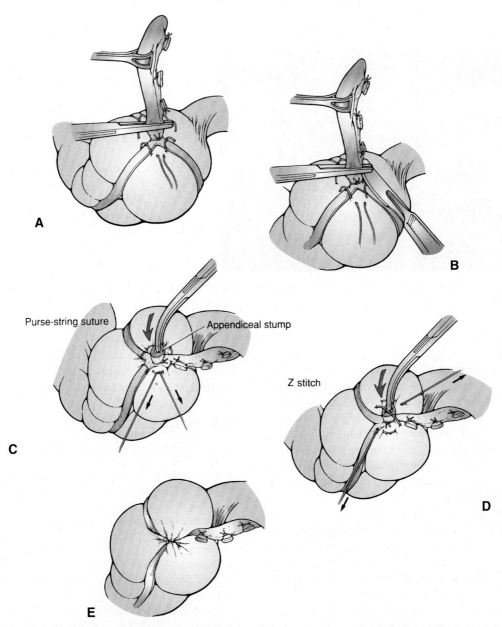

Figure 94.6 Appendectomy. **A:** Placement of purse-string suture around ligated appendix. **B:** Removal of appendix (stump previously ligated). **C:** Inverting the appendiceal stump as the purse-string suture is tightened. **D:** Alternative placement of Z-stitch automatically buries the stump under the cecum. **E:** Completed Z-stitch with appendiceal stump completely buried.

the cecal lumen. This valve may function both actively and passively. The base of the appendix is usually less than 2 cm from this valve.

Exploration in the Case of a Grossly Normal Appendix (Fig. 94.7)

Technical Points

If the appendix appears to be normal, direct your search toward adjacent organs. First, inspect the terminal ileum for signs of inflammatory bowel disease or enlarged mesenteric lymph nodes. Search for a Meckel diverticulum by "running" the small bowel carefully for a distance of at least 1.5 m (5 feet) from the ileocecal valve (Fig. 94.7A). Carefully palpate the right colon, sigmoid colon, and bladder, as well as the uterus and ovaries in female patients. The character of the peritoneal fluid on initial entry (purulent or not, foul-smelling or not, bile-stained or not) will help guide you as to the extent of your exploration. Foul-smelling, purulent fluid, bilious fluid, or succus requires a thorough search for the origin of the problem—even if that means conversion to a midline laparotomy.

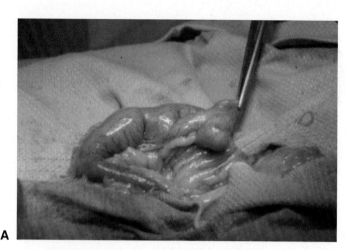
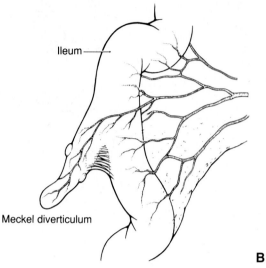

Figure 94.7 Meckel diverticulum. **A:** Prominent fatty streak indicates mesentery. **B:** Usual location is along the terminal ileum, within 1.2 m (4 feet) of the ileocecal valve.

If you find an inflamed Meckel diverticulum, excise the inflamed region by resecting a short segment of ileum and performing an end-to-end anastomosis (see Chapter 90). In some cases, simple diverticulectomy may suffice. This is easily done with a linear stapling device as shown in the chapter on Laparoscopic Appendectomy (see Chapter 95). Take care to secure the small tongue of mesentery feeding the diverticulum. This will appear as a fatty streak passing up one or both sides of the bowel (Fig. 94.7B).

Occasionally, a lesion in the upper abdomen, such as a perforated duodenal ulcer, will cause lower abdominal pain secondary to leakage of fluid down the right gutter. If pathology of the upper abdomen is suspected or confirmed, close the appendectomy incision and make a second (usually vertical midline) incision in the upper abdomen to gain adequate exposure.

Close the appendectomy incision in layers. Place drains only if a well-defined abscess cavity is encountered.

Anatomic Points

Meckel diverticulum, the most common anomaly of the gastrointestinal tract, represents a persistent remnant of the vitelline duct (embryonic yolk stalk). Typically, this diverticulum is located on the antimesenteric border of the ileum, within 50 cm of the ileocecal valve. Occasionally, such diverticula have been found as far as 170 cm from the ileocecal valve. Thus at least 200 cm of small bowel should be examined to avoid missing a Meckel diverticulum. These diverticula also vary in length from 1 to 20 cm, although most (75%) are 1 to 5 cm long. Fibrous bands sometimes run from the diverticulum to the umbilicus, mesentery, omentum, or serosa of the gut. Rarely (2%), the lumen of the duct is retained from skin to bowel, resulting in a vitelline fistula. The mucosa of a Meckel diver-

ticulum is most commonly ileal; however, gastric, pancreatic, duodenal, colonic, and bile duct mucosa have been reported.

References

1. Adams JT. Z-stitch suture for inversion of the appendiceal stump. *Surg Gynecol Obstet.* 1968;127:1321.
2. Askew AR. The Fowler–Weir approach to appendicectomy. *Br J Surg.* 1975;62:303.
3. Cullen JJ, Kelly KA, Hodge DO, et al. Surgical management of Meckel's diverticulum: An epidemiologic, population-based study. *Ann Surg.* 1994;220:564–568. (Advocates removal of asymptomatic Meckel's diverticula found at laparotomy.)
4. Delany HM, Carnevale NJ. A "bikini" incision for appendectomy. *Am J Surg.* 1976;132:126. (Presents alternative incision.)
5. Hale DA, Molloy M, Pearl RH, et al. Appendectomy: A contemporary appraisal. *Ann Surg.* 1997;225:252–261.
6. Jelenko C, Davis LP. A transverse lower abdominal appendectomy incision with minimal muscle derangement. *Surg Gynecol Obstet.* 1973;136:451. (Presents alternative incision.)
7. Lewis FR, Holcroft JW, Bowy J, et al. Appendicitis: A critical review of diagnosis and treatment in 1,000 cases. *Arch Surg.* 1975; 110:677.
8. Pepper VK, Stanfill AB, Pearl RH. Diagnosis and management of pediatric appendicitis, intussusception, and Meckel diverticulum. *Surg Clin North Am.* 2012;92:505.
9. Sandsmark M. Serious delayed rectal haemorrhage following uncomplicated appendectomy. Report of a case. *Acta Chir Scand.* 1977;143:385. (Discusses rare complication related to inversion of stump.)
10. Williamson WA, Bush RD, Williams LF. Retrocecal appendicitis. *Am J Surg.* 1981;141:507.
11. Yalchouchy EK, Marano AF, Etienne JC, et al. Meckel's diverticulum. *J Am Coll Surg.* 2001;192:658–662. (Reviews embryology and management.)

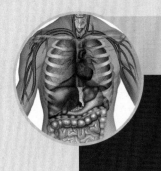

95

Laparoscopic Appendectomy and Resection of Meckel Diverticulum

This chapter describes both laparoscopic appendectomy (including mobilization of the right colon for retrocecal appendix) and laparoscopic resection of Meckel diverticulum. Two methods of laparoscopic appendectomy—with and without the use of the endoscopic stapler—are presented.

SCORE™, the Surgical Council on Resident Education, classified laparoscopic appendectomy as an "ESSENTIAL COMMON" procedure.

STEPS IN PROCEDURE

Patient position, monitors placed to facilitate access to right lower quadrant
Three trocars most commonly used
Create pneumoperitoneum and explore abdomen
Grasp appendix and elevate
Expose base of appendix
Create window in avascular "sweet spot" at base of mesentery
Divide appendix with endoscopic stapler (gastrointestinal load)
Divide mesentery with endoscopic stapler (vascular load)

Remove small appendix through 10-mm trocar
Place large appendix in endoscopic bag for removal
Irrigate field, close any trocar sites greater than 5 mm

If Appendix Normal

Check pelvic organs (female)
Run small bowel for at least 121.92 cm (4 ft) to exclude Meckel diverticulum
Be guided by character and location of any fluid

HALLMARK ANATOMIC COMPLICATIONS

Injury to bowel or vessels during peritoneal entry
Injury to cecum during mobilization for retrocecal appendix

Missed pathology because of limited ability to palpate

LIST OF STRUCTURES

Cecum

Appendix
Mesoappendix
Appendicular artery

Terminal ileum
Meckel diverticulum

Setup and Initial View (Fig. 95.1)

Technical Points

Position the patient supine with both arms tucked in. Set the room up with the primary monitor at the patient's right knee, and a secondary monitor, if desired, at the patient's left knee. Palpate the abdomen. A palpable mass in the right lower quadrant generally implies complicated appendicitis; this can be managed laparoscopically if one is experienced.

Access the abdomen through a supraumbilical port. Inspect all four quadrants, looking for confirmation of the etiology.

Aspirate and irrigate any purulent material, obtaining cultures if desired. If the appearance is consistent with appendicitis, place the operating table in Trendelenburg position with the right side elevated. The cecum should be visible in the right lower quadrant. Confirm cecum by taeniae and whiter color than adjacent loops of small intestine.

Place a working 5-mm port in the right upper quadrant at about the midclavicular line and pass an endoscopic Babcock clamp into the field. Gently retract the cecum toward the upper abdomen. The base of the appendix should roll into view. Note that the tip of the appendix is tethered by the mesoappendix, which passes

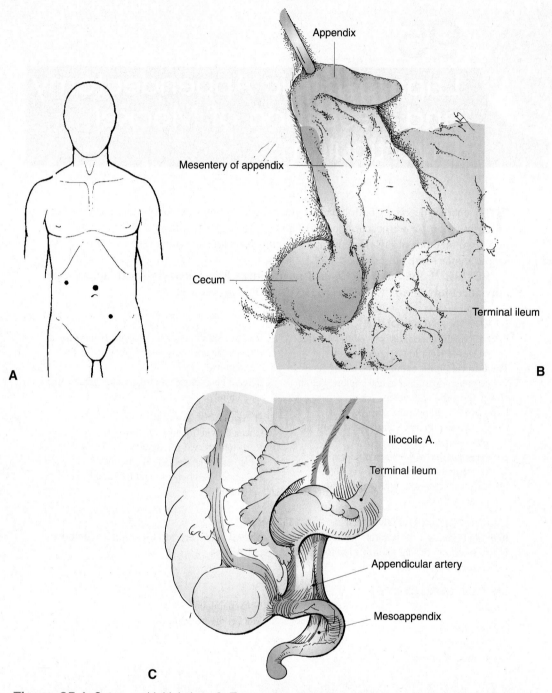

Figure 95.1 Setup and initial view. **A:** Trocar placement **B:** Initial view of appendix **C:** Regional anatomy (**B** from Scott-Conner CEH, Cuschieri A, Carter FJ, eds. Small intestine and appendix. In: *Minimal Access Surgical Anatomy.* Philadelphia, PA: Lippincott Williams & Wilkins; 2000: 165–184, with permission; **C** from Wind GG. The colon. In: *Applied Laparoscopic Anatomy: Abdomen and Pelvis.* Baltimore, MD: Williams & Wilkins; 1997:217–246, with permission).

behind the terminal ileum. Additional ports will be placed in the left lower quadrant or lower midline (12 mm), depending on the size of the patient, and optionally in the right lower quadrant for additional retraction in difficult cases (Fig. 95.1A).

Insert the 12-mm port next. If the patient is small, with a narrow abdomen, put this in the left lower quadrant, taking care to choose a site lateral to the rectus muscle to avoid the inferior epigastric vessels. If the patient is large, a lower midline site as shown will work well. As always, think in terms of working distance rather than fixed anatomic landmarks. Use an atraumatic grasper to manipulate cecum and appendix so that the appendix can be grasped by the Babcock clamp and elevated (Fig. 95.1B).

Anatomic Points

The outer muscular layer of the appendix is formed by longitudinal fibers, which are the continuation of the three taeniae of the colon. Thus the appendix may be located by seeking the convergence of the taeniae. Location of the appendix varies, but it is always tethered to some extent by the mesoappendix, which passes behind the terminal ileum (Fig. 95.1C). In many individuals, the appendix is partially or completely retrocecal.

The laparoscopic approach (base before tip) is different from that commonly used during open appendectomy. The laparoscopic surgeon has the advantage of working from within the abdomen and approaches the appendix from a vantage point cephalad and to the right. Thus as the cecum is pulled up, the base is the first part of the appendix to come into view. In all but the true retrocecal appendices (Fig. 95.4), the rest of the appendix generally then comes into view.

Appendectomy Using Endoscopic Stapling Device (Fig. 95.2)

Technical and Anatomic Points

Use a Maryland dissector to develop a window in the mesentery of the appendix at the base (Fig. 95.2A). Visualize the cecum funneling up toward the base to confirm that no residual appendiceal tissue will remain. The mesenteric window needs to be about 1.5 cm wide. Enlarge it with an endoscopic right-angled forceps. Pass an endoscopic cutting linear stapler through the left lower quadrant port and staple across the base of the appendix (Fig. 95.2B). Remove the stapler. The appendix will now be hanging by the mesoappendix. Reload the stapler with a vascular cartridge and use it to divide the mesoappendix (Fig. 95.2C). A minimally inflamed appendix can be grasped at one end (lengthwise) and withdrawn into the 12-mm trocar. Trocar and appendix can then be removed en bloc (Fig. 95.2D).

A purulent or perforated appendix is best placed in an endoscopic retrieval bag. To do this, pass the endoscopic retrieval bag through the 12-mm port and open it. Position the bag so that the opening faces the laparoscope. Maneuver the appendix

into the bag and withdraw the grasper, shaking the grasper gently to encourage the appendix to drop off the grasper into the bag (Fig. 95.2E). Exercise caution during this maneuver because the appendix commonly adheres to the grasper and is pulled back out of the bag with the grasper. After it is dropped into the pelvis among loops of bowel, the appendix may be difficult to impossible to find and recover. This is best prevented by caution during this phase of the procedure. Visually confirm that the appendix is inside of the bag before closing and withdrawing the bag through the abdominal wall.

Irrigate the operative field. If desired, place a closed-suction drain in the pelvis or in an abscess cavity.

Appendectomy Using Endoloop (Fig. 95.3)

Technical and Anatomic Points

This method works best for a minimally inflamed appendix and a mesentery that is not too fatty. Elevate the appendix and inspect the mesentery (Fig. 95.3A). It will be necessary to divide the mesentery first. Either clips or an ultrasonic scalpel can be used to secure the mesentery. To use clips, first develop a series of windows in the mesentery by dissecting with a Maryland dissector between the branches of the appendicular artery (Fig. 95.3B). Sequentially clip and divide these branches until the appendix is hanging by the base.

Pass an Endoloop through the left lower quadrant port. Extend the loop into the field, taking care not to allow the Endoloop to contact the bowel. The ligature is made of chromic catgut and will be limp (and difficult to manipulate) if it becomes wet. Shorten the loop slightly to facilitate manipulation. Pass a grasper through the Endoloop and grasp the appendix, pulling it through the loop (Fig. 95.3C). Manipulate the loop down to the base and slowly tighten the loop. Continue to adjust the position of the loop on the base of the appendix as the loop becomes smaller. Be aware that it will not be possible to open the loop and readjust it. Use the knot pusher to position the loop at the exact base and cinch the loop down. Generally, two loops are placed on the base and a third is placed above. Cut between and remove the appendix as previously described. Many surgeons place a clip over the knot of the Endoloop for added security.

Management of Retrocecal Appendix (Fig. 95.4)

Technical Points

When the appendix is retrocecal, it is necessary to mobilize the cecum to gain exposure. Using scissors and electrocautery (or ultrasonic scalpel), incise the peritoneum lateral to the cecum and roll the cecum medially. The appendix will generally be adherent to the back wall of the cecum. Identify it by feel and grasp it with an endoscopic Babcock forceps as shown. Proceed with appendectomy as previously described.

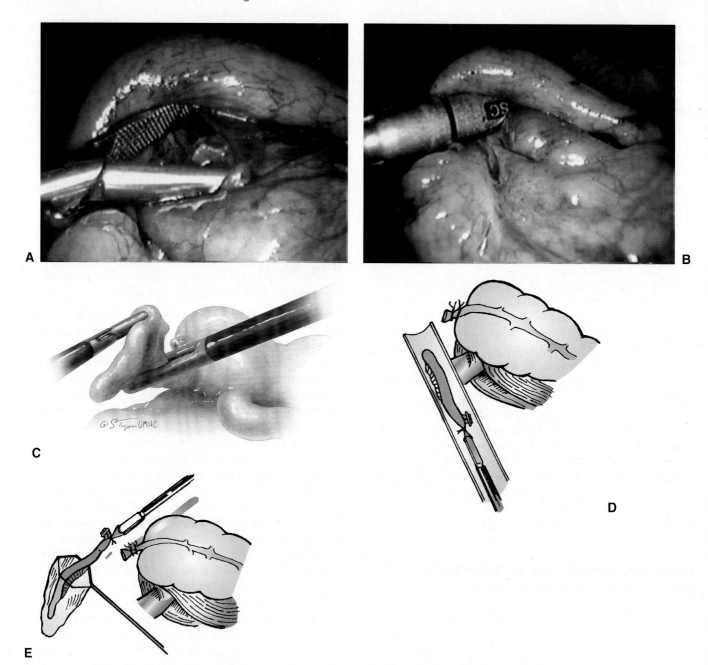

Figure 95.2 Appendectomy using endoscopic stapling device. **A:** Development of mesenteric window. **B:** Firing stapler across base of appendix. **C:** Firing stapler with vascular load across mesentery (from Fischer JE, Jones DB, Pomposelli FB, et al. Fischer's Mastery of Surgery. 6th ed. Philadelphia, PA: Lippincott Williams & Wilkins; 2012, with permission). **D:** Draw a minimally inflamed appendix up into the 12-mm trocar and remove trocar and appendix together. **E:** Place a large or purulent appendix in an endoscopic retrieval bag for removal (from Baker RJ, Fischer JE, eds. Mastery of Surgery. 4th ed. Philadelphia, PA: Lippincott Williams & Wilkins; 2001, with permission).

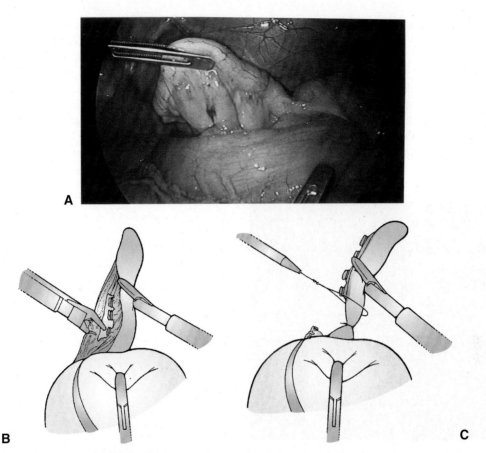

Figure 95.3 Appendectomy using Endoloop. **A:** Minimally inflamed appendix with soft mesentery, suitable for removal with endoloop. **B:** Secure the mesentery with clips as shown or Harmonic scalpel. **C:** First application of Endoloop to base (**B, C** from Scott-Conner CEH, Hall TJ, Anglin BL, et al. Laparoscopic appendectomy: Initial experience in a teaching program. *Ann Surg.* 1992;215:660–668, with permission).

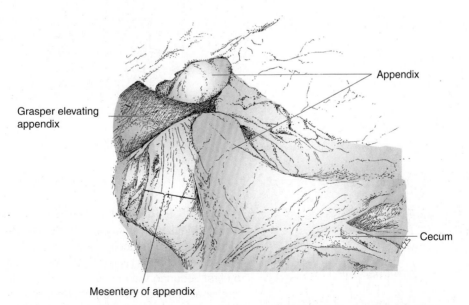

Figure 95.4 Management of retrocecal appendix (from Scott-Conner CEH, Cuschieri A, Carter FJ, eds. Small intestine and appendix. In: *Minimal Access Surgical Anatomy.* Philadelphia, PA: Lippincott Williams & Wilkins; 2000:165–184, with permission).

Removal of Meckel Diverticulum (Fig. 95.5)

Technical Points

Rarely, a normal appendix and an inflamed Meckel diverticulum are found to coexist. Inspect the region of the Meckel diverticulum (Fig. 95.5A) and decide whether simple diverticulectomy or wedge excision of the segment of ileum containing the Meckel diverticulum is required.

To perform simple diverticulectomy, first identify and control the blood vessel supplying the Meckel diverticulum. This will generally be found in a fatty stripe that runs on the cephalad surface of the ileum (Fig. 95.5B). This stripe should be visible if the loop of ileum is held in the lower abdomen (with the laparoscope looking down from above). Then pass an endoscopic stapler through the left lower quadrant port and staple across the base of the Meckel diverticulum (Fig. 95.5C).

Proceed with appendectomy as previously described, if desired.

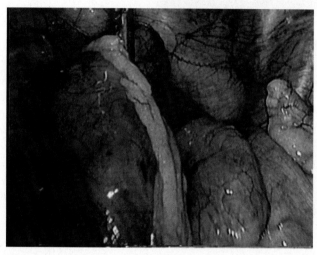

A

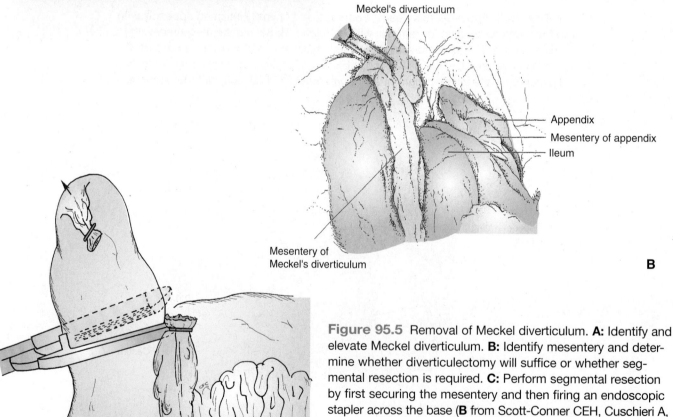

B

C

Figure 95.5 Removal of Meckel diverticulum. **A:** Identify and elevate Meckel diverticulum. **B:** Identify mesentery and determine whether diverticulectomy will suffice or whether segmental resection is required. **C:** Perform segmental resection by first securing the mesentery and then firing an endoscopic stapler across the base (**B** from Scott-Conner CEH, Cuschieri A, Carter FJ, eds. Small intestine and appendix. In: *Minimal Access Surgical Anatomy*. Philadelphia, PA: Lippincott Williams & Wilkins; 2000:165–184, with permission).

Anatomic Points

As discussed in detail in Chapter 94, a Meckel diverticulum represents a remnant of the vitelline duct. The fatty stripe containing the blood supply may be a useful landmark when the diverticulum is difficult to identify.

Acknowledgments

Laparoscopic photos in this chapter were provided by Hui Sen Chong, MD, and Evgeny V. Arshava, MD.

REFERENCES

1. Eubanks S, Phillip S. Chapter 150: Laparoscopic Appendectomy. In: Fischer JE, Jones DB, Pomposelli FB, Upchurch GR, Klimberg VS, Schwaitzberg SD, Bland KI, eds. *Fischer's Mastery of Surgery.* Philadelphia, PA: Wolters Kluwer Lippincott Williams & Wilkins; 2013:1607.
2. Moazzez A, Mason RJ, Katkhouda N. Thirty-day outcomes of laparoscopic versus open appendectomy in elderly using ACS/NSQIP database. *Surg Endosc.* 2012;27(4):1061–1071.
3. Pepper VK, Stanfill AB, Pearl RH. Diagnosis and management of pediatric appendicitis, intussusception, and Meckel diverticulum. *Surg Clin North Am.* 2012;92:505–526.
4. Scott-Conner CEH, Cuschieri A, Carter FJ, eds. Small intestine and appendix. In: *Minimal Access Surgical Anatomy.* Philadelphia, PA: Lippincott Williams & Wilkins; 2000:165–184.
5. Wilasrusmee C, Sukrat B, McEvoy M, et al. Systematic review and meta-analysis of safety of laparoscopic versus open appendicectomy for suspected appendicitis in pregnancy. *Br J Surg.* 2012; 99:1470–1478.
6. Yaghoubian A, Kaji AH, Lee SL. Laparoscopic versus open appendectomy: Outcomes analysis. *Am Surg.* 2012;78:1083–1086.

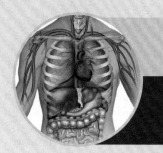

96

Colonoscopy

Colonoscopy is performed with the patient lying in the left lateral decubitus (Sims) position. Flexible sigmoidoscopy will not be discussed separately because it duplicates the initial maneuvers of colonoscopy. Concentrate on passing the scope safely and atraumatically. Inspect the region as the scope is withdrawn. Use as little air insufflation as possible to ensure patient comfort and to facilitate passage of the scope. This procedure is used to introduce the topography of the colon.

SCORE™, the Surgical Council on Resident Education, classified colonoscopy with or without biopsy or polypectomy as an "ESSENTIAL COMMON" procedure.

STEPS IN PROCEDURE

Assure intravenous access and provide sedation, if desired
Position patient in left lateral decubitus position
Perform digital rectal examination
Pass lubricated colonoscope past anal sphincters

Pass Scope Under Direct Vision to Cecum
Use as little insufflation as possible
The rectum hugs the curve of the sacrum and has three prominent valves
At the pelvic brim, angulation marks the entry into the mobile sigmoid colon

The next angulation is encountered at the splenic flexure
The three haustra of the transverse colon usually give it a triangular cross-section
The next angulation is the hepatic flexure (sometimes aspirating some air helps)
The cecum shows convergence of taeniae, appendiceal orifice and ileocecal valve may be seen
Inspect the entire bowel as you slowly withdraw the scope

HALLMARK ANATOMIC COMPLICATIONS

Missed lesions due to blind spots
Perforation

LIST OF STRUCTURES

Rectum
Transverse rectal folds (valves of Houston)
Sigmoid colon
Descending (left) colon
Splenic flexure

Transverse colon
Hepatic flexure
Ascending (right) colon
Cecum
Ileocecal valve

Rectosigmoid (Fig. 96.1)

Technical Points

Perform a digital rectal examination first to lubricate the anal canal and to confirm that no low obstructing lesions are present. If stool is encountered, consider rescheduling the examination after completion of a more adequate bowel prep.

Place the index finger of your dominant hand on the tip of the scope and press the tip, angled at about 45 degrees, against the anus. Instruct the patient to bear down. This will relax the sphincters and facilitate passage of the scope. Press the scope into the anal canal. Note that the rim of the scope is elevated, which makes insertion of the tip en face difficult, if not impossible.

The rectum curves posteriorly to hug the hollow of the sacrum. Insufflate enough air to identify its lumen. The valves of Houston may be visible.

At the pelvic brim, the relatively straight rectum blends imperceptibly with the mobile sigmoid. The length and mobility of this segment vary considerably from individual to individual and may be altered by prior surgery. Try to traverse the sigmoid using as little length of the scope and as little air insufflation as possible.

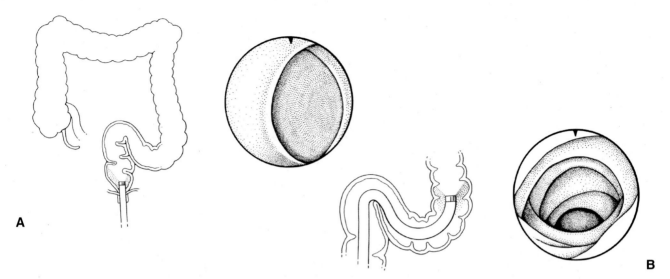

Figure 96.1 Rectosigmoid. **A:** Initial view of valves of Houston. **B:** View of circular folds of sigmoid colon.

Anatomic Points

Flexible endoscopy has significantly decreased the incidence of perforation of the rectum. However, because perforations still occur, one should be aware of the anatomy and relationships of the rectum and anal canal. As the terminal rectum penetrates the pelvic diaphragm, it makes an approximate right-angled bend. From the standpoint of the endoscopist inserting an instrument into the anus, this bend occurs about 4 cm proximal to the anal verge (here defined as the transition zone where the dry, hirsute, perianal skin changes to the moist, squamous epithelium lining the anal canal). This necessitates directing the tip of the instrument toward the concavity of the sacrum. Immediately anterior to this point of angulation are the median prostate gland and paramedian seminal vesicle in male patients, and the vagina in female patients. In male patients, more proximally, the anterior rectal wall is in contact with the urinary bladder. Still further from the anal verge (about 7.5 cm in males and 5.5 cm in females), the peritoneum is reflected from the anterior surface of the rectum to the posterior surface of the urinary bladder (in males) or the uterus (in females), forming the rectovesical or rectouterine pouch (cul-de-sac of Douglas), respectively. This is the most dependent recess of the peritoneal cavity; thus, it can fill with peritoneal fluid, pus, or loops of bowel.

The terminal large bowel is divided into a proximal rectum and terminal anal canal. From the anal verge, the anal canal extends to the pectinate line, a distance of about 1.5 cm. At this line, the stratified squamous epithelium changes to columnar cells characteristic of large bowel mucosa. At approximately this line, several changes occur: The arterial supply changes from the more caudal inferior rectal arteries to the more proximal middle and superior rectal (hemorrhoidal) arteries, the venous return changes from tributaries of the caval system to tributaries of the portal system, the lymphatic drainage pattern changes from drainage to the inguinal nodes to drainage to the internal iliac or inferior mesenteric nodes, and the nerve supply changes from somatic innervation by the pudendal nerves

to autonomic innervation (sympathetic and parasympathetic) from hypogastric plexuses.

The rectum extends from the pectinate line to the level of the third sacral vertebra, a distance of about 12 to 15 cm. The lowest part of the rectum, which is entirely below the peritoneal reflection, is significantly wider than the anal canal and is capable of great dilation; this is the rectal ampulla. It is the terminal ampulla that makes the approximate right-angled bend, termed the *perineal flexure*. The only features of note in the normal rectum are the transverse rectal folds (valves of Houston). Typically, there are three folds: The most distal one (4 to 7 cm from the anal verge) on the left, an intermediate one (8 to 10 cm from the anal verge) on the right, and the most proximal one (10 to 12 cm from the anal verge), again on the left. The number of transverse folds, however, can vary from one to five, and their placement may be reversed. Finally, it should be noted that the rectum lacks the characteristic haustra of the colon. This is a result of the dispersal of the musculature of the three taeniae coli to form a circumferential longitudinal muscle layer of uniform thickness.

Endoscopically, the sigmoid colon can be distinguished by well-marked semilunar folds. In addition, the mucosa in this region is velvety in appearance. Although the length and disposition of the sigmoid colon are variable, that it is suspended on a mesentery enables it to be somewhat straightened by the passage of the endoscope. The first part entered—the terminal sigmoid—typically lies to the right of the midline.

Descending Colon (Fig. 96.2)

Technical Points

Identify the left (descending) colon by its relative straightness compared with the tortuous sigmoid. Advancing the scope through this channel is relatively easy. If the scope does not advance easily, there is probably an excessively large loop in the sigmoid colon. Reduce this loop by simultaneously

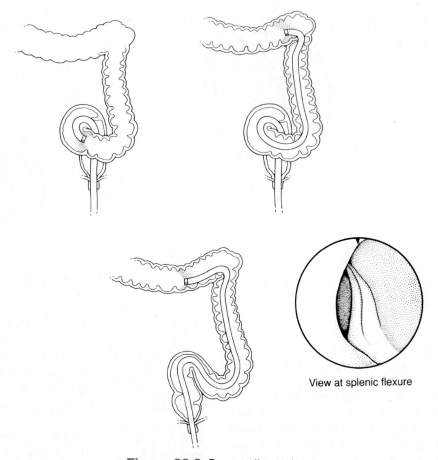

View at splenic flexure

Figure 96.2 Descending colon

withdrawing the scope while having an assistant push gently on the left lower quadrant.

At the splenic flexure, a bluish shadow (the spleen) may be visible through the bowel wall. Often, the only clue is that the lumen of the bowel disappears. To traverse the splenic flexure, hook the tip of the scope around the flexure and then straighten the scope as it is advanced.

Anatomic Points

The retroperitoneal left colon is marked by circular folds that are located at more regular intervals than are the semicircular folds of the sigmoid colon. The mucosa here is smooth, somewhat shiny, and gray-pink in color.

Transverse Colon (Fig. 96.3)

Technical Points

The transverse colon usually has a characteristically triangular lumen. It is variable in both length and mobility. Imagine the bowel being "reefed up" and shortened over the scope as it is passed.

The hepatic flexure is generally not as angulated as the splenic flexure, but it may be more difficult to pass by. Often, so

much scope has been inserted that a loop can form either in the sigmoid or in the transverse colon. Pull back on the scope and suction out some air to collapse the bowel partially. This may allow the tip to advance into the ascending (or right) colon. The bluish shadow of the liver may be visible through the bowel wall.

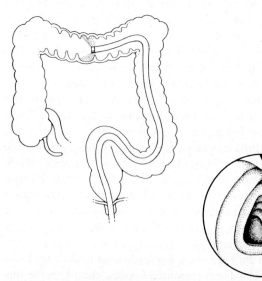

Figure 96.3 Transverse colon

Anatomic Points

The approach to the splenic flexure, the proximal end of the left colon, is recognized endoscopically by the domelike appearance of the lumen. This is the result of the sharp angulation of this flexure. The endoscope must be directed to the right and inferiorly for passage into the transverse colon.

Although quite variable in length, the transverse colon is suspended by a mesentery (transverse mesocolon), which allows it to be manipulated endoscopically. The transverse colon is characterized by its triangular lumen, which is reflected in both haustra and mucosal folds.

The hepatic flexure is not as acute as the splenic flexure, and the mucosal folds here have been described as pagoda shaped. The lumen and folds at this flexure are triangular, and the extremities of the folds overlap somewhat, rather than being continuous like those of the rest of the transverse colon.

Right Colon and Cecum (Fig. 96.4)

Technical Points

Continue to advance the scope by a series of withdrawal and advance maneuvers until the ileocecal valve and convergence of the taeniae at the cecum are visible. You must be certain that you have visualized the cecum. Many endoscopists use fluoroscopy to confirm the location of the scope within the cecal air shadow, injecting Hypaque into the bowel through the scope if necessary. If fluoroscopy is not available, confirm that the cecum has been reached on the basis of (a) endoscopic appearance, (b) the appearance of a light in the right lower quadrant, and (c) a visible indentation of the bowel wall when the right lower quadrant is palpated.

Cannulation of the terminal ileum can be achieved in many patients by angling the tip of the scope and pulling back, engaging the tip within the ileocecal valve. Several centimeters of terminal ileum can often be examined in this way.

Anatomic Points

On endoscopic examination, the retroperitoneal right (ascending) colon will be seen to have semicircular mucosal folds. Generally, it is larger in diameter than the left colon.

The cecum is greater in diameter than the rest of the colon, and its wall seems to be thinner. Because of these anatomic characteristics and LaPlace law, over-insufflation of the colon can cause the cecum to rupture more easily than other regions of the colon. The orifice of the appendix is not at the most dependent part of the cecum. Instead, it is usually on the posteromedial side of the cecum, as is the ileocecal valve. Of the two, the appendix is more caudal. It is always circular and is usually concealed by a mucosal fold.

The shape of the ileocecal valve is variable. It can present as a circular or oval protrusion into the lumen of the cecum, or it may be bilabial. In the latter case, the orientation of the lips is similar to that of the semilunar folds of the right colon. Typically, the valve is 2 to 3 cm in diameter and about 10 cm superior to the blind end of the cecum.

Completion of the Examination (Fig. 96.5)

Technical and Anatomic Points

As the colonoscope is withdrawn, carefully and systematically examine the bowel. Advance the scope to re-examine areas that are missed if the tip of the scope "jumps back" too fast for adequate inspection of the mucosa.

Note the position of any abnormalities by referring to fixed landmarks whenever possible. Distances vary from examination to examination; it is much more meaningful to state that a lesion is "just proximal to the splenic flexure" than to characterize it as being "at 100 cm."

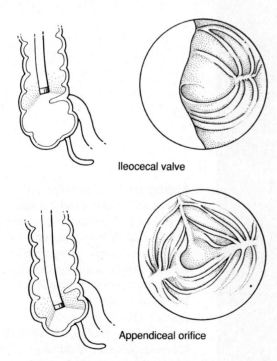

Figure 96.4 Right colon and cecum

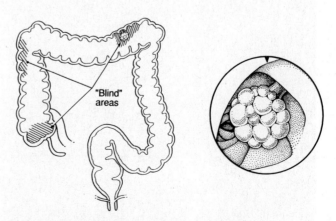

Figure 96.5 Completion of the examination

STEPS IN PROCEDURE

Biopsy

    Attain stable view of lesion

    Pass biopsy forceps

    Open forceps and impact the open jaws on the target

    Have assistant close forceps

    Withdraw forceps and retrieve sample from jaws

Polypectomy

    Attain stable view of polyp

    Pass polypectomy snare

    Maneuver snare over polyp

Have assistant slowly tighten snare as you maintain position at base of polyp

    Do not cut through base

Elevate polyp with snare to minimize chance of perforation

Have assistant slowly tighten snare as you apply cautery

    Retrieve polyp

        Polyp grasper

        Suction

    Inspect base

Biopsy and Polypectomy (Fig. 96.6)

Technical and Anatomic Points

Performance of biopsy or polypectomy significantly increases the risk of perforation. Both require an assistant and a stable view of the target. Ideally, the tip of the colonoscope should not be sharply bent, as this makes it more difficult to pass the forceps or snare.

Biopsy: Several types of biopsy forceps are available. Many have a central spike that stabilizes the lesion while the forceps close. Some can apply cauterizing current ("hot biopsy forceps"). The general principle is quite simple. First, pass the closed biopsy forceps and allow the tip to exit, visualizing the closed tip within the field of view. Note where the forceps emerge (generally this will be around 6 o'clock) and maneuver the colonoscopy to provide a straight direct path for the forceps to reach the lesion.

Have your assistant open the jaws of the forceps. Advance the open-jawed forcep until it impacts the lesion. For an exophytic lesion, such as a presumed carcinoma, push the forceps into the tissue to assure a good bite.

Have your assistant close the jaws. Withdraw the forceps and inspect the specimen. Take multiple specimens to assure adequacy of sampling. If bleeding is noted, judicious use of

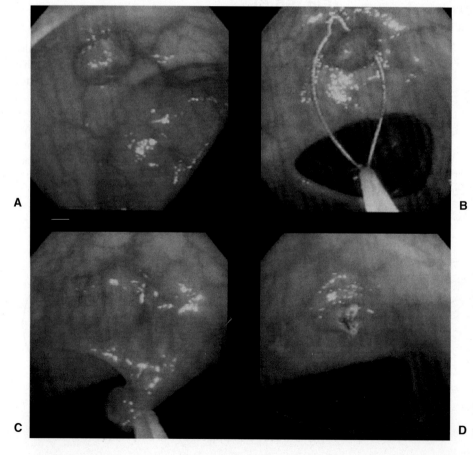

Figure 96.6 A: Small polyp visualized through colonoscope. **B:** Polypectomy snare placed in good position. **C:** Snare tightened and polyp pulled gently away from colon wall. **D:** Polypectomy base should be clean, small, and not bleeding (from Mulholland MW, Lillemoe KD, Doherty GM, et al. *Greenfield's Surgery.* Philadelphia, PA: Wolters Kluwer Lippincott Williams & Wilkins; 2013, with permission).

cautery may be required; however, most bleeding is minor and stops with observation. Use of cautery increases risk of perforation.

Polypectomy: Cautery is used for polypectomy. Assure that a grounding pad is on place. Attain a clear view of the polyp (Fig. 96.6A). Pass the polypectomy snare. Open the snare. The snare opens quite wide, and you may need a greater distance to the target in order to manipulate it. Manipulate the snare so that it encircles the polyp (Fig. 96.6B).

Have your assistant gently tighten the snare as you concentrate on maintaining position around the polyp. Be vigilant to avoid trapping mucosa around the polyp, as in extreme cases this can cause perforation. Perform this step slowly and carefully to assure that the snare is snug around the polyp, at the base, and that no extra tissue is included.

As part of this assessment, and before applying current, pull the polyp away from the wall slightly (Fig. 96.6C). This helps you to assure that the snare is in good position and, by tenting up the mucosa, minimizes the risk of full-thickness cautery injury to the bowel. Also ensure that the polyp is not touching the opposite wall, as cautery current has been reported to arc causing a burn at this location.

When you are satisfied with the location of the snare, have your assistant slowly and steadily continue to close the snare as you apply current. The goal is to have the base cut through by the current, rather than by the wire of the snare. Generally at this point the polyp will fall into the lumen. Find it!

Have your assistant withdraw the snare and pass a polyp grasper into the biopsy channel. This is a three-prong forcep that can be opened to grasp the polyp. Grasp the polyp securely, pull it up against the end of the scope, and withdraw the colonoscope and polyp together. Generally you will see a blurry orange-pink blob obscuring part or all of your view when the polyp is pulled up and secured against the scope. Carefully watch as you withdraw the scope. If you lose the view, stop and search for the polyp.

Alternatively, suck the polyp up against the end of the scope and withdraw the scope maintaining suction.

If all else fails, and you cannot retrieve the polyp, send the patient to an observation area and have the stool strained.

Check the base of the polypectomy site for bleeding (Fig. 96.6D).

REFERENCES

1. Banarjee A, Phillips MS, Marks JM. Chapter 45: Diagnostic colonoscopy. In: Soper NJ, Scott-Conner CEH eds. *The SAGES Manual.* Volume I. 3rd ed. New York, NY: Springer Verlag; 2012: 597–610.
2. Catalano MF. Normal structures on endoscopic ultrasonography: Visualization measurement data and interobserver variation. *Gastrointest Endosc Clin North Am.* 1995;5:475–486.
3. Church JM. *Endoscopy of the Colon, Rectum, and Anus.* New York, NY: Igaku-Shoin; 1995.
4. Fink AS. Therapeutic colonoscopy and its complications. In: Soper NJ, Scott-Conner CEH eds. *The SAGES Manual.* Volume I. 3rd ed. New York, NY: Springer Verlag; 2012:611–626.
5. Sugarbaker PH, Vineyard GC, Peterson LM. Anatomic localization and step by step advancement of the fiberoptic colonoscope. *Surg Gynecol Obstet.* 1976;143:457.

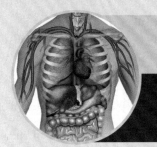

97

Loop Colostomy and Colostomy Closure

A loop colostomy is the easiest colostomy to make and to take down. It is used in situations in which temporary (often emergency) decompression or diversion of colonic contents is required. In many situations, a loop ileostomy (see Chapter 92) is preferred and used. In this chapter, the construction and closure of a right transverse colostomy is illustrated. The equivalent laparoscopic procedure is shown in Chapter 98e.

SCORE™, the Surgical Council on Resident Education, classified colostomy and colostomy closure as "ESSENTIAL COMMON" operations.

STEPS IN PROCEDURE—LOOP COLOSTOMY

Short transverse right upper quadrant incision
Deliver transverse colon into incision
Remove greater omentum from selected segment of colon
Create a window under the colon, at the antimesenteric border
Tack the loop to the fascia

Pass a colostomy bridge under the loop and secure it
Close skin around loop, if necessary
Open and mature colostomy by suturing mucosa to skin
Place appropriate colostomy bag

HALLMARK ANATOMIC COMPLICATIONS—LOOP COLOSTOMY

Failure to divert
Prolapse of defunctionalized limb

LIST OF STRUCTURES

Greater omentum
Transverse colon
Hepatic flexure
Middle colic artery

Marginal artery (of Drummond)
Rectus abdominis muscle
Anterior rectus sheath
Superior epigastric artery

The conventional terminology for various parts of the colon is shown in Figure 97.1A. The hepatic and splenic flexures are the points at which the relatively fixed ascending (sometimes called the right) colon and descending (sometimes called the left) colon transition to the mobile transverse colon. They are anchored by peritoneal bands. The transverse colon is normally covered by the greater omentum, which hangs down like a large fatty apron. The greater omentum must be lifted to expose the transverse colon. The relationships of the omentum, stomach, and transverse colon are shown in Figure 97.1B.

Isolation of Loop (Fig. 97.2)

Technical Points

Make a short (about 10 cm in length) transverse incision in the right upper quadrant. Do not make the incision too far laterally. The transverse colon becomes deeper and higher in the vicinity of the hepatic flexure (lateral) and more mobile in the midsection (medial).

Identify the colon by its overlying greater omentum. Mobilize a greatly distended and dilated colon with caution to avoid spillage of enteric contents. If the incision is not large enough to deliver the loop comfortably, enlarge the incision. Observe the character of the peritoneal fluid. If it is turbid or purulent, a colonic perforation may have occurred. In this case, proceed with a full laparotomy.

Divide the omentum to expose the colon by serially clamping and tying it. Develop a mesenteric window under the colon by passing a clamp or finger through an avascular portion of the mesocolon. Pass a Penrose drain under the colon and use it to elevate the colon.

Anatomic Points

The incision is typically made about halfway between the umbilicus and costal margin, 3 to 5 cm lateral to the linea alba. At

ORIENTATION

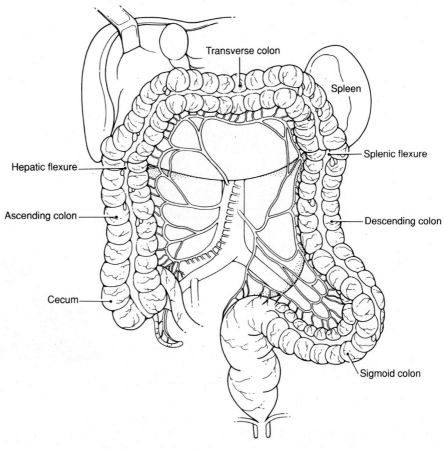

Transverse colon

Spleen

Hepatic flexure

Splenic flexure

Ascending colon

Descending colon

Cecum

Sigmoid colon

A

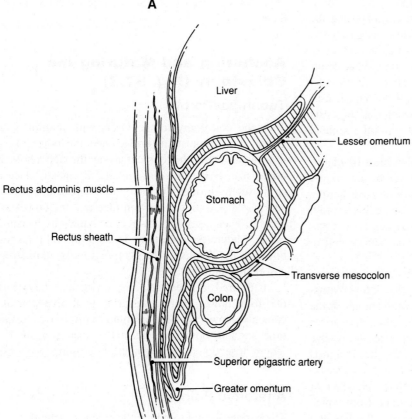

Liver

Lesser omentum

Rectus abdominis muscle

Stomach

Rectus sheath

Transverse mesocolon

Colon

Superior epigastric artery

Greater omentum

B

Figure 97.1 A: Parts of the colon. **B:** Cross-section showing relationship of greater omentum and stomach to transverse colon.

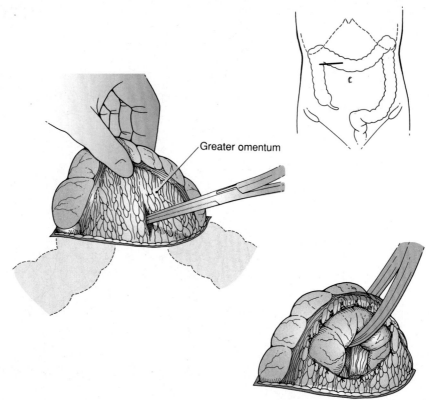

Figure 97.2 Isolation of loop

this site, all or part of the incision will cross the rectus abdominis muscle. First, cut the anterior rectus sheath, exposing the rectus fibers. Then divide the rectus fibers with electrocautery. Bleeding difficulties may result if the superior epigastric artery is not identified and controlled. This artery (and its venae comitantes) is immediately posterior to the rectus abdominis muscle, about midway between its medial and lateral borders. It usually enters the muscle, anastomosing with the inferior epigastric artery, about halfway between the umbilicus and the xiphoid cartilage.

After the peritoneum is opened, the colon must be identified with certainty. Because the anterior layer of the greater omentum forms the gastrocolic ligament, omentum overlies the colon and thus must be divided to visualize the colon clearly. Use clamps and ties to divide the omentum. Look for the distinguishing haustra, epiploic appendages, and taeniae coli to identify colon positively.

Division of the transverse mesocolon, which is necessary to encircle the colon, cannot be done blindly. Look for an avascular region and avoid trauma to the middle colic artery or the marginal artery (of Drummond). The middle colic artery arises from the superior mesenteric artery to supply the transverse colon. It should not be at risk for injury if the mesocolon is divided close to the bowel. The marginal artery, an anastomotic channel ultimately connecting the colonic branches of the inferior and superior mesenteric arteries and from which the vasa recti originate to supply the colon directly, lies at a variable distance from the wall of the colon. Its distance from

the colon has been reported to range from less than 1 cm to 8 cm.

Anchoring and Maturing the Colostomy (Fig. 97.3)

Technical Points

Tack the colostomy to the fascia with multiple interrupted sutures. Pass a colostomy bridge under the loop. Close the skin, if necessary, until the loop comes out through a hole of appropriate size. If the bowel is greatly distended, place a purse-string suture through the region to be opened. Open the bowel and pass a pool-tipped suction tube into the bowel to decompress it. Then, open the bowel more widely by incising along a taenia. Mature the colostomy by suturing full thickness of the bowel to the dermis of the skin with multiple interrupted fine absorbable sutures.

If desired, a linear stapling device may be used to close the distal bowel, thereby ensuring total diversion of colonic contents. However, keep in mind that this may recanalize in time, allowing bowel contents to flow distally again. It will also require resection of this segment for closure.

Anatomic Points

The parietal layers to which the colon is sutured, at this level, include the parietal peritoneum, fascia transversalis, rectus

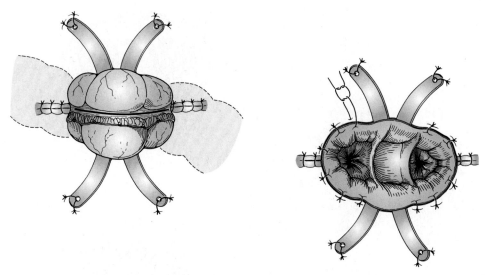

Figure 97.3 Anchoring and maturing the colostomy

abdominis muscle, and both anterior and posterior rectus sheaths. If the lateral end of the incision is lateral to the rectus abdominis muscle, then the layers included are the parietal peritoneum, fascia transversalis, and transversus abdominis muscle and the aponeuroses of the internal oblique and external oblique muscles.

The taenia selected will generally be the so-called *omental taenia,* from which the greater omentum arises. The accumulation of longitudinal muscle fibers at the taeniae coli provides additional bowel wall thickness to be included in the coloparietal suture and includes layers at right angles to each other.

Closure of a Loop Colostomy (Fig. 97.4)

Technical Points

Incise the mucocutaneous border around the colostomy. Place Allis clamps on the cut edge of the bowel and dissect in the plane between bowel and subcutaneous tissues. Identify and cut any sutures tacking the bowel to fascia. When the loop of bowel is completely free of the abdominal wall, pull sufficient bowel up to ensure that an anastomosis can be made without tension.

STEPS IN PROCEDURE—CLOSURE OF LOOP COLOSTOMY

Make incision around mucocutaneous border of colostomy

Gently Dissect to Fascia and Enter Peritoneum
Cut any sutures tacking colostomy to fascia
Fully mobilize the loop so that it can be pulled out of the abdomen

Assess Loop—If Loop has Not Been Injured During Dissection, Plastic Closure
Freshen edges of bowel to pliable normal bowel
Close transversely (suture or staple)
Bring omentum over closure and drop back into abdomen
Close fascia (do not close skin tightly)

HALLMARK ANATOMIC COMPLICATIONS—CLOSURE OF LOOP COLOSTOMY
Anastomotic leak or fistula

Under favorable conditions, the colostomy can be closed by simple suture of the open anterior wall (plastic closure) in a transverse fashion. Check the pliability and mobility of the cut ends of the bowel and carefully clean it. Place a running Connell suture of 3-0 Vicryl to invert the open bowel and then an outer layer of interrupted 3-0 silk Lembert sutures. Check the anastomosis for patency and cover with omentum if available.

Close the fascia in the usual manner. Loosely close the skin or pack it open. Tight closure of skin and subcutaneous tissue in a former ostomy site is generally ill-advised.

Anatomic Points

Here, as is true almost everywhere else in the gastrointestinal tract, inverted closures can result in significant luminal

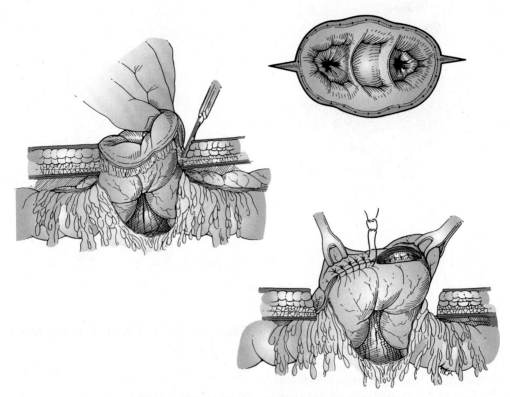

Figure 97.4 Closure of a loop colostomy

narrowing. For this reason, inverted closures of longitudinal incisions are often done in a transverse fashion.

REFERENCES

1. Abcarian H, Pearl RK. Stomas. *Surg Clin North Am.* 1988;68:1295–1305.
2. Barker WF, Benfield JR, deKernion JB, et al. The creation and care of enterocutaneous stomas. *Curr Probl Surg.* 1975;12:1–62. (Provides comprehensive review.)
3. Doberneck RC. Revision and closure of the colostomy. *Surg Clin North Am.* 1991;71:193–201. (Provides good review of complications and pitfalls.)
4. Eng K, Localio A. Simplified complementary transverse colostomy for low colorectal anastomosis. *Surg Gynecol Obstet.* 1981;153:735. (Describes simple technique that is easily constructed and closed.)
5. Keighley MRB. Ileostomy; colostomy. In: Keighley, Williams MRB, Williams NS, eds. *Surgery of the Anus, Rectum and Colon.* London: WB Saunders; 1993:139–244.
6. Kretschmer KP. *The Intestinal Stoma: Indications, Operative Methods, Care, Rehabilitation.* Philadelphia, PA: WB Saunders; 1978. (Provides good source of information about stomas and their care.)
7. Maidl L, Ohland J. Chapter 152: Care of stomas. In: *Fischer's Mastery of Surgery.* Philadelphia, PA: Wolters Kluwer Lippincott Williams & Wilkins; 2013:e37.
8. Takahashi H, Hara M, Takayama S, et al. Simple laparoscopic technique of correction of transverse loop colostomy prolapse. *Surg Laparosc Endosc Percutan Tech.* 2012;22:e263–e264.
9. Turnbull RB, Weakley FL. *Atlas of Intestinal Stomas.* St. Louis, MO: CV Mosby; 1967. (This is the classic reference.)
10. Wolff LH, Wolff WA, Wolff LH Jr. A re-evaluation of tube cecostomy. *Surg Gynecol Obstet.* 1980;151:257–259.

e98 Laparoscopic Colostomy

This chapter can be accessed online at www.lww.com/eChapter98.

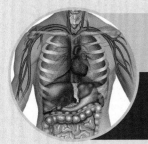

99
Right and Left Colon Resections

In this chapter, right and left hemicolectomy are discussed (as performed for malignancy), and transverse colon resection is mentioned briefly. In each case, the lymphatic drainage of the segment determines the extent of resection.

More limited resections are occasionally performed for localized perforations, ischemia, or trauma. These are done in much the same manner but require a less extensive dissection. The extensive dissection to remove lymph nodes is omitted in these circumstances. Chapter 100 describes laparoscopic colon resection. References at the end of this chapter give additional information on specialized procedures, including sentinel node biopsy, which is controversial at this time.

SCORE™, the Surgical Council on Resident Education, classified open partial colectomy as an "ESSENTIAL COMMON" procedure.

STEPS IN PROCEDURE

Right Hemicolectomy
Right transverse or midline incision
Thoroughly explore abdomen
Mobilize right colon by incising along white line of Toldt
Elevate right colon in retrocolic plane
Identify and preserve duodenum and both ureters
At hepatic flexure, take greater omentum with specimen
Extent of resection is determined by location of tumor, but will generally include terminal ileum and transverse colon to middle colic artery
Preserve middle colic artery unless extended right hemicolectomy is planned
Score peritoneum overlying mesenteric vessels down to origin of ileocolic and right colic arteries, but preserving the superior mesenteric artery
Divide mesentery between clamps and ties
Divide bowel and create anastomosis by suturing or stapling
Close mesenteric defect

Place omentum over anastomosis
Close abdomen in usual fashion without drains

Left Hemicolectomy
Midline or left paramedian incision
Thorough abdominal exploration
Mobilize left colon by incision along white line of Toldt
At splenic flexure, take omentum off colon (unless tumor is in proximity to this region)
Identify and protect both ureters
Determine extent of resection, generally preserving middle colic artery unless extended left hemicolectomy is planned
Score peritoneum over vessels, taking mesenteric resection to origin of inferior mesenteric artery
Divide peritoneum with clamps and ties
Divide bowel and create anastomosis by suturing or stapling
Place omentum over anastomosis
Close abdomen in usual fashion without drains

519

HALLMARK ANATOMIC COMPLICATIONS

Injury to ureters
Injury to superior mesenteric artery (right colon resections)

Injury to duodenum (right colon resections)
Injury to spleen (left colon resections)

LIST OF STRUCTURES

Ascending (Right) Colon
Cecum
Ileocecal valve
Hepatic flexure
Transverse colon

Descending (Left) Colon
Splenic flexure
Sigmoid colon
Rectum
White line of Toldt
Celiac artery

Superior Mesenteric Artery
Middle colic artery
Jejunal arteries
Right colic artery
Ileocolic artery

Inferior Mesenteric Artery
Left colic artery
Sigmoid arteries
Superior rectal (hemorrhoidal) artery
Middle rectal (hemorrhoidal) arteries
Marginal artery (of Drummond)
Ileum
Duodenum
Spleen
Gastrocolic omentum
Ureter
Gonadal vessels
Iliac vessels
Genitofemoral nerve

Resections of the colon are planned according to arterial supply and venous and lymphatic drainage. In general, the resection is designed to encompass the draining lymph nodes. This determines which arteries and veins must be sacrificed, which in turn determines the length of bowel that must be removed. For lesions of the cecum or ascending colon up to and including the hepatic flexure, the standard resection is a right hemicolectomy (Fig. 99.1A,B). This includes resection of the terminal ileum, ascending colon, and right transverse colon. An end-to-end anastomosis is then performed between the ileum and transverse colon.

A transverse colon lesion near one flexure is often managed by an extended hemicolectomy (e.g., a lesion of the transverse colon near the hepatic flexure would be managed by extended right hemicolectomy). Lesions involving main portion of the transverse colon can be managed by transverse colon resection, whereby the transverse colon, including both flexures, is removed and the ends are reanastomosed (Fig. 99.1C).

Left hemicolectomy (Fig. 99.1D) is performed for lesions in the sigmoid or descending colon. The colon is resected from the middle of the transverse colon to the peritoneal reflection. This wide field of resection is needed when the inferior mesenteric vein and artery are ligated at their origin in order to resect lymph nodes along the inferior mesenteric artery. An end-to-end anastomosis is then performed between the middle of the transverse colon and the rectosigmoid. In some cases, a segmental sigmoid colon resection (Fig. 99.1E) is performed instead.

The general relationship of the colon to surrounding structures, including liver and spleen, is shown in Figure 99.1F. Note how compact the right colon is, compared with the left. This allows the right colon to be resected through a short transverse incision.

Right Hemicolectomy

Incision and Exploration of the Abdomen (Fig. 99.2)

Technical Points

The hepatic flexure of the colon is quite close to the cecum, so that a right colon resection can conveniently be performed through a right transverse incision. Consider using this incision in patients who have not had previous subcostal or right lower quadrant incisions (which might compromise the vascularity of the transected rectus muscle). This incision is particularly good for obese patients. Alternatively, a midline or right paramedian incision may be chosen.

Outline a right transverse incision by palpating two landmarks: The costal margin at the anterior axillary line and the anterosuperior iliac spine. Divide the distance between these two points in half and mark it with a pen. Draw a straight transverse line from this point to a point just beyond the midline. Generally, this line will pass above the umbilicus (Fig. 99.2A), although occasionally, it will pass below. If it passes straight through the umbilicus, redraw it slightly above. Make the incision through skin and subcutaneous tissue and achieve hemostasis. Divide the muscular and fascial layers of the abdominal wall with electrocautery in a straight line with the skin incision (Fig. 99.2B). Enter the abdomen and explore it thoroughly.

A complete and thorough exploration of the abdomen is a necessary preamble to all abdominal surgery cases. In the case of colon cancer, special attention should be paid to possible sites of metastases: The liver, the lymph nodes draining the segment of colon to be resected, the pelvis, the ovaries (in women), and the peritoneal surfaces. Tumor extending beyond the field of resection does not preclude colectomy, but any such

ORIENTATION

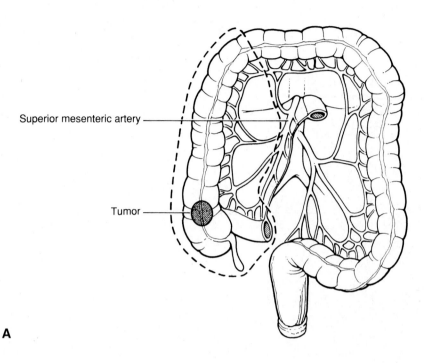

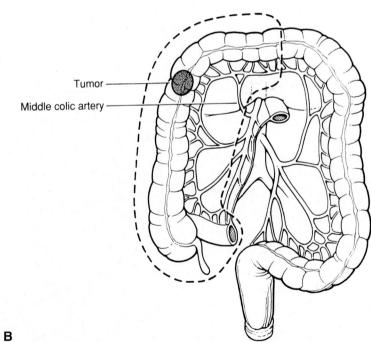

Figure 99.1 Extent of resection for lesions in various parts of the colon. The resection is planned to encompass at least 10 cm of bowel proximal and distal and to include draining mesenteric lymph nodes. **A:** Right hemicolectomy for cecal lesion. **B:** Extended right hemicolectomy for lesion of hepatic flexure. (*continued*)

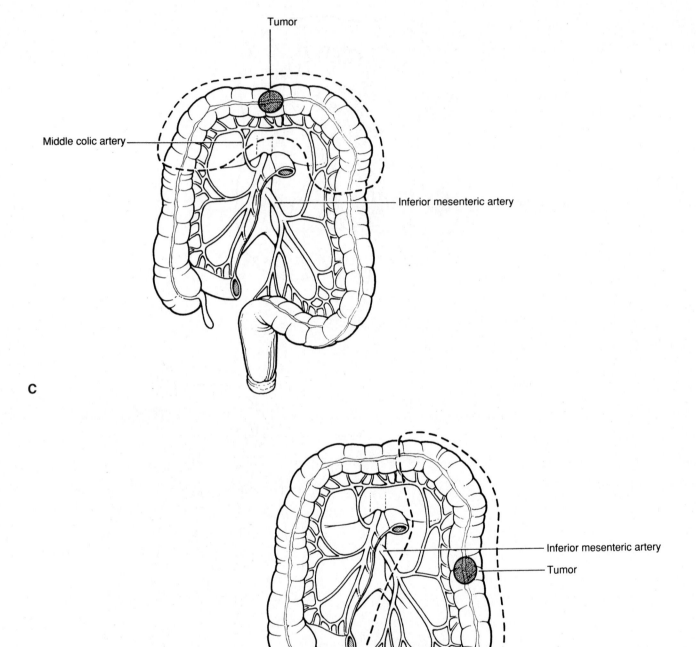

Figure 99.1 (*Continued*) **C:** Transverse colon resection. **D:** Left hemicolectomy.

ORIENTATION

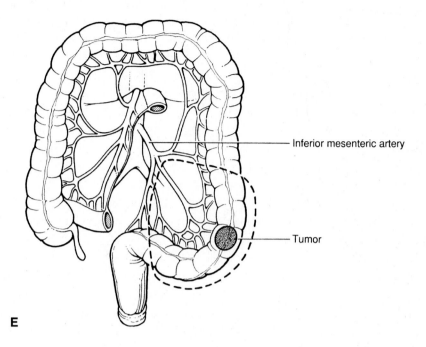

Inferior mesenteric artery

Tumor

E

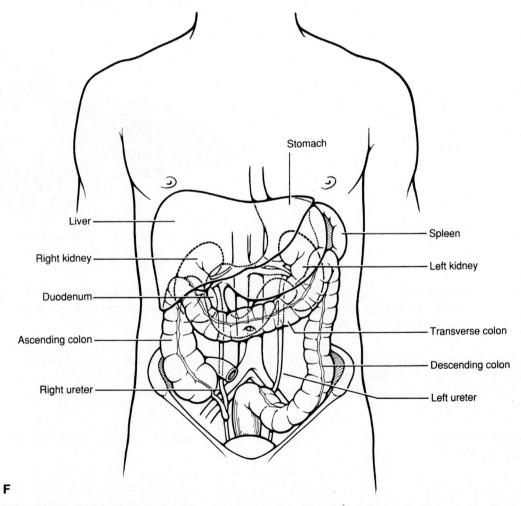

Stomach

Liver

Spleen

Right kidney

Left kidney

Duodenum

Ascending colon

Transverse colon

Right ureter

Descending colon

Left ureter

F

Figure 99.1 (*Continued*) **E:** Segmental resection of sigmoid colon. **F:** Regional anatomy.

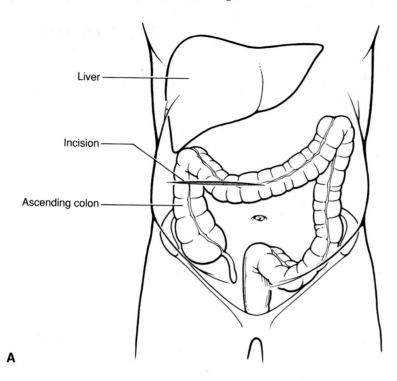

A

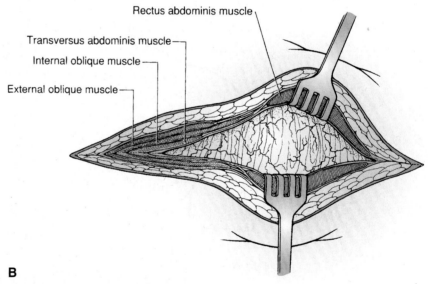

B

Figure 99.2 Incision and exploration of the abdomen. **A:** An ample transverse incision allows excellent exposure. **B:** Deepen the incision by cutting, with electrocautery, through all of the layers of the abdominal wall.

metastatic disease should be documented carefully by biopsy. Palpate the entire colon. Second primary lesions are common and may be missed on preoperative screening studies.

Anatomic Points

Transverse incisions were briefly discussed in Chapter 44. The transverse incision recommended here should not divide more than one segmental nerve and, thus, should not result in anesthesia, paresthesia, or paralysis of any part of the anterior abdominal wall, including the rectus abdominis muscle. This

incision approximates the direction of the muscle fiber bundles laterally, but is more or less transverse to the direction of rectus abdominis muscle fibers. Often, one of the tendinous inscriptions (usually the lowest) occurs at the level of the umbilicus. The incision should pass either above or below the umbilicus, thereby avoiding cutting through this tendinous inscription because segmental vessels are invariably encountered in the inscriptions and may cause bleeding. If the incision is extended across the midline above the umbilicus, the falciform ligament and ligamentum teres hepatis must be divided. This should be done between clamps, and ligatures should be placed both

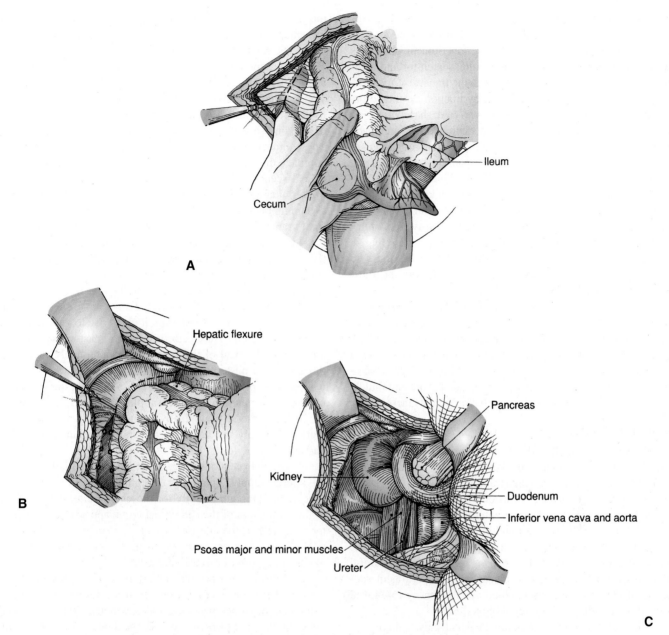

Figure 99.3 Mobilization of the right colon. **A:** Begin at the cecum. **B:** Progress up the ascending colon to the hepatic flexure. **C:** Carefully mobilize the right colon to expose the duodenum and right ureter.

proximally and distally owing to the paraumbilical veins that accompany the round ligament. These veins can be quite large if the portal system is obstructed and portal blood is shunted to the caval system.

Mobilization of the Colon (Fig. 99.3)

Technical Points

Place a self-retaining retractor, such as a Balfour, (or fixed retractors anchored to the operating table) in the incision. Elevate the cecum and pull it medially. Incise the peritoneum lateral to the cecum and pass your nondominant hand behind the colon

(Fig. 99.3A). Pass the index finger of your nondominant hand laterally to display the peritoneal reflection, thinning it out along the edge of the right colon. Incise it, using scissors or electrocautery, from the cecum to the hepatic flexure (Fig. 99.3B). In the region of the hepatic flexure, the peritoneal attachments will become increasingly thick and vascularized. Generally, these can be divided with electrocautery, although some of these vascular adhesions may require clamping and tying or clipping.

Sharply divide the filmy adhesions between the colon and retroperitoneum. Elevate the right colon up into the wound from the cecum to the hepatic flexure. As the colon is reflected medially and upward, the terminal ileum will come up as well.

Identify the right ureter where it crosses the common iliac vessels just distal to their bifurcation. The colon will come up with minimal dissection in the avascular retroperitoneal plane. As you proceed up toward the hepatic flexure, search for and identify the duodenum, which is adherent to the transverse mesocolon and frequently will be tented up by traction on the colon. Mobilize the colon off the duodenum with care, sharply incising filmy adhesions and pushing the duodenum down and back into the retroperitoneum. The completed field is shown in Figure 99.3C. Then place laparotomy pads in the bed of the colon and turn your attention to the region of the hepatic flexure.

At the hepatic flexure, one must begin taking the greater omentum with the specimen. The greater omentum connects the greater curvature of the stomach and the transverse colon.

Identify the area of the middle transverse colon that is planned for anastomosis. Preserve the middle colic artery to ensure a good blood supply to the anastomosis. Elevate the transverse colon and palpate the middle colic artery in the mesocolon. Select an area just to the right of the middle colic artery. Divide the omentum from this point up to the greater curvature of the stomach using clamps and ties. Take the greater omentum off the greater curvature of the stomach from this point distally toward the pylorus using clamps and ties. It should then be possible to elevate the entire colon, including the hepatic flexure and middle transverse colon (which will be tethered only by its mesentery).

Anatomic Points

Remember that, initially, all of the colon was intraperitoneal and that its blood supply developed during this intraperitoneal state. The ascending (right) and descending (left) colon are retroperitoneal because of fusion of apposing visceral and parietal serosal surfaces. The mesentery of the colon, with vessels derived from the superior and inferior mesenteric arteries, is retroperitoneal but lies anterior to other important retroperitoneal structures, such as the kidneys and ureters. By careful blunt dissection in the fusion plane, the retroperitoneal segments of the colon and their blood supply can be mobilized toward the midline with minimal blood loss.

Although significant variation in detail exists, there is a basic pattern of blood supply. The entire right colon, from the appendix to the junction of the middle and distal thirds of the transverse colon, is supplied by branches of the superior mesenteric artery. The superior mesenteric artery, arising just distal (1.5 cm) to the celiac trunk posterior to the pancreas, passes anterior to the third part of the duodenum to enter the root of the mesentery of the small bowel. Before it emerges from behind the pancreas, or just as it emerges, it gives rise to the middle colic artery, which usually passes into the transverse mesocolon at the inferior border of the pancreatic neck and then curves to the right. About 5 to 7 cm from the colon, the middle colic artery divides into right and left branches that parallel the transverse colon. These branches anastomose with branches of other arteries, ultimately forming the marginal artery of Drummond.

In the root of the small bowel mesentery, the superior mesenteric artery is accompanied on its right by the superior mesenteric vein. Typically, the jejunal and ileal branches arise from the left side of the superior mesenteric artery and run in the mesentery to the small bowel, which has been displaced to the right. The right colic and ileocolic arteries arise from the right side of the superior mesenteric artery and run along the posterior abdominal wall, initially posterior to the superior mesenteric vein, to the right colon. The right colic and ileocolic arteries usually divide into two main branches—an ascending and a descending branch—that approximately parallel the colon. These branches ultimately anastomose with other arteries to complete the right portion of the marginal artery of Drummond. (The descending branch of the ileocolic artery anastomoses with the termination of the superior mesenteric artery, whereas the ascending branch of the right colic artery anastomoses with the right branch of the middle colic artery.) It should be noted that it is the descending branch of the ileocolic artery that supplies the cecum, appendix, and terminal ileum. Right colon resections typically include the last few inches of the ileum in order to ensure an adequate blood supply to the area of anastomosis.

The marginal artery is located 1 to 8 cm from the bowel wall. Regardless of its formation, it gives rise to vasa recti that supply the colon. These arteries rarely anastomose because they run to the wall of the large bowel, alternately supplying the anterior or posterior side of the bowel, and enter the bowel wall in close proximity to taeniae coli. Although the vasa recti ultimately form a rich submucosal plexus, there is only limited longitudinal blood flow. Inadvertent destruction of the vasa recti that supply the anastomosis site can result in ischemia and anastomotic leak.

With few exceptions, the venous return essentially parallels the arterial supply. The major exception is the inferior mesenteric vein. Although the inferior mesenteric artery arises close to the bifurcation of the abdominal aorta, approximately at vertebral level T-4, the inferior mesenteric vein ascends to the left of the aorta and empties into the splenic vein or superior mesenteric vein posterior to the pancreas.

Lymphatics also parallel the arteries. Node located on the wall of the colon, receive afferents from the colon. Efferents from these drain into paracolic nodes, which are typically found between the marginal artery and the bowel. Efferents from these parallel the branches of the superior mesenteric artery and inferior mesenteric artery and are periodically interrupted by intermediate nodes, named according to the artery with which they are associated. Lymph vessels from the intermediate nodes ultimately drain into nodes located at the origin of the superior mesenteric artery and inferior mesenteric artery. From these principal nodes, which again are named according to the artery with which they are associated, efferents ascend to the celiac nodes or to periaortic nodes on either side of the aorta. These ultimately drain into the cisterna chyli, typically lying just to the right of the aorta and slightly inferior to the celiac artery origin.

The American Joint Commission on Cancer recognizes specific regional lymph node groups for the colon. For the cecum, these are the pericolic, anterior and posterior cecal, ileocolic, and right colic. For the ascending colon and hepatic flexure, these are the pericolic, ileocolic, right colic, and middle colic. For the transverse colon, only the pericolic and middle colic are recognized.

Resection of the terminal ileum, the cecum with its attached appendix, the ascending colon, and the proximal part of the transverse colon can be done with minimal bleeding if care is taken to enter the fusion plane immediately deep to the colon and its vasculature. Access to this plane is gained by way of a relatively avascular zone of peritoneum, called *the white line of Toldt,* which is visible when medial tension is placed on the ascending colon. As the fusion plane is entered and the colon is mobilized, care must be taken to identify other retroperitoneal structures. The largest and most lateral structure in the upper right retroperitoneal space is the kidney, whereas in the lower right retroperitoneal space, the psoas major muscle, on which the genitofemoral nerve rests, will be visualized. The ureter runs inferomedially from the renal

hilum to the pelvic brim (crossing the iliac vasculature just distal to the division of the common iliac artery into the internal and external iliac arteries). The gonadal artery and vein cross the ureter as the latter structure passes over the psoas major muscle. With continued medial reflection, the duodenum and pancreas will be visualized.

Resection of the Colon and Construction of the Anastomosis (Fig. 99.4)

Technical Points

Elevate the right colon and terminal ileum into the incision and look at the pattern of the mesenteric vascular arcades of the

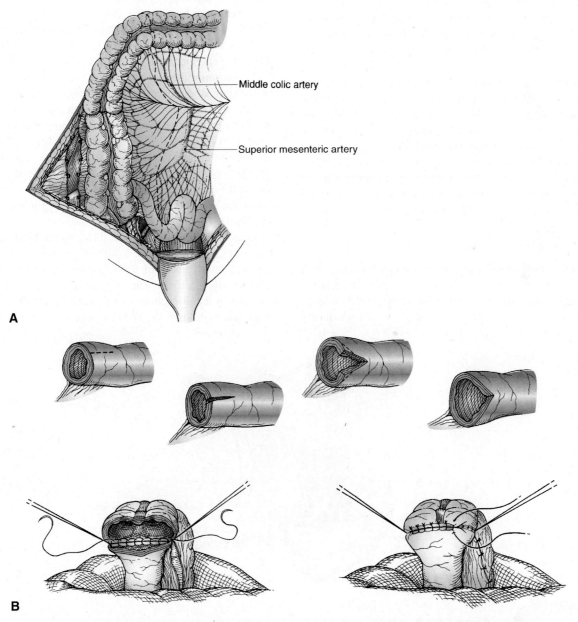

Middle colic artery

Superior mesenteric artery

Figure 99.4 Resection of the colon and construction of the anastomosis. **A:** Extent of resection for formal right hemicolectomy with lymphadenectomy. **B:** Cheatle slit and end to end anastomosis.

terminal ileum (Fig. 99.4A). Usually, about 5 to 10 cm of terminal ileum will be taken with the specimen. The length of terminal ileum is determined by its blood supply. Choose a point on the terminal ileum about 10 cm from the ileocecal valve where there appears to be good blood supply. Make a window through the ileal mesentery using hemostats. Divide the ileum with Allen clamps. Incise the peritoneum overlying the mesentery from this point to the middle transverse colon, taking the V of this peritoneal incision down to the base of the ileocolic artery. Clean the middle transverse colon and the area selected for anastomosis and divide it between Allen clamps. Then divide the mesentery of the colon serially with clamps and secure it with suture ligatures. Be sure to take the ileocolic artery and vein close to their origin to ensure that the lymph nodes associated with these vessels are taken as well. An adequate cancer operation should include 12 to 14 nodes. Operations performed for palliation are often more limited, and are tailored to the specific circumstance.

After resection is completed, check the bed of the colon for hemostasis. Construct a two-layer, sutured, end-to-end anastomosis in the usual fashion. If there is a size discrepancy between the terminal ileum and the middle transverse colon, make a Cheatle slit along the antimesenteric border of the colon (Fig. 99.4B). This will effectively lengthen the area for anastomosis and eliminate the discrepancy. Alternatively and perhaps more commonly, simply perform a stapled side-to-side (functional end-to-end) anastomosis. Close the hole in the mesentery by suturing the peritoneal surfaces of the mesentery together with a running suture of 3-0 Vicryl. Wrap omentum around the anastomosis.

Anatomic Points

The ileocolic artery divides into an ascending branch, which anastomoses with the right colic artery, and a descending branch, which supplies the terminal ileum, appendix, cecum, and proximal ascending colon. The ileal branch ultimately anastomoses with the termination of the superior mesenteric artery. Thus the surgeon must select the point of division, based on visualization and selection of appropriate vasa recti, and divide the artery only after proximal and distal control of the anastomosis is achieved.

Left Hemicolectomy

Incision and Mobilization of the Colon (Fig. 99.5)

Technical Points

Left hemicolectomy is best performed through a left paramedian or long midline incision. Alternatively, some surgeons prefer an oblique left lower quadrant incision. This incision is not generally recommended, however, because it will present difficulties if a colostomy is subsequently required.

Make a long vertical incision to provide adequate exposure of both the splenic flexure and the pelvis. Palpate the colon and assess the tumor for mobility. Place a self-retaining retractor in the incision. Begin by mobilizing the sigmoid colon.

Lift the sigmoid colon medially and in an upward direction. Incise adhesions between the left colon and lateral peritoneum. (This is generally not the true white line of Toldt, which lies beneath these adhesions.) After the colon is mobilized, the white line of Toldt, which corresponds to the peritoneal reflection, will become visible. Incise this peritoneal reflection and elevate the sigmoid colon and its mesentery up into the wound (Fig. 99.5).

Identify the left ureter where it crosses the bifurcation of the iliac artery. If you anticipate a difficult pelvic dissection because of tumor involvement or an inflammatory process, surround the ureter and place a Silastic loop around it to facilitate reference to it later in the dissection. Avoid extensive mobilization of the ureter that might strip it of its blood supply, causing ischemia and

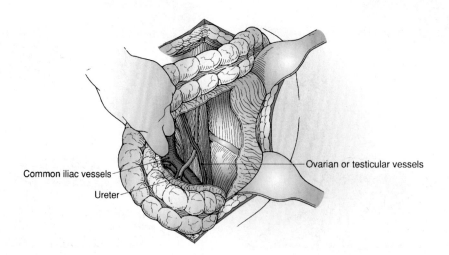

Common iliac vessels

Ureter

Ovarian or testicular vessels

Figure 99.5 Incision and mobilization of the left colon (note that the mesentery of the colon has not been divided at this point, underlying structures are shown for clarity).

stricture formation. Mobilize the colon from the distal sigmoid up to the region of the splenic flexure. Generally, mobilization will become more difficult as the splenic flexure is approached. Do not pull down on the splenic flexure—this only increases the probability of injuring the spleen. Instead, when this dissection becomes difficult, place a pack in the retrocolic space and begin dissection of the splenic flexure from the transverse colon as demonstrated below. Working thus from above and below, the splenic flexure will gradually come down into the field.

Anatomic Points

Adhesions can develop between the terminal descending colon or proximal sigmoid colon and the parietal peritoneum; frequently, these involve the epiploic appendages. Because these are lateral to the white line of Toldt, they can obscure this landmark for access to the avascular peritoneal fusion plane. Cautious dissection, coupled with medial traction of the sigmoid and descending colon, should allow identification of the proper fusion plane.

The root of the sigmoid mesocolon is variably located but typically is disposed as an inverted V, with its apex near the division of the left common iliac artery. Its left limb parallels the medial side of the psoas major muscle, whereas the right limb, which is in the true pelvis, passes inferomedially, ending in the midline at the midsacral region. This mesentery contains the sigmoid colon, sigmoid vessels, and superior rectal (hemorrhoidal) vessels. In addition, the apex of this mesentery marks the point where the left ureter enters the true pelvis. Identification and control of all vessels will facilitate mobilization; identification here (and more proximally) of the ureter will prevent iatrogenic trauma to this structure.

Skeletonization of the ureter can deprive it of its blood supply. The blood supply of the ureter, on both sides, is provided by branches from the renal artery, aorta, gonadal artery, common and internal iliac arteries, and inferior vesical arteries. Because most of its blood supply enters its medial aspect, if either side must be mobilized, it is safest to mobilize its lateral portion.

During mobilization of the descending and left colon, the following retroperitoneal structures, all of which are posterior to the colon and its blood supply, should be identified: Left kidney, left gonadal vein draining into the left renal vein, left gonadal artery, left ureter, left genitofemoral nerve on the left psoas major muscle, and the iliac vessels.

Mobilization of the Splenic Flexure (Fig. 99.6)

Technical Points

Mobilization of the splenic flexure is often the most challenging part of left hemicolectomy. Generally, the left colon dives deeply retroperitoneal and passes quite high in the vicinity of the spleen. Approach this mobilization from below (proceeding upward along the retroperitoneal reflection) and from above (proceeding from right to left along the transverse colon).

Begin by continuing to incise the white line of Toldt and elevate the colon up out of the retroperitoneum. When you have

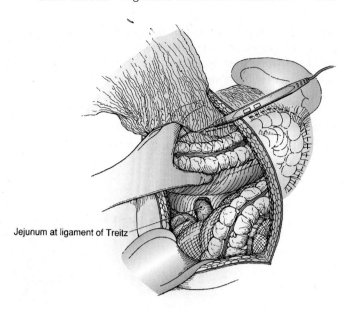

Jejunum at ligament of Treitz

Figure 99.6 Mobilization of the splenic flexure

gone as high as you can comfortably go from below, incising the peritoneal reflection from the vicinity of the descending colon, pack this area off and turn your attention to the transverse colon. Lift up on the greater omentum and separate it from the middle transverse colon by sharp dissection in the avascular fusion plane (Fig. 99.6). As this plane is developed, you can pass the fingers of your nondominant hand behind the omentum and use it to display the plane. Leave the small fat tabs that protrude 5 to 10 mm from the colon on the colon. These contain small, looping vessels that will bleed if divided. The proper plane is avascular and can be incised with Metzenbaum scissors, although many surgeons prefer to use electrocautery. In any event, be especially careful if this segment of the colon contains diverticula because diverticula may protrude into the fat tabs and be injured if the cut is too deep. Proceed up toward the region of the splenic flexure, pushing up on the omentum and down on the colon as you go. By pushing up on the omentum rather than pulling down, you minimize the risk for injuring the spleen by traction. You will soon reach a point at which it is possible to pass your nondominant hand completely around behind the splenic flexure of the colon. You can then divide the few remaining attachments with hemoclips. The attachments in the immediate vicinity of the splenic flexure frequently contain small vessels that will bleed if taken sharply. Mobilize the colon by sharp and blunt dissection into the midportion of the wound.

Anatomic Points

The anatomic relationships, as well as the peritoneal attachments, of the splenic flexure must be appreciated. The splenic flexure is quite sharp and is attached to the diaphragm by the phrenicocolic ligament. This peritoneal fold, which is continuous with the greater omentum, is inferolateral to the lower pole of the spleen and forms a "splenic shelf." Thus, the splenic flexure is typically immediately inferior and anterior to the hilum of the spleen and tail of the pancreas. This flexure is usually so sharp that the descending limb is overlaid by the terminal transverse limb. Reflection (see the previous discussion of technique) of the posterior side of the greater omentum from the anterior side of the transverse mesocolon, accomplished by dissecting in an avascular fusion plane, prevents the surgeon from placing undue traction on the spleen.

Identification of the Right Ureter and Division of the Colon Distally (Fig. 99.7)

Technical Points

Pack the sigmoid colon to the left and examine the peritoneum overlying the right common iliac artery. Often, the ureter is visible in the retroperitoneum. Incise the retroperitoneum and

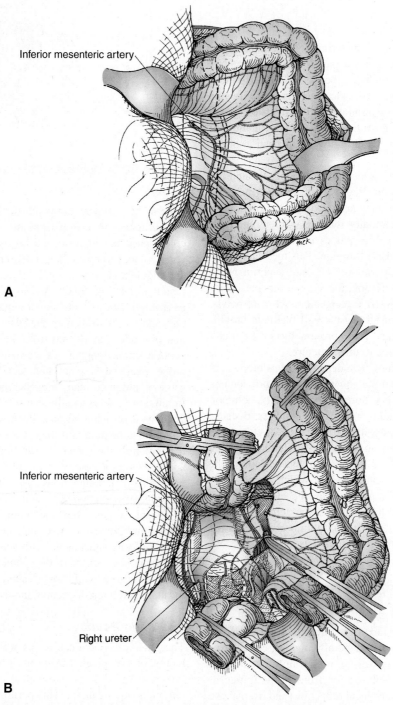

Figure 99.7 Identification of the right ureter and division of the colon distally. **A:** Extent of resection for formal left hemicolectomy. **B:** Resection, preserving both ureters.

identify the ureter where it crosses just distal to the bifurcation of the common iliac artery. If you expect difficulty dissecting in the pelvis, surround the ureter with a Silastic loop. Identify the point of the distal colon that has been chosen for resection. Generally, this will be an area just above the peritoneal reflection (Fig. 99.7A). Mobilization of the rectosigmoid below the level of the peritoneal reflection is discussed in greater detail in Chapter 101. Clean the colon circumferentially and divide it between clamps. Incise the peritoneum from the point of division of the colon up along the point of origin of the inferior mesenteric artery to a portion of the middle transverse colon just to the left of the middle colic artery (Fig. 99.7B). As with right colon resection, an adequate cancer operation should contain 12 to 14 nodes. Palliative and non-cancer resections are tailored to the specific circumstances. Clean the portion of the middle transverse colon selected for anastomosis and divide the mesentery with clamps, securing the vessels with suture ligatures of 2-0 silk. Remove the specimen.

Anatomic Points

The terminal transverse colon and left colon, to the level of the lower rectum, are supplied by the inferior mesenteric artery, which usually arises from the front of the aorta, about 3 to 4 cm distal to the origin of the superior mesenteric artery and the same distance proximal to the bifurcation of the aorta. This artery (which is directed inferiorly and to the left) and its branches are largely retroperitoneal. Within a few centimeters of its origin, it gives rise to its first major branch, the left colic artery. More distally, arteries lie lateral to their corresponding veins. The left colic artery divides into ascending and descending branches that parallel the colon. The ascending branch ultimately forms part of the marginal artery (of Drummond) before anastomosing with the left branch of the middle colic artery, whereas the descending branch anastomoses with the first sigmoid artery. Either the inferior mesenteric artery or the left colic artery passes anterior to the main trunk of the inferior mesenteric vein.

A variable number of sigmoid arteries (range of one to five, but usually two or three) next arise from the inferior mesenteric artery, enter the sigmoid colon, and, as with the arteries previously discussed, divide into ascending and descending branches. These branches anastomose with each other and with arteries derived from other branches (e.g., the descending branch of the left colic artery, the superior rectal artery), thus continuing the marginal artery (of Drummond).

The superior rectal (hemorrhoidal) artery is the termination of the inferior mesenteric artery. This artery crosses the left common iliac vessels in the base of the sigmoid mesocolon and enters the pelvis, where it lies posterior to the rectum. In this location, it soon divides into right and left branches that anastomose with branches of the paired middle rectal (hemorrhoidal) arteries. In addition, this artery usually forms an anastomosis with the last sigmoid artery, thereby negating the importance of Sudeck critical point and essentially completing a marginal artery of Drummond from the beginning of the cecum to the rectum.

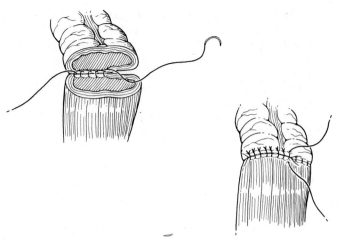

Figure 99.8 Construction of the anastomosis

As with the right colon, specific node groups are recognized by the American Joint Commission on Cancer. For the splenic flexure, these are the pericolic, middle colic, left colic, and inferior mesenteric. For the descending colon, these are the pericolic, left colic, inferior mesenteric, and sigmoid nodes. For lesions of the sigmoid, the superior rectal and sigmoid mesenteric nodes are added to those of the descending colon.

Construction of the Anastomosis (Fig. 99.8)

Technical and Anatomic Points

Generally, the transverse colon will swing easily down to anastomose without tension to the sigmoid. Occasionally, however, further mobilization is necessary. Mobility is ultimately limited by the middle colic artery and vein. Sometimes construction of an end-rectum to side-sigmoid (Baker-type) anastomosis is easier and eliminates the problem with tension and size discrepancy. Some surgeons perform a Baker-type anastomosis routinely.

If the middle transverse colon will not reach to the distal sigmoid, it may be necessary to resect back to the terminal ileum; however, this is only very rarely warranted. Construct an end-to-end anastomosis between the middle transverse colon and the sigmoid in the usual fashion. Generally, the mesenteric defect is broad and cannot be closed. If the colon has been mobilized out of the pelvis, leaving a raw surface in the hollow of the sacrum, place closed-suction drains in the pelvis.

REFERENCES

1. American Joint Committee on Cancer. Colon and rectum. In: Greene FL, Compton CC, Fritz AG, eds. *AJCC Cancer Staging Atlas*. New York, NY: Springer Verlag; 2006:107–118.
2. Baker JS. Low end to side rectosigmoidal anastomosis. *Arch Surg*. 1950;61:143.
3. Chang GJ, Kaiser AM, Mills S, et al. Practice parameters for the management of colon cancer. *Dis Colon Rectum*. 2012;55:831.
4. Dionigi G, Castano P, Rovera F, et al. The application of sentinel lymph node mapping in colon cancer. *Surg Oncol*. 2007;16: S129–S132.

5. Jordan WP, Scaljon W. Anatomic complications of abdominal surgery with special reference to the ureter. *Am Surg.* 1979;45:565.

6. Lee JF, Maurer VM, Block GE. Anatomic relations of pelvic autonomic nerves to pelvic operations. *Arch Surg.* 1973;107:324.

7. Lewis A, Akopian G, Carillo S, et al. Lymph node harvest in emergent versus elective colon resections. *Am Surg.* 2012;78:1049.

8. Lim SJ, Feig BW, Wang H, et al. Sentinel lymph node evaluation does not improve staging accuracy in colon cancer. *Ann Surg Oncol.* 2008;15:46–51.

9. Nissan A, Protic M, Bilchik AJ, et al. United States Military Cancer Institute Clinical Trials Group (USMCI GI-01) randomized controlled trial comparing targeted nodal assessment and ultrastaging with standard pathologic evaluation for colon cancer. *Ann Surg.* 2012;256:412.

10. Tajimi Y, Ishida H, Ohsawa T, et al. Three-dimensional vascular anatomy relevant to oncologic resection of right colon cancer. *Int Surg.* 2011;96:300.

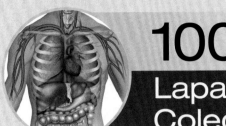

100
Laparoscopic Partial Colectomy

John C. Byrn

All benign and malignant indications for colectomy can be approached laparoscopically. Because it is difficult to palpate lesions, it is best to precisely localize the pathology before surgery (especially for smaller lesions). In contrast to open colon resection, laparoscopic colectomy is commonly performed from the "medial to lateral" approach described here. This is easier than the older "lateral to medial" approach because the mobilized colon does not obscure laparoscopic view.

SCORE™, the Surgical Council on Resident Education, classified laparoscopic partial colectomy as an "ESSENTIAL COMMON" procedure.

STEPS IN PROCEDURE

Right Colon Resection
Supine position, patient secured to bed
Trocar sites: Umbilical, suprapubic, left lateral to the umbilicus
Perform thorough laparoscopic exploration
Trendelenburg position with right side up table tilt
Place cecum and right colon mesentery on stretch to identify ileocolic artery (ICA)
Create a plane between ICA and retroperitoneum identifying duodenum
Ligate the ICA with LigaSure
Incise line of Toldt with right colon retracted medially

Mobilize colon from lateral attachments re-entering plane of medial dissection and re-identify duodenum
Place patient in reverse Trendelenburg position
Take hepatic flexure attachments medial to lateral after entering lesser sac and identifying transverse colon mesentery
Extend umbilical port incision to create a 3- to 5-cm incision
Exteriorize the right colon
Resect and control right branch of middle colic extracorporeally
Perform extracorporeal anastomosis
Return anastomosis to abdomen
Close extraction and trocar sites

HALLMARK ANATOMIC COMPLICATIONS
Ureteral injury
Injury to duodenum (right colon)

Splenic injury (left colon)
Missed lesion (resection of wrong segment)

LIST OF STRUCTURES
Colon
Inferior epigastric artery and vein

Lesser sac
Omentum

Right Colon
Cecum
Ascending colon
Hepatic flexure
Duodenum
Line of Toldt
Ileocolic artery

Transverse Colon
Right middle colic artery and vein

Left Colon
Splenic flexure
Descending colon
Sigmoid colon
Line of Toldt
Splenic flexure
Sacral promontory
Ureters
Inferior mesenteric artery and vein

Right Colon Resection—Trocar Placement and Patient Positioning

Technical Points

Place the patient in the supine position. Carefully pad and tuck both arms, placing them in a neutral "thumbs up" or slightly supinated position. This takes pressure off the ulnar nerve at the retrocondylar groove of the elbow.

Frequent, and sometimes extreme, patient positioning changes make cooperation with the anesthesia and nursing teams of utmost importance. All operating room participants should agree on positioning and padding, as the opportunity to reposition, after the patient is prepped and draped, may be limited.

Greater security in patient positioning can be obtained by using a "beanbag" (Olympus Vac Pac, Center Valley, PA). Secure this to the bed with cloth tape (to prevent rips in the beanbag). Place the beanbag flush with the perineum at the caudal extent of the operating room bed. Desufflate the bag with cranial edges "rolled" superiorly over the patient's shoulders. This allows for very secure patient positioning, even with the obese patient in the steep Trendelenburg position.

A three-trocar technique is used (Fig. 100.1). Place a 12-mm trocar at the superior aspect of the umbilicus, to accommodate a 10-mm, 30-degree laparoscope, using a Hasson technique. Place two 5-mm trocars: One in the midline suprapubic region, and the other in the left lower quadrant, but more precisely lateral to the umbilicus. True lower quadrant trocar positioning is comfortable when working on the ascending colon but will be self-limiting in terms of reach when mobilizing the hepatic flexure.

The surgeon and assistant both stand on the patient left, opposite the side of resection. Laparoscopic monitors are placed at surgeon "eye level" at about the level of the patient's umbilicus.

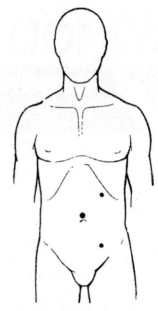

Figure 100.1 Trocar placement for laparoscopic right hemicolectomy

Right Colon Resection—Mobilizing the Colon

Technical Points

Place the patient in Trendelenburg position with slight right side up tilt. Grasp the cecum and retract it toward the anterior abdominal wall. Note that the ICA is thus placed on stretch within its mesentery, facilitating identification (Fig. 100.2A,B). Create a mesenteric window below the artery. This will allow identification of the duodenum in the retroperitoneum and ensure a safe plane prior to a "high" ligation of the ICA. It is not necessary to look for the ureter at this stage of the

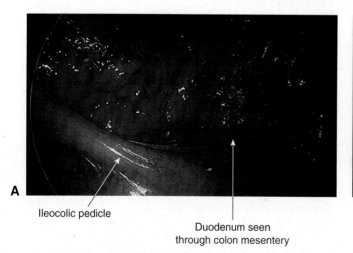

A

Ileocolic pedicle

Duodenum seen through colon mesentery

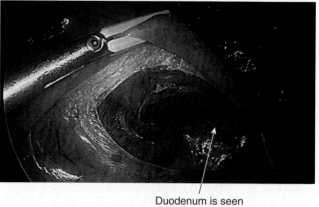

B

Duodenum is seen through incised mesentery, ileocolic pedicle on stretch

Figure 100.2 A: With the colon mobilized and the duodenum exposed, the ileocolic vascular pedicle is placed on stretch and identified as it tents up the mesentery. **B:** View behind colon with grasper elevating ileocolic vascular pedicle prior to division.

dissection. Take the major vascular pedicles of the colon preferentially with the 5-mm LigaSure (Covidien, Mansfield, MA). Carry this medial dissection cephalad toward the liver underneath the hepatic flexure and laterally to the white line of Toldt.

Next, incise the line of Toldt along the cecum or ascending colon sharply or with an energy device. The hepatic flexure can be mobilized considerably from the lateral perspective but when the dissection becomes difficult, it is best to turn one's attention to the gastrocolic omentum and enter the lesser sac. This shift to working above the transverse colon is aided by placing the position in to reverse Trendelenburg position. Enter the lesser sac and then complete the mobilization of the hepatic flexure completely from medial to lateral. The right colon should now be fully mobilized and the duodenum should be in view.

Place the transverse mesocolon on stretch and lift it up off the retroperitoneum and the root of the small bowel mesentery. The right branch of the middle colic artery is then safely taken with the duodenum in view. This vessel can also be ligated extracorporeally during specimen extraction and resection.

Anatomic Points

With the lateral attachments of the colon incised along the line of Toldt gentle medial retraction on the right colon will often lead to efficient, full mobilization. The duodenum should be viewed from lateral to medial when the plane of medial dissection is reentered during this mobilization.

When mobilizing the hepatic flexure the division of the omentum or gastrocolic omentum toward the midline allows easy entry into the lesser sac preventing inadvertent injury or uncontrolled division of the transverse mesocolon.

The duodenum should again be in view from a superior–lateral to medial vantage after the hepatic flexure is fully mobilized. This does not require ligating the right branch of the middle colic artery and vein. Identification of the duodenum medially during isolation and ligation of the ICA, lateral to medial when mobilizing the lateral right colon attachments, and then again superior–lateral to medial after hepatic flexure takedown are key views for safe right colon mobilization.

Right Colon Resection— Extracorporeal Resection and Anastomosis

Technical Points

Now extend the umbilical trocar site under direct vision to create the extraction site. Place a wound protector and use a Babcock clamp to easily grab the mobilized cecum under direct vision. Exteriorize the bowel.

Identify healthy, well-perfused transection sites on the ileum and colon where an anastomosis can be created without undue tension. For a stapled anastomosis, use a linear cutting stapling device to transect the ileum and the colon and allow removal of the surgical specimen (Fig. 100.3A) If the right branch of the middle colic artery and vein were not ligated intracorporeally, then clamp and tie these before resecting the specimen.

Next, align the antimesenteric borders of the ileum and colon (Fig. 100.3B). Excise a corner of the antimesenteric side of the staple line to allow placement of the linear cutting stapling device (Fig. 100.3C). Place one limb of the linear stapling device in the colon, the other in the small bowel (Fig. 100.3D). While closing the stapler, take care to ensure that the staple line will not incorporate the mesentery from either of the bowel limbs and that the entire length of the staple line is used to construct an adequately sized aperture (Fig. 100.3E). Fire the stapler. Inspect the staple lines for hemostasis (Fig. 100.3F). Close the enterotomy left after firing the linear cutting stapler by approximating the edge of the ileum to the colon with Allis clamps. Place these so that the previous staple lines are staggered, thus avoiding an unnecessary number of intersecting staple lines (Fig. 100.3G). Place a linear stapling device below the Allis clamps and fire it (Fig. 100.3H). Remove excess tissue distal to the staple line before removing the stapler (Fig. 100.3I). Reduce the bowel back into the abdomen and close the incisions.

STEPS IN PROCEDURE

Modified lithotomy position, patient secured to bed

Trocar sites: Umbilical, right lateral to umbilicus, left lower quadrant (2 fingerbreadths cephalad and 2 fingerbreadths left lateral from pubic symphisis)

Perform thorough laparoscopic exploration

Steep Trendelenburg position, left side up table tilt

Identify sacral promontory as a fixed reference and place sigmoid colon and its mesentery on stretch to identify inferior mesenteric artery (IMA)

Create plane between IMA and retroperitoneum and identify left ureter

Ligate IMA with LigaSure

Grasp sigmoid colon and retract toward midline

Incise line of Toldt and mobilize colon medially

Reidentify left ureter

Mobilize descending colon and splenic flexure

Divide colon distally with stapler via left lower quadrant trocar

Extend umbilical incision for specimen extraction

Transanal stapled anastomosis under laparoscopic vision

Perform leak test

Close extraction and trocar sites

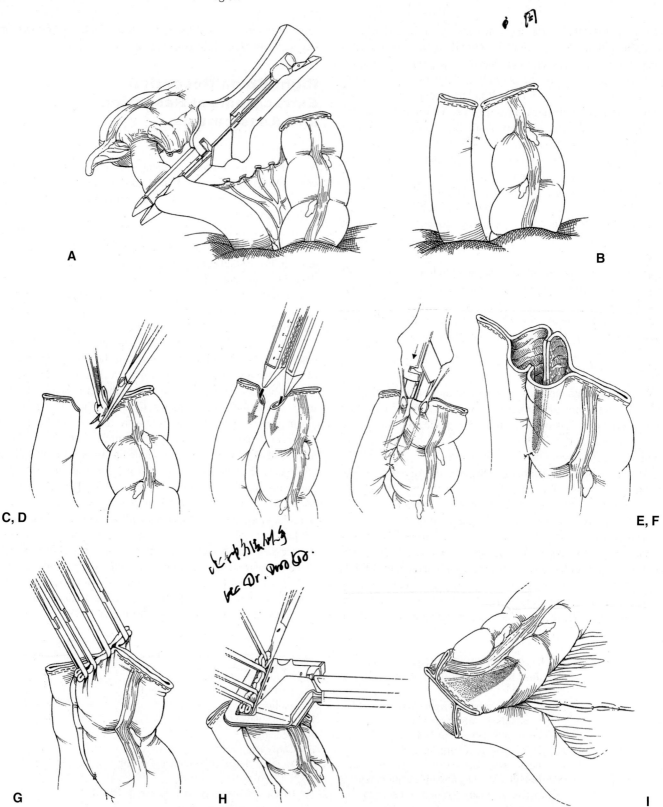

Figure 100.3 Extracorporeal division and anastomosis. **A:** Final transection of specimen by extracorporeal stapling. **B:** Two ends ready for anastomosis. **C:** Making enterotomies. **D:** Inserting stapler. **E:** Firing stapler. **F:** Inspecting staple line for bleeding. **G:** Approximation of opening (note that this method produces a triangular opening and that the two staple lines are staggered). **H:** Application of linear stapler. **I:** Completed anastomosis and closure of mesenteric defect (note wide-open triangular lumen) (from Gordon PH, Nivatvongs S. *Principles and Practice of Surgery for the Colon, Rectum, and Anus.* 2nd ed. St Louis, MO: Quality Medical Publishing; 1999:632–634, with permission).

Laparoscopic Left Hemicolectomy—Mobilization of the Left Colon and Splenic Flexure

Technical Points

Position and secure the patient as described for the laparoscopic right colectomy but use a modified, low lithotomy position with Allen stirrups. The hips need to be fully extended with the thigh level to the abdomen to prevent limitation in the range of motion of the lower abdominal trocar.

A three-trocar technique is again recommended, with a fourth optional trocar (Fig. 100.4A). Place a 12-mm trocar at the superior aspect of the umbilicus for the camera. Place a second 12-mm trocar on the right, lateral to the midline suprapubic region. A 12-mm trocar is used to accommodate the laparoscopic stapler. Place a 5-mm trocar in the right lower quadrant but more precisely lateral to the umbilicus. Again, extreme lower quadrant trocars can create difficulties (due to distance to target) when working on the splenic flexure. If necessary, place a second 5-mm trocar (four-trocar technique) on the left, lateral to the umbilicus and use this to mobilize a high splenic flexure.

The surgeon and assistant both stand on the patient right, opposite the side of resection. Laparoscopic monitors are placed at surgeon "eye level" at about the level of the patient's umbilicus.

Place the patient in Trendelenburg position and tilt the left side up. A medial to lateral dissection is then performed (Fig. 100.4B). The sacral promontory is a good fixed point of reference. Grasp the sigmoid colon and place the mesentery on stretch by retracting it toward the anterior abdominal wall and downward. The IMA will then be seen in the midline cephalad

to the sacral promontory. Create a plane between the IMA and retroperitoneum and identify the left ureter (Fig. 100.4C). The IMA is then ligated with the LigaSure.

With the left ureter identified and protected, the IMA ligated, the root of the left colon mesentery is free. The lateral mobilization of the sigmoid and descending colon can be routinely accomplished by incising the line of Toldt while supplying medial retraction on the sigmoid and descending colon. An appropriately mobilized descending colon leads to a proper plane for lateral mobilization of the splenic flexure.

When the mobilization of the splenic flexure from a lateral perspective becomes difficult, return your attention to the gastrocolic omentum and transverse colon mesentery. Place the patient in reverse Trendelenberg position. Enter the lesser sac and identify the transverse colon mesentery. Take the gastrocolic omentum from right to left until the splenic flexure is fully mobilized and the omentum has been taken down.

Anatomic Points

The root of the left colon mesentery should be essentially free of vascular structures after the high ligation of the IMA, other than the inferior mesenteric vein (IMV). The IMV will need to be ligated at the level of the duodenal–jejunal juncture, or more precisely the inferior border of the pancreas, for additional left colon mobility especially when low pelvic anastomoses are planned.

The sympathetic plexus that surrounds the IMA can be damaged during an overzealous high ligation and this should be avoided. Furthermore, if the IMA is knowingly ligated distal to the takeoff off the left colic artery, bleeding can be encountered and avoided as one mobilizes the root of the left colon mesentery.

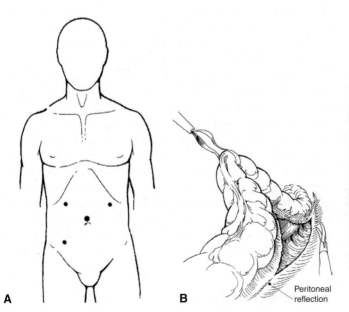

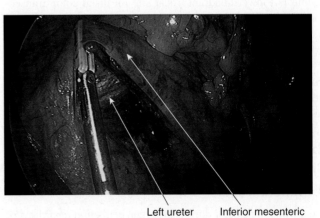

Left ureter   Inferior mesenteric artery on stretch

Peritoneal reflection

Figure 100.4 A: Trocar placement for laparoscopic left hemicolectomy. **B:** Mobilizing colon by incising peritoneum (from Wind GG. The Colon. In: *Applied Laparoscopic anatomy: Abdomen and Pelvis.* Baltimore, MD: Williams & Wilkins; 1997:217–246, with permission). **C:** Elevation of inferior mesenteric artery with exposure of left ureter.

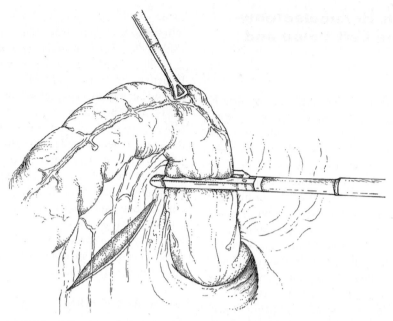

Figure 100.5 Division of the distal colon (from Weiss EG, Wexner SD. Laparoscopic segmental colectomies. In: Scott-Conner CEH, ed. *The SAGES Manual: Fundamentals of Laparoscopy and GI Endoscopy.* New York, NY: Springer-Verlag; 1999, with permission).

Resection of the Colon

Technical Points

Choose the level of distal transection based on the location of the diseased segment of colon. All other things being equal, the rectosigmoid junction provides a convenient anatomical division point as the sigmoid mesentery is easily thinned with the LigaSure at this point and the full thickness of the rectal mesentery is not encountered. This will also generally yield distal bowel that is free of diverticulae.

Pass an articulating, laparoscopic, linear stapler through the 12-mm left lower quadrant trocar site for distal colon transection (Fig. 100.5). Multiple firings may be required but take care to avoid more than three firings as this may result in excessive crossing of staple lines.

Next, grasp the stapled distal end of the colon with a noncrushing grasper, release the pneumoperitoneum, and create the extraction site by extending the umbilical trocar site incision. The proximal division is performed extracorporeally.

Extraction and Creation of the Circular Stapled Anastomosis

Technical Points

Use a wound protector during specimen extraction regardless of indication for resection. Grasp the distal end of your left-sided colon specimen with a Babcock clamp by using the laparoscopic grasper (still in place) to guide the specimen up to your extraction site under vision. Exteriorize the colon and divide the colon proximal to your diseased segment. The remaining mesentery and most notably the marginal artery will need to be ligated.

Place a purse-string suture in the proximal end of the bowel and insert the anvil of the circular stapling device (Fig. 100.6A,B). Tie the purse-string and replace the bowel into the abdominal cavity. Reestablish pneumoperitoneum. A useful technique involves cinching a slightly loosened wound protector around the Hasson 12-mm trocar with a Penrose drain and clamp. "Biting" towel clamps provide additional soft tissue approximation around the extraction site and almost always result in the restoration of excellent pneumoperitoneum.

Grasp the anvil with an anvil-grasping clamp and bring it down to the proposed anastomotic site. Take care to ensure that the bowel is not rotated as it is brought down to the anastomotic site. Pass the circular stapler transanally and advance it to the distal staple line. Extrude the trocar of the circular stapler through the staple line of the distal rectum under direct vision (Fig. 100.6C). Attach the anvil and approximate it to the cartridge under direct vision. Fire and remove the circular stapler. Inspect the donuts for completeness. Test the anastomosis by filling the pelvis with saline and occluding the bowel proximal to the anastomosis with a noncrushing bowel clamp. Next insufflate the rectum with air and observe for any bubbles, indicating a leak. Check hemostasis, irrigate the operative field, and close all port sites.

Anatomic Points

Abnormal rotation or torsion of the proximal bowel is surprisingly easy during manipulation of the anvil. If not corrected, it can lead to colonic obstruction proximal to the anastomosis. Mesenteric defects that are created during laparoscopic left-sided colon resection are not repaired.

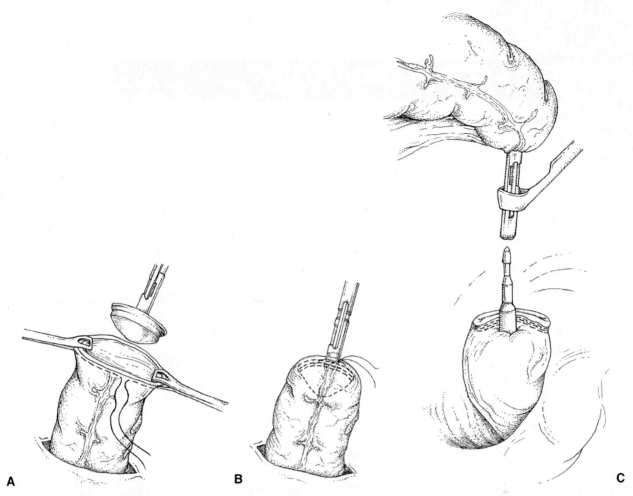

A   **B**   **C**

Figure 100.6 Construction of circular stapled anastomosis. **A:** Insertion of anvil in proximal colon. **B:** Purse-string tightened. **C:** Mating the two parts of the stapler (from Weiss EG, Wexner SD. Laparoscopic segmental colectomies. In: Scott-Conner CEH, ed. *The SAGES Manual: Fundamentals of Laparoscopy and GI Endoscopy.* New York, NY: Springer-Verlag; 1999, with permission).

REFERENCES

1. Bartels SA, D'Hoore A, Cuesta MA, et al. Significantly increased pregnancy rates after laparoscopic restorative proctocolectomy: A cross-sectional study. *Ann Surg.* 2012;256:1045–1048.
2. Braga M, Frasson M, Zuliani W, et al. Randomized clinical trial of laparoscopic versus open left colon resection. *Br J Surg.* 2010; 97:1180–1186.
3. Byrn J. Technical considerations in laparoscopic total proctocolectomy. *Surg Laparosc Endosc Percutan Tech.* 2012;22:180–182.
4. Cima RR, Pendlimari R, Holubar SD, et al. Utility and short-term outcomes of hand-assisted laparoscopic colorectal surgery: A single-institution experience in 1103 patients. *Dis Colon Rectum.* 2011;54:1076–1081.
5. Fleshman J, Sargent DJ, Green E, et al. Laparoscopic colectomy for cancer is not inferior to open surgery based on 5-year data from the COST Study Group trial. *Ann Surg.* 2007;246: 655–662.
6. Fox J, Gross CP, Longo W, et al. Laparoscopic colectomy for the treatment of cancer has been widely adopted in the United States. *Dis Colon Rectum.* 2012;55:501–508.
7. Gervaz P, Inan I, Perneger T, et al. A prospective, randomized, single-blind comparison of laparoscopic versus open sigmoid colectomy for diverticulitis. *Ann Surg.* 2010;252:3–8.
8. Jayne DG, Thorpe HC, Copeland J, et al. Five-year follow-up of the Medical Research Council CLASICC trial of laparoscopically assisted versus open surgery for colorectal cancer. *Br J Surg.* 2010; 97:1638–1645.
9. Kiran RP, Kirat HT, Ozturk E, et al. Does the learning curve during laparoscopic colectomy adversely affect costs? *Surg Endosc.* 2010;24:2718–2722.
10. Lacy AM, Delgado S, Castells A, et al. The long-term results of a randomized clinical trial of laparoscopy-assisted versus open surgery for colon cancer. *Ann Surg.* 2008;248:1–7.
11. Simorov A, Shaligram A, Shostrom V, et al. Laparoscopic colon resection trends in utilization and rate of conversion to open procedure: A national database review of academic medical centers. *Ann Surg.* 2012;256:462–468.
12. Vlug MS, Wind J, Hollmann MW, et al. Laparoscopy in combination with fast track multimodal management is the best perioperative strategy in patients undergoing colonic surgery: A randomized clinical trial (LAFA-study). *Ann Surg.* 2011;254:868–875.

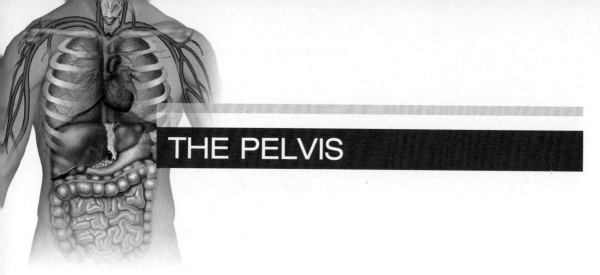

THE PELVIS

This section includes discussions on open and laparoscopic abdominoperineal resection and the related low anterior resection (Chapters 101 and 102e), continuing the discussion of colon anatomy that was begun in the previous part. More complex sphincter-sparing procedures, such as ileoanal anastomosis, are detailed in the references at the end of these chapters.

The remaining two chapters—Total Abdominal Hysterectomy and Salpingo-oophorectomy (along with related procedures) (Chapter 103) and Laparoscopic Surgery of the Female Pelvis (Chapter 104e)—present the anatomy of the female reproductive tract. The references listed at the end of these chapters provide descriptions of pelvic lymphadenectomy (both open and laparoscopic) and other, less common, pelvic operations.

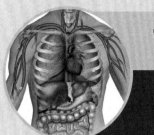

101

Abdominoperineal Resection, Low Anterior Resection

Abdominoperineal and low anterior resections are performed for carcinoma of the rectum. Wherever possible, the anal sphincters are preserved and an end-to-end anastomosis done by low anterior resection or other, more complicated, sphincter-saving procedures. Neoadjuvant therapy significantly increases the rate of sphincter preservation. The emphasis in modern cancer surgery is on total mesorectal excision, which simply means sharp dissection carried as wide as possible, removing the fatty node-containing mesentery as an intact envelope around the rectum. In contrast, operations for benign disease such as ulcerative colitis are performed as close as possible to the rectal wall (see References at the end of the chapter).

SCORE™, the Surgical Council on Resident Education, classified abdomino-perineal resection as a "COMPLEX" procedure and open partial colectomy as an "ESSENTIAL COMMON" procedure.

STEPS IN PROCEDURE

Position patient in lithotomy with access to both abdomen and perineum

Lower midline incision, explore the abdomen

Mobilize left colon by incising lateral peritoneal reflection, similarly incise peritoneum over right side, curving both peritoneal incisions down into pelvis where they continue anteriorly toward bladder or uterus

Identify both ureters, mobilize laterally in pelvis, and surround with silastic loops

Divide sigmoid with linear cutting stapler

Elevate sigmoid from pelvis and dissect sharply in presacral space

Clip any branches of middle artery as needed

Continue peritoneal incisions anteriorly over the posterior surface of the bladder (or uterus, in a female)

Male: Dissect in plane just posterior to seminal vesicles

Female: Excise portion of posterior vaginal wall if adjacent to tumor

Divide lateral attachments with clamps or clips

Assess feasibility of sphincter preservation

Abdominoperineal Resection

Complete dissection down to levator sling

Outline an elliptical incision

In male: Transverse perineal muscle forms anterior limit of dissection. In female:

Continue to excise posterior wall of vagina

Divide posterior tissues until fascia anterior to coccyx is identified; divide this sharply to enter abdominal plane of dissection

Divide puborectalis muscles with cautery

Perform anterior dissection in male with care, identifying and preserving prostate

Pass specimen out through perineum and divide remaining anterior attachments

Fashion end sigmoid colostomy

Place closed suction drains and close perineal and abdominal wounds

Low Anterior Resection

Transect distal rectum with reticulating linear stapler and divide

Place two stay sutures on each side of rectal stump

Create purse-string suture in proximal sigmoid colon and insert anvil

Create end-to-end stapled anastomosis with EEA stapler passed transanally

Test anastomosis for leaks, reinforce if needed

Consider temporary diverting loop ileostomy if any difficulty has been encountered

Closed suction drains in pelvis

Close abdomen in usual fashion

HALLMARK ANATOMIC COMPLICATIONS

Injury to ureters

Injury to male urethra or prostate

Damage to pelvic autonomic plexus, causing impotence or ejaculatory problems in men

LIST OF STRUCTURES

Sigmoid colon

Rectum
Lateral rectal ligaments
Anal canal
Ureters
Bladder
Sacrum
Coccyx
Pelvic diaphragm

Levator Ani (Levator Sling)
Iliococcygeus muscle
Pubococcygeus muscle
Coccygeus muscle
Ischiorectal fossa
Pubic symphysis
Ischial tuberosities

Perineum
Anterior (urogenital) triangle
Posterior (anal) triangle
Anococcygeal raphe
Perineal body
Pudendal nerve
Pudendal (Alcock) canal
Aorta

Inferior Mesenteric Artery
Superior rectal (hemorrhoidal) artery
Middle rectal (hemorrhoidal) arteries

Internal Pudendal Artery
Inferior rectal (hemorrhoidal) arteries
Middle sacral artery

Common Iliac Arteries
Internal iliac arteries
Presacral venous plexus
Superior hypogastric plexus

In the Male
Prostate
Seminal vesicles
Membranous urethra
Bulb of penis
Rectovesical fascia (of Denonvilliers)
Rectovesical pouch
Transverse perineal muscles

In the Female
Uterus
Ovaries
Vagina
Rectouterine pouch (of Douglas)

In this chapter, abdominoperineal resection will be considered along with the closely related low anterior resection. Figure 101.1 shows the extent of resection, including wide excision of tissues surrounding the rectum. This dissection will be described as it is done for a male patient. The modifications necessary for a female patient are described at the end of this section. The corresponding laparoscopic procedures are described in Chapter 102e.

Position of the Patient and the Incision (Fig. 101.2)

Technical Points

Position the patient supine on the operating table. Use either specially constructed leg supports or homemade outrigger "skis" to support the legs in moderate abduction with mild flexion at the hips and knees (Fig. 101.2A). The buttocks should extend slightly over the end of the operating table. Comfortable access to the perineal region should be available for the operating surgeon. Avoid the use of standard lithotomy stirrups, because these produce excessive flexion at the hip and knee and have been associated with vascular complications when used for lengthy procedures. Close the anus securely with a purse-string suture. Prepare and drape the anterior abdomen and perineal region. Place a towel over the perineum to provide temporary coverage until access is required. The initial phase of the dissection is done through the abdomen, with the second assistant standing between the legs of the patient. The instrument nurse should stand on a stool. Do not proceed with the perineal dissection unless you are certain that sphincter preservation will not be possible.

ORIENTATION

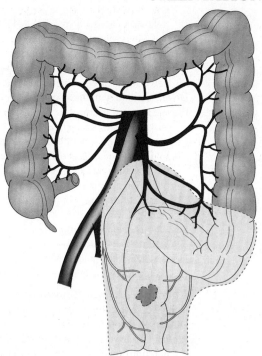

Figure 101.1 Extent of resection (from Chang AE, Morris AM. Colorectal cancer. In: Mulholland MW, Lillemoe KD, Doherty GM, Maier RV, Upchurch GR, eds. *Greenfield's Surgery: Scientific Principles and Practice.* 4th ed. Philadelphia, PA: Lippincott Williams & Wilkins; 2006, with permission).

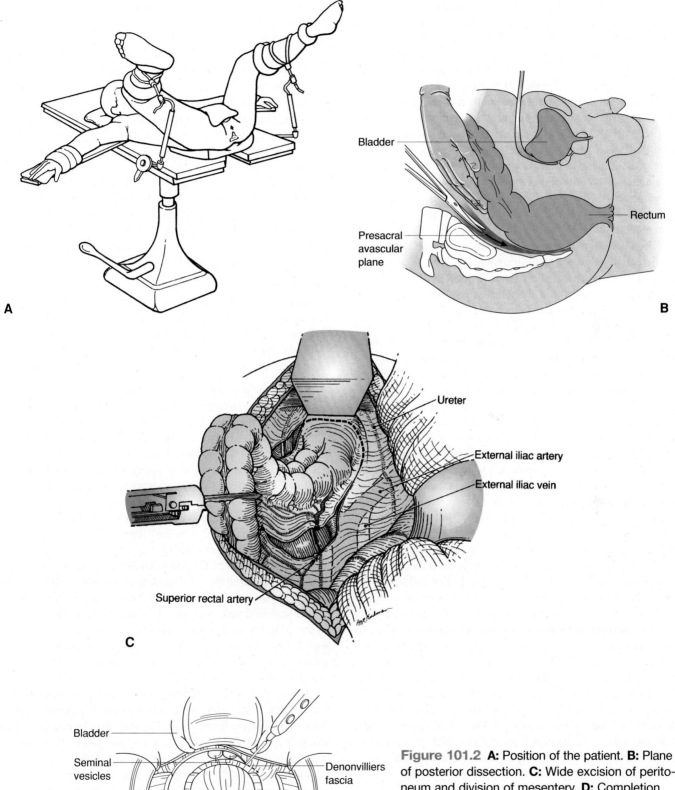

A: Position of the patient.

Bladder

Presacral avascular plane

Rectum

B

Ureter

External iliac artery

External iliac vein

Superior rectal artery

C

Bladder

Seminal vesicles

Denonvilliers fascia

D

Figure 101.2 A: Position of the patient. **B:** Plane of posterior dissection. **C:** Wide excision of peritoneum and division of mesentery. **D:** Completion of anterior incision (**B, D** from Chang AE, Morris AM. Colorectal cancer. In: Mulholland MW, Lillemoe KD, Doherty GM, Maier RV, Upchurch GR, eds. *Greenfield's Surgery: Scientific Principles and Practice.* 4th ed. Philadelphia, PA: Lippincott Williams & Wilkins; 2006, with permission).

A lower midline incision provides good exposure to the lower abdomen and pelvis. Make the incision from just above the umbilicus to the level of the pubis. Explore the abdomen. Mobilize the left colon as described in Chapter 81. Carry the peritoneal incisions anteriorly, about 1 cm up on the bladder, meeting in the midline between the bladder and the rectum.

Identify both ureters and surround them with Silastic loops. After the peritoneal incision has been completed and both ureters have been identified, divide the sigmoid colon at the point selected. Pass a hand behind the inferior mesenteric artery in the avascular plane just anterior to the vertebral bodies. Locate both ureters and confirm that they have not been included with the mesentery of the colon. Serially divide the mesentery of the colon with clamps. Using laparotomy pads, pack the proximal left colon up in the left upper quadrant.

The distal sigmoid is now completely free and can be circumferentially elevated from the pelvis, allowing access to the rectum. First, complete the posterior dissection. Elevate the sigmoid colon and initiate sharp dissection with Metzenbaum scissors in a plane just superficial to the sacrum (Fig. 101.2B). At the beginning of this dissection, you will see the aorta and common iliac vessels should be seen through a very light veil of areolar tissue. A few bands passing directly posterior between the colon and the presacral space can be divided using electrocautery or scissors. A middle sacral artery is usually present and should be secured with hemoclips. The colon should elevate easily, and a very thin glistening layer of retroperitoneal areolar tissue should be left intact over the presacral venous plexus. You should be able to dissect this plane easily by hand. If difficulty is encountered, it is possible that you are in the wrong plane; stop and reassess the situation. Torrential bleeding from the presacral venous plexus may follow inadvertent entry into this plexus. Conversely, remaining in the correct plane of dissection not only minimizes bleeding but also helps preserve autonomic nerves in the region. Dissection in the hollow of the sacrum should proceed readily until the tip of the coccyx is palpable and the rectosigmoid is elevated up on the hand. Check the hollow of the sacrum for hemostasis.

Next, turn your attention to the anterior dissection. Connect the peritoneal incisions laterally across the posterior surface of the bladder (Fig. 101.2C). Place three long hemostats, such as Crile hemostats, on the peritoneal reflection overlying the bladder. By sharp and blunt dissection, free the rectum from the posterior wall of the bladder until the seminal vesicles (in the male) are encountered (Fig. 101.2D). Carry this dissection down below the seminal vesicles, taking Denonvilliers fascia with the specimen. As noted in Figure 101.6, the posterior wall of the vagina is commonly excised with the specimen in a female. In this case, the anterior dissection need only proceed to a convenient point below the uterine cervix.

Anatomic Points

Identification of the ureters is easily accomplished if one remembers where the ureters lie as they enter the pelvis. Both left and right ureters are retroperitoneal and cross the peritoneal surface of the iliac vasculature in the vicinity of the origin of the internal iliac artery. The left ureter enters the pelvis at the apex of the sigmoid mesocolon, being crossed here by the descending limb of the mesocolon and its contained vasculature, the superior rectal (hemorrhoidal) vessels. Thus, its course in the pelvis is lateral to the pelvic limb of the sigmoid mesocolon and anterior (medial) to the internal iliac artery. The right ureter is similarly related to the internal iliac artery. Further, in the female, the ureter lies posterior to the ovarian vessels, which pass into the pelvis through the suspensory ligaments. In the female pelvis proper, the ovaries typically lie just anterior to the ureters. At this stage in the operation, it is also worthwhile to note that the blood supply of the pelvic portion of the ureters, derived from the internal iliac arteries or its branches, enters the ureter from its lateral side; hence, dissection to isolate the ureters should be done medially and the ureters gently mobilized laterally. Be careful not to skeletonize the ureters because the vascular anastomoses are tenuous at best. The ureters are at particular risk for injury during the following three phases of the operation.

1. Ligation of the inferior mesenteric artery
2. Incision of the pelvic peritoneum lateral to the rectum
3. Division of the lateral stalks of the rectum deep in the pelvis (particularly, if this phase is done from below during abdominoperineal resection)

Early identification, safe mobilization out of the operative field, and gentle marking with Silastic loops (to facilitate repeated verification of integrity) help minimize the risk for injury.

In its initial stage of development, the inferior mesenteric artery was originally located in the mesentery of the colon. However, with the fixation of the descending colon and the fusion of the left side of the mesentery with parietal peritoneum, the inferior mesenteric artery came to be primarily retroperitoneal. It can, however, be mobilized easily by blunt dissection in the fusion plane just posterior to the artery. The superior rectal (hemorrhoidal) artery, the pelvic continuation of the inferior mesenteric artery, passes into the pelvis in the base of the sigmoid mesocolon. It branches into right and left vessels approximately at the level of the rectosigmoid junction (third sacral vertebra), and these branches continue distally on the posterolateral sides of the rectum. Typically, the right branch is larger than the left. As the sigmoid and the rectum are mobilized, the superior rectal (hemorrhoidal) artery and its branches will mobilize with it.

Mobilization of the rectum from the presacral space is not without risk. If the wrong plane is entered, one can easily avulse veins of the presacral venous plexus or avulse the middle sacral artery. In 15% of individuals, the presacral venous plexus anastomoses with the vertebral plexus, usually at the level of S3 to S5. These individuals are prone to torrential bleeding if the presacral venous plexus is torn. The middle sacral artery originates from the posterior side of the aorta, just proximal to its bifurcation into the common iliac arteries. Although small, it is large enough to cause significant bleeding if not controlled. The key to avoiding this artery and the presacral venous plexus is to dissect in a plane anterior to the superior hypogastric plexus, which itself is immediately anterior to the terminal aorta, the roots of the common iliac arteries, and the middle sacral artery.

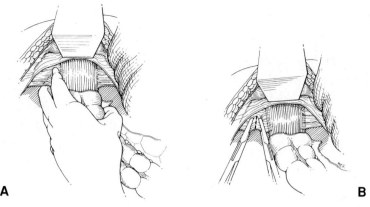

A   **B**

Figure 101.3 Division of the lateral rectal ligaments. **A:** Pull the rectum over toward to one side. **B:** Divide the ligaments between clamps or with harmonic scalpel.

The technical objective of the anterior dissection of the rectum is to dissect in the avascular plane provided by the rectovesical fascia (of Denonvilliers). This septum, located in the male between the prostate (and seminal vesicles) and the rectum, is attached above to the peritoneum of the rectovesical pouch, laterally to the pelvic diaphragm, and inferiorly to the perineal body. In the embryo, the peritoneal cavity extends inferiorly to the perineal body. As the prostate and the rectum increase in size, the peritoneum covering the posterior prostate and the anterior rectum is apposed. Subsequent fusion of the apposed serosal surfaces results in the definitive rectovesical fascia. The fusion plane is relatively avascular.

Division of the Lateral Rectal Ligaments (Fig. 101.3)

Technical Points

The remaining attachments to be taken from above are the mesentery of the rectum and the lateral rectal ligaments. These include the middle rectal (hemorrhoidal) vessels. Secure the left lateral ligament first. Place your nondominant hand on the sigmoid colon, passing two fingers anterior and two fingers posterior to the rectosigmoid. Pull the colon to the right to define a pedicle of thickened tissue between your fingers (Fig. 101.3A). Take this tissue serially with hemoclips or with sutures and ligatures (Fig. 101.3B), taking as much lateral tissue as possible. Proceed down to the pelvic diaphragm.

Next, pull the colon to the left and divide the right lateral ligament in the same fashion. The colon should now be totally free to the level of the pelvic diaphragm. At this point, it is possible to palpate the tumor to determine whether an anterior resection with anastomosis might be possible.

Anatomic Points

The ill-defined lateral rectal ligaments are often described as consisting of the connective tissue around the middle rectal (hemorrhoidal) artery and nerves. However, these ligaments are posterolateral, but the middle rectal artery approaches the rectum from a more anterolateral direction. In actuality, the ligaments consist primarily of the nerves to the rectum, accompanied by connective tissue and, in 25% of the cases, an accessory rectal artery.

The true middle rectal (hemorrhoidal) artery is quite variable in origin. It has been reported to be a branch of the internal pudendal (41%), inferior gluteal (23%), obturator, umbilical, and internal iliac arteries, among others, in the vicinity. It is rarely absent. Typically, it reaches the rectum very close to the pelvic diaphragm, not in the lateral ligaments. The middle rectal (hemorrhoidal) artery has been described as being associated with the rectovesical fascia (of Denonvilliers) in the male, and just deep to the peritoneum of the rectouterine pouch in the female. Although the middle rectal (hemorrhoidal) artery primarily supplies the muscles of the rectum, it also anastomoses freely with the superior rectal (hemorrhoidal) artery, and it may anastomose with the inferior rectal (hemorrhoidal) artery. Most surgeons and anatomists would agree that there is an arterial "watershed" at about the pectinate line of the rectum.

Low Anterior Resection (Fig. 101.4)

Technical and Anatomic Points

If, after complete mobilization of the rectum to the level of the pelvic diaphragm (levator sling), the tumor appears to be in a higher position than initially appreciated, a low anterior resection using the EEA stapling device may be performed. Place a right-angled rectal clamp across the distal rectum just above the level of transection. Place two stay sutures of 2-0 silk below the level of transection, one on each side. These will allow you to maintain control of the rectal remnant, avoiding its retraction into the perineum. Transect the rectum and remove the specimen. Have suction ready as you do this to avoid soilage. Check the pelvis for hemostasis. Place a purse-string suture of 2-0 Prolene on the distal rectum. Place this suture as a whipstitch,

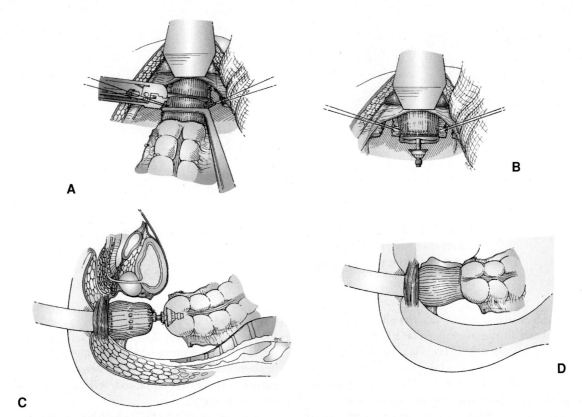

Figure 101.4 Low anterior resection. **A:** Division of rectum. **B:** Spike through staple line. **C:** Alignment of stapler. **D:** Bowel stapled, stapler still in place.

running it over and over to incorporate all layers of the bowel wall. Start from the upper surface on the outside so that it will be easy to tie the purse string over the EEA.

Alternatively, divide the distal rectum with a linear stapling device (Fig. 101.4A). This allows secure closure. The EEA can then be "spiked" through the closed rectal segment (Fig. 101.4B).

Pack off the pelvis. Place a purse-string suture on the proximal sigmoid. Check to make sure that you have sufficient mobility for the sigmoid to reach easily to the selected area of the distal rectum. If you are not certain that mobility is adequate, mobilize the splenic flexure to bring down the colon. From below, an assistant should then cut the purse-string suture that has been placed on the anus. The lubricated EEA stapling device can then be introduced through the anus. Tie both purse-string sutures securely around the instrument and close the instrument, checking to make sure that the bowel is circumferentially inverted and completely incorporated at both ends (Fig. 101.4C,D). Fire the EEA and then open it. Place a traction suture of 2-0 silk in a Lembert fashion and close the anterior wall of the anastomosis. Use this traction suture to elevate the anastomosis and remove it atraumatically from the EEA after opening the instrument. Check the anastomosis by injecting povidone-iodine solution (Betadine) into the distal rectal segment. Carefully reinforce any areas of leakage with interrupted 3-0 silk Lembert sutures. Surround the anastomosis with omentum and place closed suction drains in the pelvis.

Perineal Phase of Abdominoperineal Resection (Fig. 101.5)

Technical Points

If, even after mobilization, the tumor is too low for anterior resection, proceed with the perineal phase of the abdominopelvic resection. Remove the towel from the perineum and diagram an elliptical skin incision. In the male, palpate the transverse perineal muscle, which will form the anterior limit of the dissection. Incise the skin and subcutaneous tissues (Fig. 101.5A). Place Allis clamps on the skin edges of the specimen to approximate them. Begin the dissection laterally and posteriorly, deepening it through subcutaneous tissue (Fig. 101.5B) until the tip of the coccyx is reached. With strong scissors, cut the fascia anterior to the coccyx. Have an assistant pass a hand through the abdominal incision and down posterior to the rectum to help you identify the correct plane. Cut with scissors until you have entered the peritoneal cavity just anterior to the coccyx.

Place a finger of your nondominant hand into the peritoneal cavity and hook the puborectalis portion of the pubococcygeus muscle (Fig. 101.5C). Divide this muscle anteriorly using electrocautery, progressing upward to about 2-o'clock and 10-o'clock positions on each side.

The anterior phase of the dissection must be done with extreme care because this is the area where injury to the urethra and prostate is possible. Divide the fat anterior to the rectum carefully using Metzenbaum scissors, and look for and

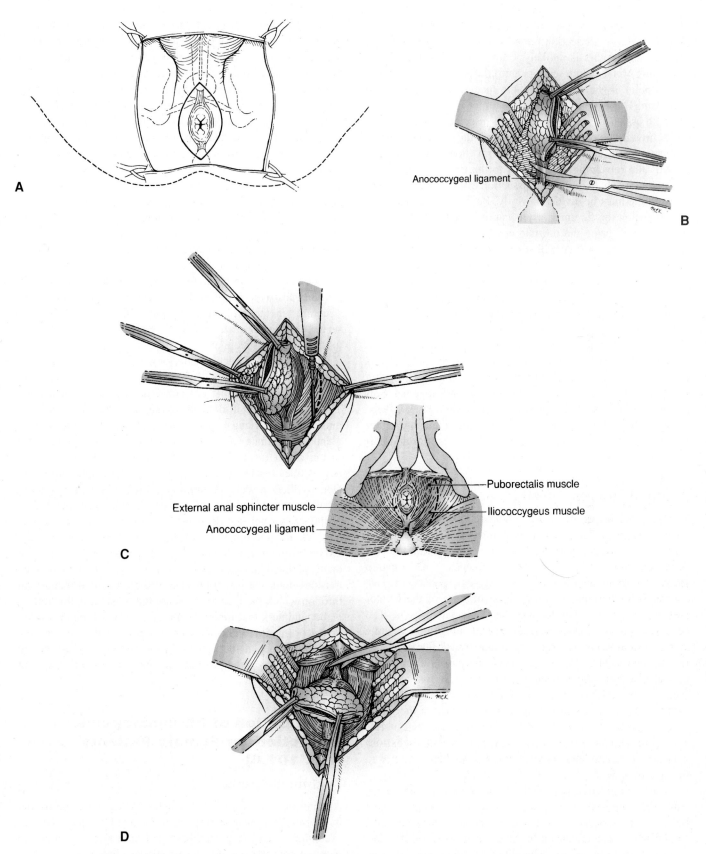

Figure 101.5 Perineal phase of abdominoperineal resection. **A:** Extent of incision. **B:** Superficial dissection through ischiorectal fat. **C:** Division of muscles. **D:** Anterior division with care to avoid urethra.

identify the transverse slips of the transverse perineal muscles (Fig. 101.5D). If dissection remains posterior to this muscle, injury to the urethra is unlikely. Carefully deepen the dissection, using Metzenbaum scissors, until the prostate is identified. At this point, it is helpful to pass the specimen out through the perineum. This is possible unless the tumor is extremely bulky. Have an assistant hand you the distal resected end of the sigmoid through the posterior opening. Roll the colon down until it is hanging out the bottom like a tail. It should be suspended only by the remaining attachments to the prostate. These can be divided by sharp and blunt dissection. Slips of the puborectalis muscle must be divided laterally. Be careful not to extend the dissection too far anteriorly because strong traction on the specimen will bring the prostate down farther than expected, and injury to the prostate will still be possible. After the specimen is removed, check hemostasis from above and below. Irrigate through with copious amounts of warm saline.

As an assistant closes the perineal wound, close the abdominal wound and fashion an end-sigmoid colostomy in the left lower quadrant of the abdomen in the usual fashion. The perineal wound is closed in layers with running 2-0 Vicryl. Generally, it is not possible to reapproximate the puborectalis muscle. With adequate tumor resection, these muscles are often taken so widely that they cannot be brought back together. Soft tissues can, however, be approximated in several layers. Place closed suction drains in the pelvis, bringing them out either lateral to the perineal incision or through the anterior abdominal wall.

Anatomic Points

The diamond-shaped perineum is bounded by imaginary lines connecting the anterior pubic symphysis, the lateral ischial tuberosities, and the posterior coccyx. The superior limit of the perineum is the pelvic diaphragm, composed of the paired levator ani (remember that the iliococcygeus, pubococcygeus, and puborectalis muscles are component parts of the levator ani) and coccygeus muscles and their associated fascia. The perineum can be divided into an anterior urogenital triangle and a posterior anal triangle by a horizontal line connecting the two ischial tuberosities. This line passes through the central tendon of the perineum (perineal body) and approximates the posterior edge of both the superficial and deep transverse perineal muscles, the latter being enclosed in the fascia of the superficial urogenital diaphragm. Because the anterior apex of the skin incision (described in the technical discussion) overlies the central tendon, the required dissection is limited to the anal triangle.

The central structure of the anal triangle is the anus. Anteriorly, the anal canal is anchored to the adjacent perineal body, and posteriorly it is anchored to the anococcygeal raphe (ligament), which attaches it to the tip of the coccyx. The lateral ischiorectal fossae are filled with fat and connective tissue. Rectal branches of the pudendal neurovascular structures pass through these spaces. Medially and superiorly, each ischiorectal fossa is limited by the pelvic diaphragm. This diaphragm is not flat, but funnel shaped. Its rim is attached to the midportion of the bony pelvis and the fascia covering the overlying obturator internus muscle, and its spout is the anus. Muscular fibers of the levator ani converge on fibers of the external anal sphincter, which some researchers consider to be an expression of the puborectalis part of the levator ani. The lateral boundary of the ischiorectal fossa is the obturator internus muscle and fascia.

Dissection in the anal triangle for removal of the rectum and anus proceeds from safe to dangerous, or from posterior to anterior. Detachment of the anococcygeal ligament from the coccyx, followed by division of the pelvic diaphragm muscles close to their insertion on this ligament and on the anal canal, preserves most of the pelvic diaphragm and the nerve supply to the retained muscle fibers because the nerves pass from posterolateral to anteromedial on the pelvic surface of these muscles. The pudendal nerve, located in a split (pudendal or Alcock canal) in the obturator fascia of the lateral wall of the ischiorectal fossa, supplies the external anal sphincter and all structures in the urogenital triangle. This nerve is also preserved if division of the pelvic diaphragm fibers is done close to the anorectal specimen.

Technically, dissection anterior to the anus is most difficult because of the proximity of the urethra and prostate gland and because of the anatomic characteristics of the perineal body. This anatomically ill-defined, pyramidal structure is a fibromuscular mass lying between the anal canal and the prostate gland (in the male) or vagina (in the female). It represents the fusion of all fascial layers in the perineum and pelvic floor (e.g., Colles fascia, both layers of urogenital diaphragm fascia, Denonvilliers fascia). In addition, muscle fibers of essentially all of the muscles in that area (such as the pubococcygeal fibers of the levator ani, the deep and superficial transverse perineal muscles, the anterior fibers of the external anal sphincter, and the bulbospongiosus fibers) have some or all of their insertion on the perineal body. Because the superficial transverse perineal muscles mark the posterior edge of the urogenital diaphragm, through which the membranous urethra must pass, this muscle is the landmark that limits the anterior extent of the dissection. Posterior traction on the anorectal specimen will allow the surgeon to dissect in the plane of Denonvilliers fascia, thereby avoiding injury to the prostate, membranous urethra, and bulb of the penis.

Modification of Abdominopelvic Resection for Female Patients (Fig. 101.6)

Technical Points

Abdominopelvic resection in the female patient is performed in essentially the same way as in the male patient. The only exception is that the posterior wall of the vagina is commonly resected with the specimen. This allows a better margin of the tumor to be obtained. Dissection in the rectovaginal septum is difficult and bloody, and a considerable amount of the posterior vaginal wall can be removed without compromising the

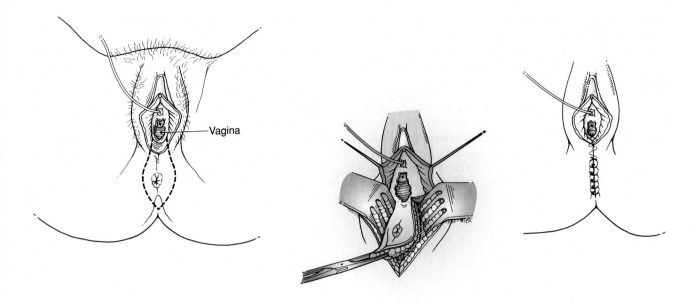

Figure 101.6 Modification of abdominopelvic resection for female patients

vaginal lumen. As dissection progresses in the perineal region, a tongue of posterior vaginal wall is excised as part of the initial skin incision. The extent of this tongue depends on the location of the tumor, but commonly it will go back 5 to 10 cm. After resection of the specimen, the vaginal epithelium is closed with a subcuticular suture of 3-0 Vicryl, and the soft tissues are approximated in the normal fashion.

Anatomic Points

The primary anatomic difference that is pertinent to the abdominal phase of this operation in the female patient is the interposition of the vagina and uterus between the rectum and the bladder. In the female patient, a rectouterine pouch (of Douglas), not a rectovesical pouch, is the lowest extent of the peritoneal cavity. In addition, a homologue to the rectovesical fascia (of Denonvilliers) is less easily demonstrated in female patients, although a cleavage plane between the rectum and posterior vaginal wall can be developed. Finally, complications can occur if one does not keep in mind that the uterine artery, a branch of the internal iliac artery (or one of its branches), passes forward, medially, and downward along the lateral wall in close proximity to the uterus. In the base of the broad ligament, lateral to the cervix, it turns medially, crossing the ureter close to the uterus. In this part of its course, it is bound to the lateral cervical ligament, contributing to this ligament's apex.

In the perineal phase of this operation, removal of part of the vaginal wall with the anorectal specimen necessitates removal of the perineal body, the more medial part of the superficial transverse perineal muscle, and a posteromedial part of the urogenital diaphragm. As in the male patient, major neurovascular structures are avoided by division of the perineal structures close to the midline.

REFERENCES

1. Allaix ME, Arezzo A, Cassoni P, et al. Metastatic lymph node ratio as a prognostic factor after laparoscopic total mesorectal excision for extraperitoneal rectal cancer. *Surg Endosc.* 2012. (epub ahead of print)
2. Bleier JL, Maykel JA. Outcomes following proctectomy. *Surg Clin North Am.* 2013;93:89–106.
3. Cherry DA, Rothenberger DA. Pelvic floor physiology. *Surg Clin North Am.* 1988;68:1217–1230.
4. Dedemadi G, Wexner SD. Complete response after neoadjuvant therapy in rectal cancer: To operate or not to operate? *Dig Dis.* 2012;30(suppl 2):109–117.
5. Dehni N, Schlegel RD, Cunningham C, et al. Influence of a defunctioning stoma on leakage rates after low colorectal anastomosis and colonic J pouch-anal anastomosis. *Br J Surg.* 1998;85:1114–1117. (Confirms protective value of defunctionalizing stoma for extremely low anastomoses.)
6. Fazio VW, Zutshi M, Remzi FH, et al. A randomized multicenter trial to compare long-term functional outcome, quality of life, and complications of surgical procedures for low rectal cancers. *Ann Surg.* 2007;246:481–490.
7. Ger R. Surgical anatomy of the pelvis. *Surg Clin North Am.* 1988;68:1201–1216. (Provides good description of anatomy and physiology along with surgical considerations.)
8. Jayne DG, Brown JM, Thorpe H, et al. Bladder and sexual function following resection for rectal cancer in a randomized clinical trial of laparoscopic versus open technique. *Br J Surg.* 2005;92:1124–1132.
9. Jeong S-Y, Chessin DB, Guillem JG. Surgical treatment of rectal cancer: Radical resection. *Surg Oncol Clin N Am.* 2006;15:95–107.
10. Marr R, Birbeck K, Garvican J, et al. The modern abdominoperineal excision: The next challenge after total mesorectal excision. *Ann Surg.* 2005;242:74–82.
11. Matthiessen P, Hallbook O, Rutegard J, et al. Intraoperative adverse events and outcome after anterior resection of the rectum. *Br J Surg.* 2004;91:1608–1612.

12. Michelassi F, Hurst R. Restorative proctocolectomy with J-pouch ilioanal anastomosis. *Arch Surg.* 2000;135:347–353.

13. Mortenson MM, Khatri VP, Bennett JJ, et al. Total mesorectal excision and pelvic node dissection for rectal cancer: an appraisal. *Surg Oncol Clin N Am.* 2007;16:177–197.

14. Perretta S, Guerrero V, Garcia-Aguilar J. Surgical treatment of rectal cancer: Local resection. *Surg Oncol Clin N Am.* 2006;15: 67–93.

15. Phillips JG, Hong TS, Ryan DP. Multidisciplinary management of early-stage rectal cancer. *J Natl Compr Canc Netw.* 2012;10: 1577–1585.

16. Schoetz DJ. Complications of surgical excision of the rectum. *Surg Clin North Am.* 1991;71:1271–1281. (Presents a good description of problems and management as well as strategies to avoid.)

17. The Standards Practice Task Force, The American Society of Colon and Rectal Surgeons. Practice parameters for the management of rectal cancer (revised). *Dis Colon Rectum.* 2005;48: 411–423.

18. Vand de Velde CJ, van den Broek CB. Quality assurance in rectal cancer treatment. *Dig Dis.* 2012;30:126–131.

19. Vignali A, Fazio VW, Lavery IC, et al. Factors associated with the occurrence of leaks in stapled rectal anastomoses: A review of 1014 patients. *J Am Coll Surg.* 1997;185:105–113.

20. Wu, JS, Fazio VW. Management of rectal cancer. *J Gastrintest Surg.* 2004;8:139–149.

ⓔ102 Laparoscopic Low Anterior and Abdominoperineal Resection

This chapter can be accessed online at www.lww.com/eChapter102.

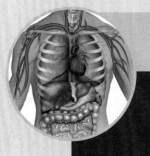

103
Total Abdominal Hysterectomy and Salpingo-Oophorectomy

Hysterectomy may be performed transabdominally or vaginally. One or both ovaries may be removed with the uterus. In this chapter, total abdominal hysterectomy with bilateral salpingo-oophorectomy is described. Modification of the technique to preserve one or both ovaries is also discussed. References at the end of the chapter describe supracervical and transvaginal hysterectomy. Chapter 104 provides an introduction to laparoscopic surgery of the female pelvis.

SCORE™, the Surgical Council on Resident Education, classified hysterectomy and salpingo-oophorectomy as "ESSENTIAL UNCOMMON" procedures.

STEPS IN PROCEDURE

Lithotomy position; empty bladder with catheter

Skin crease transverse incision

Raise flap cephalad and make vertical midline incision through fascia

Thorough abdominal exploration

Grasp uterine fundus with two Kelly clamps and elevate

Divide round ligaments with clamps and ties

If ovary is to be spared, divide uterine tube and ovarian ligament

If ovary is to be taken, incise broad ligament lateral to tube and ovary

Identify and protect ureter

Secure uterine vessels

Incise peritoneum overlying bladder and create bladder flap

Continue dissection to uterine cervix and divide

Vaginal cuff may be closed with running lock stitch or oversewn and left open

Close abdomen in usual fashion without drains

HALLMARK ANATOMIC COMPLICATIONS

Injury to ureter

Injury to bladder

LIST OF STRUCTURES

Uterus

Cervix

Vagina

Fallopian (uterine) tubes

Ovaries

Round ligament

Broad ligament

Suspensory (infundibulopelvic) ligament

Ovarian ligament

Lateral cervical (cardinal) ligament

Uterosacral ligament

Bladder

Ureter

Urachus

Vesicouterine pouch (anterior cul-de-sac)	Ovarian branch
Rectouterine pouch (posterior cul-de-sac, pouch of Douglas)	Ovarian artery
	Rectus abdominis muscle
Rectovaginal fascia	Anterior rectus sheath
Internal iliac artery	Linea alba
	Pyramidalis muscle
Uterine Artery	Transversalis fascia
Tubal branch	

Incision and Initial Exposure (Fig. 103.1)

Technical Points

Place the patient in the lithotomy position. Empty the bladder by straight catheterization or by placing an indwelling Foley catheter. After general anesthesia has been administered, perform a pelvic examination to confirm the anatomy. A Trendelenburg position of about 15 degrees will facilitate pelvic exposure.

Total abdominal hysterectomy may be performed through a lower midline incision. However, the more cosmetically appealing Pfannenstiel incision is described here.

Make a transverse incision in the natural skin crease where the skin incision will be hidden by regrowth of pubic hair.

Make the incision about 10 to 15 cm long, depending on the habitus of the patient. Carry this incision through skin and subcutaneous tissue to the underlying rectus sheath. Incise the anterior rectus sheath in line with the skin incision. Develop flaps between the anterior rectus sheath and the underlying rectus muscle until the muscle is exposed well in the midline to about the level of the umbilicus. Retract the rectus muscles laterally to expose the midline fascia and underlying peritoneum. Incise the fascia and peritoneum vertically from the umbilicus to the pubis. Identify the bladder in the inferior aspect of the incision and gently retract it downward, out of harm's way. Exposure through this incision is quite limited. Use it only when you do not anticipate a need for access to the upper abdomen.

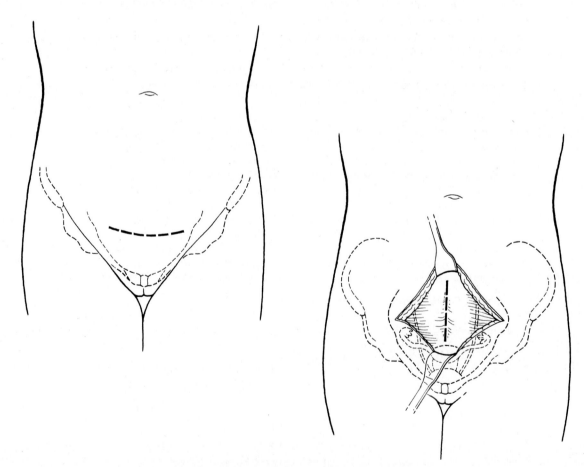

Figure 103.1 Incision and initial exposure

Anatomic Points

The infraumbilical vertical midline incision exposes a very narrow linea alba, from which fibers of the rectus abdominis muscle originate and upon which the more anterior pyramidalis muscle inserts; this makes a true midline incision technically difficult. If the exact midline is not divided, then this becomes a muscle-splitting incision through the pyramidalis and rectus abdominis muscles. Surgically, the posterior rectus sheath ends approximately halfway between the umbilicus and the pubis, at the arcuate line. Inferior to this line, the posterior surface of the rectus abdominis muscle is in contact with the transversalis fascia.

The Pfannenstiel incision, a transverse incision in the infraspinous crease, follows Langer's lines and is low enough (about 5 cm superior to the pubic symphysis) to allow the scar to be hidden by pubic hair. Retraction of the rectus sheath superiorly and inferiorly may necessitate sharp dissection because one or more infraumbilical tendinous inscriptions (where the sheath becomes adherent to the rectus muscle) may be present. When the linea alba is split vertically, caution should be used to avoid the deeper urinary bladder and the urachus. The latter is usually entirely fibrotic, but can retain a partially patent lumen in continuity with the lumen of the urinary bladder; this has been reported to occur in as many as 33% of the cases.

The uterus is positioned between the urinary bladder and the rectum. Both the uterus and the uterine tubes are invested by the broad ligament, an expression of peritoneum. Normally, the uterus is anteverted so that the fundus lies superior to the urinary bladder. Between the uterus and the bladder is a shallow recess, the vesicouterine pouch or anterior cul-de-sac, whereas posterior to the uterus, between it and the rectum, is the much deeper rectouterine pouch (of Douglas), or posterior cul-de-sac.

Immediately inferior to the junction of the uterine tube and uterus, and causing a fold on the anterior leaf of the broad ligament, is the round ligament of the uterus. The lower homolog of the gubernaculum testis runs lateral to the deep inguinal ring where it enters the inguinal canal; it then exits the superficial inguinal ring and finally blends with the connective tissue of the labium majus.

The peritoneal layers of the broad ligament are closest along its uterine attachment. As one progresses inferolaterally, the anterior and posterior leaves diverge to become continuous with peritoneum of the vesicouterine pouch and rectouterine pouch, respectively. In the lower part of the broad ligament are the ureter and uterine artery, both of which must be clearly distinguished.

Division of the Round Ligaments and Development of Pelvic Dissection (Fig. 103.2)

Technical Points

Place Kelly clamps on the uterine fundus on each side and use these to provide upward traction. Divide the round ligaments between clamps and secure the ends with suture ligatures of heavy chromic. Incise the peritoneum along the anterior and posterior surfaces of the broad ligament. If the uterine tube and ovary are to be removed with the uterus, incise the broad ligament lateral to the tube and ovary, retracting these structures medially with the uterus. If an ovary is to be spared, the uterine tube and ovarian ligament must be divided. Pass a finger behind the tube and ovary, elevating these structures with the ovarian ligament, away from the broad ligament. Clamp and suture-ligate this pedicle of tissue. Allow the ovary and distal uterine tube to retract laterally, and continue the dissection.

Identify the ureter on each side where it crosses the common iliac vessels at the bifurcation. As the dissection is carried down parallel to the cervix, the uterine vessels will be encountered at the isthmus of the uterus. Secure these with Heaney clamps and divide them. Skeletonize these vascular pedicles so that they can be securely divided and secured with suture ligatures.

Place retractors to expose the bladder and the anterior cul-de-sac. Continue the anterior incision of the broad ligament across the peritoneum overlying the bladder. By sharp and blunt dissection, develop the flap of bladder and free this from the underlying uterus and cervix.

Anatomic Points

The uterine tubes, which occupy the superior free edge of the broad ligament curve, pass laterally from the body of the uterus, loop superiorly over the ovary, and then curve downward and posteriorly to allow the fimbriae to "embrace" the ovary. The suspensory ligaments run from the bend of the uterine tube to the lateral pelvic wall, transmitting the ovarian vessels. From the medial end of the ovary, and visible on the posterior surface of the broad ligament, the ovarian ligament runs from the ovary, between the two peritoneal layers of the broad ligament, to the lateral border of the uterus just inferior to the uterine tube. This fibrous cord is the upper homolog of the male gubernaculum testis. The angle made by the ovarian ligament and the uterine tube is quite acute.

Tubal and ovarian branches of the uterine artery are also located in the broad ligament close to both the uterine tube and the ovarian ligament. The ovarian branch has a functional anastomosis with the ovarian artery.

As the ureter crosses the iliac vessels, it is in close proximity to the more lateral suspensory ligament. Thus incision of the peritoneum in this area should be done with some caution.

The origin of the uterine arteries is variable, although, in all cases, it ultimately is derived from the internal iliac artery. From its origin, it courses inferomedially along the lateral pelvic wall in close proximity to the ureter. Lateral to the cervix of the uterus, this medially directed artery crosses over the ureter to reach the lateral aspect of the uterus at the level of the uterine isthmus. Here, it divides into ascending and descending trunks that parallel the uterus and vagina and, through short branches, supply these organs. The ascending trunk has broad anastomoses with the ovarian artery. Typically, the point where the uterine artery crosses the ureter is about 1.5 to 2 cm lateral to

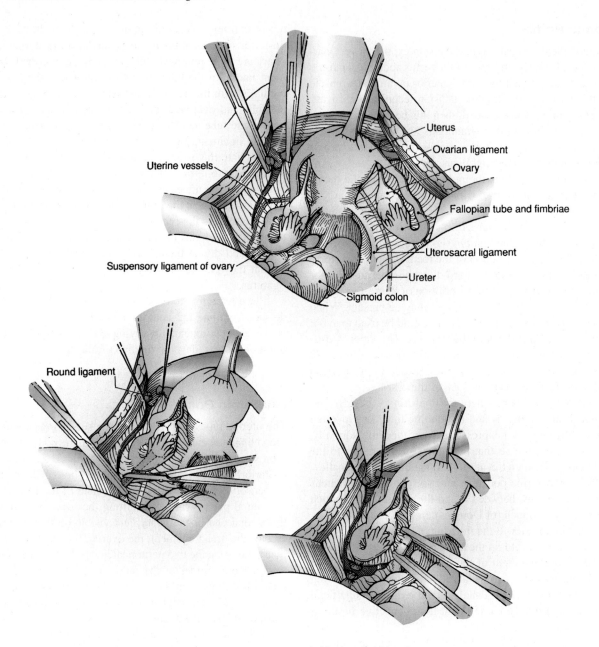

Figure 103.2 Division of the round ligaments and development of pelvic dissection

the cervix, but this can be quite variable. Further, the oblique course of the ureter with respect to the uterine artery renders the two structures in contact or closely adjacent to each other for a distance of 1 to 2.5 cm. These two facts make a meticulous dissection of the uterine artery mandatory.

Completion of the Hysterectomy (Fig. 103.3)

Technical Points

Retract the uterus upward to expose the rectovaginal fascia. Incise the peritoneum overlying the uterosacral ligaments and

free the vagina from the rectum, especially on the medial aspect of these ligaments. The rectovaginal fascia should dissect easily. Divide any remaining lateral attachments and secure them with suture ligatures. Palpate the cervix and divide the vagina just below the cervix. Place clamps on the two lateral corners of the vagina and suture-ligate them.

Anatomic Points

Between the anterior wall of the rectum and the posterior wall of the vagina, the rectovaginal fascia extends from the peritoneum to the pelvic floor and laterally to the pelvic walls. This fascia, the homolog of the male rectovesical fascia, is attached,

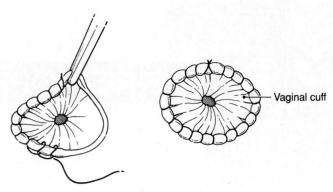

Figure 103.4 Closure of the peritoneum

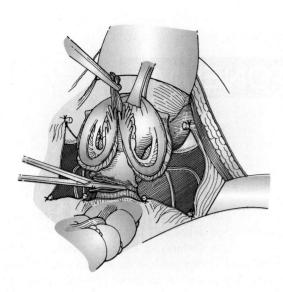

Figure 103.3 Completion of the hysterectomy

but separable, from the vagina; it is easily separable from the rectum. This fascia provides a plane of dissection between the rectum and the vagina.

The fibromuscular uterosacral ligaments—the more posterior and medial parts of the extraperitoneal pelvic supporting tissue—are broadly continuous with the lateral cervical or cardinal ligaments. The uterosacral ligaments attach to the cervix and upper vagina and, with a gentle lateral curve, course posteriorly to attach to the sacrum on either side of the rectum. They form the rectouterine folds (of Douglas), which are the lateral boundaries of the rectouterine pouch (of Douglas) or posterior cul-de-sac. The rectouterine folds contain smooth muscle, fibroelastic connective tissue, and neurovascular structures.

Closure of the Peritoneum (Fig. 103.4)

Technical and Anatomic Points

The vaginal cuff may be closed with a running lock stitch or left open for drainage. To leave the cuff open, overrun the edge of the cuff with a running lock stitch of absorbable suture to ensure hemostasis. Reperitonealize the pelvic floor with a running suture of 2-0 Vicryl. Close the abdominal incision in the usual fashion.

REFERENCES

1. Aslan P, Brooks A, Drummond M, et al. Incidence and management of gynaecological-related ureteric injuries. *Aust N Z J Obstet Gynaecol.* 1999;39:178–181.
2. Blikkendaal MD, Twijnstra AR, Pacquee SC, et al. Vaginal cuff dehiscence in laparoscopic hysterectomy: Influence of various suturing methods of the vaginal vault. *Gynecol Surg.* 2012;9: 393–400.
3. Brubaker LT, Wilbanks GD. Urinary tract injuries in pelvic surgery. *Surg Clin North Am.* 1991;71:963–976.
4. Daly JW, Higgins KA. Injury to the ureter during gynecologic surgical procedures. *Surg Gynecol Obstet.* 1988;167:19–22.
5. Grainger DA, Soderstrom RM, Schiff SF, et al. Ureteral injuries at laparoscopy: Insights into diagnosis, management, and prevention. *Obstet Gynecol.* 1990;75:839–843.
6. Harkki-Siren P, Sjoberg J, Tiitinen A. Urinary tract injuries after hysterectomy. *Obstet Gynecol.* 1998;92:113–118. (Risk for ureteral injury is higher with laparoscopic than with conventional hysterectomy.)
7. Learman LA, Summitt RL Jr, Varner RE, et al. A randomized comparison of total or supracervical hysterectomy: Surgical complications and clinical outcomes. *Obstet Gynecol.* 2003;102:453–462. (Supracervical hysterectomy is emerging as a less invasive alternative in selected patients with benign disease.)
8. Lethaby A, Mukhopadhyay A, Naik R. Total versus subtotal hysterectomy for benign gynaecological conditions. *Cochrane Database Syst Rev.* 2012;4:CD004993.
9. Masterson BJ. Selection of incisions for gynecologic procedures. *Surg Clin North Am.* 1991;71:1041–1052.
10. Radley S, Keighley MR, Radley SC, et al. Bowel dysfunction following hysterectomy. *Br J Obstet Gynaecol.* 1999;106: 1120–1125.
11. Summitt RL Jr. Laparoscopic-assisted vaginal hysterectomy: A review of usefulness and outcomes. *Clin Obstet Gynecol.* 2000; 43:584–593.

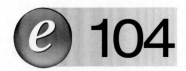

104 Laparoscopic Surgery of the Female Pelvis

This chapter can be accessed online at www.lww.com/eChapter104.

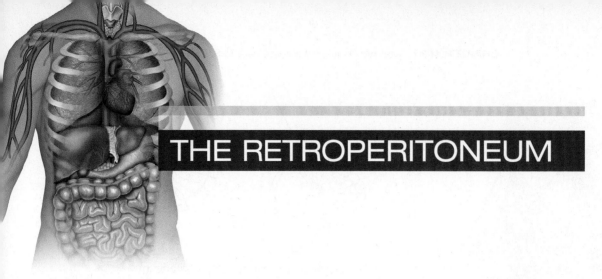

THE RETROPERITONEUM

The complex retroperitoneum technically includes anything that is not suspended on a mesentery. To the surgeon, only the genitourinary tract, major vascular structures, and sympathetic chain are generally considered to be retroperitoneal because of the way in which these structures are approached. The pancreas, also a retroperitoneal organ, has been discussed in previous chapters (Chapters 84 to 87).

The general approach to structures in this region involves mobilizing portions of overlying gastrointestinal tract by returning them to their original midline (embryonic) location. The complex anatomy of the underlying structures is first described by presenting the genitourinary tract. Chapters 105 and 106 describe the anatomy of the adrenal (suprarenal) glands through a discussion of adrenalectomy, performed by (open) anterior and posterior approaches and laparoscopically. Chapter 105 also presents some anatomy of the back muscles in the section on the posterior approach to the adrenals. Renal anatomy is then described through a discussion of renal trauma, radical nephrectomy, and renal transplantation (Chapters 107 to 110e).

Open and endovascular approaches to the abdominal aorta are described next (Chapters 111 and 112). Lumbar sympathectomy (Chapter 113e) is rarely performed now, but is included to show the anatomy of the sympathetic chain and to illustrate the manner in which deep structures can be approached through a lateral extraperitoneal route. A new chapter on placement of an inferior vena cava filter (Chapter 115) concludes this section.

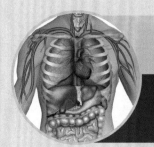

105

Adrenalectomy

The optimal choice of surgical approach in adrenal surgery depends on many factors including the dimensions of the mass, its location and size, functional status, the patient's preoperative condition, and the surgeon's experience. Laparoscopic adrenalectomy has become the "gold standard" for treatment of benign adrenal tumors over the last 2 decades. Current indications for open adrenalectomy are limited to large tumors (>6 to 10 cm), malignant or possibly malignant tumors, or conditions hostile to a laparoscopic approach. In this chapter, the open transabdominal approach to the adrenal glands is described because it is appropriate for bilateral tumors, such as pheochromocytomas, allows for complete examination of the abdominal cavity, as well as resection of extraadrenal lesions.

The posterior approach to the adrenals is rarely performed. In the past, it was performed for endocrine ablation or for resection of a small, isolated aldosteronoma. It is described at the end of this chapter because it is still occasionally used when the anterior laparoscopic or open approaches are contraindicated. It also provides the anatomic basis for posterior minimally invasive approaches to the glands.

A lateral or flank approach provides excellent exposure, especially for the right adrenal gland. However, it is rarely used except in conversion from the laparoscopic approach. References at the end of this chapter provide details of exposure using this method. Occasionally, large adrenal tumors require a thoracoabdominal incision for adequate exposure. Again, this is rare.

Laparoscopic adrenalectomy is described in Chapter 106.

SCORE™, the Surgical Council on Resident Education, classified open adrenalectomy as a "COMPLEX" procedure.

STEPS IN PROCEDURE

Transabdominal Adrenalectomy
Supine position, roll under lower costal margin
Bilateral subcostal or midline incision
Thorough abdominal exploration

Left Adrenalectomy
Divide gastrocolic omentum and retract stomach
    cephalad
Incise peritoneum along inferior border of
    pancreas and gently retract cephalad
Reflect transverse colon inferiorly
Palpate kidney and incise Gerota fascia just
    medial to superior aspect of kidney
Identify adrenal gland and left renal vein
Expose anterior surface of left renal vein
Identify left adrenal vein; divide now or later
Identify and divide small branches from
    inferior phrenic artery and vein
Divide adrenal vein if not already taken

Right Adrenalectomy
Reflect hepatic flexure downward and fully
    mobilize duodenum

Retract liver cephalad
Palpate right kidney and identify adrenal
    gland just medial to inferior vena cava
    at superior pole of kidney
Expose adrenal gland
Identify and secure right adrenal vein
Secure small vessels along medial aspect of
    gland and remove it

Posterior Adrenalectomy
Patient is positioned prone with slight
    break to straighten the curvature of
    the spine
Incision straight from tenth rib downward,
    then curving laterally toward iliac
    crest
Divide attachments of erector spinae muscle to
    twelfth rib and resect rib (subperiosteally)
Expose Gerota fascia and elevate diaphragm
    and pleura
Pull downward on kidney to expose adrenal
    gland

Posterior Adrenalectomy (*Continued*)

Divide attachments of adrenal gland, leaving vein for last step (both sides)

Ligate adrenal vein and divide it

Obtain hemostasis and close without drains

HALLMARK ANATOMIC COMPLICATIONS

Injury to inferior vena cava (right)

Entry into pleural space (posterior adrenalectomy)

LIST OF STRUCTURES

Adrenal (Suprarenal) Glands

Left and right suprarenal veins
Inferior phrenic vein
Inferior phrenic artery
Superior suprarenal arteries
Middle suprarenal artery
Inferior suprarenal artery

Kidneys

Left renal vein
Left gonadal vein

Gerota fascia
Inferior vena cava
Organ of Zuckerkandl
Trapezius muscle
Latissimus dorsi muscle
Erector spinae muscles
Internal oblique muscle
Transversus abdominis muscle
Quadratus lumborum muscle
Lumbodorsal fascia
Eleventh and twelfth ribs

The right adrenal gland nestles close to the inferior vena cava, and the left adrenal gland is located relatively higher and more lateral, close to the renal vein, but relatively far from the aorta and inferior vena cava (Fig. 105.1). Differences in relative location and nature of blood supply and venous drainage necessitate modifications in technique depending upon which gland is being approached. Here, left adrenalectomy is described first, followed by right adrenalectomy.

ORIENTATION

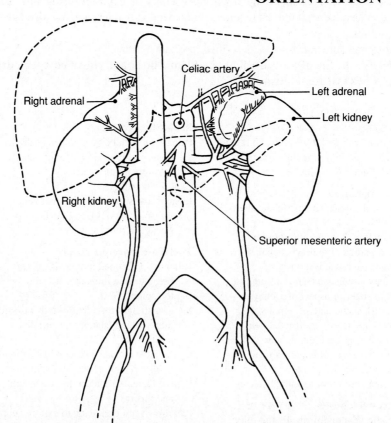

Figure 105.1 Regional anatomy of the adrenal glands

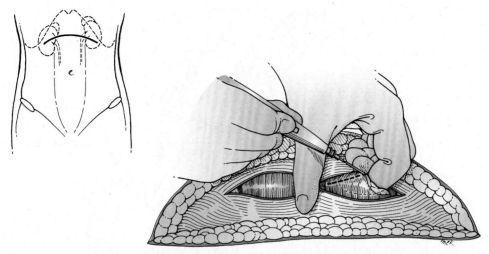

Figure 105.2 Transabdominal adrenalectomy incision

Transabdominal Adrenalectomy Incision (Fig. 105.2)

Technical Points

Position the patient supine on the operating table with a roll under the lower costal margin, or break the operating table slightly to elevate the upper abdomen. Plan a bilateral subcostal or midline incision, depending on the physical habitus of the patient. For most patients, a subcostal approach is best. It may be necessary to make this incision quite long to obtain adequate exposure, especially in obese patients. Thoroughly explore the abdomen in the usual fashion.

Anatomic Points

The right adrenal lies slightly lower than the left and is conveniently approached through a right subcostal incision. Access to the left adrenal is more difficult because the gland occupies a more cephalad position. Although both adrenal glands are covered by overlying structures of the gastrointestinal tract, mobilization of these structures is easier on the right than on the left.

Left Adrenalectomy (Fig. 105.3)

Technical Points

Divide the gastrocolic omentum widely by taking the omentum off the greater curvature of the stomach. Serially control and divide the multiple branches of the gastroepiploic artery and vein that extend from the omentum to the greater curvature. Elevate the stomach cephalad with a retractor. Incise the peritoneum lying along the inferior border of the pancreas and gently elevate the pancreas by blunt dissection. Place a Harrington retractor on a moist laparotomy pad to elevate the pancreas. Reflect the transverse colon downward to improve exposure (Fig. 105.3A). Rarely, it may be necessary to mobilize the splenic flexure to achieve adequate exposure. Generally, the adrenal gland lies far enough medially that simple downward traction on the colon suffices.

Exposure obtained through the lesser sac is limited and is appropriate only for small or superiorly located tumors. If wider exposure is required, fully mobilize the spleen and tail of the pancreas up into the midline to expose the underlying retroperitoneal structures.

Palpate the kidney and use this as a guide to the left adrenal, which lies just cephalad and medial. Incise Gerota fascia just medial to the superior aspect of the left kidney. The adrenal gland should be palpable and visible in this region. Identify the left renal vein and open the tissues overlying it to expose its anterior surface. The left gonadal vein is a useful landmark. The left adrenal vein generally lies just medial to it, on the superior aspect of the left renal vein. Begin to mobilize the adrenal gland by clipping small branches from the inferior phrenic artery and vein, which may enter the superior and medial borders of the adrenal. Secure these with hemoclips and divide them. The harmonic scalpel facilitates divison of these branches, which are often embedded in retroperitoneal fat. It should then be possible to slip a finger behind the adrenal and elevate it. This posterior plane is generally avascular. Downward mobilization of the adrenal gland is facilitated by keeping the attachments to the kidney intact until the vein is approached.

The adrenal vein passes inferiorly. Trace the superior aspect of the left renal vein to identify the relatively long adrenal vein passing off the superior surface just medial to the entrance of the gonadal vein. Ligate it in continuity and divide it (Fig. 105.3B). Leave the tie on the adrenal side long and use it to further elevate the adrenal into the field. Divide any remaining connections at the superior aspect of the gland hemostatically (Fig. 105.3C). Because these contain only multiple, small arterial twigs, no major structures are at risk for injury.

Anatomic Points

The middle colic artery may be at risk for injury when the peritoneum along the caudal border of the pancreas is divided, or when the transverse colon is retracted inferiorly. This artery, an early branch of the superior mesenteric artery, usually arises

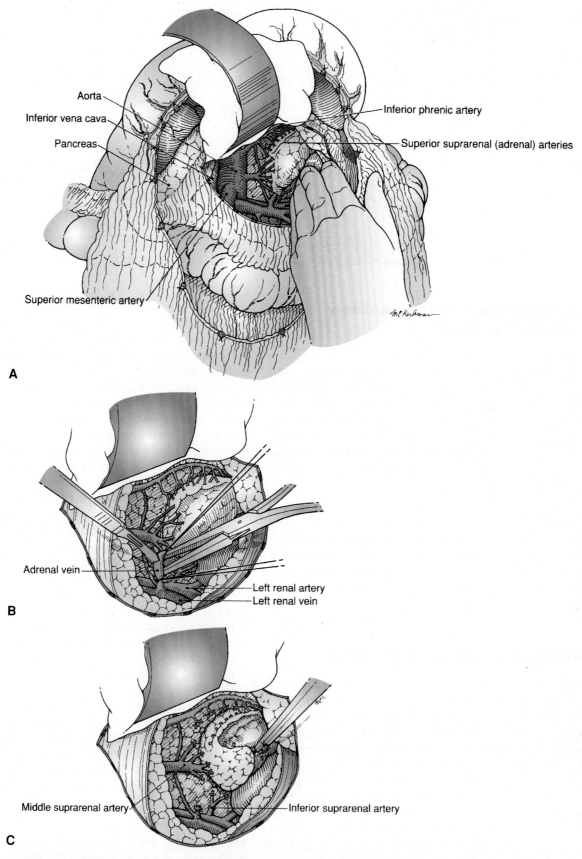

Figure 105.3 Left adrenalectomy. **A:** Exposure by creating a large window into the lesser sac. **B:** Division of adrenal vein. **C:** Division of remaining attachments may be completed with ties or Harmonic scalpel.

posterior or just inferior to the neck of the pancreas and passes to the right. However, it can divide into left and right branches shortly after its origin, with the left branch then being in potential danger; alternatively, an accessory middle colic artery passing toward the splenic flexure can be present (occurring about 10% of the time). The inferior or transverse pancreatic artery runs along, or in, the caudal border of the pancreas, giving off posterior epiploic arteries that run in the anterior leaf of the transverse mesocolon, or sometimes giving off a fairly significant colic branch to the left colic flexure.

The left adrenal (suprarenal) gland is located within a subdivision of Gerota fascia and is surrounded by perirenal fat and connective tissue. In contrast to the pyramidal right adrenal gland, the left gland is semilunar or leaf shaped, flattened, and broadly in contact (through its posterior surface) with the medial surface of the kidney, superior to the renal vasculature and to the left crus of the diaphragm. The anterior surface of this gland is related to the posterior wall of the omental bursa and, more inferiorly, to the body of the pancreas. Inferiorly, the gland may be in contact with the renal vasculature. Laterally, it can be in contact with the renal surface of the spleen. Medially, it is closely related to the left greater splanchnic nerve and celiac ganglion.

The arterial supply of the left adrenal gland is derived from three different sources. The superior suprarenal arteries, which are always multiple (ranging in number from 3 to 30), arise from the inferior phrenic artery as this artery passes close to the medial and superior borders of the gland. The middle suprarenal artery arises as a single vessel from the anterolateral aspect of the aorta, superior to the origin of the renal artery. The inferior suprarenal artery arises from the superior aspect of the renal artery. The middle and inferior suprarenal arteries may be multiple or may have branches, especially at the periphery of the suprarenal gland. In addition to these constant sources, the suprarenal gland can also receive blood from accessory renal arteries, the upper ureteric artery, and the gonadal artery. Almost all of the arteries, regardless of their origin, enter the periphery of the gland. These multiple, small vessels are not individually ligated, but are secured in clips together with a mass of surrounding soft tissue, or divided with a harmonic scalpel.

The venous drainage of the left suprarenal gland is usually through a single, comparatively large vein that emerges from the central region of the anterior surface of the gland. From here, it passes inferiorly, joins the inferior phrenic vein, and empties into the superior aspect of the left renal vein. Typically, its termination is medial to the termination of the left gonadal vein.

Right Adrenalectomy (Fig. 105.4)

Technical Points

Reflect the hepatic flexure of the colon downward. Fully mobilize the duodenum with a wide Kocher maneuver and expose the inferior vena cava. Retract the liver cephalad with a Harrington retractor. The right adrenal gland should be palpable just above and medial to the kidney in the region between the superior pole of the kidney and the inferior vena cava as shown diagrammatically in Figure 105.4A. Make a peritoneal incision overlying the adrenal and expose it (Fig. 105.4B). Free the lateral border of the adrenal by serially clamping and tying or dividing with electrocautery. The medial border is dissected next. This dissection should be done directly on the vena cava, without the use of heat-generating instruments.

Anatomic Points

The right adrenal gland is pyramidal in shape and is located, like its counterpart, in a subcompartment within Gerota fascia. It is related to the anteromedial aspect of the upper pole of the kidney. Anteriorly, its upper part is in contact with the bare area of the liver, and frequently, with the inferior vena cava, whereas its lower part is covered by the parietal peritoneum lateral to the duodenum. Posteriorly, it is related to the right crus of the diaphragm.

The blood supply to the right adrenal gland is similar to that of the left, in that it receives a multitude of branches derived from the inferior phrenic artery, aorta, and renal artery. These branches enter the periphery of the gland. Dissection along the lateral side of the gland should be relatively avascular because the small arterial branches tend to enter superiorly, inferiorly, and medially.

Division of the Right Adrenal Vein (Fig. 105.5)

Technical Points

The right adrenal vein is short and fat and enters directly into the vena cava. It may be difficult to secure this vein, and it is important to avoid injuring the vena cava. Gently skeletonize the vein and divide it in continuity. If bleeding occurs in the course of this dissection, avoid the temptation to apply a clamp blindly. The vena cava is fragile and easily torn, and a small hole can rapidly enlarge into a disastrous rent. Control the bleeding with your finger until you can either suture the tear directly or apply a partial occlusion vascular clamp (such as a Satinsky clamp) to the inferior vena cava as shown in the inset. Divide the remaining attachments to the adrenal with hemoclips or harmonic scalpel.

Anatomic Points

Right adrenalectomy is comparatively difficult because part of the gland may be posterior to the inferior vena cava and because the single right suprarenal vein typically drains directly into the posterior aspect of the inferior vena cava. The right adrenal vein may enter the inferior vena cava at the angle between the renal vein and the inferior vena cava or may terminate directly into the inferior vena cava at the level of the adrenal. To expose the right adrenal vein, it is usually necessary to retract the

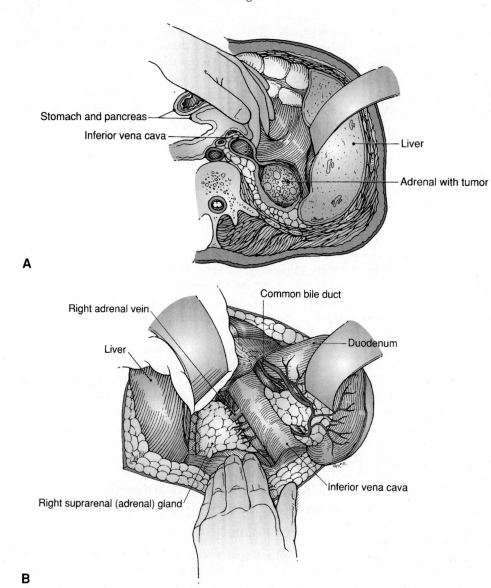

Stomach and pancreas

Inferior vena cava

Liver

Adrenal with tumor

A

Common bile duct

Right adrenal vein

Duodenum

Liver

Inferior vena cava

Right suprarenal (adrenal) gland

B

Figure 105.4 Right adrenal-ectomy. **A:** Cross-section showing principles of exposure. **B:** Adequate exposure of right adrenal after full mobilization of duodenum and head of pancreas and cephalad retraction of liver.

inferior vena cava carefully to the left. The surgeon should be aware that this vein is usually less than 1 cm in length and that its diameter, which measures about 3 mm, is unexpectedly large. In addition, it is said to be particularly fragile, as is this segment of the vena cava. To further complicate exposure of the right suprarenal vein, frequently, small hepatic tributaries drain directly into the vena cava, and these, too, can be avulsed. Because of the anatomic relationships of the structures in this area, especially the liver, hemorrhage in this region is difficult to control.

Exploration of the Retroperitoneum (Fig. 105.6)

Technical Points

Bilateral or extra-adrenal pheochromocytomas are not rare, especially in familial syndromes. With current CT imaging,

extra-adrenal tumors are often identified preoperatively. Therefore, both adrenal glands and the retroperitoneum should be palpated when an adrenalectomy is being performed in patients with known familial endocrinopathies. Incise the peritoneum overlying the aorta and the bifurcation of the common iliac arteries, and palpate the region of the para-aortic and para-iliac lymph nodes for tumor masses. Also check the region of the bladder for tumor masses. Achieve hemostasis in the operative field and close the incision in the usual fashion, without drains.

Anatomic Points

A logical plan for exploration of the retroperitoneum must be based on an understanding of the development of the suprarenal glands. The adrenal cortex develops from mesoderm. Initially, the elongated primordium develops bilaterally on either side of the midline dorsal mesentery adjacent to the cranial end

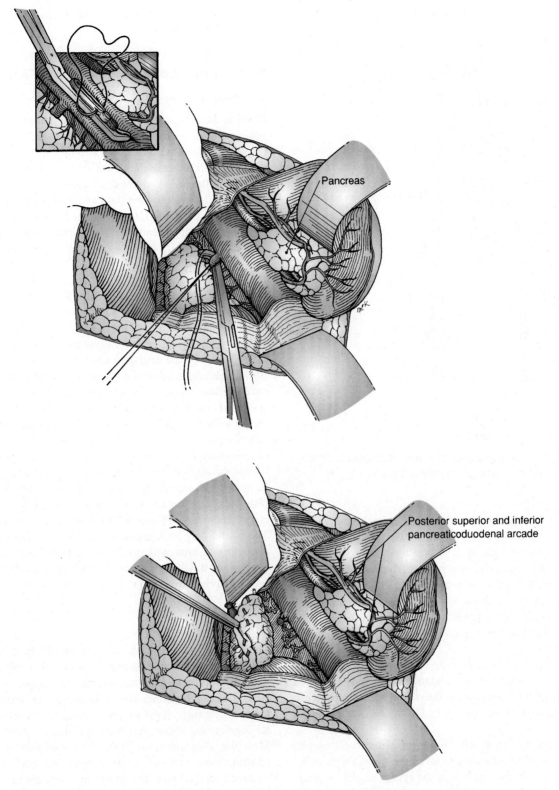

Figure 105.5 Division of the right adrenal vein. Inset shows management of tear or avulsion from vena cava. Note control has been achieved with a vascular clamp.

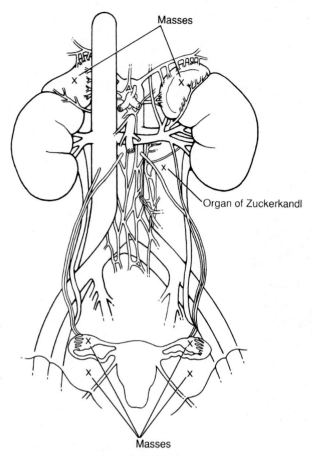

Figure 105.6 Exploration of the retroperitoneum. Sites of accessory adrenal tissue are marked by an ×

of the mesonephros. As the developing metanephric kidney "ascends," it contacts the lower pole of the suprarenal gland; later ascent causes the glands to assume their definitive shapes.

The primordia of the adrenal medullae develop at the same time. These are derived from neural crest cells associated with future ganglia from T-6 through T-12. As the peripheral neural tissue develops, the future medullary cells (or chromaffin cells) migrate into the developing adrenal cortex, assuming a central position.

Accessory adrenocortical tissue of mesodermal origin can occur almost anywhere in the abdomen. The most frequent locations for cortical nodules are deep to the renal capsule, in the broad ligament of the female, and in the spermatic cord of the male.

Extramedullary chromaffin tissue (of neural crest origin) is normally found in proximity to all of the sympathetic chain ganglia and in discrete masses in the region of the abdominal sympathetic plexuses. The largest of these—the organ of Zuckerkandl—is located at about the origin of the inferior mesenteric artery or at the aortic bifurcation. These extramedullary chromaffin cells, especially those of the organ of Zuckerkandl, occur normally. They are, however, subject to the same disease processes (e.g., pheochromocytoma) as the adrenal medulla; hence, exploration of the retroperitoneum

may be considered when familial diseases of the adrenal medulla are diagnosed.

Posterior Adrenalectomy (Fig. 105.7)

Technical Points

Position the patient face down on the operating table with rolls beneath the hips and the chest to allow the abdomen to sag (Fig. 105.7A). This will avoid placing pressure on the vena cava and will increase the distance from the posterior abdominal wall to the intra-abdominal viscera. Jackknife the operating table slightly to straighten the curvature of the spine. Plan an incision that extends straight from the tenth rib downward, parallel to the midline, and that then curves gently down toward the iliac crest. Carry this down through fascia and through the latissimus dorsi muscle.

Divide the attachments of the erector spinae muscle to the twelfth rib and resect this rib subperiosteally. Open the lumbodorsal fascia longitudinally along the lateral margin of the quadratus lumborum. Expose Gerota fascia. Clamp and tie the subcostal artery and vein, if necessary, and retract the subcostal nerve out of the operative field. Avoid injury to the nerve. Bluntly elevate the diaphragm and pleura off of the underlying retroperitoneal tissues. Gently push the pleura out of the way, and divide the diaphragm with clamps and ties. Pull downward on the kidney to expose the adrenal gland. Divide lateral and superior attachments with hemoclips until only the adrenal vein (inferior on the right, medial on the left) remains (Fig. 105.7B). Ligate the adrenal vein in continuity with 2-0 silk and divide it. Secure the remaining attachments and remove the adrenal (Fig. 105.7C, D). Achieve hemostasis and close the incision in layers. If the pleura is entered, the parenchyma is rarely injured. The pleura may be repaired by suturing the opening closed in a running fashion with a catheter in place. Air in the pleural cavity may then be evacuated by pulling the catheter out after a valsalva maneuver and tying down the suture.

Anatomic Points

The incision, as described, will first divide those fibers of the trapezius muscle that originate from the eleventh and twelfth thoracic vertebrae and that overlap the upper fibers of the latissimus dorsi muscle. The latter muscle originates from the lower six thoracic vertebrae and, through an aponeurosis, from all lumbar and sacral vertebrae and the posterior iliac crest. Muscular slips also arise from the lower three or four ribs, interdigitating with slips of the external oblique muscle. Thus, as the incision is carried inferiorly, fibers of the latissimus dorsi muscle will be divided, as will sensory branches of the posterior primary divisions of spinal nerves superiorly and the anterior divisions inferiorly.

The lumbodorsal (thoracolumbar) fascia is the investing (deep) fascia of the back. It is composed of the fused aponeuroses of the latissimus dorsi, internal oblique, and transversus abdominis muscles. The aponeuroses of the two abdominal

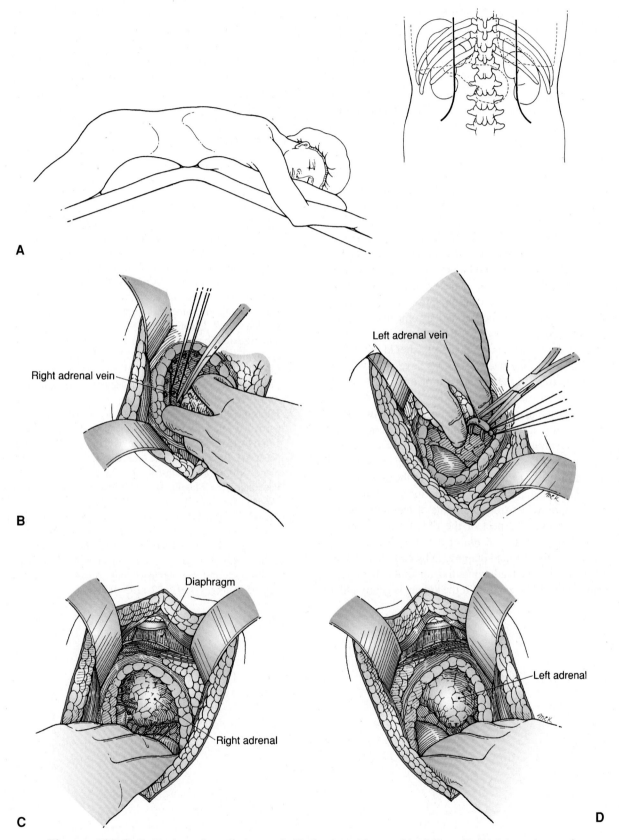

Figure 105.7 Posterior adrenalectomy. **A:** Patient position and incisions. **B:** Division of adrenal vein. **C:** Conclusion of dissection on right. **D:** Conclusion of dissection on left.

muscles fuse at the lateral edge of the erector spinae muscle mass, then split to encompass both anterior and posterior surfaces of the erector spinae, ultimately attaching to both spinous and transverse processes of the lumbar vertebrae. Fibers of the internal oblique muscle begin close to the site of fusion, whereas the transversus abdominis muscle fibers remain aponeurotic for some distance laterally. Thus recognition of muscle fibers can afford the surgeon an indication of the depth of the incision because all else should be aponeurotic.

The quadratus lumborum muscle lies anterior to the anterior lamella of the lumbodorsal fascia. Branches of the spinal nerves that may be encountered in this dissection (subcostal, iliohypogastric, and ilioinguinal) pass laterally, anterior to the quadratus lumborum muscle. At variable distances laterally, they gain access to the plane between the transversus abdominis and internal oblique muscles to continue their course to the anterior midline. Because the kidney and suprarenal gland, within Gerota fascia, lie in tissue planes anterior (deep) to the quadratus lumborum muscle, caution must be exercised to avoid traumatic injury to the nerves and accompanying vascular structures.

Division of the latissimus dorsi muscle should expose the twelfth rib. Because some twelve muscles have at least a partial origin or insertion to the periosteum of this rib, it is most expedient to resect it subperiosteally.

In this region, the diaphragm originates from the twelfth rib and the lateral lumbocostal arch, a fibrous fascial thickening over the quadratus lumborum muscle that extends from the tip of the transverse process of vertebra L-2 to the tip of the twelfth rib. Resection of the last rib allows access to the superior side of the diaphragm medially and to its inferior aspect laterally. The parietal pleura reflect from the dome of the diaphragm to the posterior and lateral aspect of the ribs, forming the costodiaphragmatic recess. The pleura of the costodiaphragmatic recess, attached to the ribs and diaphragm by endothoracic fascia, can be gently elevated, allowing division of the diaphragm. The adrenal gland will be exposed if the kidney is gently pulled inferiorly. This latter maneuver is necessary because the upper pole of the kidney, and thus the adrenal gland, lies superior to the T-12 vertebra and the last rib.

Because the adrenal gland lies cephalad to this incision, some prefer more direct exposure through the bed of the eleventh rib. In this case, more of the diaphragm must be divided and the pleura may be entered.

REFERENCES

1. Atmaca AF, Akbulut Z, Altinova S, et al. Routine postoperative chest radiography is not needed after flank incisions with eleventh rib resection. *Can J Urol.* 2008;15:3986–3989.
2. Avisse C, Marcus C, Patey M, et al. Surgical anatomy and embryology of the adrenal glands. *Surg Clin North Am.* 2000;80:403–415.
3. Carey LC, Ellison EH. Adrenalectomy: Technique, errors, and pitfalls. *Surg Clin North Am.* 1966;46:1283–1292. (Emphasizes potential problems and how to avoid them.)
4. Chino ES, Thomas CG. An extended Kocher incision for bilateral adrenalectomy. *Am J Surg.* 1985;149:292–294. (Describes extended bilateral subcostal approach.)
5. Geelhoed GW, Dunnick NR, Doppman JL. Management of intravenous extensions of endocrine tumors and prognosis after surgical treatment. *Am J Surg.* 1980;139:844–848.
6. Godellas CV, Prinz RA. Surgical approach to adrenal neoplasms: Laparoscopic versus open adrenalectomy. *Surg Oncol Clin North Am.* 1998;7:807–817.
7. Johnstone FRC. The surgical anatomy of the adrenal glands with particular reference to the suprarenal vein. *Surg Clin North Am.* 1964;44:1315. (Presents good review of vascular anatomy.)
8. Nash AG, Robbins GF. The operative approach to the left adrenal gland. *Surg Gynecol Obstet.* 1973;137:670–672.
9. Pezzulich RA, Mannix H. Immediate complications of adrenal surgery. *Ann Surg.* 1970;172:125–130.
10. Russell CF, Hamberger B, van Heerden JA, et al. Adrenalectomy: Anterior or posterior approach? *Am J Surg.* 1982;144:322–324. (Discusses pros and cons of two approaches.)
11. Thompson GB, Grant CS, van Heerden JA, et al. Laparoscopic versus open posterior adrenalectomy: A case-control study of 100 patients. *Surgery.* 1997;122:1132–1136.

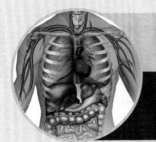

106

Laparoscopic Adrenalectomy

J.C. Carr and James R. Howe

Adrenalectomy is performed for primary and metastatic tumors of the adrenal gland as well as for adrenal hyperplasia. In the past, most procedures were performed in an open fashion, by transabdominal, flank, posterior, or thoracoabdominal approaches, as described in Chapter 105. Laparoscopic adrenalectomy was first described in 1992, and over the last decade this has become the most commonly used approach for adrenal neoplasms.

Variations on the lateral transabdominal (LT) approach described here, including retroperitoneal, robotic, and single-port have also been gaining in popularity. The principal advantages of the laparoscopic approach are the same as those described for other laparoscopic procedures, which include smaller incisions, a magnified view of the operative field, less postoperative pain, shorter hospital stay, and a quicker return to work. The laparoscopic approach; however, is more technically demanding in terms of equipment and the experience of the surgeon. In addition, bilateral adrenalectomy requires repositioning the patient. Finally, the laparoscopic approach is not recommended for larger lesions or the treatment of malignant neoplasms.

There are two general approaches to laparoscopic removal of the adrenal gland, the lateral transabdominal (or transperitoneal), and retroperitoneal, where the patient is placed prone. In the transperitoneal approach, the anatomical relationships are more familiar to most surgeons, as insufflation of the peritoneal cavity allows for visualization of the liver, spleen, colon, and stomach, which are helpful anatomic landmarks. In the retroperitoneal approach, the intraperitoneal organs can be left undisturbed, and the challenge is to create a working space in the retroperitoneum. This chapter will describe the lateral transabdominal approach to adrenalectomy. References at the end describe alternative approaches.

The adrenal glands have two components: The outer cortex, which gives rise to cortical adenomas and carcinomas; and the inner medulla, which is the site of development of pheochromocytomas. The cortex develops from coelomic mesenchyme from the urogenital ridge during embryogenesis. The medulla develops from neural crest ectodermal cells, which migrate into the adrenal cortex during week 7 to 8 of development. These glands come to lie superomedial to each kidney, and thus the older designation, "suprarenal glands." The right gland tends to be more triangular in shape, while the left is more crescentic (see Figure 105.1). The average size is 3 to 5 cm in length and 5 to 10 mm in width, with a weight of 3 to 6 g. The color of the adrenal is yellow-orange, which is distinct from the paler yellow appearance of the perinephric fat.

SCORE™, the Surgical Council on Resident Education, classified laparoscopic adrenalectomy as a "COMPLEX" procedure.

STEPS IN PROCEDURE

Lateral position, with kidney rest
  elevated
Four ports distributed two fingerbreadths
  below the costal margin from the midline
  (10 to 15 cm caudad to xiphoid) to the
  anterior flank (between 11th rib and
  anterior superior iliac spine)

Left Adrenalectomy
30-degree laparoscope
Thorough abdominal exploration
Mobilize splenic flexure of colon
Place fourth port under direct vision
Retract spleen, colon, and peritoneal reflection
  medially

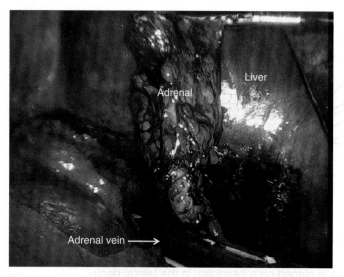

Figure 106.4 Dividing the adrenal vein. An EndoGIA stapler with a 2.5-mm-vascular load is positioned with one fork posterior and one anterior to the adrenal vein.

anteriorly, and confirm it by palpation with the tip of a grasper or harmonic scalpel.

Move the camera to the fourth port at this point, and use the other two ports for a grasper and the harmonic scalpel. Open Gerota fascia vertically starting at the midpole, and clear the anterior surface of the kidney by dividing the overlying perinephric fat (Fig. 106.2). Next, pull upward on the medial border of the fascia, and dissect Gerota fascia from the underlying perinephric fat and rotate it medially.

Pass a fan retractor through the first port, and use it to retract the spleen and peritoneal edge medially. Since the adrenal gland is superomedial to the upper pole of the kidney, divide the perinephric fat just above the superior pole, and then work toward the diaphragm, separating the lateral perinephric fat from the medial fat and adrenal gland. Next, carry the dissection medially and posteriorly in the general direction of the aorta. During this dissection, larger tumors (>2 cm) will be readily visible as orange-yellow rounded masses if cortical adenomas (or gray if pheochromocytomas), while smaller tumors will be difficult to distinguish from the pale yellow fat. The adrenal is more solid and flat than the surrounding fat, but palpation alone is not of much help in revealing the gland. Some surgeons use laparoscopic ultrasonography to help localize the position of the adrenal, but this is not generally necessary. Dissection along the superior aspect of the perinephric fat and superomedial edge of the kidney will eventually uncover an area of yellow-orange tissue which can be recognized as the adrenal gland (Fig. 106.3). This dissection requires occasional switching of grasper and harmonic scalpel in ports 2 and 3 to optimize traction.

Next, dissect along the lateral and superior borders of the gland, leaving some adjacent fat that can be used to grasp the gland. Retract the gland anteriorly, which facilitates clearing the superomedial attachments. Divide this tissue with the harmonic scalpel, as it contains tiny arterial branches (which are usually not even visualized).

We prefer to approach the adrenal vein last, because misadventure in this region is the most likely cause for conversion to an open approach. Not only can the adrenal vein be torn, but the superior pole vessels to the kidney can be injured if the dissection is carried out 1 to 2 cm inferiorly or medially. Once a plane along the aorta is developed medially, and also between the adrenal and kidney inferiorly, divide the remaining tissue at the inferior border of the adrenal using an EndoGIA stapler with a 2.5-mm load, or simply doubly clip and divide the vein (Fig. 106.4).

The adrenal gland should now be free. Pass an endoscopic retrieval bag into the field through port 2, and place the adrenal in it. Remove the bag. Check the operative bed for hemostasis, observe the color of the superior pole of the kidney, and check the region for presence of residual or accessory adrenal tissue. Irrigate the area and close the port sites in the usual fashion with 0 Vicryl sutures.

Anatomic Points

The arterial blood supply to each adrenal is derived from three sources: (1) branches from the aorta, (2) renal artery, and (3) inferior phrenic artery. These vessels are not generally seen during the dissection, and are adequately controlled with the harmonic scalpel. The left adrenal vein drains into the left renal vein. Care must be taken to not encroach upon the superior pole vessels of the kidney when ligating the left adrenal vein, which will manifest as a purple demarcation of the superior renal pole from the normal pink parenchyma. We divide the vein last, preferring to have as complete a dissection as possible prior to ligation. This requires that patients with pheochromocytoma are well blocked prior to the procedure, and most patients who have received 2 weeks of gradually increasing alpha-blockade preoperatively will generally not have dramatic fluctuations in blood pressure. Care must be taken to avoid the pancreas, by incising Gerota fascia and reflecting it with the spleen. Care must also be taken not to injure the spleen while retracting it medially, nor to get into the splenic vein posterior to the pancreas by dissecting in the wrong plane. If it is difficult to find the adrenal gland or if troublesome bleeding is encountered, consider placing a hand port to palpate the adrenal or apply direct pressure without having to convert to an open procedure. Here, an 8-cm incision is made by extending either the incision of port 1 or 4.

Right Adrenalectomy

Technical Points

The ports are placed in the same positions and sequence as described for left adrenalectomy, except on the right side. The hepatic flexure is visualized while pushing down on the abdominal wall from proposed the fourth port site. If there is adequate free abdominal wall, then introduce the port under direct vision. If not, mobilize the hepatic flexure to obtain more working space on the abdominal wall. Place the 30-degree camera through port 2, and a fan retractor through port 1. Retract the liver. Use a grasping clamp to pick up the lateral peritoneum, and the peritoneal reflection of the right triangular ligament is

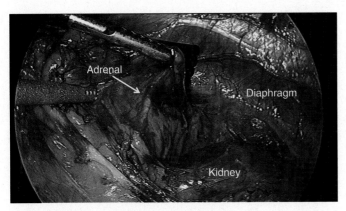

Figure 106.5 Superomedial dissection of the adrenal. This is facilitated by gently retracting the spleen and lateral peritoneum medially with the fan retractor.

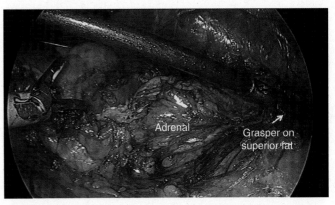

Figure 106.6 Dissection along the superolateral aspect of the gland with the harmonic scalpel. The superior adrenal fat is used to rotate the gland anteriorly for optimal exposure and takedown of the superomedial attachments.

divided with the harmonic scalpel as high as possible. As the dissection proceeds, medial retraction and elevation of the liver improves the exposure of the kidney and adrenal gland.

Open Gerota fascia vertically over the midportion of the kidney to a point 4 to 6 cm above the superior pole of the kidney. Bisect the perinephric fat vertically beginning at the superior pole of the kidney. Then dissect the fascia medially over this entire vertical length until the vena cava is visualized, which is the medial extent of the dissection. Place the fan retractor on this fascial edge and the liver, elevating it and rotating it medially. Larger adrenal tumors may be visible at this time, and this facilitates finding the edge of the adrenal gland.

Once the flattened edge of the yellow-orange adrenal gland is seen, dissect the superior and lateral surfaces first with the harmonic scalpel, freeing the gland from the surrounding fat

(Fig. 106.5). If the gland is not visualized, continue to dissect through the perinephric fat in a superior and medial direction from the earlier point of bisection. The edge of the adrenal will eventually be encountered. If the lateral edge is not found, then dissect in the plane between the vena cava and above the superior pole of the kidney until it is encountered (Fig. 106.6). Once the superior and lateral portions of the adrenal are dissected, carefully clear the groove between the kidney and the adrenal. Do not dissect too far inferomedially, where the superior pole renal vessels are located.

Once this is achieved, then the gland can be gently retracted laterally, and carefully divide the areolar tissue between the inferior aspect of the adrenal and vena cava using the harmonic scalpel. Also clear the areolar tissue from the superomedial

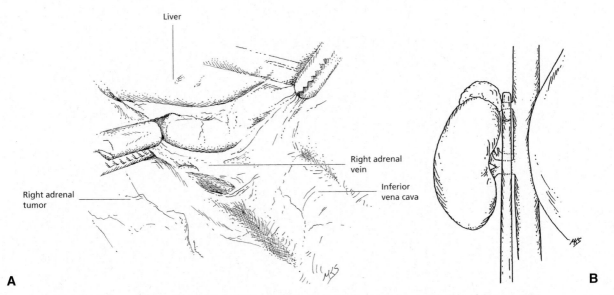

Figure 106.7 A: Exposure of right adrenal vein in groove between adrenal gland and inferior vena cava. **B:** Division of the right adrenal vein using an EndoGIA stapler (**A** from Hedican SP. Kidneys and adrenal glands. In: Scott-Conner CEH, Cuashieri A, Carter FJ, eds. *Minimal Access Surgical Anatomy.* Philadelphia, PA: Lippincott Williams & Wilkins; 2000:267–292, with permission).

border of the adrenal, being careful to stay at the level of the top of the gland, so that you do not inadvertently injure the adrenal vein.

The last remaining connection between the openings created inferiorly and superiorly on the lateral side of the vena cava will be areolar tissue containing the adrenal vein. Divide this with an EndoGIA 2.5-mm-vascular stapler placed adjacent and parallel to the vena cava through these openings (Fig. 106.7). Place the adrenal gland in an endoscopic bag, and remove it through port 2. Inspect the area of dissection for hemostasis, irrigate and close as previously described for left adrenalectomy.

Anatomic Points

In order to expose the superior aspects of the right adrenal and vena cava, the liver must be well mobilized. Once this is achieved, the fan retractor can be used to suspend the liver out of the way, above the adrenal. As on the left side, the three arteries are divided using the harmonic scalpel and are seldom visualized. The adrenal vein on the right is extremely short (~1 cm), wide, and drains directly into the vena cava. Any misadventure with this vein will result in significant blood loss, which will be difficult or impossible to control laparoscopically. These events can be minimized if one uses the EndoGIA stapler and dissects out the inferior and superomedial aspects of the adrenal gland. Care should be taken not to encroach upon the lateral wall of the vena cava using this technique.

REFERENCES

1. Assalia A, Gagner M. Laparoscopic adrenalectomy. *Br J Surg.* 2004;91(10):1259–1274.
2. Berber E, Tellioglu G, Harvey A, et al. Comparison of laparoscopic transabdominal lateral versus posterior retroperitoneal adrenalectomy. *Surgery.* 2009;146(4):621–625.
3. Gagner M, Pomp A, Heniford BT, et al. Laparoscopic adrenalectomy: Lessons learned from 100 consecutive procedures. *Ann Surg.* 1997;226(3):238–246; discussion 246–247.
4. Gonzalez R, Smith CD, McClusky DA 3rd, et al. Laparoscopic approach reduces likelihood of perioperative complications in patients undergoing adrenalectomy. *Am Surg.* 2004;70(8):668–674.
5. Lee J, El-Tamer M, Schifftner T, et al. Open and laparoscopic adrenalectomy: Analysis of the National Surgical Quality Improvement Program. *J Am Coll Surg.* 2008;206(5):953–959; discussion 959–961.
6. Rubinstein M, Gill IS, Aron M, et al. Prospective, randomized comparison of transperitoneal versus retroperitoneal laparoscopic adrenalectomy. *J Urol.* 2005;174(2):442–445.
7. Walz MK, Alesina PF, Wenger FA, et al. Posterior retroperitoneoscopic adrenalectomy—results of 560 procedures in 520 patients. *Surgery.* 2006;140(6):943–948.
8. Walz MK, Groeben H, Alesina PF. Single-access retroperitoneoscopic adrenalectomy (SARA) versus conventional retroperitoneoscopic adrenalectomy (CORA): A case-control study. *World J Surg.* 2010;34(6):1386–1390.
9. Winter JM, Talamini MA, Stanfield CL, et al. Thirty robotic adrenalectomies: A single institution's experience. *Surg Endosc.* 2006;20(1):119–124.

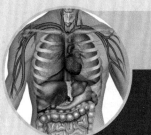

107

Management of Injuries to Kidneys, Ureter, or Bladder

This chapter describes techniques that are useful for management of injuries to the urinary system. Many renal injuries are managed nonoperatively; however, when an operative approach is required it is important to have a plan for approach and management as described here. Ureteral injuries are sometimes iatrogenic, but may also result from external trauma. Simple repair is described here and more complex techniques are referenced. Bladder repair is an essential tool for management of colovesical fistula as well as trauma and is described in this chapter.

SCORE™, the Surgical Council on Resident Education, classified repair of renal, ureteral, or bladder injuries as "ESSENTIAL UNCOMMON" procedures.

STEPS IN PROCEDURE—OPERATIVE APPROACH TO RENAL TRAUMA

Preliminary vascular control
Mobilize bowel to expose renal vein and
    artery in midline
Isolate renal artery and place Silastic loops
    for rapid control
Isolate renal vein and place Silastic loops for
    rapid control
Mobilize bowel to expose perinephric hematoma
Enter hematoma and rapidly but atraumatically
    mobilize kidney
Take care not to strip capsule from renal
    parenchyma
Occlude renal artery and vein if major
    hemorrhage is encountered
Identify injury and determine if collecting
    system has been entered

Simple laceration
Close collecting system with running
    absorbable suture
Close parenchyma with interrupted sutures,
    using pledgets
Place drain
Major injury limited to lower or upper pole
Perform partial nephrectomy
Ligate branch of renal artery and vein
    entering pole
Sharply amputate devascularized portion
Obtain hemostasis in remnant
Close collecting system with running
    absorbable suture
Close parenchyma with pledgeted sutures
Place drain

HALLMARK ANATOMIC COMPLICATIONS
Urinary leak
Ureteral stricture

LIST OF STRUCTURES
Kidney
Renal artery
Renal vein
Ureter

Adrenal gland
Inferior vena cava
Aorta
Bladder

Exposure of Kidney and Suture of Laceration (Fig. 107.1)

Penetrating injuries to the perinephric region require exploration and repair. It is crucial that the initial mobilization be done efficiently with minimal blood loss, and that no additional damage be done to the kidney during mobilization. The capsule is easily stripped from the renal parenchyma. Take

care to preserve the capsule, as it is the part that best holds the suture.

Mobilize overlying colon by incising the avascular line and allowing the colon and its mesentery to come to the midline. Carefully inspect the colon and mesentery for injuries as you do this. This should expose the underlying perinephric hematoma.

Decide whether or not to perform preliminary vascular control by isolating the renal artery and renal vein in the midline,

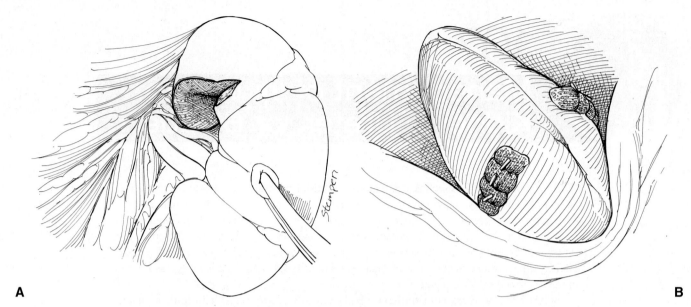

A

B

Figure 107.1 Exposure and repair of simple renal laceration. **A:** Exposure of renal injury. **B:** Pledgeted repair of simple laceration (from Graham SD Jr, Keane TE, eds. *Glenn's Urologic Surgery.* 7th ed. Philadelphia, PA: Lippincott Williams & Wilkins; 2010, with permission).

away from the hematoma. Some surgeons routinely obtain preliminary control and others do it selectively. Preliminary vascular control allows the perinephric hematoma to be explored with minimal additional blood loss; however, it may require significant additional time (and associated continued blood loss into the hematoma). Many surgeons use preliminary vascular control selectively, employing it when the nature of the injury or the appearance of the hematoma suggests that major arterial bleeding will be encountered on exploring the injury.

To obtain preliminary vascular control, isolate the renal artery and vein outside the hematoma in the midline. See Chapters 108e and 109 for a discussion of the relevant anatomy.

Open Gerota fascia to expose the kidney and rapidly mobilize the kidney from lateral to medial, taking care not to damage the kidney further (Fig. 107.1A). Take great care not to strip the capsule from the kidney. At the end of this mobilization, the kidney and hilar vessels should be accessible. If necessary, place a vascular clamp across the hilar vessels to control hemorrhage. Assess the nature of the damage.

A simple laceration such as that shown in Figure 107.1B can be managed by simple suture. Take care to assure that the collecting system is intact. Place small retractors (such as Army–Navy retractors) into the parenchymal injury to expose the depths. The collecting system is whitish. If it is injured, you will see the edges of the injury in the depths of the laceration and will also note a hole into a cavity lined with shiny white epithelium (the collecting system). It may be necessary to extend the parenchymal injury slightly to adequately expose the injury.

Close the collecting system with a running absorbable suture. Then close the parenchyma with interrupted sutures, tied over pledgets of Teflon, perinephric fat, or a buttress of omentum. Place a drain in proximity to the injury and check hemostasis.

Always remember that in reaching the kidney, the missile (whether bullet or knife blade) may have traversed colon or small bowel or other viscera. After dealing with the renal injury, check again for missed visceral injuries. Return colon to its anatomic position and close.

Partial Nephrectomy (Fig. 107.2)

Mobilize and expose the kidney as described above. Determine that the injury is too severe for simple closure. Always remember that a basic principle of management of renal injuries is

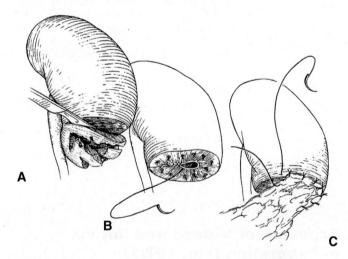

A

B

C

Figure 107.2 Partial nephrectomy. **A:** Amputation of injured lower pole. **B:** Closure of collecting system. **C:** Omental pack placed to buttress repair (from Graham SD Jr, Keane TE, eds. *Glenn's Urologic Surgery.* 7th ed. Philadelphia, PA: Lippincott Williams & Wilkins; 2010, with permission).

preservation of renal volume if possible. Partial nephrectomy allows a severely damaged upper or lower pole to be resected while preserving the rest of the kidney.

Identify, if possible, renal polar vessels supplying the injured pole and place Silastic loops around these. Amputate the injured pole (Fig. 107.2A). Obtain hemostasis and close the collecting system with a running absorbable suture (Fig. 107.2B). Close the injury with pledgets and buttress the renal remnant with a tongue of omentum (Fig. 107.2C). Place drains.

In rare circumstances, a kidney may be shattered beyond repair or there may be such significant damage to the renal hilum

that nephrectomy is needed as an emergency life-saving procedure. Ligate the renal artery and vein. Trace the ureter down to its termination at the bladder and ligate it low with an absorbable tie. Be aware that this leaves a segment of ureter within the wall of the bladder. Inform the patient that this remnant exists, as very rare instances of urothelial carcinoma have occurred in these remnants. Some advocate dissecting out the intramural portion of the ureter for this reason, but this significantly adds operative time in a patient that may be hemodynamically unstable.

As before, take care not to miss injuries to overlying bowel. Obtain final hemostasis and close.

STEPS IN PROCEDURE—REPAIR OF URETER

Expose the ureter by mobilizing overlying colon	Proximal into the renal pelvis
Incise peritoneum over ureter	Distal into the bladder
Freshen the edges of the ureter	Close the ureter with multiple interrupted
Spatulate the ends	sutures of fine absorbable material
Pass a double-J ureteral stent through the	Place drain
injured ends	

Repair of Ureter (Fig. 107.3)

Injuries to the midportion of the ureter are repaired by spatulation and simple suture over a stent. There are several more complex ways of handling distal ureteral injuries such as the psoas hitch, and these are referenced at the end of the chapter. Simple repair is a useful skill that will suffice for a majority of situations.

Expose the injured ureter by mobilizing the colon as above. Incise the peritoneum parallel to the ureter, to expose a

segment proximal and distal to the injury. Take care not to strip the periureteral tissue as this contains the blood supply.

Freshen the ends of the ureter. Spatulate the injured segments. Place a double-J stent into the injured segment, feeding it proximal into the renal pelvis, and distal into the bladder. Close the ureter with multiple fine interrupted sutures. Cover with omentum and place a closed suction drain. As always, double check for associated visceral injuries.

Repair of Bladder (Fig. 107.4)

Identify the extent of injury. Place retractors and look inside the bladder to determine the relationship of the injury to the trigone, where the ureters enter the bladder and the urethra leaves. Identify the trigone in its normal relatively low posterior location and shiny flat surface with three orifices. If necessary, use a dye such as indigo carmine (given intravenously) to more easily identify the ureteral orifices. Remember that the ureters pass through the wall of the bladder on their way to the trigone. Injuries in proximity to the trigone or involving the trigone require specialized expertise to manage. Fortunately, the vast majority of injuries involve the dome of the bladder and are remote from the trigone.

Freshen the edges of the injury and define a defect that can be closed as a simple linear laceration. Close with an initial layer of running 2-0 or 3-0 absorbable suture. Then place an outer layer of running or interrupted sutures in such a manner as to invert and reperitonealize the first suture line. Do this in the same way that you might close bowel, but use a synthetic absorbable suture for this second layer as well.

Leave a Foley catheter in place for drainage. Suprapubic catheters are no longer routinely used and should be avoided. Place omentum over the repair. Check for other injuries and close.

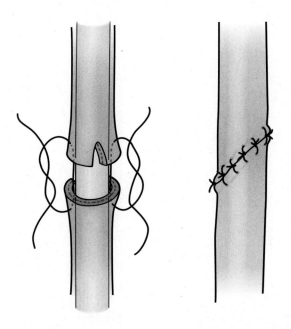

Figure 107.3 Spatulated repair of ureter (from Delacroix SE Jr, Winters JC, eds. Urinary tract injuries: Recognition and management. *Clin Colon Rectal Surg.* 2010;23:104–111, with permission).

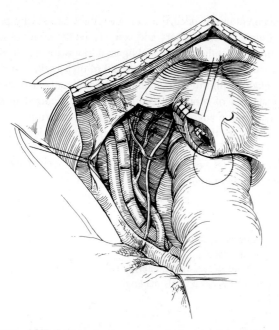

Figure 107.4 Two-layer repair of bladder injury (from Graham SD Jr, Keane TE, eds. *Glenn's Urologic Surgery.* 7th ed. Philadelphia, PA: Lippincott Williams & Wilkins; 2010, with permission).

REFERENCES

1. Buckely JC, McAninch JW. Chapter 9. Renal trauma. In: Graham SD Jr, Keane TE, eds. *Glenn's Urologic Surgery.* 7th ed., Philadelphia, PA: Lippincott Wolters Kluwer; 2010:59.
2. Delacroix SE Jr, Winters JC. Urinary tract injuries: Recognition and management. *Clin Colon Rectal Surg.* 2010;23:104–111.
3. Frober R. Surgical anatomy of the ureter. *BJU Int.* 2007;100:949–965.
4. Myers JB, Taylor MB, Brant WO, et al. Process improvement in trauma: Traumatic bladder injuries and compliance with recommended imaging evaluation. *J Trauma Acute Care Surg.* 2013;74: 264–269.
5. Riedmiller H, Becht E, Hertle L, et al. Psoas-hitch ureteroneocystostomy: Experience with 181 cases. *Eur Urol.* 1984;10:145–150. (Alternative to primary repair for low ureteral injuries.)
6. Shariat SF, Trinh QD, Morey AF, et al. Development of a highly accurate nomogram for prediction of the need for exploration in patients with renal trauma. *J Trauma.* 2008;64:1451–1458.
7. Yeung LL, Brandes SB. Contemporary management of renal trauma: Differences between urologists and trauma surgeons. *J Trauma Acute Care Surg.* 2012;72:68–75.

e **108** Radical Nephrectomy

This chapter can be accessed online at www.lww.com/eChapter108.

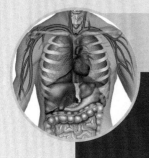

109

Cadaveric Donor Nephrectomy and Renal Transplantation

Daniel A. Katz and Rajesh Shetty

In this chapter, harvesting of kidneys and renal transplantation are described as a means of illustrating the anatomy of the retroperitoneum. The en bloc nephrectomy specimen consists of a segment of aorta, a segment of vena cava, the kidneys and their vessels, the ureters, and a generous amount of perinephric tissue, including the adrenal glands.

SCORE™, the Surgical Council on Resident Education, classified en bloc abdominal organ retrieval and kidney transplant as "COMPLEX" procedures.

STEPS IN PROCEDURE

Cadaveric Donor Nephrectomy

Longitudinal midline incision from suprasternal notch to symphysis pubis

Median sternotomy

Chest and abdominal teams work simultaneously

Kidneys dissected free and easily removed after harvest of liver and pancreas

Dissect terminal aorta free, divide inferior mesenteric artery and place two umbilical tapes around aorta

Isolate supraceliac aorta

Heparinize

Insert aortic cannula into terminal aorta

Clamp supraceliac aorta

Place vent in vena cava, usually just above the diaphragm

Perfuse kidneys with 2 L of cold preservation solution

Identify both ureters and divide near the bladder

Tag ureters

Mobilize kidneys medially with Gerota fascia

Divide the aorta and vena cava distally, at the level of the aortic cannula insertion

Mobilize en bloc specimen cephalad while dividing prevertebral fascia

Remove en bloc specimen and complete preparation with separation of kidneys on back table

Renal Transplantation

Foley catheter, instill neomycin solution into bladder

Curvilinear Gibson type pelvic incision

Divide inferior epigastric vessels

Extraperitoneal dissection to expose external iliac artery and vein

Venous anastomosis to external iliac vein

Arterial anastomosis (generally with cuff of aorta) to external iliac artery

Ureteroneocystostomy to dome of bladder

Expose bladder mucosa

Anastomose ureter to bladder mucosa

Close second layer of bladder wall over ureter to create muscular tunnel

Obtain hemostasis and close incision in layers

HALLMARK ANATOMIC COMPLICATIONS
Devascularization of ureter

LIST OF STRUCTURES

Kidneys
Renal artery and vein
Ureter
Bladder
Gerota fascia
Gonadal artery and vein

Adrenal (Suprarenal) Gland
Right adrenal (suprarenal) vein

Aorta
Celiac artery
Superior mesenteric artery
Inferior mesenteric artery (and vein)

Common iliac artery (and vein)
Internal iliac artery (and vein)
External iliac artery (and vein)

Diaphragm
Left and right crura
Inferior phrenic artery
Stomach
Duodenum
Pancreas
Spleen
Colon

Cadaveric Donor Nephrectomy

Cadaveric Donor Nephrectomy: Incision and Exposure of the Chest and Abdomen (Figs. 109.1 and 109.2)

Technical and Anatomic Points

Donor and recipient blood types are confirmed. Time-out is performed according to current UNOS guidelines. After con-

sent is achieved, the donor is placed on the operating table in the supine position and ventilated with 100% oxygen. Exposure for organ harvesting is provided by a longitudinal midline incision that extends from the suprasternal notch to the symphysis pubis (Fig. 109.1A). This incision provides sufficient exposure of and access to the heart, lungs, and abdominal viscera.

The sternum is split with an electric saw or a Lebsche knife; hemostasis of the cut surface is achieved with electrocautery

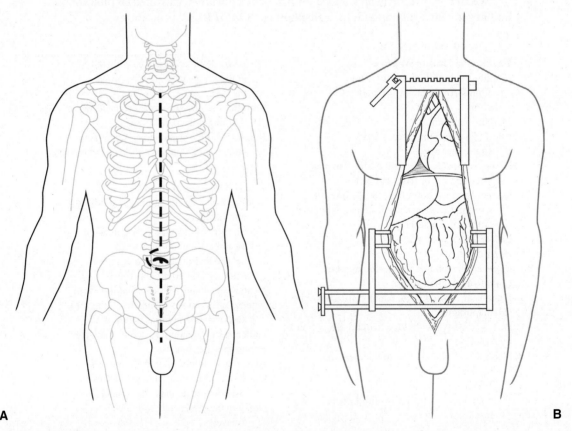

A

B

Figure 109.1 A: Cadaveric donor nephrectomy: Incision. **B:** Placement of retractors and initial exposure.

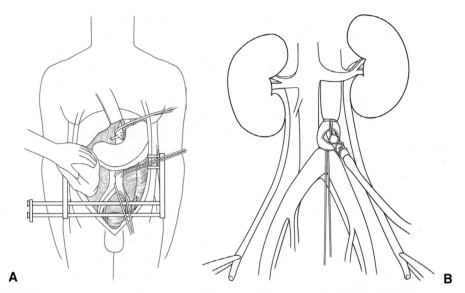

Figure 109.2 A: Isolation of supraceliac and infrarenal aorta with tapes.
B: Insertion of cannula for perfusion and flushing.

and bone wax. A sternal retractor with spikes is placed in the lower third of the sternum and spread laterally. A special large Balfour retractor with teeth is used for the abdomen (Fig. 109.1B). The heart and liver teams usually start the dissection simultaneously. The kidneys can be dissected free and easily removed after flushing of the graft and the liver and pancreas are removed.

Preparation and Flushing of the Graft (Fig. 109.2)

Technical Points

Generally, left and right medial visceral rotations will already have been completed by teams procuring liver, pancreas, or bowel. However, if not done, Mattox maneuver and Kocher–Cattell maneuver at this stage (prior to heparinization) facilitate kidney dissection later in the procedure. Dissection to expose the left renal vein insertion into the inferior vena cava is desirable. Dissect the terminal aorta free. Divide the inferior mesenteric artery between ligatures and place two umbilical tapes around the terminal aorta (Fig. 109.2A). As a last step in the preparatory dissection, encircle the supraceliac aorta with an umbilical tape after separating the muscle fibers of the diaphragmatic crura longitudinally in a blunt fashion and incising the preaortic fascia. This step is omitted if the heart is not procured because the descending aorta can be cross-clamped in the left pleural cavity without preliminary dissection.

Heparin at a dose of 300 to 500 U/kg should be administered intravenously 3 minutes before cross-clamping. For a nonheart-beating donor, the dosage of heparin should be doubled. Tie the terminal aorta with an umbilical tape. Insert the aortic cannula into the terminal aorta (Fig. 109.2B) while controlling the aorta with the left hand proximal to the aortotomy.

Position the tip of the aortic cannula below the renal artery to avoid blocking perfusion of renal artery. Secure the aortic cannula with the other, more proximal umbilical tape.

Apply a vascular clamp on the supraceliac aorta and perfuse the kidneys through the terminal aortic cannula with 2 L of preservation solution. At the same time, vent the supradiaphragmatic vena cava, to prevent venous engorgement and to drain flush solution from the operative field. Apply slush to the abdominal and thoracic cavities to cool the organs.

Anatomic Points

The paracolic gutters lie lateral to the colon and are limited medially by the retroperitoneal colon (ascending or descending) and its serosal covering, which became fused with parietal peritoneum during development. The white line of Toldt, visible in the angle between the parietal peritoneum and the lateral colon, marks the location of the fusion plane between original serosa or mesocolon and parietal peritoneum. Dissection in the fusion plane, from colon to midline, results in no damage to structures and minimal blood loss.

The gonadal vessels are the first major retroperitoneal structures encountered just superior to the pelvic brim. The right gonadal vein (a tributary of the inferior vena cava) and artery (an anterolateral branch of the aorta slightly inferior to the renal arteries) should be encountered as they cross the external iliac vessels somewhat lateral to the ureter. The ureter is just medial to these vessels.

More superiorly, Gerota fascia (enclosing the right kidney, suprarenal gland, and perirenal fat) will be exposed as the hepatic flexure is mobilized. Further medial mobilization of the colon will expose the C-loop of the duodenum, encompassing the head of the pancreas. These retroperitoneal structures are in direct contact with the anterior surface of Gerota fascia. Further medial mobilization of the right colon, terminal ileum, duodenum, and head of the pancreas will expose the entire infrahepatic inferior vena cava lying to the right of the midline.

Encirclement of the distal aorta, just proximal to its bifurcation, is aided by lateral retraction of the inferior mesenteric artery because this parallels, to the left, the distal aorta. Skeletonization of the distal aorta; however, should be done with some care to avoid inadvertent laceration of the left fourth lumbar vein, which passes to the left posterior to the aorta.

As the abdominal aorta is skeletonized from inferior to superior, the first structure to be encountered should be the inferior mesenteric artery. More superiorly, again from the anterior surface of the aorta, small gonadal arteries can be identified. These may arise as a common trunk, separately and at the same or different levels, or they may arise from a renal or suprarenal artery. The next structure to be encountered should be the left renal vein, which typically crosses the anterior surface of the aorta just inferior to the origins of the superior mesenteric artery and left renal artery. However, retroaortic left renal veins or circumaortic left renal veins do occur, as commonly as 6% of the time. The superior mesenteric artery usually originates about 1 cm distal to the celiac artery; however, both of these major arteries can arise from a common trunk. Rarely, one or more of the three celiac artery branches (left gastric, splenic, or common hepatic) arise independently from the aorta and the procurement surgeon needs to be aware of these anatomic variations.

Nephrectomy (Fig. 109.3)

Technical Points

After the hepatectomy and pancreatectomy are complete, dissection is carried out in a bloodless field. The kidneys have already been flushed in situ. The colon, duodenum, and pancreas will generally have been mobilized by the team procuring the liver. If performing a kidney only retrieval, it is helpful to divide the entire mesocolon to the level of the midsigmoid colon and reflect the entire colon (still in continuity with the small bowel) off the field. If still in situ, mobilize the spleen and pancreas medially to expose the anterior left Gerota fascia. Mobilize both kidneys medially with Gerota fascia, using sharp dissection. Identify both ureters and transect these in the midpelvis in order to provide at least 15 cm of ureter length in adult donors. Tag and dissect the ureters to several centimeters above the level of the aortic bifurcation (further dissection is generally accomplished on the back table). Divide the inferior vena cava and aorta just below the level of the aortic cannula. Complete the en bloc excision by incising the prevertebral fascia cephalad with a pair of heavy scissors, while the aorta and the inferior vena cava are retracted upward together with the kidneys and ureters (Fig. 109.3A). Five to ten minutes are required for this en bloc dissection.

Once removed, immerse the kidneys in an ice basin and separate them. Divide the left renal vein first (Fig. 109.3B), including a cuff of the inferior vena cava. Of note, the entire inferior vena cava is left with the right kidney. Turn the kidneys posteriorly and incise the aorta between the paired lumbar arteries (Fig. 109.3C). After identifying the renal arteries from within, split the aorta anteriorly and separate the kidneys. Insert a fistula tip in each renal artery and flush a total of 250 to 300 mL of chilled preservation solution through each kidney. Split Gerota fascia along the convex surface of the kidney and partially dissect it off the kidney, particularly if there is a considerable amount of perinephric fat, to ensure good cooling. Package the kidneys separately and store them in preservation solution. All remaining back table preparation is left for the recipient surgeon.

The kidneys are not separated if the donor is younger than 2 years of age—they are recovered and transplanted en bloc.

Anatomic Points

The blood supply to the right ureter is provided by branches from the renal arteries, aorta, gonadal arteries, iliac (common or internal) arteries, and vesical arteries. The longitudinal anastomosis between these vessels, on the surface of the ureter, is usually good. Typically, ureteric branches of arteries superior to the pelvic brim approach the ureter from its medial side. In the pelvis, because the ureters lie medial to the internal iliac arteries, the blood supply approaches from its lateral side. This is essentially true for as far as the ureters can be exposed in the pelvis.

Mobilization of the kidneys and ureters is facilitated by a conceptual understanding of Gerota fascia. This perirenal fascia has been variously interpreted as being either continuous with the transversalis fascia or a "condensation" of retroperitoneal tissue. Regardless of its derivation, this facial layer encloses the kidney, suprarenal gland, and perirenal fat. The anterior layer of Gerota fascia is rather poorly developed, whereas the posterior layer is significantly thicker. Anterior and posterior layers fuse around the lateral and superior aspects of the kidney and suprarenal gland. Medially and inferiorly, anterior and posterior layers do not fuse (or at least not firmly), so that the capsule is continuous with pericaval and periaortic tissues across the midline and is "open" inferiorly, essentially anterior and posterior to the ureter. Mobilization of the kidney is easiest if the plane posterior to the posterior layer of Gerota fascia is developed, rather than trying to develop a plane between the true capsule of the kidney and Gerota fascia.

Exposure of the left kidney and ureter follows most of the colon mobilization procedures done with performing a left hemicolectomy. On the antimesenteric side of the colon, incision along the white line of Toldt, a comparatively avascular line formed by embryonic fusion of the serosa and parietal peritoneum, enables entrance to the relatively avascular plane that results from fusion of the descending mesocolon and parietal peritoneum. Blunt dissection to the midline in this plane allows complete mobilization of the descending colon. As the peritoneum and inferior mesenteric vessels are elevated and mobilized, it is important to identify the ureter; frequently, this adheres to the peritoneum and can be inadvertently reflected with the colon and its vasculature. The ureter should be identified as it passes into the pelvis in the vicinity of the apex of

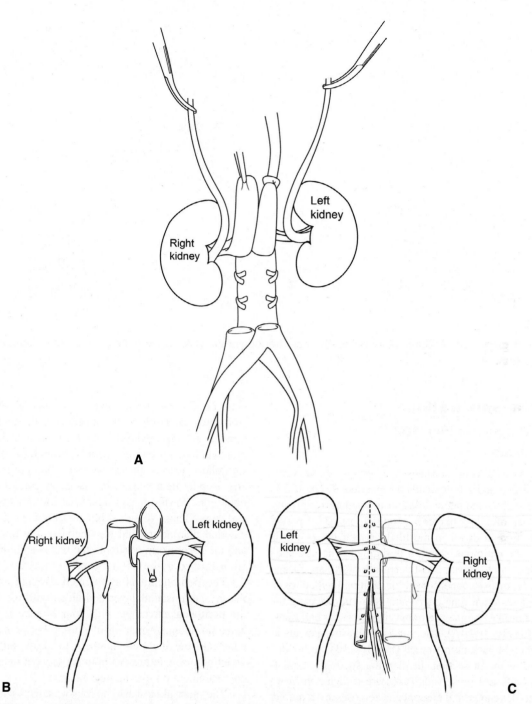

Figure 109.3 Nephrectomy. **A:** En bloc removal begins inferiorly and progresses cephalad. **B:** The kidneys and ureters are removed en bloc with segments of the inferior vena cava and aorta. The left vein is first detached from the cava with a thin rim of caval cuff. **C:** The bloc has been flipped over and the posterior aspect of the aorta is opened vertically between the paired lumbar arteries.

the root of the sigmoid mesocolon. Remember that the upper (lateral) limb of this inverted V is lateral to the ureter, whereas the lower (medial) limb is medial to the ureter.

When the left crus of the diaphragm is exposed, the inferior phrenic artery, which courses superiorly on the crus, should be identified and controlled before division of the crus. In addition, the first two lumbar arteries, which arise from the posterior aspect of the aorta, pass through or behind the diaphragmatic crura; their division, if uncontrolled, can be a source of hemorrhage that can obscure the operative field. Division of the crus is necessary because it allows control of the aorta superior to the celiac artery, which typically arises between the left crus and the right crus just as the aorta enters the abdomen.

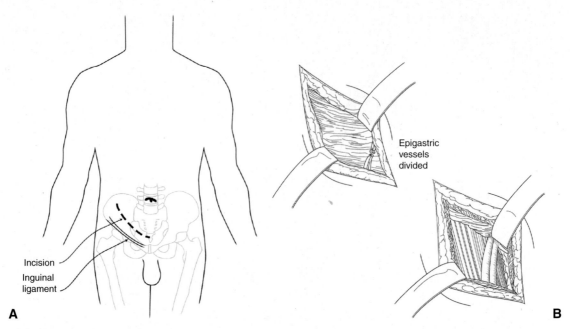

A

B

Figure 109.4 Surgical technique of renal transplantation. **A:** Incision. **B:** Ligation of epigastric vessels.

Renal Transplantation

Surgical Technique (Fig. 109.4)

Technical Points

After induction of general anesthesia, a central venous pressure line is placed and a Foley catheter inserted. Then, 150 to 200 mL of a 0.25% neomycin solution is instilled by gravity into the bladder, and the catheter is clamped for a short period to allow the fluid to dwell in the bladder then the clamp is released and the antibiotic solution is drained. The abdomen is then prepped and draped. Most renal allografts are placed heterotopically, in an extraperitoneal location in the iliac fossa.

Expose the external iliac artery and vein after incising the external and internal oblique and transversus muscles and transversalis fascia (Fig. 109.4A). The inferior epigastric vessels as well as the round ligament in women (Fig. 109.4B) are divided in the course of the dissection. In men the spermatic cord is reflected medially and preserved. Take care to ligate the lymphatics. Arterial, venous, and ureteral anastomoses are required.

Anatomic Points

This skin incision approximates the direction of Langer lines and heals with comparatively minimal scarring. The skin incision is curvilinear starting approximately one or two finger breadths above the symphysis pubis and ending two finger breadths medial to the anterior superior iliac crest. Incision of the superficial fascia, here typically divisible into a fatty superficial layer (Camper fascia) and a deeper, more fibrous layer (Scarpa fascia), follows the same line as the skin incision. Only cutaneous nerves—branches of spinal nerves T11 through L1—are encountered during this stage of the dissection. The major branches of these cutaneous nerves are at the interface between Camper fascia and Scarpa fascia. The fascial incision starts inferiorly at the junction of the rectus and oblique muscle and fascial layers. As the fascial incision progresses more cephalad it curves laterally through the oblique muscles. The plane deep to the transversus abdominis muscle is actually deep to the transversalis fascia. To enter this properitoneal plane, one must cut and ligate the inferior epigastric arteries and veins. These vessels originate from the terminal part of the external iliac artery and pass between the transversalis fascia and the peritoneum to supply the rectus abdominis muscle and are identified in the inferior aspect of the dissection.

The peritoneum is swept medially and the remainder of the fascial/muscular layer is divided with the cautery. Protect the peritoneal envelope with your fingers. It is important to leave an adequate margin of muscle between the inferior cut edge and the inguinal ligament to allow sufficient tissue in which to place sutures without subsequent muscle ischemia or encroachment on the inguinal ligament.

The interval between the transversalis fascia and the peritoneum is truly the retroperitoneal plane, where all retroperitoneal organs are located. Thus, dissection along this plane should lead one to the urogenital and vascular structures necessary to complete this procedure. As this space is developed, one will readily realize that no major nerves or vessels need be damaged.

Vascular Anastomosis (Fig. 109.5)

Technical Points

With the retroperitoneal dissection developed, the retraction system is placed. A Fast Track Wishbone Omni is shown (Fig. 109.5A), although Balfour and Bookwalter systems also work well.

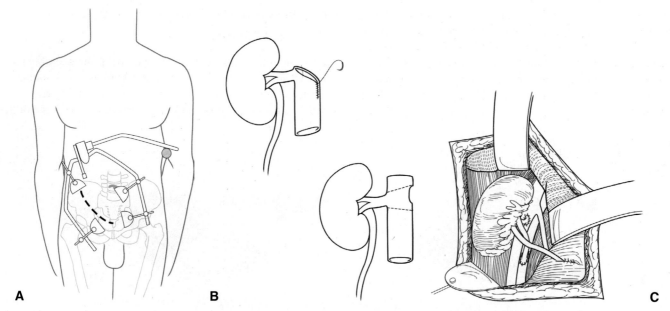

Figure 109.5 Vascular anastomosis. **A:** Position of retractor blades for optimum exposure. **B:** Techniques for attaining greater right renal vein length. "Dogleg" and "straight" extensions are shown. **C:** Grafted kidney in situ showing anastomoses.

The venous anastomosis is generally performed first. For a left kidney, the renal vein usually is anastomosed with a cuff of vena cava end-to-side to the external iliac vein. For a right kidney, the venous anastomosis can present some difficulty. The right renal vein can be anastomosed directly, usually with a cuff of vena cava. The vein is short on the right, however, and some surgeons prefer to increase the length. Several options exist and two popular options are shown in Figure 109.5B. A segment of vena cava attached to the vein often is successfully used by oversewing the left renal vein orifice and superior caval opening thus creating a "dogleg" extension. It helps to create the proper orientation for implantation by trimming the distal open cava at an angle. Another option is to use a transverse section of vena cava extending straight out from the renal vein by using a vascular linear stapler to close the proximal and distal caval openings and enlarging the left vein orifice so that the entire lateral caval sidewall is open between staple lines. This option has the advantage of being simple and quick; however, it is important to flange the cava so that it is wider on the left renal vein side than the right. Finally, a donor iliac vein or caval graft may be sutured end-to-end to the renal vein to gain length (not shown). Multiple veins tend not to be a problem; a bifurcated vein graft can be used, or one vein can be ligated.

In some arterial or venous reconstructions, a "growth factor" is used while tying, on completion of the anastomosis, to prevent stricture. For the artery and vein, continuous nonabsorbable monofilament suture is used.

The renal artery usually is anastomosed with a cuff of aorta end-to-side to the external iliac artery, although it may also be sewn end-to-end to the internal iliac artery (Fig. 109.5C). In the case of multiple arteries, there are several options. If the arteries are close together on a cuff of aorta, it may be sim-

plest to use a long cuff containing both arteries. If there is a large gap between the arterial takeoffs, then the intervening segment of aorta can be removed and the separate patches are sewn together to form a common patch. Sometimes it is necessary to sew separate arterial vascular anastomoses. If a polar artery has been transected, it may be anastomosed on the back table to the side of the main renal artery. If there are two transected vessels, they may be either implanted separately or partially anastomosed in pantaloon fashion to form a single vessel that can be sutured to the iliac artery. Alternately, they can be lengthened by an arterial graft from the same donor. The latter solution also may be effective when the donor aortic cuff is atherosclerotic and the orifice of the renal artery is narrowed.

Anatomic Points

The shape of the pelvis, which may be classified as gynecoid, anthropoid, or android, is highly variable. In fact, some studies indicate that more than 50% of all females have an android or anthropoid pelvis, classifications supposedly characteristic of male pelvis.

Reflection of the peritoneal sac reveals the common iliac vessels, which are crossed, on their peritoneal aspect, by the ureter. This occurs approximately at the point where the common iliac artery bifurcates into external and internal iliac arteries. It is also in this vicinity that the right common iliac and external iliac arterial trunk, which initially is medial to the corresponding veins, crosses the peritoneal surface of the veins to lie lateral to the vein. On the left, the arterial trunk is always lateral to the corresponding veins. In the male, the testicular artery lies on the peritoneal surface of the distal external iliac artery. Genital branches of the genitofemoral nerve will also be seen to cross the distal external iliac artery, exiting through the deep inguinal ring. The obturator artery (usually a branch of the internal iliac artery) and the obturator nerve lie medial to the external iliac vein, in the groove between the psoas major muscle and the iliacus muscle. The artery can be ligated, but care should be taken not to damage this motor nerve to the hip adductors.

Ureteroneocystostomy (Fig. 109.6)

Technical Points

This part of the procedure is perhaps the most problematic and least standardized. Dozens of variations exist, although the most popular derive from three or four basic types. The extravesical ureteroneocystostomy is placed at the dome of the

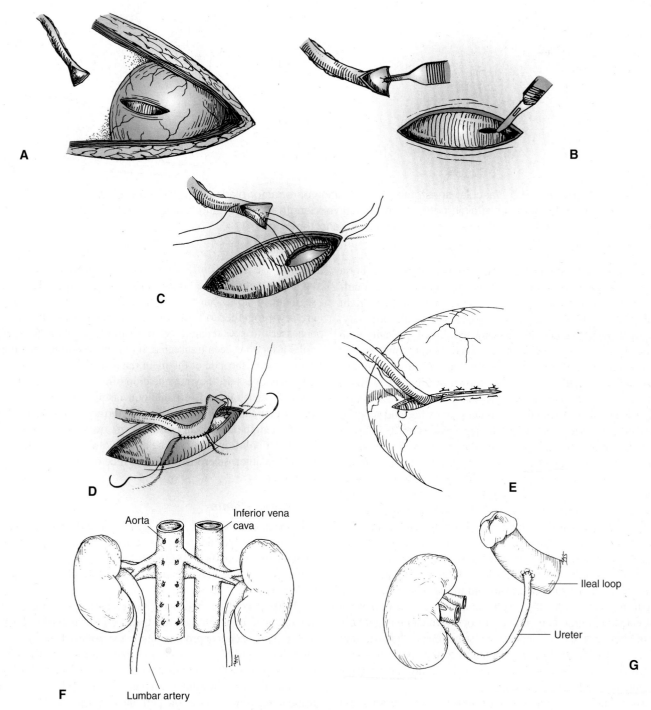

Figure 109.6 A: Ureteroneocystostomy—incision in bladder. **B:** Exposure of mucosa. **C:** Placement of spatulated end of ureter. **D:** Completion of mucosal anastomosis. **E:** Closure of bladder wall. **F:** Ligation of lumbars for en bloc transplant of both kidneys from a pediatric donor. **G:** Use of ileal loop as urinary conduit.

bladder. The bladder mucosa is exposed through a 2.5- to 3-cm incision in the muscle, and full-thickness ureter is sutured to the mucosa with interrupted or continuous absorbable sutures. A second layer of bladder wall muscle is then approximated over the first layer to create a submucosal tunnel. This is shown in Figure 109.6A–E.

In the case of ureters whose blood supply has been stripped, it may be necessary to perform a ureteroureterostomy or pyelo-ureterostomy to the ureter of the native kidney. Double ureters can be reimplanted separately or partially anastomosed and transplanted as one. Care should be taken not to disrupt what is usually a common blood supply.

In the case of pediatric kidneys transplanted en bloc, the donor aorta and vena cava are used for the vascular anastomoses. It is important to ligate all the lumbar and gonadal branches on the back table (Fig. 109.6F). Separate ureteral reimplantations can be performed. Alternately, the ureters can be partially anastomosed and reimplanted together.

Ureteral reimplantation into an ileal loop is performed in one layer, anastomosing full-thickness ureter to full-thickness bowel with interrupted absorbable sutures, as demonstrated in Figure 109.6G.

In most cases, the venous anastomosis is performed first, followed by the arterial anastomosis. As the vessels are sutured, the patient should be hydrated and given furosemide, 1 mg/kg, and mannitol, 0.2 g/kg. The systolic blood pressure should be 140 mm Hg at the time of cross-clamp release. Immunosuppression is given as the operation begins. The ureteral anastomosis is performed last. After hemostasis is achieved, the wound is closed in layers.

Anatomic Points

The rectovesical fascia (of Denonvilliers), located between the rectum and the urinary bladder (and prostate), is significant to this part of the procedure only in the male. In females, this homologous structure is interposed between the rectum and the vagina; in both sexes, it is formed by fusion of the caudal-most part of the embryonic peritoneal sac.

The blood supply of the ureter is provided by branches from the renal artery, aorta, gonadal artery, iliac (common, external, or internal) artery, and vesical artery. These arteries anastomose and lie on the ureter itself; thus, meticulous skeletonization of the ureter, with removal of the periureteral sheath and ureteric arteries, is not indicated and, in fact, can jeopardize the transplantation. Obviously, the supply from the renal artery is most important because that will serve as the sole blood supply to the donor ureter until neovascularization occurs following its anastomosis to the urinary bladder.

REFERENCES

1. Dunkin BJ, Johnson LB, Kuo PC. A technical modification eliminates early ureteral complications after laparoscopic donor nephrectomy. *J Am Coll Surg.* 2000;190:96–97.
2. Ko DSC, Cosimi AD. The donor and donor nephrectomy. In: Morris PJ, ed. *Kidney Transplantation: Principles and Practice.* 5th ed. Philadelphia, PA: WB Saunders; 2001:89–105.
3. Kuo PC, Cho ES, Flowers JL, et al. Laparoscopic living donor nephrectomy and multiple renal arteries. *Am J Surg.* 1998;176:559–563.
4. Montgomery RA. The laparoscopic donor nephrectomy. In: Morris PJ, ed. *Kidney Transplantation: Principles and Practice.* 5th ed. Philadelphia, PA: WB Saunders; 2001:106–112.
5. Yanaga K, Podesta LG, Byoznick B, et al. Multiple organ recovery for transplantation. In: Starzl TE, Shapiro R, Simmons RI, eds. *Atlas of Organ Transplantation.* Philadelphia, PA: JB Lippincott; 1991:3.1–3.49.

e110 Laparoscopic Donor Nephrectomy

This chapter can be accessed online at www.lww.com/eChapter110.

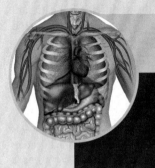

111

Abdominal Aortic Aneurysm Repair and Aortofemoral Bypass

Lilja Thyri Bjornsdottir and W. John Sharp

Many aortic aneurysms are now repaired by an endovascular route. The classic open operation is still required in some circumstances. In this chapter, the anatomy of the abdominal aorta and iliac vessels is explored through the procedure of abdominal aortic aneurysm repair. The femoral region is then introduced through the closely related procedure of aortofemoral bypass grafting.

SCORE™, the Surgical Council on Resident Education, classified abdominal aortic aneurysm repair (open) and aortofemoral bypass as "ESSENTIAL UNCOMMON" procedures.

STEPS IN PROCEDURE

Abdominal Aortic Aneurysm Repair— Transperitoneal Approach

Midline incision from xiphoid to below umbilicus

Reflect transverse colon cephalad

Reflect duodenum and small bowel cephalad and to the right

Retract descending colon and sigmoid to the left

Preclot graft, if necessary

Isolate proximal and distal neck of aneurysm in preparation for clamping

Heparinize patient

Clamp aorta proximally and distally

Open the anterior wall of the aneurysm (longitudinal incision, T-ed across at superior and inferior ends)

Remove mural thrombus and suture-ligate any back-bleeding lumbar vessels

Suture-ligate the inferior mesenteric artery (from inside the aneurysm wall) if it is back bleeding

Anastomose graft to proximal aorta using running suture

Flush and then clamp the graft distally; inspect suture line for leaks

Complete distal anastomosis and flush before opening clamps

Close the aneurysm sac over the graft after obtaining hemostasis

Abdominal Aortic Aneurysm Repair— Retroperitoneal Approach

Supine position with chest in right lateral decubitus position

Incision from the tip of eleventh rib to midhypogastrium

Divide all muscular and fascial layers in the direction of the incision (not their fibers)

Mobilize the peritoneal sac medially to expose the aorta and both iliac vessels

Proceed as outlined above

Aortobifemoral Bypass

Expose femoral vessels by incision over each femoral pulse (inguinal ligament downward for approximately 10 cm)

Isolate and control the femoral arteries and branches

Create retroperitoneal tunnels over the anterior surface of the iliac and femoral arteries

Midline incision and exposure of the aorta as outlined above

Place clamp on proximal aorta, taking care not to fracture plaque

Clamp common, superficial, and profunda femoris arteries

Anastomosis to aorta can be performed as end (aorta)-to-end (graft) or as side (aorta)-to-end (graft)

Anastomosis to femoral vessels is end (graft)-to-side (vessel)

Obtain hemostasis and close

HALLMARK ANATOMIC COMPLICATIONS

Left colonic ischemia from inadequate collaterals

Injury to ureters

Injury to left renal vein

Injury to hypogastric nerve plexus

Seroma (lymphocele) formation in groin incisions

LIST OF STRUCTURES

Aorta

Left and right renal arteries

Left and right gonadal arteries

Inferior mesenteric artery

Lumbar arteries

Left and right common iliac arteries

Left and right internal iliac (hypogastric) arteries

Left and right external iliac arteries

Left and right common femoral arteries

Superficial circumflex iliac artery

Superficial epigastric artery

Superficial external pudendal artery

Profunda femoris artery

Medial femoral circumflex artery

Lateral femoral circumflex artery

Inferior Vena Cava

Left renal vein

Left and right common iliac veins

Left and right internal iliac veins

Left and right external iliac veins

Femoral vein

Profunda femoris vein

Hypogastric nerve plexus

Duodenum

Ligament of Treitz (suspensory muscle of the duodenum)

Ureters

External oblique muscle

Internal oblique muscle

Transversus abdominis muscle

Anterior rectus sheath

Rectus abdominis muscle

Inguinal ligament

Femoral sheath

Femoral triangle

Femoral Nerve

Cutaneous branch

Muscular branch

Genitofemoral nerve

Saphenous nerve

Adductor canal (of Hunter)

Abdominal Aortic Aneurysm Repair

Skin Incision (Fig. 111.1)

Technical Points

Many surgeons prefer a midline transperitoneal incision, as shown in Figures 111.1 to 111.4. Position the patient supine. Prepare and drape the abdomen from the nipples to the knees to allow a midline incision with the possibility of extending the bypass to the femoral arteries in the groin if necessary. Place a sterile towel over the genitalia and an iodophor-impregnated plastic adhesive drape over all exposed skin to protect the prosthetic graft from skin flora. Make a midline incision from the xiphoid to the midhypogastrium or symphysis pubis (Fig. 111.1A). Cover the transverse colon and omentum with a moist lap and elevate superiorly out of the abdominal cavity. Sharply mobilize the third and fourth portion of the duodenum to the right and off the infrarenal aorta by dividing the ligament of Treitz (Fig. 111.1B). Pack the small bowel in a moist towel and retract to the right. Pack and retract the descending and sigmoid colon laterally and inferiorly if necessary. The aneurysm should now

be well exposed. Self-retaining retractors such as the Omni are very helpful. An alternative retroperitoneal approach is presented in Figures 111.5 and 111.6.

Anatomic Points

The midline incision has many anatomic advantages if a transperitoneal approach is used. In addition to providing maximal exposure of the peritoneal cavity, it affords a strong closure because several fascial and aponeurotic layers fuse as the linea alba. Retraction of the transverse colon superiorly displaces the transverse mesocolon superiorly, exposing the superior aspect of the root of the mesentery, which begins at the duodenojejunal flexure. Direct visualization and palpation of the ligament of Treitz (suspensory muscle of the duodenum) is then possible. This fibromuscular band arises from the right crus of the diaphragm and then passes posterior to the pancreas and splenic veins and anterior to the left renal vasculature. It may contain numerous small vessels. Reflection of the duodenum and small bowel to the right, and of the descending and sigmoid colon to the left, exposes the aneurysm, which is covered with parietal peritoneum.

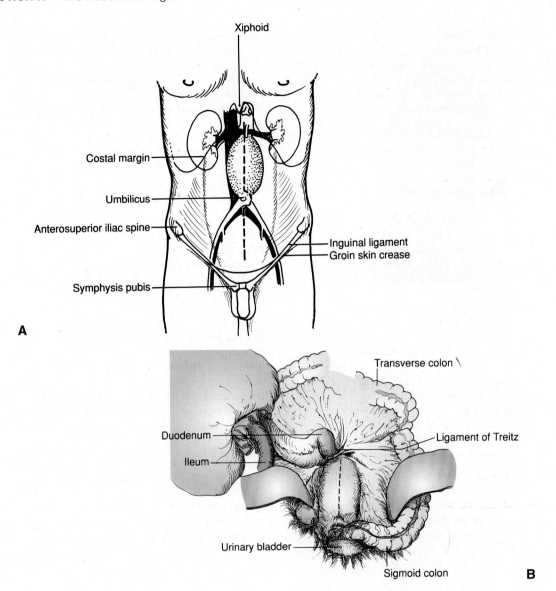

Figure 111.1 Skin incision. **A:** Skin incision. **B:** Initial exposure of aneurysm.

Exposure of the Infrarenal Aorta and Iliac Arteries (Fig. 111.2)

Technical Points

Open the peritoneum over the aneurysm staying slightly to the right of the midline (Fig. 111.2A). More than 90% of abdominal aortic aneurysms are infrarenal. The superior neck of the aneurysm (area of normal aorta just proximal to where the aneurysmal widening begins) then lies just distal to the renal arteries and posterior to where the renal vein crosses over the aorta. Exercise care to avoid injury to these vessels in dissecting the neck of the aneurysm for clamping. The left renal vein may be dissected circumferentially and retracted proximally with a vein retractor. Dividing the left gonadal vein, lumbar vein and adrenal vein branches will allow further retraction of the left renal vein for better visualization of the juxtarenal aorta. Rather than risk tearing the left renal vein during an unusually

difficult exposure, it may be intentionally divided at the onset and oversewn adjacent to the vena cava while preserving the above branches. On reviewing films prior to surgery, look for the retroaortic left renal vein anatomic variant as it is highly susceptible to accidental injury during clamping and subsequent massive, difficult-to-control hemorrhage.

The ureters lie close to the aneurysm and are most susceptible to dissection or retraction injury where they cross anterior to the iliac bifurcation to enter the pelvis. The common iliac veins adhere closely to the arteries and should be carefully separated from them only for a distance that is sufficient to allow clamping of the arteries (Fig. 111.2B).

Aspirate blood from the inferior vena cava or aorta for preclotting of knitted Dacron grafts. Preclotting of woven, "presealed" knitted, or PTFE grafts is unnecessary. Then have the anesthesiologist administer 100-U/kg heparin intravenously. Clamp all vessels gently to avoid dislodging atheroma or thrombus

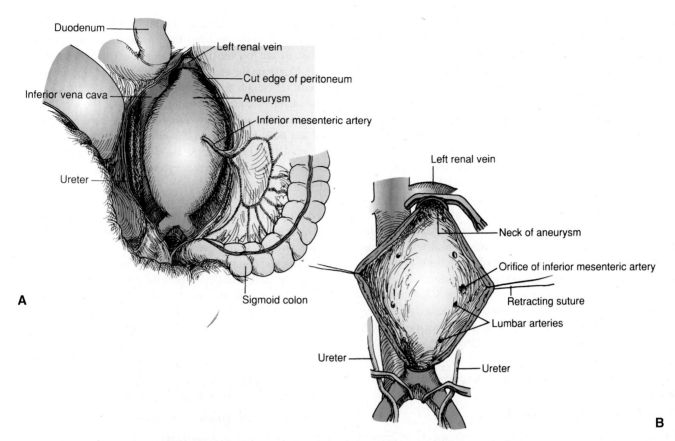

Figure 111.2 Exposure of the infrarenal aorta and iliac arteries

as emboli. Open the anterior wall of the aneurysm longitudinally staying to the right of the origin of the inferior mesenteric artery. Remove mural thrombus and suture-ligate bleeding lumbar arteries. At the superior and inferior necks of the aneurysm, extend the incision transversely in a T pattern through the anterior half of the wall. Leave the posterior portion intact for strong purchase of sutures. Retracting sutures or a self-retaining retractor placed in the wall of the aneurysm may be helpful. Remove any debris from both necks of the aneurysm.

If the inferior mesenteric artery is back bleeding, suture-ligate it from inside the aneurysm to avoid disturbing the collateral circulation to the distal inferior mesenteric artery. Carefully inspect the bowel for signs of ischemia before closure of the abdomen. If there is concern regarding the viability of the colon, reimplant the inferior mesenteric artery with a cuff of aortic wall into the graft.

Anatomic Points

The hypogastric nerve plexus contains postganglionic sympathetic fibers from spinal cord segments L1 to L2 or L3 and parasympathetic fibers from spinal cord segments S2 to S4. This plexus is located just inferior to the bifurcation of the aorta into the common iliac arteries. Fibers connecting this plexus to more superior plexuses ascend anterior to the common iliac arteries (especially on the left) and continue to predominate on the left side of the aorta. Although those parasympathetic

fibers mediating erection are not endangered, whereas the sympathetic fibers controlling emission and ejaculation are, successful erection apparently demands the integrated function of both sympathetic and parasympathetic systems. For this reason, many surgeons prefer to open the aneurysm on the right side of the aorta, rather than in the midline or on the left in the male. Obviously, extensive circumferential dissection of the aorta is not only unnecessary but also is contraindicated.

The renal arteries usually arise from the aorta in the upper half of the body of vertebra L2, slightly inferior to the origin of the superior mesenteric artery. Variations in the level of origin of the renal arteries can occur, and the displacement is usually more caudal than cranial. Moreover, supernumerary renal arteries, which typically are end arteries to kidney segments, can arise from the aorta inferior to the level of origin of the renal arteries. Should these be occluded or interrupted, a zone of renal necrosis can result.

The left renal vein, which typically crosses the peritoneal aspect of the aorta at the level of the left renal artery, is always at risk for injury. This is particularly true if the course of this vein is anomalous (e.g., retroaortic). If the vein is ligated, this should be done as close as possible to its termination in the inferior vena cava. Collateral venous pathways draining the left kidney, including the left gonadal and suprarenal veins, will thus be preserved.

The gonadal arteries (spermatic or ovarian) arise from the anterolateral aspect of the aorta 2 to 5 cm caudal to the origin of the renal arteries. The collateral circulation of the testis in the male (the deferential artery, derived from the umbilical artery near the latter's origin from the internal iliac artery, and the cremasteric artery, a branch of the inferior epigastric artery) and the ovary in the female (a branch of the uterine artery) usually permits ligation of the gonadal artery with little to no morbidity.

Finally, care must be taken to avoid injury to the ureters or their blood supply. The ureters are most susceptible to trauma where they cross the peritoneal surface of the common or external iliac arteries. This is also the site where their blood supply (derived from the renal arteries, aorta, gonadal artery, common or external iliac artery, and vesical arteries) is at greatest risk.

The inferior mesenteric artery arises from the aorta about one vertebral level superior to the bifurcation of the aorta into the common iliac arteries. It is frequently completely occluded. Theoretically, it can be ligated and divided close to its origin with no ill effect; however, because the anastomoses (collateral pathways) shown in texts are not always functional, the descending and sigmoid colon should be inspected for signs of ischemia. A widely patent inferior mesenteric artery that is not briskly back bleeding should be reimplanted.

Construction of a Vascular Anastomosis (Fig. 111.3)

Technical and Anatomic Points

All aortic anastomoses are made with continuous, or running, 3-0 polypropylene suture. It helps to view the proximal aortic circumference as a clock. Starting at the 3-o'clock position, place the first suture from the outside to in on the graft and inside to out on the uncut double-thickness posterior aortic wall. Continue the anastomosis in a running fashion around the face of this clock at "hourly intervals," ideally taking six bites to complete the posterior suture line to the 9-o'clock position. The posterior sutures are left loose in a parachute-like fashion and pulled tight when the posterior half of the anastomosis is completed (Fig. 111.3A, B). This technique minimizes any existing aorta/graft size discrepancies and facilitates symmetry of the anastomosis.

Complete the anterior suture line using the same suture from the 9-o'clock position at the corner opposite you across the anterior wall and complete the anastomosis where it began. Make sure the suture line is taut.

After you complete the proximal anastomosis, flush and then clamp the graft distally. Inspect the anastomosis for leaks. Cut the graft to length and anastomose to the aortic bifurcation in similar fashion. If you are using a bifurcated graft to the iliacs, spatulate the ends and use 4-0 polypropylene for the distal anastomoses (see Figures 111.7 and 111.8).

Closure of the Aneurysm Wall and Posterior Peritoneum Over the Graft (Fig. 111.4)

Technical and Anatomic Points

Perigraft infection and aortoenteric fistulas are extremely difficult and morbid complications of aortic surgery. In addition

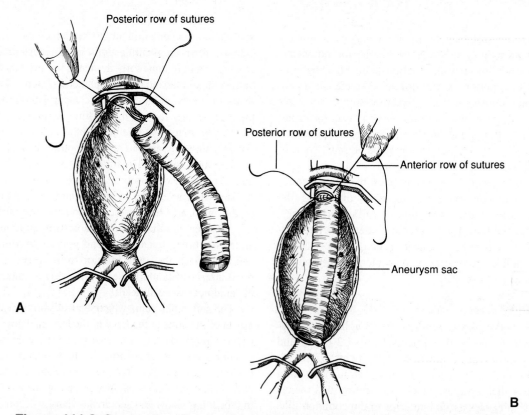

Figure 111.3 Construction of a vascular anastomosis. **A:** Exposure of infrarenal artery. **B:** Aneurysm has been opened. Note ostea of inferior mesenteric artery and lumbar arteries.

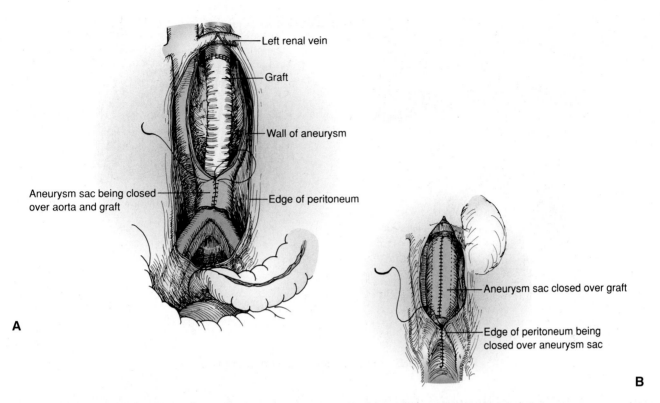

Left renal vein

Graft

Wall of aneurysm

Aneurysm sac being closed
over aorta and graft

Edge of peritoneum

A

Aneurysm sac closed over graft

Edge of peritoneum being
closed over aneurysm sac

B

Figure 111.4 Closure of the aneurysm wall and posterior peritoneum over the graft

to the use of prophylactic antibiotics, these complications are best prevented by closing the aneurysm sac and peritoneum over the graft and anastomosis with two layers of 2-0 Vicryl, thus placing viable tissue between the bowel and the graft (Fig. 111.4A, B). The abdominal incision is then closed in a routine fashion. Drains are not used because of their potential for introducing contamination and initiating infection.

Retroperitoneal Approach to the Aorta (Fig. 111.5)

Technical Points

The aorta can also be well exposed by a left flank retroperitoneal approach, which is easily extended superiorly within the intercostal spaces to provide access to the suprarenal and thoracic aortas. This approach may be associated with a decreased incidence of ileus and pulmonary dysfunction as well as a shorter hospitalization.

Place the patient supine on a bean bag with the central portion of the trunk over the table break. Rotate the chest in a near right lateral decubitus position with the left arm supported on an armrest, as for a left thoracotomy. Rotate the hips back 30 to 45 degrees to allow access to the groin area if needed. Flex the table to open up the left flank and use the bean bag to maintain the position. The patient is then prepared and draped from the axilla to the knees. For exposure of the infrarenal and juxtarenal aortas, extend the incision from the tip of the eleventh rib or the tenth intercostal interspace

toward the midhypogastrium (Fig. 111.5A). Tailor this incision to the intercostal space most appropriate to the level of proximal aortic exposure required.

Divide the external oblique, internal oblique, and transversus abdominis muscles in the direction of the incision. Occasionally, the anterior rectus sheath and rectus abdominis muscle must be partially divided to provide adequate exposure (Fig. 111.5B, C). Enter the retroperitoneal space posteriorly by the tip of the eleventh rib. If the peritoneal cavity is entered, close the peritoneal rent with continuous absorbable sutures.

Anatomic Points

This incision closely approximates both Langer lines and the course of the major trunks of the intercostal nerves, which in this region provide motor and sensory innervations to the anterior and anterolateral abdominal wall. After the external and internal oblique muscles are divided, the neurovascular layer of the abdominal wall is exposed; it is in this interval that the neurovascular bundles supplying the rectus abdominis and anterolateral muscles are located. When the rectus abdominis muscle is approached, caution is warranted to avoid injuring the inferior epigastric artery (a branch of the external iliac artery), which enters the lateral aspect of the rectus sheath somewhat inferior to the incision. Although this artery can be ligated and divided with no ill effect owing to collaterals provided by segmental arteries and the superior epigastric artery, one should be careful not to cut it inadvertently.

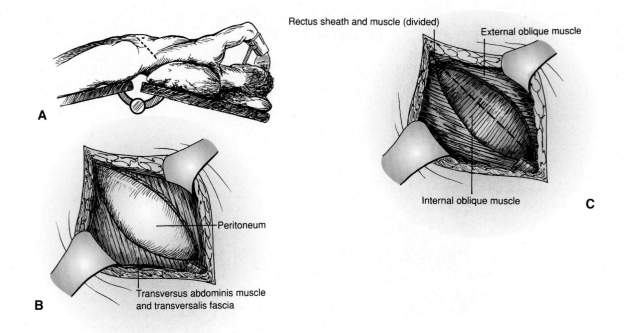

Figure 111.5 Retroperitoneal approach to the aorta

Exposure of the Retroperitoneum (Fig. 111.6)

Technical Points

Enter the retroperitoneal space by blunt dissection, sweeping the left colon, ureter, and Gerota fascia off the anterior surface of the psoas muscle and aorta. The lumbar branch of the left renal vein usually requires ligation and division to provide adequate exposure without tearing the vein during retraction. The suprarenal and infrarenal aortas, common iliac arteries, and left renal artery and vein are easily exposed. The internal iliac arteries and the left external iliac artery are usually accessible.

The right renal artery distal to the vena cava is not easily exposed by this approach.

Control of the distal right external iliac artery through the left retroperitoneal approach is also problematic and may require occlusion by an intraluminal balloon catheter or a separate right lower quadrant retroperitoneal incision; however, these measures are rarely necessary. The femoral vessels may be accessed through separate groin incisions.

Anatomic Points

Entering the retroperitoneal space without entering the peritoneal cavity is probably easiest by blunt dissection posterolaterally because, here, there is typically an accumulation of retroperitoneal fat between the transversalis fascia and the

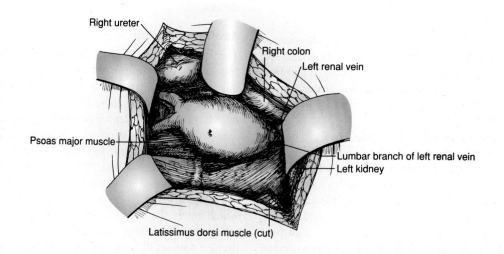

Figure 111.6 Exposure of the retroperitoneum

parietal peritoneum. After the appropriate plane is entered, blunt dissection can be carried anteriorly, displacing the descending colon, lower pole of the kidneys, renal vein, left gonadal vein, and retroperitoneal tissues from the flank muscles and aorta. Any communication between the left renal vein and either a segmental lumbar vein, an ascending lumbar vein, or the beginning of the azygos vein (all of which aid in the drainage of the posterior body wall) should be identified and ligated to prevent avulsion.

This technique has several anatomic advantages, including excellent exposure of the major arteries (aorta; left common, external, and internal iliac arteries; and left renal arteries), displacement of the ureter with minimal damage to its blood supply (because the blood supply to the ureter enters from its medial aspect), and easy retraction and visualization of the left renal vein and its tributaries. The primary disadvantage of this

approach is that exposure of the right common, external, and internal iliac arteries is somewhat compromised, as is exposure of the right renal artery.

Aortofemoral Bypass Graft

Groin Incisions (Fig. 111.7)

Technical Points

If aortobifemoral bypass is planned, expose the femoral vessels before entering the abdomen. This minimizes heat and fluid loss from the peritoneal cavity.

In each groin, make a 10-cm long, longitudinal incision over the femoral pulse. To adequately expose the common femoral artery, the incision should start at the level of the inguinal ligament which is about 4 cm proximal to the groin crease.

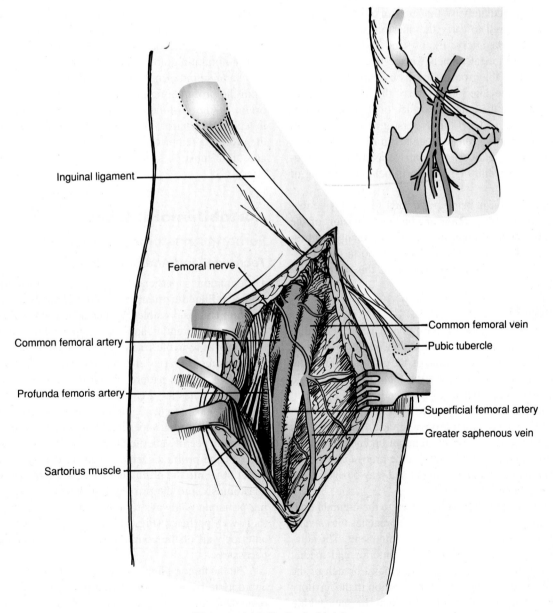

Figure 111.7 Groin incisions

If femoral pulses are absent, base your incision on bony landmarks beginning midway between the anterosuperior iliac spine and the pubic tubercle.

Figure 111.7 shows the exposed femoral arteries. Injury of the femoral nerve by excessive lateral dissection or retraction will result in quadriceps weakness and sensory loss of the anterior thigh. The femoral vein and its tributaries may be adherent to the arteries, especially during redo operations, and thus are susceptible to injury during dissection. The common femoral artery has several branches at the level of the inguinal ligament that may need to be dissected and temporarily controlled to expose a sufficient length of the femoral artery for clamping and arteriotomy. When dissecting the femoral bifurcation, look out for the circumflex femoral vein that crosses the origin of the profunda artery on its way to the femoral vein medially. This needs to be ligated and divided to expose the proximal profunda. The profunda femoris artery frequently branches almost immediately, so that control of more than one branch may be required to carry the anastomosis down over the proximal profunda artery. Expose the abdominal aorta. Then create retroperitoneal tunnels for the limbs of the graft from the abdomen to the groins. Do this by careful blunt finger dissection over the anterior surface of the femoral arteries from below and over the anterior surface of the iliac arteries from above. Be sure to keep the ureters anterior to the tunnels to avoid their obstruction between the graft and the native artery and to prevent tearing any small veins that could produce troublesome bleeding. Give heparin before clamping of vessels.

When the operation is being performed for occlusive disease, the surgeon has the option of complete division of the aorta with end-to-end anastomosis or, less commonly, end-to-side anastomosis to the anterior wall of the aorta (not illustrated). The completed abdominal portion of this operation is shown in Figure 111.7.

Anatomic Points

The femoral artery lies between the femoral nerve (laterally) and the femoral vein (medially) and within the femoral triangle, approximately at the midpoint of the inguinal ligament. Hence a vertical incision to expose the femoral artery should be located approximately halfway along the inguinal ligament, regardless of the presence or absence of a pulse in this area. Keep in mind that the inguinal groove (crease) is a cutaneous and subcutaneous reflection of the inguinal ligament. Because of the pendulous nature of these tissues, the groove is typically 3 to 4 cm distal to the inguinal ligament and may be even more distal in obese patients.

Almost immediately after passing deep to the inguinal ligament to enter the thigh, the femoral nerve branches into a variable number of cutaneous and muscular components. The cutaneous branches provide sensation to the anterior and medial thigh distal to the incision, whereas the femoral branch of the genitofemoral nerve is responsible for sensation in the territory of the incision. The genitofemoral nerve may be seen within the femoral sheath, superficial and lateral to the femoral artery.

Retract the nerve laterally when exposing the artery. Two branches of the femoral nerve (the saphenous nerve, which provides sensation to the medial leg and posteromedial foot, and the nerve to the vastus medialis muscle) may be injured in skeletonizing the femoral artery. These nerves are also within the femoral sheath and lie lateral to the femoral artery in the area of dissection. The saphenous nerve crosses the femoral artery within the adductor canal (of Hunter). Other important branches of the femoral nerve provide innervation to the anterior thigh muscles. Again, these nerves remain lateral to the artery, so that they are endangered by excessive lateral dissection or retraction.

Typically, three superficial branches of the femoral artery—the superficial epigastric, superficial circumflex iliac, and superficial external pudendal arteries—originate just distal to the inguinal ligament. Although these all anastomose with other arteries and thus can be sacrificed, a reasonable effort should be made to preserve them for their potential contribution to collateral circulation. The branches of the profunda femoris artery that may create problems are the medial and lateral femoral circumflex arteries. Either or both of these arteries can arise independently from the femoral artery instead of from the profunda femoris artery, or they may be so near the origin of the profunda femoris artery as to necessitate their independent control. The profunda femoris vein lies anterior to the profunda femoris artery and posterior to the femoral artery and often must be sacrificed to expose the profunda femoris artery.

Aortobifemoral Graft

Femoral Anastomoses (Fig. 111.8)

Technical and Anatomic Points

The common, superficial, and profunda femoris arteries are all clamped. Plan the orientations of these clamps so that they are as atraumatic as possible. When plaque is present, it frequently is not circumferential, and the clamp should be placed in such a manner as to avoid fracturing the plaque. The type of femoral anastomosis varies and depends on the peculiarities of the individual disease pattern. When the common femoral artery and its branches are free of disease, it is acceptable to place the anastomosis to the common femoral artery, often overriding the origin of the superficial femoral artery. Because of the high incidence of superficial femoral artery occlusion and stenosis of the profunda femoris orifice, it may be necessary to direct flow into the profunda by extending the arteriotomy and anastomosis into the proximal profunda femoris. An overriding principle is always to make sure that the profunda femoris is well perfused (Fig. 111.8). Begin the arteriotomy in the anterior wall of the common femoral artery and extend it as necessary.

Cut the femoral limbs of the graft obliquely, making them an appropriate length to provide tension-free anastomosis without redundant graft. A preferred approach is to use 5-0 continuous polypropylene suture and parachute the anastomosis beginning

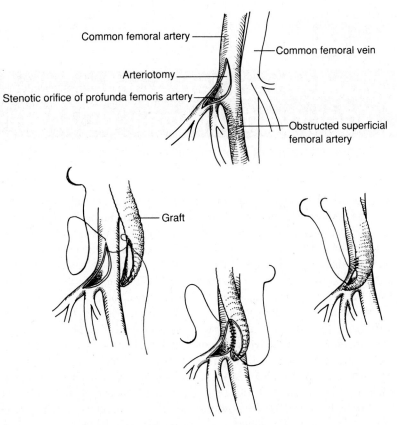

Figure 111.8 Femoral anastomoses

outside to in on the graft two bites away from the heel on the side away. This is continued toward the operator for two bites around the heel and then pulled down. The anastomosis is continued with the same needle toward the toe of the graft and completed where it was begun. This method allows the heel and toe of the anastomosis (the critical portion) to be done open under direct vision and minimizes needle and suture changing. Allow the arteries to back bleed. Flush the graft before completing the anastomosis and removing all clamps.

In vascular surgery, the groin is the most common site for wound separation and infection. To provide maximum tissue coverage over the grafts, close the wound in three layers.

REFERENCES

1. AbuRahma AF, Robinson PA, Boland JP, et al. The risk of ligation of the left renal vein in resection of the abdominal aortic aneurysm. *Surg Gynecol Obstet.* 1991;173(1):33–36.
2. Cambria RP, Brewster DC, Abbott WM, et al. Transperitoneal versus retroperitoneal approach for aortic reconstruction: A randomized prospective study. *J Vasc Surg.* 1990;11(2):314–324.
3. Ferguson LRJ, Bergan JJ, Conn J Jr, et al. Spinal ischemia following abdominal aortic surgery. *Ann Surg.* 1975;181:267–272.
4. Sharp WJ, Bashir M, Word R, et al. Suprarenal clamping is a safe method of aortic control when infrarenal clamping is not desirable. *Ann Vasc Surg.* 2008;22(4):534–540.
5. Sharp WJ, Hoballah JJ, Mohan CR, et al. The management of the infected aortic prosthesis: A current decade of experience. *J Vasc Surg.* 1994;19(5):844–850.
6. Sicard GA, Allen BT, Munn JS, et al. Retroperitoneal versus transperitoneal approach for repair of abdominal aortic aneurysms. *Surg Clin North Am.* 1989;69:795–806.
7. Truty MJ, Bower TC. Congenital anomalies of the inferior vena cava and left renal vein: Implications during open abdominal aortic aneurysm reconstruction. *Ann Vasc Surg.* 2007;21(2):186–197.
8. Veith FJ, Gupta S, Daly V. Technique for occluding the supraceliac aorta through the abdomen. *Surg Gynecol Obstet.* 1980;151:426–428. (Provides clear description of emergency exposure and control of the aorta at the hiatus.)
9. de Virgilio C, Gloviczki P. Aortic reconstruction in patients with horseshoe or ectopic kidneys. *Semin Vasc Surg.* 1996;9(3):245–252.

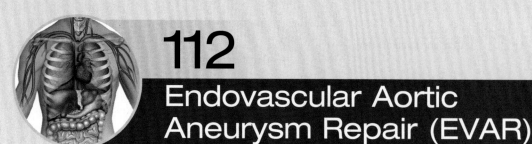

112

Endovascular Aortic Aneurysm Repair (EVAR)

Kristine Clodfelter Orion and Rachael Nicholson

Indications for aneurysm repair remain the same for both open and endovascular techniques. However, the choice of technique is dependent upon morphologic characteristics of the patient's aneurysm. When determining whether or not a patient is a candidate for endovascular repair of an abdominal aortic aneurysm (EVAR), anatomic criteria that need to be evaluated include the diameter and length of the normal aortic segment between the lowest renal artery and the proximal extent of the aneurysm (the neck), angulation of the neck, adequacy of the distal landing site, patency and degree of aneurysmal and/or occlusive disease within iliac and femoral arteries. The exact anatomic dimensions vary slightly by device manufacturer. Currently there are several companies producing stent grafts for aneurysm repair with many variations in their individual product design. As devices have evolved, anatomic requirements have changed and will continue to transform as technology advances.

The technique for performing EVAR has also progressed, so that the procedure can now be performed completely percutaneously, in well-chosen patients (as shown here), rather than through the standard exposure of the common femoral arteries through two transverse groin incisions. Detailed analysis of preoperative imaging is essential for the determination of a patient's EVAR candidacy, choice of stent graft, as well as operative approach. The following is a description of the basic steps of a percutaneous, two-piece endograft placement for an isolated infrarenal abdominal aortic aneurysm with normal iliac and common femoral arteries.

SCORE™, the Surgical Council on Resident Education, classified endovascular repair of aortic aneurysm as a "COMPLEX" procedure.

LIST OF STRUCTURES

Aorta
Common, external, and internal iliac arteries
Common femoral, superficial femoral,
    profunda arteries
Femoral nerve
Renal arteries
Celiac artery

Superior mesenteric artery
Inferior mesenteric artery
Lumbar arteries
Pubic tubercle
Anterosuperior iliac spine
Inguinal ligament

STEPS IN PROCEDURE

Mark bilateral pedal pulses
Use ultrasound to mark the common femoral
    artery bifurcation
Prep the patient from nipple to knees
Obtain bilateral common femoral arterial
    access
Exchange micropuncture sheath and place
    guidewire
Position two percutaneous closure devices and
    replace these with 9-Fr sheaths
Systemic heparinization (100 U/kg)
Place guidewire and catheter into the proximal
    descending thoracic aorta and exchange
    wire

Mark distal extent of wire on the table to
    avoid inadvertent advancement of the
    wire during the remainder of the case
Under fluoroscopy exchange 9-Fr sheaths for
    large bore sheaths
Obtain lateral fluoroscopic view
Select the main body of endograft.
Advance the main body into the pararenal
    aorta and pull sheath back
Aortogram through a marking pigtail catheter
    near the renal arteries under magnified
    views
Position endograft to deploy just below the
    lowest renal artery and deploy

Deploy the main body of the stent graft

Inflate coda Balloon

Cannulate the contralateral gate of the main body and perform exchange for stiff wire

Place stiff wire back into the proximal descending thoracic aorta through the pigtail catheter

Pull contralateral sheath to a location distal to the hypogastric artery

Perform an angiogram

Advance contralateral sheath *with its dilator* into contralateral gate

Advance contralateral limb into the main body

Pull contralateral sheath into the external iliac artery and deploy the limb

Angioplasty area of graft-to-graft overlap (mandatory) as well as the distal landing sites (optional)

Perform completion angiogram to ensure no endoleak

Remove sheaths and close arteriotomies with percutaneous closure devices

Assess distal lower extremities for ischemia and distal embolization

Pitfalls and complications

Endoleak

Vascular injury due to advancing wires/catheters without direct fluoroscopic visualization

Embolization secondary to wire/catheter/graft manipulation

Thrombosis because of inadequate anticoagulation

Groin hematoma/lymphocele

Migration of endograft

Arteriovenous fistula

Renal failure

Bowel ischemia

Spinal cord ischemia

Stroke

Initial Access to the Femoral Artery (Fig. 112.1)

Technical Points

This procedure may be performed under general anesthesia, with a spinal block or with local anesthetic and monitored sedation depending on the surgeon and patient's preferences and overall surgical risk. It is vital that the patient be comfortable enough to prevent aberrant motion and disruption during fluoroscopy. Mark the pedal pulses bilaterally, and prep the patient from nipples to knees.

If performing the procedure percutaneously, take extreme care to ensure a clean puncture in the common femoral artery (Fig. 112.1A). Use fluoroscopy to mark the middle of the femoral head with a hemostat. In addition, use ultrasound to note the level of the femoral bifurcation (Fig. 112.1B). Ultrasound may be used to guide puncture of the common femoral artery as well. If after employing these measures, concerns remain about the quality and location of the puncture, inject contrast through the small caliber micropuncture sheath, confirming the accuracy of the puncture in the common femoral artery before committing to the large bore sheaths that will eventually be needed for the stent graft. Obtain bilateral common femoral arterial access using a micropuncture kit.

Exchange micropuncture sheath for 6-Fr sheaths. Place a Bentson guidewire, 150 cm (Cook, Inc., Bloomington, IN) through sheaths into distal aorta/proximal common iliac arteries. For the preclose technique using two devices, place these in the 10-o'clock and 2-o'clock positions. Replace percutaneous closure devices with 9-Fr sheaths.

At this point, initiate systemic heparinization (100 U/kg). Place Glidewire (Terumo Medical Corporation, Somerset, NJ) and Glidecath (Terumo Medical Corporation, Somerset, NJ)

into the proximal descending thoracic aorta. Exchange Glidewire through Glidecath for an exchange length stiff wire, such as Amplatz Super Stiff Guide Wire, 260 cm (Boston Scientific, Natick, MA). Mark the distal extent of wire on the table to avoid inadvertent advancement of the wire during the remainder of the case.

Utilization of large bore sheaths demands attentiveness in all patients, but particularly in patients with diseased iliac arteries and/or previously stented iliac arteries to avoid iliac rupture or iliac avulsion. Avoid retrograde advancements of such sheaths without their dilators. Resistance to sheath advancement should be a warning to consider alternative approaches. Balloon angioplasty or serial dilatation with vascular dilators can be performed in a controlled fashion. Alternatively, if iliac access remains difficult serious thought should be given to either an open surgical conduit through a small retroperitoneal incision or an endovascular conduit utilizing a large caliber stent graft to purposely rupture the common and external iliac arteries to the point of access in the common femoral arteries. Concern about sheath access or hemodynamic compromise of the patient should prompt rapid angiographic assessment to evaluate for arterial disruption.

Anatomic Points

The common femoral artery is the continuation of the external iliac artery below the inguinal ligament. It lies in the lateral to the common femoral vein and medial to the femoral nerve and bifurcates into the superficial femoral artery and the profunda femoris artery. There is usually a notable decrease in caliber at the bifurcation. Mistaken puncture of the external iliac, superficial femoral, or profunda arteries leads to higher rates of access-related complications such as pseudoaneurysms, dissections, hematomas, extravasation, and thrombosis.

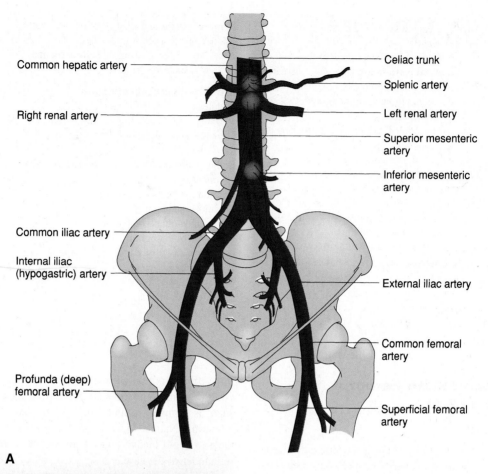

Common hepatic artery

Right renal artery

Common iliac artery

Internal iliac
(hypogastric) artery

Profunda (deep)
femoral artery

Celiac trunk

Splenic artery

Left renal artery

Superior mesenteric
artery

Inferior mesenteric
artery

External iliac artery

Common femoral
artery

Superficial femoral
artery

A

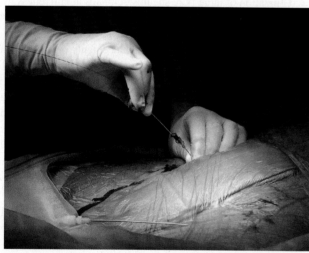

B

Figure 112.1 A: Anatomy of the abdominal aorta and iliac branches (from Greenfield's Textbook of Surgery, Philadelphia, PA, 2013, with permission). **B:** Percutaneous access of the common femoral artery using a micropuncture kit after fluoroscopic localization of the femoral head. Note on left groin, the marking of the common femoral artery bifurcation by ultrasound.

Particularly with the use of the large sheaths required for EVAR, it is important to avoid puncture of vessels other than the common femoral artery. In obese and even overweight patients, the inguinal crease can be misleading often resulting in a puncture below the femoral bifurcation in either the profunda femoris or the superficial femoral artery. Bony landmarks are more liable. Therefore, palpate the anterosuperior iliac spine and pubic tubercle to determine the location of the inguinal ligament. As described earlier, fluoroscopic localization of the femoral head and ultrasound determination of the femoral bifurcation can avoid this complication.

The nerve is the most lateral structure in the femoral sheath. Traveling lateral to medial are the artery and vein, respectively. Injury to the femoral nerve can occur with compression from hematoma or direct injury during the course of a groin dissection. The Mackiewicz sign to evaluate for femoral nerve injury can be tested with the patient prone by lifting the thigh in one hand and bending the knee slowly with the other to see if severe pain in the anterior thigh and groin can be elicited.

In addition to using preoperative imaging to assess an aneurysm to determine if it meets the morphologic criteria for EVAR, the CT scan should also be thoroughly studied to gather information about the patient's mesenteric and hypogastric arteries. For example, performing an EVAR in the setting of an occluded or severely stenotic superior mesenteric artery with a patent inferior mesenteric artery and a large meandering branch in a patient with poor collateral through the celiac artery or hypogastric arteries could lead to catastrophic small bowel infarct.

Spinal cord ischemia is a rare, but devastating complication of endovascular infrarenal aortic aneurysm repair. It can occur immediate following repair or in a delayed fashion. Although the mechanism is not completely understood, atheroembolization, disruption of collateral circulation to the spinal cord, and intraoperative hypotension are thought to play significant roles.

The blood supply to the spinal cord is provided by longitudinal arteries which originate from the vertebral arteries, one large anterior spinal artery and two smaller posterolateral spinal arteries. The anterior spinal artery resides in the anterior median sulcus and supplies 75% of the spinal cord. The anterior spinal artery is supplied by intercostal and lumbar arteries which come directly from the aorta. The artery of Adamkiewicz is the largest feeding vessel which comes off the aorta most commonly between T9 and T12, although it can arise between T7 and L4.

In most patients, the renal arteries originate from the aorta between T12 and L2. So repair of an infrarenal aortic aneurysm usually does not involve occluding the artery of Adamkiewicz, unless it has an aberrantly low takeoff from the aorta. However, deployment of an infrarenal stent graft does cover the origins of the inferior mesenteric artery and infrarenal lumbar arteries which can be important collaterals for the spinal cord. In addition, patients with aneurysmal disease can have diseased hypogastric arteries which serve as collateral arterial supply to the spine. At times, a hypogastric artery might need to be embolized in order to successfully place an endograft which interrupts this potential arterial pathway.

Placement of Graft (Fig. 112.2)

Technical and Anatomic Points

Under fluoroscopy, exchange the 9-Fr sheaths for large bore sheaths (18 to 24 Fr for the main body and 12 to 20 Fr for the contralateral limb). Obtain lateral fluoroscopic view to define anterior/posterior orientation of each sheath.

If preoperative imaging is adequate to determine length of graft needed, advance selected main body of endograft into the pararenal aorta and pull sheath back to ensure the stent graft will not deploy within the sheath. If preoperative imaging is inadequate to determine length of graft needed, perform an angiogram of aorta through a marking pigtail catheter (Cook, Inc., Bloomington, IN) to measure the distance from lowest renal artery to the hypogastric artery. Select the appropriate endograft.

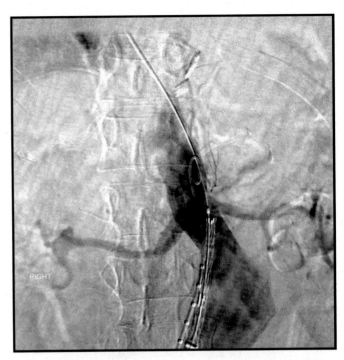

Figure 112.2 Magnified view of the renal arteries with the main body stent graft nearby just prior to deployment.

Advance the main body of the endograft into the pararenal aorta and pull the sheath back. Perform an aortogram through a marking pigtail catheter near the renal arteries under magnified views.

Position the endograft to deploy just below the lowest renal artery. Deploy the main body of the stent graft. Inflate coda Balloon (Cook Inc., Bloomington, IN) to specified diameter in the neck of the endograft. Cannulate the contralateral gate of the main body with a Glidewire and angled catheter (e.g., multipurpose catheter). Exchange the catheter for pigtail catheter, turning formed catheter within the main body to confirm intraluminal cannulation. Place stiff wire back into the proximal descending thoracic aorta through the pigtail catheter. Pull contralateral sheath to a location distal to the hypogastric artery.

Perform an angiogram with the image intensifier at a 30- to 45-degree angle to mark location of hypogastric origin and to measure the distance from contralateral gate to the hypogastric artery in order to choose the length of the contralateral limb. Advance contralateral sheath with its dilator into contralateral gate. Advance the contralateral limb into the main body, overlapping according to manufacturer's specifications. Pull the contralateral sheath into the external iliac artery and deploy the limb. Use noncompliant balloon angioplasty to the area of graft-to-graft overlap (mandatory) as well as the distal landing sites (optional).

Completion of Procedure (Fig. 112.3)

Technical and Anatomic Points

Perform a completion angiogram to ensure that there is no endoleak. Remove sheaths and close arteriotomies with percutaneous closure devices.

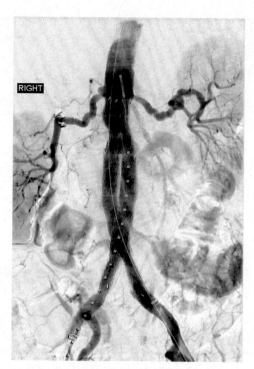

Figure 112.3 Completion angiogram of EVAR demonstrating filling in both renal arteries and hypogastric arteries.

When closing the arteriotomies with percutaneous closure devices, have your assistant hold pressure above the puncture site by an assistant while you tighten the sutures. Maintain wire access until closure success is considered likely. If there is apprehension about hemostasis, an additional closure device can be placed if the wire is retained until the very end. Should there be any doubt about the adequacy of hemostasis, consider cutting down on the femoral artery.

Assess distal lower extremities for ischemia and distal embolization.

Renal artery compromise can occur as a result of embolization of mural thrombus, dissection from vagrant wires, or the unintentional deployment of the stent graft over the renal artery orifice. In the setting of embolization, attempts at suction thrombectomy should be made. If wire access can be achieved in the case of a dissection, the artery can be stented. If the renal artery orifice is covered by the endograft, an attempt to bring the graft to a more distal location can be done by inflating a coda balloon and pulling the graft toward the aortic bifurcation. Clearly this should be done only with prudence as it carries the risk of aortic rupture, especially if the graft has proximal barbs. If the origin of the renal artery is only partially covered, attempts should be made to gain wire entry into the renal artery and to place a stent or stent graft in a chimney- or snorkel-style fashion to ensure adequate flow into the kidney. Antegrade access from the brachial artery might be needed in order for this maneuver to be successful. If both renal arteries are inadvertently covered in a reasonable surgical candidate, open revascularization should be contemplated rather than commit the patient to permanent dialysis.

REFERENCES

1. Anson BJ, McVay CB. The vertebral column and spinal cord. In: *Anson and McVay's Surgical Anatomy,* 6th ed. Philadelphia, PA: Saunders. 1984:990–992.
2. Bajwa A, Davis M, Moawad M, et al. "Paraplegia Following Elective Endovascular Repair of Abdominal Aortic Aneurysm: Reversal with Cerebrospinal Fluid Drainage" *Eur J Vasc Endovasc Surg.* 2008;35:46–48.
3. Kouvelos GN, Papa N, Nassis C, et al. "Spinal Cord Ischemia After Endovascular Repair of Infrarenal Abdominal Aortic Aneurysm: A Rare Complication." Case Reports in Medicine Vol 2011, Article ID 953472, pp. 1–4.
4. Ohryi A. "Dr. Jacob Mackiewica (1887-1966) and his sign." *J Med Biogr.* 2007;15(2):102–103.
5. Reid JA, Mole DJ, Johnston LC, et al. "Delayed paraplegia after endovascular repair of abdominal aortic aneurysm" *J Vasc Surg.* 2003;37:1322–1323.
6. Hinchliffe RJ, Hopkinson BR. Mastery of endovascular surgical treatment of abdominal aortic aneurysm. In: Zewlenock GB, Huber TS, Messina LM, et al., eds. *Mastery of Vascular and Endovascular Surgery.* Philadelphia, PA: Lippincott Williams & Wilkins; 2006: 139–145.

e 113 Lumbar Sympathectomy

This chapter can be accessed online at www.lww.com/eChapter113.

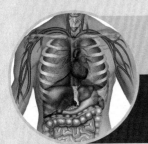

114

Insertion of Inferior Vena Cava Filters

Parth B. Amin and Joss D. Fernandez

Inferior vena cava filters have supplanted surgical interruption of the vena cava in the prevention of venous thrombotic embolic events. The ease of implantation has resulted in an increase and varied use despite very specific role they play in the management of patients with venous thromboembolic (VTE) disease. At present, the only absolute indications for placement include patient populations with (1) the development of a pulmonary embolus (PE) while on therapeutic anticoagulation and (2) an absolute contraindication to anticoagulation in patients with deep venous thrombosis (DVT). Relative indications include prophylaxis in patient who cannot be anticoagulated but are at high risk for DVT and those patients who have had a PE with continued residual DVT and may not tolerate another PE event. It is important to note that IVC filters may reduce episodes of pulmonary embolism, but have not been shown to reduce mortality. Long term, IVC filters are associated with an increased risk of lower extremity venous insufficiency. Other complications of IVC filters include migration, perforation of the vena cava or bowel, and complete thrombosis.

The two preferred routes of access are a right transfemoral venous approach and right transjugular venous approach. Alternative access sites include the left femoral and jugular veins and the left or right subclavian veins. Fluoroscopic guidance is the primary method used and will be the primary focus of this chapter. Both transabdominal and intravascular ultrasound have been used to guide successful placement of IVC filters. A brief discussion of suprarenal filters, congenital venous anomalies, and other special situations are also included in this text.

SCORE™, the Surgical Council on Resident Education, classified insertion of inferior vena cava filter as an "ESSENTIAL COMMON" procedure.

STEPS IN PROCEDURE

Choose approach
Transfemoral approach versus internal jugular
   approach
Access the vein percutaneously and dilate it
Perform cavogram

Measure IVC diameter
Identify renal veins
Deploy device
Withdraw wires and delivery device

HALLMARK ANATOMIC COMPLICATIONS

Femoral arterial puncture
Carotid arterial puncture
Groin hematoma
Neck hematoma

Pneumothorax
Hemothorax
Deep venous thrombosis
Iliac vein perforation

IVC thrombosis
Renal vein thrombosis

LIST OF STRUCTURES
Anterior superior iliac spine
Pubic tubercle
Inguinal ligament
Femoral artery
Superficial femoral artery
Profunda femoris artery
Femoral vein
Right and left iliac veins
Inferior vena cava
Hepatic veins

Filter migration
Filter erosion

Right atrium
Right and left renal veins
Lumbar veins
Carotid artery
Sternocleidomastoid muscle
Sternal head
Clavicular head
Subclavian vein
Superior vena cava
Innominate vein

Placement of Inferior Vena Cava Filter (Fig. 114.1)

Multiple devices have been approved by the Food and Drug Administration for prevention of VTE disease (Table 114.1). Some examples are shown in Figure 114.1. Although the specific mechanisms by which different manufacturers design deployment devices varies, the basic principles of placement are similar. Familiarize yourself with the device that you plan to use.

A right transjugular approach or right transfemoral approach is most often selected. Identification of anatomic landmarks is paramount and can be facilitated by ultrasound in difficult situations.

Femoral Vein Approach (Fig. 114.2)

Local anesthetic is administered in the skin overlying the planned puncture site. Initial percutaneous access is then performed. This can be done using a standard Seldinger-type needle. A Micropuncture introducer set (Cook Incorporated, Bloomington, Indiana) is often used for initial percutaneous entry. This allows for the placement of a low-profile 0.018-inch wire into a 21-gauge Seldinger-type needle. Exchange can then be performed for a 4-French coaxial catheter, which allows for a 0.035-inch wire to be placed into the vena cava. Inadvertent arterial puncture is better tolerated with this system than a standard 18-gauge needle, although in experienced hands, complication rates are low with both methods even when patients are fully anticoagulated.

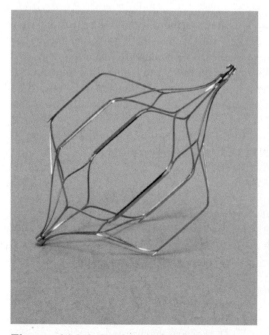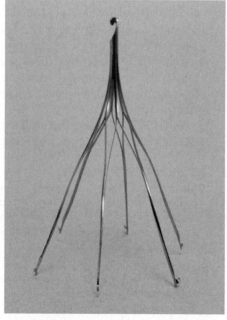

Figure 114.1 Representative types of vena cava filter devices (from Fischer's Mastery of Surgery, with permission).

Table 114.1 Characteristics of IVC Filter Devices Available in the United States

	Initial FDA Approval	Updated Approval	Temporary or Permanent	Maximum IVC Size	Access Route	MRI Compatible
B Braun Medical Inc. (Bethlehem, PA, USA)						
VenaTech(TM) LP IVC filter	2001	N/A	Permanent	35 mm	IJ/Fem	Yes
VenaTech(TM) LGM IVC filter	1989	2001	Retrievable	28 mm	IJ/Fem	Yes
CR Bard, Inc. (Murray Hill, NJ, USA)						
G2	2005	2008	Permanent	28 mm	IJ/SC/Fem	Yes
G2X	2005	2008	Both available	28 mm	IJ/SC/Fem	Yes
Eclipse	2010	N/A	Both available	28 mm	IJ/Fem	Yes
Simon Nitinol	1990	N/A	Permanent	28 mm	IJ/SC/Fem/ Brach	
ALN Implants Chirurgicaux (Ghisonaccia, France)						
ALN Optional	2008	N/A	Retrievable	28 mm	IJ/Fem/Brach	Yes
Boston Scientific (Natick, MA, USA)						
Titanium Greenfield	1989	N/A	Permanent	28 mm	IJ/Fem	Yes
Cordis Corp. (Bridgewater, NJ, USA)						
TrapEase	2001	2002	Permanent	30 mm	Fem	Yes
OptEase	2002	2010	Both	28 mm	Fem	Yes
Cook Medical, Inc. (Bloomington, IN, USA)						
Celect	2008	2009	Temporary	30 mm	IJ/Fem	Yes
Gunther-Tulip	2003	2009	Temporary	30 mm	IJ/Fem	Yes
Gianturco-Roehm Bird's Nest	1989	2008	Permanent	40 mm	IJ/Fem	MRI Conditional
Rex Medical, L.P. (Conshohocken, PA, USA)						
Rex Medical Option	2009	N/A	Retrievable	30 mm	IJ/Fem	Yes
Rafael Medical Technologies, Inc. (Dover, DE, USA)						
SafeFlo	2009	N/A	Permanent	27 mm	IJ/Fem	Yes

Once a 0.035-inch wire is advanced under fluoroscopy from the femoral vein, into the iliac venous system, and eventually into the inferior vena cava (IVC). It is preferable to begin with a wire which the IVC filter delivery device will track over. A small transverse skin incision should then be made around the wire to facilitate placement of an angiographic catheter into the femoral vein. Under fluoroscopic guidance this is advanced into the IVC.

The approximate level of the renal veins is just above the junction of the second and third lumbar vertebrae interspace. This can be found radiographically, by using the twelfth rib as a landmark for the twelfth thoracic vertebra. The lumbar vertebra simply needs to be counted to arrive at the approximate level of the renal veins. This approximation needs confirmation with venography. Approximately 10 mL of diluted contrast is then injected into the vena cava using digital subtraction angiography. The contrast can be immediately followed by heparinized saline. Once the renal veins are identified and the size of the vena cava is measured (Fig. 114.2A), the IVC filter deployment device can be inserted through the femoral vein.

A series of dilators is often necessary for the larger delivery devices (12 French). Advance the delivery device into the IVC and deploy it according the instructions for use for each respective device. Take care to deploy below the renal veins. Perform a completion venogram to assure proper deployment, orientation, and location (Fig. 114.2B). Remove the wires and catheters, hold manual pressure, and place a sterile dressing on the wound.

Anatomic Points

The inguinal ligament can be envisioned by drawing a line from the anterior superior iliac spine to the pubic tubercle. This ligament forms the anatomic boundary where the external iliac artery becomes the common femoral artery. The common femoral artery generally bisects the inguinal ligament and can be used as a landmark for the common femoral vein. By finding the midpoint of the inguinal ligament, the femoral pulsation is identified. The common femoral vein is identified 1 cm distally and 1 cm medial to this bisection point.

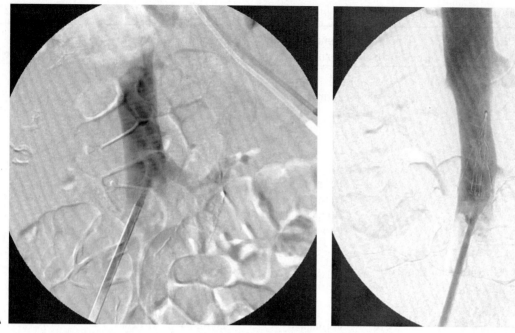

Figure 114.2 A: Cavogram from the right femoral venous approach identifying left renal vein. **B:** Proper deployment in inferior vena cava below both renal veins.

The superficial femoral vein, so-named as it accompanies the corresponding artery, and the profunda femoris vein join to drain into the common femoral vein. The superficial femoral vein is currently referred to as the femoral vein to minimize confusion regarding its status as a deep vein. The great saphenous vein, in addition to multiple tributaries, also drains into the common femoral vein. Again, at the inguinal ligament, the external iliac vein arises and continues to drain into the common iliac vein as the internal iliac vein joins it. The common iliac venous confluence into the IVC is formed at the fifth lumbar vertebra. Posteriorly, the ascending lumbar vein drains into the IVC. The gonadal vein drains into the IVC at around L2, the renal veins at around L1, and the hepatic veins at around T8 before emptying into the right atrium.

Internal Jugular Vein Approach (Fig. 114.3)

Technical Points

An internal jugular approach can also be performed. The right internal jugular is the preferred route of access in these cases, and ultrasound guidance is becoming more commonplace as is low-profile Seldinger needle systems, due to the potential for inadvertent carotid puncture. Similarly, a cavogram needs to be performed. If an IVC filter is placed from the jugular method, confirmation of wire access into the IVC needs to be the rule and some advocate wire access into an iliac vein to avoid tracking the device into the right atrium. Manufacturers specify the route of access in the indications for use materials (IFU) provided with each device.

Anatomic Points

The right internal jugular vein is found lateral to the common carotid artery and posteromedial to the sternocleidomastoid muscle (SCM). It is often paralleled to the external jugular vein, which is located more superficially. The medial border of the sternocleidomastoid muscle is easily palpable and exposure is

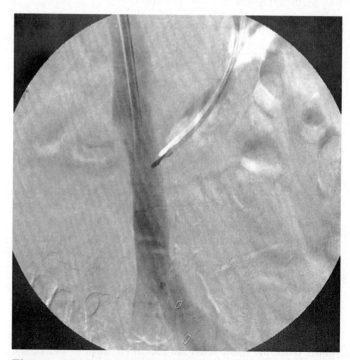

Figure 114.3 Cavogram from internal jugular approach identifying both iliac veins.

facilitated by positioning the head in slight extension and turned toward the left side. As the SCM is followed from the upper neck to the root of the neck, the sternal head and clavicular head arise and attach to the corresponding bony landmarks. The junction of the SCM with its two heads is the ideal place for internal jugular vein access. This is primarily due to the fact that the gap in musculature allows for access without going through the SCM, as might be required further up in the neck. The internal jugular vein will be lateral to the carotid artery at this level.

The right internal jugular vein drainage meets the right subclavian vein to drain into the right brachiocephalic vein. The right brachiocephalic vein and left brachiocephalic vein meet to drain into the superior vena cava (SVC) at the level of the first costal cartilage. Multiple smaller veins drain into each brachiocephalic vein along the way, including the respective internal mammary veins, inferior thyroidal veins, vertebral veins, and supreme intercostal veins. At the level of the third costal cartilage, the SVC drains into the right atrium.

The venous drainage of spinal column drains into the ascending lumbar veins and eventually into the azygous system, which serves as an indirect pathway connecting the SVC and IVC via respective separate large tributaries. The main draining tributary to the SVC is just beyond the confluence of both brachiocephalic veins. The course of the draining vein to the IVC is more variable, but is often just above the location of the renal veins.

Special Circumstances

Megacava

Although a minority of cases, there are certain anatomic and clinical situations which require an alternate approach to IVC filter placement. The most common issue constraint is the presence of a megacava. This is defined as an IVC diameter greater than or equal to 28 mm. Usually, it is much larger, and there are multiple options for IVC filter placement in this setting. The Bird's Nest Filter (Cook Medical Inc., Bloomington, IN) is most commonly used, although there are multiple IVC filters available for 30-mm diameter veins. Another option is to place a standard IVC filter in each iliac vein.

Duplicated IVC

A duplicated IVC results from failure of regression of the left supracardinal vein during development and occurs in up to 3% of the population. A right and left IVC are present and converge at the level of the renal veins. It requires a filter in both the right and left IVC. Alternatively, a suprarenal filter can be placed with the same technique described, but deployment is just above the superior-most renal vein.

IVC Thrombus

A suprarenal filter also needs to be placed if there is thrombus in the IVC. The approach is usually through the right internal jugular approach, although devices which can be advanced

through brachial, left internal jugular, and either subclavian routes are manufactured. A similar principle can be applied if there are bilateral iliofemoral DVT.

Circumaortic Renal Collar

A circumaortic renal vein can be present and can act as a separate pathway from the IVC for embolic phenomenon. A suprarenal IVC filter can be placed in this situation so as to place it just below the renal collar. Alternatively an IVC filter can be placed in each iliac limb.

SVC Filter Placement

SVC filter placement has also been described for upper extremity DVT, although the orientation of the filter needs to be reversed. This can be accomplished by the placement of a standard jugular approach filter through the femoral vein and vice-versa. Filters placed in the SVC position may compromise future placement of upper extremity central lines.

Pregnancy

IVC filters that were placed prior to pregnancy are generally safe to patient and fetus. Patients with acute thromboembolic events during pregnancy may benefit from suprarenal placement of the fetal to prevent compression and tilting due to the gravid uterus and to protect against gonadal vein thromboembolic events.

Temporary and Retrievable Filters

In order to prevent the long-term complications of IVC filters, a family of temporary or retrievable filters has been designed for patients with transient indications for filter placement. Temporary filters often have tether wires that allow extraction of the filter. Retrievable filters are designed to be recaptured into sheaths and often have a hook or other mechanism to allow snaring. These filters are engineered to prolong dwell time in the IVC which is limited by neointimal formation around the filter struts.

REFERENCES

1. Crowther MA. Inferior vena cava filters in the management of venous thromboembolism. *Am J Med.* 2007;120(10 suppl 2):S13–S17.
2. Joels CS, Sing RF, Heniford BT. Complications of inferior vena cava filters. *Am Surg.* 2003;69(8):654–659.
3. Malgor RD, Oropallo A, Wood E, et al. Filter placement for duplicated cava. *Vasc Endovascular Surg.* 2011;45(3):269–273.
4. PREPIC Study Group. Eight-year follow-up of patients with permanent vena cava filters in the prevention of pulmonary embolism: The PREPIC (Prevention du Risque d'Embolie Pulmonaire par Interruption Cave) randomized study. *Circulation.* 2005;112(3):416–422.
5. Streiff MB. Vena caval filters: A comprehensive review. *Blood.* 2000;95(12):3669–3677.
6. Young T, Tang H, Hughes R. Vena caval filters for the prevention of pulmonary embolism. *Cochrane Database Syst Rev.* 2010;(2):CD006212.

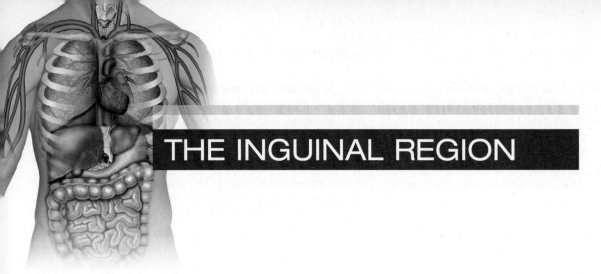

THE INGUINAL REGION

This anatomically complex region has been the subject of many books. In this part, inguinal and femoral hernia repairs and hydrocelectomy (Chapters 115 to 118) are illustrated. Inguinal lymph node dissection (Chapter 119) and sentinel node biopsy for melanoma of the trunk (Chapter 120) conclude the part, which serves as a transition to the next two sections: *The Sacral Region and Perineum* (Chapters 121 to 125) and *The Lower Extremity* (Chapters 126 to 134).

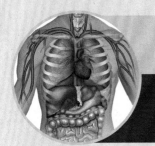

115

Repair of Inguinal and Femoral Hernias

The muscular and aponeurotic layers of the abdominal wall form a strong continuous barrier that supports and contains the intra-abdominal viscera. This continuous barrier is breached in the groin by the inguinal canal, an oblique passage from the abdomen to the scrotum (in the male) or to the labium majus (in the female). This anatomically complex area is a frequent site of hernia formation.

SCORE™, the Surgical Council on Resident Education, classified open repair of inguinal and femoral hernias as "ESSENTIAL COMMON" procedures.

STEPS IN PROCEDURE

Inguinal Hernia Repair

Skin crease incision

Incise aponeurosis of external oblique muscle from external ring laterally

Identify and preserve ilioinguinal nerve

Mobilize spermatic cord (or round ligament, in females)

Incise cremaster muscle fibers to expose spermatic cord fully

Seek indirect sac

If one is found, separate sac from cord structures, twist, and suture ligate (resecting redundant sac)

In female, divide and ligate round ligament with sac

Assess floor of canal and choose method of repair

Bassini Repair

Place Allis clamps on conjoined tendon and pull down

Create relaxing incision on fascia

Suture conjoined tendon to inguinal ligament with multiple interrupted sutures

In male, internal ring should admit Kelly clamp; in female, close internal ring completely

McVay Repair

Place Allis clamps on conjoined tendon and create relaxing incision as above

Clean Cooper ligament of overlying fatty and fibrous tissue

Suture conjoined tendon to Cooper ligament with multiple interrupted sutures

In vicinity of femoral vein, transition to inguinal ligament

Shouldice Repair

Incise transversalis fascia in direction of its fibers

Reflect superior leaf of transversalis fascia and clean underside, identify arch of aponeurosis of transversus abdominis muscle

Running monofilament suture from pubic tubercle toward internal ring; suture arch of aponeurosis to iliopubic tract

At internal ring, run suture line back toward pubic tubercle, suturing free edge of superior leaf to inguinal ligament and tie suture to itself

Begin third suture line at internal ring; suture conjoined tendon to inguinal ligament; at pubic tubercle, return suture line back to internal ring and tie suture to itself

Plug-and-Patch Repair

Define edges of any defect in transversalis fascia

Place preformed plug into the defect and tack it in place

Overly the patch over the floor of the canal, bringing the tails around the spermatic cord

Suture the patch in place

Closure of Canal after Repair

Check hemostasis and close external oblique aponeurosis with running suture (taking care to avoid iliohypogastric nerve)

Close fascia and skin

Femoral hernia repair

Repair from Below

Incision directly over femoral hernia, parallel to inguinal ligament

Isolate sac and open it

Reduce any contents (check for viability)

If necessary, incise inguinal ligament vertically to enlarge canal

Twist, suture ligate, and amputate the sac

Create a rolled "cigarette" of permanent mesh and insert it into the canal, suture in place
Suture inguinal ligament back together if necessary
Close subcutaneous tissues and skin

Repair from Above
Widely expose floor of inguinal canal as for inguinal hernia repair

Open floor of canal to expose femoral region
Identify sac as diverticulum of peritoneum extending down into leg
Open the sac and reduce the contents
Perform McVay repair as outlined above

HALLMARK ANATOMIC COMPLICATIONS

Missed hernia
Injury to ilioinguinal nerve
Injury to iliohypogastric nerve
Injury to genitofemoral nerve

Testicular edema or ischemia
Injury to femoral vein
Postherniorrhaphy pain

LIST OF STRUCTURES

Inguinal region
Processus vaginalis

External (Superficial) Inguinal Ring
Medial and lateral crura
Intercrural fibers
Internal (deep) inguinal ring
Hesselbach triangle

Inferior Epigastric Artery and Vein
Pubic branch of artery (accessory obturator artery)
Obturator artery
Superficial (Camper and Scarpa) fascia
Innominate fascia
External oblique muscle and aponeurosis
Internal oblique muscle and aponeurosis
Transversus abdominis muscle

Transversalis Fascia
Iliopubic tract
Transversalis fascial sling
Preperitoneal tissue
Peritoneum
Pubic tubercle
Inguinal ligament
Pectineal (Cooper) ligament
Lacunar ligament

Conjoined tendon
Interfoveolar ligament
Ilioinguinal nerve
Iliohypogastric nerve

Genitofemoral Nerve
Genital branch
Femoral canal
Femoral sheath

Femoral Artery and Vein
Greater saphenous vein
Saphenous hiatus
Fascia lata

Male
Spermatic cord
External spermatic fascia
Cremasteric muscle and fascia
Internal spermatic fascia
Vas deferens
Scrotum
Testis
Testicular vessels

Female
Round ligament
Labium majus

Three types of groin hernias are distinguishable clinically: Indirect inguinal, direct inguinal, and femoral. An individual may have one, two, or (occasionally) all three hernias within the same groin.

Indirect inguinal hernia is the most common hernia in both males and females. In the male, indirect inguinal hernia is associated with persistent patency of the processus vaginalis. Communicating hydroceles are closely related. The spermatic cord traverses the abdominal wall as it passes from the internal to the external ring to supply the testis. This produces an area of natural weakness in the male. In the female, the round ligament exits the abdomen to anchor in the labia majora and mons

pubis. Indirect hernias in females form in much the same way as do those seen in males.

Direct hernias are generally acquired as a result of weakness in the floor of the inguinal canal that allows intra-abdominal pressure to produce a bulge through the thinned-out transversalis fascia. Indirect hernias occur lateral to the inferior epigastric vessels, whereas direct hernias project straight through the floor of the canal in the region of Hesselbach triangle (Fig. 115.1), medial to the inferior epigastric vessels.

The femoral canal is inferior to the inguinal ligament. A *femoral hernia* occurs when weakness in the femoral canal allows herniation of peritoneum, followed by intra-abdominal

ORIENTATION

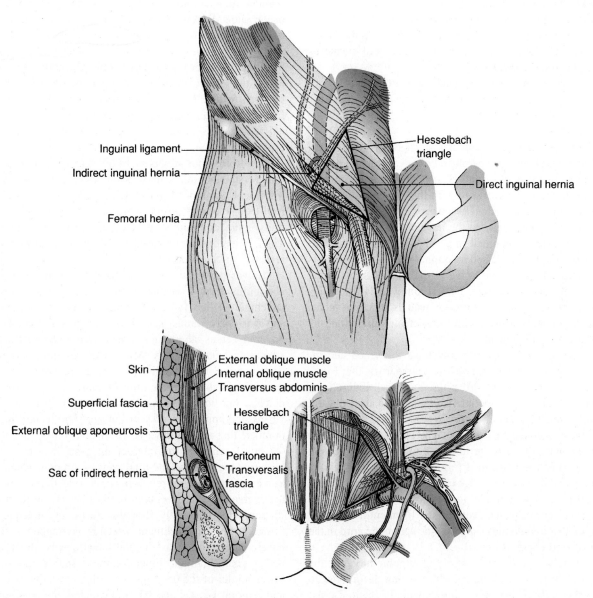

Figure 115.1 Regional anatomy

viscera, into the canal. Femoral hernias are seen most commonly in elderly patients. Small, incarcerated femoral hernias may feel exactly like enlarged lymph nodes. The combination of small bowel obstruction and palpable adenopathy in one groin should lead one to suspect an incarcerated femoral hernia.

In this chapter, four types of inguinal hernia repair—the Bassini, McVay, Shouldice, and plug-and-patch methods—are described. Femoral hernia repair from both below and above is described. References at the end of the chapter give details of other techniques, and laparoscopic herniorrhaphy is described in Chapter 116. Chapter 118 describes how to repair an inguinal hernia in an infant or young child.

Descriptions of the anatomy of the inguinal region are confusing, in part because the standard texts of anatomy are based on dissection of the embalmed cadaver (in which tissue planes are not nearly as definable as in fresh tissues) and in part because of the plethora of synonyms applied to structures in this region. Here, the terminology commonly used by surgeons is presented. (Because of the inherent complexity, a long orientation section is given here.)

The abdominal wall is multilayered. These layers can be classified as either superficial or deep, and they are mirror images of each other, with the reflecting plane being the internal oblique muscle. Thus, from superficial to deep, the following layers are encountered.

1. Skin
2. Superficial (Camper and Scarpa) fascia
3. "Outer" investing (innominate) fascia
4. External oblique muscle and aponeurosis
5. Internal oblique muscle and aponeurosis (Note: In the inguinal canal, the spermatic cord or round ligament of the uterus substitutes for this layer.)
6. Transversus abdominis muscle and aponeurosis
7. "Inner" investing or endoabdominal (transversalis) fascia
8. Preperitoneal tissue
9. Peritoneum

The inguinal canal is a triangular passageway through the body wall in which lies the spermatic cord or its female homolog, the round ligament of the uterus. Its entrance is the internal inguinal ring, which is associated with the transversalis fascia and which is located immediately superior to the middle of the inguinal ligament and lateral to the inferior epigastric vessels. Its exit is the external inguinal ring, which is associated with the external oblique muscle and innominate fascia and which is located immediately superior to the medial end of the inguinal ligament at the pubic tubercle. Its anterior wall is the external oblique aponeurosis, its posterior wall is the transversus abdominis aponeurosis fused with transversalis fascia, and its base is the inguinal ligament.

The inguinal ligament is the somewhat thickened and inrolled free edge of the external oblique aponeurosis that forms the inferior "shelving edge" of the inguinal canal. Laterally, it is attached to the anterosuperior iliac spine and the adjacent iliac fascia. Medially, it attaches to the pubic tubercle and adjacent pectineal ligament (of Cooper). The parallel fibers of the inguinal ligament that fan out to attach to the pubic tubercle and adjacent pectineal ligament form the lacunar ligament. It should be noted that the free edge of the lacunar ligament does not extend far enough laterally to participate in the formation of the normal femoral canal. The lacunar ligament does; however, lie inferior to (and thus supports) the spermatic cord in the medial part of the inguinal canal.

Immediately superior and lateral to the pubic tubercle, the aponeurotic fibers of the external oblique muscle diverge to attach to the body of the pubis superomedially (medial crus) and to the pubic tubercle inferolaterally (lateral crus). The triangular interval between the two crura, through which the spermatic cord or round ligament of the uterus passes, is the superficial or external inguinal ring. Intercrural fibers, which are derived from innominate fascia, are oriented at right angles to the external oblique fibers, convert the triangular hiatus into an oval, and usually prevent spreading of the crura. External spermatic fascia, the outer covering of the spermatic cord, is also derived from innominate fascia.

When fibers of the external oblique aponeurosis are split superolaterally from the superficial inguinal ring, the inguinal canal is opened. The somewhat transversely oriented muscular fibers of the internal oblique muscle can then be seen arching over the spermatic cord. The cremasteric muscle and fascia, which constitute the middle covering of the spermatic cord, are in continuity with the internal oblique muscle and its investing

fascia. Internal oblique fibers in this region originate from iliac fascia, pass superficial to the spermatic cord and deep (internal) inguinal ring, and attach to the rectus sheath and adjacent body of the pubis. Rarely (3% of cases), the lowest internal oblique fibers are aponeurotic, join aponeurotic fibers of the transversus abdominis muscle, and insert into the pubic tubercle and pectineal ligament (of Cooper) as a conjoint tendon. However, typically, the lowest fibers are muscular and do not extend below the arch formed by the deeper transversus abdominis muscle. Because the internal oblique is primarily muscular in the inguinal region, it is of little importance in the surgical repair of groin hernias.

The third musculoaponeurotic layer is composed of the transversus abdominis muscle and aponeurosis and its investing fascia, the inner layer of which is transversalis fascia. By itself, transversalis fascia, which is intimately attached to the transversus abdominis muscle, has little intrinsic strength. Thus, it is considered with the muscle layer rather than as a separate, distinct entity.

Lower muscular or aponeurotic fibers of the transversus abdominis form a distinct arch extending from their lateral attachment (iliac fascia) to their medial attachment on the superior pubic ramus, lateral to the rectus abdominis muscle. As transversus abdominis fibers arch over spermatic cord structures laterally, they define the superior margin of the deep inguinal ring. Medial to the deep inguinal ring, the distinct arch is the superior limit of most direct inguinal hernia defects. Inferior to this arch, aponeurotic fibers of the transversus abdominis are present but are significantly reduced in number; these fibers diverge from each other, and the transversalis fascia fills the intervening gaps. It is this area—the posterior wall of the inguinal canal—through which a direct hernia occurs. Still more inferiorly, a collection of aponeurotic transversus and transversalis fascia fibers form the important iliopubic tract. Laterally, iliopubic tract fibers attach to the iliac fascia. From this attachment, which is overlapped by the inguinal ligament, fibers pass medially and deeply, diverging from the inguinal ligament. Fibers of the iliopubic tract define the lower border of the deep inguinal ring, cross the external iliac and femoral vessels and femoral canal as the anterior wall of the femoral sheath, and then fan out to attach to the pectineal ligament (of Cooper). Medial to the femoral canal, some fibers recurve inferolaterally, forming the medial wall of the femoral sheath. Thus, it is the iliopubic tract, not the more superficial and medial lacunar ligament, that forms the medial border of the femoral canal. Further, it should be noted that the iliopubic tract is often confused with the inguinal ligament because it more or less parallels the course of this ligament.

Although the transversus abdominis and transversalis fascia are considered as a unit, some attention must be paid to regional expressions that are unique to transversalis fascia only. One of these regional expressions is the transversalis fascial sling and its reinforcement by the interfoveolar ligament, which together form the medial boundary of the deep inguinal ring. The transversalis fascial sling results from the obliquity of the inguinal canal with respect to the plane of the deep inguinal ring. Abdominopelvic structures destined to become spermatic cord structures are located in preperitoneal tissue. When these evaginate the transversalis fascia covering the deep inguinal ring (creating the internal spermatic fascia) to enter the inguinal canal, the axis of this tubular prolongation creates a redundancy of transversalis fascia at the medial side of the deep inguinal ring. This sling, which is intimately attached to the transversus abdominis muscle, is mobile and probably represents the so-called shutter mechanism thought to operate at the deep inguinal ring when lateral abdominal muscles contract.

Remember that, during the embryologic descent of the testes, the first structure to pass out of the deep inguinal ring into the inguinal canal, and finally out of the superficial ring into the incipient scrotum, is the processus vaginalis, a tubular evagination of the peritoneal sac. Failure of fusion and subsequent fibrosis of this evagination provide a route for indirect hernias.

The femoral sheath and canal are located inferior to the inguinal ligament. The femoral sheath is a continuation of the transversalis fascia into the thigh. Lateral to medial, it contains the femoral artery, femoral vein, and femoral canal. The femoral canal contains areolar tissue and lymphatic structures. The internal mouth of this canal—the *femoral ring*—is bounded anteriorly and medially by the iliopubic tract, laterally by peri-

adventitial tissue medial to the femoral vein, and posteriorly by the pectineal ligament (of Cooper).

In summary, it is the transversus abdominis and transversalis fascia layer that normally prevents inguinal and femoral hernias. Variations or defects in this layer allow groin hernias to occur.

Inguinal Hernia Repair

Incision and Exposure of the Spermatic Cord (Fig. 115.2)

Technical Points

The traditional hernia incision lies in a straight line from the anterosuperior iliac spine to the pubic tubercle. A more cosmetic incision can be made in a natural skin crease. The most important consideration is to make the incision directly over the pubic tubercle so that exposure in this area is good. Often, the incision can be completely hidden within the hair-bearing area of the pubis. Deepen the incision until the external oblique aponeurosis is identified.

Palpate the external ring. Verify the position of the external ring by passing your finger through it. Use Metzenbaum scissors to extend the incision of the external oblique aponeurosis in its midportion in the direction of its fibers through the

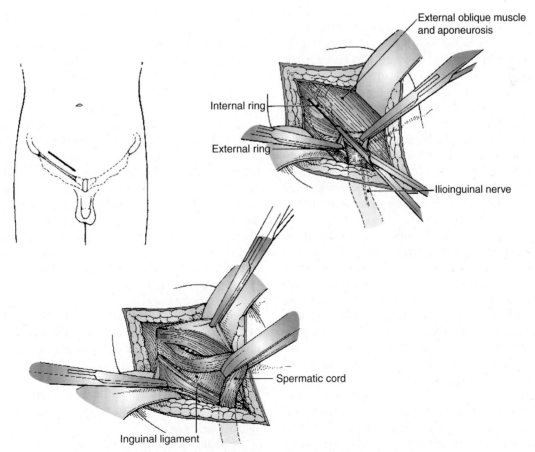

Figure 115.2 Incision and exposure of the spermatic cord

external ring. Place hemostats on the two leaves of the external oblique aponeurosis and lift up. Look underneath and be careful to identify and protect from injury the ilioinguinal nerve. This nerve generally lies just under the external oblique muscle but is somewhat variable in its location.

By sharp and blunt dissection, separate the spermatic cord from the underside of the external oblique aponeurosis. Inferiorly, the inguinal ligament should come into view. Free the spermatic cord circumferentially at the pubic tubercle. Dissection is easiest here because the bony pubic tubercle protects the floor of the canal from injury and provides a constant deep reference point. Pass a Penrose drain around the spermatic cord and lift up. Free the cord to the level of the internal ring. Place a self-retaining retractor within the leaves of the external oblique aponeurosis to hold the canal open.

Anatomic Points

The aponeuroses and ligaments involved in the inguinal canal converge on bone at the pubic tubercle, making this end of the canal relatively fixed. Superficial circumflex iliac vessels coursing superolaterally near the lateral end of the incision, as well as superficial external pudendal vessels crossing anterior to the superficial ring and spermatic cord, probably will be encountered in this stage of the dissection.

After the skin incision is made, fascial layers are encountered. The superficial fascia here is divisible into the more superficial, fatty Camper fascia and the deeper, fibrous Scarpa fascia. Deep to Scarpa fascia is innominate fascia, the deep fascia of the abdomen. The thickness and complexity of the superficial fascia is dependent on the body habitus of the patient. In the obese patient, the fat lobules of Camper fascia are large and irregular. A fat layer can occur deep to Scarpa fascia, but here, the fat lobules are smaller. No fat is present deep to the innominate fascia, through which the fibers of the external oblique aponeurosis are visible. In the dissection through superficial fascia, named vessels that will be encountered include the superficial epigastrics coursing superomedially from the vicinity of the deep inguinal ring, the superficial circumflex iliacs coursing superolaterally near the lateral end of the incision, and the superficial external pudendals running medially anterior to the superficial ring or spermatic cord.

The external ring is immediately superolateral to the pubic tubercle. The outer covering of the cord—the external spermatic fascia—is continuous with innominate fascia and must be incised when the external ring is opened. Exercise caution in this, though, for just deep to the external oblique aponeurosis, typically on the anterior side of the spermatic cord, the ilioinguinal nerve (L1) exits the external ring to lie immediately deep to the external spermatic fascia. The iliohypogastric nerve (L1 and sometimes T12) does not pass through the external ring, but instead is usually slightly superior to this landmark.

As the spermatic cord is mobilized, the inguinal ligament and its medial expansion (lacunar ligament) will be visible. At this point in the dissection, vascular structures should not be encountered because these are deep to transversalis fascia or its spermatic cord continuity.

Inspection of the Spermatic Cord and Identification and Ligation of the Indirect Hernia Sac (Fig. 115.3)

Technical Points

Stretch the spermatic cord slightly and use forceps to pick up on the longitudinally running cremasteric fibers. Incise these in the direction of their fibers for a distance of several centimeters. Place hemostats on the two leaves of the cremaster muscle. Gently shell the cord from its surrounding cremasteric fibers. Try to keep intact the internal spermatic fascia because this will help to protect the cord and cord structures from injury. The cord should "shell out" cleanly, surrounded by its enveloping fascia. Palpate the vas deferens, which will feel like a piece of whipcord running within the structures of the cord. Place the Penrose drain around the cord, excluding the cremaster muscle.

Often, the cremasteric layer is quite fatty and bulky. If this is the case, it is advisable to excise it to skeletonize the cord sufficiently to attain a good repair. Skeletonizing the cord will interfere with the ability of the testis to retract into the scrotum and may be objectionable to some men. It should be done only when necessary to achieve a sound repair. To skeletonize the cord, divide the leaves of cremasteric fibers into two or three pedicles that can then be clamped above and below and excised. Ligate these with 2-0 silk. The proximal pedicle will generally disappear into the peritoneal cavity when the tension on the cord is relaxed. The object is to thin the cord out sufficiently at the level of the internal ring to allow a sound repair to be performed. Spread out the cord and its contents over your finger and look for a hernia sac. This will be visible as a whitish, moon-shaped structure protruding from the internal ring. A sac that extends all the way down into the scrotum will be a cylindrical structure, the termination of which will not be able to be identified. If you do not see a sac, place traction on the cord until a lappet of peritoneum is pulled up into the cord. The appearance of this peritoneal lappet confirms that there is no sac.

If a sac is identified within the cord, place hemostats on the sac and separate it from other cord structures by sharp and blunt dissection. A sac that continues all the way into the scrotum can be transected and a small amount of distal sac left in situ. Divide the sac with electrocautery. Take care to secure hemostasis. Leave the sac open. Dissect the proximal sac circumferentially all the way to the internal ring. The vas deferens at the internal ring will often be quite adherent and close to the sac; therefore, you must be especially careful to avoid injuring it.

Place strong traction on the cord so that a good high ligation of the sac can be performed. Open the sac and inspect it to be sure that it is empty. Reduce any contained viscera or omentum. Twist the sac to milk its contents down out of the way and transfix it with a suture ligature of 2-0 silk. Amputate the sac and allow it to retract. Alternatively, place a purse-string suture in the neck of the sac with the sac open. This approach has the advantage of being done under direct vision and may be most suitable for large sacs.

A sliding hernia is one in which part of the wall of the sac is composed of one of the viscera—generally, the bladder,

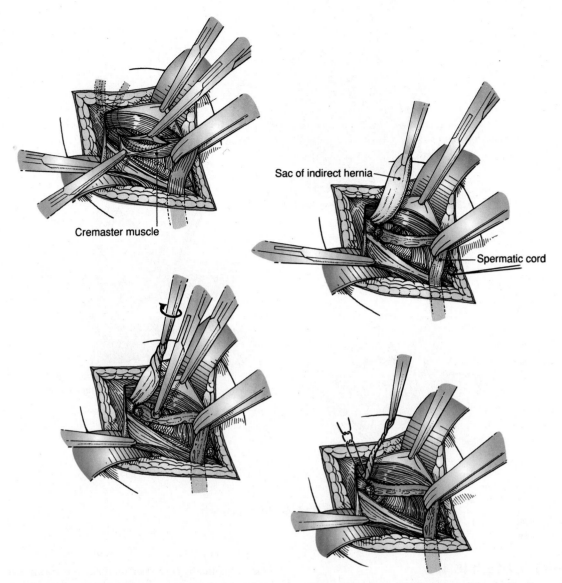

Figure 115.3 Inspection of the spermatic cord and identification and ligation of the indirect hernia sac

sigmoid colon, or cecum. Do not attempt to dissect the sac from the viscus in such cases. Rather, amputate the sac just above the attachment of the viscus and close it just above the attachment. Separate the sac fully from the cord and reduce the viscus and sac into the abdomen. This will prevent any remaining finger of peritoneum from acting as a lead point for recurrent hernia.

Check hemostasis in the cord and the floor of the canal. Secure small bleeding veins on the cord by suture ligature with fine silk or with ties. If a tight repair is done, swelling in the immediate postoperative period may create a "venous tourniquet" effect, causing otherwise insignificant vessels to bleed. A painful scrotal hematoma may result.

Anatomic Points

The cremasteric muscle and fascia are continuous with the internal oblique muscle and its investing fascia. Deep to this layer, and on the posterior side of the spermatic cord, is the genital branch of the genitofemoral nerve (L1, L2). This nerve supplies the cremaster muscle. Severance of the nerve can best be avoided by separation, rather than division, of cremasteric fibers. If you must divide cremaster fibers, be careful not to entrap the nerve.

In indirect inguinal hernias, a hernia sac passes through the deep inguinal ring, following the route of testicular descent. As a consequence, the indirect inguinal hernia sac becomes a cord constituent and is covered by external spermatic fascia, cremasteric fascia, and internal spermatic fascia (continuous with the transversalis fascia). By contrast, a direct inguinal hernia, although covered by attenuated transversalis fascia of the posterior wall of the inguinal canal, lies adjacent to the spermatic cord, not within it. If it progresses to the point of exiting the external ring, it will be covered by external spermatic fascia, but it will remain outside the cremasteric fascia.

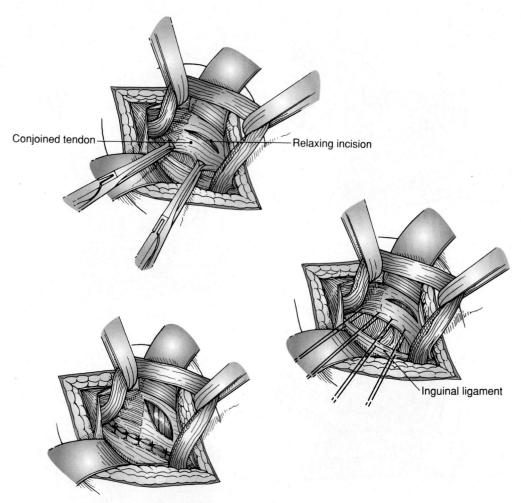

Conjoined tendon —

— Relaxing incision

Inguinal ligament

Figure 115.4 Bassini repair

Bassini Repair (Fig. 115.4)

Technical Points

Assess the strength of the floor of the canal. High ligation of the sac is all that is required for a simple indirect hernia in an infant (Chapter 118) or young male. Often, the presence of the hernia has dilated the internal ring and may have partially weakened the floor. The floor is basically sound, but the anatomy may have been distorted by the hernia sliding through the internal ring. In this case, a Bassini repair is a good option because it does not require opening of the floor of the canal and does not risk weakening what is basically already a strong structure.

A Bassini repair is performed by suturing conjoint tendon to inguinal ligament. Elevate the upper flap of the external oblique muscle. Make a relaxing incision in the medial superior aspect of the conjoined tendon using electrocautery. Be careful to check hemostasis in this incision. Place Allis clamps on the conjoined tendon, seen here as a muscular and aponeurotic arc spanning the superior aspect of the floor of the canal. Test the mobility of the conjoined tendon by pulling it down to the inguinal ligament. It should pull down easily with minimal tension as the relaxing incision opens up. Extend the relaxing incision superiorly if nec-

essary. Suture the conjoined tendon to the inguinal ligament with interrupted heavy sutures; 0-0 silk on a Mayo needle is particularly convenient for this purpose. Place the sutures no more than 3 to 4 mm apart. Tie the sutures snugly, but not so tightly as to necrose tissue. Tighten the internal ring so that it will no longer accept the tip of your finger. A Kelly clamp should slide easily down along the cord. Recheck hemostasis.

Anatomic Points

Although a true conjoined tendon is seldom seen, there is nevertheless a continuous musculoaponeurotic arch formed by the lower fibers of the transversus abdominis muscle. Relaxing incisions medial to the conjoined tendon area are necessary because aponeurotic fibers of the internal oblique and transversus abdominis muscles continue to the midline as part of the anterior rectus sheath. Because the Bassini repair does not require violation of the transversalis fascia layer, no named vessels should be encountered. Hemostasis can be achieved using electrocautery only.

As the internal ring is approached and as it is tightened, remember that the inferior epigastric vessels lie deep to the

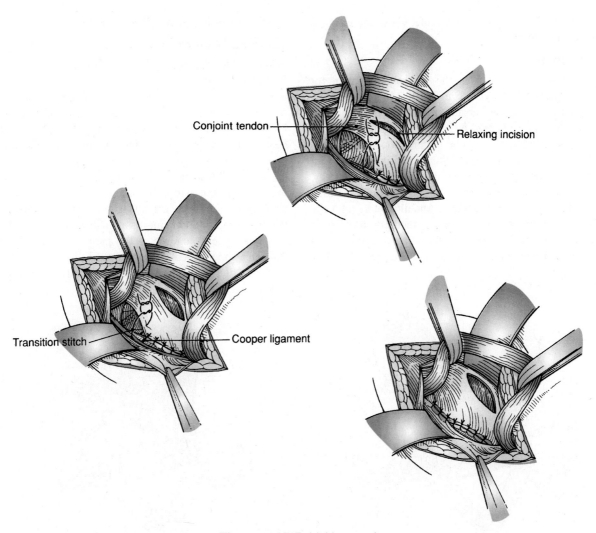

Conjoint tendon

Relaxing incision

Transition stitch

Cooper ligament

Figure 115.5 McVay repair

transversalis fascia, immediately medial to the internal ring. Care should be taken to avoid these vessels when placing sutures near the internal ring.

McVay Repair (Fig. 115.5)

Technical Points

When the floor of the canal is weak, a McVay repair may be preferred over a Bassini repair. Use the McVay repair when a good conjoined tendon that is strong and largely aponeurotic is identified in the floor of the canal. The McVay repair involves suturing conjoined tendon to the pectineal ligament (of Cooper), which is a fixed and unyielding structure. An adequate relaxing incision is necessary to allow the conjoined tendon sufficient mobility to extend down to Cooper ligament without tension. Make this relaxing incision as described previously.

Beginning at the pubic tubercle, break through the floor of the canal, which generally will be thin and tenuous. Just deep to the inguinal ligament, identify Cooper ligament, a whit-ish, shining structure. Push fatty and areolar tissue away from Cooper ligament and clean it laterally. Identify the sheath of the femoral vein in the lateral region of the dissection, taking care not to damage the vein. Place Allis clamps on the conjoined tendon and pull it down to determine whether adequate mobility has been achieved to bring it to Cooper ligament without tension.

Suture the conjoined tendon to Cooper ligament with multiple interrupted sutures; 0-0 Nurolon on a Mayo needle is particularly convenient for this. The heavy Mayo needle is especially important for a Cooper ligament repair because the tip will not be damaged or bent by the tough periosteum underlying Cooper ligament. Begin at the pubic tubercle and commence laterally. As the femoral vein is approached and the repair progresses from the deep plane of Cooper ligament to the more superficial plane of the inguinal ligament, place a transition stitch midway between the Cooper ligament and the inguinal ligament. Take care not to injure the vein or to constrict it. Place the last suture between the conjoined tendon and the inguinal ligament at the level of the internal ring. Tie all sutures and test the strength of the repair and the size of the internal ring. Close the canal as previously described.

Anatomic Points

The McVay repair demands that the pectineal ligament (of Cooper) be visualized. To visualize this ligament, the transversus aponeurosis and transversalis fascia layer must be violated because Cooper ligament is on a deeper plane than the inguinal ligament and pubic tubercle. After Cooper ligament is exposed, be aware of the potential for comparatively large vessels, such as the pubic branch of the inferior epigastric artery, to be present in this area. This artery lies on the iliopubic tract, runs inferiorly across Cooper ligament, and ultimately joins the obturator artery; a branch of this courses medially on Cooper ligament. In about 25% of patients, the pubic branch is 2 to 3 mm in diameter and is referred to as an *accessory obturator artery.*

Shouldice Repair (Fig. 115.6)

Technical Points

When the floor is significantly weakened but some transversalis fascia is identifiable, especially within the iliopubic tract, a Shouldice repair is a good option. Carefully clean the floor of the canal, but do not break through it. Identify the iliopubic tract, which is a thickening of the transversalis fascia adjacent to and adherent to the inguinal ligament. Generally, it is about 2 to 3 mm wide and is identifiable as a slightly whitish, glistening, fibrous band. Incise the transversalis fascia next to the iliopubic tract from the internal ring to the pubic tubercle (Fig. 115.6A). Take care not to injure the inferior epigastric vessels at the internal ring or a small branching vessel that is occasionally encountered at the pubic tubercle. Place hemostats on a superior leaf of transversalis fascia and elevate it. By sharp and blunt dissection, separate the underlying preperitoneal

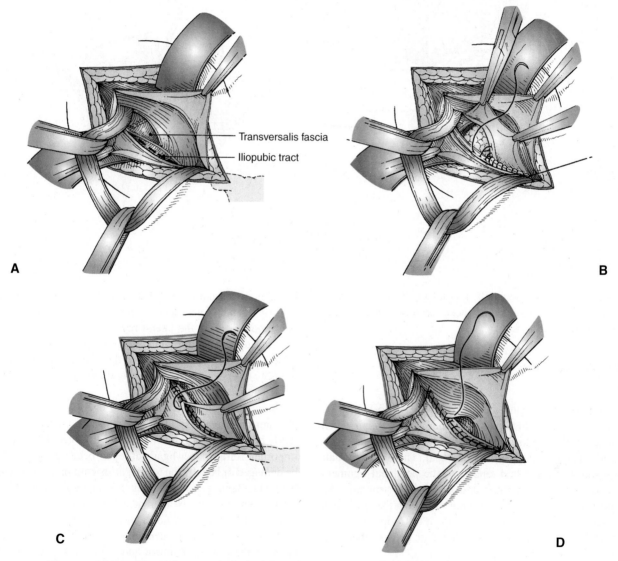

Transversalis fascia

Iliopubic tract

A

B

C

D

Figure 115.6 Shouldice repair. **A:** Incision along iliopubic tract. **B:** Start of first suture line. **C:** This suture turns back at the internal ring and continues as the second suture line. **D:** Placement of third (and fourth) suture line.

fat from the transversalis fascia. The arch of the transversus abdominis aponeurosis should be readily visible as a shiny, white area of thickening on the underside of this tissue layer.

Place a sponge stick in the floor of the canal to hold the contents of the floor out of your way as you proceed with the repair. Use 2-0 or 3-0 monofilament suture; prolene is a good choice for this suture. Begin your suture line at the pubic tubercle and sew the underside of the arch of the transversus abdominis aponeurosis to the free edge of the iliopubic tract (Fig. 115.6B). The suture line runs from the pubic tubercle to the internal ring. Do not try to tighten the internal ring. Four overlapping suture lines will progressively tighten, and it will be quite snug by the end of the repair. At this point, it should be loose.

At the internal ring, bring your suture up through the free edge of the upper leaf of transversalis fascia and commence suturing it to the inguinal ligament with a running suture. This suture line continues from the internal ring laterally to the pubic tubercle medially and is tied to itself (Fig. 115.6C). This concludes the first and second suture lines. At the conclusion of this, the floor should be closed, and the internal ring should be approximated, but not tight.

The third and fourth suture lines bring conjoined tendon to inguinal ligament. Begin a suture at the internal ring and bring conjoined tendon down to the inguinal ligament using a running suture from the internal ring to the pubic tubercle (Fig. 115.6D). At the pubic tubercle, turn the suture line around and reinforce it by crisscrossing over the previous suture. At the internal ring, check the snugness of the fit around the cord. It should be possible to place a Kelly clamp down through the internal ring next to the cord, but it should not be possible to pass the tip of your finger down next to the cord. Tie the suture. Check hemostasis in the floor.

Anatomic Points

The deepest fibrous tissue immediately adjacent to the inguinal ligament is often loosely considered to be part of the inguinal ligament. This is the iliopubic tract, an expression of the transversus abdominis aponeurosis and transversalis fascia. This relatively flimsy structure is used for the first suture line of the Shouldice repair because it is mobile, allowing the relatively high arch of the transversus abdominis aponeurosis to be sutured without tension.

Plug-and-Patch Repair (Fig. 115.7)

Technical and Anatomic Points

Identify, dissect, and perform high ligation of the sac of any indirect hernia present. Define the edges of the any defect in the transversalis fascia. Circumferentially excise it, exposing the preperitoneal fat. There are several kinds of preformed plug-and-patch kits, or you can make your own. The essential common elements are shown here. Place a preformed plug into this defect in such a manner that the leaflets of the plug expand underneath the transversalis fascia, sort of like a partially opened umbrella. Tack it in place with one or two sutures of 3-0 Vicryl.

Take the patch and place it around the spermatic cord. Suture it to conjoined tendon superiorly and inguinal ligament inferiorly.

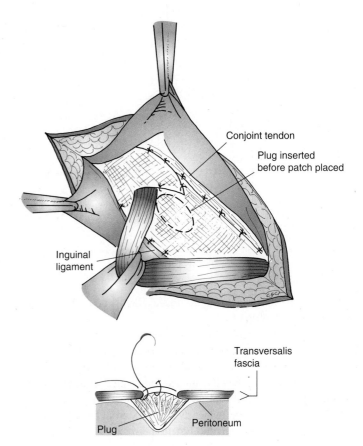

Figure 115.7 Plug-and-patch repair

Closure of the Canal (Fig. 115.8)

Technical and Anatomic Points

Close the canal by suturing the external oblique aponeurosis together using a running suture of 3-0 Vicryl. Reapproximate the external ring if possible. Place a few sutures of 3-0 Vicryl in the subcutaneous tissue and close the skin with a running

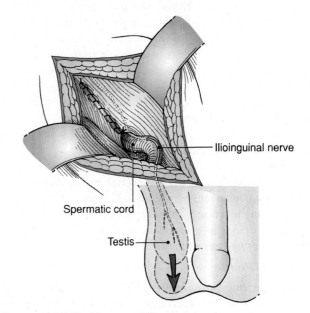

Figure 115.8 Closure of the canal

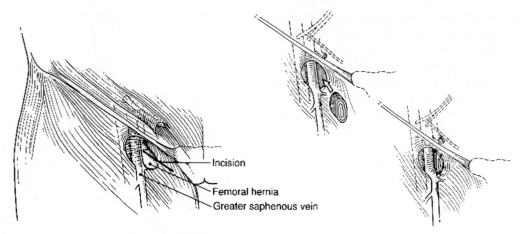

Incision
Femoral hernia
Greater saphenous vein

Figure 115.9 Femoral hernia repair from below

subcuticular absorbable suture. Place a dressing on the incision and remove the drapes.

At the conclusion of the operation, it is important to palpate the testis in the scrotum and to pull it back down into the scrotum. Generally, traction on the cord will have elevated the testis almost to the level of the external ring during the course of the dissection. If it is allowed to remain in this position, scar tissue may tether it permanently at the external ring, producing an undesirable cosmetic and functional result.

Femoral Hernia Repair

Femoral Hernia Repair from Below (Fig. 115.9)

Technical Points

Repair of the femoral hernia from below does not allow a good anatomic repair. However, this procedure can be done under local anesthesia and is sometimes performed in extremely frail, elderly, or debilitated patients.

Make an incision directly over the femoral hernia. This incision should be parallel to the inguinal ligament and will generally lie about 2 cm below it. Identify the sac of the hernia and, by sharp and blunt dissection, free it from the surrounding soft tissues. Open the sac and reduce any contents into the abdominal cavity. It may be necessary to incise the inguinal ligament vertically, retracting the spermatic cord upward, to enlarge the canal sufficiently to reduce the contents of the sac. Twist the sac and ligate it with a suture ligature. Amputate the sac and reduce the stump into the abdomen.

Closure of the femoral canal from below is best achieved by inserting a patch of prosthetic material, such as Marlex. Roll the Marlex patch up into a small ball and place it in the femoral canal, suturing it in place. Take care not to injure or impinge on the femoral vein. Close subcutaneous tissues with interrupted Vicryl sutures and close the skin.

Anatomic Points

Repair of a femoral hernia from below necessitates ligation and division of several veins that either join the upper end of the saphenous vein or run through the saphenous hiatus of the femoral sheath and fascia lata to drain directly into the femoral vein. The anatomic key to repair from below is to remember that the femoral ring is bounded by the iliopubic tract anteriorly and medially, by Cooper ligament posteriorly, and by venous periadventitial tissue laterally. It is to these structures that the prosthetic material is sutured. Of these boundaries, the lateral wall of periadventitial tissue is the least fixed. Therefore, compression of the femoral vein is easily possible, as is needle trauma to the vein if sutures are placed too deeply.

The entrance to the femoral canal is about 1 cm deep to the external opening of the canal, through which the hernia protrudes. Adequate closure of the opening of this canal is difficult from below; for this reason, closure with a plug of mesh may be simpler than attempting suture closure.

Femoral Hernia Repair from Above (Fig. 115.10)

Technical Points

Repair of the femoral hernia through the floor of the inguinal canal not only is more anatomically appropriate, but also permits controlled reduction of incarcerated sac contents as well as resection of infarcted bowel, if necessary. This approach involves dissection through an otherwise intact inguinal floor. Despite this single disadvantage, this method is generally the preferred approach for most femoral hernias.

Open the inguinal canal in the manner described for inguinal hernias. Open the floor of the canal by sharp and blunt dissection to identify Cooper ligament. The repair of the floor that will be done is the McVay repair. The neck of the femoral hernia sac will be identifiable as a diverticulum of peritoneum extending down from the abdomen through the femoral canal, a space medial to the femoral vein. Open the femoral hernia sac and reduce its contents into the inguinal incision (see Chapter 88, Figure 88.4). It may be necessary to cut the inguinal ligament to do this. Note that a vessel—the so-called artery of death—frequently runs along the underside of the inguinal ligament; this must be identified and ligated before division of the inguinal ligament. Ligate and divide the sac of the femoral hernia.

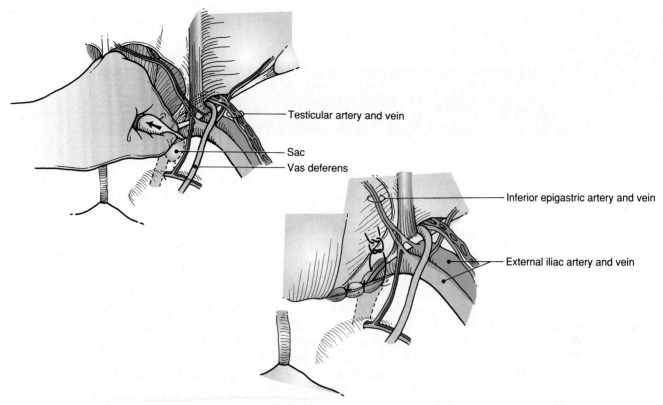

Testicular artery and vein

Sac

Vas deferens

Inferior epigastric artery and vein

External iliac artery and vein

Figure 115.10 Femoral hernia repair from above

Close the floor of the canal in the McVay fashion, obliterating the femoral canal and excluding it from the abdomen. Take care not to impinge on the femoral vein.

Anatomic Points

This is a classic Cooper ligament repair. The only anatomic point that has not been previously covered is the artery of death. This artery arises from the pubic branch of the inferior epigastric artery and, if left uncontrolled, can cause serious morbidity. The vessel is at greatest risk when a femoral hernia is repaired from below. From that approach, it is invisible, and injury to it during division of the inguinal ligament may not be immediately obvious, resulting in delayed, possibly occult, retroperitoneal bleeding.

REFERENCES

1. Amid PK, Chen DC. Surgical treatment of chronic groin and testicular pain after laparoscopic and open preperitoneal inguinal hernia repair. *J Am Coll Surg.* 2011;213:531.
2. Buhck H, Untied M, Bechstein WO. Evidence-based assessment of the period of physical inactivity required after inguinal herniotomy. *Langenbecks Arch Surg* 2012;397:1209.
3. Condon RE. Surgical anatomy of the transversus abdominis and transversalis fascia. *Ann Surg.* 1971;173:1.
4. DeBord JR. The historical development of prosthetics in hernia surgery. *Surg Clin North Am.* 1998;78:973–1006.
5. Henry AK. Operation for femoral hernia: By a midline extraperitoneal approach. *Lancet.* 1936;230:531.
6. Koning GG, Adang EM, Stalmeier PF, et al. TIPP and Lichtenstein modalities for inguinal hernia repair: A cost minimization analysis alongside a randomized trial. *Eur J Health Econ.* 2012; Dec 28 (Epub ahead of print).
7. Lichtenstein IL. Herniorrhaphy: A personal experience with 6321 cases. *Am J Surg.* 1987;153:53.
8. Lichtenstein IL, Shulman AG, Amid PK, et al. The tension-free hernioplasty. *Am J Surg.* 1989;157:188. (Describes mesh inguinal hernioplasty.)
9. McVay CB. The anatomic basis for inguinal and femoral hernioplasty. *Surg Gynecol Obstet.* 1974;139:931.
10. Milone M, Di Minno MN, Musella M, et al. Outpatient inguinal hernia repair under local anaesthesia: Feasibility and efficacy of ultrasound-guided transversus abdominis plane block. *Hernia.* 2012; Nov 16 (Epub ahead of print).
11. Mizrachy B, Kark AE. The anatomy and repair of the posterior inguinal wall. *Surg Gynecol Obstet.* 1973;137:253. (Describes Shouldice technique.)
12. O'Dwyer PJ, Alani A, McConnachie A. Groin hernia repair: Postherniorrhaphy pain. *World J Surg.* 2005;29:1062–1065.
13. Ponka JL. Seven steps to local anesthesia for inguinofemoral hernia repair. *Surg Gynecol Obstet.* 1963;117:115.
14. Rutkow IM, Robbins AW. Classification systems and groin hernias. *Surg Clin North Am.* 1998;78:1117–1127.
15. Starling JR, Harms BA, Schroeder ME, et al. Diagnosis and treatment of genitofemoral and ilioinguinal entrapment neuralgia. *Surgery.* 1987;102:581. (Provides good review of presenting symptoms, possible causes, and management.)

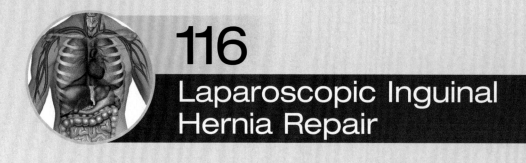

116

Laparoscopic Inguinal Hernia Repair

Laparoscopic inguinal hernia repair takes a totally different approach from open repair. It is most nearly analogous to a preperitoneal open repair, sometimes termed the *Nyhus repair,* performed with mesh. The logic is similar to that employed during laparoscopic ventral herniorrhaphy: Because the problem is a weakness in the transversalis fascia (or a persistently patent processus vaginalis), approach the defect from inside. Peritoneum is stripped from the region, and the defect is repaired with a large sheet of prosthetic mesh. Intra-abdominal pressure holds the mesh buttressed against the muscular and aponeurotic layers of the abdominal wall, which are not dissected. Tacks are placed to secure the mesh in place. The anatomy that is stressed for this repair is very different than that stressed in Chapter 115. There is little emphasis on the muscular and aponeurotic layers of the abdominal wall, because these layers are not encountered. Rather, avoiding complications during these procedures requires intimate knowledge of the anatomy of crucial nerves and blood vessels that must be avoided when the mesh is secured. Major complications of the procedure include vascular injury and neurapraxia. The procedure may be done transabdominal preperitoneal (TAPP) or totally extraperitoneal (TEP). In this chapter, the transabdominal approach is shown first, followed by the modification employed for TEP.

SCORE™, the Surgical Council on Resident Education, classified laparoscopic inguinal or femoral hernia repair as "ESSENTIAL COMMON" procedures.

STEPS IN PROCEDURE

Transabdominal Preperitoneal (TAPP) Approach
Supine position
Trocars at umbilicus and left and right paraumbilical
Abdominal exploration
Confirm presence of hernia defect or defects
Incise peritoneum from median umbilical ligament to anterosuperior iliac spine, approximately 2 cm cephalad to hernia
Develop flaps and reduce sac
Tailor large piece of mesh and pass into abdomen

Secure mesh with staples or tacks along superior edge of mesh
Close peritoneum over mesh
Close trocar sites in usual fashion

Total Extraperitoneal Repair (TEP)
Initial entry into preperitoneal space via open technique
Bluntly dissect preperitoneal fat from fascia
Use dissecting balloon to develop the space
Place additional trocars
Separate sac from underlying structures; ligate large indirect sac if necessary
Place mesh as noted above
Close trocar sites in usual fashion

HALLMARK ANATOMIC COMPLICATIONS

Injury to lateral femoral cutaneous nerve
Injury to anterior femoral cutaneous nerve
Injury to femoral nerve
Injury to genitofemoral nerve (femoral or genital branches)

Injury to external iliac artery or vein
Injury to aberrant obturator arteries
Injury to bladder (if prior surgery in the preperitoneal space)

LIST OF STRUCTURES

Peritoneum
Transversalis fascia
Patent processus vaginalis
Ductus deferens

Seminal vesicles
Round ligament of uterus
Bladder
Deep (internal) inguinal ring

Medial Umbilical Ligament (Fold)
Urachus
Median umbilical ligaments (folds)
Obliterated umbilical artery

Lateral Umbilical Ligaments (Folds)
Inferior epigastric artery and vein
Supravesical fossa
Medial umbilical fossa
Lateral umbilical fossa
Hesselbach triangle
Iliopubic tract
Femoral canal
Cooper ligament
Conjoint tendon
Arch of aponeurosis of transversus abdominis

Lateral femoral cutaneous nerve
Anterior femoral cutaneous nerve
Femoral nerve
Genitofemoral nerve
Femoral branch
Genital branch
Ilioinguinal nerve
Iliohypogastric nerve
External iliac artery and vein
Femoral artery and vein
Internal iliac artery and vein

Obturator Artery
Aberrant obturator artery
Prevesical space (of Retzius)

The muscular and aponeurotic structures of the anterior abdominal wall appear different when viewed from inside with the peritoneum removed (Fig. 116.1A). Note how the ductus (or vas) deferens enters through the deep inguinal ring and then passes inferiorly and medially to join the seminal vesicles in the region of the base of the bladder. The internal spermatic vessels pass from lateral to medial and ascend to pass through the deep inguinal ring. The inferior epigastric vessels ascend and pass medially, defining the lateral border of Hesselbach triangle. The medial umbilical ligaments, the obliterated remnants of the umbilical arteries, form useful visual landmarks. The median umbilical landmark is rarely seen. Figure 116.1B shows peritoneum intact on the right side, demonstrating the peritoneal folds and visual landmarks with peritoneum intact. On the left side, the peritoneum has been removed to reveal underlying structures of significance. Note the iliopubic tract, the femoral canal, Cooper ligament, and the arch of the aponeurosis of the transversus abdominis. Contrast this view with the anterior and posterior views shown in Chapter 115, Figure 115.1.

Multiple nerves and vessels, most never encountered during open inguinal or femoral herniorrhaphy, are at risk during laparoscopic repair. Nerves include the lateral femoral cutaneous nerve, the anterior femoral cutaneous nerve, the femoral nerve, the femoral branch of the genitofemoral nerve, and the genital branch of the genitofemoral nerve. The vascular structures at risk include the external iliac artery and vein and aberrant obturator arteries. The latter, also termed the "artery of death," is a potential pitfall when a femoral hernia is repaired from above (see Figure 115.9 in Chapter 115).

Two triangles, which lie together to form a rough trapezoid, encompass the majority of these structures and form a useful mnemonic device (Fig. 116.1C). The "triangle of pain" is bounded by the iliopubic tract superiorly, the testicular vessels medially, and the cut edge of the peritoneum inferiorly. It contains most of the nerves previously mentioned. The "triangle of doom," bounded by the testicular vessels laterally, the ductus

deferens medially, and the cut peritoneal edge inferiorly, contains the vessels. Extreme care must be exercised while dissecting in these triangles, and no staples or other fixation devices should be placed in these regions.

TAPP—Orientation and Initial View of Male and Female Pelvis (Fig. 116.2)

Technical Points

Position the patient supine. Place three ports as shown (Fig. 116.2A). Use an angled (30- or 45-degree) laparoscope for better visualization of the inguinal region. Note that in the male, the ductus deferens and inferior spermatic vessels form the apex of a triangle that points to the internal inguinal ring (Fig. 116.2B). Normally, the peritoneum over this region is smooth, or, at most, a tiny dimple or crescentic fold will be seen at the internal ring. In the female, the round ligament is seen to terminate in the internal ring (Fig. 116.2C). Confirm the presence of a hernia or of multiple defects by noting outpouchings in the peritoneum either medial (direct) or lateral (indirect) to the inferior epigastric vessels (Fig. 116.2D, E).

Anatomic Points

As the parietal peritoneum covers the undersurface of the anterior abdominal wall and pelvis, underlying structures tent it up, creating five peritoneal folds. These form visual landmarks useful to the laparoscopic surgeon.

In the midline, the remnant of the obliterated urachus links the umbilicus with the dome of the bladder. Although this median umbilical fold is shown in parts A and B of the Figure 116.1, it is rarely actually visible to the laparoscopic surgeon, perhaps because it is so close to the umbilically placed laparoscope. The space above the bladder is termed the *supravesical fossa*.

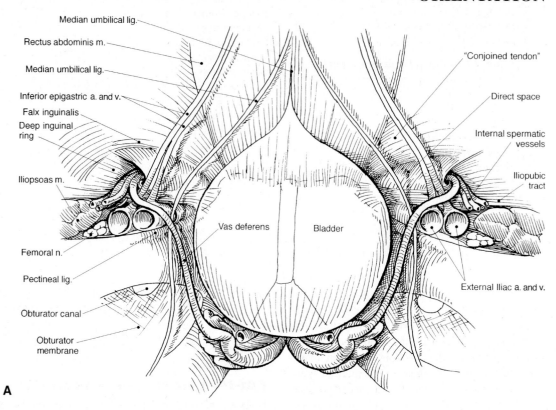

Median umbilical lig.

Rectus abdominis m.

Median umbilical lig.

Inferior epigastric a. and v.

Falx inguinalis

Deep inguinal ring

Iliopsoas m.

Femoral n.

Pectineal lig.

Obturator canal

Obturator membrane

"Conjoined tendon"

Direct space

Internal spermatic vessels

Iliopubic tract

Vas deferens

Bladder

External Iliac a. and v.

A

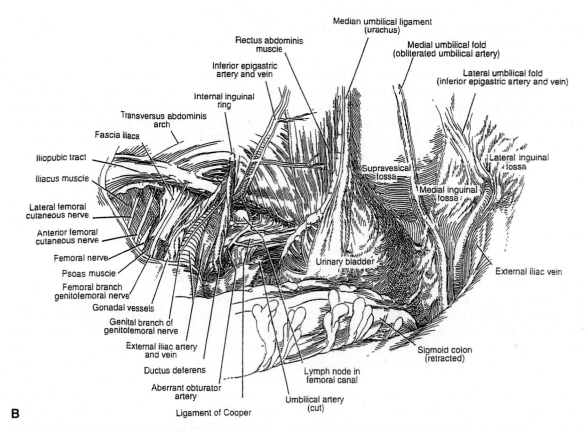

Median umbilical ligament (urachus)

Rectus abdominis muscle

Medial umbilical fold (obliterated umbilical artery)

Inferior epigastric artery and vein

Lateral umbilical fold (inferior epigastric artery and vein)

Internal inguinal ring

Transversus abdominis arch

Fascia iliaca

Iliopubic tract

Iliacus muscle

Lateral femoral cutaneous nerve

Anterior femoral cutaneous nerve

Femoral nerve

Psoas muscle

Femoral branch genitofemoral nerve

Gonadal vessels

Genital branch of genitofemoral nerve

External iliac artery and vein

Ductus deferens

Aberrant obturator artery

Ligament of Cooper

Supravesical fossa

Medial inguinal fossa

Lateral inguinal fossa

Urinary bladder

External iliac vein

Sigmoid colon (retracted)

Lymph node in femoral canal

Umbilical artery (cut)

B

Figure 116.1 Laparoscopic view of pelvis and inguinal region. **A:** Peritoneum stripped to reveal underlying structures. **B:** Peritoneum intact on right side, stripped on left.

ORIENTATION (Continued)

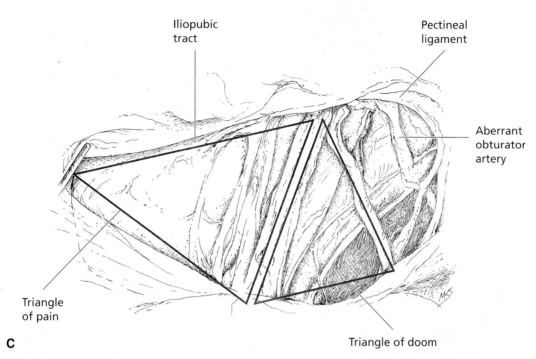

Iliopubic tract

Pectineal ligament

Aberrant obturator artery

Triangle of pain

Triangle of doom

C

Figure 116.1 *Continued.* **C:** Triangles of doom and pain.

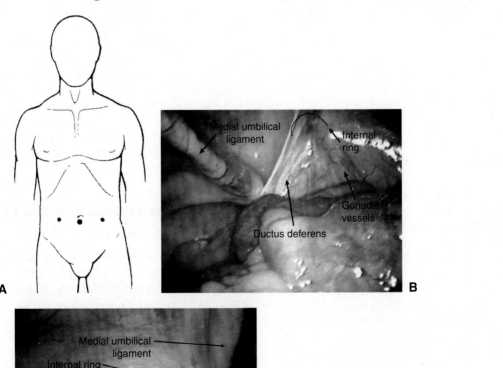

Medial umbilical ligament

Internal ring

Gonadal vessels

Ductus deferens

A

B

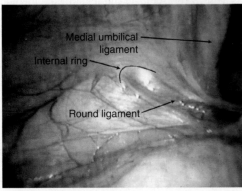

Medial umbilical ligament

Internal ring

Round ligament

C

Figure 116.2 TAPP—orientation and initial view of male and female pelvis. **A:** Trocar placement. **B:** Normal male groin from peritoneum. **C:** Normal female groin from peritoneum. (*continued*)

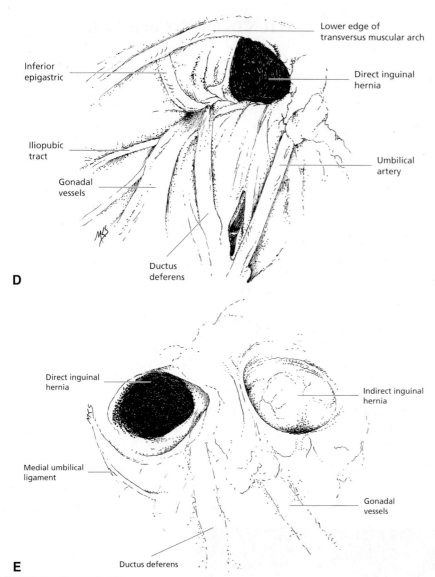

Figure 116.2 *Continued*. **D:** Direct inguinal hernia from peritoneum. **E:** Direct and indirect inguinal hernias seen from peritoneum (**B, D, E** from Colborn GL, Brick WG. Inguinal region. In: Scott-Conner CEH, Cuschieri A, Carter FJ, eds. *Minimal Access Surgical Anatomy.* Philadelphia, PA: Lippincott Williams & Wilkins; 2000:239–266, with permission; **C** from Hedican SP. Pelvis. In: Scott-Conner CEH, Cuschieri A, Carter FJ, eds. *Minimal Access Surgical Anatomy.* Philadelphia, PA: Lippincott Williams & Wilkins; 2000:211–238, with permission).

The paired medial umbilical ligaments are much more obvious. These contain the obliterated remnants of the umbilical arteries. They lead from the umbilicus to the internal iliac arteries bilaterally. The region of interest to the laparoscopic hernia surgeon lies just lateral to the medial umbilical ligaments.

In the male, a very obvious triangle marks the convergence of the testicular vessels and ductus deferens on the internal (deep) inguinal ring. In the female, the corresponding gonadal (ovarian) vessels do not traverse the internal inguinal ring; thus, the triangle is incomplete, and only the round ligament points the way to the internal ring.

Of the landmarks that delineate Hesselbach triangle, only the inferior epigastric vessels (contained in the lateral umbilical folds) are visible. The space between the medial and lateral umbilical folds is termed the *medial umbilical fossa*. Similarly, the region lateral to the lateral umbilical folds (i.e., lateral to the inferior epigastric vessels), is the *lateral umbilical fossa*.

TAPP—Peritoneal Incision (Fig. 116.3)

Technical Points

Identify the medial umbilical ligament visually and the anterosuperior iliac spine (by palpation on the outside of the abdomen, if necessary). Make an incision in the peritoneum (Fig. 116.3A) from the level of the median umbilical ligament to the anterosuperior iliac spine about 2 cm cephalad to the upper edge of the hernia. Develop flaps in the superior and inferior direction. In particular, carefully reflect the inferior flap of peritoneum to expose the muscular and aponeurotic structures of the inguinal region, including the femoral canal, from within (Fig. 116.3B).

Anatomic Points

In contrast to open hernia repair, in which muscular and aponeurotic structures are divided from superficial to deep, only

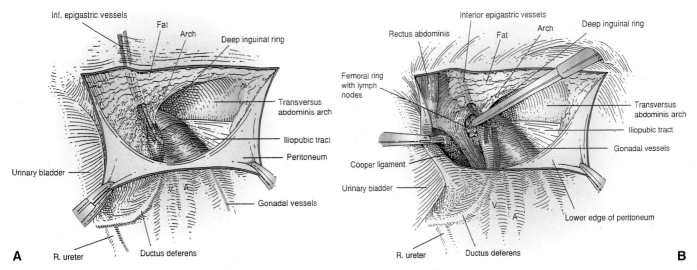

Figure 116.3 TAPP—peritoneal incision and initial exposure. **A:** Peritoneum incised and peeled down. **B:** Location of femoral ring (**A, B** from Colborn GL, Skandalakis JE. Laparoscopic cadaveric anatomy of the inguinal area. *Probl Gen Surg.* 1995;12:13–20, with permission).

the deepest structures are seen during laparoscopic surgery, and none of these are actually divided. The iliopubic tract, a condensation of the transversalis fascia, may be seen, indicating the position of the (unseen) inguinal ligament. The arch of the aponeurosis of the transversus abdominis muscle can be seen passing from lateral to medial as the muscular fibers of the transversus abdominis give way to aponeurosis. This aponeurosis contributes to the formation of the conjoint tendon and blends with the linea alba medially. Medially, the rectus abdominis muscle may be seen.

TAPP—Reducing Sac of Hernia and Defining Anatomy (Fig. 116.4)

Technical Points

Gently tease fat and peritoneum from the region of Hesselbach triangle and the iliopubic tract (Fig. 116.4A). The sac of a direct hernia will generally reduce as the peritoneal flap is developed (Fig. 116.4B). An indirect sac must be reduced from within the spermatic cord (if the sac is not very long) or amputated and allowed to remain (if a large sac). To amputate a large sac, begin dissection on the side opposite the cord structures and work toward the cord (Fig. 116.4C). Only when the cord structures are seen to be separate from the sac should it be amputated.

Anatomic Points

The entire region of interest should now be exposed. Identify the pubic tubercle, Cooper ligament, the iliac artery and vein, and the inferior epigastric vessels (Fig. 116.4C).

TAPP—Placement of Mesh (Fig. 116.5)

Technical Points

Carefully check the region for hemostasis because access will be lost after the mesh is placed. The field should resemble Figure 116.5A. Tailor a large piece of mesh (at least 11 × 6 cm) to cover the internal ring completely, including direct, indirect, and femoral hernial orifices. Roll the mesh into a narrow cylinder and introduce it into the peritoneal cavity. Unroll it and place it under the peritoneal flaps. Position it with care so that the area of potential and actual weakness is covered with good overlap.

Place staples along the upper edge of the mesh (Fig. 116.5B) and along the iliopubic tract medially. Never place staples in the triangle of doom or pain (Fig. 116.1C).

Anatomic Points

Several nerves and vessels are vulnerable during this dissection. Although the nerves are primarily encountered in the triangle of pain and the vessels in the triangle of doom, the entire area inferior to the iliopubic tract and lateral to the ductus deferens should be considered to be "off limits" for staples, tacks, or overly vigorous dissection (Fig. 116.5C).

The femoral nerve, the single largest branch of the lumbar plexus, emerges from the lateral border of the psoas major muscle about 6 cm above the iliopubic tract. It then passes behind the inguinal ligament to enter the thigh. Pain and weakness of the anterior thigh result from injury.

The anterior cutaneous branch of the femoral nerve (Fig. 116.5D) arises early and may be encountered near or beneath the iliopubic tract just lateral to the external iliac vessels.

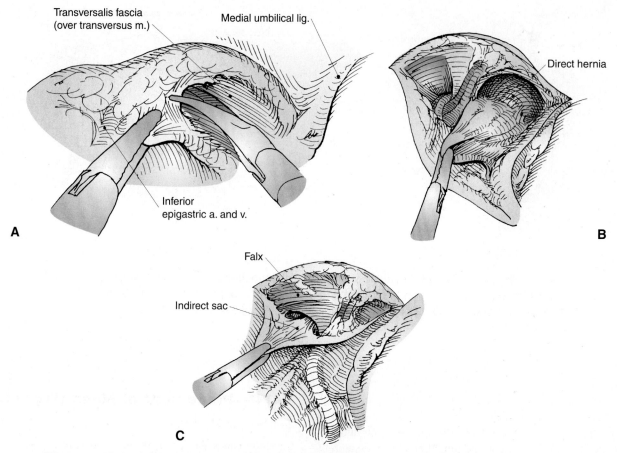

Figure 116.4 TAPP—reducing sac of hernia and defining anatomy. **A:** Developing exposure. **B:** Pulling sac of direct hernia into field **C:** Pulling sac of indirect hernia into field (**A–C** from Wind GG. The inguinal region. In: *Applied Laparoscopic Anatomy: Abdomen and Pelvis.* Baltimore, MD: Williams & Wilkins; 1997:85–140, with permission).

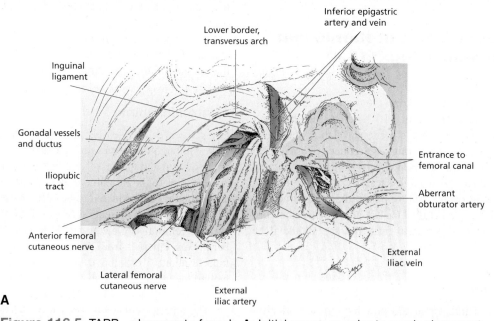

Figure 116.5 TAPP—placement of mesh. **A:** Initial exposure prior to mesh placement.

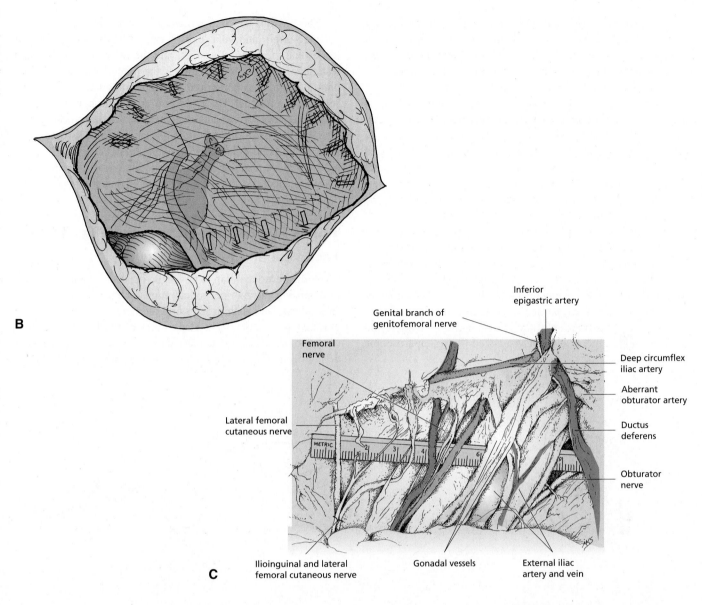

B

C

Inferior
epigastric artery

Genital branch of
genitofemoral nerve

Femoral
nerve

Deep circumflex
iliac artery

Aberrant
obturator artery

Ductus
deferens

Lateral femoral
cutaneous nerve

METRIC

Obturator
nerve

Ilioinguinal and lateral
femoral cutaneous nerve

Gonadal vessels

External iliac
artery and vein

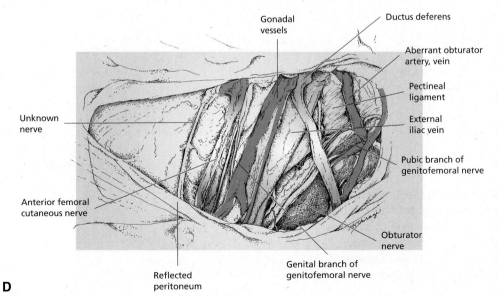

D

Gonadal
vessels

Ductus deferens

Aberrant obturator
artery, vein

Pectineal
ligament

External
iliac vein

Pubic branch of
genitofemoral nerve

Obturator
nerve

Genital branch of
genitofemoral nerve

Reflected
peritoneum

Anterior femoral
cutaneous nerve

Unknown
nerve

Figure 116.5 *Continued.*
B: Mesh tailored to cover all
defects and potential hernia ori-
fices. **C:** Regional anatomy and
nerves. **D:** Regional anatomy
including aberrant obturator
artery (**A, C, D** from Colborn GL,
Brick WG. Inguinal region. In:
Scott-Conner CEH, Cuschieri A,
Carter FJ, eds. *Minimal Access
Surgical Anatomy.* Philadelphia,
PA: Lippincott Williams &
Wilkins; 2000:239–266, with
permission; **B** from Wind
GG. The inguinal region. In:
*Applied Laparoscopic Anatomy:
Abdomen and Pelvis.* Baltimore,
MD: Williams & Wilkins;
1997:85–140, with permission).

The lateral femoral cutaneous nerve is one of the two nerves most commonly injured during laparoscopic herniorrhaphy. It emerges from the lateral border of the psoas major muscle and exits the pelvis by passing beneath the inguinal ligament, usually within 1 cm of the anterosuperior iliac spine.

The genitofemoral nerve passes down along the psoas major muscle, crosses behind the ureter, and divides into the genital and femoral branches. The exact site of bifurcation varies. In one common variant, the genital branch of the genitofemoral nerve passes below the iliopubic tract to enter the inguinal canal from below, placing it at risk during laparoscopic herniorrhaphy (Fig. 116.5D). Burning pain and numbness in the labium or scrotum and medial thigh result from injury.

The ilioinguinal and iliohypogastric nerves lie in a plane superficial to the plane in which laparoscopic hernia surgery is performed. These nerves are not seen but can be injured if counterpressure (with one hand from outside the abdomen) is used to facilitate placement of deep staples or tacks in the vicinity of the iliopubic tract, particularly lateral to the internal ring.

The actual distribution of the individual nerves varies, and these nerves are generally not visualized during laparoscopic herniorrhaphy.

The obvious vascular structures at peril include the external iliac artery and vein, exiting below the inguinal ligament to become the femoral vessels, and the inferior epigastric and testicular vessels. Less obvious is the potential for an aberrant obturator artery to be injured. These common anomalous vessels link the internal iliac artery with the obturator artery.

These numerous vascular and neural structures must be protected from rough dissection or placement of tacks or staples. A simple rule articulated by Seid and Amos (see references) is never to place a staple below the iliopubic tract anywhere lateral to the ductus (all the way to the anterosuperior iliac spine).

TAPP—Peritoneal Closure (Fig. 116.6)

Technical and Anatomic Points

Close the peritoneal flap to cover the mesh completely. Do this by apposing the two peritoneal edges at the point where tension is least and then progressing along the incision until full closure has been obtained. Staples may be used for this purpose (Fig. 116.6A). Take care to place these sufficiently close that gaps do not occur. Clips are used by some surgeons (Fig. 116.6B) to

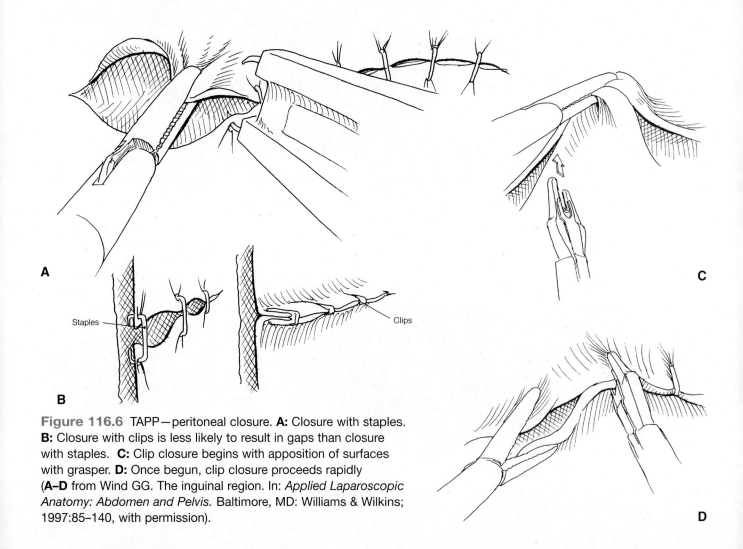

Figure 116.6 TAPP—peritoneal closure. **A:** Closure with staples. **B:** Closure with clips is less likely to result in gaps than closure with staples. **C:** Clip closure begins with apposition of surfaces with grasper. **D:** Once begun, clip closure proceeds rapidly (**A–D** from Wind GG. The inguinal region. In: *Applied Laparoscopic Anatomy: Abdomen and Pelvis.* Baltimore, MD: Williams & Wilkins; 1997:85–140, with permission).

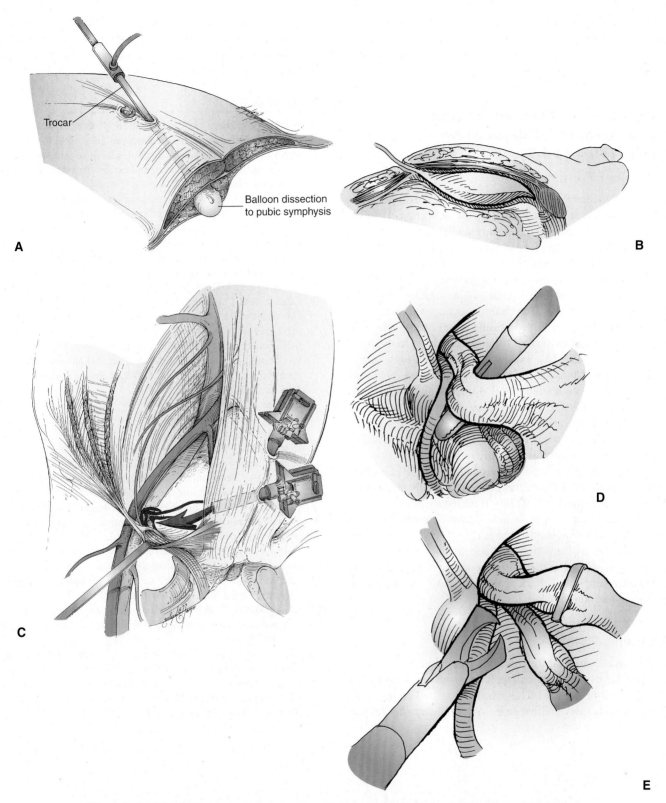

Figure 116.7 TEP—trocar placement and development of dissection plane. **A:** Initial placement of balloon at symphysis pubis. **B:** Balloon expanded to develop plane. **C:** Trocar placement. **D:** Sac dissected from cord structures. **E:** Sac amputated (**A, C** from Crawford DL, Phillips EH. Totally extraperitoneal laparoscopic herniorrhaphy. In: Zucker KA, ed. *Surgical Laparoscopy.* 2nd ed. Philadelphia, PA: Lippincott Williams & Wilkins; 2001:571–584, with permission; **B, D, E** from Wind GG. The inguinal region. In: *Applied Laparoscopic Anatomy: Abdomen and Pelvis.* Baltimore, MD: Williams & Wilkins; 1997:85–140, with permission).

diminish this problem by providing greater peritoneal overlap (Fig. 116.6C,D).

Desufflate the abdomen, check hemostasis, and close the trocar sites in the usual fashion.

TEP—Trocar Placement and Development of Dissection Plane (Fig. 116.7)

Technical Points

The crucial maneuver is developing a plane in the proper extra-peritoneal space at the beginning of the dissection. If this is done properly, the rest of the repair is similar to that previously described. If the wrong plane is entered or if a hole is made in the peritoneum, dissection may be more difficult.

Make initial entry into the preperitoneal space with an open technique. After incising the fascia, visualize the fat of the preperitoneal space. Use blunt dissection with a finger to establish an initial plane progressing toward the pubic symphysis. Introduce a dissecting balloon and pass it to the pubic symphysis (Fig. 116.7A), expanding the balloon to develop a working space. Note that the bladder is mobilized downward (Fig. 116.7B). Do not attempt this dissection in a patient who has had previous surgery in the space of Retzius because the plane may be obliterated.

Place additional trocars as shown (Fig. 116.7C). As during TAPP, a direct sac will generally reduce as dissection progresses laterally. An indirect sac may cause difficulty. Carefully separate the sac from the ductus deferens medially and testicular vessels laterally (Fig. 116.7D). If necessary, divide the sac, taking extreme care not to include ductus deferens, testicular vessels, or intraperitoneal structures (Fig. 116.7E).

Identification of structures and placement of mesh proceeds exactly as described earlier. At the end of the procedure, the peritoneum simply falls back against the mesh, and there is no peritoneal incision to repair.

Anatomic Points

The prevesical space of Retzius gives free entry, through loose fatty areolar tissue, to the extraperitoneal anterior bladder and ultimately to the prostate. This space is accessed during retropubic prostatectomy and hence becomes obliterated with scar tissue. The only significant structures that should be encountered are the pubic symphysis, visible as a large white transversely oriented structure, and the urinary bladder. The bladder is displaced posteriorly as dissection progresses and is not seen.

REFERENCES

1. Brick WG, Colborn GL, Gadacz TR, et al. Crucial anatomic lessons for laparoscopic herniorrhaphy. *Am Surg.* 1995;61:172–177.
2. Broin EO, Horner C, Mealy K, et al. Meralgia paraesthetica following laparoscopic inguinal hernia repair: An anatomical analysis. *Surg Endosc.* 1995;9:76–78.
3. Colborn GL, Brick WG. Inguinal region. In: Scott-Conner CEH, Cuschieri A, Carter FJ, eds. *Minimal Access Surgical Anatomy.* Philadelphia, PA: Lippincott Williams & Wilkins; 2000:239–266. (Gives more details of anatomy.)
4. Colborn GL, Skandalakis JE. Laparoscopic cadaveric anatomy of the inguinal area. *Probl Gen Surg.* 1995;12:13–20.
5. Crawford DL, Phillips EH. Laparoscopic repair and groin hernia surgery. *Surg Clin North Am.* 1998;78:1047–1062.
6. Dibenedetto LM, Lei Q, Gilroy AM, et al. Variations in the inferior pelvic pathway of the lateral femoral cutaneous nerve: Implications for laparoscopic hernia repair. *Clin Anat.* 1996;9:232–236.
7. El-Dhuwaib Y, Corless D, Emmett C, et al. Laparoscopic versus open repair of inguinal hernia: A longitudinal cohort study. *Surg Endosc.* 2013;27:936–945.
8. Eubanks S, Newman L 3rd, Goehring L, et al. Meralgia paresthetica: A complication of laparoscopic herniorrhaphy. *Surg Laparosc Endosc.* 1993;3:381–385.
9. Keating JP, Morgan A. Femoral nerve palsy following laparoscopic inguinal herniorrhaphy. *J Laparoendosc Surg.* 1993;3:557–559.
10. Kraus MA. Nerve injury during laparoscopic inguinal hernia repair. *Surg Laparosc Endosc.* 1993;3:342–345.
11. Ladwa N, Sajid MS, Sains P, et al. Suture mesh fixation versus glue mesh fixation in open inguinal hernia repair: A systematic review and meta-analysis. *Int J Surg.* 2013;11:128–135.
12. Sampath P, Yeo CJ, Campbell JN. Nerve injury associated with laparoscopic inguinal herniorrhaphy. *Surgery.* 1995;118:829–833.
13. Seid AS, Amos E. Entrapment neuropathy in laparoscopic herniorrhaphy. *Surg Endosc.* 1994;8:1050–1053.
14. Skandalakis JE, Colborn GL, Androulakis JA, et al. Embryologic and anatomic basis of inguinal herniorrhaphy. *Surg Clin North Am.* 1993;73:799–836.
15. Woods S, Polglase A. Ilioinguinal nerve entrapment from laparoscopic hernia repair. *Aust N Z J Surg.* 1993;63:823–824.
16. Yang J, Tong da N, Yao J, et al. Laparoscopic or Lichtenstein repair for recurrent inguinal hernia: A meta-analysis of randomized controlled trials. *ANZ J Surg.* 2013;83:312–318.

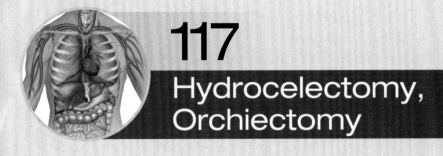

117

Hydrocelectomy, Orchiectomy

Hydroceles are collections of fluid between the parietal and visceral layers of the tunica vaginalis. Communicating hydroceles, in which this space communicates with the peritoneal cavity, are often encountered during repair of indirect inguinal hernias. These are simply managed by amputating the distal portion of the hernia sac. In noncommunicating hydroceles, the balance between fluid generation and absorption in this space becomes uneven and fluid accumulates.

A variety of conditions can cause noncommunicating hydroceles. The most important thing is to exclude testicular malignancy. High-resolution scrotal ultrasound can help exclude malignancy.

As with most cancers, testicular malignancy is most appropriately treated by an experienced multidisciplinary team. The surgical treatment of testicular malignancy consists of radical orchiectomy through an inguinal approach. This chapter describes two common procedures for hydrocelectomy as well as inguinal orchiectomy. The precautions used in cases of possible malignancy are also described.

SCORE™, the Surgical Council on Resident Education, did not classify hydrocelectomy and orchiectomy but included hydroceles and testicular tumors in the recommended curriculum under the "Broad" and "Focused" categories, respectively.

STEPS IN PROCEDURE

Inguinal incision
Identify and protect ilioinguinal nerve
Identify spermatic cord at external ring
Surround spermatic cord with Penrose drain
    Place noncrushing clamp on cord, if
        malignancy suspected
Deliver testis and cord into surgical field
    Identify vas, epididymis, and vessels

Hydrocelectomy

Open hydrocele in an area remote from testis
    and supporting structures
Biopsy and obtain frozen section of any
    suspicious areas
    If negative, release clamp
    If positive, consult urology or proceed
        with orchiectomy (below)
For simple excision:
    Excise redundant tissue of hydrocele,
        leaving cuff around testis (one
        fingerbreadth)

Oversew the cut edge of hydrocele
    with running lock stitch, absorbable
    suture
For bottle operation:
    Excise redundant tissue of hydrocele,
        leaving generous cuff around
        testis
    Invert tissue around testis and suture
        cuff to itself, leaving loose closure at
        top to allow exit of cord structures
Return cord and testis to scrotum
Check hemostasis and close inguinal
    incision

Orchiectomy

Individually clamp and tie vas and vessels
Ligate remaining structures
Remove cord and testis together
Release clamp
Check hemostasis and close inguinal
    incision

HALLMARK ANATOMIC COMPLICATIONS

Ischemic orchitis
Injury to vas
Failure to identify malignancy

LIST OF STRUCTURES

Camper and Scarpa fasciae
External oblique aponeurosis
Ilioinguinal nerve
Spermatic cord
Processus vaginalis
Tunica vaginalis

Vas deferens
Epididymis
Testis
Testicular artery
Pampiniform plexus

The testis lies posterior in the scrotum as shown in Figure 117.1A. Anterior to the testis there is a potential space lined by tunica vaginalis (termed visceral, where it is adherent to the testis; and parietal, where it is adherent to the scrotum). This space covers approximately the anterior two-thirds of the testis. When fluid accumulates in this space, it is termed a hydrocele. Figure 117.1B shows the situation when the processus vaginalis seals off distally, but does not completely seal proximally, and an indi-rect inguinal hernia forms (see Chapter 115). When the processus vaginalis does not seal off at all, a communicating hydrocele (Fig. 117.1C) forms. This type of hydrocele is generally encountered and repaired during management of the associated inguinal hernia. Related situations are shown in Figure 117.1D and F. These are primarily encountered in infants and children.

The most common type of hydrocele requiring intervention in adults is the noncommunicating hydrocele (Fig. 117.1E).

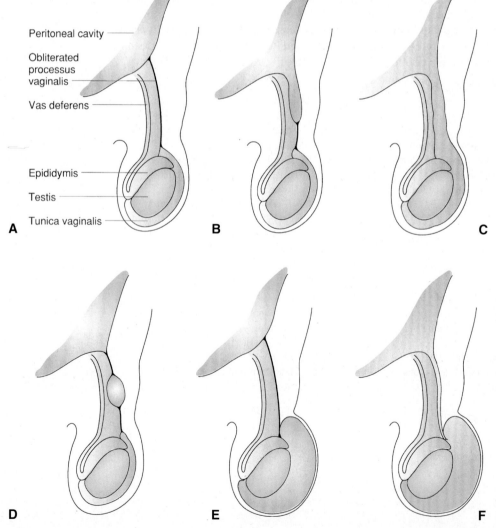

Peritoneal cavity

Obliterated processus vaginalis

Vas deferens

Epididymis

Testis

Tunica vaginalis

A   B   C

D   E   F

Figure 117.1 Terminology used for various sorts of inguinal her-nias and hydroceles. **A:** Normal anatomy. **B:** Indirect inguinal her-nia. **C:** Communicating hydrocele associated with indirect inguinal hernia. **D:** Hydrocele of cord and scrotum. **E:** Noncommunicating hydrocele. **F:** Communicating hydrocele with patent processus vaginalis, no clinically appar-ent indirect inguinal hernia (from *Greenfield's Surgery.* 5th ed. Philadelphia, PA: Lippincott Williams & Wilkins: 2011, with permission).

The fluid may accumulate for a variety of reasons, and it is important to exclude malignancy as a possible cause.

Hydrocelectomy (Fig. 117.2)

Technical Points

When the diagnosis of hydrocele is certain and neither associated hernia nor tumor is suspected, a small incision may be made in the midline of the scrotum. The inguinal approach described here allows any associated hernia to be repaired, and also avoids violating the skin of the scrotum if malignancy is encountered.

Make a long oblique incision or one in a natural skin crease, ending at the pubic tubercle (see Chapter 116, Figure 116.1). Deepen this incision through Camper and Scarpa fasciae until the aponeurosis of the external oblique muscle is encountered. At the external ring, palpate the spermatic cord.

Palpate the pubic tubercle. With a peanut sponge and your index finger, gently develop the avascular plane deep to the spermatic cord. By keeping your dissection on the pubic tubercle, avoid entering the spermatic cord. Pass a Penrose drain around the spermatic cord.

If there is any question of possible malignancy, tighten the Penrose drain or place a noncrushing clamp across the spermatic

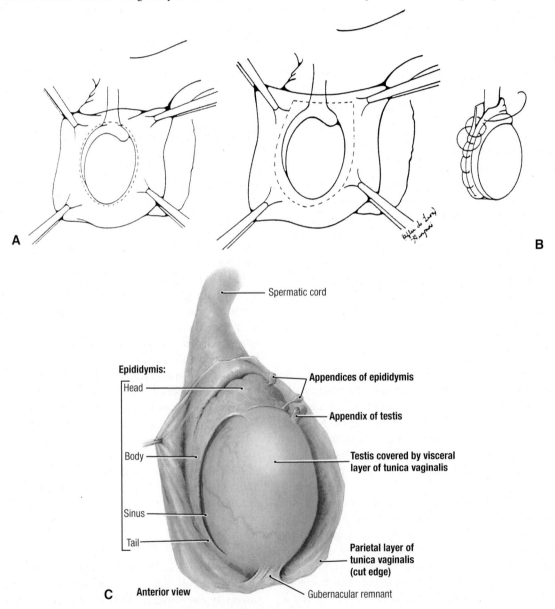

Figure 117.2 Surgery for hydrocele. **A:** Simple excision of hydrocele. **B:** Bottle operation showing eversion of hydrocele sac. **C:** Anatomy of testis showing relationship of tunica vaginalis to testis (**A** and **B** from Graham SD Jr, Keane TE, eds. *Glenn's Urologic Surgery.* 7th ed. Philadelphia, PA: Lippincott Williams & Wilkins; 2010, with permission. **C** from Agur AMR, Dalley AF. *Grant's Atlas of Anatomy.* 12th ed. Philadelphia, PA: Lippincott Williams & Wilkins; 2009, with permission).

cord to avoid tumor emboli during the manipulation of the testis. Note the clamp time.

Deliver the distal cord and testis into the incision, by gentle traction and division of avascular attachments to the scrotum. Inspect the hydrocele sac and testis.

Carefully identify the testis, epididymis, and cord structures. Normally, these will be posterior, but very large hydroceles may distort the anatomy. Transilluminate the sac, if necessary, to find a safe area (opposite the testis and associated structures) to open the hydrocele.

Biopsy and obtain frozen section of any suspicious areas. Note that you can extend the clamp time, if necessary, by icing the testis.

If these biopsies are negative, remove the clamp. If these are positive, obtain urology consultation or proceed to inguinal orchiectomy (see below).

Simple excision: Fully open the hydrocele. Excise the redundant sac, leaving a cuff of tissue approximately one fingerbreadth in width to avoid injury to cord structures. Most commonly, it is enough to simply oversew the resulting cuff of tissue for hemostasis (Fig. 117.2A). If the sac is flimsy and there is concern about potential recurrence, perform a bottle operation.

Bottle operation: This procedure requires a cuff of tissue sufficient to approximate in an inside-out fashion behind the testis. Excise the redundant sac as noted above. Then approximate the edges of the sac behind the testis and approximate these with a running lock stitch (Fig. 117.2B). Leave a wide opening at the top for cord structures to enter and exit.

Check hemostasis carefully and return testis and cord to normal anatomic position. Close the incision in the usual fashion. Ensure that the testis is fully returned to its normal position without twisting.

Anatomic Points

The ovoid, paired testes lie in separate pouches of the scrotum. Each testis lies in a vertical orientation (and a horizontally lying testis may be a clue to testicular torsion). The testis is anchored by the remnants of the gubernaculum, which should not be divided during this procedure. Posterior and cephalad to the testis is the epididymis which is normally separately palpable. The normal testis feels smooth and relatively soft. Any nodules may indicate tumor.

During the third month of gestation, the testes descend from the retroperitoneum, traverse the inguinal canal, and ultimately come to their final position in the testis. A finger of peritoneum, the processus vaginalis, follows each testis down into the scrotum. Normally, the processus vaginalis is obliterated proximally. The portion that is adherent to the testis becomes the tunica vaginalis. The tunica vaginalis has a visceral and a parietal component.

The visceral tunica vaginalis is closely applied to the testis except posteriorly, where the body and tail of the epididymis and associated structures exit to ascend to the spermatic cord (Fig. 117.2C). The parietal tunica vaginalis is closely applied to the dartos muscle of the scrotum. The tunica vaginalis normally contains a small amount of fluid. When an abnormal amount of fluid accumulates, the result is a hydrocele. Note that the bottle operation cannot fully surround the testis with a sutured cuff of inverted hydrocele sac because of the need to accommodate the exiting epididymis and vascular supply to testis.

The arterial blood supply and venous drainage of the testis come down through the inguinal canal with the testis and are encountered in the spermatic cord rather than in the plane between the testis and the scrotum. The testis is anchored in the scrotum by the relatively avascular gubernaculum.

The primary blood supply to the testis is the testicular artery. A smaller artery supplies the ductus deferens and smaller branches go to the epididymis.

The venous drainage forms the pampiniform plexus of veins which ascend along the spermatic cord, where they may be encountered during inguinal hernia repair. When these veins become enlarged, a varicocele results.

Orchiectomy (Fig. 117.3)

Technical Points

It is important to recognize that many alternatives to orchiectomy exist, and that careful evaluation by a specialist is important in choosing the appropriate alternatives (see References). The procedure described here is the basic procedure for inguinal orchiectomy with radical excision of the spermatic cord.

Make an inguinal incision and obtain control of the spermatic cord with a noncrushing clamp or Penrose drain as noted above. Note that radical inguinal orchiectomy requires ligation of the spermatic cord at the internal ring. If this procedure is intended, open the inguinal canal by incising the aponeurosis of the external oblique muscle and obtain control of the spermatic cord at the internal ring (Fig. 117.3A). Deliver the testis and cord into the operative field.

Divide the gubernaculum of the testis at the inferior pole. Doubly clamp, divide, and ligate the spermatic cord at the internal ring. Remove the testis and cord from the surgical field.

Obtain hemostasis. An appropriately sized testicular prosthesis may then be placed in the scrotum. Close the incision in the usual fashion.

Anatomic Points

As the testis descends into the scrotum, it carries with it not only its blood supply but also lymphatics. Testicular cancer metastasizes to the lumbar nodes, bypassing the superficial inguinal nodes. The skin of the scrotum drains in the usual fashion to lymphatics in the superficial inguinal region (Fig. 117.3B). Approaching testicular tumors through the groin rather than through the scrotum allows the surgeon to obtain proximal control, avoiding potential tumor emboli in the venous or lymphatic system.

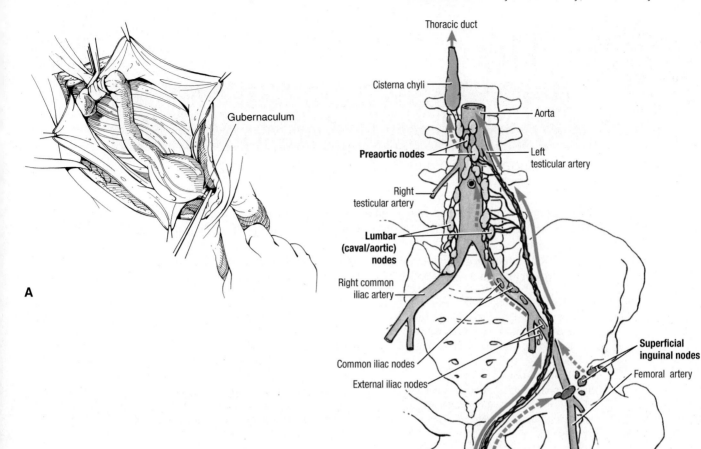

Figure 117.3 A: Radical orchiectomy. Note control of cord structures at internal inguinal ring. **B:** Anatomic basis of inguinal approach to testicular tumors. Note that the lymphatic drainage of the testis follows the spermatic cord to the lumbar nodes (**A** from Graham SD Jr, Keane TE, eds. *Glenn's Urologic Surgery,* 7th ed. Philadelphia, PA: Lippincott Williams & Wilkins; 2010, with permission. **B** from Agur AMR, Dalley AF. *Grant's Atlas of Anatomy.* 12th ed. Philadelphia, PA: Lippincott Williams & Wilkins; 2009, with permission).

REFERENCES

1. Carver BS, Donat SM. Simple orchiectomy. In: Graham SD Jr, Keane TE, eds. *Glenn's Urologic Surgery.* 7th ed. Philadelphia, PA: Wolters Kluwer Lippincott Williams & Wilkins; 2010:428 ff. (Includes scrotal approach and details on placement of testicular prostheses.)
2. Chandak P, Shah A, Taghizadeh A, et al. Testis-sparing surgery for benign and malignant testicular tumours. *Int J Clin Pract.* 2003; 57:912.
3. Connolly SS, D'Arcy FT, Bredin HC, et al. Value of frozen section analysis with suspected testicular malignancy. *Urology.* 2006; 67:167.
4. Emir L, Sunay M, Dadli M, et al. Endoscopic versus open hydrocelectomy for the treatment of adult hydroceles: A randomized controlled clinical trial. *Int Urol Nephrol.* 2011;43:55–59.
5. Francis JJ, Levine LA. Aspiration and sclerotherapy: A non-surgical treatment option for hydroceles. *J Urol.* 2012;189:1725–1729.
6. Gottesman JE. Hydrocelectomy: Evaluation of technique. *Urology.* 1976;7:386–387.
7. Kirkham AP, Kumar P, Minhas S, et al. Targeted testicular excision biopsy: When and how should we try to avoid radical orchidectomy? *Clin Radiol.* 2009;64:1158–1165.
8. Swanson DA. Inguinal orchiectomy. In: Graham SD Jr, Keane TE, eds. *Glenn's Urologic Surgery.* 7th ed. Philadelphia, PA: Wolters Kluwer Lippincott Williams & Wilkins; 2010:433 ff.

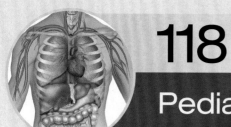

118

Pediatric Inguinal Hernia

Raphael C. Sun and Graeme J. Pitcher

Inguinal hernias in infants and young children represent pure indirect hernias. Correction involves high ligation of the sac. The floor of the inguinal canal is left along and does not require repair.

SCORE™, the Surgical Council on Resident Education, classified inguinal herniorrhaphy in children as an "ESSENTIAL COMMON" procedure.

STEPS IN PROCEDURE

Skin crease incision centered over the mid-inguinal point (halfway between anterior superior iliac spine and pubic tubercle)

Divide Scarpa fascia

Incise aponeurosis of external oblique

Identify and preserve ilioinguinal nerve

Identify sac by separating cremaster fibers from sac

Identify cord and cord structures and dissect the sac away

In females, divide and ligate round ligament and sac simultaneously

In males, once sac separated from cord structures, transect sac and suture ligate

Pull scrotal contents into scrotum

Close external oblique, Scarpa fascia and skin in layers with absorbable sutures

HALLMARK ANATOMIC COMPLICATIONS

Injury to spermatic cord

LIST OF STRUCTURES

External oblique muscle and aponeurosis

Inguinal canal

Processus vaginalis

External (superficial) inguinal ring

Superficial (Scarpa) fascia

Spermatic cord (male)

Round ligament and ovary (female)

Background

Inguinal hernia in pediatric patients commonly require surgical repair. These are indirect hernias, and they develop from a processus vaginalis that remains patent after birth.

Inguinal hernias are more common in males than females. They are also more common in preterm than in full-term infants. Inguinal hernias occur more on the right (60%) compared to the left (25% to 30%), and 10% to 15% are bilateral.

Incision (Fig. 118.1)

Technical Points

The traditional adult hernia repair involves an incision from the anterior superior iliac spine (ASIS) to the pubic tubercle. However, for pediatric patients a curvilinear incision in the skin crease over the mid-inguinal point provides proper exposure to the structures of the inguinal canal and is better cosmetically (Fig. 118.1).

Deepen the incision down to the external oblique aponeurosis. This may be done with the use of electrocautery, blunt, or sharp dissection. The method is optional. The key is to locate the relatively avascular tissue plane superficial to the external oblique aponeurosis.

Anatomic Points

The incision should be made along the skin crease. In pediatric patients, the incision ends up being more transverse than a traditional adult inguinal hernia repair incision. The inguinal canal will be well exposed if the incision is centered over the mid-inguinal point as the important steps of the operation take place at the internal ring. It is important to define the lower border of the inguinal ligament to ensure that the canal is entered over its anterior border. If the external oblique incision is made too cranially, the surgeon will struggle to locate the sac and the patient will be put at risk for iatrogenic injury.

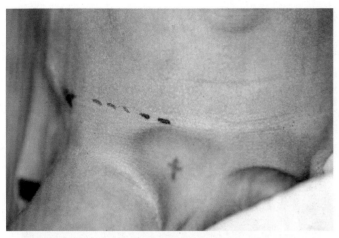

Figure 118.1 Location of incision for right inguinal repair in an infant. Note that the most prominent skin crease centered over the mid-inguinal point is used. This allows good access to the internal ring. In this case, the crease is cranial to the mid-inguinal point but because of the mobility of the skin will afford excellent access and still preserve excellent cosmesis.

The subcutaneous tissue, fat, and Scarpa fascia can be quite dense. The thickness of the fascia before reaching the level of the external oblique varies based on body habitus.

Identification of External Oblique (Fig. 118.2)

Technical Points

It is important to visualize the inguinal ligament and external ring to rule out the rare femoral hernia and to ensure that the inguinal canal is opened in the correct place (just above the inguinal ligament). Once the external oblique is identified,

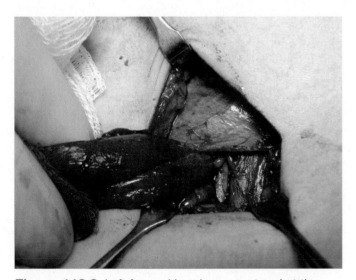

Figure 118.2 Left femoral hernia encountered at the time of groin exploration. Note the anatomic configuration with the hernia emerging beneath the inguinal ligament and medial to the femoral vein.

use a no. 15 blade to open the aponeurosis. Use Metzenbaum scissors to extend the incision toward the external ring. The external ring does not need to be opened unless orchidopexy is planned.

Next, mobilize the external oblique to identify the cord structures. In larger children, a hemostat on the fascial edge may facilitate this dissection. The hernial sac should be anteromedial to the cord and cord structures. Downward pressure on the abdominal wall assists with the identification of the sac. Dissect the hernial sac away from the cremaster fibers with an atraumatic forceps or with blunt sponge dissection. Once the sac is isolated you need to decide whether to proceed by opening the sac deliberately or keeping the sac closed. It is advisable to open the sac if the patient is a small baby with a large sac or if the patient is a female. Always open the hernial sac in a female to ensure that a fallopian tube is not present in the sac.

Anatomic Points

The external ring is superolateral to the pubic tubercle. The hernial sac usually is anteromedial to the cord structures. The cord is covered with cremasteric muscle and fascia, which is continuity with the internal oblique.

Management of Hernial Sac (Fig. 118.3)

Technical Points

Once the hernial sac is dissected free, clamp the proximal portion with a hemostat. The distal sac should be left without further dissection, which is meddlesome and may predispose to postoperative scrotal hematoma. A high ligation is the standard inguinal hernia repair in the pediatric patient. To ensure that a high ligation is achieved, the sac must be dissected to the retroperitoneum. This point is reached at the point when preperitoneal fat is seen and the vas starts to veer medially (Fig. 118.3A). The sac is typically twisted after ensuring that it is empty and suture ligated with 3-0 or 4-0 Vicryl sutures (Fig. 118.3B). High-risk hernias can be double ligated. The hernial sac is transected and the stump should retract. Pull the testicles and scrotal contents into the scrotum and ensure that they are not entrapped in the scar tissue of the repair causing a so-called ascending testis.

For girls, the round ligament can be ligated with the same suture as the sac. The distal portion of the round ligament is usually ligated for hemostasis.

Close the external oblique aponeurosis starting at the external ring. Take care not to suture or entrap the ilioinguinal nerve. Close in layers with absorbable sutures.

Anatomic Points

In children, the operation is more properly referred to as a herniotomy as no reparative operation (as in herniorrhaphy) is performed on the inguinal canal.

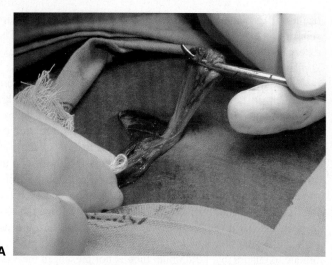
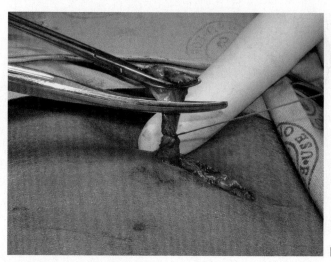

Figure 118.3 **A:** Patient undergoing right inguinal hernia repair showing the anatomical position at which high ligation is performed. **B:** High ligation performed.

In newborns and infants, you will find that the external and internal rings are almost superimposed upon each other resulting in a shorter inguinal canal than in an adult. In babies with extremely large internal rings expanded by giant hernias, it may be necessary to bolster the fascia transversalis with some fine polypropylene sutures (in the form of a medial interfoveolar ligament or Marcy repair) to minimize recurrence. This is controversial.

If a truly undescended testicle (either in a position of incomplete or ectopic descent) is encountered at the time of repair of a symptomatic hernia then it is correct to perform an orchidopexy at that time rather than to commit the patient to a subsequent operation in a scarred field.

When dissecting to identify the sac, the surgeon should avoid dissecting in a deep plane below the internal oblique muscle as this puts the fascia transversalis at risk of injury and iatrogenic direct inguinal hernia which will present as a recurrence.

REFERENCE

1. Ein SH, Njere I, Ein A. Six thousand three hundred sixty-one pediatric inguinal hernias: A 35-year review *J Pediatr Surg.* 2006:41; 980–986.

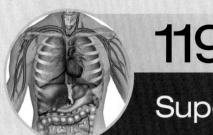

119

Superficial Groin Dissection

Laura A. Adam and Neal Wilkinson

A variety of terms are used to describe lymphadenectomy of the inguinal and ilioinguinal regions. In this chapter, we will use the terms *superficial* and *deep*. A superficial dissection includes the lymph node basins of the inguinal ligament, saphenous vein, and femoral vessels. Cloquet's node is typically removed during a superficial dissection (Fig. 119.1). A deep dissection includes the lymph node basins extending along the course of external, internal, and common iliac vessels. In addition, deep dissection may include lymph nodes within the obturator canal.

SCORE™, the Surgical Council on Resident Education, classified ilioinguinal–femoral lymphadenectomy as a "COMPLEX" procedure.

SUPERFICIAL REGION

Inguinal   Femoral
Saphenous   Cloquet's node

DEEP REGION

External iliac   Common iliac
Internal iliac   Obturator

When both the superficial and deep regions are removed, we will refer to a superficial and deep dissection, realizing that the term *radical* is occasionally used in this setting. The proximal extent or pelvic component of the dissection may vary depending on the pathology being treated and must be clearly stated in the operative note instead of using vague terms such as deep or radical.

STEPS IN PROCEDURE

Superficial Inguinal Dissection

Supine position with leg externally rotated and knee slightly flexed

Lazy S–shaped incision from anterosuperior iliac spine to medial thigh

Proximal extent used primarily for deep dissection or in obese patients

Develop flaps medially and laterally just above superficial fascia; to lateral border of sartorius muscle and medial border of gracilis muscle

Avoid lateral femoral cutaneous nerve

Ligate tributaries of saphenous vein entering field and saphenous vein itself entering inferior aspect of field

Sweep fatty node-bearing tissue cephalad to saphenofemoral junction and ligate and divide saphenous vein (oversew femoral end)

Divide or retract inguinal ligament to expose femoral canal

Remove nodal tissue; label the highest node as Cloquet's node and submit separately

Deep Inguinal Ligament

Place deep self-retaining retractors and divide external oblique aponeurosis

Divide inguinal ligament

Displace spermatic cord (in males) medially and divide the inferior epigastric vessels

Gently displace peritoneum medially to expose retroperitoneal structures

Begin laterally on the pelvic sidewall and sweep nodes and associated tissues medial

Mobilize rectum and bladder medially and retract these behind moist packs

Obturator node dissection can be performed by following the obturator nerve and artery

Obtain hemostasis and reapproximate the inguinal ligament and abdominal wall structures

Detach sartorius high on the anterosuperior
iliac spine
Mobilize it, rotating it to fit into the space over
the femoral vessels
Suture the sartorius muscle to the inguinal
ligament

Place closed-suction drains and close
Close incision in layers

HALLMARK ANATOMIC COMPLICATIONS

Injury to lateral femoral cutaneous nerve
Injury to femoral vein or femoral nerve
Injury to obturator nerve

Injury to pelvic nerve plexus
Lymphocele or lymphedema
Skin necrosis

LIST OF STRUCTURES

Inguinal Lymph Nodes
Superficial inguinal lymph nodes
Deep inguinal lymph nodes
Node of Cloquet
Iliac lymph nodes

Obturator Lymph Nodes
Obturator foramen
Obturator canal
Anterosuperior iliac spine
Lateral femoral cutaneous nerve
Inguinal ligament

Pubic tubercle
External oblique aponeurosis
Fascia lata

Femoral Triangle
Femoral nerve
Femoral artery
Femoral vein

Saphenous Vein
Saphenofemoral junction
Adductor longus muscle
Sartorius muscle

ORIENTATION

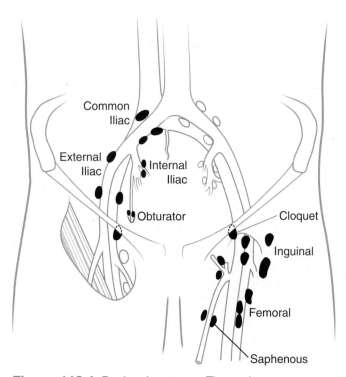

Figure 119.1 Regional anatomy. The nodes encompassed during a superficial dissection are shown on the right-hand side of the figure, and the nodes taken during deep dissection are shown on the left.

The superficial and deep inguinal lymph node dissection is most commonly performed for cutaneous malignancies of the lower extremity, lower abdomen, and flank. Melanoma remains the most common indication and the majority will have been localized to the region by sentinel node mapping techniques. Additional indications include penile, distal urethral, scrotal, vulvar, anal, and anal canal cancers. The pelvic lymphadenectomy for gynecologic pathology may include many of the same regional lymph node basins, but is approached through a lower midline incision and will not be covered in this chapter.

These procedures carry a significant risk of local morbidity, including skin flap necrosis, wound infection, seroma formation, and lymphedema. For melanoma, the procedure should only be performed for documented disease in the region commonly described as a "therapeutic" lymphadenectomy. Sentinel lymph node staging, computed tomography, or ultrasound-directed fine-needle aspiration, and now positron emission tomography can be used to preoperatively stage the region and has replaced elective nodal dissection for melanoma.

Incision and Elevation of Flaps: Superficial and Deep Regions (Fig. 119.2)

Technical Points

After induction of anesthesia, the patient is positioned supine with the leg externally rotated and the knee slightly flexed to

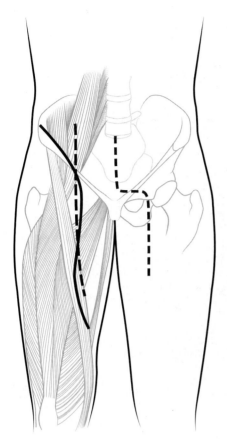

Figure 119.2 Incision and elevation of flaps: Superficial and deep regions

improve medial exposure. In larger patients, placing a bump under the thigh may further facilitate exposure. Preoperative antibiotics are frequently given despite the procedure being a Class I (infection classification) case. Most wound complications are related to skin flap necrosis and lymphedema. These are not likely to be influenced by antibiotics, and randomized controlled trials have questioned their efficacy in preventing wound complications. However, because of these high wound complication rates, it is reasonable to provide a short course of antibiotics directed toward common skin flora. A Foley catheter and sequential compression devices are typically used. Muscle paralysis should be minimized until the femoral nerve is clearly identified. The skin preparation and draping should include lower abdomen to knee with wide medial and lateral exposure.

The inferior aspect of the incision is placed directly over the femoral vessels and should extend inferiorly to the convergence of the sartorius and femoral vessels. The superior aspect of the incision may vary based on surgeon choice, patient body habitus, and anticipated proximal extent of the dissection. We prefer a lazy S–shaped incision from the anterosuperior iliac spine to the medial thigh with the middle portion overlying the bottom of the inguinal ligament. The abdominal pannus in large body habitus patients can be rotated medially and elevated superiorly to provide better visualization. An alternate straight vertical incision traversing the inguinal ligament onto

the lower abdomen works well in thin patients. If a previous sentinel lymph node biopsy site exists, it should be included in the incision. The proximal extent of the incision can vary depending on the proximal extent of the dissection and will need to be longer if a deep dissection is to be done. The abdominoinguinal incision is seldom indicated to gain wider access to the pelvis but can provide wide exposure of the entire internal pelvis when clinically indicated: Proximal control of vessels, difficult bleeding, or bulky adenopathy.

Develop skin flaps medially and laterally using every attempt to ensure viable flaps for closure by using gentle traction with skin hooks, minimizing cautery damage, and ensuring proper flap thickness. Below the inguinal ligament the skin flaps should be just above the level of the superficial fascia to assure both a complete specimen and decrease the risk of flap necrosis. Extend the flaps to the medial border of the gracilis muscle and to the lateral edge of the sartorius. Avoid injury to the lateral femoral cutaneous nerve during lateral dissection. The lateral femoral cutaneous nerve lies just below the anterosuperior iliac spine and supplies sensory distribution to the lateral thigh. Above the inguinal ligament, skin flaps are developed approximately 5 cm superiorly to the level of the external oblique aponeurosis. Skin flaps superior to the inguinal ligament may be thicker if site of the primary is distal on the extremity because the lymphatic chain is deep to this level. If, on the other hand, the primary lesion is on flank or abdominal wall, skin flaps may need to include the subcutaneous lymphatics.

Superficial Lymph Node Dissection (Fig. 119.3)

Technical Points

The lymph node chains follow the course of the major vasculature structures: Saphenous vein, femoral artery and vein, and iliac artery and vein. Carefully watching the thickness of the medial and lateral skin flaps will provide adequate exposure and ensure viable tissue for closure. The saphenous vein has numerous proximal tributaries as it enters the saphenofemoral junction. Ligate these tributaries distally and include them within the specimen. The superficial dissection includes all subcutaneous and nodal tissues within the boundaries of the sartorius and gracilus muscles (Fig. 119.3A), which is delineated during skin flap formation. Identify the deep tissue plane either proximally at the inguinal ligament or distally where the sartorius and gracilus converge. The femoral pulse can be used to identify the neurovascular bundle and ensuring that the dissection does not injure the nerve laterally or vein medially. The femoral vein, artery, and nerve form the floor of the dissection and need to be clearly visualized to adequately remove the lymphatics. The saphenous vein crosses through the subcutaneous tissue on the inferior and medial aspects of the dissection. Ligate the vessel distally and include the proximal vessel up to the saphenofemoral junction within the specimen (Fig. 119.3B). Extend the dissection along the superficial surface of the femoral vein until the saphenofemoral junction

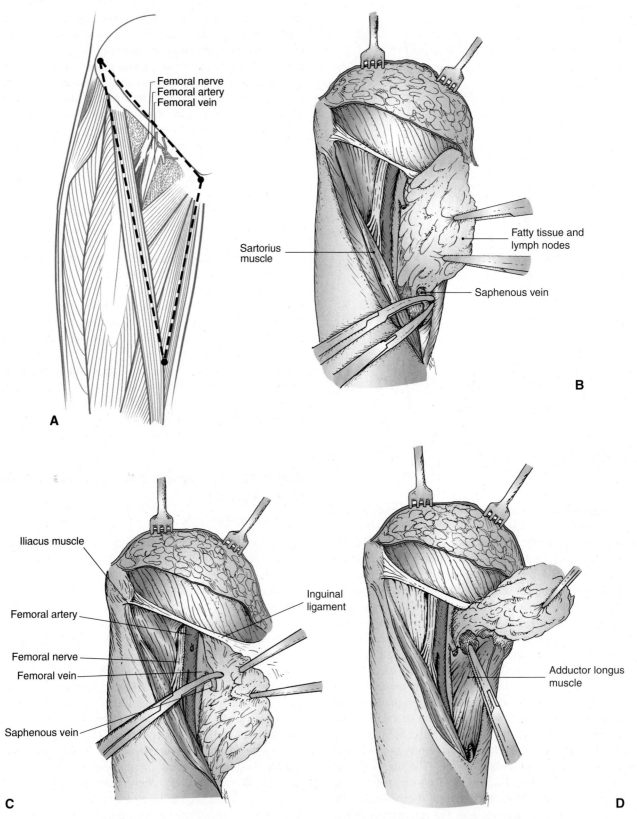

Figure 119.3 Superficial lymph node dissection. **A:** Boundaries of dissection (femoral triangle). **B:** Saphenous vein is divided at inferior boundary and fatty tissue swept upward. **C:** Saphenous vein is divided at cephalad aspect as tissue is swept medially. **D:** Final dissection of fatty tongue at upper aspect (Cloquet's node will be found at the apex of this dissection).

is reached. The saphenous vein is divided for a second time at the saphenofemoral junction (Fig. 119.3C). The femoral vein should be oversewn with a polypropylene suture in a running fashion to avoid stenosis or ligature slippage. The superficial surface of the femoral vessels and nerve make up the deepest part of the dissection. Circumferential control of the vessels within the femoral triangle is not needed and iatrogenic injury to the nerve must be avoided.

At the proximal aspect of the superficial dissection, the inguinal ligament must be retracted or divided to exposure the femoral canal. The vessels enter the femoral canal below the inguinal ligament and become the external iliac vessels. The highest node within the canal should be removed and identified as Cloquet's node (Fig. 119.3D). The highest lymph node removed should be marked for pathology if this information will have clinical implications. When complete, this procedure creates an en bloc resection of the regional nodes to include all subcutaneous tissues following the distal saphenous vein to the saphenofemoral junction and all lymphatics parallel to the femoral artery, vein, and nerve.

Anatomic Points

A safe therapeutic operation hinges on a clear understanding of the anatomy of the femoral triangle. The boundaries of the femoral triangle are the sartorius muscle, the gracilus muscle, and the inguinal ligament (Fig. 119.3A). The inguinal ligament forms the superior border of the femoral triangle and stretches from the pubic tubercle to the anterosuperior iliac spine. The gracilus muscle stretches from the pubic tubercle to medial condyle of the tibia (only the proximal and lateral aspects to the muscle needs to be identified). The adductor muscles run from insertion at the pubis to the linea aspera on the back of the femur (some advocate using these muscles as the medial margin). Laterally, the sartorius muscle runs at an oblique angle from its origin at the anterosuperior iliac spine to its insertion in the medial shaft of the tibia. The sartorius muscle will be divided proximally if a sartorius flap is created to cover the vessels. Distal dissection need only extend to adductor or gracilus muscles.

The fascia lata of the anterior thigh contains many of the superficial veins and lymphatics. This fascia runs in continuity with the external oblique aponeurosis and inferiorly it becomes the deep fascia of the leg. It covers and protects the femoral vessels and nerves except where fossa ovalis allows vascular and lymphatic entry at the saphenofemoral junction. The investing facial with the saphenous vein and tributaries will be removed with the dissection. The fascia covering the adductor muscles can be used to strip and clear all lymphatics medially up to the femoral vessels.

The femoral triangle includes from lateral to medial the femoral nerve, the femoral artery, and the femoral vein. The femoral nerve is made of branches of L2, L3, and L4 of the lumbar plexus. It runs in the retroperitoneum along the psoas muscle until passing under the inguinal ligament. It supplies the pectineus, sartorius, and quadriceps muscles as well as cutaneous sensation to the anteromedial thigh.

As with the femoral nerve, the femoral vessels also arise from just underneath the inguinal ligament. The femoral vein and artery are encased within the femoral sheath for the first few centimeters of their course. The common femoral artery is a direct extension of the external iliac artery, and likewise, the common femoral vein drains into the external iliac vein. Medially, the saphenous vein drains into the femoral vein at the saphenofemoral junction. The femoral canal forms a channel behind the inguinal ligament that encircles the femoral vessels. It is deep within this canal that the node of Cloquet is located. This node is the highest inguinal node and should be considered a part of the superficial dissection. In select texts, this node is described as a "deep superficial node," but should not be confused with nodes removed in a deep dissection. The node of Cloquet represents the transition node where the lymphatics gain access to the pelvis and is frequently used as an indicator of proximal disease.

Deep Lymph Node Dissection (Fig. 119.4)

The decision to perform a deep dissection (external, internal, common iliac, and obturator lymphadenectomy) is best made before embarking on a superficial dissection. A combined superficial and deep dissection if easier than a staged procedure and there is little added morbidity with the additional lymphadenectomy. Intraoperative assessment of Cloquet's node (see Figure 119.1 for location of this node), finding four or more positive superficial nodes, or preoperative imaging such as positron emission tomography or computed tomography have all been used to determine whether to proceed with a deep dissection but the validity of each of these modalities is beyond the scope of this chapter. Unfortunately, intraoperative

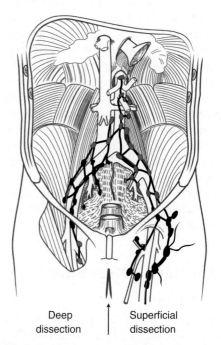

Figure 119.4 Deep lymph node dissection

decisions based on frozen section analysis may not be confirmed in the final pathology report. A false-negative intraoperative pathology report may mean that the patient is subjected to a second surgery or less rigorous lymphatic clearance if only a superficial dissection is done.

Technical Points

To obtain adequate visualization, self-retaining retractors with deep malleable blades are ideal. Skin and soft tissues can be held out of the way and deep tissues protected behind moist packing. Divide the external oblique aponeurosis toward the anterior iliac spine followed by dividing the inguinal ligament. Next, divide the internal oblique and transversalis layers to expose the femoral canal and follow its contents into the retroperitoneum. Displace the spermatic cord medially and then divide the inferior epigastric vessels to allow wide exposure. Expose the retroperitoneal structures by gently pushing the peritoneum medially. If the peritoneum is inadvertently opened, close it with an absorbable suture to keep bowel contents from disrupting your visualization. It is easier to mobilize the lymphatics into the specimen by beginning lateral on the pelvic sidewall and sweep the lymphatic tissue medial. Work along the lateral pelvic sidewall proximally to the desired level; ideally, the common iliac and, if indicated, to the aorta. To achieve exposure of the internal iliac region, the bladder and rectum are mobilized medially and retracted behind moist packing on deep malleable retractors. Only those tissues adequately visualized should be swept into the specimen to avoid iatrogenic injury to pelvic veins. Preservation of one side of the pelvic nerves should be adequate to maintain bladder and sphincter control. Every effort should be made to preserve bilateral nerve function. Divide lymphatic channels sharply using clips or suture to control small vessels and lymphatics. Sweep the fibrofatty tissue and nodes into the specimen using gentle traction while protecting major vessels, ureter, and nerves. The external iliac vessels and the ureter can be circumferentially controlled with vessel loops to assist with mobilization and exposure during the deep regional dissection (recall that circumferential control is not needed during the superficial dissection within the femoral triangle). The pelvis should be cleared of all lymphatic tissues without entering or injuring any major structures during the procedure. The deep specimen is removed en bloc with superficial specimen using the described technique. Separating the specimen (superficial and deep) theoretically will divide potentially involved lymphatics. But if the superficial specimen hinders visualization (large or bulky tissue), dividing the specimen will improve exposure and make for a safer, more thorough deep dissection.

Obturator Canal Dissection (Fig. 119.5)

Technical Points

The obturator lymph nodes can be dissected without extending the incision. Visualize the canal medially on the pelvic floor by following the obturator nerve and artery. These structures

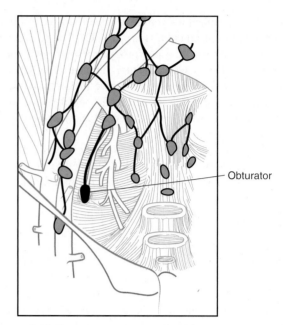

Figure 119.5 Obturator canal dissection

travel down from the upper medial pelvis and exit the pelvic floor through the foramen. Gently sweep the lymphatic tissues of the obturator canal into the specimen without injuring the artery and nerve.

Anatomic Points

The obturator canal is a small opening in the obturator foramen, the largest foramen in the body. The foramen is formed by rami of the ischium and pubis with the canal representing the anterosuperior aspect of the foramen where there is an obturator membrane defect. The canal runs 2 to 3 cm long and 1 cm in diameter within the medial thigh. It contains the obturator nerve, artery, and vein. The obturator artery is typically a branch of the internal iliac artery, and the obturator nerve is a branch of L3–L4, which runs along the psoas muscle until it passes behind the iliac vessels to enter the obturator canal. The obturator nerve leaves the pelvis to innervate the adductor musculature and should be preserved.

Sartorius Transposition Flap and Wound Closure (Fig. 119.6)

Technical Points

Irrigate the entire wound and complete hemostasis. Reapproximate the layers of the inguinal ligament (external and internal obliques and transversalis aponeurosis) with a heavy nonabsorbable suture to prevent herniation of the abdominal contents through the disrupted inguinal and femoral canals.

Release the sartorius muscle high on the anterosuperior iliac spine while protecting the lateral femoral cutaneous nerve. Mobilize it without excess devascularization until it will cover the exposed neurovascular structures. Rotate the muscle from lateral to medial and cover the nerves and vessels (inset). Secure

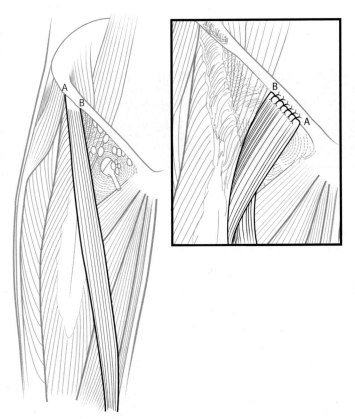

Figure 119.6 Sartorius transposition flap and wound closure. Note that point A (lateral) is flipped over and sutured medial to point B to achieve best coverage.

the muscle to the inguinal ligament with interrupted horizontal mattress sutures. Further securing of the sartorius medially and laterally along the length of its dissection is performed with simple interrupted sutures.

Approaches differ for skin approximation because of the high risk of flap necrosis. At this point, the skin flaps are resected sharply for 3 to 5 mm to ensure healthy tissue for skin closure. This limited skin loss will not compromise wound reapproximation. Place drains along the medial and lateral aspects of the thigh and bring ends out through the skin at the inferior thigh aspect. Skin is brought together with interrupted deep dermal sutures followed by a running subcuticular closure. Others advocate placing interrupted, vertical mattress nylon sutures. Wrap the leg from the foot to the thigh with an elastic bandage and elevate while in bed. Ambulation can begin with assistance immediately after surgery.

REFERENCES

1. Essner R, Scheri R, Kavanagh M, et al. Surgical management of the groin lymph nodes in melanoma in the era of sentinel lymph node dissection. *Arch Surg.* 2006;141:877–884.
2. Hoang D, Roberts KE, Teng E, et al. Laparoscopic iliac and iliofemoral lymph node resection for melanoma. *Surg Endosc.* 2012;26:3686–3687. (Application of minimally invasive techniques to deep node dissection.)
3. Hughes TM, Thomas JM. Combined inguinal and pelvic lymph node dissection for stage III melanoma. *Br J Surg.* 1999;86:1493–1498.
4. Karakousis CP. Therapeutic node dissections in malignant melanoma. *Ann Surg Oncol.* 1998;5:473–482.
5. Rapaport DP, Stadelmann WK, Reintgen DS. Inguinal lymphadenectomy. In: Balch CM, Houghton AN, Sober AJ, et al., eds. *Cutaneous Melanoma.* St Louis, MO: Quality Medical Publishing; 1998:269–280.
6. Swan MC, Furniss D, Cassell OC. Surgical management of metastatic inguinal lymphadenopathy. *BMJ.* 2004;329:1272–1276.
7. Wevers KP, Bastieannet E, Poos HP, et al. Therapeutic lymph node dissection in melanoma: Different prognosis for different macrometastasis sites? *Ann Surg Oncol.* 2012;19:3913–3918.

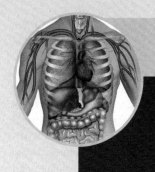

120

Sentinel Node Biopsy for Melanoma of the Trunk; Wide Local Excision

Scott K. Sherman and James R. Howe

The lymphatic drainage patterns from lesions located on the trunk are less predictable than those of the extremities. Therefore, when sentinel node biopsy for melanoma is indicated, it is important that lymphoscintigraphy be performed to include imaging through the inguinal, axillary, and cervical nodal basins. It is not uncommon to see drainage to more than one of these areas, which will require multiple sentinel lymph node biopsies. The location of these nodal basins and the primary tumor will then determine whether all areas can be addressed in one position, or whether the patient will need to be repositioned (such as a midback lesion that drains to bilateral axillae).

STEPS IN PROCEDURE

Sentinel Node Biopsy

Send patient to nuclear medicine for injection of Tc-99m–labeled sulfur colloid in four quadrants around lesion/previous biopsy site

Review lymphoscintigrams and discuss results with nuclear medicine staff; determine nodal basins with accumulation of Tc-99m

In the operating room, use hand-held gamma counter to identify sites of nodes

Inject 0.5-mL isosulfan blue dye in each of four quadrants around lesion/previous biopsy site

Position patient appropriately for removal of primary and/or sentinel nodes

Prep and drape these sites

Make 2- to 3-cm incision directly over area with highest counts in nodal basin, oriented so that it could be excised should complete node dissection be performed later

Dissect through subcutaneous tissues, directed by gamma probe and blue dye; take in situ count

Identify hot or blue nodes, remove, take ex vivo count and post excision count in basin; if >10% of in situ, then search for additional node(s) with probe

Close incision in two layers

Wide Excision

For 0.75- to 1-mm lesions, 1-cm margins, orient along Langer lines to reduce tension

For 1- to 4-mm Breslow depth, 2-cm margins

Make ellipse around lesion to facilitate primary closure

Excise skin and fat down to or to include muscle fascia

Close primarily in two layers

HALLMARK ANATOMIC COMPLICATIONS

Missed sentinel node
Lymphocele
Wound infection/disruption

LIST OF STRUCTURES

Axillary lymph nodes
Inguinal lymph nodes
Cervical lymph nodes

Biopsy of Suspected Melanoma

The diagnosis of melanoma begins with an adequate biopsy. Current guidelines recommend complete excisional biopsy whenever possible. For large or cosmetically important areas, punch biopsy is acceptable, but is associated with higher rates of both sampling error and understaging. Shave biopsy does not accurately assess the depth of invasion, and is not recommended. For excisional biopsy, the entire lesion is excised sharply to a depth of approximately 10 mm, with 1- to 3-mm lateral margins of normal appearing tissue. The orientation of the biopsy incision is important to facilitate closure after wide local excision (should this be necessary), and the incision is closed primarily.

Sentinel Node Biopsy (Fig. 120.1)

Technical Points

In addition to wide local excision, sentinel node biopsy is currently recommended for melanomas with depth 0.75 to 1 mm

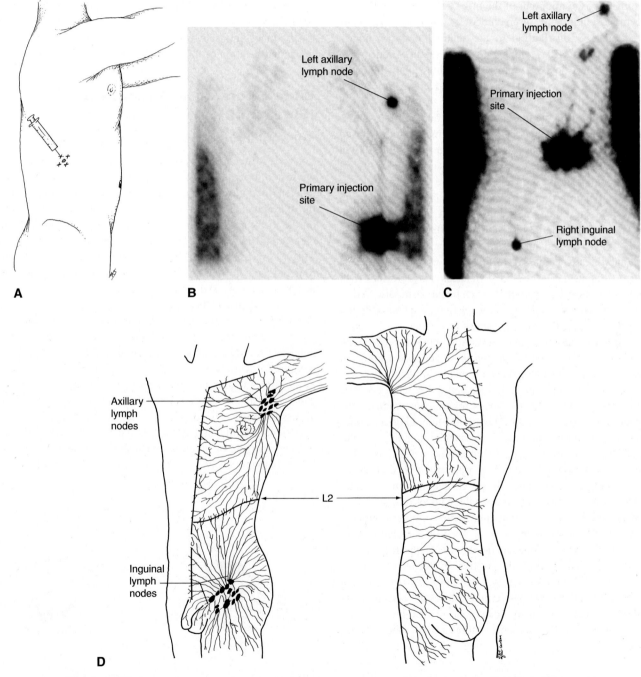

Figure 120.1 Sentinel node biopsy. **A:** Injection of tracer at site of primary lesion. **B:** Scintigram showing drainage to ipsilateral axillary node. **C:** Scintigram showing drainage to left axillary and right inguinal nodes. **D:** Typical drainage patterns indicate dividing lines at the midline and at L2, but there is considerable individual variation.

with high-risk features such as ulceration or mitotic rate ≥1/mm², and for all intermediate thickness melanomas 1 to 4 mm in depth. Sentinel lymph node biopsy may also be indicated for staging thick melanomas (with depth greater than 4 mm).

Just prior to surgery (1 to 24 hours), intradermal injection of 0.5 mCi of Tc-99m sulfur colloid is performed with a small (25-gauge) needle in the nuclear medicine suite. If the primary lesion had an incisional or punch biopsy, injection is done in four quadrants surrounding the lesion (Fig. 120.1A). If the lesion was biopsied by complete excision, four-quadrant injection surrounds the midpoint of the biopsy scar.

Lymphoscintigraphy is recorded at intervals to follow the radiotracer's distribution to the sentinel node or nodes. Truncal melanomas have higher rates of sentinel node positivity than other locations, and require whole body imaging, as sentinel nodes may reside in unexpected or multiple nodal basins. Figure 120.1B shows a lesion near the umbilicus with drainage to the axilla, while Figure 120.1C demonstrates drainage to both the inguinal and the axillary. Imaging is reviewed with the nuclear medicine physician to determine all areas of radiotracer accumulation, as lymph node sampling from each positive nodal basin is required.

In the operating room, a gamma probe is used to confirm the sites of greatest radiotracer accumulation, and a pre-excision count is taken. Intradermal injection with 0.5 mL of isosulfan blue dye is performed in four quadrants around the primary lesion, and the area is massaged for several minutes to promote lymphatic drainage. Next, a 2- to 3-cm incision is performed over the area of greatest radioactivity in each nodal basin, oriented so that it could easily be excised if a completion lymphadenectomy becomes necessary. Prior to excision of any nodes, a 10-second in situ gamma emission count of the hottest area is recorded with the probe in the incision. Dissection is carried down until hot or blue nodes are encountered. The principle sentinel node and any adjacent hot nodes are removed, and an ex vivo count is performed to confirm that the nodes removed are radioactive. Hot nodes are labeled as sentinel nodes, and nonradioactive ones as nonsentinel nodes, then sent for permanent pathology evaluation (with the containers marked with radioactive stickers). The probe is returned to the incision for a post excision count of the hottest area that can be found; if the post excision count is greater than 10% of the in situ count, additional hot nodes remain, which should be sought with the probe and removed, unless they are distant from the nodal basin (such as along the subclavian vein outside of the axilla). Enlarged or abnormal appearing nodes should also be excised, regardless of their dye or uptake.

We generally do not perform touch prep or frozen section of the excised nodes because micrometastases are common and will not be detected on cursory examination. The incisions are closed primarily with absorbable sutures in the subcutaneous layer and skin.

Anatomic Points

Lymphatic drainage of the trunk generally flows in the distribution illustrated in Figure 120.1D. Lymphatics above *Sappey*

line (from the umbilicus anteriorly to L2 posteriorly) tend to drain to ipsilateral axillary nodes, and those below drain to ipsilateral inguinal nodes. However, there is wide variability to these drainage patterns, and lymphoscintigraphy is important to accurately define the nodal basins at risk. One such example is shown in Figure 120.1C, where a lesion above the umbilicus and to the left of midline drains across both Sappey line and the midline to end up in the right inguinal region (as well as the left axilla, as expected). In Figure 120.1B, the lateral primary site at the level of the umbilicus sits at the border of the different drainage distributions demonstrated in Figure 120.1D, making prediction of the drainage pattern impossible. In both cases, the lymphoscintigram resolves uncertainty by demonstrating the actual location of the sentinel nodes.

Wide Excision of Primary Site (Fig. 120.2)

Technical and Anatomic Points

For wide local excision, an elliptical incision is planned around the lesion, oriented to permit both skin closure under the least tension (along Langer lines), and further excision if needed. On the extremities, longitudinal incisions are preferred. Depending on the location of the primary lesion and sentinel node basins, the patient may require repositioning prior to wide excision. This is especially true for lesions on the back that drain to regional nodes on both the left and right sides; most other lesions can be excised using one position.

The margins of the wide excision depend on the Breslow depth of the primary cancer. For lesions up to 1 mm, 1-cm margins are preferred, and for those 1 to 4 mm in depth, 2-cm margins should be employed. Margins of 2 cm are also recommended for lesions deeper than 4 mm, but prospective data on these thick melanomas are lacking. Dissection proceeds perpendicular to the skin surface to the level of the fascia, and all tissue above it is completely excised. Removing the fascia is optional. While melanomas of the face or extremities can present cosmetic or functional obstacles to wide excision, truncal melanoma can usually be excised with sufficient margins

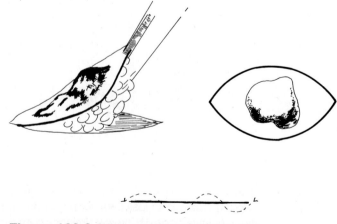

Figure 120.2 Wide excision of primary site

and closed primarily; skin grafts are rarely necessary even with 2-cm margins. To reduce tension, closure is assisted by elevation of skin flaps just below Scarpa fascia. This layer is closed with interrupted 2-0 or 3-0 absorbable sutures, and the skin with vertical mattress 3-0 nylon sutures, which are removed after 2 weeks.

Acknowledgment

This chapter was contributed by Dr. Peter R. Jochimsen in the previous edition.

REFERENCES

1. Callender GG, Egger ME, Burton AL, et al. Prognostic implications of anatomic location of primary cutaneous melanoma of 1 mm or thicker. *Am J Surg.* 2011;202(6):659–664; discussion 664–665.
2. Coit DG, Andtbacka R, Bichakjian CK, et al. Melanoma. *J Natl Compr Canc Netw.* 2009;7(3):250–275.
3. Federico AC, Chagpar AB, Ross MI, et al. Effect of multiple-nodal basin drainage on cutaneous melanoma. *Arch Surg.* 2008; 143(7):632–637; discussion 637–638.
4. Morton DL, Thompson JF, Cochran AJ, et al. Sentinel-node biopsy or nodal observation in melanoma. *N Engl J Med.* 2006; 355(13):1307–1317.
5. Sladden MJ, Balch C, Barzilai DA, et al. Surgical excision margins for primary cutaneous melanoma. *Cochrane Database Syst Rev.* 2009;7(4):CD004835.
6. Steen ST, Kargozaran H, Moran CJ, et al. Management of popliteal sentinel nodes in melanoma. *J Am Coll Surg.* 2011;213:180–186.
7. Uren RF, Howman-Giles R, Thompson JF. Patterns of lymphatic drainage from the skin in patients with melanoma. *J Nucl Med.* 2003;44:570–582.
8. Wong SL, Balch CM, Hurley P, et al. Sentinel lymph node biopsy for melanoma: American Society of Clinical Oncology and Society of Surgical Oncology joint clinical practice guideline. *Ann Surg Oncol.* 2012; 19(11):3313–3324.
9. Wrightson WR, Wong SL, Edwards MJ, et al. Complications associated with sentinel lymph node biopsy for melanoma. *Ann Surg Oncol.* 2003;10(6):676–680.

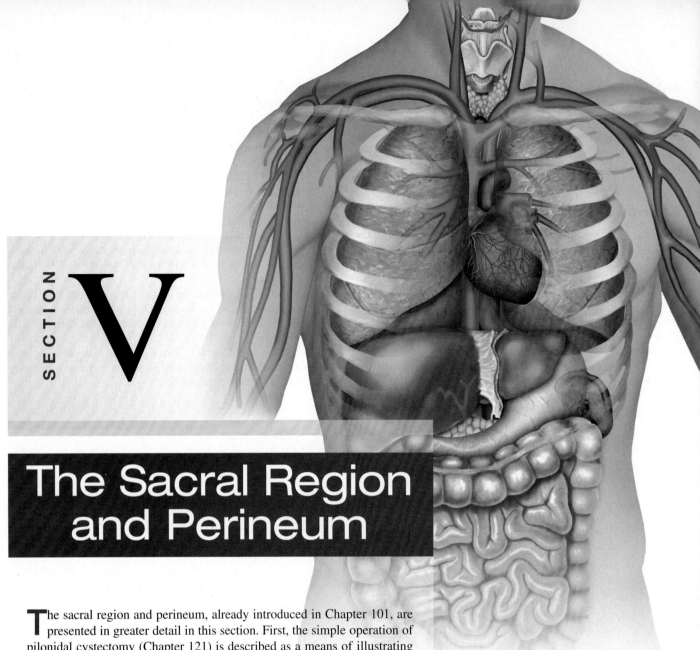

The Sacral Region and Perineum

The sacral region and perineum, already introduced in Chapter 101, are presented in greater detail in this section. First, the simple operation of pilonidal cystectomy (Chapter 121) is described as a means of illustrating the anatomy of the sacrum and the presacral region. This is often one of the first operations performed by the beginning surgeon, yet results are often less than perfect, and numerous modifications of the operation exist. Two of these, marsupialization and Z-plasty, have emerged as dominant and are described in this chapter.

The anorectum is then described through the procedure of hemorrhoidectomy (Chapter 122) and other minor rectal procedures (Chapter 123). Although these are considered to be minor procedures, surgery in this area can cause considerable pain and disability; hence, careful attention to operative technique is important.

The transsacral approach to rectal lesions is described in Chapter 124e. This uncommon approach provides excellent exposure of the lower rectum and is useful in a variety of situations. Finally, rigid sigmoidoscopy is described in Chapter 125.

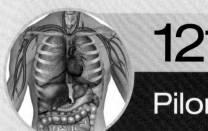

121

Pilonidal Cystectomy

Whether pilonidal cysts are congenital or acquired lesions remains a topic of debate. The frequent appearance of an epithelialized tract in the midline, leading to a cyst that may or may not contain hair, suggests a congenital origin. A pilonidal cyst (or sinus) characteristically occurs in the posterior midline skin overlying the sacrum. Secondary infection within the cyst or sinus causes pain, drawing attention to the cyst. Incision and drainage may be needed, but are not definitive treatment, and recurrent bouts of infection are typical. Definitive treatment involves either marsupialization or excision of the cyst.

The variety of techniques that are available for dealing with pilonidal cysts indicates that complications have occurred with all approaches. Marsupialization, the simplest procedure, is described in this chapter. A more complex procedure for primary closure, Z-plasty, may be used in some circumstances. Consult the references at the end for alternative approaches.

Whenever possible, avoid operating if the cyst is acutely infected. Treat the patient with antibiotics and aspiration (or incision and drainage), and operate only after allowing the inflammation to subside.

SCORE™, the Surgical Council on Resident Education, classified pilonidal cystectomy as an "ESSENTIAL COMMON" procedure.

STEPS IN PROCEDURE

Prone jackknife position
Tape buttocks open to enhance exposure
Cannulate tract
Inject mixture of 50% methylene blue and
    50% hydrogen peroxide

Marsupialization
Completely open all tracts
Excise overlying skin to saucerize the
    wound
Curette the base of the cyst to healthy
    tissue

Suture skin edges to edges of cyst
Pack wound open

Z-Plasty
Excise median tract with overlying skin
Include any side tracts—if extensive side tracts
    are encountered, consider marsupialization
Carry excision down to fascia
Outline top and bottom bars of Z
Elevate flaps at fascial level
Transpose flaps and close skin over a closed-
    suction drain

HALLMARK ANATOMIC COMPLICATIONS

Recurrence
Delayed wound healing

LIST OF STRUCTURES

Sacrum
Lateral sacral crest
Intermediate sacral crest
Median sacral crest
Posterior sacral foramina
    Sacral promontory
Ilium
Sacroiliac joint
Coccyx
Lumbodorsal fascia
Gluteus maximus muscle

Gluteus medius muscle
Gluteus minimus muscle
Intergluteal cleft
Gluteal aponeurosis
Sacral nerves
Posterior femoral cutaneous nerve
Gluteal branches
Anus
Rectum
Anococcygeal ligament
Levator ani muscles

Positioning the Patient (Fig. 121.1)

Technical Points

Place the patient in a prone jackknife position. Use tincture of benzoin on the lateral buttocks to prepare the skin. Place tape on the lateral buttocks and use this tape to pull laterally, spreading the intergluteal cleft. Shave the region of the cyst and the gluteal region.

Anatomic Points

The prominent and important structures in this area are all musculoskeletal. The bony sacrum forms the posterior part of the bony pelvic ring and is the distal continuation of the vertebral column. Formed by the fusion of the five sacral vertebrae (the number of vertebrae that fuse to form the sacrum varies from four to six, but is commonly five), the sacrum is a complexly curved and heavy bone that is shield shaped when viewed from behind. The posterior surface is roughened and has two paramedian crests—the lateral sacral and intermediate crests—which, with the prominent midline median sacral crest, form points of attachment for fascial and aponeurotic structures. Four broad posterior sacral foramina between the five fused vertebrae are points of ingress and egress for the dorsal rami of the sacral spinal nerves. Viewed from the side, a prominent anterior concavity, commonly termed the *hollow of the sacrum,* is obvious. This forms a space in which lie the rectum, muscles of the pelvic diaphragm, neurovascular structures, and a variable amount of fat. At the top of this concavity, the sacral promontory (located at the point of articulation of the body of the lowest lumbar vertebra with the sacrum) forms an easily palpable bony landmark for the surgeon operating within the pelvis. The sacrum is shorter and wider in the female pelvis than in the male pelvis, contributing to the wider, rounder gynecoid shape that is designed to accommodate the head of a full-term infant at the time of delivery.

The coccyx is composed of three to five remaining vertebrae (commonly, four). These small, nubbin-like, rudimentary vertebrae articulate with the sacrum. Only the first coccygeal vertebra possesses identifiable transverse processes and homologues of pedicles (coccygeal cornua). No vertebral canal is present. The mobility of the coccygeal vertebrae varies considerably from individual to individual, and the terminal three coccygeal vertebrae are commonly fused.

Recall that the perineum is diamond shaped, bounded anteriorly by the pubic symphysis, laterally by the two ischial tuberosities, and posteriorly by the tip of the coccyx. It may be divided into two triangles—the anterior or urogenital triangle and the posterior or anal triangle—by drawing a transverse line that passes just anterior to the anus and connects the ischial tuberosities. Thus, the tip of the coccyx marks the end of the gluteal region and the beginning of the perineal (anal triangle) region. This is an important distinction because of the differences in the pathologic processes found in each region. The tip of the coccyx, therefore, is a critical, easily palpated landmark for the surgeon. The anococcygeal ligament extends from the tip of the coccyx to the anus. This fibrous band is formed by the decussation of fibers of the two levator ani muscles, two broad flat muscles that form the main part of the pelvic diaphragm.

The gluteus maximus is a large muscle that plays an important role in extension of the hip; it is inactive in standing. It originates primarily from the sacrum, along a roughly diagonal line extending from the tip of the coccyx to the iliac crest, although it also takes its origin from the aponeurosis of the sacrospinous and sacrotuberous ligaments. The gluteal aponeurosis, which is the fascia covering the gluteus medius,

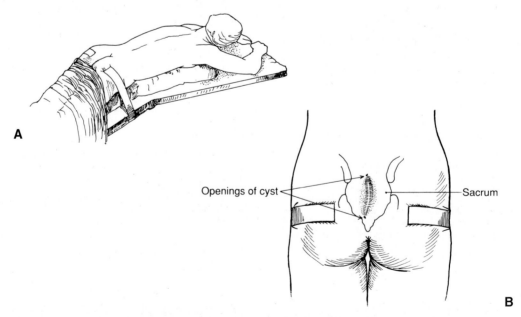

Figure 121.1 Positioning the patient. **A:** Prone position. **B:** Tape the lateral buttocks to provide optimum exposure of the gluteal cleft.

from which the most cephalad part of this muscle, the gluteus maximus, arises, extends from the region of the sacroiliac joint anteriorly, along the crest of the ilium. The gluteus medius lies lateral, deep to the gluteal aponeurosis and gluteus maximus. Whereas the gluteus maximus extends and laterally rotates the thigh, the gluteus medius abducts and medially rotates it; its primary function is to prevent pelvic sag on the unsupported side during walking. The gluteus minimus, which lies deep to the gluteus medius, has similar functions.

The midline intergluteal cleft is formed by the infolding of skin and fatty tissue enveloping the gluteal muscles. It extends from the midsacral level to the anus, blending imperceptibly with the perineum in the region of the anus. The skin of this region is thick (although thinner than the skin of the back or buttocks) and is covered with a variable amount of hair. Abnormalities of the skin of the intergluteal cleft may provide a clue to underlying sacral anomalies, which are relatively common. Particularly in hirsute individuals, an increased amount of hair may be present in the intergluteal cleft normally, which may account for the formation of pilonidal cysts in this area. Moreover, a localized patch of hair, a dimple, or a lipoma-like mass may be the only external clue to an underlying spina bifida occulta, which is an asymptomatic anomaly of fusion of the lower vertebral column.

Sensory innervation in the region of the intergluteal cleft is derived from branches of the sacral and coccygeal nerves. The skin overlying the lower and lateral portions of the gluteal muscles is innervated by gluteal branches of the posterior femoral cutaneous nerve.

Delineation of the Cyst and Incision of Tracts (Fig. 121.2)

Technical Points

Look for an external opening of the tract. This is most likely to be found in the midline. Cannulate this opening with a blunt-tipped needle and gently inject a mixture of 50% hydrogen peroxide and 50% methylene blue. This will help to define the tracts and stain the tissues involved by the burrowing process. Several lateral openings may be identified as the methylene blue exits the tissues. These are often visible externally as small, inflamed openings.

Insert a probe into the external opening and define the main tract. Generally, this will track in the midline superiorly or inferiorly. Take care not to go below the coccyx. Extension into the perianal region is extremely unusual and is usually indicative of other pathology. Place a grooved director over the probe and incise the tissue overlying the tract with electrocautery. Look for and cannulate any lateral satellite extensions of the tract, opening these in continuity with the primary tract.

Anatomic Points

The sacral nerves that provide sensory innervation to the skin of the intergluteal cleft emerge from the laterally placed

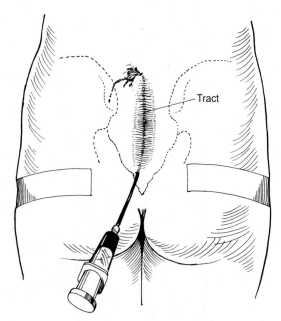

Figure 121.2 Delineation of the cyst and incision of tracts

posterior sacral foramina and turn medially and downward. In the midline, no nerves are cut, and no significant structures occupy the space between the skin of the intergluteal cleft and the underlying fascia. Although a network of superficial veins exists here, as elsewhere in the body, it is rare to encounter even small veins in the midline. Hence, dissection can proceed swiftly and is attended by little risk.

The fascia overlying the sacrum is a continuation of the lumbodorsal fascia and lies relatively deep to the skin, under a variable amount of fatty connective tissue. Although the fatty layer is typically less than that encountered laterally over the gluteal muscles, it may be several centimeters thick in obese individuals. Pilonidal sinuses are located relatively superficially (typically within 1 to 1.5 cm of the skin) in this region.

Excision of Overlying Skin and Marsupialization of Tracts (Fig. 121.3)

Technical and Anatomic Points

After all of the tracts have been incised, place Allis clamps on the edges of the overhanging skin and excise the excess skin. The objective here is to convert the incision into a wide, flat depression. Curette the base of the cyst to remove gelatinous material, granulation tissue, and hair. Do not disrupt the posterior wall of the cyst.

Conclusion of Marsupialization (Fig. 121.4)

Technical and Anatomic Points

Place interrupted sutures of 2-0 Vicryl from the dermal layer of the skin down to the back wall of the cyst in such a way as

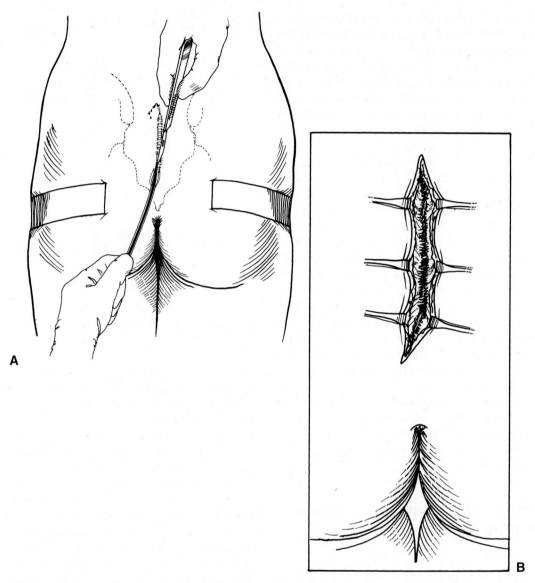

Figure 121.3 Excision of overlying skin and marsupialization of tracts. **A:** Pass a probe into the tract and incise the overlying skin and soft tissues. **B:** Completely open the tract.

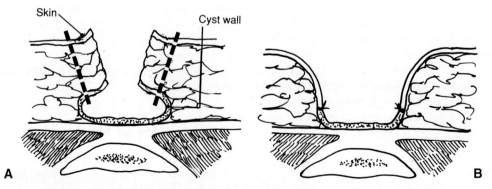

Figure 121.4 Conclusion of marsupialization. **A:** Excise overhanging skin and soft tissues. **B:** Suture skin down to presacral fascia or back wall of cyst.

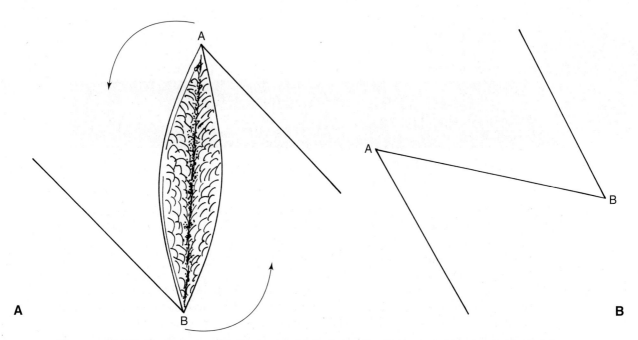

Figure 121.5 Z-plasty for pilonidal cyst. **A:** Outline a Z with the crossbar incorporating the excision site. **B:** Transpose the tips so that the scar now crosses the gluteal cleft instead of lying within it.

to cover the intervening subcutaneous fat. The objective is to bring the skin down to the back wall of the cyst. At the conclusion of the procedure, a narrow, open area, consisting of the back wall of the cyst, should still be visible. This small area is left to heal by secondary intention.

Check hemostasis and pack the incision with dry, sterile gauze.

Z-Plasty for Pilonidal Cyst (Fig. 121.5)

Technical and Anatomic Points

This technique affords primary closure but avoids an incision in the midline. When properly performed, it substitutes a broad flat defect for the narrow gluteal crease that contributed to the original cyst formation. Meticulous attention to technique and careful patient selection is essential. When this method fails, a larger open wound results than that created by simple marsupialization.

Position the patient and identify the tract as described in Figures 121.1 and 121.2. Completely excise the cyst and tract with a narrow ribbon of overlying midline skin. Take this excision down to fascia. All cyst material and lateral tracts must be excised to healthy fat.

Create a Z by outlining an incision at the upper and lower poles of the incision, extending out for approximately the length of the original incision at an angle of approximately 30 degrees as shown in Figure 121.5A. You should have a Z with the top and bottom of the Z extending at an angle and the diagonal limb of the Z created by the vertical limb. Elevate the two resulting triangular flaps at the level of the fascia.

Transpose the Z-plasty flaps to create a new Z, with the diagonal limb running at an angle across the intergluteal cleft rather than vertically (Fig. 121.5B). Close the incision over a small closed-suction drain.

REFERENCES

1. Allen-Mersh TG. Pilonidal sinus: Finding the right track for treatment. *Br J Surg*. 1990;77:123–132. (Presents excellent review of alternatives.)
2. Bendewald FP, Cima RR, Metcalf DR, et al. Using negative pressure wound therapy following surgery for complex pilonidal disease: A case series. *Ostomy Wound Manage*. 2007;53:40–46. (Describes use of negative pressure dressing after marsupialization.)
3. Camazine BM, Williams C. The z-plasty solution for pilonidal disease. *Contemp Surg*. 2007;63:70–71.
4. Rabie ME. Methylene blue in pilonidal sinus surgery. *ANZ J Surg*. 2007;77:600.
5. Toubanakis G. Treatment of pilonidal sinus disease with the Z-plasty procedure (modified). *Am Surg*. 1986;52:611–612.
6. Zimmerman CE. Outpatient excision and primary closure of pilonidal cysts and sinuses. *Am J Surg*. 1978;136:640–642. (Describes primary closure for simple cases.)

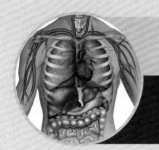

122

Hemorrhoid Management

Andreas M. Kaiser

Hemorrhoids are a pathologic engorgement of the hemorrhoidal plexus. The latter are part of the normal anatomy of the anal canal and form soft cushions that contribute to fine-tuning the anal seal. Hemorrhoids are classified as *internal* (if they occur above the dentate line), *external* (if found below), or *mixed* (if both).

The true etiology of hemorrhoids remains a matter of speculation: Apart from an individual/familial predisposition, they have been associated with the Western culture and diet, constipation with straining, and pregnancy with impaired venous return. In contrast to common opinion, liver cirrhosis and portal hypertension are not associated with a higher incidence of hemorrhoids, but can result in rectal varices (typically located in mid to upper rectum).

Hemorrhoid symptoms are nonspecific in nature. *Internal hemorrhoids* can cause bleeding and, with increasing size, tend to prolapse. Hemorrhoids do not itch, but a prolapse may result in chronic moisture which then triggers an itching sensation. *External hemorrhoids* are most commonly asymptomatic (innocent bystanders); occasionally, they cause difficulty with the local hygiene (if very large), or they may develop an acute painful thrombosis. Pain otherwise is rare and only occurs in nonreducible, potentially gangrenous prolapsed hemorrhoids. Complaints of recurring/persistent pain and "painful hemorrhoids" should therefore direct the examination to look for a fissure with a sentinel skin tag. Be careful to exclude other pathology before ascribing rectal bleeding to "hemorrhoids."

SCORE™, the Surgical Council on Resident Education, classified hemorrhoidectomy and banding for internal hemorrhoids as "ESSENTIAL COMMON" procedures. SCORE™ classified stapled hemorrhoidectomy as a "COMPLEX" procedure.

STEPS IN PROCEDURES

Excisional Hemorrhoidectomy (Internal and External Hemorrhoids)

Prone jackknife or lithotomy position

Avoid unnecessary anal dilation

Place retractor, inspect the three hemorrhoidal pedicles, and identify the number of hemorrhoidectomies to be carried out (generally 1–3)

Place one Kelly clamp on the first target pedicle and pull outward, place second Kelly clamp on inner aspect of pedicle thus exposed

Place absorbable suture ligature at apex of hemorrhoidal pedicle

Make a V-shaped incision to the external skin and extend it to a narrow eye-shaped mucocutaneous incision toward the ligated vascular pedicle

Lift the external angle of the "eye" and dissect it off the underlying external and internal sphincter structures (transverse fibers), using blunt dissection, sharp scissors, electrocautery, or more expensive but not more effective energy devices/lasers

Once the ligated pedicle is reached, amputate the hemorrhoid (send for pathology)

Bury the ligated stump, and close the mucocutaneous defect (Ferguson technique) with running absorbable sutures, leaving only the most external portion open. Alternatively, the wound may be left open (Milligan–Morgan technique)

Repeat for up to two more pedicles, making sure that sufficient epithelial bridge is preserved between the excision sites

HALLMARK COMPLICATIONS

Bleeding

Urinary retention

Recurrence

Sphincter injury and dysfunction

Pelvic sepsis

Stricture

LIST OF ANATOMIC STRUCTURES

Inspection/palpation landmarks:

    Perineum

    Anterior or urogenital triangle

    Posterior or anal triangle

    Symphysis pubis

    Ischial tuberosities

    Coccyx

    Anus, anal verge, four perianal

        quadrants (left/right, anterior/

        posterior)

Dentate line (pectinate line):

    Anal crypts

    Anal columns (of Morgagni)

Blood supply:

    Internal iliac arteries

        Inferior rectal (hemorrhoidal) arteries

    Inferior mesenteric vein

        Superior rectal (hemorrhoidal) vein

    Internal iliac vein

        Middle rectal (hemorrhoidal) vein

        Rectal (hemorrhoidal) plexus of veins

Muscular structures:

Internal anal sphincter (smooth muscle, white)

External anal sphincter (skeletal muscle, red)

Intersphincteric groove

Puborectalis muscle (skeletal muscle)

Evaluation and Decision Making

Modern management of hemorrhoids depends on the acuity of presentation, the degree, type and evolution of symptoms, and the clinical findings. Under elective circumstances, conservative measures should be initiated, and additional interventions tailored to the specific needs.

Internal hemorrhoids are classified on a largely patient-reported scale from I–IV. Grade I hemorrhoids are enlarged cushions and may bleed but do not prolapse through the anal canal. Grade II hemorrhoids protrude during straining, but spontaneously reduce on relaxation. Grade III hemorrhoids protrude and require manual reduction, which is usually easily accomplished. Grade IV hemorrhoids are irreducible protrusions of internal (mucosa-covered) hemorrhoids. The most frequent confusions include incorrect interpretation of a large external (skin-covered) hemorrhoid component with any internal degree as grade IV, or confusion of a true rectal prolapse with prolapsing hemorrhoids. Note that a true mucosal rectal prolapse will show concentric folds of mucosa, and prolapsing hemorrhoids present with a radial pattern of mucosal protrusions.

If previously grade II or III internal hemorrhoids do not reduce quickly enough, edema rapidly occurs because the anal sphincter acts as a tourniquet. Increasing swelling and pain prevent reduction, and a vicious circle starts which may lead to tissue gangrene. This acute prolapse (grade IV) is typically very painful and therefore an emergency. Rarely, grade IV hemorrhoids are chronically prolapsing and not painful, often in the context of a lax anal sphincter that is unable to retain the hemorrhoids in a reduced position and does not strangulate the prolapsed tissue.

An *excisional hemorrhoidectomy,* typically performed under general or spinal anesthesia, is still the gold standard but it is generally more painful than the alternatives. It is the standard approach for (A) emergency situations (grade IV incarcerated

internal hemorrhoids with/without gangrene), or (B) electively for large, mixed internal and external hemorrhoids (grades I–III) if the patient desires a removal of the external component as well. If a patient is only symptomatic from the internal hemorrhoids and not annoyed by any degree of external component, treatment should focus on the internal hemorrhoids only. In addition to conservative measures, an *office procedure* (banding, sclerosing, infrared coagulation) is simple, well tolerated, avoids anesthesia, and might provide adequate relief after a single or repeated applications. Cryotherapy for hemorrhoids is considered obsolete. However, a *stapled hemorrhoidectomy* (aka hemorrhoidopexy), performed under general or spinal anesthesia, is an excellent solution for very voluminous internal hemorrhoids (grades II/III, occasionally grade I) or if office procedures have failed.

Age- and risk-adjusted colon evaluation is mandatory before all elective hemorrhoid interventions.

In this chapter, classic excisional hemorrhoidectomy, stapled hemorrhoidectomy, and rubber band ligation are described. The references at the end list a number of systematic reviews and reference texts.

Excisional Hemorrhoidectomy

Patient Positioning and Setup (Fig. 122.1)

Technical Points

The procedure may be performed in the prone jackknife or lithotomy position—a debate that largely remains a matter of personal preference. The prone jackknife position is more convenient for the surgeons and reduces the venous congestion in the hemorrhoids. The lithotomy position is preferred by some because it is quickly set up (Fig. 122.1A) and provides better control of the airway. In high-risk patients (e.g., super-obesity, ankylosing spondylitis), the lithotomy position may be

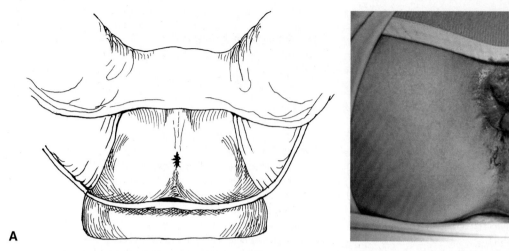

A   **B**

Figure 122.1 **A:** Patient in lithotomy position. **B:** Grade IV hemorrhoids (from Wexner SD, Fleshman JW, eds. *Master Techniques in General Surgery: Colon and Rectal Surgery: Anorectal Operations.* Philadelphia, PA: Lippincott Williams & Wilkins; 2012, with permission).

somewhat safer. Addition of local anesthesia helps with sphincter relaxation and postoperative pain control.

After adequate anesthesia has been induced, the anus is again carefully examined and a digital examination performed (Fig. 122.1B). However, the historically recommended finger dilation should be avoided as it may cause damage to the sphincter complex. Use of povidone–iodine solution (Betadine) for lubrication rather than water-soluble lubricant keeps the operative field less slippery during the procedure.

Anatomic Points

The perineum is a diamond-shaped region bounded by the pubic symphysis anteriorly, the coccyx posteriorly, and the two ischial tuberosities laterally. A transverse line connecting the anterior edge of the ischial tuberosities and passing just anterior to the anus divides the region into two triangles: An anterior urogenital triangle and a posterior anal triangle. The detailed anatomy of the perineum is discussed in Chapter 101 and hence is only briefly be reviewed here. The posterior triangle contains the anus and associated musculature as well as neurovascular structures. Specific locations around the anus are best described by assigning them to one of four quadrants (left/right, anterior/posterior), whereas the clock as orientation is confusing if the patient's position changes.

The anus links the terminal part of the gastrointestinal tract (endodermal origin) with the outside (ectodermal origin). The dentate line or pectinate line represents this important embryologic and anatomical landmark where epithelium, vascular, lymphatic, and neural anatomy switch from visceral to somatic.

■ Above the dentate line
   ■ Epithelium: Mucosa with anal transitional zone (ATZ) changing from multilayer cuboidal cells to the regular columnar epithelium of the rectum.

   ■ Arterial blood supply: From visceral (inferior mesenteric artery) and somatic (internal iliac arteries) to superior and middle hemorrhoidal arteries and plexus.
   ■ Venous drainage predominantly upward, following the drainage of the lower rectum to the portal system (inferior mesenteric vein) and through the internal iliac veins to the caval system.
   ■ Lymphatics: Following venous drainage.
   ■ Sensation: Visceral sensation, poorly localized, dull and diffuse, mediated by autonomic nervous system.
■ Below the dentate line
   ■ Epithelium: Squamous cell (i.e., skin-type) with full skin appendages present outside the anal canal.
   ■ Arterial blood supply: From iliac arteries via inferior pudendal arteries to inferior hemorrhoidal plexus.
   ■ Venous drainage: Superficial rich network from the inferior rectal (hemorrhoidal) veins, which drain into the inferior pudendal veins and hence into the iliac veins (caval system), and to lesser degree via connections to superior hemorrhoidal plexus to internal iliacs and portal vein system.
   ■ Lymphatics: Drain into the inguinal lymph nodes.
   ■ Sensation: Somatic sensory neurons branches of the pudendal nerves with fast pain fibers (sharp, intense, and well-localized pain). The anal region has been described by some surgeons as the second most sensitive structure in the body, with the eye rated the most sensitive.

The distinction between internal and external hemorrhoids is important for both patient and surgeon. Internal hemorrhoids, predominantly dilatations of the superior and middle rectal (hemorrhoidal) venous plexus, are mucosa covered; pain in the region of internal hemorrhoids is dull, poorly localized, and often less intense. Because of this relatively poor sensory innervation, internal hemorrhoids may be treated in the office by rubber band ligation, injection, infrared coagulation, or laser therapy, with little or no need for anesthesia. External hemorrhoids are skin covered and exquisitely sensitive; manipulations are not tolerated without any type of anesthesia.

Definition of Hemorrhoidal Pedicles (Fig. 122.2)

Technical Points

Place a retractor and define the hemorrhoidal pedicles to be addressed: Generally, they are located in the left lateral, right anterior, and right posterior quadrant, defining a triangle. Place a Kelly clamp on the outside of each pedicle and pull laterally (Fig. 122.2A). Place a second pair of Kelly clamp on the pedicle near the dentate line to pull internal hemorrhoidal tissue further out of the anus (Fig. 122.2B). Start with the biggest hemorrhoid first (Fig. 122.2C); as needed, the other hemorrhoid pedicles are subsequently addressed in similar fashion; thus, only one will be described.

Anatomic Points

The common pattern of three hemorrhoidal pedicles has been postulated to result from the typical pattern of termination of the superior rectal (hemorrhoidal) arteries. The right superior rectal (hemorrhoidal) artery generally splits into an anterior and posterior division, whereas the left superior rectal (hemorrhoidal) artery remains single. Arteriovenous communication has been demonstrated, and the common observation of arterial bleeding at a hemorrhoidectomy site supports this etiology. When more than three hemorrhoidal pedicles are present, the surgeon may still be able to define three major groups, obliterating smaller hemorrhoids through the three major incisions. The hemorrhoidal plexus may serve a physiologic role by forming a cushion that distends and fine-tunes the anal canal sealing, hence preventing leakage of stool. Hemorrhoidectomy may have a negative impact on this physiologic hemorrhoid function as well on the sphincter complex (stretching, injury), such that fecal soilage may occur, particularly if too much tissue has been removed, the anus dilated, or the sphincter muscles directly injured.

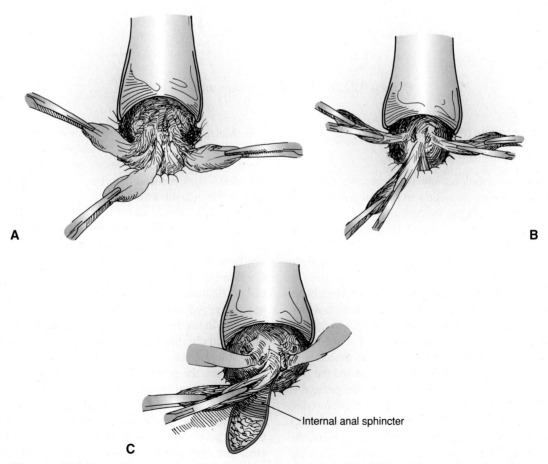

Internal anal sphincter

Figure 122.2 A: Traction on three hemorrhoidal pedicles. **B:** Additional hemostats placed to assure all redundant mucosa is included. **C:** Beginning of excision. Note preservation of internal anal sphincter.

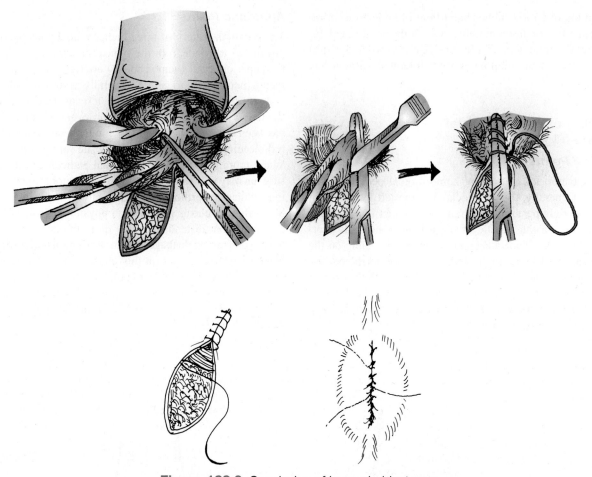

Figure 122.3 Conclusion of hemorrhoidectomy

Hemorrhoidectomy (Fig. 122.3)

Technical and Anatomic Points

The objective of hemorrhoidectomy is to preserve sufficient epithelium between the excision sites to prevent postoperative stricture, while excising all the subcutaneous venous tissues, ligating the hemorrhoidal pedicles, and restoring near-normal anatomy.

Insert the anal retractor (e.g., bullet retractor, Ferguson retractor). Retract the previously placed Kelly clamp to expose the hemorrhoidal pedicle and place an absorbable suture ligature (e.g., 2-0 Vicryl) to its apex. Doing this step before rather than after dissecting the hemorrhoidal tissue will help to reduce unnecessary bleeding. Make a V-shaped incision outside the more external Kelly clamp and extend it as a narrow eye-shaped mucocutaneous incision toward the previously ligated vascular pedicle. If more than one pedicle is to be excised, it is crucial to leave enough epithelium (skin and mucosa) between each site in order because an anal stricture may result. If large, external hemorrhoids are present, the redundant skin allows for a more generous excision. Develop flaps laterally just under the skin and mucosa. Starting at the external angle of the "eye," lift the hemorrhoidal veins off the underlying sphincter muscle, moving toward the central liga-

tion. Metzenbaum scissors are a very effective tool, but the step can also be achieved with scalpel, electrocautery, or any other tool (energy device, laser), the latter of which may be associated with reduced pain but otherwise do not provide a measurable benefit while substantially increasing the cost of the procedure.

As the dissection progresses, the sphincter muscles with the red external and white internal muscles should be clearly visible and preserved by moving down any transverse fibers. Continue until the hemorrhoidal pedicle with the previously placed ligature comes down to a small base. The suture is again wrapped around and tied. Amputate the hemorrhoid and send the tissue for pathology. Check hemostasis in the base of the pedicle. Secure small bleeders with electrocautery or with suture ligature. Use the needle end of the suture ligature to bury the pedicle stump and close the wound as a running suture from inside out. Avoid a loose space underneath the closure by making sure that each bite not only grasps the wound edges but runs below the bottom of the wound to achieve good compression and reduce hematoma formation. Once the anal verge is reached, assess the remainder of the external skin wound and excise any redundant tissue to avoid large "dog ears" or skin tags. Minor redundancies will generally smooth out and can be ignored. Continue the closure but leave the most external part of the wound open for possible drainage.

If deemed necessary, one or both of the hemorrhoids should be dealt with in a similar fashion. At the conclusion of the procedure, there will be a linear radial suture line in each excision site. Check hemostasis. Use suture ligatures to address bleeding sites. Once hemostasis is good, roll up and place a Gelfoam in the anal canal to ensure hemostasis. This is not; however, a substitute for surgical hemostasis. Additional boost injection of the perianal skin with long-acting local anesthetic such as bupivacaine hydrochloride (Marcaine) supports the postoperative pain control.

Banding (Internal Hemorrhoids Only)

Prone jackknife, lithotomy, or lateral decubitus position

Preload at least three rubber rings onto loading cone, load one rubber ring to banding device (suction vs. grasping technique)

Insert large diameter anoscope and identify three hemorrhoidal pedicles

Band largest hemorrhoid first: Place ligator to the apex of the target hemorrhoid, well above the dentate line; suction or pull it with a grasper into the device and deploy the loaded rubber band

Expose next pedicle and repeat for two more pedicles

If patient complains of severe pain, use L-shaped rubber band cutting removal hook to remove band and repeat procedure at higher level

---

Rubber Band Ligation (Fig. 122.4)

Technical Points

This is an office procedure. Because there is minimal sensation above the dentate line, anesthesia is not required. It is appropriate for grades I–III internal hemorrhoids if there is no need or desire to also address an external component. Any position is acceptable, for example, prone jackknife, lithotomy, or lateral decubitus position. In preparation, preload at least three rubber rings onto loading cone, load one rubber ring to banding device. There are different devices types (suction vs. grasping technique), but the suction bander is more convenient as it can be applied single-handed.

Perform a digital rectal examination. Lubricate the anus and gently insert a large diameter anoscope to identify three hemorrhoidal pedicles and define which one should be banded. Select the largest hemorrhoid first: Place the ligator to the apex of the target hemorrhoid, well above the dentate line; suction or pull it with a grasper into the device and deploy the loaded rubber band. Expose next pedicle and repeat for up to two more pedicles. This procedure should be painless even if it may leave the patient with a sense of urgency. If the patient complains of severe pain, the hemorrhoid has been banded too low down. In this case, use the L-shaped rubber band cutting removal hook to remove band. A repeat procedure should target a higher level.

Complications are uncommon, most frequently delayed bleeding. Rarely, pelvic sepsis may follow this procedure. Suspect this potentially life-threatening complication if the patient develops fever, pain, urinary retention, or systemic symptoms.

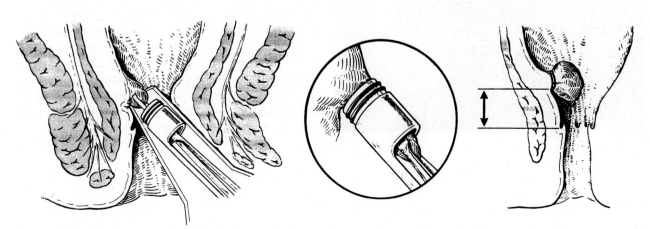

Figure 122.4 Rubber band procedure for internal hemorrhoids (Keighley MRS, Williams NS. *Surgery of the Anus Rectum, and Colon.* Philadelphia, PA: WB Saunders; 1993, with permission).

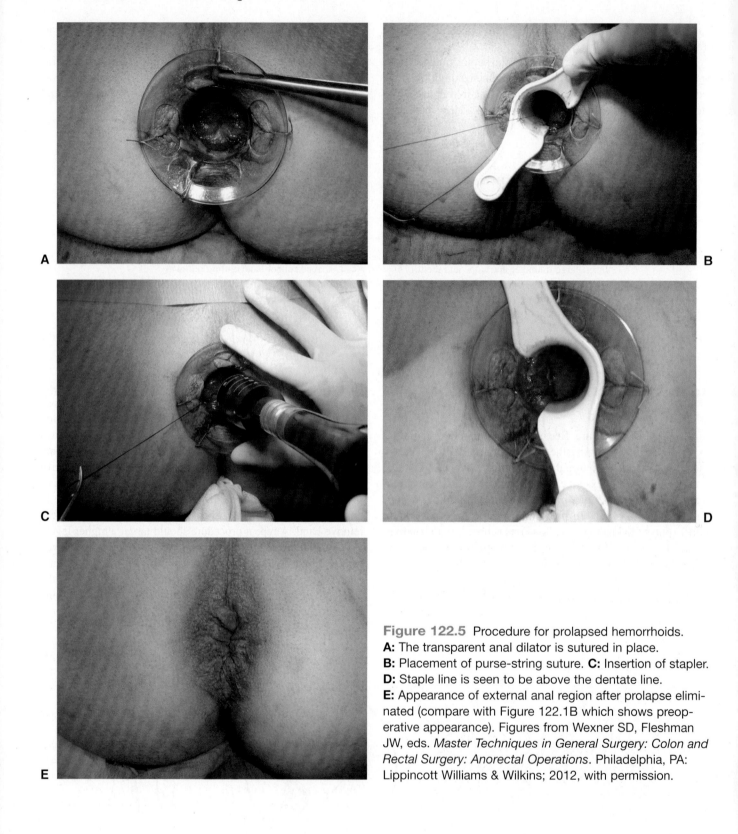

Figure 122.5 Procedure for prolapsed hemorrhoids.
A: The transparent anal dilator is sutured in place.
B: Placement of purse-string suture. **C:** Insertion of stapler.
D: Staple line is seen to be above the dentate line.
E: Appearance of external anal region after prolapse elimi-
nated (compare with Figure 122.1B which shows preop-
erative appearance). Figures from Wexner SD, Fleshman
JW, eds. *Master Techniques in General Surgery: Colon and
Rectal Surgery: Anorectal Operations*. Philadelphia, PA:
Lippincott Williams & Wilkins; 2012, with permission.

Stapled Hemorrhoidectomy (Hemorrhoidopexy, Internal Hemorrhoids Only)

Prone jackknife or lithotomy position

Avoid unnecessary anal dilation

Place anal dilator/retractor set and suture the transparent retractor to the perianal skin

Inspect the anal canal: The dentate line should be protected underneath the retractor

Insert the suture anoscope and place a mucosal purse-string suture about 3–4 cm above the dentate line

Insert the fully opened stapling device, avoid any force

Tie the purse-string suture to the rod and guide its two ends through the lateral openings in the stapler

Close the stapler under continued traction on the sutures until the maximum has been reached

Before firing the stapler, verify that neither the posterior vaginal wall nor the anoderm have been tethered into the stapler

Fire the stapler and wait 2 minutes, then open it 1½ turns and gently it; verify the donut

Check the staple line for its position above the dentate line and for hemostasis: Use electrocautery or suture ligatures for bleeding sites

Stapled Hemorrhoidectomy (Also Termed Hemorrhoidopexy, or Procedure for Prolapsing Hemorrhoids) (Fig. 122.5)

Technical Points

The procedure may be performed in the prone jackknife or lithotomy position (see discussion in previous section). The patient should have received at least two enemas in preparation and standard colorectal antibiotic prophylaxis. Once the patient is prepped and draped, inject local anesthesia into the ischioanal fossa on either side and as a subcutaneous block around the anus.

Avoid unnecessary anal dilation as it may cause damage to the sphincter complex. Gently insert the anal dilator with the transparent retractor and suture the latter with a strong Vicryl suture temporarily to the perianal skin (Fig. 122.5A). Remove the obturator and inspect the anal canal: The dentate line should be protected underneath the transparent retractor. Insert the suture anoscope and place a mucosal purse-string suture (e.g., 2/0 Prolene) about 3 to 4 cm above the dentate line (Fig. 122.5B). Care has to be taken to not move closer to the dentate line with every stitch. The bites should only grasp the mucosa and not leave any gaps between the out- and following in-stitch as the mucosa is otherwise not circumferentially pulled into the stapler. Verify the completeness of the purse string with a digital examination. Insert the fully opened stapling device past the purse-string suture (Fig. 122.5C). Make sure to avoid any undue force. Cut the needle off, tie the purse-string suture to the rod, and guide its two ends through the lateral openings in the stapler. These two suture ends are continuously pulled away from the anus as the stapler is closed to its maximum. During the stapler closure, its measuring scale on the stapler body moves into the anal canal.

Before firing the stapler, you should always do two safety stops and verify that neither the posterior vaginal wall nor the anoderm have been tethered into the stapler. Fire the stapler

and wait 2 or more minutes. Normal bleeding time is more than 6 minutes. A waiting time of 5 minutes with the stapler closed is well-invested time as the incidence of staple line bleeding is very low; the time that would have to be spent for hemostasis if the stapler was removed too soon clearly exceeds these few minutes. The stapler is then opened with 1½ turns and gently removed. The donut should be verified and is a substantially larger piece of tissue than after a conventional stapling. Before terminating the procedure, check the staple line for its correct position above the dentate line (Fig. 122.5D) and for hemostasis. Use electrocautery or suture ligatures for bleeding sites. No prolapse should be visible at conclusion of the procedure, as shown in Figure 122.5E. Once hemostasis is good, roll up and place a Gelfoam in the anal canal to ensure hemostasis. This is not; however, a substitute for surgical hemostasis.

REFERENCES

1. Beck DE, Roberts PL, Saclarides TJ, Senagore AJ, Stamos MJ, Wexner SD, eds. *The ASCRS Textbook of Colon and Rectal Surgery.* 2nd ed. New York, NY: Springer Publisher; 2011.
2. Balasubramaniam S, Kaiser AM. Management options for symptomatic hemorrhoids. *Curr Gastroenterol Rep.* 2003;5(5):431–437.
3. Burch J, Epstein D, Sari AB-A, et al. Stapled haemorrhoidopexy for the treatment of haemorrhoids: A systematic review. *Colorectal Dis.* 2009;11(3):233–243; discussion 43.
4. Corman ML. *Corman's Colon and Rectal Surgery.* 6th ed. New York, NY: Lippincott Williams & Wilkins; 2012.
5. Gordon PH. *Principles and Practice of Surgery for the Colon, Rectum, and Anus.* 3rd ed. New York, NY: Informa Healthcare; 2007.
6. Infantino A, Altomare DF, Bottini C, et al. Prospective randomized multicentre study comparing stapler haemorrhoidopexy with Doppler-guided transanal haemorrhoid dearterialization for third-degree haemorrhoids. *Colorectal Dis.* 2012;14(2):205–211.
7. Jayaraman S, Colquhoun PHD, Malthaner RA. Stapled versus conventional surgery for hemorrhoids. *Cochrane Database Syst Rev.* 2006;(4):CD005393.
8. Jayaraman S, Colquhoun PH, Malthaner RA. Stapled hemorrhoidopexy is associated with a higher long-term recurrence rate

of internal hemorrhoids compared with conventional excisional hemorrhoid surgery. *Dis Colon Rectum.* 2007;50(9):1297–1305.

9. Joshi GP, Neugebauer EAM, PROSPECT Collaboration. Evidence-based management of pain after haemorrhoidectomy surgery. *Br J Surg.* 2010;97(8):1155–1168.

10. Kaiser AM. *McGraw-Hill Manual Colorectal Surgery.* 1st ed. New York, NY: McGraw-Hill Publishers; 2009.

11. Katdare MV, Ricciardi R. Anal stenosis. *Surg Clin N Am.* 2010; 90(1):137–145.

12. Laughlan K, Jayne DG, Jackson D, et al. Stapled haemorrhoidopexy compared to Milligan-Morgan and Ferguson haemorrhoidectomy: A systematic review. *Int J Colorect Dis.* 2009;24(3): 335–344.

13. Milito G, Cadeddu F, Muzi MG, et al. Haemorrhoidectomy with Ligasure vs. conventional excisional techniques: Meta-analysis of randomized controlled trials. *Colorectal Dis.* 2010;12(2):85–93.

14. Nienhuijs S, de Hingh I. Conventional versus LigaSure hemorrhoidectomy for patients with symptomatic hemorrhoids. *Cochrane Database Syst Rev.* 2009;(1):CD006761.

15. Nunoo-Mensah JW, Kaiser AM. Stapled hemorrhoidectomy. *Am J Surg.* 2005;190(1):127–130.

16. Nystrom PO, Qvist N, Raahave D, et al. Randomized clinical trial of symptom control after stapled anopexy or diathermy excision for haemorrhoid prolapse. *Br J Surg.* 2010;97(2):167–176.

17. Shanmugam V, Thaha MA, Rabindranath KS, et al. Systematic review of randomized trials comparing rubber band ligation with excisional haemorrhoidectomy. *Br J Surg.* 2005;92(12): 1481–1487.

18. Shao WJ, Li GCH, Zhang ZHK, et al. Systematic review and meta-analysis of randomized controlled trials comparing stapled haemorrhoidopexy with conventional haemorrhoidectomy. *Br J Surg.* 2008;95(2):147–160.

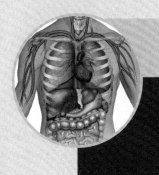

123

Management of Perirectal Abscesses, Anal Fistulas, and Chronic Anal Fissure

Andreas M. Kaiser

*P*erirectal abscesses* and anal fissures are among the most frequent causes of anorectal pain. Cryptoglandular abscesses characteristically originate in one of 8 to 12 anal glands that empty in the crypt at the dentate line. The infection spreads along anatomical paths, tracking laterally into the soft tissues of defined perirectal spaces. The abscess is defined by its location, the depth and size, and the relation to sphincter and pelvic floor muscles. The increase in pressure in a limited space in conjunction with a dense sensory neural network leads to the characteristic progressive painful swelling. Surgical drainage is the treatment of choice.

Perirectal/anal fistulas are intertwined with abscesses through their common pathogenesis and anatomy. The fistula is a chronic condition that may be initiated by or aggravated by acute episodes (abscesses). A perirectal fistula represents a communication between at least two sites that are not naturally connected. The primary opening represents the origin of the fistula in the anal gland; the secondary opening(s) is/are the result of either a spontaneous perforation of an infection or abscess or of a surgical incision and drainage procedure (see below). The course of the fistula tract in regard to the sphincter complex forms the basis for categorizations into superficial, transsphincteric, intersphincteric, extrasphincteric, and complex fistulas. The treatment is surgical and aims at the best compromise between curing the fistula and avoiding excessive sphincter damage with fecal incontinence.

An *anal fissure* is a longitudinal tear at the anal verge, typically located in the midline (posterior > anterior) and associated with a high anal sphincter tone. Symptoms include pain with and after defecation as well as minor bleeding. Treatment aims at normalizing stool regularity and decreasing sphincter tone. While pharmacologic tools (topical nitroglycerin or calcium channel blockers, botulinum toxin injection) are available, the most reliable tool is a surgical lateral internal sphincterotomy, which is the core of surgical management to achieve a reduction of the resting anal sphincter tone. The sphincterotomy may be combined with excision of sentinel skin tag (external end of fissure) and/or hypertrophic anal papilla (internal end of fissure), or formal fissurectomy.

In this chapter, the anatomy of the anal sphincter mechanism is presented through the operations for perirectal abscess and anal fistula as well as through the discussion of lateral internal sphincterotomy.

SCORE™, the Surgical Council on Resident Education, classified anorectal abscess drainage, and anal sphincterotomy—internal as "ESSENTIAL COMMON" procedures.

STEPS IN PROCEDURES

Drainage of Perirectal Abscess
Prone jackknife, lithotomy, or lateral position.
Perform careful and gentle bidigital rectal examination. Palpate the perianal tissues including the deep postanal space in order to clinically define the extent of the abscess.

Unless procedure done under anesthesia, anesthetize the skin overlying the abscess with local anesthetic.
If electrocautery is available, excise a skin disk over the abscess maximum. Alternatively, make a cruciate incision with a scalpel and the edges are removed

(to avoid premature closure of the skin). A submucosal abscess should be drained into the rectum.

As soon as the abscess cavity is reached, pus should flow immediately; otherwise the correct level has not been reached and the procedure has not yet achieved its goal.

Digital break-down of loculations is not only painful but has also been associated with a higher incidence of incontinence. It should nowadays be used with caution for select circumstances and not be routine; in absence of general anesthesia it should be avoided.

Management of underlying the fistula is only of secondary priority: If the procedure

is performed under general anesthesia, excision of the cryptoglandular origin and a definitive fistula procedure may be reasonable, but due to the inflamed tissue carries an increased risk of creating false tracts.

A horseshoe abscess that involves the deep postanal space and both ischioanal fossae is accessed in the posterior midline (modified Hanley procedure); two counter incisions in the anterolateral quadrants are made to place a drain looped to itself (e.g., Penrose drain).

Major packing is not needed and prevents emptying of the abscess cavity; loose insertion of iodoform gauze is acceptable.

HALLMARK ANATOMIC COMPLICATIONS

Pain
Bleeding
Urinary retention
Insufficient drainage with persistence/recurrence

Pelvic sepsis
Sphincter injury and dysfunction (incontinence to stool/gas)

LIST OF ANATOMIC STRUCTURES

Inspection/Palpation Landmarks

Anus, anal verge, four perianal quadrants (left/right, anterior/posterior)
Dentate line (pectinate line):
    Anal crypts
    Anal columns (of Morgagni)
Muscular structures:
    Internal anal sphincter (IAS, smooth muscle, white, 1 to 2 mm thick; on ultrasound hypoechogenic/black)

External anal sphincter (EAS, skeletal muscle, red, 7 to 10 mm thick; on ultrasound hyperechogenic/white)
Intersphincteric groove
Puborectalis muscle (skeletal muscle; on ultrasound hyperechogenic/white)
Perirectal spaces:
    Ischioanal fossa
    Deep postanal space of Courtney
    Intersphincteric space

Drainage of Perirectal Abscess (Fig. 123.1)

Technical Points

Even though the drainage procedure may be performed in any position (depending on the overall setting in clinic, emergency room, or the operating room), the prone jackknife allows best access to all perirectal spaces including the deep postanal space.

The anus is again carefully examined with visual inspection, external palpation, and a (bi) digital examination. The perirectal and ischioanal tissue are gently palpated between the inserted index finger (inside the rectum) and the external thumb in order to define areas of thickening/induration, relation to sphincters, and (if patient awake) pain (Fig. 123.1A). "Fluctuance" is not a prerequisite for treatment as it may be absent even if an abscess is quite large.

After administration of adequate anesthesia (local or general), the area is disinfected with povidone-iodine solution (Betadine). Perform (at least) proctoscopy as part of the pre- or intraoperative evaluation to assess for obvious signs of malignancy or inflammatory bowel disease. The goal of the

procedure is to create a sufficient size opening to allow drainage of pus and debris, and avoid premature skin closure. Make the opening as close as possible to the anal verge to ensure that the resulting fistula tract will be short (Fig. 123.1B). If the abscess location in uncertain, an 18-gauge needle on an aspirating syringe can be used before drainage to confirm the presence/location of pus. If electrocautery is available, excise a skin disk over the maximum of the abscess; alternatively, perform a cruciate incision and remove the edges. As soon as the abscess cavity is reached, pus should flow abundantly; otherwise the incision needs to be deepened with a clamp until the correct level is reached. In contrast to past recommendations, digital breakdown of loculations should be avoided if possible (particularly in absence of general anesthesia) as it has been associated with a higher incidence of incontinence.

Management of an underlying fistula is only of secondary priority: If the procedure is performed under general anesthesia, it may be reasonable to excise the cryptoglandular origin and place a seton (as outlined in the next section); however, the inflamed tissue carries an increased risk of creating false passages and is not well suited for flap procedures or the plug.

Types of abscesses

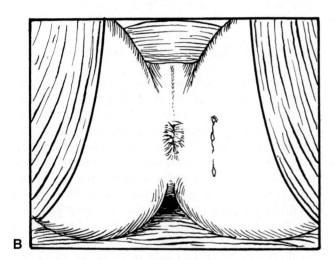

A   Perianal   Ischiorectal   Submucous   Transsphincteric

Levator ani

Puborectalis

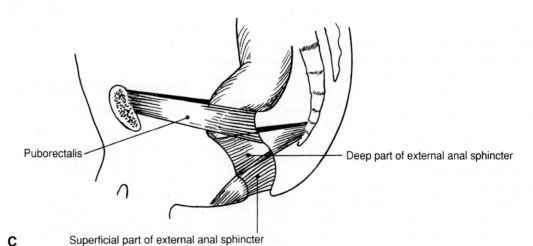

Puborectalis   Deep part of external anal sphincter

C   Superficial part of external anal sphincter

Figure 123.1 Drainage of perirectal abscess. **A:** Types of abscesses. **B:** Opening into abscess releases pus. **C:** Relationship of sphincters.

A horseshoe abscess involving the deep postanal space and both ischioanal fossae should be accessed through a radial incision in the posterior midline between coccyx and anal verge (modified Hanley procedure); two counter incisions in the anterolateral quadrants are made to place lateral Penrose drains that are secured by looping them.

Submucosal abscesses are drained into the rectum, rather than externally. For this purpose, an anal retractor is placed to expose the abscess. The location is confirmed by aspiration with a needle and syringe. Incise the mucosa overlying the abscess and allow it to drain into the rectum. If the cavity is large, place a Penrose drain or mushroom catheter into the abscess cavity to keep it open. Generally, such a drain will be passed within 1 to 2 days.

Antibiotics alone do not resolve a perirectal abscess and are not routinely needed; they may be given in support if there is a substantial phlegmonous component or if the patient is immunocompromised.

Anatomic Points

Specific locations around the anus are best described by assigning them to one of four quadrants (left/right, anterior/posterior). The alternative "clock-face" nomenclature is confusing if the patient's position changes. Abscesses and fistulas are commonly classified according to the path taken by the burrowing infection relative to the external anal sphincter and the pelvic floor muscles (Fig. 123.1A,C).

- Perianal abscess: Most common type with superficial infection tracking down the intersphincteric plane to the perianal skin. These abscesses are fairly small and typically very close to the anal verge. Drainage in local anesthesia in the office is appropriate. The resulting fistula will at most affect part of the internal sphincter and can be opened without fear of incontinence.
- Transsphincteric abscess/fistula: When the infection tracks laterally across the internal and external sphincters into the ischioanal fat, an ischioanal abscess results. Drainage in local anesthesia in the office is appropriate.
- Deep postanal space abscess and horseshoe abscess: Transsphincteric spread of infection from the posterior midline into the deep postanal space of Courtney with bilateral extension into the ischioanal fossae. Surgery more appropriate for general anesthesia.
- Intersphincteric abscess: Infection tracks from the intersphincteric groove in cephalad direction. Due to the lack of space, this form is associated with extreme pain and a lack of clinical swelling. Evaluation and surgical treatment typically require anesthesia.
- Supralevator abscess: Very rare form of abscess, often associated with a primary abdominal pathology that tracks down.

The IAS is a circular smooth muscle of whitish color and is the direct continuation of the muscularis propria (smooth muscle layer) of the rectum. Just above its distal end at the intersphincteric groove, this muscle layer becomes consider-

ably thickened, forming a visible and palpable band around the anal canal. On endorectal ultrasound, the IAS is visible as a hypoechogenic ring.

The EAS and the pelvic floor (levator ani) muscles are skeletal muscles of pink-red color. The latter consists of several subunits and forms a funnel-shaped musculotendinous pelvic diaphragm that is anchored in the bony pelvis at the arcus tendineus of the obturator fascia, extending from the pubic bone to the anococcygeal raphe. At its caudad and most medial portion, the puborectalis muscle forms a U-shaped sling with anterior traction that angulates the anorectum (anorectal angle, Fig. 123.1C). Below that, the muscle fibers reconstitute to a circumferential structure and form the EAS. On endorectal ultrasound, the puborectalis muscle and the EAS have a hyperechogenic appearance. The levator ani muscles are innervated by branches of the ventral primary rami of the spinal nerves S3 to S4; the EAS also receives input from the inferior rectal branch of the pudendal nerve. The EAS is a fatigue-resistant slow-twitch muscle which together with the puborectalis sling contributes the majority of active sphincter control.

The levator ani divides the pelvis into the supralevator space (between peritoneum and pelvic diaphragm) and the infralevator (extrapelvic) spaces. The ischioanal fossa is bounded superiorly by the levator ani, medially by the EAS complex, laterally by the obturator fascia, and inferiorly by the thin transverse fascia separating it from perianal space. It predominantly consists of fat, but contains neurovascular structures including pudendal nerve and internal pudendal vessels, which enter through pudendal (Alcock) canal. The deep postanal spaces of Courtney are located behind anal canal between the anococcygeal ligament and the skin (superficial postanal space) and between the anococcygeal ligament and the anococcygeal raphe (deep postanal space). It bilaterally communicates with the ischioanal fossae and hence forms a route for development of a horseshoe abscess.

Surgery for Anal Fistula (Fig. 123.2)

Technical Points

Position the patient preferably into prone jackknife position as it gives best access to all perirectal spaces including the deep postanal space; alternatively, the lithotomy position may be used in selected patients.

Identify the secondary external openings of the fistula, which may be multiple. Apply Goodsall's rule for an educated guess about the likely location of the primary (internal) opening. Goodsall's rule states that if the external orifice lies anterior to a transverse line through the anus, the tract will run directly to an internal opening in the anterior hemicircumference; fistulas with an external opening posterior to this line have curved tracts that enter the anus in the posterior midline (Fig. 123.2A). If the primary external opening lies more than 3 cm from the anal verge, even an anterior tract will curve and track to a posterior midline position.

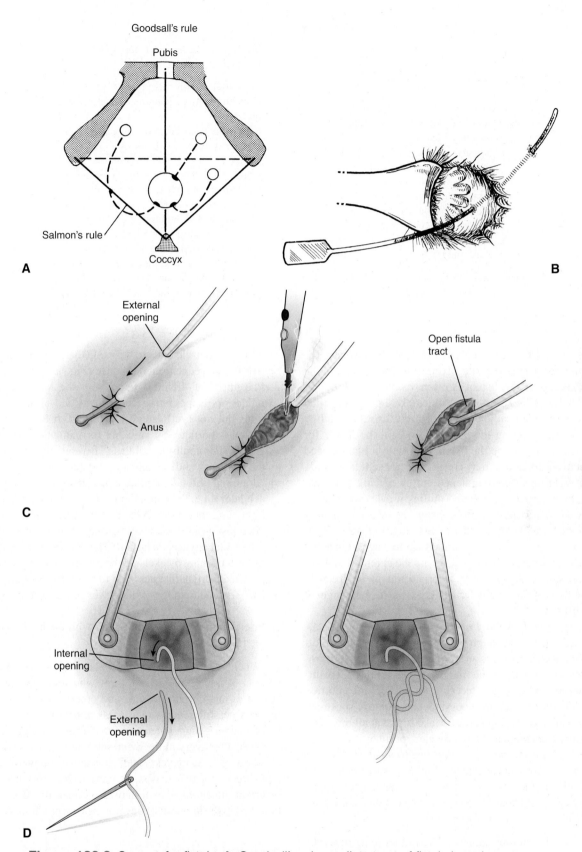

Figure 123.2 Surgery for fistula. **A:** Goodsall's rule predicts tract of fistula based upon location of opening. **B:** Identifying tract of fistula by passing a probe through the fistula. **C:** Fistulotomy. **D:** Seton placement (from Wexner SD, Fleshman JW, eds. *Colon and Rectal Surgery: Anorectal Operations.* Philadelphia, PA: Lippincott Williams & Wilkins; 2012, with permission).

STEPS IN PROCEDURE

Preferably prone jackknife, alternatively lithotomy position

Identification of secondary opening(s) and educated guess on the expected site of the primary opening (Goodsall's rule)

Insertion of anal retractor and circumferential evaluation of dentate line for possible site of primary opening. If it is not visible, injection of peroxide into secondary opening and look for bubbling on the inside

Careful probing of fistula tract with a blunt-tipped probe, avoid creating false tracts. Fistula tract may be straightened by placement of Kocher clamp to external opening and traction away from anus

Once fistula tract successfully probed, assess the extent of sphincter

involvement to decide on appropriate treatment:

1. Minor sphincter involvement (<20%): Fistulotomy by dividing the tissue over the probe
2. Substantial sphincter involvement (>20%): Options include: (1) placement of cutting seton (e.g., vessel loop) to sit on the muscle portion after dividing the epithelial layer and connective tissue between primary and secondary fistula openings; (2) placement of draining seton, leaving the epithelial layer between primary and secondary openings intact; (3) endorectal advancement flap; (4) ligation of intersphincteric fistula tract (LIFT procedure); and (5) insertion of fistula plug

Insert an anal retractor and circumferentially evaluate the dentate line for a possible site of the primary opening. The internal opening of the fistula is often visible near a hypertrophied anal papilla. If it is not visible, take a peroxide-filled syringe with an angiocatheter tip and insert it to the external opening: While injecting the peroxide observe the inside for bubbling. Carefully probe the fistula tract with a blunt-tipped probe, but avoid force as it may create false tracts. If necessary, the fistula tract may be straightened out by placing a Kocher clamp to the external opening and pulling it away from anus. Alternatively, try to pass a probe from the internal opening through the tract and out the external opening (Fig. 123.2B). It may be necessary to open the external tract in stages. Once the fistula tract is successfully probed, assess the extent of sphincter involvement to decide on appropriate treatment. Keep in mind that the regular sphincter thickness is in the range of only 5 to 10 mm.

Very superficial fistula tracts with only minor sphincter involvement (<20%) are appropriately treated with a fistulotomy. Divide the soft tissues overlying the tract using electrocautery and excise part of the margin to convert the deep slit-like defect into a V-shaped defect (Fig. 123.2C). Send a portion of the margin of the tract for biopsy. Obtain a biopsy specimen from any suspicious-looking areas. Make sure that all tracts are fully opened. Achieve hemostasis by electrocautery.

If there is substantial sphincter involvement (>20%) or multiple tracts, the management is more complicated. The treatment aims at the best compromise between curing the fistula and avoiding excessive sphincter damage with fecal incontinence. Options include the following.

1. Placement of a cutting seton (e.g., vessel loop) to sit on the muscle portion after dividing the epithelial layer and connective tissue between the primary and secondary fistula openings. The seton is tightened in the office in regular intervals to result in a delayed fistulotomy that is so slow to

allow the muscle ends to scar together, thus minimizing the risk for subsequent incontinence (Fig. 123.2D).
2. Placement of draining seton with the intent to primarily reduce the suppurative component and abscess complications but not (yet) intend to cure the fistula as such. This option is particularly valuable for patients with Crohn disease and/or multiple fistulas. The epithelial layer between the primary and secondary openings is left intact. If a "draining" seton should be converted into a "cutting" seton at a later time, the epithelial layer needs to be opened before tightening that seton. Note that the insertion of the seton is done just as shown above, but the seton is not tightened.
3. Endorectal advancement flap: The concept is to close off the internal opening by excising the primary opening and raising a proximal partial thickness flap to be pulled over that opening.
4. LIFT procedure: One of the newer concepts that failed in the past.
5. Insertion of collagen fistula plug with the hope to obliterate the tract.

When dealing with fistulas, one should keep in mind a number of issues. We do not know why some patients develop abscesses and chronic fistulae and others do not. Even an initially successful treatment has a risk of recurrence. Incontinence is the patient's biggest fear, and the surgeon's biggest liability. It is seen after every of the mentioned surgical methods but may not show until many years later. It is unwise; however, to avoid any surgery for that reason, as chronic fistulae carry a risk of recurrent infections (which may also impair the sphincter function) and in the long run of developing cancer within the fistulas.

Anatomic Points

The anal canal is the terminal portion of the gastrointestinal tract. Among the significant anatomic structures is the dentate (pectinate) line, which is typically 1 to 2 cm proximal to anal verge and represents the embryologic fusion point between endoderm and ectoderm. Proximal to it, the rectum transitions into the anal canal with a change of smooth mucosal lining to a plicated appearance that forms the columns of Morgagni. At their base in-between are the crypts into which 8 to 12 anal glands open. Most anal fistulas and perirectal abscesses begin in these sinuses. The intersphincteric groove marks the distal end of the internal smooth muscle cone, at which point only the external (striated muscle) anal sphincter is left. This groove can be palpated but not seen.

STEPS IN PROCEDURE

Prone jackknife or lithotomy position

Visualization and assessment of the fissure (posterior or anterior midline): Bare sphincter muscle fibers, elevated wound edges, formation of a sentinel skin tag, and hypertrophic anal papillae represent signs of chronicity

Palpation of the intersphincteric groove typically easy due to the hypertrophic internal sphincter

Right lateral incision at the intersphincteric groove and division of connective tissue overlaying the sphincter complex

Identification of the white fibers of IAS, to be distinguished from the pink fibers of the EAS

Loading of IAS fibers onto clamp and division of its fibers (e.g., with electrocautery) up to the level of the proximal end of the fissure

Wound irrigation and closure

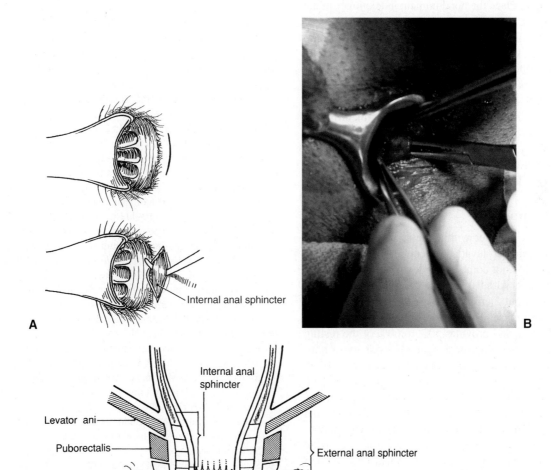

Figure 123.3 Lateral internal sphincterotomy. **A:** Lateral incision and elevation of sphincter. **B:** Elevation of sphincter using right angle clamp (from Wexner SD, Fleshman JW, eds. *Colon and Rectal Surgery: Anorectal Operations.* Philadelphia, PA: Lippincott Williams & Wilkins; 2012, with permission). **C:** Cross section of sphincters.

Lateral Internal Sphincterotomy (Fig. 123.3)

Technical Points

Position the patient in the prone jackknife or lithotomy position. Visualize and assess the fissure which is typically located in the posterior or anterior midline: Bare sphincter muscle fibers, elevated wound edges, formation of a sentinel skin tag (outside), and hypertrophic anal papillae (inside) represent signs of chronicity. Gently place a retractor.

■ Open technique: Palpate the intersphincteric groove and make a lateral 5- to 10-mm incision (Fig. 123.3A). Using a hemostat, gently dissect down until the white internal sphincter is identified. Use a clamp to hook up and elevate the internal sphincter (Fig. 123.3B). Electrocautery works well to divide the sphincter fibers up to the level of the proximal end of the fissure. Use palpation to confirm that the internal sphincter has been divided.

■ Closed technique: Place the nondominant index finger in the anal canal. At the lateral position, insert a Beaver blade or number 11 blade in parallel direction to the internal sphincter through the skin and into the intersphincteric groove. Turn the blade 90 degrees toward the anal canal and divide the sphincter carefully without damaging the mucosa or the finger. You will know when the sphincter is completely divided when there is a sensation of the last fibers giving way as they are cut. The sphincter will then seem much more open. Apply pressure to this area from within the anal canal for a couple of minutes to ensure hemostasis. The incision can then be closed with an absorbable suture.

Anatomic Points

The IAS lies like a cylinder within the spout of the funnel-shaped external sphincter–levator ani complex (Figs. 123.1C and 123.3C), but does not come as far down as the EAS does. Particularly in patients with fissures, the intersphincteric groove is easily palpable about 2 cm into the anal canal as the IAS is very prominent and tense. The internal sphincter as a smooth muscle is involuntary and provides 50% to 60% of the resting tone; it is largely responsible for the pathophysiology of nonhealing anal fissures as the tone is much higher than normal. The external sphincter and puborectalis muscles as skeletal muscles have an involuntary resting tone, but can be actively contracted (squeeze) and contribute with the overall tone, anal canal length and angulation to the maintenance of normal continence. This is not altered in any way by controlled division of the internal sphincter only; however, manual anal dilation (a former and now largely abandoned treatment for anal fissures) induces damage to both the internal and external sphincter structures.

REFERENCES

1. David EB, Patricia LR, Theodore JS, Anthony JS, Michael JS, Steven DW. *The ASCRS Textbook of Colon and Rectal Surgery.* 2nd ed. New York, NY: Springer Publisher; 2011.
2. Browder LK, Sweet S, Kaiser AM. Modified Hanley procedure for management of complex horseshoe fistulae. *Techn Coloproctol.* 2009;13(4):301–306.
3. Corman ML. *Corman's Colon and Rectal Surgery.* 6th ed. New York, NY: Lippincott Williams & Wilkins; 2012.
4. Garg P, Song J, Bhatia A, et al. The efficacy of anal fistula plug in fistula-in-ano: A systematic review. *Colorectal Dis.* 2010; 12(10):965–970.
5. Gordon PH. *Principles and Practice of Surgery for the Colon, Rectum, and Anus.* 3rd ed. New York, NY: Informa Healthcare; 2007.
6. Iesalnieks I, Gaertner WB, Glass H, et al. Fistula-associated anal adenocarcinoma in Crohn's disease. *Inflamm Bowel Dis.* 2010; 16(10):1643–1648.
7. Kaiser AM. *McGraw-Hill Manual Colorectal Surgery.* 1st ed. New York, NY: McGraw-Hill Publishers; 2009.
8. Kaiser AM, Ortega AE. Anorectal anatomy. *Surg Clin North Am.* 2002;82(6):1125–1138.
9. Malik AI, Nelson RL. Surgical management of anal fistulae: A systematic review. *Colorectal Dis.* 2008;10(5):420–430.
10. Malik AI, Nelson RL, Tou S. Incision and drainage of perianal abscess with or without treatment of anal fistula. *Cochrane Database Syst Rev.* 2010;(7):CD006827.
11. McCourtney JS, Finlay IG. Setons in the surgical management of fistula in ano. *Br J Surg.* 1995;82(4):448–452.
12. Parks AG, Gordon PH, Hardcastle JD. A classification of fistula-in-ano. *Br J Surg.* 1976;63(1):1–12.
13. Perry WB, Dykes SL, Standards Practice Task Force of the American Society of Colon and Rectal S, et al. Practice parameters for the management of anal fissures (3rd Revision). *Dis Colon Rectum.* 2010;53(8):1110–1115. 10.007/DCR.0b013e3181e23dfe.
14. Sajid MS, Hunte S, Hippolyte S, et al. Comparison of surgical vs chemical sphincterotomy using botulinum toxin for the treatment of chronic anal fissure: A meta-analysis. *Colorectal Dis.* 2008;10(6):547–552.
15. Shao WJ, Li GC, Zhang ZK. Systematic review and meta-analysis of randomized controlled trials comparing botulinum toxin injection with lateral internal sphincterotomy for chronic anal fissure. *Int J Colorectal Dis.* 2009;24(9):995–1000.
16. Siddiqui MRS, Ashrafian H, Tozer P, et al. A diagnostic accuracy meta-analysis of endoanal ultrasound and MRI for perianal fistula assessment. *Dis Colon Rectum.* 2012;55(5):576–585.
17. Sinha R, Kaiser AM. Efficacy of management algorithm for reducing need for sphincterotomy in chronic anal fissures. *Colorectal Dis.* 2012;14(6):760–764.
18. Soltani A, Kaiser AM. Endorectal advancement flap for cryptoglandular or Crohn's fistula-in-ano. *Dis Colon Rectum.* 2010; 53(4):486–495.
19. Steele SR, Kumar R, Feingold DL, et al. Practice parameters for the management of perianal abscess and fistula-in-Ano. *Dis Colon Rectum.* 2011;54(12):1465–1474. 10.097/DCR.0b013e 31823122b3.

ⓔ **124** Transsacral Approach to Rectal Lesions

This chapter can be accessed online at www.lww.com/eChapter124.

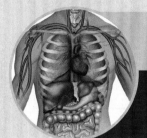

125

Proctoscopy

This chapter deals with the performance of rigid proctoscopy (sometimes called rigid sigmoidoscopy). Flexible fiberoptic sigmoidoscopy is performed essentially as detailed in Chapter 96, except that the distance to be traversed is not as great. Rigid proctoscopy is indicated in patients who have poorly prepped colons or who are being examined for foreign bodies or massive lower gastrointestinal bleeding. In these cases, the fiberoptic scope may not permit an adequate examination. The figures in this chapter detail the sequence of maneuvers necessary to pass the rigid proctoscope and to examine the rectosigmoid colon thoroughly.

SCORE™, the Surgical Council on Resident Education, classified proctoscopy as an "ESSENTIAL COMMON" procedure.

STEPS IN PROCEDURE

Left lateral decubitus or prone jackknife position (knee–chest position)
Digital rectal examination
Gently introduce scope with obturator in place
Anal canal angles forward, then directly back
Remove obturator when sphincters have been crossed
Use gently insufflation to open the lumen

Pass the scope under direct vision
Angle the scope from side to side to traverse the rectal valves
At about 15 cm, an angulation at the peritoneal reflection will be encountered
Do not pass the scope beyond this point unless it goes easily under direct vision

HALLMARK ANATOMIC PROCEDURES
Perforation
Missed lesion

LIST OF STRUCTURES
Anal canal
Rectum
Sigmoid colon

Peritoneal reflection
Rectal valves (of Houston)

Positioning of the Patient and Insertion of the Scope (Fig. 125.1)

Technical Points

Place the patient on a proctoscopy table in the knee–chest position. If such a table is not available, the left lateral decubitus or Sims

position is a useful alternative. If the patient is in the Sims position, make sure that the buttocks extend over the edge of the table. This will allow you to maneuver the scope fully and to move your head around as needed to get a good view of the entire lower bowel.

First, perform a digital rectal examination to confirm that there is no pathologic lesion within the immediate anorectal

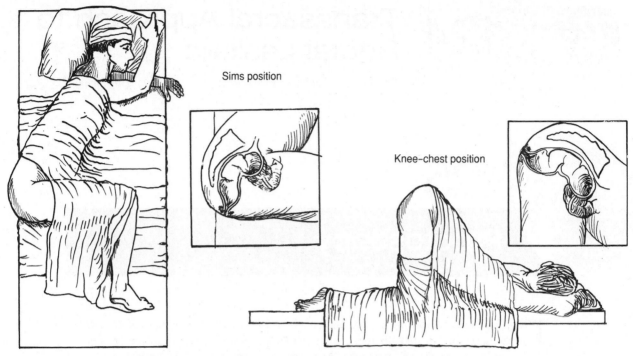

Figure 125.1 Positioning of the patient and insertion of the scope

area and to determine the angle of the rectal canal. Place the obturator within the proctoscope and introduce the scope by gentle pressure.

The anal canal first passes anteriorly and then angles sharply back toward the hollow of the sacrum. Therefore, the scope must initially be passed in a direction pointing toward the patient's umbilicus, and then almost immediately angled back toward the small of the back after the sphincter mechanism has been traversed. As soon as you feel the scope traverse the sphincter mechanism, remove the obturator and pass the scope under direct vision. On the way in, concentrate on passing the scope safely and atraumatically. On the way out, concentrate on visualizing and examining the entire rectosigmoid colon for any signs of pathology.

The first few centimeters of the scope in the lower rectum should take you straight back toward the hollow of the sacrum. It will then be necessary to pass the scope more anteriorly. Insufflate air as you proceed in order to open up the bowel enough to see where you are headed. Angle the scope from side to side to traverse the rectal valves (of Houston), of which there are generally three. When you have inserted the scope to a depth of about 15 cm, you will have reached the peritoneal reflection and the bowel will angle sharply, usually to the left. At this point, you must angle the tip of the scope sharply to pass by it. Often, it is not possible to pass the scope deeper than 15 to 18 cm. If you cannot advance it safely under direct vision, do not attempt to do so.

Anatomic Points

The embryology of the terminal gastrointestinal tract helps to explain the anatomy of this region. Initially, the terminal hindgut or cloaca, an endodermally lined cavity, is common to the reproductive, excretory, and digestive systems. The ventral aspect of the cloaca is continuous with the allantois, a small cloacal diverticulum that is the forerunner of the urachus. Distally, at the cloacal membrane, cloacal endoderm and surface ectoderm are in contact. Externally, the cloacal membrane is located in the proctodeum (anal pit), a caudal depression that results from the proliferation of mesoderm surrounding the cloacal membrane. (Because there is no mesoderm in the cloacal membrane, there is no mesodermal proliferation.) Relatively early, a coronally oriented wedge of mesenchyme—the urorectal septum—develops in the interval between the posterior hindgut and the ventrally located allantois, growing caudally until it makes contact with the cloacal membrane. This divides the cloaca into a posterior terminal gastrointestinal tract and a ventral urogenital sinus. The point of contact between the urorectal septum and the cloacal membrane becomes the central perineal tendon (perineal body). During this time, the cloacal membrane, both anterior and posterior to the central perineal tendon, degenerates and ruptures, establishing communication of the terminal gastrointestinal tract and urogenital system with the environment (at this time, the amniotic cavity).

The events just described, which result in the formation of the anal canal, explain many peculiarities of the anal canal. The location of the cloacal membrane is approximately indicated by the pectinate line. Proximal to this line, the epithelium of the anal canal is derived from hindgut, whereas distal to this line, it is derived from surface ectoderm. Superior to the pectinate line, the predominant blood supply stems from the superior rectal (hemorrhoidal) artery, the terminal branch of the inferior mesenteric artery, which supplies the hindgut structures. Inferior to this line, the blood supply is provided by the middle and inferior rectal (hemorrhoidal) arteries, which ultimately are branches of the internal iliac (hypogastric) artery, basically a parietal artery. Venous drainage of the anal canal proximal to the pectinate line is accomplished by the superior rectal (hemorrhoidal) vein, a tributary of the portal system, whereas distally, venous drainage is a function of the middle and inferior rectal (hemorrhoidal) veins, which are tributaries of the caval system. The lymphatic drainage of the anal canal is indicative of its dual origin: Proximal to the pectinate line, the lymphatics tend to drain to the preaortic and para-aortic nodes, whereas distal to this line, the lymphatics drain to the inguinal nodes. Proximal to the pectinate line, sensory innervation is provided by visceral nerves, whereas distally, sensory innervation is a function of somatic nerves. Finally, although there is spatial overlap, the more proximal internal anal sphincter is in continuity with the smooth muscle of the gut (innervated by parasympathetic fibers), whereas the external anal sphincter is in continuity with striated muscle fibers of the levator ani (somatic motor innervation).

With respect to the surgical anatomy relating to rigid proctoscopy, the most important thing to remember is the almost

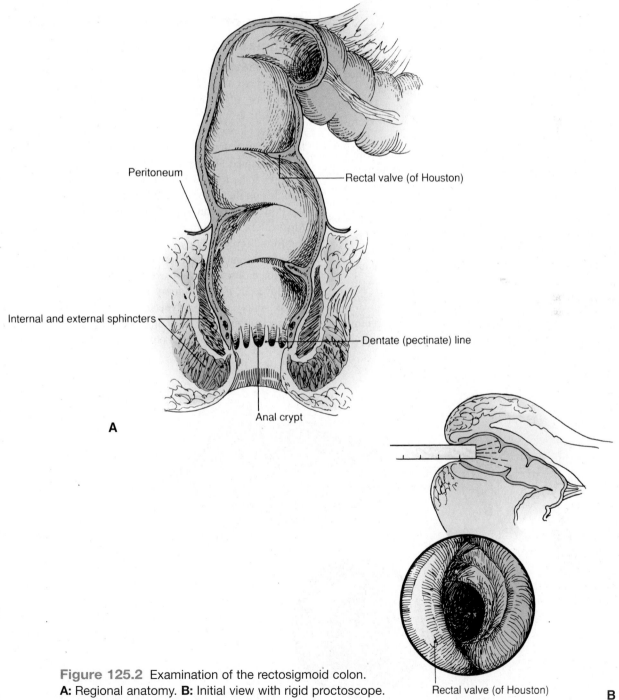

Figure 125.2 Examination of the rectosigmoid colon.
A: Regional anatomy. **B:** Initial view with rigid proctoscope.

right-angled bend between the lumen of the anal canal and that of the rectum. This severe angle dictates that the proctoscope must be first directed toward the umbilicus for a distance of 4 to 5 cm, then superoposteriorly toward the lumbar vertebrae. The angle between the anal canal and the rectum is maintained by the puborectalis muscle, the thickest and most medial part of the levator ani. Its fibers arise from the inner surface of the body of the pubis and blend with the deep fibers of the external anal sphincter posterior to the anal canal. This voluntary muscle is essential to anal continence.

Examination of the Rectosigmoid Colon (Fig. 125.2)

Technical Points

The sigmoid is identifiable by its tendency to collapse, the angulation that occurs at 15 cm, and the concentric appearance of its folds. After passing the scope to its maximum safe extent, gently withdraw it using a turning motion to ensure that the bowel is adequately inspected in each direction. At the rectosigmoid juncture, the rectum, in comparison to the sigmoid, will appear as a larger, more commodious hollow viscus, with less of a tendency to collapse. The rectal valves (of Houston) will appear at intervals. It is necessary to angle the scope carefully to inspect behind the valves, where small lesions may be hidden. Carefully withdraw the scope, allowing the bowel to collapse as you do so. In the lower rectum, take care to inspect the entire rectal ampulla, particularly the area adjacent to the anus. An anoscope may allow improved visualization of the anal area.

Anatomic Points

The junction between the sigmoid colon and the rectum is ill-defined at best. This has resulted in the use of a purely arbi-

trary point—the level of the third sacral element—to delineate between these two portions of the gastrointestinal tract. Clinically, it is perhaps better to consider the rectosigmoid as a unit. Despite the ambiguities surrounding the terminal colon and beginning rectum, there are several anatomic changes that characterize this boundary. These include a change in peritoneal relationships, the disappearance of haustra, "dispersal" of taeniae coli into a layer of longitudinal muscle completely surrounding the viscus, division of the superior rectal (hemorrhoidal) artery into its left and right branches, and presence of the highest transverse rectal fold (valve of Houston).

Biopsy or Polypectomy (Fig. 125.3)

Technical and Anatomic Points

Because the biopsy forceps that are used through the rigid proctoscope take a large bite of tissue, they should be used only in the case of obvious polypoid growths protruding into the mucosa or lesions on the valves of Houston. Inadvertent full-thickness biopsy of normal bowel wall can result in bowel perforation. Visualize the lesion from which a biopsy specimen is to be obtained and pass the biopsy forceps through the proctoscope. Take a good bite of the lesion to obtain an adequate sample and then check for bleeding.

Polypectomy can be performed through a rigid proctoscope. Most often, if a polyp is seen, that is considered an indication for formal colonoscopy (since there may be other polyps or even frank cancer elsewhere in the bowel), and polypectomy is performed during that subsequent colonoscopy.

However, *if* polypectomy is to be performed with the rigid scope, simply pass a polypectomy snare around the polyp and tighten it around the base of the polyp. Use electrocautery to coagulate the base and then pull the polyp through. As previously

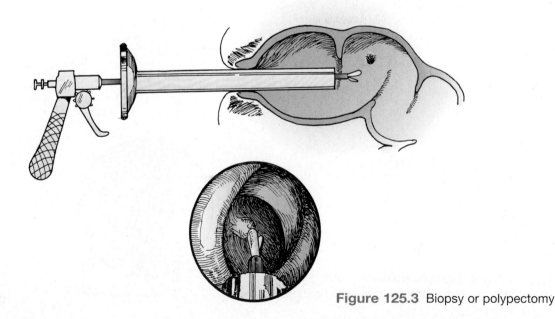

Figure 125.3 Biopsy or polypectomy

noted, polypectomy is most commonly performed through the flexible colonoscope (see Chapter 96) because the examination of the entire colon for other polyps is necessary and visualization is often improved with the use of this instrument.

REFERENCES

1. Goligher JC. Diagnosis of diseases of the anus, rectum and colon. In: Goligher JC, ed. *Surgery of the Anus, Rectum and Colon.* 4th ed. London: Bailliere Tindall; 1980:48. (This book is old, but it remains a classic. It contains an excellent description of physical examination and performance of rigid proctoscopy.)

2. Jagelman DG. Anoscopy. In: Sivak MV, ed. *Gastroenterologic Endoscopy.* Philadelphia, PA: WB Saunders; 1987:960.

3. Keighley MRB. Injuries to the colon and rectum. In: Keighley MRB, Williams NS, eds. *Surgery of the Anus, Rectum, and Colon.* London: WB Saunders; 1993:1909–1912. (Discusses causes of iatrogenic perforation and management.)

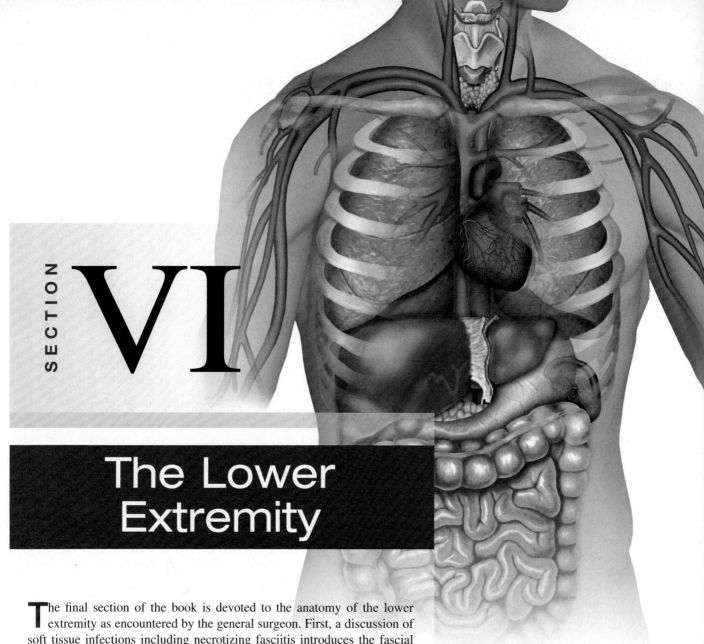

SECTION VI

The Lower Extremity

The final section of the book is devoted to the anatomy of the lower extremity as encountered by the general surgeon. First, a discussion of soft tissue infections including necrotizing fasciitis introduces the fascial and fatty layers of the region. Next, a series of chapters on amputations introduce the muscle groups and neurovascular structures. Chapter 127 details techniques for the so-called minor amputations of the digits and forefoot. These are often performed by junior residents, yet meticulous attention to patient selection and technique is imperative for proper healing. This is also true for major amputations—the below-knee amputation (Chapter 128) and the above-knee amputation (Chapter 129). Amputation at other levels, such as the Syme amputation, knee or hip disarticulation, and hemipelvectomy, are detailed in the references.

The next few chapters deal with vascular surgery of the lower extremity. Venous anatomy is given first, in two related chapters. Chapter 130 describes the great saphenous vein through the operations of venous stripping and ligation (and the related topic of harvesting the saphenous vein for vascular conduit). The related minor procedures of saphenous vein cutdown at the ankle and the groin are presented in Chapter 131. The femoral artery was first introduced in Chapter 36e and is explored in greater detail in Chapter 133, which is devoted to femoropopliteal bypass grafting.

Finally, Chapter 134 details fasciotomy of the lower extremity and reinforces the anatomy of the section.

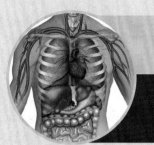

126

Debridement and Split-Thickness Skin Graft

This chapter describes two strategies for debridement of burns or necrotizing soft tissue infections. It also details the technique of split-thickness skin graft. Skin grafting is an extremely versatile method for closure of wounds that are too large for primary closure, when local flap closure is impractical or to be avoided.

SCORE™, the Surgical Council on Resident Education, classified burn debridement or grafting as "COMPLEX" procedures and skin grafting as an "ESSENTIAL COMMON" procedure.

STEPS IN PROCEDURE

Tangential excision
Consider use of tourniquet if area is large
Ensure area to be excised is held taut
Use a Weck knife or similar device
Use a rapid back-and-forth sawing motion to advance the knife
Plan to excise in several passes until bleeding tissue is obtained
If tourniquet is used, tissue will not bleed
Look for shiny, white fresh-appearing tissue
Obtain hemostasis by pressure or electrocautery
Excision to fascia
Start at edge of area to be excised
Outline the area with electrocautery
Cut down to deep fascia
Elevate the debrided tissue as a single plaque
Obtain hemostasis with electrocautery
Split-thickness skin graft
Choose recipient site

Prepare with sterile mineral oil or saline
Set appropriate width and depth on dermatome
Test dermatome
Start at the near edge of the donor site and push the dermatome away from you
Observe for a uniform thickness ribbon of translucent graft
Have an assistant pull this up to avoid jamming, if necessary
Terminate the cut when sufficient length has been obtained
Aim dermatome sharply up to cut through skin
Alternatively, turn dermatome off and cut graft free with scalpel or scissors
Obtain hemostasis in donor site with pressure
Secure graft to recipient site with interrupted sutures, staples, or Steri-strips
Immobilize graft with pressure dressing, bolster, or suction dressing
Dress donor site with occlusive dressing

HALLMARK ANATOMIC COMPLICATIONS

Inadequate debridement
Cutting the graft too thick, thus creating a full-thickness defect at the donor site

LIST OF STRUCTURES

Skin
Epidermis
Dermis
Subcutaneous tissue
Skin appendages

Hair follicles
Sebaceous glands
Superficial fascia
Deep fascia

Tangential Excision of Burn Wounds (Fig. 126.1)

Technical Points

When the burn wound is deep partial thickness (Fig. 126.1A), it may be possible to preserve some dermis by performing tangential excision. This provides an excellent bed for skin grafting while maintaining the underlying structure of the skin. It is absolutely essential that a clean viable bed be achieved. Classically, this is done by observing punctate bleeding from the excision bed, and this may result in considerable blood loss. Tangential excision is commonly limited to small cosmetically or functionally sensitive areas such as hands and fingers.

Perform tangential excision with a handheld dermatome such as a Weck knife. Guards are available for various thicknesses. Place the knife at the farthest margin of the patch to be excised. Rapidly move it from side to side, producing a sawing motion that enables the knife to cut a slab of dead tissue off with minimal force. Progress down through the area to be excised (Fig. 126.1B). Generally multiple passes are required to excise the entire area. The goal is not to excise the full depth of the burned area in the first pass (although this may occasionally happen), but rather to sequentially excise all of the burned tissue in several layers for maximal control.

Wipe the dead tissue off the knife and insert a new blade when the one you are using becomes dull.

Carefully progress, excising layer by layer until clean, viable, bleeding tissue is seen. All burned and devitalized areas must be removed to provide a good bed for skin graft. If you are using a tourniquet to limit blood loss, you will not see bleeding but should note clean glistening moist white tissue. More practice is required to recognize the correct depth of excision in this situation.

Obtain hemostasis with pressure and electrocautery. Place a moist laparotomy pad over the prepared recipient site while you obtain the graft (see Figure 126.4).

Anatomic Points

The epidermis is the portion of skin superficial to the basement membrane. This layer is the primary barrier against evaporative water loss and injury from the outside world. All burns injure this layer. The epidermis is avascular and is divided into five layers. From superficial to deep these are stratum corneum (the outermost layer of dead cells), stratum lucidum, stratum granulosum, stratum spinosum, and stratum basale (the layer in which new cells are formed). Cells in the stratum basale divide, producing new epidermal cells that are pushed upward through the various layers to eventually die and form the stratum corneum. The dead cells of the stratum corneum are shed in approximately 2 weeks. In addition to the epithelial cells, the epidermis contains Langerhans cells (a crucial part of the immune system), melanocytes, and Merkel cells.

The dermis contains collagen and elastin as well as reticular fibers. It is divided into two layers: The upper papillary layer and the lower reticular layer. The dermis provides structural support for the epidermis. It contains hair follicles and their associated erector pili muscles. Numerous blood vessels and nerves traverse this layer. Glands (sebaceous, apocrine, and eccrine) are found here. Regeneration of deep partial thickness burns occurs by re-epithelialization from these deep structures. Specialized nerve cells that sense pressure and touch are also located here. Burn injuries that completely destroy this layer are classified as full-thickness (or third degree). Because the nerve injuries are destroyed, these full-thickness burned areas are anesthetic and may be surprisingly painless.

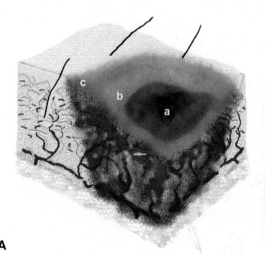
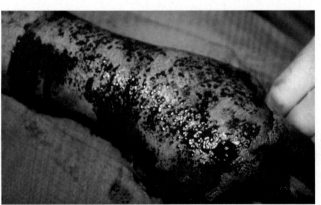

A   **B**

Figure 126.1 A: Zones of burn injury. "a" demarcates the central zone of necrosis, "b" is a surrounding zone of questionable viability termed the zone of stasis, and "c" is a zone of hyperemia where tissue may survive unless infection supravenes. **B:** Tangential excision of burn wound (from Mulholland MW, ed. *Greenfield's Surgery,* 5th ed. Philadelphia, PA: Lippincott Williams & Wilkins; 2011, with permission).

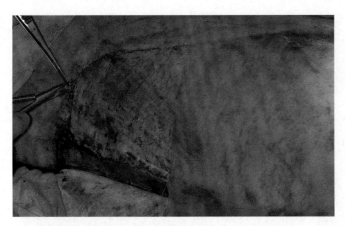

Figure 126.2 Fascial excision of burn wound (from Mulholland MW, ed. *Greenfield's Surgery,* 5th ed. Philadelphia, PA: Lippincott Williams & Wilkins; 2011, with permission).

Subcutaneous tissue is primarily fat and conveys larger blood vessels and nerves. When the burn extends down into the subcutaneous tissue, thrombosed veins may be visible through the translucent surface of the burn.

Fascial Excision of Burn (Fig. 126.2)

Technical and Anatomic Points

Obvious full-thickness burn injuries to large parts of the body (such as the anterior chest or anterior abdominal wall) are best excised by removing all tissue down to fascia. This is also the technique that would be used for excision of necrotizing soft tissue infections of these areas.

Fascial excision allows removal of the entire area with far less bleeding than tangential excision. The fascia provides a better surface for skin grafting than would the relatively poorly vascularized subcutaneous fat.

Begin at the periphery of the burned or infected area and cut down to deep fascia overlying the muscles with electrocautery. Peel the skin and fatty subcutaneous tissues off, securing bleeders with electrocautery. Obtain hemostasis and cover the recipient site with a moist laparotomy pad as previously mentioned.

Split-thickness Skin Graft—Principles (Fig. 126.3)

Technical and Anatomic Points

Split-thickness skin grafts are used to close defects that are too large to close primarily (or by local flaps) and for coverage of burn wounds after excision. The ability to cut a uniform graft of the desired thickness is a crucial skill.

In general, if the graft is cut thin, the donor site regenerates more rapidly. These very thin grafts are used primarily when a donor site must be harvested repeatedly; for example, during treatment of patients with large body surface area burns. Because the graft contains relatively little dermal collagen, the resulting coverage is more fragile and may not be cosmetically as appealing as that obtained from a thicker graft.

If the graft is cut more thickly, it will include more dermal collagen and be more durable and possibly cosmetically more appealing. The trade-off is that the donor site will take longer to regenerate and may scar.

Harvesting the Skin Graft (Fig. 126.4)

Technical and Anatomic Points

Become familiar with the dermatome that you are going to use. Most dermatomes are either electrically or pneumatically driven. They allow the user to set the width of the graft to be harvested, and to control the thickness of the graft. Make sure that the blade is set correctly and that the dermatome is set

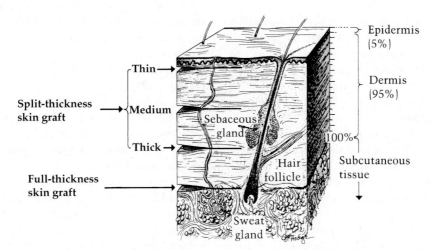

Figure 126.3 Depths of split-thickness skin grafts (from Thorne CH, ed. *Grabb and Smith's Plastic Surgery,* 6th ed. Philadelphia, PA: Lippincott Wolters Kluwer; 2007, with permission).

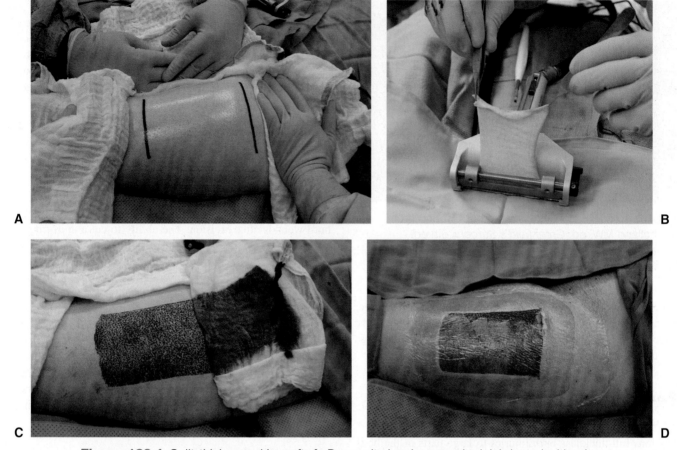

Figure 126.4 Split-thickness skin graft. **A:** Donor site has been marked, lubricated with mineral oil, and is being stabilized by assistant. **B:** Graft should be translucent and uniform in color. **C:** The donor site should show uniform petechial bleeding. **D:** Dress the donor site with a plastic occlusive dressing to minimize pain. (Figures courtesy of Wei F Chen MD, University of Iowa Carver College of Medicine.)

for the width and thickness of the graft that you plan to cut. The length of the graft is controlled by the surgeon and by the geometry of the donor site.

If a small graft is needed in an elective case, choose a donor site that will be hidden under clothes. A large flat surface is ideal, thus the anterior or lateral thigh is often used; but be mindful that this site is visible when the patient wears shorts. When large amounts of skin must be harvested for burn wound coverage, all available donor sites may be utilized and even reused after skin has regrown.

Have an assistant apply pressure (or, sometimes, elevate the donor site with towel clips) to produce as flat a surface as possible (Fig. 126.4A). Position yourself so that you have an easy pass with the dermatome, pushing it forward away from you. Lower the operating table, if necessary, to have comfortable access.

Many surgeons lubricate the donor skin with sterile mineral oil or saline, to enable the dermatome to slide easily.

Position the dermatome at the nearest point of the donor site and turn it on. Gently but firmly push forward. A common mistake is to push the dermatome down into the skin too hard,

so that it digs into the tissue. This should not be necessary. As you push the dermatome slowly forward, you should see a ribbon of skin, uniform in color (indicating uniform thickness) coming out of the slot (Fig. 126.4B). You may have an assistant pull this ribbon back to avoid jamming in the slot, but generally this is not necessary.

The donor bed should be white and shiny and show petechial bleeding (Fig. 126.4C). If fat is exposed, the graft is generally too thick. If it does not bleed, the graft is very thin.

When you have harvested the length of graft that you need, terminate the cut by aiming the dermatome sharply up at the ceiling so that it cuts through the graft, or stop the dermatome and amputate the graft.

Place a moist laparotomy pad over the donor site.

Carefully put the skin on an opened moist sponge. Be careful to maintain the orientation of the graft! If the graft is applied wrong side down, it will die. If you are not certain which side is the living side of the graft (i.e., the freshly cut side, which is the side that goes onto the recipient bed), look carefully at the skin and observe the following clues: The live side is moist and wet, the dead side has a finely reticulated pattern and is dull.

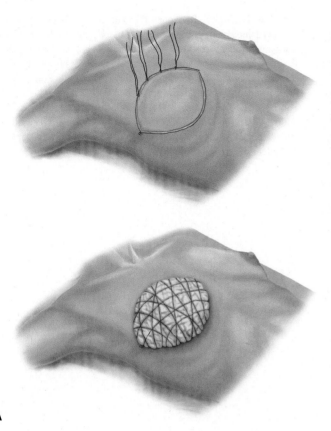

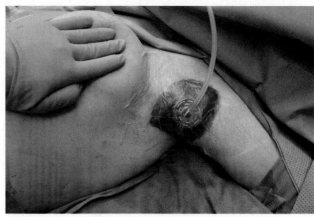

Figure 126.5 Methods of securing the skin graft. **A:** Skin graft secured to small recipient site (after radical mastectomy) with a tie-over bolster. Note that the graft is sutured to the intact skin at the edges of the defect and the tails are left long. The tails are then tied over the bolster in a crisscross fashion (from Bland KI, Klimberg VS, eds. *Master Techniques in General Surgery: Breast Surgery,* Philadelphia, PA: Lippincott Williams & Wilkins; 2010, with permission). **B:** Commercial vacuum dressing applied to axillary site after excision and grafting for hidradenitis (Figure courtesy of Wei F chem MD, University of Iowa Carver College of Medicine).

The live side is usually shiny white, and the dead side shows the natural skin color. The graft, if thick enough, will tend to curl up with the live side inside and the dead side outside. It is best to avoid this problem altogether by always placing the graft on a gauze in a particular orientation (e.g., live side down).

Dress the donor site with Tegaderm after obtaining hemostasis (Fig. 126.4D).

Securing the Graft on the Recipient Site (Fig. 126.5)

During the initial phase of healing, the graft is completely supported by diffusion of oxygen and nutrients from the recipient bed tissue below. It is therefore crucial that blood or serum not be allowed to accumulate under the graft. It is common practice to perforate the graft in several places and place some kind of pressure dressing to ensure that it is immobilized and protected.

Trim the graft to size and secure it to the recipient site with Steri-strips, sutures, or staples. A common way to do this is to allow the graft to overlap the recipient defect slightly and trim the overlap after placing some anchoring sutures.

Small grafts (e.g., at the site of excision of skin lesions) may be secured with tie-over dressings (called bolsters) as shown in this figure. To secure a tie-down bolster, place sutures around the periphery of the graft (through the graft into the intact skin at the edge of the defect), tie these but leave the tails long. Create a bolster from sterile foam covered with sterile Vaseline gauze, or from cotton balls over a nonadherent dressing such as Vaseline gauze. The cotton balls may be dipped in sterile mineral oil and squeezed out before placing them on the Vaseline gauze. This allows them to conform, but the mineral oil does not readily support bacterial growth. Tie the long tails across the bolster in a crisscross fashion, securing it in place (Fig. 126.5A).

Grafts on the extremities may be secured with elastic dressings. Some surgeons prefer to use a commercial vacuum dressing, particularly on an irregularly contoured surface (Fig. 126.5B).

After the graft adheres, capillaries will begin to grow into the graft and provide permanent adhesion and blood supply. This takes several days. The graft will still be vulnerable to mechanical trauma or infection until it is fully healed and vascularized. This usually takes at least a week.

REFERENCES

1. Boyce ST, Kagan RJ, Greenhalgh DG, et al. Cultured skin substitutes reduce requirements for harvesting of skin autograft for closure of excised, full-thickness burns. *J Trauma.* 2006;60: 821–829.
2. Branski LK, Herndon DN, Pereira C, et al. Longitudinal assessment of Integra in primary burn management: A randomized pediatric clinical trial. *Crit Care Med.* 2007;35:2615–2623.

3. Harte D, Gordon J, Shaw M, et al. The use of pressure and silicone in hypertrophic scar management in burns patients: A pilot randomized controlled trial. *J Burn Care Res.* 2009;30: 632–642.

4. Llanos S, Danilla S, Barraza C, et al. Effectiveness of negative pressure closure in the integration of split thickness skin grafts: A randomized, double-masked, controlled trial. *Ann Surg.* 2006;244:700–705.

5. Orgill DP. Excision and skin grafting of thermal burns. *N Engl J Med.* 2009;360:893–901.

6. Papp AA, Usaro AV, Ruokonen ET. The effect of topical epinephrine on haemodynamics and markers of tissue perfusion in burned and non-burned patients requiring skin grafting. *Burns.* 2009;35:832–839.

7. Taylor GI. The blood supply of the skin. In: Thorne CH, ed-in-chief. *Grabb and Smith's Plastic Surgery.* 6th ed. Philadelphia, PA: Lippincott Wolters Kluwer; 2007:33–41, Chapter 4.

8. Thorne CH. Techniques and principles in plastic surgery. In: Thorne CH, ed-in-chief. *Grabb and Smith's Plastic Surgery.* 6th ed. Philadelphia, PA: Lippincott Wolters Kluwer; 2007:3–14, Chapter 4. (Excellent discussion of flaps as well.)

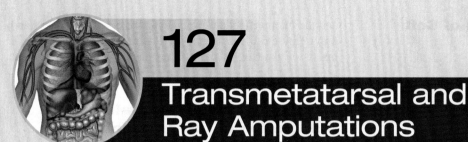

127

Transmetatarsal and Ray Amputations

Transmetatarsal and ray amputations require meticulous patient selection and attention to surgical technique when performed in patients with peripheral vascular disease. Transmetatarsal amputation is performed for gangrene, trauma, or rarely, tumors limited to the distal part of the foot. Part or all of the foot may be resected at the midmetatarsal level. In this chapter, the standard full transmetatarsal amputation is described, followed by a discussion of both partial transmetatarsal and ray amputations.

SCORE™, the Surgical Council on Resident Education, classified toe amputations as "ESSENTIAL UNCOMMON" procedures.

STEPS IN PROCEDURE

Transmetatarsal Amputation

Incision at level of metatarsal heads; longer posterior flap

Divide soft tissues to level of bone

Secure digital arteries with suture ligatures or ties

Periosteal elevator to clear soft tissues from the bone to point of division

Divide metatarsals just beyond the heads

Smooth the bone ends

Divide plantar fascia and remaining soft tissues

Meticulous hemostasis and closure

Ray Amputation

Tennis racquet–shaped incision around base of affected toe

Clear soft tissues from bone

Take care to spare digital artery to next digit

Divide metatarsal in midshaft

Smooth the bone ends

Meticulous hemostasis and closure

HALLMARK ANATOMIC COMPLICATIONS

Ischemia from choice of incorrect level of amputation

Injury to digital artery to adjacent digit causing digital ischemia

LIST OF STRUCTURES

Metatarsal bones

Phalanges

Tarsal Bones

Cuboid

Superficial fascia

Deep fascia of the foot

Plantar aponeurosis

Dorsal Venous Arch

Great saphenous vein

Lesser saphenous vein

Superficial peroneal nerve

Deep peroneal nerve

Sural nerve

Anterior Tibial Artery

Dorsalis pedis artery

First dorsal metatarsal artery

Arcuate artery

Lateral plantar artery

Plantar arterial arch

Dorsal Arterial Arch

Digital arteries

Extensor hallucis longus muscle

Extensor hallucis brevis muscle

Inferior extensor retinaculum

Extensor digitorum longus muscle

Extensor digitorum brevis muscle

Peroneus tertius muscle

Interosseous muscles (dorsal and plantar)

Adductor hallucis muscle

Skin Incision and Division of Soft Tissues (Fig. 127.1)

Technical Points

Plan a gently curved skin incision that is longer on the plantar surface than on the dorsal surface of the foot. The skin of the plantar surface is stronger and can be pulled up to form a good flap over the tips of the metatarsals. Make the skin incision at about the level of the metatarsal heads (Fig. 127.1A). Divide the soft tissues down to the level of the bone. Secure the digital arteries with suture ligatures (Fig. 127.1B).

Anatomic Points

Division of the skin and superficial fascia of the dorsum of the foot will expose the superficial veins and nerves that occupy the plane between superficial and deep fasciae. The anatomy of the superficial venous network varies; however, recall that the great and lesser (small) saphenous veins begin as continuations of the medial and lateral ends of the dorsal venous arch, respectively. The dorsal venous arch is located roughly over the middle of the second through the fifth metatarsals. The great saphenous vein begins over the proximal end of the first metatarsal, and the lesser saphenous vein begins over the cuboid. The branches of two sensory nerves—the superficial peroneal and sural nerves—lie relatively superficial and may be encountered. The superficial peroneal nerve supplies most of the skin of the dorsum of the foot and toes, except for the first interdigital space and apposing sides of digits 1 and 2 (supplied by a branch of the deep peroneal nerve). The sural nerve provides cutaneous innervation to the lateral side of the foot. The nerves are crossed superficially by the superficial veins.

When the deep fascia of the dorsum of the foot is divided, the dorsalis pedis artery, a continuation of the anterior tibial artery, should be identified and ligated (if necessary) before its division. This artery, accompanied by the deep peroneal nerve, lies lateral to the extensor hallucis longus tendon, passes deep to the inferior extensor retinaculum, and is crossed by the extensor hallucis brevis (Fig. 127.1C). At the proximal end of the first intermetatarsal space, it turns plantarward, between the interosseous muscles of this space, to anastomose with the deep branch of the lateral plantar artery, forming the plantar arterial arch. Branches of the dorsalis pedis artery that must be considered in amputations include the first dorsal metatarsal artery. This artery bifurcates, in the cleft between the first two digits at the level of the metatarsophalangeal joint, into two dorsal digital arteries, which supply the contiguous sides of these two digits. The arcuate artery, a lateral branch of the dorsalis pedis artery that lies deep to the intrinsic extensor musculature and that gives rise to the remaining three dorsal metatarsal arteries, crosses the bases of all metatarsals except the first.

In addition to neurovascular structures on the dorsum of the foot, several extensor muscles or tendons have to be divided to provide unobstructed access to the periosteum. These include the tendons of the extensor hallucis longus and brevis muscles

and the multiple tendons of the extensor digitorum longus and brevis muscles. The tendon of the peroneus tertius muscle inserts on the base of the fifth metatarsal and is at that point proximal to the line of resection.

Division of the Metatarsals and Completion of the Amputation (Fig. 127.2)

Technical Points

Use a periosteal elevator to elevate periosteum and soft tissues from the metatarsals at the point of division (Fig. 127.2A). Divide the metatarsals cleanly just behind their heads, using a pneumatic bone saw or bone cutters. A pneumatic saw is preferable because it cuts cleanly without splintering. If you use bone cutters, be careful to smooth the metatarsal shafts after division and remove any splinters of bone. A rongeur is convenient for this.

Be careful not to strip back past the level of amputation because this would separate soft tissue from bone and create dead space.

The amputation may then be rapidly completed by transecting the plantar tendons and remaining soft tissues posteriorly. Divide the tendons flush with the surrounding soft tissues (Fig. 127.2B).

Irrigate the stump and secure meticulous hemostasis.

Anatomic Points

Elevation of the periosteum of the metatarsals will detach the origins and insertions of the muscles that attach to the shafts of these bones. This includes the four dorsal interossei muscles, which lie in the dorsal aspect of each intermetatarsal space, as well as the three plantar interossei muscles that lie just deep to the former muscles (there is no plantar interosseous muscle in the first intermetatarsal space).

Subsequent division (from dorsal to plantar) of the soft tissues of the plantar aspect of the foot will first divide the dorsal and plantar interosseous muscles, the intrinsic plantar muscles of the little toe (the flexor digiti minimi brevis and abductor digiti minimi), and two of the three intrinsic plantar muscles of the great toe (the flexor hallucis brevis and adductor hallucis). Division of these muscles exposes the fascial plane in which lie the plantar metatarsal arteries that arise from the plantar arterial arch (from the most lateral intermetatarsal space to the most medial metatarsal space) and the medial plantar artery. Because of the proximal location of the plantar arch, the metatarsal arteries and the medial plantar artery will be divided; these are large enough to require ligation. The digital nerves (branches of the medial and lateral plantar nerves) that accompany these arteries will also be divided.

After division of the neurovascular structures, the soft tissues of the oblique head of the adductor hallucis and tendons of the flexor digitorum longus and hallucis longus (including the attached lumbrical muscles) are next divided. This exposes the fascial plane that contains branches of the medial plantar

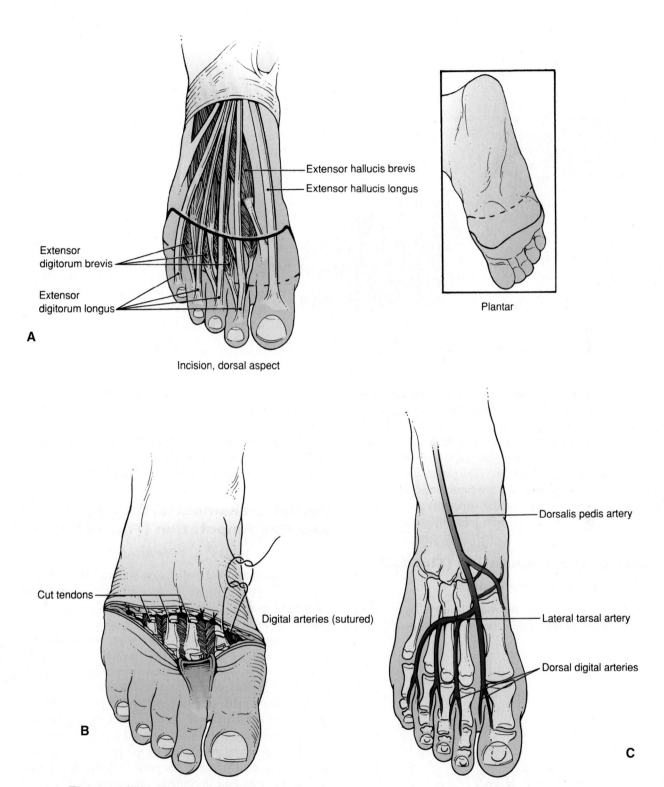

Figure 127.1 Transmetatarsal amputation. **A:** Skin incision. **B:** Division of soft tissues. **C:** Branches of dorsalis pedis artery.

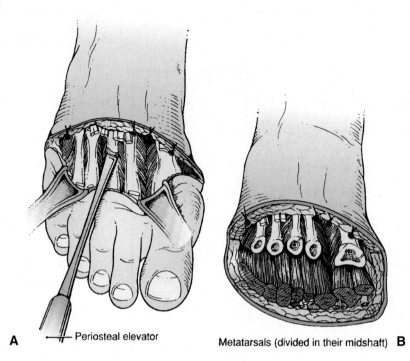

A —/— Periosteal elevator

Metatarsals (divided in their midshaft) **B**

Figure 127.2 Division of the metatarsals and completion of the amputation. **A:** Stripping the periosteum. **B:** Completed amputation (with anterior flap pulled back to show metatarsals clearly).

and lateral plantar nerves, which are also divided. These are primarily sensory branches. Division of these nerves and the accompanying connective tissue exposes the flexor digitorum brevis, the last muscle that must be divided. When this muscle is divided, the deep surface of the plantar aponeurosis, an expression of deep fascia, is exposed. The plantar aponeurosis, superficial fascia, and plantar skin are firmly attached to each other, and because no major vascular structures are present in these layers, they can be divided with impunity.

Closure of the Amputation (Fig. 127.3)

Technical and Anatomic Points

Close the soft tissues over the metatarsal heads in layers, using interrupted Vicryl sutures. Tailor the flap so that there are no

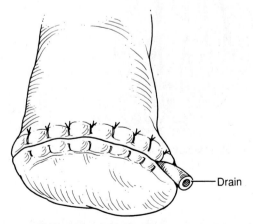

Tailored flap (completed)

Figure 127.3 Closure of the amputation. Drain is optional.

"dog ears" and so that it can be brought together without tension. If the flaps come together under tension, resect additional metatarsal bone to allow comfortable closure.

Approximate the skin carefully. Handle the skin edges with care to avoid traumatizing tissues that are probably ischemic. A drain may be placed under the flap, if desired.

Partial Transmetatarsal Amputation and Ray Amputation (Fig. 127.4)

Technical Points

Partial transmetatarsal amputation is occasionally performed when one or two digits are involved and the rest of the foot is thought to be salvageable. It can be done as an open or closed procedure, but is more commonly done open.

The skin incision in this case passes down between the toes along a line between the two metatarsal shafts and then crosses over the head of the metatarsals. Again, the posterior flap should be made longer than the anterior one.

It is important to spare the digital artery going to the adjacent toe that is to remain. If this artery is ligated or traumatized, the ischemia may progress to involve this digit as well.

Clean the metatarsal heads of the periosteum and divide the bones in their midshaft, as previously described. Closure is similar to that done in complete transmetatarsal amputation.

Alternatively, the flap may be left open to granulate. It may then be closed secondarily, or covered by split-thickness skin grafts. This approach is slow and requires meticulous wound care during the postoperative period; however, it may result in salvage of part of the foot when infection is present, particularly if arterial inflow can be improved after the infection clears.

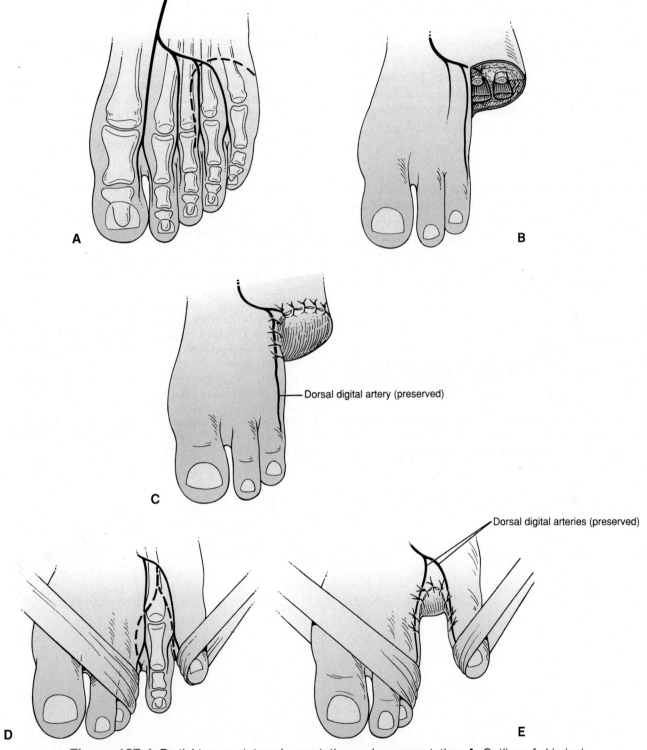

Figure 127.4 Partial transmetatarsal amputation and ray amputation. **A:** Outline of skin incision for partial transmetatarsal amputation. **B:** Preservation of dorsal digital artery as amputation proceeds. **C:** Completed amputation stressing preservation of dorsal digital artery. **D:** Ray amputation—skin incision (*dotted lines*). **E:** Completed ray amputation showing preservation of dorsal digital arteries.

Ray amputation is performed when only one digit needs to be removed. Outline a tennis racquet–shaped incision around the base of the affected toe. Divide the soft tissues as described earlier, being careful to spare the digital vessels to the neighboring toes. Divide the metatarsal in its midshaft portion. In this case, it is safest to use bone cutters, which can be placed precisely around the bone in a relatively small working space. Smooth the end of the metatarsal with a rongeur. Close the small incision in layers.

Anatomic Points

Remember that there are both dorsal and plantar digital arteries and that of the two, the plantar arteries are larger. Dorsal and plantar digital arteries are branches of dorsal and plantar metatarsal arteries, respectively. Digital arteries actually arise quite distally in the interdigital space, so that it is necessary to preserve the metatarsal artery in its entirety, with ligation and division of only the digital arteries supplying the digits to be removed.

REFERENCES

1. Chang BB, Jacobs RL, Darling RC III, et al. Foot amputations. *Surg Clin North Am.* 1995;75:773–782. (Discusses alternatives, emphasizing management of patients with peripheral vascular disease.)
2. Clark N, Sherman R. Soft-tissue reconstruction of the foot and ankle. *Orthop Clin North Am.* 1993;24:489–503. (Presents thorough discussion of management options for trauma.)
3. DeCotiis MA. Lisfranc and Chopart amputations. *Clin Podiatr Med Surg.* 2005;22:385–393. (Presents alternatives to standard levels of amputation.)
4. Early JS. Transmetatarsal and midfoot amputations. *Clin Orthop Relat Res.* 1999;361:85–90. (Discusses patient selection, technique, alternative approaches.)
5. Faglia E, Clerici G, Caminiti M, et al. Feasibility and effectiveness of internal pedal amputation of phalanx or metatarsal head in diabetic patients with forefoot osteomyelitis. *J Foot Ankle Surg.* 2012;51:593.
6. Ger R, Angus G, Scott P. Transmetatarsal amputation of the toe: An analytic study of ischemic complications. *Clin Anat.* 1999;12:407–411.
7. Kono Y, Muder RR. Identifying the incidence of and risk factors for reamputation among patients who underwent foot amputation. *Ann Vasc Surg.* 2012;26:1120.
8. Little JM. Transmetatarsal amputation. In: Malt RA, ed. *Surgical Techniques Illustrated: A Comparative Atlas.* Philadelphia, PA: WB Saunders; 1985:578.
9. Stone PA, Back MR, Armstrong PA, et al. Midfoot amputations expand limb salvage rates for diabetic foot infections. *Ann Vasc Surg.* 2005;19:805–811.
10. Wagner FW. The Syme amputation. In: American Academy of Orthopaedic Surgeons. *Atlas of Limb Prosthetics: Surgical and Prosthetic Principles.* St. Louis: CV Mosby; 1981:326. (Provides a clear description of an alternative to below-knee amputation in selected patients.)
11. Wheelock FC. Amputation of individual toes. In: Malt RA, ed. *Surgical Techniques Illustrated: A Comparative Atlas.* Philadelphia, PA: WB Saunders; 1985:582.
12. Wheelock FC. Transmetatarsal amputation. In: Malt RA, ed. *Surgical Techniques Illustrated: A Comparative Atlas.* Philadelphia, PA: WB Saunders; 1985:572.

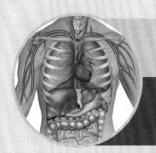

128

Below-Knee Amputation

Most amputations are performed for ischemia. The choice of the level of amputation requires mature judgment. Although it is important to salvage as much length as possible, a poor initial choice of level may doom the patient to a second amputation, often at a significantly higher level. References at the end discuss factors to consider in selecting an amputation site as well as the utility of several commonly performed tests.

When below-knee amputation is performed for ischemia, the stump should be made long enough to allow fitting of a prosthesis, but not so long that viability is sacrificed. Below-knee amputation that is performed for trauma, in the presence of normal arteries, may be performed at a lower level.

In this chapter, the standard procedure for below-knee amputation, as performed for ischemia, is described. References at the end of the chapter detail alternative techniques, including amputation for trauma or tumor.

SCORE™, the Surgical Council on Resident Education, classified below-knee amputation as an "ESSENTIAL UNCOMMON" procedure.

STEPS IN PROCEDURE

Skin incision should provide longer posterior flap than anterior flap
Incise anteriorly and laterally, but not posteriorly at this stage, to limit blood loss
Preserve as much length as possible
Ligate and divide greater saphenous vein
Divide all soft tissues to tibia anteriorly and through fascia of muscles laterally
Strip periosteum from tibia circumferentially
Divide tibia 1 to 2 cm above level of skin incision
Divide fibula several centimeters higher than tibia

Smooth ends of bone
Suture-ligate and divide posterior tibial artery and vein
Divide common peroneal nerve cleanly and allow to retract
Develop posterior flap
Complete posterior skin incision
Ligate and divide lesser saphenous vein
Obtain hemostasis and tailor skin flaps
Close in layers

HALLMARK ANATOMIC COMPLICATIONS

Ischemia of stump
Neuroma formation

LIST OF STRUCTURES

Tibia
Tibial tuberosity
Fibula
Greater saphenous vein
Lesser saphenous vein
Saphenous nerve
Common peroneal nerve
Superficial fascia
Deep fascia
Interosseous membrane
Gastrocnemius muscle
Soleus muscle

Tibialis anterior muscle
Extensor digitorum longus muscle
Extensor hallucis longus muscle
Peroneus longus muscle
Tibialis posterior muscle
Tendon of plantaris muscle

Popliteal Artery and Vein
Anterior tibial artery and vein
Posterior tibial artery and vein
Peroneal artery and vein

Skin Incision and Development of Flaps (Fig. 128.1)

Technical Points

Plan a skin incision with a long posterior flap. The length of the posterior flap should approximate the transverse diameter of the leg. As extra length of flap can always be trimmed; it is advisable to make the flap too long at the initial incision. Divide the minimal soft tissues anterior to the tibia. Plan to divide the tibia about four fingerbreadths below the tibial tuberosity. If the amputation is being performed for trauma, a longer stump may be tailored. Generally, when amputation is done for ischemia, a shorter stump is desirable.

Identify and ligate the greater saphenous vein in the medial aspect of the anterior incision. Divide all soft tissues down to the tibia anteriorly and through the fascia of the muscles laterally.

To limit blood loss, do not create the posterior skin incision at this point.

Anatomic Points

The division of the tibia about four fingerbreadths inferior to the tibial tuberosity corresponds to approximately the level of the greatest circumference of the leg. At this location, the greater saphenous vein and accompanying saphenous nerve are located in the superficial fascia just posterior to the medial border of the tibia—that is, in the fascia overlying the tibial origin of the soleus muscle. No important structures lie in the superficial fascia anterior to the greater saphenous vein. The anteromedial surface of the tibia lies just deep to the superficial fascia. Hence, the anterior border of the tibia is a useful landmark, and no muscles must be divided to expose it.

Lateral to the anterior border of the tibia, the deep fascia covering the muscles of the anterior compartment of the leg must be divided. At the usual level of amputation, the muscle most closely associated with the tibia is the tibialis anterior; posterior to this is the belly of the extensor digitorum longus muscle. The belly of the extensor hallucis longus may be encountered between the extensor digitorum longus and the tibialis anterior if a low below-knee amputation is performed.

When the fascia is divided still more posterolaterally, the anterior intermuscular septum will be encountered; this forms the anterior wall of the lateral compartment. Division of the deep fascia of the lateral compartment exposes the belly of the peroneus longus muscle. Continued circumferential division of the deep fascia should allow visualization of the posterior intermuscular septum, which separates the lateral compartment muscles from the posterior compartment muscles.

Division of the Tibia and Fibula (Fig. 128.2)

Technical Points

Strip the periosteum from the tibia circumferentially with a periosteal elevator. Divide the tibia with a pneumatic bone saw 1 to 2 cm above the level of the skin incision. If a pneumatic

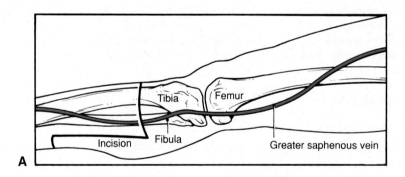

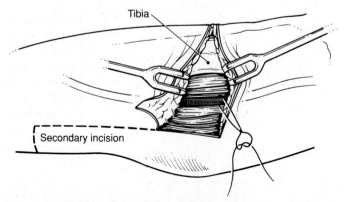

Figure 128.1 Skin incision and development of flaps

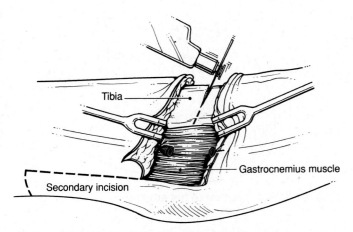

Figure 128.2 Division of the tibia and fibula

saw is not available, a Gigli wire saw works well. Angle the cut on the tibia upward as you progress anteriorly so that the anterior edge of the tibia does not form a sharp projection that could traumatize the stump.

Divide the fibula several centimeters higher than the tibia. It is often convenient to do this with bone cutters, so that the bone can be divided high up within the soft tissues of the stump. Carefully smooth the end of the fibula with a rongeur and remove any spicules of bone that are left in the wound after the fibula has been divided.

Anatomic Points

Elevation of the tibial periosteum does not require division of any muscles because the periosteum can be entered on the anteromedial surface of the tibia. Exposure of the fibula; however, demands division or detachment of the origins of the extensor digitorum longus muscle in the anterior compartment, the peroneus longus muscle in the lateral compartment, and the soleus and tibialis posterior muscles in the posterior compartment. As you expose the fibula, be careful to avoid inadvertent injury to the vessels in the region. Anterior to the interosseus membrane, in close proximity to the fibula, are the anterior tibial vessels. The posterior tibial vessels, as well as the peroneal vessels, lie in the plane between the superficial and deep posterior compartments—that is, deep to the soleus and superficial to the tibialis posterior muscles. The peroneal vessels are in close proximity to the fibula.

Completion of the Amputation (Fig. 128.3)

Technical Points

Behind the tibia, identify the posterior tibial artery and vein and suture-ligate them. Identify the common peroneal nerve, ligate it, and transect it cleanly under traction, allowing it to retract into the depths of the stump.

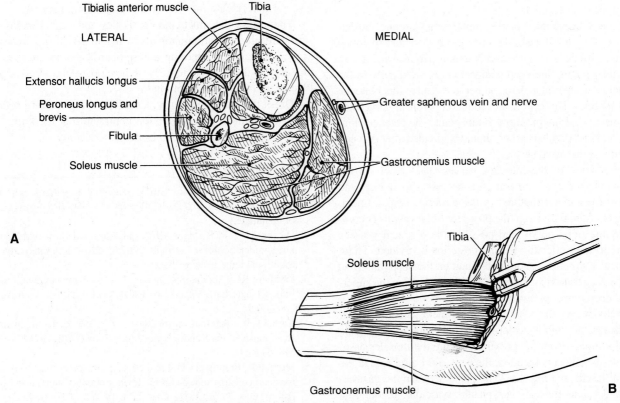

Figure 128.3 Completion of the amputation

Within the deep flexor muscle compartment, identify and suture-ligate the deep vessels. The level of amputation and the variable level of trifurcation of the popliteal artery into anterior tibial, posterior tibial, and peroneal branches influence the number and exact location of these neurovascular bundles. The tibial nerve accompanies the posterior tibial vessels and must be ligated and divided under tension.

Develop the posterior flap to include the soleus muscle. Enter the plane between the gastrocnemius and soleus muscles by dividing the posterior crural septum laterally. The plane between the gastrocnemius and soleus muscles is generally avascular and can rapidly be developed by blunt dissection. Laterally and medially, it is necessary to incise the fascial attachments that anchor the two muscles together.

Complete the posterior skin incision. Identify and ligate the lesser saphenous vein. Transect the soleus muscle and remaining soft tissues at the level of the skin incision to complete the amputation.

Anatomic Points

The anterior tibial vessels pass into the anterior compartment through a gap in the interosseus membrane just inferior to the proximal tibiofibular joint. To expose these vessels, and as a necessary part of the amputation, the tibialis anterior, extensor digitorum longus, and extensor hallucis longus should be divided. The nerve that accompanies these vessels in the anterior compartment is the deep peroneal nerve, a branch of the common peroneal nerve. It is not necessary to divide the deep peroneal nerve at this level because the common peroneal nerve will be divided next.

The common peroneal nerve, which wraps around the lateral aspect of the fibula just inferior to its head, should be found deep to the peroneus longus. The common peroneal nerve can be located by tracing the deep peroneal nerve proximally to the point where the superficial peroneal nerve is seen to innervate the peroneal muscles. Division of the common peroneal nerve then involves nerve division proximal to this point. The peroneus longus muscle, if not divided earlier, should be divided after division of the common peroneal nerve.

After division of the muscles, nerves, and vessels in the anterior and lateral compartments, it is necessary to identify and divide neurovascular structures in the posterior compartment. At the level of tibial division, the posterior tibial vessels accompanied by the tibial nerve, and possibly the peroneal vessels, should be located after the tibialis posterior is divided. These neurovascular structures should be found on the deep (anterior) side of the deep transverse fascia, a septum separating the superficial and deep posterior compartments.

After division of the posterior compartment's neurovascular structures and the tibialis posterior, all that remains connecting the distal segment from the proximal leg are the muscles associated with the calcaneal tendon, the posterior crural fascia, the superficial fascia, and the skin. The plane between the gastrocnemius and soleus muscles is typically avascular. Frequently, the small saphenous vein, which ascends in the superficial fascia

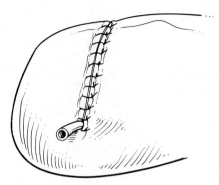

Figure 128.4 Closure of the stump

or a deep fascia compartment in the midline of the calf, passes between the two heads of the gastrocnemius muscle to enter the popliteal vein posterior to the knee joint. As the plane between the gastrocnemius and soleus muscles is developed, the tendon of the plantaris muscle can be observed passing from lateral to medial on the superficial surface of the soleus muscle.

Closure of the Stump (Fig. 128.4)

Technical and Anatomic Points

Irrigate the stump carefully and secure hemostasis. If bleeding from the marrow cavity of the tibia is a problem, use bone wax to close the cavity. Use only the minimal amount necessary because this acts as a foreign body and may potentiate infection. Pull the posterior flap up and suture it to the anterior flap. Tailor the flap in such a way that there are no "dog ears." Close the fascia securely with interrupted 2-0 Dexon sutures first.

Then close the subcutaneous tissues and skin. Handle the skin carefully and atraumatically. Particularly in the presence of ischemia, rough handling may jeopardize subsequent healing of the flaps. Meticulously approximate the skin edges. Placement of a drain is optional.

Dress the stump carefully. Consider using a well-padded, posterior splint to prevent flexion contracture at the knee. Do not use tape on the skin of an ischemic extremity.

REFERENCES

1. Allcock PA, Jain AS. Revisiting transtibial amputation with the long posterior flap. *Br J Surg.* 2001;88:683–686. (Reaffirms value of technique.)
2. Dwyer AJ, Paul R, Mam MK, et al. Modified skew-flap below-knee amputation. *Am J Orthop.* 2007;36:123–126. (Alternative to traditional long posterior flap.)
3. Frykberg RG, Abraham S, Tierney E, et al. Syme amputation for limb salvage: Early experience with 26 cases. *J Foot Ankle Surg.* 2007;46:93.
4. Kaufam JL. Alternative methods for below-knee amputation: Reappraisal of the Kendrick procedure. *J Am Coll Surg.* 1995;181: 511–516.
5. Morgan K, Brantigan CO, Field CJ, et al. Reverse sural artery flap for the reconstruction of chronic lower extremity wounds in high-risk patients. *J Foot Ankle Surg.* 2006;45:417–423. (Alternative to avoid amputation in highly selected patients.)

6. Rush DS, Huston CC, Bivins BA, et al. Operative and late mortality rates of above-knee and below-knee amputations. *Am Surg.* 1981;47:36.

7. Smith DG, Fergason JR. Transtibial amputations. *Clin Orthop Relat Res.* 1999;361:108–115. (Reviews alternative techniques and outcomes.)

8. Song EK, Moon ES, Rowe SM, et al. Below knee stump reconstruction by turn-up technique: Report of 2 cases. *Clin Orthop Relat Res.* 1994;307:229–234.

9. Wheelock FC, Little JM, Dale WA, et al. Below knee amputation. In: Malt RA, ed. *Surgical Techniques Illustrated: A Comparative Atlas.* Philadelphia, PA: WB Saunders; 1985:544.

10. Winburn GB, Wood MC, Hawkins ML, et al. Current role of cryo-amputation. *Am J Surg.* 1991;162:647–650. (Describes temporizing maneuver in infected cases.)

11. Yu GV, Schinke TL, Meszaros A. Syme's amputation: A retrospective review of 10 cases. *Clin Podiatr Med Surg.* 2005;22:395–427.

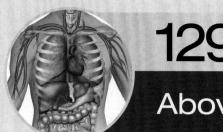

129

Above-Knee Amputation

Above-knee amputation is performed when it is not possible to save the knee joint because of the extent of injury or ischemic damage. Generally, the longer the stump, the better. The limiting factor is usually the condition of the skin and the soft tissues above the knee. If there is a question about the extent of gangrene or infection in the subcutaneous tissues in the skin, perform a guillotine amputation at the lowest possible level, leaving the stump open. When the infection is controlled, revise the amputation.

SCORE™, the Surgical Council on Resident Education, classified above knee amputation as an "ESSENTIAL UNCOMMON" procedure.

STEPS IN PROCEDURE

Symmetric fishmouth-type incision, preserving as much length as possible
Identify and ligate the greater saphenous vein
Divide muscles anteromedially to expose the femoral artery and vein
Suture-ligate and divide femoral artery and vein separately
Divide remaining muscles to expose femur

Use periosteal elevator to clean bone at site of division
Divide bone and smooth the ends
Ligate and divide profunda femoris artery and vein
Divide sciatic nerve and allow it to retract
Divide remaining muscles and soft tissues
Achieve meticulous hemostasis
Close in layers

HALLMARK ANATOMIC COMPLICATIONS

Recurrent ischemia
Neuroma

LIST OF STRUCTURES

Superficial fascia of the thigh
Fascia lata (deep fascia of the thigh)
Iliotibial tract
Lateral intermuscular septum
Anteromedial intermuscular septum
Posteromedial intermuscular septum
Femoral nerve
Obturator nerve
Sciatic nerve
Saphenous nerve

Femoral Vein
Greater saphenous vein (great saphenous vein)
Lesser saphenous vein (small saphenous vein)
Popliteal vein

Femoral Artery
Superficial femoral artery
Profunda femoris artery
Popliteal artery

Inferior Gluteal Artery
Ischiadic artery
Femur
Adductor (Hunter) canal
Adductor longus muscle
Adductor brevis muscle
Adductor magnus muscle
Gracilis muscle
Semimembranosus muscle
Semitendinosus muscle
Gluteus maximus muscle
Sartorius muscle
Tensor fascia lata muscle
Biceps femoris muscle

Quadriceps Femoris Muscle
Vastus lateralis muscle
Vastus medialis muscle
Vastus intermedius muscle
Rectus femoris muscle

Incision

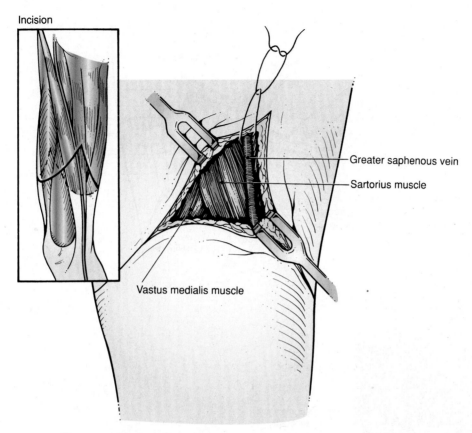

Greater saphenous vein

Sartorius muscle

Vastus medialis muscle

Figure 129.1 Position of the patient and development of flaps

Position of the Patient and Development of Flaps (Fig. 129.1)

Technical Points

Position the patient supine with the leg draped free and allow the leg to fall into external rotation to facilitate access to the greater saphenous vein and underlying structures. Plan symmetric fishmouth skin flaps anteriorly and posteriorly. The flaps should be of approximately the same size and length. Gently curve the fishmouth to avoid interfering with the blood supply to the tip of the flap.

Make a skin incision and deepen the incision down to the fascia overlying the muscle groups. Identify and ligate the greater saphenous vein in the medial portion of the anterior flap. Incise the fascia sharply.

Anatomic Points

The greater saphenous vein and a variable number of tributaries are the only structures of consequence in the superficial fascia of the thigh. The course of the greater saphenous vein can be approximated by a line running from a point 8 to 10 cm posterior to the medial side of the patella to a second point that is level with, and 4 cm lateral to, the pubic tubercle. Note that, in the thigh, the larger veins of this system are in a plane between two layers of superficial fascia. Frequently, a large communicating branch between the lesser and greater saphenous veins

ascends obliquely around the medial side of the thigh; other large tributaries join the greater saphenous vein on its anterolateral side. One fairly common variant of the greater saphenous system that would necessitate additional vein ligations is duplication of the greater saphenous vein in the more distal part of the thigh. When such duplication occurs, one of the vessels is typically deeper than the other, although both are still within the superficial fascia.

The deep fascia of the thigh, or fascia lata, is not of equal thickness throughout. It is thicker proximally and especially laterally, where it is reinforced by the iliotibial tract, which is actually the long, flat tendon of insertion (to the lateral condyle of the tibia) of the tensor fascia lata and most of the gluteus maximus. In addition, the fascia lata is thickened distally about the knee joint, where it is reinforced by fibrous expansions from the biceps femoris muscle laterally, the sartorius muscle medially, and the quadriceps femoris muscle anteriorly.

Division of the Anterior Muscles and Femoral Vessels (Fig. 129.2)

Technical Points

Divide the sartorius, rectus femoris, and vastus lateralis muscles sharply. The femoral artery and vein lie between the sartorius and vastus medialis muscles and are surrounded by soft

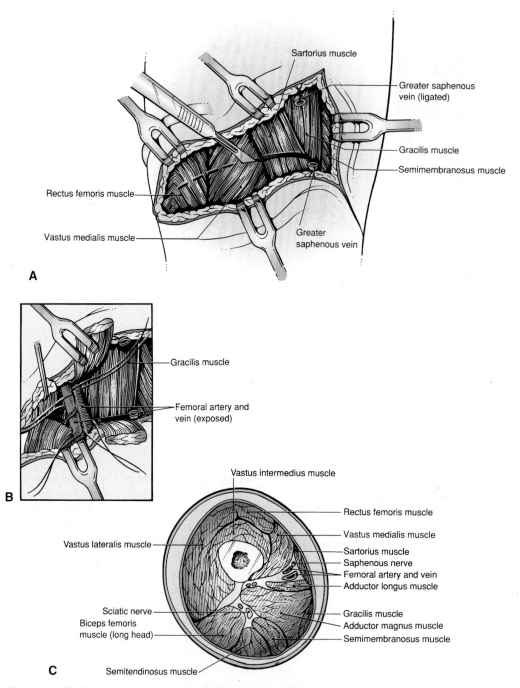

Figure 129.2 Division of the anterior muscles and femoral vessels. **A:** After securing the greater saphenous vein, divide the sartorius, rectus femoris, and vastus medialis muscles to expose the femoral artery and vein. **B:** Exposure of femoral artery and vein in preparation for ligation. **C:** Structures shown in cross-section.

tissue. They will be encountered in the medial aspect of the dissection after the muscles have been divided. It is safest to divide first all the muscles lying directly anterior to the femur, then to progress medially, working carefully to identify and protect from harm the femoral artery and vein. Suture-ligate and divide each vessel individually. Continue to divide the medial muscles, working posteriorly until the medial aspect of the femur is accessible.

Laterally, only the vastus lateralis and vastus intermedius muscles need to be divided to expose the femur. No major neurovascular structures should be encountered.

Anatomic Points

A conceptual scheme of the compartmentalization of the thigh is helpful to visualize throughout the procedure. At the levels where most above-knee amputations are made, there are three compartments in the thigh, each separated by intermuscular septa. The anterior compartment is bounded by the lateral intermuscular septum, lying between the vastus lateralis muscle and the short head of the biceps femoris muscle and attached to the fascia lata and linea aspera of the femur, and an anterior medial intermuscular septum, lying between the vastus medialis and adductor muscles and likewise attached to the fascia lata and linea aspera of the femur. Muscles in this compartment are all innervated by the femoral nerve and include both the sartorius and the quadriceps femoris. The *quadriceps femoris muscle* is the collective term for the vastus lateralis, vastus medialis, vastus intermedius, and rectus femoris muscles. The anterior boundary of the medial or adductor compartment is the anteromedial intermuscular septum. The posterior boundary is a posteromedial intermuscular septum, perhaps more theoretical than actual, which lies between the adductor magnus muscle and the hamstring muscles. Muscles in this compartment, innervated by the obturator nerve, include (at amputation levels) the adductor longus, adductor brevis, and adductor magnus muscles as well as the gracilis muscle. The posterior compartment is bounded by the lateral and posteromedial intermuscular septa. The muscles in this compartment include the semimembranosus, semitendinosus, and biceps femoris. These muscles are innervated by the sciatic nerve. A fourth compartment includes muscles (gluteus maximus and tensor fascia lata) innervated by the gluteal nerves; however, the neuromuscular structures of this compartment are seldom encountered in a typical amputation.

The sartorius muscle arises from the anterosuperior iliac spine and spirals inferomedially to insert on the medial aspect of the tibia. In the proximal third of the thigh, it forms the lateral boundary of the femoral triangle and is thus lateral to the femoral vessels and nerves. In the middle third of the thigh, it forms the roof of the adductor (subsartorial or Hunter) canal. This triangular intermuscular canal, whose other boundaries are the vastus medialis muscle laterally and the adductor longus and magnus muscles medially, contains the (superficial) femoral artery and vein, the saphenous nerve, and the nerve to the vastus medialis muscle.

The rectus femoris muscle, the most anterior division of the quadriceps femoris muscle, arises from the anteroinferior iliac spine and from a groove superior to the acetabulum. As its name implies, the muscle then passes straight down the thigh to insert, through the patellar ligament, on the tibial tuberosity. In the upper thigh, it is essentially deep to the sartorius. In the middle third of the thigh, it is primarily lateral to the sartorius, whereas in the distal third of the thigh, it is immediately lateral to the vastus medialis muscle.

Lateral to the rectus femoris muscle is the vastus lateralis muscle, which originates from the intertrochanteric line, greater trochanter, lateral tip of the gluteal tuberosity, and proximal half of the lateral lip of the linea aspera. The largest component of the quadriceps femoris muscle, the vastus lateralis, is superficial to the vastus intermedius muscle. Quite proximally, it is deep to the tensor fascia lata. Its fibers are directed inferomedially, inserting onto a strong aponeurosis and tendon that ultimately contributes to the patellar ligament.

The vastus medialis muscle, which originates primarily from the medial lip of the linea aspera, is covered in the middle third of the thigh by the sartorius muscle. In the distal third of the thigh, it lies between the sartorius and rectus femoris muscles. As with the vastus lateralis muscle, it is superficial to part of the vastus intermedius muscle. From its long origin, its fibers are directed inferolaterally to insert on the common aponeurosis and tendon that ultimately contributes to the patellar ligament. Remember that this muscle forms the lateral wall of the adductor canal.

The final anterior compartment muscle to be divided is the vastus intermedius. This deep, thin muscle has a fleshy origin from the proximal two-thirds of the anterior and lateral shaft of the femur. These muscular fibers run anteroinferiorly to attach to the deep part of the common quadriceps tendon.

Division of the muscles within the medial compartment necessitates identification and protection of the contents of the adductor canal. If the level of amputation is at or above the midthigh, this will include the nerve to the vastus medialis muscle, which lies lateral to the femoral artery.

Regardless of the level of amputation, two medial compartment muscles—the gracilis and adductor magnus—will be divided. The gracilis muscle, the most superficial of the medial compartment muscles, originates from the ischiopubic ramus and inserts on the medial aspect of the tibia posterior to the insertion of the sartorius muscle. The adductor magnus muscle also arises from the ischiopubic ramus and the ischial tuberosity. From this origin, it fans out to insert along the entire medial lip of the linea aspera, medial supracondylar line, and adductor tubercle. This extensive insertion is interrupted by five osseoaponeurotic openings. The most distal of these openings, located approximately at the junction of the middle and distal thirds of the thigh, is the adductor hiatus. The femoral artery and vein pass into the popliteal fossa through this hiatus, becoming the popliteal artery and vein. The more proximal four openings, which are much smaller, transmit the perforating branches of the profunda femoris artery, the last of which is the termination of this artery. The openings, the most distal of which is approximately at the midthigh level, are posterior to the adductor longus muscle.

In amputations involving the proximal third of the femur, the adductor longus muscle must also be divided. This muscle arises from the body of the pubis, and its fibers fan out to its insertion on the linea aspera. It lies anterior to the adductor brevis and adductor magnus muscles. The anterior branch of the obturator nerve, along with the corresponding branch of the obturator artery and, more inferiorly, the profunda femoris artery, lies in the plane between the adductor longus and the more posterior adductor muscles.

Division of the Femur and Completion of the Amputation (Fig. 129.3)

Technical Points

When a sufficient amount of muscle has been divided, circumferentially strip the periosteum from the femur with a

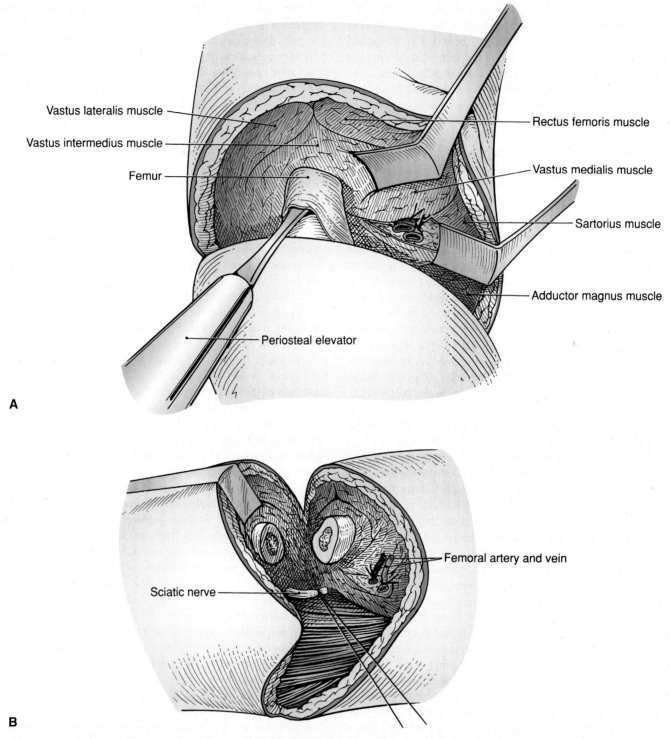

Figure 129.3 Division of the femur and completion of the amputation. **A:** After ligating the femoral artery and vein, elevate the periosteum from the proximal tibia. **B:** Divide the sciatic nerve.

periosteal elevator. Retract the muscles and soft tissues of the stump and divide the femur obliquely with a pneumatic or Gigli saw. Angle the cut so that the anterior surface is slightly shorter than the posterior surface. Use a rasp to smooth the cut surface of the bone. If the cavity of the marrow tends to ooze, apply bone wax to seal the cavity.

The profunda femoris artery and vein lie close on the bone and may be encountered as the bone is divided. Careful stripping of the periosteum should elevate these vessels, which can then be ligated.

The sciatic nerve lies medially and posteriorly, between the biceps femoris and semitendinosus muscles. Ligate and cleanly

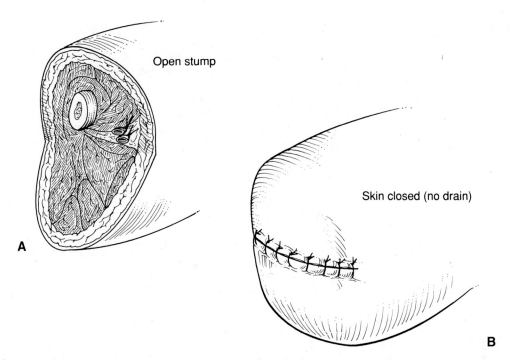

Figure 129.4 Closure of the stump. **A:** Tibia and ligated vessels prior to closure. **B:** Skin closed without a drain.

divide the sciatic nerve under tension, allowing it to retract. Cut the sciatic nerve and then clamp and tie it with a heavy nonabsorbable suture. Allow it to retract into the stump.

Divide the remaining muscles and soft tissues rapidly, achieving temporary hemostasis by applying pressure. Definitive hemostasis is more easily obtained after the amputation is completed.

Anatomic Points

After division of the femur, the structures in the posterior compartment of the thigh must be divided. If the femur is divided distal to the level of the adductor hiatus, the popliteal artery and vein will be encountered. Posterior to these, but with varying degrees of approximation to vascular structures (depending on the level of amputation), the sciatic nerve will be encountered. This nerve is posteromedial and can present as a medial tibial nerve and a lateral common peroneal nerve. In the more distal part of the thigh, the sciatic nerve is located in the connective tissue posterolateral to the biceps femoris muscle. More superiorly, the long head of the biceps femoris muscle (which arises from the ischial tuberosity) crosses posterior to the sciatic nerve to join the short head of the biceps femoris (which arises from most of the lateral lip of the linea aspera) to insert on the lateral femoral condyle and head of the fibula. It should be noted that the sciatic nerve is accompanied by the slender ischiadic artery, typically a branch of the inferior gluteal artery. This artery represents the proximal part of the original axial artery of the extremity and occasionally can be the primary vascular supply to the lower extremity.

Two other muscles, both of which lie in the posterior compartment, must be divided to complete the amputation.

These posteromedial muscles are closely related, spatially and functionally, to each other. Of the two, the semitendinosus muscle is most superficial. It arises from the ischial tuberosity by a tendon in common with the long head of the biceps femoris. It presents as a fleshy, fusiform muscle belly that ends about midthigh in a long, rounded tendon inserting on the medial tibial surface posterior to the insertions of the sartorius and gracilis muscles. The other muscle is the semimembranosus muscle, which arises by a flat tendon from the ischial tuberosity that rapidly develops into an aponeurosis. About midthigh, fleshy fibers arise to constitute the belly of the semimembranosus muscle. These fibers converge on a distal aponeurosis slightly proximal to the knee, and this aponeurosis changes to a complex tendon that basically inserts into the medial tibial condyle.

Closure of the Stump (Fig. 129.4)

Technical and Anatomic Points

Check hemostasis in the stump and irrigate it to remove fragments of bone and foreign material. Approximate the muscles over the bone and close the fascia with multiple interrupted 2-0 Vicryl sutures.

Trim the skin flaps so that they oppose each other without "dog ears" and without tension. If the flaps are under tension, revise the stump by shortening the femur. Close the skin with multiple interrupted fine sutures. Place a soft, bulky dressing on the stump.

REFERENCES

1. Berardi RS, Keonin Y. Amputations in peripheral vascular occlusive disease. *Am J Surg.* 1978;135:231.
2. Burgess EM. General principles of amputation surgery. In: American Academy of Orthopaedic Surgeons. *Atlas of Limb Prosthetics: Surgical and Prosthetic Principles.* St Louis: CV Mosby; 1981: 14.
3. Gottschalk F. Transfemoral amputation: Biomechanics and surgery. *Clin Orthop Relat Res.* 1999;361:15–22. (Presents excellent review.)
4. Medhat MA. Rehabilitation of the vascular amputee. *Orthop Rev.* 1983;12:51.
5. Morse BC, Cull DL, Kalbaugh C, et al. Through-knee amputation in patients with peripheral arterial disease: A review of 50 cases. *J Vasc Surg.* 2008;48:638. (An attractive alternative in selected patients.)
6. Shea JD. Surgical techniques of lower extremity amputation. *Orthop Clin North Am.* 1972;3:287.
7. Wheelock FC, Dale WA, Jamieson CW, et al. Above-knee amputation. In: Malt RA, ed. *Surgical Techniques Illustrated: A Comparative Atlas.* Philadelphia, PA: WB Saunders; 1985:528.

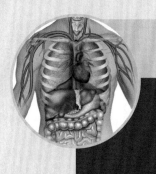

130

Ligation, Stripping, and Harvesting of the Saphenous Vein

Amir F. Sleiman and Jamal J. Hoballah

This chapter first covers excision of the greater and lesser saphenous veins for management of varicosities, and then harvesting for use as a vascular conduit.

Superficial venous insufficiency and varicose vein formation can develop in the trunk of the greater or lesser saphenous veins and their respective branches. The resulting varicose veins may be asymptomatic or cause a variety of symptoms, including heaviness in the leg, itching or burning sensation, and venous stasis ulcerations. Compression stockings are often used as the first line of therapy, but symptoms may persist. Difficulties with compliance, particularly during hot weather, and dissatisfaction with the cosmetic appearance of the legs cause many patients to seek other therapy. Surgical removal, described here, has stood the test of time as an effective management. The key principle remains to remove all varicose veins using the smallest skin incisions possible and to minimize complications. Endovascular ablation using radiofrequency or laser catheters have gained popularity as a less invasive treatment option. The procedure can be performed in the office under local tumescent anesthesia with mild sedation. Nevertheless, many patients may opt for the surgical removal especially when the saphenous vein is very dilated or very superficial.

The saphenous vein is usually stripped by inserting a stripper from one end of the vein toward the other. The stripper is usually passed from the distal end toward the groin to avoid catching on valve cusps. The distal end of the vein is then ligated around the stripper, divided, and then pulled out. The branch veins are usually excised using very small incisions through which the branch may be grasped and avulsed—the so-called "stab incision and vein avulsion or stab phlebectomy" technique. Traditionally, the greater saphenous vein was stripped from the ankle to the groin. However, this approach was found to be associated with saphenous nerve injury, resulting in loss of cutaneous sensation in the medial leg and ankle, because of proximity and adherence of the saphenous nerve to the greater saphenous vein in the lower leg. In addition, the posterior arch vein is usually the main pathway of incompetence in the leg rather than the saphenous vein. Consequently, it is recommended to strip the greater saphenous vein from just below the knee level to the groin. The lowest recurrence rates in the surgical options are obtained by combining stripping of the saphenous vein with excision of the associated branches.

Frequently, varicosities are limited to these branches, and the main trunks are relatively normal and of small caliber. Stripping the trunk in this situation may deprive the patient of a vein that could be a useful conduit in the future, should the need for lower extremity or coronary revascularization arise. Thus, some surgeons recommend avoiding stripping the saphenous veins when the varicosities are limited to the branches and the duplex ultrasound shows no evidence of significant reflux in the greater saphenous vein. In this situation, only stab avulsion of the varicosities is performed. This procedure may be complemented by ligation and division of the saphenofemoral junction if this is proved incompetent by duplex ultrasound evaluation.

SCORE™, the Surgical Council on Resident Education, classified operation for varicose veins as an "ESSENTIAL COMMON" procedure.

STEPS IN PROCEDURE

Stripping Greater Saphenous Vein

A 3- to 4-cm transverse incision in the inguinal crease centered 1 cm medial to the femoral pulse

If preoperative vein mapping was performed, center incision over vein

Skeletonize saphenofemoral junction

Ligate and divide all veins draining into it

Ligate and divide the greater saphenous vein 2 cm distal to saphenofemoral junction

Suture-ligate the saphenofemoral junction with 2-0 silk

Make 1-cm incision over marked greater saphenous vein few centimeters below the knee

Ligate distal end of vein

Introduce stripper, guide it to the groin, and allow it to exit the ligated end of the vein

Apply olive-shaped head to distal end of stripper and secure with tie

Pull the stripper to extract vein and stripper from groin incision

If you plan it to strip to ankle, make small incision 1 cm anterior and superior to medial malleolus

Identify and preserve the saphenous nerve

Pass stripper and remove vein as previously described

Irrigate wounds and close

Apply compressive dressing

Stab Avulsion of Branch Varicosities

Mark all branches with patient standing upright

A 2- to 3-mm stab incision along side of branch

Introduce crochet hook and hook up the vein

Clamp segment of vein and divide it

Avulse as much of each segment of vein as possible

Harvesting Greater Saphenous Vein for Reverse or Nonreverse Bypass Procedures

Small incisions over vein (preoperative vein marking helps)

Alternatively, harvest endoscopically

Carefully ligate all branches flush with vein

Gently flush with chilled whole blood, cold Ringer's lactate, or other solution

Avoid overdistension by monitoring pressure

HALLMARK ANATOMIC COMPLICATIONS

Injury to saphenous nerve

Injury to femoral vein

Recurrence of varicosities

LIST OF STRUCTURES

Femoral artery

Common femoral vein

Greater (great) saphenous vein; saphenofemoral junction

Lesser saphenous vein

Femoral Nerve

Saphenous nerve

Medial femoral cutaneous nerve

Posterior femoral cutaneous nerve

Sural nerve

Lateral cutaneous nerve

Musculocutaneous nerve

Patella

Lateral malleolus

Medial malleolus

Inguinal crease

Pubic tubercle

Fascia Lata

Saphenous hiatus (fossa ovalis)

Adductor canal

Sartorius muscle

Gastrocnemius muscle

Stripping the Greater Saphenous Vein: Exposure of the Saphenofemoral Junction (Fig. 130.1)

Technical Points

A 3- to 4-cm transverse incision in the inguinal crease has an excellent cosmetic result. Preoperative duplex ultrasonography allows precise mapping of the veins, including the saphenofemoral junction. It can be especially helpful in determining the location of the greater saphenous vein just below the knee when the leg is large or the patient is overweight. If preoperative mapping was performed, center the skin incision over the saphenofemoral junction. Alternatively, use anatomic landmarks and begin the inguinal crease incision 1 cm medial to the femoral pulse and extend it medially for 3 to 4 cm (Fig. 130.1A). If the femoral pulse is not palpable, identify a point midway between the pubic tubercle and the anterosuperior iliac spine and begin the skin incision 1 cm medial to this point. Deepen the incision through the subcutaneous tissues and Scarpa fascia to expose the vein. Often, one of the branches draining into the saphenofemoral junction is encountered first; trace

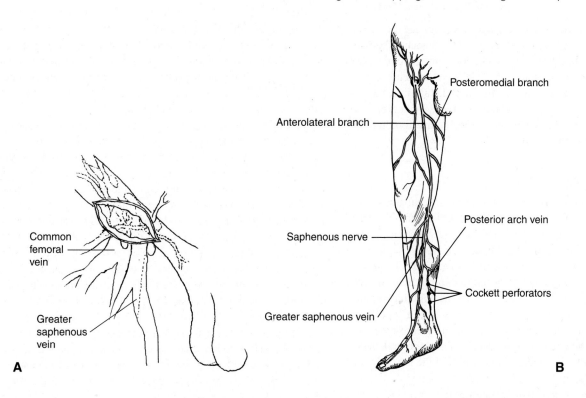

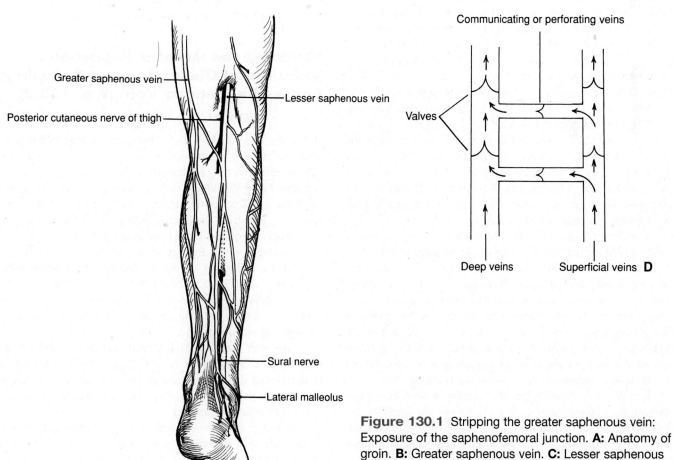

Figure 130.1 Stripping the greater saphenous vein: Exposure of the saphenofemoral junction. **A:** Anatomy of groin. **B:** Greater saphenous vein. **C:** Lesser saphenous vein. **D:** Arrangement of valves in deep and superficial systems and role of perforating veins.

this branch to the saphenofemoral junction. Skeletonize the saphenofemoral junction, and ligate and divide all the branches draining into it. These branches include the epigastric vein, the circumflex iliac vein, the external pudendal vein, and the anterolateral vein.

Ligate the greater saphenous vein 2 cm distal to the saphenofemoral junction. Apply a clamp to the saphenofemoral junction and divide the saphenous vein, suture-ligating the saphenofemoral junction with 2-0 silk.

Anatomic Points

The greater saphenous vein originates on the medial side of the arch of the dorsum of the foot (Fig. 130.1B). It ascends anterior to the tip of the medial malleolus and then over the subcutaneous surface of the lower end of the tibia. The greater saphenous vein continues up to the knee, where it moves posterior to the back part of the internal condyle of the femur and then follows the course of the sartorius muscle up to the inguinal region. Below the knee, the greater saphenous vein lies in a superficial subcutaneous plane and is accompanied by the great saphenous nerve. The saphenous nerve is a branch of the femoral nerve transmitting sensation from the medial aspect of the leg and foot. Above the knee, the greater saphenous vein gradually moves into a deeper subcutaneous plane and penetrates the fascia lata in the upper thigh through the fossa ovalis to join the common femoral vein. In the thigh, the greater saphenous vein is accompanied by branches of the medial femoral cutaneous nerve. The length of the greater saphenous vein in an adult male is estimated to be 60 cm. Frequently, a duplicate system can be found in the thigh (35%) or in the leg. The vein contains approximately 8 to 12 valves, with more valves present in the below-knee segment.

The greater saphenous vein has several important branches. The anterolateral and the posteromedial veins represent the main branches in the thigh. The posterior arch vein (vein of Leonardo) is the main branch in the leg, and deserves special attention because it has numerous perforators. It runs parallel and posterior to the saphenous vein in the leg and usually joins the saphenous vein just below the knee.

The lesser saphenous vein starts posterior to the lateral malleolus along the lateral border of the Achilles tendon (Fig. 130.1C). It crosses above the Achilles tendon and reaches the midline of the posterior aspect of the leg. The lesser saphenous vein continues upward in the subcutaneous tissues and usually penetrates the muscular fascia at the level where the tendon of the gastrocnemius muscle starts. The vein runs just below the fascia to join the popliteal vein between the heads of the gastrocnemius muscle. The lesser saphenous vein is accompanied by the lesser saphenous nerve and measures about 30 cm.

In addition to draining into the femoral and popliteal veins through the saphenofemoral and saphenopopliteal junctions, the greater and lesser saphenous veins and their branches communicate with the deep veins through communicating veins that perforate the deep fascia to join the deep venous system. These perforating veins are frequently paired, are spread throughout the lower extremity, and may be as numerous as 60 perforators per extremity. Typically, when lying supine, the superficial venous

system empties the blood into the deep venous system through the saphenofemoral or saphenopopliteal junction. During standing or walking, the perforating veins become the major route of blood flow from the superficial to the deep system. Except for those smaller than 2 mm in diameter, perforators tend to have valves that help prevent the blood refluxing from the deep to the superficial venous system during muscle contractions (Fig. 130.1D). In the presence of deep venous obstruction, the perforators become an important collateral route, diverting the flow from the deep to the superficial system. Although most perforators are unnamed, some carry the names of those who described them. May or Kuster perforators connect the greater saphenous vein in the ankle and foot to posterior tibial and plantar veins. Bassi perforators connect the lesser saphenous vein to the posterior tibial and peroneal veins posteriorly in the lower leg. Cockett perforators are three sets of veins connecting the posterior arch vein to the posterior tibial veins and are located proximal to the medial malleolus. It is worth mentioning that in the leg, most of the perforators draining to the gastrocnemius, soleus, and posterior tibial veins originate from the posterior arch vein of Leonardo rather than the greater saphenous vein. Boyd perforators connect the greater saphenous vein to the gastrocnemius vein just below the knee. Dodd perforators connect the greater saphenous vein to the femoral vein in the distal thigh and the Hunterian perforators do the same in the proximal thigh.

Stripping the Greater Saphenous Vein: Distal Dissection and Stripping; Lesser Saphenous Vein (Fig. 130.2)

Technical Points

Below the knee, make a 1-cm transverse or longitudinal incision over the marked greater saphenous vein. The vein is usually identified directly beneath the skin. Ligate the distal end of the vein (Fig. 130.2A) and make a small venotomy proximal to the ligature. Introduce the stripper, guide it up to the groin, and allow it to exit from the ligated inguinal end of the saphenous vein. Apply an olive-shaped head to the distal end of the stripper, securing it with a ligature around the vein. Divide the vein distal to the venotomy. Apply the handle on the inguinal end of the stripper (Fig. 130.2B,C). Steadily and firmly pull the stripper, applying mild pressure on the stripper head and gentle countertraction on the skin, to extract stripper and vein from the inguinal incision (Fig. 130.2D).

If the vein is to be stripped from the ankle, make a 1-cm transverse or longitudinal incision 1 cm anterior and superior to the medial malleolus. Identify and mobilize the saphenous nerve away from the vein. Pass the stripper and remove the vein as previously described.

After stripping the vein, roll a towel over the medial aspect of the extremity to express any blood collecting in the track of the stripped vein. Irrigate the wound and close it with 3-0 absorbable sutures for the subcutaneous tissue and 4-0 absorbable subcuticular sutures for the skin. Apply elastic bandages from the ankle to the upper thigh.

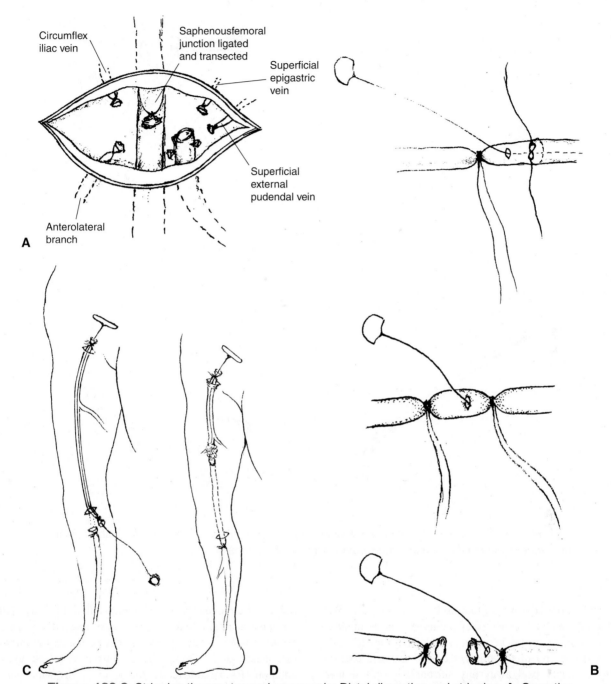

Figure 130.2 Stripping the greater saphenous vein: Distal dissection and stripping. **A:** Operative field with branches ligated in preparation for stripping. Saphenofemoral junction has been ligated and transected. **B:** Passage of stripper. **C:** Stripping greater saphenous vein. **D:** Removal of vein.

To strip the lesser saphenous vein, place the patient in the prone position. Make a 2- to 3-cm transverse skin incision behind the knee over the marked vein. Identify the lesser saphenous vein just beneath the skin and trace it to the saphenopopliteal junction. Next, make a 1-cm transverse or longitudinal incision over the lateral aspect of the ankle to identify the distal end of the vein. Identify and separate the sural nerve from the distal vein. Strip the vein as described previously.

Excision of Branch Varicosities Using Stab Avulsion Technique (Fig. 130.3)

Technical Points

It is essential that all the branches be accurately marked with the patient standing upright using marking ink. Make a 1- to 2-mm stab incision along the side of the branch to be removed using a number 11 blade or a 14-gauge needle. Introduce a crochet hook and pass it under the anticipated location of the vein.

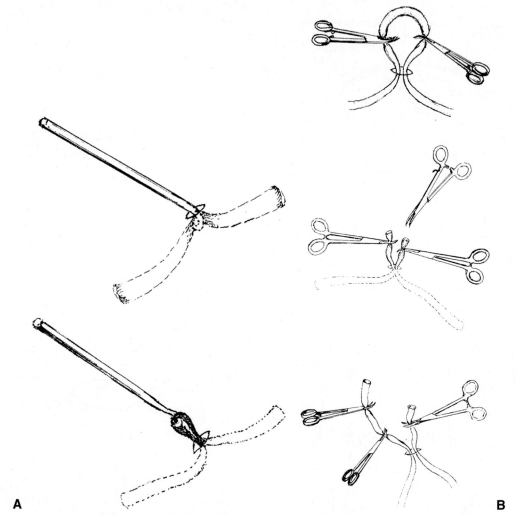

Figure 130.3 Excision of branch varicosities using stab avulsion technique. **A:** Stab incision and access of vein. **B:** Ligation and excision of branch varicosity.

Withdraw the hook, catching a loop of the vein (Fig. 130.3A). Grasp the loop with a fine hemostat and tease it out of the incision. Divide the vein loop between two clamps (Fig. 130.3B). Gently pull one end of the transected vein, using a rotating movement. Gently peel away any surrounding soft tissues. Reapply the clamp closer to the skin and again pull the vein until it is avulsed. Repeat the technique with the other end of the transected vein. Make another stab incision 6 to 8 cm from the prior incision along the anticipated course of the vein and repeat. Continue this procedure until all the branches have been excised.

Endovascular Radiofrequency Ablation of the Greater Saphenous Vein

Technical and Anatomic Points

Evaluate the greater saphenous vein from below the knee to the saphenofemoral junction by duplex ultrasonography. Using Seldinger technique, and under ultrasound guidance, puncture the most accessible site of the greater saphenous vein below the knee using a micropuncture set. Exchange the micropuncture sheath for a 7-French sheath. Introduce the radiofrequency ablation (RFA) catheter to the level of the saphenofemoral junction just distal to the epigastric branch. Place the patient in a Trendelenburg position. Infiltrate tumescent anesthesia under ultrasound guidance in the subfascial plane, pushing the vein 2 cm deeper to the skin. After the tumescent anesthesia is completely infiltrated, check the position of the RFA catheter: It should be just distal to the epigastric vein.

Begin the ablation from the saphenofemoral junction level for two 20 second ablations for the first 7 cm and then 20 second ablation for all the remaining vein in 7 cm segments. Once at the level of the sheath, retract the sheath to allow the most distal segment of vein to be ablated. Recheck the saphenous vein by ultrasound to ensure complete ablation and absence of thrombus in the common femoral vein. Then remove the sheath and catheter.

Exposure and Harvesting of the Greater Saphenous Vein for Bypass Procedures (Fig. 130.4)

Technical and Anatomic Points

The greater saphenous vein is considered the gold standard with which all other conduits are compared when performing infrainguinal reconstructions. It is also the most commonly used conduit in coronary revascularization. When used for infrainguinal revascularization, the greater saphenous vein is either harvested or kept in its bed (in situ bypass; see Chapter 133), a procedure that requires disruption of its valves to allow for blood flow. When harvested, the vein is either reversed (reversed vein bypass) or used nonreversed, which also necessitates disruption of its valves (nonreversed vein bypass). Valve disruption is usually performed using a valvulotome. Improper valvulotomy may injure the vein or fail to disrupt the valves completely. A good-quality saphenous vein that measures 3 cm or greater in diameter will perform equally well as a reversed, nonreversed, or in situ bypass. Small veins (<3 cm in diameter) tend to perform better if used in an in situ or nonreversed fashion.

It is essential to use proper technique to avoid injury, which may occur by one of several mechanisms. First, the vein wall can be crushed with the forceps during dissection. Consequently, try to grasp only the adventitia with the forceps. Excessive traction applied to a Silastic loop passed around the vein may injure the

conduit. Injury can also occur if small branches are inadvertently avulsed during the dissection or if branches are ligated very close to the body of the graft, thus narrowing the lumen. Overdistention of the vein may result in significant endothelial damage. Avoid this by monitoring intraluminal pressure and keeping it below 300 mm Hg. Chilled whole blood, or a cold solution of Ringer's lactate (1 L) or dextran 40 (1 L) mixed with 5,000 U of heparin and 60 mg of papaverine, can be used to distend the vein or to run through the conduit while harvesting. This maintains flow and helps avoid the formation of intraluminal thrombi. Finally, it is important to keep the exposed or harvested vein moist and avoid desiccation injury. Avoid this by covering the vein with gauze soaked with warm saline. Adding papaverine (60 mg/500 mL) may help decrease spasm in the conduit.

Preoperative evaluation of the greater saphenous vein with duplex ultrasonography allows the location to be mapped. The skin incision can then be made over the marked skin. Alternatively, use anatomic landmarks. At the ankle level, make a longitudinal incision 1 cm anterior and superior to the medial malleolus. Identify the vein directly beneath the skin. At the inguinal region, begin the incision 1.5 cm medial to the femoral pulse and extend it at a 30-degree angle to the vertical axis of the lower extremity. If the femoral pulse is not palpable, begin the incision 1.5 cm medial to a point midway between the pubic tubercle and the anterosuperior iliac spine. Deepen the incision through the subcutaneous tissues and Scarpa fascia to expose the vein.

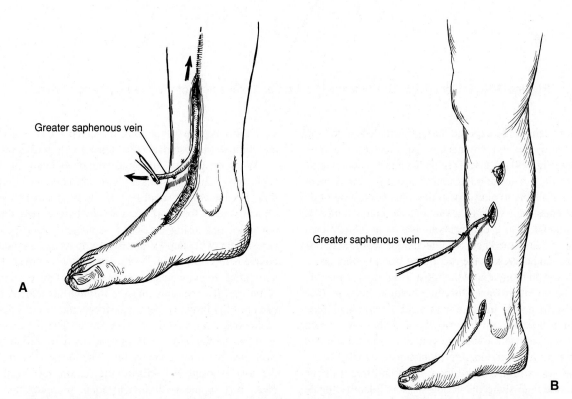

Figure 130.4 Exposure and harvesting of the greater saphenous vein for bypass procedures. **A:** Access of distal greater saphenous vein. **B:** Multiple small incisions permit access and minimize morbidity. (*continued*)

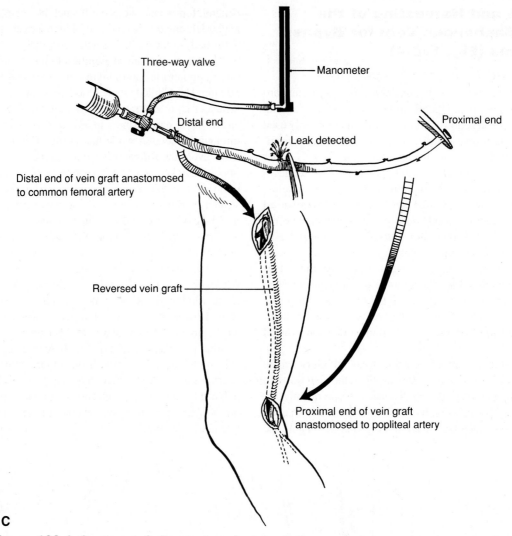

Figure 130.4 *Continued.* **C:** Preparation of vein and placement of reversed saphenous vein.

The entire vein can be exposed through a single long incision or through multiple 6- to 8-cm incisions separated by 4- to 6-cm skin bridges (Fig. 130.4A and B) in an attempt to minimize the morbidity of the single long incision. Currently, various methods are also available to allow for endoscopic harvesting of the greater saphenous vein through a single small inguinal incision and or additional 1- to 2-cm incisions placed at various locations above or below the knee. Such technique was found to be safe, reliable, and decreases the risk of leg wound infections.

Identify a side branch near the most distal part of the vein and introduce a blunt-tipped needle through this site (Fig. 130.4C). Tie the needle in place with a silk ligature and allow the distention solution to drip slowly into the vein lumen. Alternatively, ligate and divide the vein at its most distal end, and use this site to introduce the blunt-tipped needle. Gently encircle the vein with a Silastic loop; lift it and free it of surrounding tissue with sharp dissecting scissors. Identify, ligate, and divide all tributaries.

If the conduit is to be used in the nonreversed fashion, leave long 3-mm stumps on several branches along the body of the

vein. Introduce the valvulotome through the distal end of the vein and through these stumps (see Figure 133.5 in Chapter 133e).

When the greater saphenous vein is not available, the lesser saphenous vein represents a good alternative autogenous conduit. Because of its small length, the lesser saphenous vein is typically used for short bypasses or bypass revisions. When contemplating using the lesser saphenous vein, preoperative assessment with duplex ultrasonography and mapping of its course is recommended. If vein mapping is not available, begin a longitudinal skin incision in the middle of the posterior aspect of the calf. Deepen this incision through the subcutaneous tissue until the fascia is identified. Incise the fascia, exposing the saphenous vein directly underneath it. The lesser saphenous vein can be harvested with the patient lying prone or supine. Both involve some compromise. The prone position provides the best exposure but will usually require turning the patient back to a supine position and again prepping and draping. When the patient is lying supine, external rotation of the leg and the gastrocnemius muscle will allow access to the lesser saphenous vein. However, the junction to the popliteal vein remains challenging to expose from this approach. The lesser saphenous vein can also be approached through a medial skin incision; however, this requires the creation of large skin flaps and allows access to only a short segment of the vein.

REFERENCES

1. Allen KB, Shaar CJ. Endoscopic saphenous vein harvesting. *Ann Thorac Surg.* 1997;64:265–266.
2. Crane C. The surgery of varicose veins. *Surg Clin North Am.* 1979;59:737.
3. Goren G, Yellin AE. Ambulatory stab avulsion phlebectomy for truncal varicose veins. *Am J Surg.* 1991;162:166–174.
4. Jimenez JC, Lawrence PF, Rigberg DA, et al. Technical modifications in endoscopic vein harvest techniques facilitate their use in lower extremity limb salvage procedures. *J Vasc Surg.* 2007;45(3):549–553.
5. Large J. Surgical treatment of saphenous varices, with preservation of the main great saphenous trunk. *J Vasc Surg.* 1985;2: 887.
6. Nabatoff RA. The short saphenous vein. *Surg Gynecol Obstet.* 1979;149:49.
7. Ouzounian M, Hassan A, Buth KJ, et al. Impact of endoscopic versus open saphenous vein harvest techniques on outcomes after coronary artery bypass grafting. *Ann Thorac Surg.* 2010;89(2):403–408. doi: 10.1016/j.athoracsur.2009.09.061.
8. Samuels PB. Technique of varicose vein surgery. *Am J Surg.* 1981; 142:239.
9. Thomson H. The surgical anatomy of the superficial and perforator veins of the lower limb. *Ann R Coll Surg Engl.* 1979;61:198.

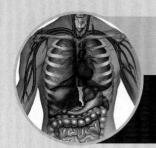

131

Venous Access: Saphenous Vein Cutdown

The greater saphenous vein is an anatomically constant vein that is easily cannulated for emergency venous access. The saphenous vein at the ankle is constant, although it may be involved by varicose vein disease in elderly patients. Although the interosseus route is faster in children, this remains a useful route of access, especially because it is somewhat removed from the central area and thus out of the way of resuscitative attempts. Bony landmarks render the vein easy to find.

The greater saphenous vein at the groin is sometimes used for introduction of an extremely large catheter, such as a sterile oxygen flow catheter, through which blood and intravenous fluids can be infused rapidly in a patient with traumatic injuries. The techniques of saphenous vein cutdown at the ankle and the groin are described in this chapter. Alternatives are discussed in the references at the end.

SCORE™, the Surgical Council on Resident Education, did not classify saphenous vein cutdown.

STEPS IN PROCEDURE

Cutdown at Ankle

Local anesthesia two fingerbreadths above and two fingerbreadths medial to medial malleolus

Transverse skin incision

Spread tissues in longitudinal direction until vein is seen

Elevate the saphenous vein into field

Identify and protect saphenous nerve

Place ligatures proximally and distally

Cannulate vein and tie ligature around cannula

Ligate distal vein

Secure catheter and close incision

Cutdown at Groin

Moderate external rotation

Local anesthesia medial to femoral pulse, two fingerbreadths below inguinal crease

Incision parallel to inguinal crease

Dissect in subcutaneous fat

Identify the saphenous vein and elevate into incision

Cannulate as described above

Use Seldinger technique to avoid ligating vein, if desired

HALLMARK ANATOMIC COMPLICATIONS

Injury to saphenous nerve

Injury to femoral vein

LIST OF STRUCTURES

Common Femoral Vein

Greater saphenous vein

Saphenofemoral junction

Superficial epigastric vein

Superficial circumflex iliac vein

Superficial external pudendal vein

Medial malleolus

Patella

Inguinal ligament

Superficial fascia

Fascia Lata

Saphenous hiatus (fossa ovalis)

Femoral Nerve

Saphenous nerve

Medial femoral cutaneous nerve

Anterior femoral cutaneous nerve

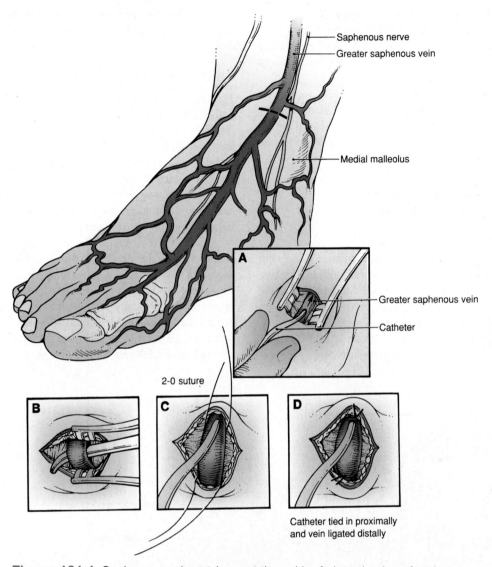

Figure 131.1 Saphenous vein cutdown at the ankle. **A:** Introduction of catheter into vein without ligation of vein. **B:** Isolation of vein. **C:** Insertion of catheter with vascular control of vein. **D:** Vein ligated distally and catheter tied in proximally.

Saphenous Vein Cutdown at the Ankle (Fig. 131.1)

Technical Points

Place the leg in external rotation and prep the medial aspect of the ankle from the medial malleolus around to the anterior aspect of the ankle. Infiltrate the area of the proposed skin incision, which will be two fingerbreadths above and two fingerbreadths medial to the medial malleolus. Make a transverse incision through the skin. The greater saphenous vein will lie immediately under the skin. Take great care not to enter the vein while making the initial skin incision. Spread tissues in a longitudinal fashion as you look for the saphenous vein. The saphenous vein is usually at least 3 to 5 mm in diameter and often is even larger.

Elevate the saphenous vein into the field and clean it by sharp and blunt dissection. Identify and protect the saphenous nerve. Place ligatures proximally and distally and make a venotomy on the anterior surface of the vein. Introduce the catheter and secure it, tying the catheter into place proximally and ligating the vein distally.

Anatomic Points

The greater saphenous vein is typically the largest and, in most cases, anatomically the most consistent of the superficial veins. It starts on the medial side of the dorsal venous arch of the foot, passing from there 2.5 to 3 cm anterior to the medial-most projection of the medial malleolus. From there, it courses up the medial side of the leg, passing posterior to the knee joint, about

8 to 10 cm posterior to the anteromedial border of the patella. It then ascends in the superficial fascia of the thigh to a point about 2.5 cm distal to the inguinal ligament, where it passes through the saphenous hiatus (fossa ovalis) of the fascia lata to terminate in the common femoral vein.

At the ankle, the greater saphenous vein is very superficial and thus can be injured when making the initial skin incision. The saphenous nerve is a sensory branch of the femoral nerve. It typically runs immediately anterior to the greater saphenous vein.

Saphenous Vein Cutdown at the Groin (Fig. 131.2)

Technical Points

Place the extremity in moderate external rotation. The skin incision will be made medial to the femoral pulse, about two fingerbreadths below the inguinal crease. Make a transverse incision about 4 cm in length. The saphenous vein will lie on the subcutaneous fat and will be relatively superficial.

Identify the saphenous vein and elevate it into the incision. Make a venotomy on the anterior surface of the vein

and introduce the catheter as previously described. Secure the catheter in place and close the incision with absorbable suture material.

Anatomic Points

The inguinal skin crease does not always directly correspond with the location of the deeper inguinal ligament. In thin people, the skin crease is immediately superficial to the ligament, but in most people, it is 2 to 3 cm distal. Because the saphenous hiatus (fossa ovalis) is located about 2.5 to 3 cm distal to the inguinal ligament, the initial skin incision for exposure of this vein should always be distal to the skin crease (i.e., one should attempt to gain access to the vein while it is in the superficial fascia, not at the hiatus itself).

In its course through the thigh, the saphenous vein lies deeper than it does in the lower leg. Typically, it is located between two layers of superficial fascia, its depth being dependent on the amount of adipose tissue in the thigh. In its upper part, it typically receives large tributaries draining the posteromedial and anterolateral thigh as well as the smaller peri-inguinal veins (superficial epigastric, circumflex iliac, and external pudendal veins). In addition, it frequently is closely

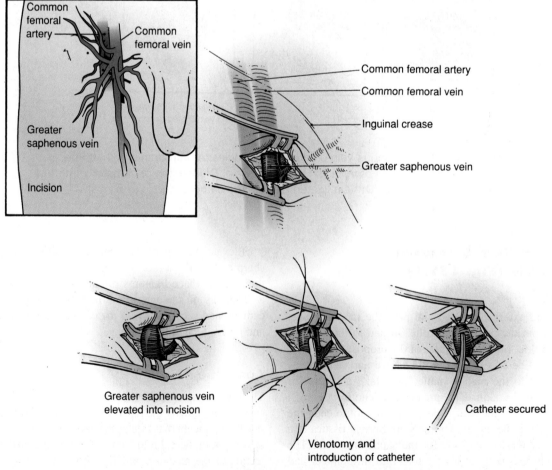

Figure 131.2 Saphenous vein cutdown at the groin

related to branches of the medial femoral cutaneous nerve, or to other sensory branches (e.g., anterior femoral cutaneous nerve) of the femoral nerve.

REFERENCES

1. American College of Surgeons Committee on Trauma. Shock. In: *Advanced Trauma Life Support Manual.* 7th ed. Chicago: American College of Surgeons; 2004:69–102. (Presents excellent discussion of alternatives, including percutaneous femoral line placement and interosseous infusion.)
2. Chappell S, Vilke GM, Chan TC, et al. Peripheral venous cutdown. *J Emerg Med.* 2006;31:411–416.
3. Cole I, Glass C, Norton JH, et al. Ultrasound measurements of the saphenous vein in the pediatric emergency department population with comparison to i.v. catheter size. *J Emerg Med.* 2012;43:87.
4. Haas NA. Clinical review: Vascular access for fluid infusion in children. *Crit Care.* 2004;8:478.
5. Hansbrough JF, Cain RL, Millikan JS. Placement of 10-gauge catheter by cutdown for rapid fluid replacement. *J Trauma.* 1983;23:231. (Provides classic description of rapid infusion line placement.)
6. Klofas E. A quicker saphenous vein cutdown and a better way to teach it. *J Rheum.* 1997;43:985–987. (Discusses Seldinger technique application to cutdown.)

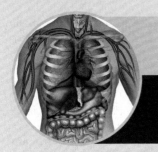

132

Peripheral Embolectomy

Parth B. Amin and Rachael Nicholson

Acute peripheral arterial ischemia is commonly a result of cardioembolic phenomenon. History and physical examination can adequately diagnose this problem and allow for the appropriate operative exposure. Embolic occlusions very often occur at major arterial branch points and accordingly, exposures are best planned with this understanding. Upper extremity embolic phenomenon can best be approached through a brachial exposure, whereas lower extremity can be approached from either the femoral artery or the below knee popliteal artery. Heparin should be initiated at the time of suspected ischemia, prior to the patient being in the operating room. Activated clotting times can be monitored intraoperatively to assess the adequacy of anticoagulation.

SCORE™, the Surgical Council on Resident Education, classified embolectomy of artery as an "ESSENTIAL UNCOMMON" procedure.

STEPS IN PROCEDURE

Brachial Thromboembolectomy
Transverse incision one fingerbreadth distal to the antecubital crease
Mobilize superficial veins
Incise the bicipital aponeurosis
Dissect distal brachial, proximal ulnar, and proximal radial arteries
Transverse arteriotomy
Embolectomy with antegrade and retrograde passage of Fogarty catheters
Arteriotomy closure
Skin closure

Femoral Thromboembolectomy
Longitudinal incision one fingerbreadth distal inguinal ligament
Mobilize the inguinal ligament
Incise femoral sheath
Dissect common femoral, superficial femoral, and profunda femoris arteries
Transverse arteriotomy; unless there is severely diseased common femoral artery, in which case consider

longitudinal arteriotomy with patch angioplasty
Embolectomy with antegrade and retrograde passage of Fogarty catheters
Primary arteriotomy closure for transverse arteriotomy and patch angioplasty for longitudinal arteriotomy
Wound closure

Popliteal Thromboembolectomy
Longitudinal incision 1 cm posterior to tibia
Incise fascia
Divide pes anserinus, (if further exposure needed)
Isolate popliteal artery
Divide soleus
Isolate tibial vessels
Transverse arteriotomy
Embolectomy with antegrade and retrograde passage of Fogarty catheters
Primary arteriotomy closure for transverse arteriotomy
Wound closure

HALLMARK ANATOMIC COMPLICATIONS
Retained thrombus
Lymphocele

Wound breakdown
Saphenous nerve injury

LIST OF STRUCTURES
Inguinal ligament
Pubic tubercle
Anterior superior iliac spine
Femur
Medial femoral condyle
Superficial circumflex iliac artery and vein

Inferior epigastric artery
Superficial external pudendal artery and vein
Inguinal lymph nodes
Femoral sheath
Fascia lata
Common femoral artery

Superficial femoral artery	Adductor longus muscle
Profunda femoris artery	Adductor magnus muscle
Femoral vein	Adductor tubercle
Greater saphenous vein	Adductor canal
Femoral nerve	Sartorius muscle
Saphenous nerve	Semimembranosus
Fossa ovalis	Semitendinosus muscle
Inguinal lymph nodes	Vastus medialis muscle
Iliopsoas muscle	Popliteal fossa
Pectineus muscle	Soleus muscle
Adductor brevis muscle	Gastrocnemius muscle

Upper Extremity (Fig. 132.1)

Technical Points

Thrombectomy for a presumed embolus to the brachial artery is best approached through a transverse incision one fingerbreadth distal to skin crease at the antecubital fossa (Fig. 132.1A). Mobilize the superficial veins. Incise the bicipital aponeurosis to expose the brachial artery. Begin sharp dissection of the brachial artery on its anterior surface and proceed to obtain circumferential proximal control. Continue the dissection distally until the brachial artery bifurcates into the radial and ulnar arteries. Place Silastic loops around the brachial, ulnar, and radial arteries (Fig. 132.1B). Loops can be placed in a double-looped or Potts fashion, or single-looped with the addition of small, atraumatic vascular clamps which are used for control once the embolus is removed.

On the anterior surface of the brachial artery use an 11-blade knife at a 45-degree angle to start a transverse arteriotomy. Once completely through the anterior surface of the arterial wall and into the lumen, extend the arteriotomy transversely with Potts scissors. Pass a Fogarty embolectomy catheter (Edwards Lifescience, Irvine, CA) in a retrograde fashion past the proximal extent of the thrombus, gently inflate the balloon to the point that there is a small amount of tension as the catheter is pulled back (Fig. 132.1C,D), then extract the thrombus. More than one pass might be needed to obtain brisk antegrade flow. Use the markings on the catheter to assess the distance needed to advance the catheter before inserting it into the vessel. To minimize bleeding from the vessel once the clot is removed, be ready to retract gently on the vessel loop as the catheter balloon approaches the arteriotomy site. Sizes of the catheters range from 2F to 7F with the corresponding maximal inflation diameters between 4 and 12 mm. Close the vessel with fine 6-0 or 7-0 polypropylene suture. Assess Doppler signals of the distal vessels.

If the blind passage of the Fogarty catheter does not yield satisfactory revascularization, perform an angiogram. If there is a significant amount of residual clot, reopen the arteriotomy. Place a sheath in an antegrade fashion toward the hand. Use intraoperative fluoroscopy to guide a 0.018-inch wire into the distal radial and ulnar arteries and use an over-the-wire Fogarty catheter to perform the thrombectomy. Inject small amounts of contrast as needed to assess progress of the thrombectomy. Once flow has been restored into the hand, remove the sheath and close the arteriotomy with interrupted sutures (Fig. 132.1E).

Anatomic Points

The muscles of the arm are divided into the flexor and extensor compartments by the medial and lateral intermuscular septa and the humerus. The flexor compartments include the biceps brachii muscle, the brachialis muscle, and the coracobrachialis. The brachialis muscle originates from the anterior surface of the humerus and inserts onto the ulnar tuberosity. The biceps brachii has two heads. The long head originates onto the supraglenoid tubercle of the scapula, while the short head originates on the coracoid process of the scapula. The posterior compartment contains only one muscle, the triceps brachii.

A discussion of venous structures begins with identification of the deltoid muscle and pectoralis major muscles. The junction of the shoulder and arm, in between the deltoid muscle and the pectoralis major muscle is where the cephalic vein is located. The vein travels on the lateral surface of the arm within the confines of the deltopectoral groove. The median cubital vein drains into the cephalic vein at the level of the antecubital fossa. Toward the medial surface of the arm, the median cubital vein drains into the basilic vein at the antecubital fossa. The location of the basilic vein is found by palpating the groove between the biceps brachii medially and the triceps muscle and entering the fascia.

The major arterial supply to the upper limb is via the brachial artery. The axillary artery becomes the brachial artery at the inferior border of the teres major. Its distal course lies within the bicipital groove which can be palpated. The course of the brachial artery throughout the upper arm is quite superficial and lies beneath a strong, protective fascial layer which must be incised for exposure. Care must be taken to avoid confusing the bicipital groove for the groove between the two heads of the biceps brachii when planning an incision. The brachial artery course ends in the cubital fossa prior to its division as the radial and ulnar arteries.

The other key structure amidst the vasculature that must be identified is the median nerve, which is located just anterior to the brachial artery. The median nerve travels on the medial

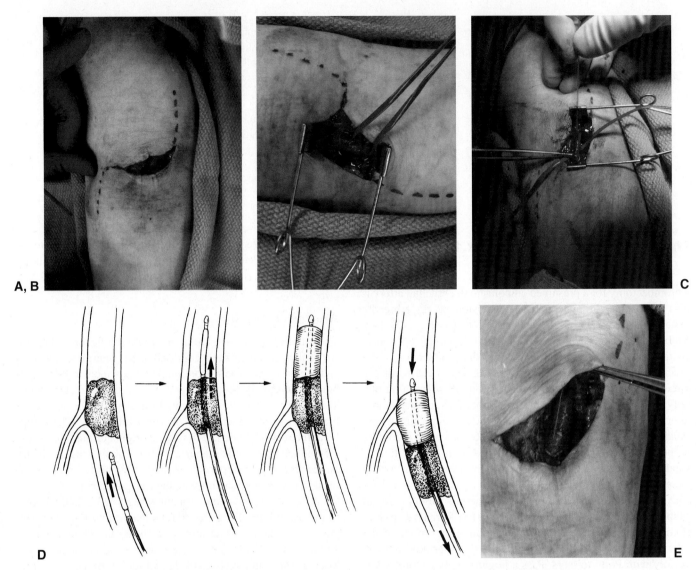

Figure 132.1 A: Incision for brachial embolectomy. **B:** Control of brachial artery and its branches. **C:** Passage of embolectomy catheter through transverse incision. **D:** Schematic of embolectomy catheter removing embolus (figure from Fischer JE, ed. *Fischer's Mastery of Surgery.* 6th ed. Philadelphia, PA: Lippincott Wolters Kluwer; 2012, with permission). **E:** Incision closed with simple interrupted sutures.

head of the triceps brachii, then on the coracobrachialis, and finally, on the brachialis. The basilic vein lies on its medial side, but is separated from it in the lower part of the arm by the deep fascia. The cubital fossa is, however, the primary site of exposure for brachial artery.

The boundaries of the cubital fossa are as follows: The brachioradialis muscle laterally, the pronator teres muscle medially, and the antecubital skin crease proximally. The median cubital vein is superficial to the flexor retinaculum. Deep to the median cubital vein, the flexor retinaculum must be incised. Once the brachial artery is identified and the median nerve protected, the ulnar and radial arteries are exposed distally in the arm. As a reference point, the ulnar artery runs between the flexor digitorum superficialis and the flexor digitorum profun-

dus. The radial artery, on the other hand, can be found lateral to the tendon of the flexor carpi radialis muscle.

Lower Extremity

Common Femoral Exposure and Embolectomy (Fig. 132.2)

Technical Points

Identify the inguinal ligament along a line connecting the anterior superior iliac spine and the pubic tubercle. Create a longitudinal incision 1 cm distal to the inguinal ligament overlying the common femoral artery. Divide the superficial subcutaneous tissues sharply or with cautery. Ligate and tie visible

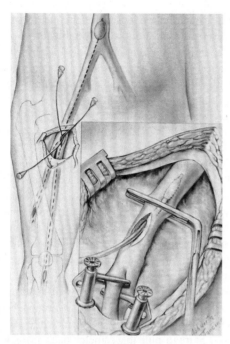

Figure 132.2 Femoral arteriotomy (transverse) and passage of Fogarty catheter (figure from Fischer JE, ed. *Fischer's Mastery of Surgery.* 6th ed. Philadelphia, PA: Lippincott Wolters Kluwer; 2012, with permission).

lymphatic channels. Mobilize the inguinal ligament off the femoral sheath along its oblique course in the wound. Sharply incise the femoral sheath longitudinally, directly over the proximal common femoral artery (see Chapter 133, Figure 133.1B,C). Although the pulsation is likely absent, the tubular structure of the artery can often be palpated at this point. Dissect the anterior surface of the common femoral artery first and then proceed to the medial, lateral, and posterior sides of the artery to obtain circumferential control. Avoid ligating any arterial branches. Extend the dissection distally, exposing the superficial femoral and the profunda femoris arteries, and place Silastic loops around them for control.

When the common femoral artery is relatively disease free, make a transverse arteriotomy near the bifurcation so that a Fogarty catheter can be directed easily into either the profunda or superficial femoral arteries (Fig. 132.2). If there is a significant amount of occlusive disease in the common femoral artery, consider a longitudinal arteriotomy and patch closure. A 3- or 4-French Fogarty is generally used for the popliteal and superficial femoral arteries. A 2- or 3-French Fogarty is used for the tibial vessels. The marks on the catheter are used before performing thromboembolectomy to estimate the length of the catheter needed to reach the distal popliteal and tibial vessels. The catheter should be pulled retrograde just prior to the start of balloon inflation in the tibial arteries as these vessels easily rupture, dissect, or spasm with over inflation.

If the arteriotomy is transverse, close the vessel primarily with 5-0 or 6-0 polypropylene after confirming adequate forward and back bleeding and flushing with heparinized saline.

Assess the circulation in the foot. When the blind passage of the Fogarty catheter does not yield satisfactory revascularization, perform an angiogram. If there is a significant amount of residual clot, reopen the arteriotomy. Place a sheath in an antegrade fashion toward the foot. Use intraoperative fluoroscopy to guide a 0.018-inch wire into the distal tibial arteries and use an over-the-wire Fogarty catheter to perform the thrombectomy. Inject contrast as needed to assess the progress of the thrombectomy. Once flow has been restored into the foot, remove the sheath and close the arteriotomy as before.

Anatomic Points

The common femoral artery begins as an extension of the external iliac artery below the inguinal ligament. Posterior to the inguinal ligament, the femoral sheath is identified, wherein, the major neurovascular structures which supply the lower limb originate. The common femoral artery extends for several centimeters before bifurcating into the profunda femoris and superficial femoral arteries. In the setting of an acute embolic event, there might be a water-hammer pulsation in the very proximal portion of the common femoral artery which will make the dissection easier. However, there often is no palpable pulse to guide the incision in which case a longitudinal incision one-third the distance from the pubic tubercle along the line of the inguinal ligament will place the operator directly over the common femoral artery. During the dissection of the common femoral artery, take care not to inadvertently injure the superficial external pudendal, superficial epigastric, and superficial iliac circumflex arteries as they originate from the medial and lateral sides of the proximal artery.

The takeoff of the profunda femoris can be identified when the diameter of the femoral artery changes abruptly. The superficial femoral artery is sometimes mistaken for the common femoral artery because the course of this major branch is in direct continuity with the common femoral artery. This is particularly true if exposure of the common femoral artery is attempted at the groin crease. The superficial femoral artery then continues posterior to the sartorius muscle. At the adductor hiatus, the superficial femoral artery becomes the popliteal artery.

The profunda femoris comes off the common femoral artery most often posterolaterally. More distally in the leg, it can be found directly behind the superficial femoral artery. The medial circumflex artery is a branch that is often in close proximity to the takeoff of the profunda femoris. This arterial branch, along with the lateral femoral circumflex artery, usually comes off the profunda femoris artery prior to the plethora of perforating branches which continue to come off down the leg. The medial or lateral circumflex artery can often be large collaterals in patients and can directly come off the common femoral artery. Care must be taken when obtaining circumferential control of the profunda as the circumflex femoral vein crosses between the superficial femoral and profunda just past the bifurcation and can be a source of difficult to control bleeding if unintentionally entered. Exposure of the mid-to-distal profunda femoris requires division of this vein.

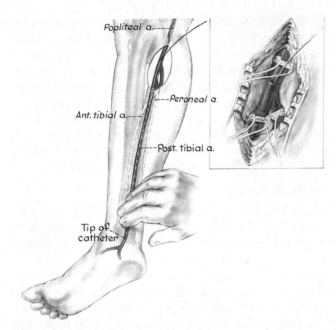

Figure 132.3 Infrageniculate approach to popliteal and tibial vessels (figure from Fischer JE, ed. *Fischer's Mastery of Surgery.* 6th ed. Philadelphia, PA: Lippincott Wolters Kluwer; 2012, with permission).

Infrageniculate Popliteal Artery Exposure (Fig. 132.3)

Technical and Anatomic Points

Successful thromboembolectomy of the lower extremity, including the distal tibial vessels, can often be done solely through a groin incision. However at times exposure of the below knee popliteal artery is required. Create a longitudinal incision one fingerbreadth posterior to the tibia as shown in Chapter 133, Figure 133.4. Extend the incision through the subcutaneous tissue. Avoid injury or ligation of the greater saphenous vein. Incise the deep fascia longitudinally to gain access to the popliteal vessels. Reflect the soleus and gastrocnemius muscles posteriorly to expose the distal popliteal artery and vein. Further exposure can be obtained by dividing portions of the pes anserinus, which include the tendons of the gracilis, semitendinosus, and sartorius. Encircle the popliteal artery with a vessel loop. Continue the dissection distally along the popliteal artery until the soleus muscle is encountered. Divide the soleus muscle attachments to the tibia over a right

angle clamp to facilitate exposure of the anterior tibial artery and tibioperoneal trunk. Follow the popliteal distally until the origin of the anterior tibial artery is noted anteriorly and laterally and encircle it with a vessel loop. Dissect distally dissection along the tibioperoneal trunk for approximately 2.5 cm until the origins of the posterior tibial and peroneal arteries are seen and encircle them with vessel loops. Small crossing veins should be carefully ligated as exposure becomes greatly limited when small venous branches retract and bleed.

Once proximal control of the popliteal artery and distal control of the three tibial vessels are obtained (Fig. 132.3), place Yasargil clamps on each vessel. A larger clamp might be needed for the popliteal artery. Create a transverse arteriotomy in the distal popliteal artery near the takeoff of the anterior tibial artery. If inflow has not been yet established, place a 3 or 4 Fogarty catheter in a retrograde fashion into the popliteal and guide it into the superficial femoral artery. Inflate the balloon and remove the clot. Flush the vessel with heparinized saline and replace the clamp. Guide a 2- or 3-French Fogarty balloon individually down each tibial vessel while the other two are clamped. Start to pull the catheter back prior to inflation of the balloon. Once the clot is removed and back bleeding is achieved, flush the vessel with heparinized saline and replace the clamp. Repeat this step with the remaining two tibial vessels and then close the arteriotomy with interrupted Prolene sutures. Again, use caution with embolectomy in the tibial vessels as they are very prone to rupture, dissection, and spasm with over inflation.

REFERENCES

1. Goss CM. The arteries. In: Goss CM, ed. *Gray's Anatomy of the Human Body.* Philadelphia, PA: Lea & Febiger; 1973:561–672.
2. Haimovici H. The upper extremity. In: Haimovici H, ed. *Vascular Surgery: Principles and Techniques.* Norwalk, CT: Appleton-Century Crofts; 1984:203–217.
3. Hellerstein HK, Martin JW. Incidence of thromboembolic lesions accompanying myocardial infarction. *Am Heart J.* 1947;33:443.
4. Sheiner NM, Zeltzer J, Macintosh E. Arterial embolectomy in the modern era. *Can J Surg.* 1982;25:373.
5. Singer A. Anatomy of the femoropopliteal system. In: Nyhus LM, Baker RJ, eds. *Mastery of Surgery.* 1st ed. Boston: Little Brown; 1988:1477–1484.
6. Stanley JC, Henke PK. The treatment of acute embolic lower extremity ischemia. *Adv Surg.* 2004;38:281–291.
7. Tawes RL Jr, Harris EJ, Brown WH, et al. Arterial thromboembolism: A 20-year prospective. *Arch Surg.* 1985;120:595.

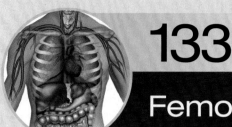

133

Femoral to Popliteal Bypass

Parth B. Amin and Melhem J. Sharafuddin

A number of conduits have been used to bypass obstructed segments of the femoropopliteal system. Autogenous saphenous vein has the best patency and avoids the potential for prosthetic graft infection. Furthermore, primary assisted patency can be improved substantially with surveillance duplex examination. This chapter will focus on femoropopliteal bypass using saphenous vein as a conduit.

SCORE™, the Surgical Council on Resident Education, classified femoral–popliteal bypass as an "ESSENTIAL UNCOMMON" procedure.

STEPS IN PROCEDURE

Expose greater saphenous vein
Expose common femoral artery from vein harvest incision
Dissect common femoral artery, profunda femoris, and superficial femoral artery
Exposure of suprageniculate popliteal artery
From vein harvest incision, enter popliteal fossa anterior to sartorius
Continue dissection posterior to the femur
Identify the popliteal artery and vein
Divide venous tributaries crossing over the popliteal artery
Exposure of infrageniculate popliteal artery
Approach incision 1 cm posterior to tibia and 2 cm distal to medial femoral condyle
Incise fascia and retract soleus and gastrocnemius to get into popliteal space
Divide crossing veins on top of popliteal artery
Measure length of vein needed for bypass
Divide vein at saphenofemoral junction
Mobilize saphenous vein by dividing branches
Prepare vein using retrograde valvulotome or used reversed vein
Create proximal anastomosis
Tunnel vein subsartorially into popliteal fossa
For infrageniculate bypass, tunnel from suprageniculate to infrageniculate popliteal compartment
Perform distal anastomosis
Doppler evaluation and completion angiogram

HALLMARK ANATOMIC COMPLICATIONS

Bypass graft thrombosis
Lymphocele
Wound breakdown
Saphenous nerve injury

LIST OF STRUCTURES

Inguinal ligament
Pubic tubercle
Anterior superior iliac spine
Femur
Medial femoral condyle
Superficial circumflex iliac artery and vein
Inferior epigastric artery
Superficial external pudendal artery and vein
Inguinal lymph nodes
Femoral sheath
Fascia lata
Common femoral artery
Superficial femoral artery
Profunda femoris artery
Femoral vein
Greater saphenous vein
Femoral nerve
Saphenous nerve
Fossa ovalis
Inguinal lymph nodes
Iliopsoas muscle
Pectineus muscle
Adductor brevis muscle
Adductor longus muscle

Adductor magnus muscle	Semitendinosus muscle
Adductor tubercle	Vastus medialis muscle
Adductor canal	Popliteal fossa
Sartorius muscle	Soleus muscle
Semimembranosus	Gastrocnemius muscle

Exposure of Saphenous Vein

The greater saphenous vein is superficial and medial to the common femoral artery (see Chapters 130 and 131 for discussion of the anatomy of this vein). A preoperative saphenous vein marking using ultrasound may help reduce complications from skin flaps and also diagram larger tributaries. The greater saphenous vein is the largest vascular structure in the superficial fascia and essentially overlies the proximal femoral vein. In its course in the upper thigh, it lies between two layers of superficial fascia and is, therefore, not as obvious as it is in the lower leg. In addition to receiving the small tributaries mentioned earlier, typically, one or more larger tributaries draining the thigh or communicating with the lesser saphenous vein also drain into the greater saphenous vein.

Place the patient supine on the operating table with the thigh mildly externally rotated, flexed, and elevated at the level of the knee joint. Expose the vein first to assure adequate conduit for bypass. Use either a long continuous incision or several interrupted incisions along the course of the greater saphenous vein to perform an in situ bypass. Minimize handling of the edges of the skin incision and avoid making the skin flaps too thin. Skin flaps that are thin or traumatized with forceps, especially in patients with ischemia or occlusive vascular disease, usually result in wound problems. Complications such as wound infections, sloughing of skin flap edges, or sloughing of the skin flap (particularly the posterior flap) often arise in such cases. A gentle, meticulous technique is therefore critical when creating the skin flaps.

Once adequate length has been exposed, attention is then turned to arterial exposure. The proximal and distal arterial vessels are exposed and sites of anastomoses decided upon. After measuring this distance, a slightly longer segment of saphenous vein is harvested. The saphenous vein can be used in a reversed fashion particularly if there is no substantial size mismatch between the ends of the vein, and the respective arterial segment to which anastomosis will be performed. A nonreversed vein can be used as well for concerns regarding size mismatch. Valvulotome usage is described after proximal and distal arterial exposure.

Sites of Groin Incision (Fig. 133.1)

Technical Points

Palpate the inguinal ligament and identify the pubic tubercle and anterosuperior iliac spine. Often, a short flap can be created, such that exposure of the common femoral artery can be obtained using the saphenous vein harvest site. If this is not feasible, place a longitudinal skin incision centered over the femoral artery. This skin incision should extend from 1 to 2 cm above the inguinal ligament to about 10 cm below the inguinal ligament. If separate incisions are used, the saphenous vein harvest incision should be started distally to the inferior most aspect of the femoral artery exposure. Often, there is substantial disease in the mid-to-distal common femoral artery. More proximal exposure can be obtained by retraction of the inguinal ligament cephalad, or by simply dividing a portion of the inguinal ligament. Care must be taken when dissecting at the junction of the external iliac and common femoral arteries as two major collateral branches, the superficial circumflex iliac artery and the inferior epigastric artery. Furthermore, the circumflex iliac veins are often seen crossing transversely under the inguinal ligament. Dissection here must be taken with great care as exposure can be limited.

The profunda femoris artery usually takes off from the common femoral artery about 1 to 3 cm distal to the inguinal ligament. The skin incision must, therefore, extend above the inguinal ligament to expose the common femoral artery adequately. If the incision or dissection is below the usual anatomic bifurcation of the common femoral artery, only the superficial femoral artery will be seen. The profunda femoris artery can also be used as a source of inflow, and so exposure of this vessel can be paramount. Suitable exposure of the profunda femoris as an inflow vessel most often requires division of the later circumflex femoral vein, which crosses the artery in a transverse manner. Once divided, care must be taken to avoid injuring smaller branches. Two larger branches off the profunda femoris, the medial and lateral circumflex femoral arteries, serve as important collaterals for patients with severe ischemia. These two collaterals can often arise directly off the common femoral artery and care should be taken to look for this variation.

Several lymph nodes will be found anterior to the femoral artery in the femoral canal. Be careful to avoid injury to the lymphatic channels and lymph nodes in this area. Disruption of the lymphatic system can result in lymphocele formation and wound problems. Dissect the common femoral, profunda femoris, and superficial femoral arteries gently. A small venous branch courses over the profunda femoris artery. If necessary, ligate and divide this vein to allow access to the profunda femoris distal to its first perforating branch. Obtain proximal control of the common femoral artery and distal control of both the superficial femoral and profunda femoris arteries using Silastic loops.

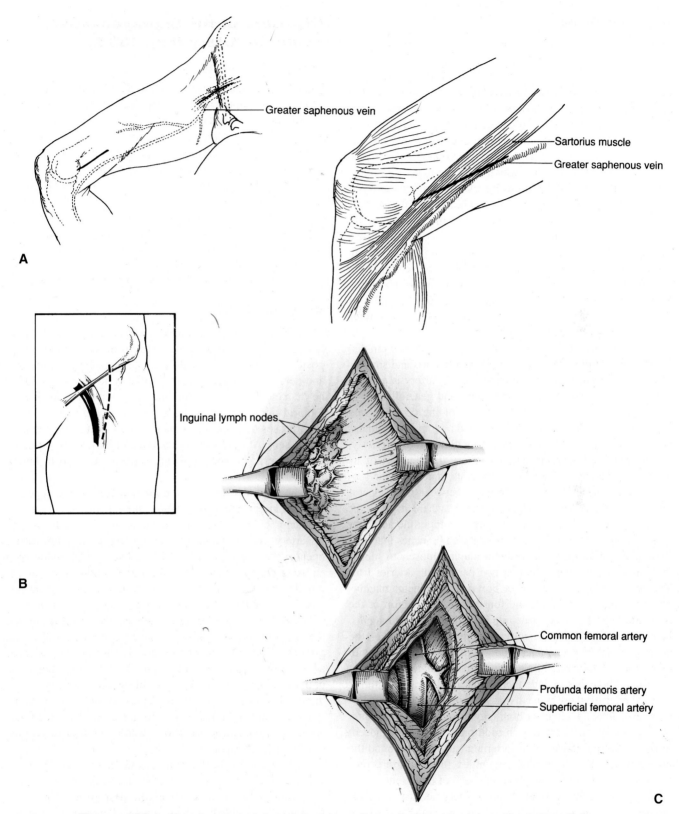

Figure 133.1 Site of groin incision. **A:** Incisions. **B:** Inguinal lymph nodes reflected medially with soft tissues. **C:** Exposure of femoral artery.

Anatomic Points

The common femoral artery is the most lateral structure in the femoral sheath. It reliably bisects the inguinal ligament. This relationship can be used to locate the femoral artery, even when occlusive disease prevents location of a palpable pulse. The femoral nerve lies immediately lateral to the femoral artery, whereas the femoral vein is immediately medial to the artery.

Several superficial inguinal lymph nodes are found in this area. These constitute two groups: Horizontal and vertical nodes. The horizontal nodes (which drain the lower trunk) and their vessels parallel the inguinal ligament and are just inferior to the ligament. The vertical nodes, which drain the inferior extremity, lie in the superficial fascia over the femoral artery. Efferents from these nodes pass through the cribriform fascia and drain into nodes closely associated with the femoral canal, a space in the femoral sheath just medial to the femoral vein through which the lymphatics pass to drain into iliac nodes. Reflection of the lymph node mass from lateral to medial with division of lymphatic tissue bundles between fine silk sutures helps minimize the chance of lymphatic leak.

Typically, the common femoral artery passes 4 to 5 cm distally before it bifurcates into the profunda femoris and superficial femoral arteries. The superficial femoral artery is a direct extension of the common femoral artery and generally lies in the same axis. With respect to the axis of the common and superficial femoral arteries, the profunda femoris originates posterolaterally, then curves posteromedially and inferiorly, posterior to the superficial femoral artery. In this part of its course, it crosses the iliopsoas, pectineus, and adductor brevis muscles. It then passes in the plane between the adductor longus and the adductor magnus muscles, where it gives off several branches. Although most of these supply the adductor muscles, typically there are four perforating branches that pass through the insertion of the adductor magnus muscle to supply the hamstring muscles. The first two perforating arteries usually penetrate both the adductor brevis and adductor magnus muscles, whereas the third and fourth (the termination of the profunda femoris artery) penetrate only the adductor magnus. In addition to supplying the posterior compartment muscles, the penetrating arteries also anastomose with each other and with other arteries, thus providing an important collateral network. Additional branches include the medial and lateral circumflex femoral arteries; these typically arise from the profunda femoris artery, although either or both may arise from the common femoral artery. These arteries, in addition to supplying adjacent muscles, also participate in the arterial anastomosis around the hip joint. Further, the medial circumflex femoral artery provides most of the blood supply to the head of the femur.

Exposure of the profunda femoris artery necessitates skeletonization of the common femoral and proximal part of the superficial femoral arteries. When the profunda femoris artery is exposed and skeletonized, caution should be exercised because the profunda femoris vein and any of its lateral tributaries are anterior to the artery. In fact, the circumflex femoral branch is noted in a transverse orientation needs to be divided to allow exposure beyond the first order branches of the profunda.

Exposure of the Suprageniculate Popliteal Artery (Fig. 133.2)

Technical Points

Flex the knee and externally rotate the knee and thigh. When exposing the suprageniculate popliteal artery, the roll should be placed slightly distal to the knee joint. Make a 4- to 5-inch long longitudinal incision 1 inch proximal and inferior to the adductor tubercle. The greater saphenous vein is superficial in this location and should already be exposed.

Retract the sartorius muscle posteriorly and the tendons of the adductor magnus, semimembranosus, and semitendinosus muscles anteriorly. Identify the popliteal artery and vein along the posterior medial borders of the femur. Meticulous dissection is required to avoid injuring the venous plexus that surrounds the popliteal artery. Secure the branches of the venous plexus with Silastic loops or divide them fine silk suture.

Anatomic Points

The popliteal artery is exposed through an incision that parallels the anterior border of the sartorius muscle and passes just posterior to the medial condyle. The greater saphenous vein and nerve lie posterior to the medial condyle and should not be damaged. The saphenous nerve, a sensory branch of the femoral nerve that provides sensation to the medial leg and foot, passes through the adductor canal along with the femoral vessels. At the level of the adductor hiatus, the saphenous nerve emerges posterior to the sartorius muscle to become superficial.

The popliteal artery is the continuation of the superficial femoral artery after its passage through the adductor canal (adductor hiatus). Exposure of the terminal superficial femoral artery and proximal popliteal artery is accomplished by opening the distal adductor canal, dividing the tendon of the adductor magnus (which forms part of the adductor hiatus), and mobilizing the distal gracilis and medial hamstring muscles. The distal adductor canal is opened by division of the intermuscular fascia between the vastus medialis and sartorius muscles, thereby allowing the sartorius muscle to be retracted posteriorly. Division of the tendon of the adductor magnus opens the adductor hiatus, the anatomic point where the (superficial) femoral artery becomes the popliteal artery. Posterior retraction of the gracilis muscle, as well as of those muscles (semitendinosus and semimembranosus) that form the superomedial boundary of the popliteal fossa, allows visualization of the contents of the popliteal fossa.

After exposure of the structures in the popliteal space, one will find the popliteal vein to be superficial to the popliteal artery, and both of these vessels lie deep to the tibial nerve. Note that the popliteal artery is somewhat more medial than the vein and that the vein is somewhat more medial than the nerve.

In addition to preserving the network of small veins surrounding the popliteal artery, which are almost venular in size, it is important to preserve the genicular arteries, of which there are three in the popliteal fossa. The superior medial and superior lateral genicular arteries arise from the proximal popliteal

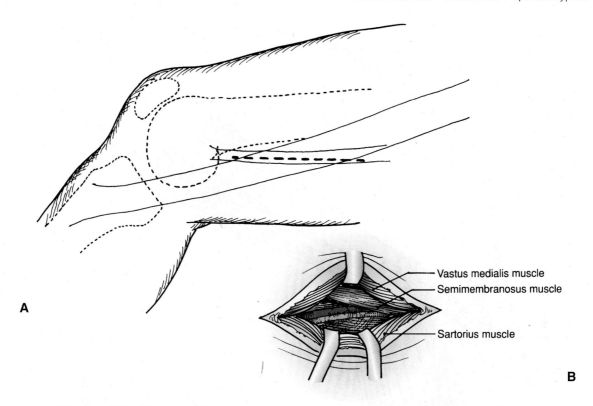

Figure 133.2 Suprageniculate popliteal exposure. **A:** Incision. **B:** Exposure of artery.

artery and pass along the floor of the popliteal space to encircle the femur, just above the respective epicondyles. Ultimately, these arteries participate in an arterial plexus around the patella, thus constituting part of the collateral circulation around the knee joint. The small middle genicular artery arises from the deep surface of the popliteal artery, quickly piercing the capsule of the knee joint to supply intrinsic ligaments and the synovial membrane of this joint.

Exposure of the Infrageniculate Popliteal Artery (Figs. 133.3 and 133.4)

Technical Points

Flex the knee and externally rotate and elevate the leg using rolls or a pillow. Make an incision, measuring about 7 to 10 cm in length. The incision should begin 1 cm posterior to the tibia, and 1 to 2 cm distal to the medial femoral condyle.

Anatomic Points

As on the thigh, the greater saphenous vein and nerve must be identified. The location of the vein can be closely approximated by a line connecting the anterior side of the medial malleolus with a point about one handbreadth (8 to 10 cm) posterior to the medial side of the patella. The saphenous nerve accompanies the vein through the superficial fascia.

Incise the deep fascia to gain entrance to the popliteal vessels. Retract the soleus and gastrocnemius muscles to expose

the distal popliteal artery and vein. Again, be gentle when freeing up the venous tributaries from the popliteal artery. Obtain proximal and distal control of the popliteal artery using vessel loops. Further exposure can be obtained by dividing portions of the pes anserinus, which include the tendons of the gracilis, semitendinosus, and sartorius.

Tunneling and Performance of Anastomoses

Technical Points

Create the graft tunnel prior to heparinization by connecting the course of the superficial femoral artery to the popliteal fossa, subsartorially. After securing proximal and distal hemostasis of the femoral artery and its branches, as well as of the popliteal artery, heparinize the patient with 100 U/kg of heparin. The area of the arteriotomy on the inflow vessel (common femoral artery, superficial femoral artery, or profunda femoris) should be relatively free of disease. Ideally, if there is plaque on the side of the inflow vessel, the arteriotomy will be made directly opposite the disease. This will allow a more technically anastomosis. If endarterectomy is absolutely essentially, a smooth tapering endpoint should be attempted for improve flow dynamics.

The segment of saphenous vein being used on this area should be harvested with this anastomosis in mind. The saphenofemoral junction can serve as a hood if a nonreversed vein graft is performed. Alternatively, a vein branch can be used as a "T" junction from which a hood can be formed if a reversed

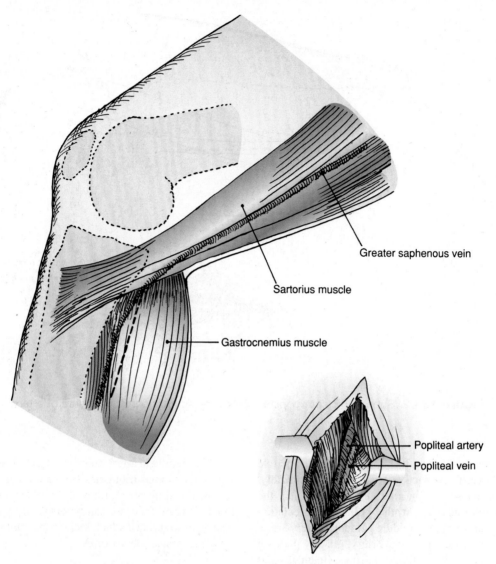

Greater saphenous vein

Sartorius muscle

Gastrocnemius muscle

Popliteal artery
Popliteal vein

Figure 133.3 Infrageniculate popliteal exposure—regional anatomy

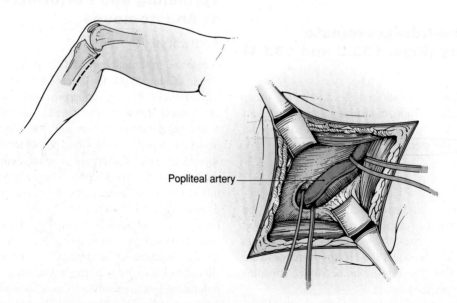

Popliteal artery

Figure 133.4 Incision and isolation of infrageniculate popliteal artery

saphenous vein graft is performed. The proximal anastomosis (i.e., the anastomosis of the saphenous vein to the common femoral artery) is performed using 6-0 polypropylene suture and a continuous running stitch.

Anatomic Points

To open the lower popliteal space, it is necessary first to open the crural fascia. After this is done, the semimembranosus and semitendinosus tendons must either be divided close to their tibial insertions or mobilized anteriorly. Likewise, the medial head of the gastrocnemius muscle, which originates in the medial femoral condyle and capsule of the knee joint, must be mobilized from these fibrous and bony structures as well as from the popliteus muscle; this may require division of the medial head of the gastrocnemius muscle. The soleus muscle, the deepest of the three muscles whose tendons form the calcaneal tendon, takes part of its origin from the soleal line of the tibia, just distal to the insertion of the popliteus muscle. If necessary, this muscle may be partially reflected from its origin to expose the distal-most part of the popliteal artery and the beginnings of the anterior and posterior tibial arteries.

After these muscles have been mobilized, divided, or both, the distal popliteal vessels should be apparent, wrapped in a common fibrous sheath. Frequently, the distal popliteal vein is represented by anterior and posterior tibial veins that have

not yet joined to form a single popliteal vein. Regardless of whether the popliteal vein is single or multiple, the location of the largest vessels is medial to the popliteal artery.

Exposure of the anterior and posterior tibial arteries demands division of the tibial origin of the soleus muscle. If the anterior tibial artery is to be visualized posteriorly, it is also necessary to divide the anterior tibial vein because this lies medial to the artery as these vessels pass through the interosseus membrane. Exposure of the peroneal vessels usually requires complete detachment of the soleus muscle from its tibial origin because the peroneal artery usually arises from the posterior tibial artery some 2.5 to 3 cm distal to the bifurcation of the popliteal artery into anterior and posterior tibial arteries.

Throughout the exposure of the peroneal artery and its branches, care must be taken to avoid the tibial nerve. This nerve accompanies the popliteal vessels and the posterior tibial artery in its course through the leg. Typically, it is more superficial than the artery. Because it is a large nerve, its location is seldom in question.

Passage of a Valvulotome (Fig. 133.5)

Technical Points

Because valves are located anteriorly and posteriorly in the greater saphenous vein, a valvulotome must be passed in a

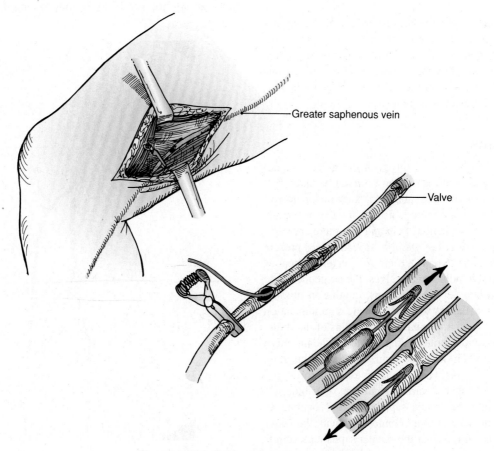

Figure 133.5 Passage of valvulotome

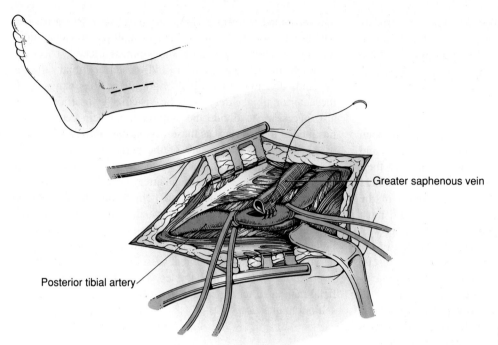

Greater saphenous vein

Posterior tibial artery

Figure 133.6 Distal anastomosis

retrograde fashion to remove them. Use a distal venous tributary of the greater saphenous vein to pass the Mills or Leather valvulotome. Flow should be evident through the distal end of the greater saphenous vein once the venous valves are incompetent.

Use a large clip to occlude the distal end of the greater saphenous vein after completion of the proximal anastomosis. This will allow passage of the vein graft subsartorially while maintaining distension, allowing a more precise maintenance of the graft's orientation. Tailor the distal end of the saphenous vein as a hood for the distal anastomosis.

Anatomic Points

The number and distribution of valves in the greater saphenous vein are variable, although it can be reliably stated that there are fewer valves in the vein above the knee than below it. Researchers have found that there is usually a valve at the termination of the greater saphenous vein and that there are varying numbers (range, 0 to 11) of variably spaced valves present (averaging one for every 6.6 to 8.8 cm of greater saphenous vein length present). In addition to valves, the surgeon should be aware that there are perforating veins, ranging in number from one to six (but usually two), that provide communication between the greater saphenous and the deep veins of the thigh, with the most constant perforator being located at the midthigh level. Finally, the surgeon should recognize that, with this vein, as with all superficial veins, variation is the rule. Accordingly, the surgeon may find that a variable number of tributaries, some large, drain into the greater saphenous vein, or that the greater saphenous has one or more connections with the lesser (smaller) saphenous vein, or that the greater saphenous vein is doubled in all or part of its course.

Distal Anastomosis (Fig. 133.6)

Technical and Anatomic Points

Secure proximal and distal control of the popliteal artery and make an arteriotomy 10 to 15 mm in length. Anastomose the

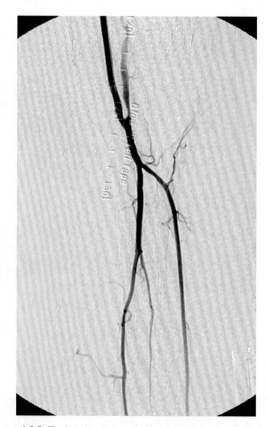

Figure 133.7 Angiogram of distal anastomosis

greater saphenous vein in an end-to-side fashion using 7-0 polypropylene suture and a continuous running stitch (Fig. 133.6).

Obtain an intraoperative angiogram at the completion of the procedure to assess for any potential technical problems (Fig. 133.7). Inject a 50% concentration of contrast media into the saphenous vein just distal to the proximal anastomosis through a 22-gauge needle.

Alternatively, after completion of the distal anastomosis, check the graft and the distal native artery using a sterile Doppler flow detector. This modality is an accurate, effective means of evaluating for technical problems, but it often requires more operator experience than does angiography.

Irrigate all wounds with antibiotic-containing solution. Then close the subcutaneous tissue in two layers using absorbable suture. Close the skin using either skin staples or 4-0 absorbable sutures placed with a running subcuticular stitch.

Acknowledgment

This chapter was contributed by Dr. Kenneth B. Simon in the previous edition.

REFERENCES

1. Abbott WM. Prosthetic above-knee femoral-popliteal bypass: Indications and choice of graft. *Semin Vasc Surg.* 1997;10:3–7.
2. Ascer E, Veith JF, Flores SAW. Infrapopliteal bypass to heavily calcified, rock-like arteries: Management and results. *Am J Surg.* 1986;152:220.
3. Belkin M. Secondary bypass after infrainguinal bypass graft failure. *Semin Vasc Surg.* 2009;22(4):234–239.
4. Donaldson MC, Mannick JA, Whitemore AD. Femoral-distal bypass with in situ greater saphenous vein. Long-term results using the Mills valvulotome. *Ann Surg.* 1991;213(5):457–464.
5. Karmody AM, Leather RP, Shah DM, et al. Peroneal artery bypass: A reappraisal of its value in limb salvage. *J Vasc Surg.* 1984;1:809.
6. Leather RP, Shah DM, Corson JD, et al. Instrumental evolution of the valve incision method of in situ saphenous vein bypass. *J Vasc Surg.* 1984;1:113. (Reviews techniques of valve destruction for in situ bypass.)
7. Mitchell RA, Bone GE, Bridges R, et al. Patient selection for isolated profundaplasty: Arteriographic correlates of operative results. *Am J Surg.* 1979;138:912.
8. Pomposelli FB Jr, Jepsen SJ, Gibbons GW, et al. A flexible approach to infrapopliteal vein grafts in patients with diabetes mellitus. *Arch Surg.* 1991;126:724–727; discussion, 727–729.
9. Schulman ML, Badhey MR, Yatco R. Superficial femoral-popliteal veins and reversed saphenous veins as femoropopliteal bypass grafts: A randomized comparative study. *J Vasc Surg.* 1987; 6:1–10.
10. Skudder PA Jr, Rhodes GA. Hemodynamics of in situ vein bypass: The role of side branch fistulae. *Ann Vasc Surg.* 1986;1: 335–339.
11. Tiefenbrun J, Beckerman M, Singer A. Surgical anatomy in bypass of the distal part of the lower limb. *Surg Gynecol Obstet.* 1975;141:528.
12. Tilson MD, Baue AE. Obturator canal bypass graft for infection of the femoral artery. *Surg Rounds.* 1981:14.

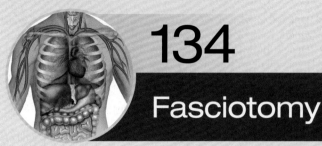

134

Fasciotomy

Parth B. Amin and W. John Sharp

Fascial envelopes surround the major muscle groups in the leg, dividing them into compartments. Arterial bleeding, venous hemorrhage, or severe edema within a compartment can cause the pressure within this close space to rise rapidly. If severe enough, neuromuscular function can be threatened, and fasciotomy indicated. Burns, electrical injury, crush injuries, reperfusion injury, and venous outflow obstruction can all result in increased compartment pressures. Most commonly, this occurs within the four muscle compartments below the knee. Clinical suspicion should be balanced with intracompartmental pressure measurements. Substantial data suggests that a difference between systemic diastolic pressure and intracompartmental pressure less than 30 mm Hg, should warrant a fasciotomy. Four-compartment fasciotomy is described in this chapter.

SCORE™, the Surgical Council on Resident Education, classified fasciotomy for injury as an "ESSENTIAL UNCOMMON" procedure.

STEPS IN PROCEDURE

Four-compartment fasciotomy
Medial incision along the posterior edge of tibia
Identify and preserve the greater saphenous
    vein and saphenous nerve
Decompress superficial and posterior
    compartments

Lateral incision along the anterior edge
    of the fibula
Identify and preserve saphenous vein and
    peroneal nerve

HALLMARK ANATOMIC COMPLICATIONS

Inadequate fasciotomy
Injury to the lesser or greater saphenous vein

Injury to the superficial peroneal nerve
Injury to the saphenous nerve

LIST OF STRUCTURES

Anterior compartment
Boundaries
    Tibia
    Interosseous membrane
    Fibula
    Anterior intermuscular septum
    Deep fascia
Contents
    Tibialis anterior muscle
    Extensor digitorum longus muscle
    Peroneus tertius muscle
Extensor hallucis longus muscle
    Deep peroneal nerve
    Anterior tibial artery
Lateral compartment

Boundaries
    Anterior intermuscular septum
    Fibula
    Posterior intermuscular septum
    Deep fascia
Contents
    Peroneus longus muscle
Peroneus brevis muscle
    Common peroneal nerve
    Superficial peroneal nerve
Superficial posterior compartment
Boundaries
    Posterior intermuscular septum
    Transverse crural septum
    Deep fascia

Contents
 Gastrocnemius muscle
 Soleus muscle
 Plantaris muscle
Deep posterior compartment
Boundaries
 Tibia
 Interosseous membrane
 Fibula
 Transverse crural septum

Contents
 Popliteus muscle
 Flexor hallucis longus muscle
 Flexor digitorum longus muscle
 Tibialis posterior muscle
 Tibial nerve
 Posterior tibial artery
 Peroneal artery

Four-Compartment Fasciotomy Through Two Incisions (Fig. 134.1)

Technical Points

The double-incision technique allows decompression of all four compartments through two skin incisions. Prep and drape the leg circumferentially in the usual sterile fashion. Make a medial incision, starting about 1 cm posterior to the edge of the tibia (Fig. 134.1A). Identify the greater saphenous vein and nerve to avoid injury to these structures when incising the fas-

cia. The medial incision will provide access to the superficial and deep posterior compartments. The deep posterior compartment is often missed altogether or inadequately decompressed. Expose the fascia enclosing the gastrocnemius muscle and incise it along its length. Separate the fibers of the gastrocnemius and soleus muscles to gain entrance to the deep posterior compartment. Decompress the deep posterior compartment by incision of its fascia.

The lateral incision provides access to the lateral and anterior compartments. The incision should extend along the

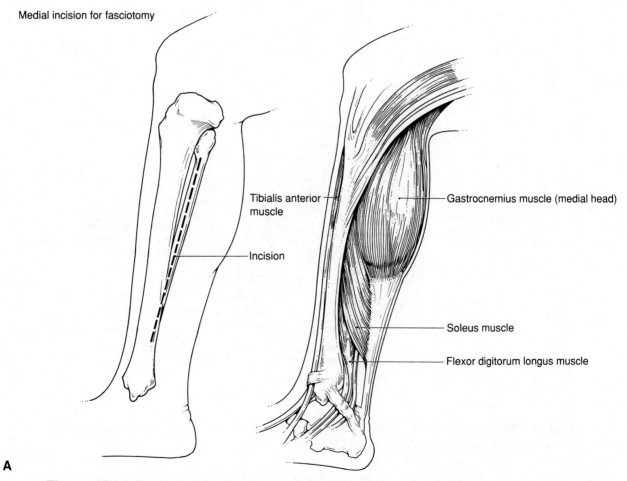

Medial incision for fasciotomy

Tibialis anterior muscle

Incision

Gastrocnemius muscle (medial head)

Soleus muscle

Flexor digitorum longus muscle

A

Figure 134.1 Double-incision fasciotomy. **A:** Medial incision and underlying muscles. (*continued*)

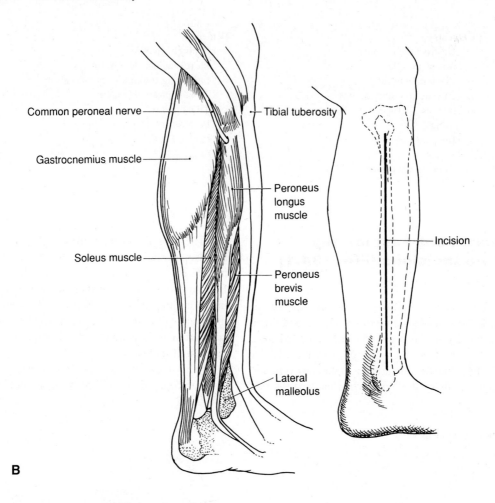

B

1. Tibialis anterior muscle
2. Extensor hallucis longus muscle
3. Extensor digitorum longus muscle *Anterior tibial artery and deep peroneal nerve

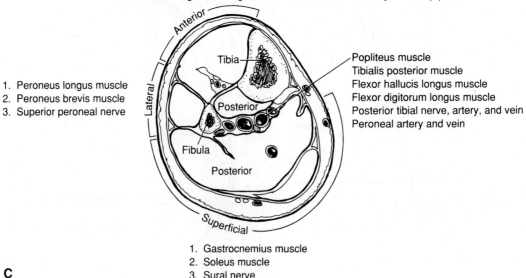

1. Peroneus longus muscle
2. Peroneus brevis muscle
3. Superior peroneal nerve

Popliteus muscle
Tibialis posterior muscle
Flexor hallucis longus muscle
Flexor digitorum longus muscle
Posterior tibial nerve, artery, and vein
Peroneal artery and vein

1. Gastrocnemius muscle
2. Soleus muscle
3. Sural nerve

C

Figure 134.1 *Continued.* **B:** Lateral incision and underlying muscles. **C:** Cross-section of calf showing compartments and contents.

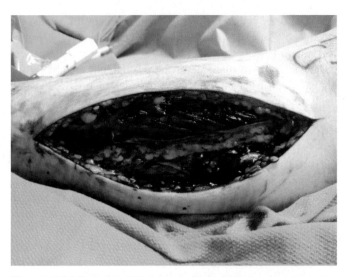

Figure 134.2 Lateral incision and underlying muscle.

anterior edge of the fibula (Fig. 134.1B). Incise the fascia of the lateral compartment from the knee down to the ankle. Undermine the anterior skin flap to gain exposure to the anterior compartment (Fig. 134.2). The underside of the tibia needs to be felt in order for the anterior compartment to be adequately decompressed.

Assess muscle viability in all compartments. Dress the incisions with moistened gauze or nonadherent dressings. Interrupted nylon sutures may be placed through the skin and subcutaneous tissue to approximate the skin edges once the edema resolves.

Anatomic Points

The superficial fascia overlying the lateral aspect of the fibula contains but a few structures of surgical importance. The lesser saphenous vein, which starts on the lateral side of the dorsal venous arch of the foot, passes posterior to the lateral malleolus and peroneal muscle tendons and then ascends for a short distance in the superficial fascia lateral to the calcaneal tendon. It then runs superomedially so that, by midcalf, it lies in the posterior midline. The point where it pierces the deep fascia can be at the level of the popliteal space or lower.

Frequently, comparatively large tributaries connect the lesser and greater saphenous veins, extending diagonally in a superomedial direction from the lesser to the greater saphenous vein. In addition, six or seven perforating veins connect the lesser saphenous vein with the peroneal veins. Typically, the lesser saphenous vein is accompanied by the posterior femoral cutaneous nerve (which provides sensation to the posteromedial thigh, popliteal region, and a variable amount of the posteromedial calf) proximally, and by the sural nerve (which provides sensation to the lower lateral leg and lateral and dorsolateral aspect of the foot) more distally. An incision over the lateral aspect of the leg, extending from the head of the fibula to the lateral malleolus, should avoid these large superficial veins and the major cutaneous nerves.

The four compartments of the leg are formed by the skeletal elements and attached fibrous intermuscular septa (Fig. 134.1C). Osteofascial boundaries of the *anterior compartment* include the tibia, interosseous membrane, fibula, anterior intermuscular septum, and deep fascia. Osteofascial boundaries of the *lateral compartment* include the anterior intermuscular septum, fibula, posterior intermuscular septum, and deep fascia. Osteofascial boundaries of the *superficial posterior compartment* are the posterior intermuscular septum, transverse crural septum, and deep fascia. Osteofascial boundaries of the *deep posterior compartment* are the tibia, interosseous membrane, fibula, posterior intermuscular septum, and transverse crural septum.

Although all four compartments of the leg contain muscles, thereby necessitating a neurovascular supply, only three of the four compartments contain major named nerves, and only two of the four contain major named vessels. Contents of the four compartments are described next.

Anterior Compartment

Muscles in the anterior compartment, all of which are involved with dorsiflexion of the foot, include the tibialis anterior, extensor digitorum longus, peroneus tertius, and extensor hallucis longus. They are all innervated by the deep peroneal nerve, a terminal branch of the common peroneal nerve.

The deep peroneal nerve enters the compartment by piercing the anterior intermuscular septum just inferior to the neck of the fibula. It accompanies the anterior tibial vessels, which lie on the interosseous membrane. In addition to supplying all muscles in the anterior compartment and dorsum of the foot, this nerve also provides sensory innervation to the apposing sides of the first and second toes and the first interspace.

The anterior tibial artery, which arises in the lower popliteal region as one of the terminal branches of the popliteal artery, enters the anterior compartment through a gap in the interosseous membrane just inferior to the proximal tibiofibular joint. In its distal course through the anterior compartment, it lies on the interosseous membrane, and through most of its course, it is medial to the deep peroneal nerve. When this artery crosses the ankle joint, it becomes the dorsalis pedis artery.

Lateral Compartment

The only two muscles in the lateral compartment are the peroneus longus and peroneus brevis muscles, both of which are innervated by the superficial peroneal nerve. The superficial peroneal nerve is one of the two terminal branches of the common peroneal nerve. This nerve typically arises at the point where the common peroneal nerve pierces the posterior intermuscular septum, at the neck of the fibula, to enter the lateral compartment. The superficial peroneal nerve runs downward, at first lying between the peroneus longus muscle and the fibula, and then passes distally between the two peroneal muscles and the extensor digitorum longus muscle, giving off muscular branches. In the lower third of the leg, it pierces the deep fascia to supply the skin of the lower lateral leg and of the dorsum of the foot, except for the first interspace and adjacent sides of the first two digits.

There are no named arteries in the lateral compartment. The peroneal muscles are supplied by perforating branches of the peroneal artery, which lies in the deep posterior compartment.

Superficial Posterior Compartment

Muscles in the superficial posterior compartment are those plantar flexors that attach to the tuberosity of the calcaneus. These include the gastrocnemius, soleus, and plantaris muscles.

There are no named neurovascular structures in the superficial posterior compartment. The muscles are innervated by branches of the tibial nerve as it passes through the popliteal fossa (although the soleus muscle does receive some innervation from the tibial nerve more distally). Likewise, the primary branches supplying the muscles arise from the popliteal artery, rather than its more distal posterior tibial artery.

Deep Posterior Compartment

Muscles in the deep posterior compartment include the popliteus, flexor hallucis longus, flexor digitorum longus, and tibialis posterior. The latter muscle is basically deep to the two flexors; some clinicians consider it to be a fifth compartment.

The tibial nerve enters this compartment by passing deep to the soleus muscle. Within the posterior compartment, this nerve remains on the deep surface of the transverse crural septum. It is thus superficial to the popliteus muscle, then superficial to the tibialis posterior muscle. Ultimately, it passes posterior to the medial malleolus, between the tendons of the flexor digitorum longus and flexor hallucis longus muscles, to enter the foot, where it innervates all of the intrinsic muscles of the plantar aspect and provides cutaneous innervation to the sole.

The posterior tibial artery, which begins at the distal border of the popliteus muscle, accompanies the tibial nerve through the thigh and into the foot. In its course through the leg, it has numerous muscular, nutrient, and anastomotic branches. Its largest branch is the peroneal (fibular) artery. Typically, the peroneal artery arises 2 to 3 cm distal to the origin of the posterior tibial artery. It passes laterally across the tibialis posterior muscle, ultimately descending within a fibrous canal formed by the fibula, tibialis posterior muscle, and flexor hallucis longus muscle. Here, it supplies the muscles nearby, including the soleus and peroneus muscles, through perforating branches.

The superficial fascia on the medial side of the leg contains the greater saphenous vein and the accompanying saphenous nerve. The greater saphenous vein starts at the medial end of the dorsal venous arch of the foot and ultimately passes through the saphenous hiatus of the fascia lata to empty into the femoral vein 2 to 3 cm inferior to the inguinal ligament. In its passage through the superficial fascia of the lower extremity, it passes just anterior to the medial malleolus, then about 8 to 10 cm posterior to the medial side of the patella, and then along the medial side of the thigh to the saphenous hiatus. Its location in the leg can be approximated by a straight line connecting a point on the anterior side of the medial malleolus to a point lying about 10 cm posterior to the medial side of the patella. The saphenous nerve is a branch of the femoral nerve that provides sensation to the medial leg and foot distally to the level of the first metatarsophalangeal joint. Because the course of the greater saphenous vein and saphenous nerve lies very close to the medial margin of the tibia, caution should be exercised after the skin has been incised.

Medially, the deep posterior compartment is exposed by splitting fibers of the gastrocnemius and soleus muscles or, alternatively, by detaching soleus muscle fibers from their origin on the middle third of the medial border of the tibia. One should remember that soleus muscle fibers also arise from the soleal line of the tibia, the head and proximal quarter of the fibula, and a fibrous arch superficial to the tibial vessels and nerve.

REFERENCES

1. Burns JB, Frykberg ER. Management of extremity compartment syndrome. In: Cameron JL, ed. *Current Surgical Therapy.* 10th ed. Philadelphia, PA: Elsevier Saunders; 2011:1028–1031.
2. Finklestein JA, Hunter GA, Hu RW. Lower limb compartment syndrome: Course after delayed fasciotomy. *J Trauma.* 1996; 40(3):342–344.
3. Mabee JR, Bostwick TL. Pathophysiology and mechanisms of compartment syndrome. *Orthop Rev.* 1993;22(2):175–181.
4. Mubarak SJ, Owen CA. Double-incision fasciotomy of the leg for decompression in compartment syndromes. *J Bone Joint Surg Am.* 1977;59(2):184–187.
5. Patman RD, Thompson JE. Fasciotomy in peripheral vascular surgery. Report of 164 patients. *Arch Surg.* 1970;101(6):663–672.
6. Rollins DL, Bernhard VM, Towne JB. Fasciotomy: An appraisal of controversial issues. *Arch Surg.* 1981;116(11):1474–1481.
7. Rorabeck CH. The treatment of compartment syndromes of the leg. *J Bone Joint Surg Br.* 1984;66(1):93–97.
8. Shadgan B, Menon M, O'Brien PJ, et al. Diagnostic techniques in acute compartment syndrome of the leg. *J Orthop Trauma.* 2008; 22(8):581–587.
9. Ulmer T. The clinical diagnosis of compartment syndrome of the lower leg: Are clinic findings predictive of the disorder? *J Orthop Trauma.* 2002;16(8):572–577.

Index

Note: Page number followed by e indicates page numbers from Web-only chapters, f indicates figure and t indicates table.